Pediatric Neuropsychiatry

Pediatric Neuropsychiatry

EDITORS

C. EDWARD COFFEY, MD, FANPA

Kathleen and Earl Ward Professor and Chair of Psychiatry, Professor of Neurology
Vice President, Behavioral Health Services
Henry Ford Health System
Detroit, Michigan

ROGER A. BRUMBACK, MD

Professor of Pathology and Psychiatry
Chair, Department of Pathology
Editor-in-Chief, *Journal of Child Neurology*
Creighton University Medical Center
Omaha, Nebraska

ASSOCIATE EDITORS

DAVID R. ROSENBERG, MD

Miriam L. Hamburger Endowed Chair of Child Psychiatry
Children's Hospital of Michigan
Professor and Chief of Child Psychiatry and Psychology
Department of Psychiatry and Behavioral Neurosciences
Wayne State University School of Medicine
Detroit, Michigan

KYTJA K.S. VOELLER, MD

Director, Western Institute for Neurodevelopmental Studies and Interventions
Boulder, Colorado

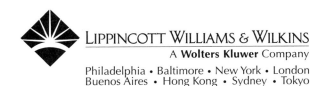

LIPPINCOTT WILLIAMS & WILKINS
A **Wolters Kluwer** Company
Philadelphia • Baltimore • New York • London
Buenos Aires • Hong Kong • Sydney • Tokyo

Acquisitions Editor: Charles W. Mitchell
Managing Editor: Lisa Kairis
Production Manager: Bridgett Dougherty
Senior Manufacturing Manager: Benjamin Rivera
Associate Director Of Marketing: Adam Glazer
Design Coordinator: Holly McLaughlin
Production Services: Schawk, Inc.
Printer: Edwards Brothers

© 2006 by **LIPPINCOTT WILLIAMS & WILKINS**
530 Walnut Street
Philadelphia, PA 19106 USA
351 West Camden Street
Baltimore, Maryland 21201-2436 USA
LWW.com

Printed in the USA

Library of Congress Cataloging-in-Publication Data

Pediatric neuropsychiatry / editors, C. Edward Coffey ... [et al.].
    p. ; cm.
        Includes bibliographical references and index.
        ISBN-13: 978-0-7817-5191-9 (alk. paper)
        ISBN-10: 0-7817-5191-8 (alk. paper)
        1. Pediatric neuropsychiatry. I. Coffey, C. Edward, 1952- .
        [DNLM: 1. Nervous System Diseases—Child. 2. Nervous System Diseases
    —Infant. 3. Child Development. 4. Developmental Disabilities —Child.
        5. Developmental Disabilities—Infant. 6. Mental Disorders—Child.
        7. Mental Disorders—Infant. 8. Neurobehavioral Manifestations—Child.
        9. Neurobehavioral Manifestations—Infant. 10. Neuropsychology—methods
    —Child. 11. Neuropsychology—methods—Infant.
        WS 340 P371345 2006]
        RJ486.5.P38 2006
        618.92'8—dc22

                                                                    2005028170

Care has been taken to confirm the accuracy of the information presented and to describe generally accepted practices. However, the authors, editors, and publisher are not responsible for errors or omissions or for any consequences from application of the information in this book and make no warranty, expressed or implied, with respect to the currency, completeness, or accuracy of the contents of the publication. Application of this information in a particular situation remains the professional responsibility of the practitioner.

The authors, editors, and publisher have exerted every effort to ensure that drug selection and dosage set forth in this text are in accordance with current recommendations and practice at the time of publication. However, in view of ongoing research, changes in government regulations, and the constant flow of information relating to drug therapy and drug reactions, the reader is urged to check the package insert for each drug for any change in indications and dosage and for added warnings and precautions. This is particularly important when the recommended agent is a new or infrequently employed drug.

Some drugs and medical devices presented in this publication have Food and Drug Administration (FDA) clearance for limited use in restricted research settings. It is the responsibility of the health care provider to ascertain the FDA status of each drug or device planned for use in their clinical practice.

To purchase additional copies of this book, call our customer service department at (800) 639-3030 or fax orders to (301) 223-2320. International customers should call (301) 223-2300. Visit Lippincott Williams & Wilkins on the Internet: at LWW.com. Lippincott Williams & Wilkins customer service representatives are available from 8:30 am to 6pm, EST.

                                                        10 9 8 7 6 5 4 3 2

Contributors

NATACHA AKSHOOMOFF, PHD Assistant Professor, Department of Psychiatry, School of Medicine, University of California, San Diego; Research Scientist, Child & Adolescent Services Research Center, Children's Hospital, San Diego, California.

ROBERT T. AMMERMAN, PHD Professor, Department of Pediatrics, University of Cincinnati College of Medicine; Scientific Director, Every Child Succeeds, Division of Behavioral Medicine and Clinical Psychology, Cincinnati Children's Hospital Medical Center, Cincinnati, Ohio.

CAROL E. ANDERSON, MD Associate Professor of Pediatrics, Drexel University College of Medicine; Chief, Section of Clinical Genetics, Department of Pediatrics, St. Christopher's Hospital for Children, Philadelphia, Pennsylvania

PETER E. ANDERSON, PHD Psychologist, Department of Psychology, Children's Hospital of Eastern Ontario, Ottawa, Ontario, Canada

SHARON ARFFA, PHD, MPPM Assistant Professor, Department of Psychiatry, Drexel University, Allegheny Campus; Chief of Neuropsychology, Department of Psychology, The Watson Institute, Sewickley, Pennsylvania

MARILYN AUGUSTYN, MD Associate Professor, Department of Pediatrics, Boston University School of Medicine, Boston, Massachusetts; Assistant Director, Division of DBP, Boston Medical Center, Boston, Massachusetts.

STEPHEN BAGNATO, EDD, NCSP Professor of Pediatrics and Psychology, Department of Pediatrics, School of Medicine, Applied Developmental Psychology, School of Education, The UCLID Center, University of Pittsburgh; Director, Early Childhood Partnerships, Children's Hospital of Pittsburgh, Pittsburgh, Pennsylvania.

ISABELLE BEAULIEU, PHD Senior Bioscientific Staff, Department of Psychiatry, Division of Neuropsychology, Henry Ford Health System, Detroit, Michigan.

MARTHA ANN BELL, PHD Associate Professor, Department of Psychology, Virginia Polytechnic Institute and State University, Blacksburg, Virginia.

NAOMI BRESLAU, PHD Professor, Department of Epidemiology, College of Human Medicine, Michigan State University, East Lansing, Michigan.

ROGER A. BRUMBACK, MD Professor and Chairman, Department of Pathology, Creighton University, Omaha, Nebraska; Department of Pathology, Creighton University Medical Center, Omaha, Nebraska.

OSCAR G. BUKSTEIN, MD, MPH Associate Professor, Department of Psychiatry, University of Pittsburgh; Western Psychiatric Institute and Clinic, Pittsburgh, Pennsylvania.

SARA BULGHERONI Department of Child Neurology and Psychiatry, Istituto Neurologico C. Besta, Milan, Italy.

ROCHELLE CAPLAN, MD Professor, Pediatric Neuropsychiatry Program, Department of Psychiatry and Behavioral Sciences, University of California (UCLA), Los Angeles, California.

LESLIE J. CARVER, PHD Assistant Professor, Department of Psychology and Human Development, University of California–San Diego, La Jolla, California.

HARRY T. CHUGANI, MD Rosalie and Bruce Rosen Professor, Carman and Ann Adams Department of Pediatrics, Department of Neurology and Radiology, Wayne State University School of Medicine; Chief, Division of Pediatric Neurology, Director, PET Center, Children's Hospital of Michigan, Detroit, Michigan.

MARIAH E. COE, PHD Post-Doctoral Fellow, Division of Behavioral Medicine and Clinical Psychology, Cincinnati Children's Hospital Medical Center, Cincinnati, Ohio.

C. EDWARD COFFEY, MD, FANPA Professor and Chair, Department of Psychiatry, Professor of Neurology, Henry Ford Health System, Detroit, Michigan.

STEFANO D'ARRIGO, MD Assistant, Department of Developmental Neurology, Istituto Neurologico C. Besta, Milan, Italy.

MELISSA P. DELBELLO, MD Associate Professor, Psychiatry and Pediatrics, Co-Director, Center for Bipolar Disorders Research, Department of Psychiatry, University of Cincinnati College of Medicine, Cincinnati, Ohio.

GABRIELLE A. DEVEBER, MD, MHSC Associate Professor, Department of Pediatrics, Division of Neurology, University of Toronto; Director, Children's Stroke Program, Division of Neurology, Hospital for Sick Children, Toronto, Ontario, Canada .

PATRICIA K. DUFFNER, MD Professor of Neurology and Pediatrics, Neurology and Pediatrics Department, State University of New York at Buffalo School of Medicine & Biomedical Sciences, Buffalo, New York; Attending Neurologist, Department of Neurology, Women & Children's Hospital, Buffalo, New York.

CARL J. DUNST, PHD Research Scientist, Orelena Hawks Puckett Institute, Asheville, North Carolina.

JUDITH F. FELDMAN, PHD Lecturer, Department of Psychiatry, Columbia University, 1051 Riverside Drive, New York, New York; Research Scientist, Division of Child Psychiatry, New York State Psychiatric Institute, New York, New York.

LAURA FLORES-SARNAT, MD Pediatric Neurologist, Alberta Children's Hospital, Calgary, Alberta Canada.

DANIEL A. GELLER, MD, MBBS, FRACP Assistant Professor, Department of Psychiatry, Harvard Medical School; Director Pediatric OCD Program, Pediatric Psychopharmacology Program, Massachusetts General Hospital, Boston, Massachusetts.

JAY N. GIEDD, MD Chief, Brain Imaging Unit, Child Psychiatry Branch, National Institute of Mental Health, Bethesda, Maryland.

KEVIN M. GRAY, MD Assistant Professor, Department of Psychiatry and Behavioral Sciences, Youth Division, Medical University of South Carolina, Charleston, South Carolina; Clinical Director for Dual Diagnosis Day Treatment Programming, Department of Psychiatry and Behavioral Sciences, Youth Division, Medical University of South Carolina, Charleston, South Carolina.

PAUL G. HAMMERNESS, MD Instructor in Psychiatry, Department of Psychiatry, Harvard University Medical School; Massachusetts General Hospital, Cambridge, Massachusetts.

PETER C. HAUSER, PHD Assistant Professor of Psychology, Department of Psychology, College of Liberal Arts, Rochester Institute of Technology, Rochester, New York; Clinical Neuropsychologist, College Health Enterprises Psychological Services, Rochester, New York.

PETER K. ISQUITH, PHD Assistant Professor of Psychiatry and Pediatrics, Dartmouth Medical School, One Medical Center Drive, Lebanon, New Hampshire.

DAVID C. JIMERSON, MD Department of Psychiatry, Beth Israel Deaconess Medical Center & Harvard Medical School, Boston, Massachusetts.

CSABA JUHÁSZ, MD, PHD Assistant Professor, Carman and Ann Adams Department of Pediatrics and Department of Neurology, Wayne State University School of Medicine; Assistant Professor, PET Center, Children's Hospital of Michigan, Detroit, Michigan.

DAVID L. KAYE, MD Professor of Clinical Psychiatry, Department of Psychiatry State University of New York at Buffalo; Children's Psychiatry Clinic, Women and Children's Hospital, Buffalo, New York; Children's Psychiatry Clinic, Millard Fillmore Hospital, Buffalo, New York.

BETH D. KENNARD, PSYD Graduate School of Biomedical Sciences, University of Texas Southwestern Medical Center, Dallas, Texas.

BRYAN H. KING, MD Professor and Vice Chair for Child and Adolescent Psychiatry, Department of Behavioral Sciences, University of Washington, Seattle, Washington; Director, Child Psychiatry and Mental Health, Children's Hospital and Regional Medical Center, Seattle, Washington.

ROBERT A. KOWATCH, MD Professor of Psychiatry and Pediatrics, Department of Psychiatry, University of Cincinnati Medical Center, Cincinnati, Ohio; Cincinnati Children's Hospital Medical Center, Cincinnati, Ohio.

MARKUS J.P. KRUESI, MD Professor, Department of Psychiatry and Behavioral Sciences, Medical University of South Carolina, Charleston, South Carolina.

RENÉE LAJINESS-O'NEILL, PHD Assistant Professor, Department of Psychology, Eastern Michigan University, Ypsilanti, Michigan; Senior Bioscientific Staff, Department of Behavioral Health, Division of Neuropsychology, Henry Ford Health System, Detroit, Michigan.

ERIN LANPHIER, PHD Assistant Research Psychologist, Department of Psychiatry, UCLA Semel Institute of Neuroscience and Human Behavior, Los Angeles, California.

PAUL D. LARSEN, MD Professor of Pediatrics and Neurological Sciences, Division Head, Pediatric Neurology, University of Nebraska College of Medicine, Nebraska Medical Center, Omaha, Nebraska; Division Head, Pediatric Neurology, University of Nebraska Medical Center, Omaha, Nebraska.

PATRICIA HORAN LATHAM, JD Latham & Latham, The Watergate, Washington, D.C.

PETER S. LATHAM, JD Latham & Latham, The Watergate, Washington, D.C.

GREGORY S. LIPTAK, MD, MPH Professor, Department of Pediatrics, University of Rochester Medical Center, Rochester, New York; Attending Pediatrician, Department of Pediatrics, Strong Memorial Hospital, Rochester, New York.

MARIA-CECILIA LOPES, MD Research Fellow, Sleep Disorders Clinic, Department of Psychiatry, Stanford University, Stanford, California; Departamento de Psicobiologia, Universidade Federal de São Paulo, São Paulo, Brazil.

JOHN M. LORENZ, MD Professor of Clinical Pediatrics, College of Physicians and Surgeons, Columbia University, New York, New York; Attending Neonatologist, Department of Pediatrics, Morgan Stanley Children's Hospital of New York-Presbyterian, New York, New York.

HILLARY MANGIS, MED Department of Counseling, Psychology and Special Education, Duquesne University, Pittsburgh, Pennsylvania.

TARYN MAYES, MS Department of Psychiatry, University of Texas Southwestern Medical Center, Dallas, Texas.

JEFFREY A. MILLER, PHD Associate Professor, School of Education, Duquesne University, Pittsburgh, Pennsylvania.

RUTH MIZE MYERS, MD Associate Professor, Department of Psychiatry, University of Colorado Health Sciences Center, Denver, Colorado; Chief Clinical Officer, Grafton Hospital, Winchester, Virginia.

SILKE NAAB MD Klinik Roseneck, Prien am Chiemsee, Germany.

NIGEL PANETH, MD MPH Professor of Epidemiology and Pediatrics and Human Development, Department of Epidemiology and Pediatrics and Human Development, College of Human Medicine, Michigan State University, East Lansing, Michigan.

CHIARA PANTALEONI, MD Senior Executive, Developmental Neurology Division, Istituto Neurologico C. Besta, Milan, Italy.

SANJEEV PATHAK, MD Assistant Professor of Psychiatry and Pediatrics, Department of Psychiatry and Pediatrics, Cincinnati Children's Hospital Medical Center, University of Cincinnati College of Medicine, Cincinnati, Ohio.

RAFAEL PELAYO, MD Department of Pediatric Neuropsychiatry, Stanford University, Stanford, California.

BRUCE D. PERRY, MD, PHD Senior Fellow, The ChildTrauma Academy, Houston, Texas.

DARIA RIVA, MD Department of Child Neurology and Psychiatry, Istituto Neurologico C. Besta, Milan, Italy.

ROBERT L. RODNITZKY, MD Professor and Interim Head, Department of Neurology, Carver College of Medicine, University of Iowa, Iowa City, Iowa; Professor and Interim Head, Department of Neurology, University of Iowa Hospitals and Clinics, Iowa City, Iowa.

DAVID ROSENBERG, MD Professor and Chief of Child Psychiatry and Psychology, Department of Psychiatry and Behavioral Neurosciences, Wayne State University, Detroit, Michigan; Miriam L. Hamburger Endowed Chair of Child Psychiatry, Department of Psychiatry and Psychology, Children's Hospital of Michigan, Detroit, Michigan.

HARVEY B. SARNAT, MD, FRCPC Professor of Paediatrics, Pathology (Neuropathology) and Clinical Neurosciences, University of Calgary Faculty of Medicine; Division Chief Paediatric Neurology, Calgary Health Region Alberta Children's Hospital, Calgary, Alberta Canada.

THOMAS SPENCER MD Associate Professor of Psychiatry, Harvard Medical School, Cambridge, Massachusetts.

SUZANNE T.P.V. SUNDHEIM, MD WINSI, Boulder, Colorado; Department of Psychiatry, Boulder Community Hospital, Boulder, Colorado.

RALPH E. TARTER, PHD Professor of Pharmaceutical Sciences, Psychiatry and Psychology, Department of Pharmaceutical Sciences, University of Pittsburgh, Pittsburgh, Pennsylvania.

ERGUN Y. UC, MD Assistant Professor of Neurology, Department of Neurology, Carver College of Medicine, University of Iowa, Iowa City, Iowa.

KYTJA K.S. VOELLER, MD Director, Western Institute for Neurodevelopmental Studies and Interventions, Boulder, Colorado.

AGNES WHITAKER Clinical Professor of Psychiatry, Department of Child and Adolescent Psychiatry, Columbia University, New York, New York; Director, Developmental Neuropsychiatry Program, New York Presbyterian Hospital-Columbia University Medical Center, New York, New York.

JAMES WINDE, MD Medical Examiner, La Grande, Oregon.

BARBARA E. WOLFE, PHD, RN, CS, Klinik Roseneck, Prien am Chiemsee, Germany.

KIN YUEN American Academy of Sleep Medicine, Westchester, Illinois.

Preface

The recent and rapid expansion of our knowledge of neurobiology and human nervous system development has resulted in considerable interest in the study of behavioral disorders associated with normal and "abnormal" brain maturation. Pediatric neuropsychiatry is an evolving clinical discipline devoted to the diagnosis and treatment of psychiatric or behavioral disorders in children and adolescents who have disturbances of brain function.

Our first attempt to systematize the discipline of pediatric neuropsychiatry culminated in the publication in 1998 of *The American Psychiatric Press Textbook of Pediatric Neuropsychiatry*. While this tome received critical acclaim, its comprehensiveness resulted in a volume that was quite large, relatively expensive, and thus inaccessible to some readers. Its publication also generated considerable correspondence from readers with appreciation for our efforts and suggestions for improvements to future editions.

Pediatric Neuropsychiatry takes to heart this advice and incorporates the very latest in neuroscience research in an updated and streamlined text designed for clinicians interested in brain-behavior relations. *Pediatric Neuropsychiatry* bridges the fields of pediatric medicine, pediatric neurology, pediatric neuropsychology, child and adolescent psychiatry, and clinical pediatric neuroscience, and emphasizes the relations between neuropsychiatric illness and the developing nervous system. This book is intended for health care professionals—child neurologists, child and adolescent psychiatrists, psychologists, pediatricians, and other clinicians—who desire to understand and ameliorate disturbed behavior associated with diseases of the brain through a comprehensive approach based on a thorough knowledge of contemporary neuroscience. *Pediatric Neuropsychiatry* endeavors to establish a link between the neurobiology of major psychiatric illness and the neurobiology of brain disorders that cause disturbed behavior in children and adolescents, and in so doing stimulate consideration of fundamental brain-behavior relationships as they evolve upon a backdrop of the developing nervous system.

Pediatric Neuropsychiatry is organized into four sections, each edited by one or more of the book's editors or associate editors. The section editors have assembled an outstanding collection of world-renowned neuropsychiatrists, clinical neuroscientists, and scholars, who in turn have endeavored to produce chapters that impart clinically relevant information within the context of the very latest research in developmental neuroscience.

Section I, "Neuropsychiatric Assessment of the Child and Adolescent," begins with an overview of normal and abnormal brain development, followed by two practical chapters on bedside, neuropsychological, and psychoeducational assessment of the pediatric patient; and three chapters on the role of advanced brain imaging technologies (computed tomography, magnetic resonance imaging, positron emission computed tomography, quantitative electroencephalography, and evoked potentials) in the evaluation of the child and adolescent. This section accomplishes the essential and fundamental task of defining the acceptable limits of "normal brain development" as assessed at the bedside and in the clinical neuroscience laboratory.

Sections II and III provide the clinical core of *Pediatric Neuropsychiatry* and focus upon the neuropsychiatric aspects of psychiatric and neurological disorders, respectively, in children and adolescents. The comprehensive chapters in these sections highlight the influence of the developing nervous system on the pathophysiology, neuropsychiatric manifestations, clinical course, treatment, and prognosis of psychiatric and neurological illness in the child and adolescent.

Section IV, "Principles of Treatment of Pediatric Neuropsychiatry," emphasizes the special considerations that are essential for safe and effective treatment of neuropsychiatric disorders in children and adolescents. This final section features up-to-date chapters on neuropsychopharmacology, electroconvulsive therapy, genetic interventions, psychosocial and family therapies, educational interventions, and residential facilities. The section also includes a chapter on the special legal considerations that impact the provision of care for these patients. The discussions and recommendations for treatment are anchored as much as possible in a firm foundation of clinical neuroscience research.

Acknowledgments

We thank the associate editors, David R. Rosenberg, MD, and Kytja K.S. Voeller, MD, for the amazing effort they devoted to *Pediatric Neuropsychiatry*. They join us in thanking each of the chapter authors for their impressive contributions—such quality work requires thought, time, and energy, all of which must be redirected from other pressing demands including those of managed care. Stacey Sebring, Lisa Kairis, and Charley Mitchell of Lippincott Williams & Wilkins provided much guidance and were always available to assist with the many issues that invariably arise with a project of this scale. We are grateful that all of these collaborators—the associate editors, chapter authors, and LWW—shared our vision and made this text a priority.

We also acknowledge with special appreciation Mark Kelley, MD, and the Henry Ford Medical Group, as well as the Board of Trustees of Henry Ford Behavioral Health Services, all of whom understand and value the importance of art and science in the enterprise of clinical medicine. Further, we acknowledge Creighton University, which in the Jesuit tradition of supporting educational efforts (particularly in the sciences), provided encouragement during the tasks of compiling this text. Finally, this project was ultimately made possible by the understanding, patience, and support of our families.

C. Edward Coffey, MD
Roger A. Brumback, MD

Contents

Neuropsychiatric Assessment of the Child and Adolescent

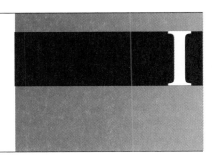

Normal Development of the Nervous System

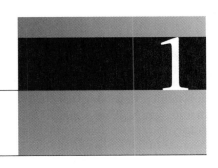

Harvey B. Sarnat, MD FRCPC   **Laura Flores-Sarnat, MD**

Embryology, the traditional term for ontogeny, has been the basis for understanding development for three centuries. Until recently, embryology was limited to descriptive morphogenesis, both macroscopic and microscopic. Two major advances, beginning in the late 1980s, continue to provide insight with new discoveries of importance almost daily. The first was the discovery of genetic programming as the basis of early development of the neural tube. The second was the recognition that neuroembryology cannot be restricted to the central, or even the central and peripheral, nervous systems, because the developing neuroepithelium and its derivatives, particularly neural crest tissue, induce and regulate the formation of many nonneural tissues. This phenomenon is well demonstrated in craniofacial development and its disorders associated with CNS malformations. Examples of the latter are the midfacial hypoplasia in many cases of holoprosencephaly and the hypertelorism that accompanies many cases of agenesis of the corpus callosum. These facial anomalies, previously recognized only as useful clinical diagnostic markers, can be explained in much more depth than ever before. The *New Neuroembryology* is, therefore, an integration of classical morphogenesis with molecular genetic programming and includes the induction of other tissues by the nervous system during embryonic and fetal life.

Maturation may be further defined by molecular genetics in terms of autocrine, paracrine, and endocrine influences of neurotrophins and other secretory molecules. Specific receptors on the plasma membranes of even "undifferentiated" neuroepithelial cells have been identified. The maintenance of mature neuronal and glial identity in the adult by many of these same genetic transcripts of fetal life provides a further basis for the continuity of development and maturity.

The new neuroembryology in no way invalidates or renders obsolete the classical meticulous observations of central nervous system (CNS) histogenesis, beginning with those of Santiago de Ramón y Cajal (1909–1911) and continuing to this day with ongoing major contributions by such distinguished neuroembryologists as Pasco Rakic, Miguel Marín-Padilla, Ronan O'Rahilly, and Fabiola Müller. Developmental neuropathologists, such as Paul Yakovlev, Reinhard L. Friede, Ellsworth C. Alvord Jr., Lucy Rorke, Margaret G. Norman, and Laurence E. Becker, also have contributed much by applying neuroembryological principles to the explanation of cerebral malformations. Without such a framework, molecular biology would consist of nothing more than a meaningless list of identified gene products. Modern neuroembryology thus encompasses classical embryology to demonstrate maturational change and molecular biology to provide insight into how and why such change occurs.

Embryological development is most readily understood as a sequence of distinct processes with considerable spatial and temporal overlap (Pinter and Sarnat 2004; Sarnat 1992a): (1) genetic patterning, the establishment of the axes of the neuroepithelium, and neural induction; (2) neurulation; (3) neural crest separation and migration; (4) neuroepithelial cell proliferation and differentiation; (5) apoptosis, or programmed cell death; (6) neuroblast migration; (7) axonal pathfinding; (8) membrane excitability; (9) dendritic sprouting and synaptogenesis; (10) biosynthesis of neurotransmitters; and (11) myelination.

An important additional principle of neuroembryology is *initial redundancy*. More neuroblasts are generated than are needed as mature neurons; surplus cells survive for a finite period and are then deleted through the mechanism of programmed cell death. Axonal collaterals are often numerous during development but later retract, so that diffuse projections become more specific. Transient synapses form that are later deleted. Finally, some cells of the immature brain are functionally important only during fetal life, after which time they disappear or change into another mature cell (e.g., cells that form the boundaries between embryonic segments of the neural tube; Cajal-Retzius neurons of the molecular layer of the cerebral cortex; radial glial cells of the cerebrum). Such cells provide transitional synaptic circuitry, and some contribute "pioneer axons" in long pathways to help guide the first permanent axons of those tracts (e.g., the subplate neurons that form the first descending fibers of the internal capsule before the appearance of pyramidal cell axons from deep cortical layers).

Although cerebral vasculature is not of neuroectodermal origin, the vascular supply and blood-brain barrier are intimately linked to many of the processes of neural development and should be recognized as important aspects of neuroembryology. The formation of the cranium, meninges, and other neural crest derivatives, including facial structures, is also closely associated with neural development, both normal and abnormal.

EARLIEST EMBRYOGENESIS

Cleavage and Blastulation

Even before the first mitotic division, the fertilized ovum shows a tendency toward axis polarity in the rotation and asymmetrical distribution of microtubules in its cytoplasm, producing animal and vegetal poles. The assembly of microtubules is encoded by a maternal gene and remains stable during cleavage (Gong and Brandhorst 1988); this gene is expressed by microtubule growth during mitotic spindle elongation (Shelden and Wadsworth 1990). The first mitosis yields a pair of daughter cells called *blastomeres;* each subsequent division doubles the number of cells. If the second tetrad of cells lies directly above the first, the arrangement is known as *radial cleavage;* if the second tetrad is rotated so that its cells are staggered above and between cells of the bottom tetrad, the arrangement is called *spiral cleavage.* Like all other vertebrates and some invertebrates, humans follow a radial cleavage pattern. The majority of invertebrates begin embryonic life with spiral cleavages; a few follow unique cleavages that are neither radial nor spiral. Most spiral cleavages are *determinate:* by the eight-cell stage, each cell is already programmed to form certain tissues and no others; for example, the cell of insect embryos forms all mesodermal derivatives, and selective removal of these cells is not compensated as the larva develops. Humans and other animals exhibiting radial cleavages are *indeterminate:* cells are not so rigidly programmed that others cannot compensate, and thus the destruction of one does not produce a defective embryo.

Further mitoses and an increased number of blastomeres produce a hollow sphere of cells, the *blastula,* which in birds and mammals is flattened into a bilaminar disk. The bottom sheet of the disk is known as the *hypoblast,* and the upper is called the *epiblast.* The hypoblast becomes endoderm, and the epiblast will form ectoderm, from which the neural plate and also the mesoderm will differentiate at a later stage. The *blastula* cavity, the *blastocoel* of spherical blastulas, is a potential space between the cellular sheets of hypoblast and epiblast. The *blastocyst* comprises the *embryonic disk* of the flat epiblast and hypoblast, together with the *trophoblast,* or peripheral epithelium, that forms the amnionic and chorionic membranes but is not part of the embryo proper. The blastocyst cavity is therefore not the same as the blastocoel. Both cellular proliferation and apoptosis occur in the blastocyst before and after implantation (Hardy et al. 1989).

GASTRULATION

The next developmental stage in early ontogenesis, gastrulation, is the most crucial because it is during this stage that the body axes establish anatomic form and *induction*—the process whereby one layer of embryonic tissue influences another to cause the affected cells to differentiate in a direction other than that of the inducing cells—begins. Morphological development of the organism depends on normal gastrulation, and any error at this stage is lethal or produces gross defects.

In simple animals with a spherical blastula, such as the frog, gastrulation begins with a small dimple or invagination—the *blastopore*—at one site of the hollow ball of cells. The blastopore deepens, becoming not a hole in the blastula but an invaginated finger lined with surface cells protruding into the blastocoel. The new cavity formed within this finger is the *archenteron,* the lumen of the future gut. The archenteron compresses and eventually obliterates the earlier blastocoel.

NORMAL DEVELOPMENT OF THE NERVOUS SYSTEM

Because the human blastula is flattened, the site of invagination appears as an elongated pair of parallel cellular ridges flanking a central groove. This ridged groove, *the primitive streak,* is the first morphological marker to define the dorsal surface of the embryo; it also establishes the rostrocaudal axis and bilateral symmetry. The day of gastrulation not only is a landmark of the establishment of the axes of the body, but also is the "birthday of the nervous system" because it is the first time that a neuroepithelium can be distinguished as a neural placode on each side of the primitive streak.

Classical embryology attributed great importance to the correlation of spiral cleavage with *prostomes* and of radial cleavage with *deuterostomes;* in prostomes, the site of the blastopore becomes the mouth, and in deuterostomes, it becomes the anus. This distinction may be less important in evolution than was previously thought, however (Willmer 1990). The primitive streak elongates through cellular proliferation at one end, designated caudal, while its other end, designated rostral, becomes enlarged as *Hensen's node,* also sometimes called the *primitive node* or *primitive knot.* A shallow depression on the surface of Hensen's node, the *primitive pit,* corresponds to the original blastopore. Cells from the surface of the primitive streak move inward and laterally to form the *mesoderm.* The classical embryological notion of three germ layers—ectoderm, mesoderm, and endoderm—that acquire identity during gastrulation is an oversimplification; molecular genetic studies suggest that this distinction of germ layers may be an outdated concept (Willmer 1990). Neural crest tissue contains the primordia of both ectodermal and mesodermal derivatives. Cells of the neural tube may be experimentally induced to change their fate to mesodermal differentiation (Bronner-Fraser 1995). Myogenic genes influence neural as well as muscle development (Tajbakhsh and Buckingham 1995).

NOTOCHORD FORMATION

The notochord is an unsegmented transitory embryonic structure, regarded as mesodermal in origin, that helps establish body axes. It is the principal inductor of the overlying neural plate to form the neural tube. The notochord also induces formation of the sclerotomes, the precursors of the vertebral bodies.

The notochord itself undergoes considerable embryological development before it is ready to serve as an inductor. It originates from Hensen's node as a solid cellular strand or column, the *notochordal* process, that grows rostrally between the ectodermal and endodermal layers of epiblast and hypoblast until it reaches a small oval of columnar endodermal cells known as the *prochordal plate.* This plate acts as a barrier to further growth of the notochordal process. The point of attachment of the prochordal plate to the epiblastic ectoderm is the *buccopharyngeal membrane,* the site of the future mouth. The primitive pit extends into the notochordal process to create a tubular lumen, the *notochordal canal.* The primitive streak shortens as the notochordal process elongates. The ventral surface of the notochordal process then fuses with the underlying endoderm and degenerates. The remaining dorsal half of the notochordal process forms a flattened, grooved, elongated plate that remolds itself into the solid cylinder of the "mature" notochord. Mesodermal tissue grows between the notochord and the endoderm and also between the notochord and the neural plate dorsally, but this intervening tissue—the *mesenchyme*—does not impede the transport of secretory induction molecules (e.g., the gene product of *Sonic hedgehog* [see discussion later in this chapter]) from the notochord to the neural plate. The notochord also secretes other diffusible molecules, including trypsin, to repel migratory cells of the neural crest (Pettway et al. 1990). The mesenchyme forming the sheath of the notochord even-

tually contributes to the formation of the meninges—in particular, the dura mater and tentorium cerebelli. The cranial leptomeninges are mesencephalic neural crest derivatives, but the spinal leptomeninges are derived from paraxial mesoderm.

GENETIC PATTERNING AND NEURAL INDUCTION

The genes that program development of the nervous system consist of a specific series of deoxyribonucleic acid (DNA) base pairs linked to small proteins known as *transcription factors.* A common structure of many transcription factors is the *basic helix-loop-helix* (bHLH), a configuration so primordial in evolution that it first appears in bacteria (Boncinelli et al. 1988). The ribonucleic acid (RNA) transcript translates a peptide, a glycoprotein, or other molecules that mediate induction or serve as trophic factors.

In situ hybridization is a method that allows histological identification of individual cells in which a precise nucleic acid sequence or a product of that sequence is expressed. This method involves the "hybridization" of a nucleic acid probe with a specific target nucleic acid to be recognized within the tissue section and represents a histochemical extension of the older method, liquid phase hybridization. Two single-stranded nucleic acid molecules recognize each other and form hydrogen bonds of complementary base pairs: DNA-DNA, RNA-RNA, or DNA-RNA duplexes. The most common application of in situ hybridization in studies of the developing nervous system is in the detection of specific messenger RNA (mRNA) molecules that are expressed only at precise times and in specific cells during embryogenesis. DNA or RNA probes used for in situ hybridization must be linked to a *reporter,* a means of making the localization within the tissue detectable. The traditional reporters—autoradiographic labels—are now seldom used and have largely been replaced by nonisotope reporters. These include biotin (vitamin H of the B complex), which binds with high affinity to the glycoprotein avidin and may then be demonstrated histochemically as a colored precipitate (the avidin-biotin method). Alternative methods use digoxigenin and enzyme-labeled reporters such as tyrosine kinase, alkaline phosphatase, 3-glucuronidase, or horseradish peroxidase, which may be demonstrated in tissues by either fluorescence or light microscopy (Tecott et al. 1994).

The three main classes of hybridization probes in current use are complementary DNA (cDNA), RNA (riboprobes), and oligonucleotide probes (for a limited segment of the RNA molecule; these require dependence on published nucleic acid sequences). The cDNA probe is double stranded, and the insert (the region complementary to mRNA) is usually contained within a plasmid or bacteriophage. Riboprobes are single-stranded RNA molecules produced from cloned cDNA that was previously introduced into a specifically designed plasmid transcription system. RNA-RNA hybrids are more stable than corresponding DNA-RNA hybrids, but riboprobes are "stickier" than DNA probes and produce a higher degree of nonspecific binding to tissue; this nonspecific background may be reduced by posthybridization treatment with ribonuclease.

Induction is the process whereby one type of embryonic tissue influences another, causing the affected cells to differentiate in a direction other than that of the inducing cells. Induction often takes place between germ layers, as when the notochord (mesoderm) induces the floor plate of the neural tube (ectoderm). Induction may also occur within a germ layer; for example, the optic cup (neuroepithelium) induces the overlying surface ectoderm to form a lens placode and cornea rather than simply more epidermis.

Induction was discovered in 1924 by Hans Spemann and Hilda Mangold, who showed that in newts the dorsal lip of the gastrula was capable of inducing the formation of an ectopic second nervous system when it was transplanted to a different region of a host embryo. This dorsal lip of the amphibian gastrula is homologous with the primitive node (Hensen's node) in avian and mammalian embryos, and transplantation of this node yields similar results. The regulatory gene *Cnot*, with major domains in Hensen's node, the notochord, and the prenodal and postnodal neural plate, is probably responsible for this induction (Stein and Kessel 1995).

Neural induction is the maturation of nervous system structures in response to signaling molecules secreted in the vicinity by other tissues of either mesodermal or ectodermal origin. It is the receptors in the membrane of the induced cell, not the inductive molecule that determines the specific type of tissue that the affected cell will become. These membrane receptors are responsive to the effects of the inductive molecules only during a precise period of time known as the *competence* of the induced cell. A gene called *Notch* regulates the competence of response to more specific inductive cues in the CNS and in many other embryonic tissues (Fortini and Artavanis-Tsakonas 1993). Some mesodermal tissues (e.g., smooth muscle of fetal gut) may act as mitogens on the neuroepithelium by increasing the rate of cellular proliferation (Fontain-Perus 1993), but this phenomenon does not represent true neural induction because the proliferating cells do not differentiate. Some regulatory genes, such as *Wnt-1* (see discussion later in this chapter), also have mitogenic effects (Dickson et al. 1994).

ORGANIZER GENES AND HOMEOBOXES

In all vertebrates and most invertebrates, the fundamental body plan is established early in embryonic development and is defined by bilateral symmetry and axes of polarity—cephalocaudal and dorsoventral gradients of differentiation and growth. The radial symmetry exhibited by some invertebrates, such as sponges, coelenterates (e.g., sea anemone, hydra, jellyfish), and echinoderms (e.g., starfish), often is secondarily achieved or represents an exceptional alteration of early programming (Sarnat 1992a). From a phylogenetic perspective, the fundamental body plan became firmly established in the Cambrian Period, 570 million years ago, although various other body models have been discovered in long-extinct multicellular organisms dating from the earlier Ediacara Epoch (Seilacher 1984). Bilateral symmetry as a body plan is more ancient than previously thought. A simple marine invertebrate with a bilaterally symmetrical body, named Vernanimalcula, from the pre-Cambrian period of 580-600 million years ago, recently was discovered in Guizhou Province, China, from microfossils with excellent preservation (Bottjer 2005).

Organizer genes are the earliest to be expressed in ontogenesis. They continue to regulate polarity and body axes beyond the gastrula state; they also establish growth gradients as embryonic cells multiply. The transcription products of these genes may be expressed in several differentiating organ systems but not necessarily in all; some of these products are integral to neural development.

The early formation of the neural plate is accomplished not only by mitotic proliferation of neuroepithelial cells but also by conversion of surrounding cells to a neural fate. In amphibians, a gene known as *achaete-scute (XASH-3)* is expressed very early in the dorsal part of the embryo from the time of gastrulation and acts as a molecular switch to change the fate of undifferentiated cells to become neuroepithelial rather than surface ectodermal or mesodermal cells (Turner and Weintraub 1994). Inhibitor genes also play a major role in controlling cell fate; some cells differentiate as specific types because they are inhibited from developing as others.

Each gene of the developing nervous system has a specific site of expression along the rostrocaudal and dorsoventral axes. Some genes determine the patterning of particular segments of the neural tube, such as the midbrain. A dorsal or ventral gradient of expression may or may not be associated with influence on adjacent regions. A *dorsalizing* gene not only has a dorsal distribution of expression but will also cause ventral regions of the neural tube to differentiate as dorsal regions if the influence of *ventralizing* genes is insufficiently expressed. This principle is well demonstrated in the development of the somite, in which the sclerotome normally lies ventral to the myotome and dermatome; implantation of ectopic floor-plate cells next to the somite in chick embryos causes ventralization of the somite, so that excessive amounts of sclerotome (cartilage and bone) and insufficient amounts of myotome (muscle) and dermatome (dermis) are formed (Brand-Saberi et al. 1993; Pourquie et al. 1993). The floor plate in this case functions as a ventralizing inductor of the mesodermal somite, and the gene product probably responsible is one known as *Sonic hedgehog*, which also exerts a ventralizing effect in the neural tube (see "*Sonic Hedgehog [Shh] Family*," on page 9). Genes have often been assigned bizarre names, and vertebrate and invertebrate homologues may have similar but not identical names even if their nucleotide sequences are identical.

Table 1.1 summarizes several of the important genes and gene families that program the nervous systems of all

TABLE 1.1

PARTIAL LIST OF ORGANIZER GENES AND HOMEOBOXES THAT PATTERN EARLY DEVELOPMENT OF THE MAMMALIAN NERVOUS SYSTEM

Gene	Site(s) of Expression	Function(s)
Lim-1	Rostral progenitor cells	Head organizer, mesenchyme and neural placode
twist	Rostral progenitor cells	Head organizer, mesenchyme only
XASH-3 (achaete-scute)	Epiblast, neural plate	Induces neuroepithelial differentiation, mediolateral gradient
Notch	All embryonic cells	Determines competence of cells to respond to induction
Delta	All neural precursor cells	Antagonizes *Notch*; prevents adjacent cells from undergoing neural differentiation
Numb	All embryonic cells	Antagonizes *Notch* during mitotic cycling
Cnot (Xnot)	Primitive node, notochord, prenodal diencephalon, postnodal neural plate caudal to hindbrain in a decreasing gradient	Responsible for specification of notochord and prechordal mesoderm; early induction of neural plate
goosecoid	Cells rostral to notochord	Induces prenotochordal mesoderm and forebrain
Sonic hedgehog	Ventral midline of neural plate and neural tube; posterior and distal limb buds	Mediates early induction from Hensen's node, notochord, and floor plate; exerts strong ventralizing polarity gradient; initiates differentiation of motor neurons
HNF-3 (forkhead)	Ventral neural tube	Patterns ventral midline of neural tube
Islet-1,2	Ventral neural plate	Promotes differentiation of motor neurons
Hox-1.5	Neural crest	Programs mesenchymal neural crest, thymus, parathyroids
Hox-1.6 (Hoxa-1)	r4 through r7	Contributes to rostrocaudal patterning and segmentation of hindbrain
Hox-2.1	r8, spinal cord	Contributes to rostrocaudal patterning and segmentation of hindbrain
Hox-2.6	Spinal cord to r6/r7 boundary	Contributes to rostrocaudal patterning and segmentation of hindbrain
Hox-2.7	Spinal cord to r4/r5 boundary	Contributes to rostrocaudal patterning and segmentation of hindbrain
Hox-2.8	Spinal cord to r2/r3 boundary	Contributes to rostrocaudal patterning and segmentation of hindbrain; regulatory axonal pathfinding at r3
Hox-2.9 (Hoxb-1)	r4 only	Contributes to rostrocaudal patterning and segmentation of hindbrain; cranial neural crest formation
Hox-3.1 (Hoxc-8)	Spinal cord (r8), especially brachial (cervical) region	Contributes to patterning of spinal cord
Krox-20 (zinc finger)	r3, r5	Regulates expression of *Hox* genes; myelination by Schwann cells
Zic (zinc finger)	r1	Programs differentiation and maintenance of cerebellar granule cells
En-1 (engrailed)	Midbrain, r1	Programs differentiation of midbrain, cerebellum, and rostral metencephalon (pons)
En-2	Midbrain, r1	Regulates differentiation of midbrain, cerebellum, and rostral metencephalon (pons)
Wnt-1 (wingless)	Midbrain, r1, lateral margins of neural plate of r3 to spinal cord; diffusely and weakly in forebrain	Maintains expression of *En-1* redundant with *Wnt-3* in hindbrain; mitogenic
Wnt-3	r3 through r8; Purkinje cells of cerebellum	Exerts dorsalizing polarity gradient for differentiation of hindbrain structures; maintains integrity of Purkinje cells
Pax-2 (paired)	r2 through r8 in ventricular zone adjacent to sulcus limitans; spinal cord; ventral half of optic up and stalk	Regulated by signals from notochord and floor plate; plays adjunctive role in segmentation of hindbrain; exerts dorsalizing polarity gradient
Pax-3	Spinal cord; Bergmann glia of cerebellum	Maintains integrity of Bergmann cells
Pax-6	Hindbrain; granule cells of cerebellum; forebrain; eye; pituitary; olfactory nasal epithelium	Maintains integrity of granule cells
Dlx-1, 2 ,3	Forebrain	Provides positional information for somatotopic organization
BF-1,2	Forebrain, retina	Provides positional information for somatotopic organization
Nkx-2.2	Forebrain, neural tube	Induces forebrain compartmentalization; defines longitudinal columns of neural cells along entire neuraxis

Note: Genes are listed in general order of time of expression. r = rhombomere.

vertebrates. The gene locations of known human mutations causing specific CNS malformations are summarized in a recent table (Sarnat 2005). Homologues of vertebrate genes in the fruit fly *Drosophila* perform parallel though often more extensive functions in invertebrates, and gene products of the fly and the mouse are so similar that they can be experimentally interchanged to achieve the expected effect. Most of these genes are also functionally active in other systems of the body, such as in programming the gradient of anteroposterior differentiation of the limb buds.

Although *homeoboxes* and *regulator genes* overlap considerably with organizer genes and, in some of their expressions, could be dually listed under the "organizer" rubric, homeoboxes generally program the stage of CNS development subsequent to that in which the polarity gradients of the neural plate are established. Homeoboxes establish embryonic segmentation of the neural tube and invoke limits on cellular migration between successive compartments (Fig. 1.1); they initiate the differentiation of specific neuronal and glial cells and later help to maintain the morphological and metabolic identities of those cells even into adult life. These genes also provide for receptors on the cell membrane to receive specific inductive and neurotrophic molecules. From a molecular genetic perspective, homeoboxes consist of specific nucleotide sequences that encode a DNA-binding sequence, the *homeodomain* that is found in many transcriptional regulator proteins involved in development. Some human malformations are likely the result of failure of segmentation, with ectopic or deficient expression of homeoboxes to form normal neuromeres. Examples include congenital absence of the mesencephalon and metencephalon with cerebellar hypoplasia, probably due to an *EN=2* mutation (Sarnat et al. 2002) and perhaps the Chiari malformations (Sarnat et al. 2004a).

The evolutionary biologists and theorists of the late nineteenth century, led by Thomas Huxley in England, were constantly seeking "missing links" in evolution—between humans and great apes, between primates and other mammals, between mammals and reptiles, and, most perplexing of all, between vertebrates and invertebrates, whose bodies and central nervous systems differ so greatly that evidence of homology between structures often is elusive when one must depend solely on anatomic and histological examination. *Homeoboxes are the missing link*, because nucleic acid sequences *identical* to those that serve as segment polarity genes in larval arthropods and worms also program embryonic segmentation of the vertebrate brain (De Pomerai 1990).

Homeoboxes are restricted DNA sequences composed of 183 base pairs of nucleotides that encode a class of proteins sharing a common or very similar 60-amino-acid motif, the *homeodomain* (McGinnis and Krumlauf 1992). Homeodomains contain sequence-specific DNA binding sites and are components of larger regulatory proteins, the transcription factors. Homeoboxes, or homeotic genes, are classified into various families having a common molecular structure

and similar general expression in ontogenesis. A set of some 13 *Hox*genes determines the rostrocaudal gradient of differentiation of the neural tube and also creates *neuromeres*, segments that restrict cellular migration in the longitudinal axis (Keynes and Krumlauf 1994). A series of eight such segments, or *rhombomeres*, each of which forms predictable structures, has been identified in the hindbrain (Keynes and Lumsden 1990; Lumsden 1990). Rhombomeres are identified morphologically as a series of transverse ridges and ringlike constrictions at the dorsal or ventricular surface of the hindbrain. The eighth rhombomere is continuous with the spinal cord. Apparent segmentation of the spinal cord is

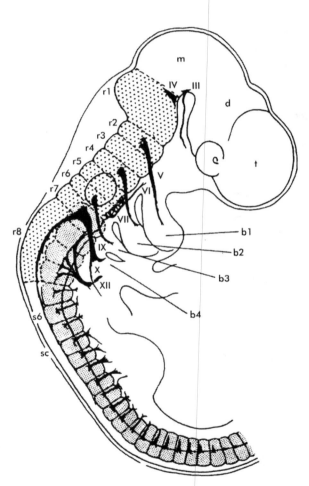

Figure 1.1 Drawing of parasagittal section of a 3-day chick embryo to illustrate hindbrain rhombomeres (rl–r8) as a primary segmentation of the developing central nervous system. These compartments are mainly programmed by *Hox* homeobox genes. The spinal cord *(sc)* is really a caudal continuation of r8, and its segmentation is secondary, imposed by surrounding mesodermal somites. The midbrain *(m)* neuromere and diencephalic *(d)* and telencephalic *(t)* neuromeres are rostral continuations of the series; the forebrain actually consists of at least three distinct neuromeres. The cranial motor nerves *(III–XII)* are shown, but not the cranial ganglia. The exit points of branchial motor nerves *(V, VII, IX)* are in alternate rhombomeres, in register with the first three branchial arches (bl–b3). The entire cerebellum is derived from rl. (Reproduced from Lumsden A. The cellular basis of segmentation in the developing hindbrain. *Trends in Neuroscience* 13:329–335, 1990. Copyright 1990, Elsevier Science, Ltd. Used with permission.)

actually a phenomenon of changes between somites adjacent to the spinal cord (Stern et al. 1991).The spinal cord does show distinctions in different regions, for example parasympathetic preganglionic neurons confined to the cervical and sacral regions and sympathetic neurons in the thoracolumbar region, and the presence of the column of Clarke, neurons of origin of the dorsal spinocerebellar tract, only at T1 to L2 levels, but these regional differences do not denote distinct compartments separated by neuromeric boundaries in embryonic life, hence are not true segments or distinct neuromeres.

In traditional neuroembryology the CNS is divided into two components, the brain and the spinal cord. However, the organization of the spinal cord is merely a continuation of fundamental brainstem architecture; molecular biology and comparative vertebrate neuroanatomy suggest that the spinal cord is nothing more than an elongated single rhombomere. It appears segmental only because of extrinsic groupings of nerve roots imposed by the primary segmentation of adjacent somites and of bony neural arches. A few intrinsic regional differences do occur, however, such as the autonomic relay nuclei of the intermediolateral columns and the column of Clarke for spinocerebellar relay.

The entire cerebellum is derived from rhombomere 1 (rl), though the deep cerebellar nuclei arise from r2. (Fig. 1.1). Each cranial nerve originates from a pair of sequential rhombomeres lying in register with an adjacent branchial arch. Thus, the neurons of the trigeminal nerve derive from r2 and r3, opposite the first branchial arch; the facial nucleus arises from r4 and r5, opposite the second arch; and the glossopharyngeal nerve emerges from r6 and r7, opposite the third arch. Furthermore, the rostral member of each rhombomere pair produces motor axons earlier than does the caudal member and contains the motor nerve root. The mesencephalic neural crest develops and migrates not only from the mesencephalic neuromere (r0), but also from r1 and r2' (the rostral half of r2, which together with r1, produces the metencephalon or rostral pons, in addition to the cerebellum).

The intermitotic to-and-fro movement of proliferating neuroepithelial cell nuclei within their own radial cytoplasmic processes, between the ventricular and pial surfaces, is active within rhombomeres but is reduced or absent at rhombomere boundaries. Although cells continue to divide at the ventricular surface at boundaries, their nuclei remain close to this surface throughout the cell cycle; this relative stasis and increased cell-cell adhesion contributes to the formation of barriers to cellular movement from one rhombomere to the next (Guthrie et al. 1991).

Certain genes are essential to segmentation of the neural tube and, if not expressed at the proper time, specific neuromeres fail to form (Sarnat and Menkes 2000). For example, agenesis of the midbrain and metencephalon (rostral pons) with cerebellar agenesis or hypoplasia may be caused by mutations in the WNT1, EN1 or EN2 homeobox genes (Sarnat et al 2004).

FAMILIES OF REGULATORY GENES OF EARLY NEURAL DEVELOPMENT

Fundamental Organizer Genes (Notch, Delta, Numb, Lim, islet, twist, Cnot, goosecoid)

These organizer genes establish the fundamental axes of differentiation and growth of the neuroepithelium from the time of gastrulation and also are important in determining cell fate, including to which germ layer a cell belongs. The expression of achaete-scute converts ectodermal cells to a neural fate (Turner and Weintraub 1994) and provides for neural induction and position along the mediallateral axis of the neural plate (Zimmerman et al. 1993). Notch regulates the competence of cells to induction. Notch is expressed in virtually all embryonic cells, in contrast to achaete-scute genes, whose expression is restricted to small territories from which neurons arise (Fortini and Artavanis-Tsakonas 1993). Neural precursors, by expressing the "antagonistic" gene Delta, inhibit neighboring Notch expressing cells from becoming committed to a neural fate. Interference with Delta activity results in overproduction of primary neurons; thus, commitment to a neural fate is regulated by Delta-s-Notch signaling (Chitnis et al. 1995; Henrique et al. 1995).

Notch is symmetrically expressed during the mitotic cycling of the neuroepithelial cell, and its gene products are concentrated on one side of the cell; an antagonistic gene, Numb, is associated with Delta and is expressed on the side of the cell opposite to Notch expression. The orientation of the cleavage plane or mitotic spindle, whether parallel with or perpendicular to the ventricular surface, determines the fate of the pair of daughter cells; if the cleavage plane is perpendicular to the ventricular wall, Notch and Numb are equally divided between the two daughter cells; if the cleavage is parallel, however, one cell inherits nearly all of the Notch and the other inherits nearly all of the Numb. One of these cells is at the ventricular surface and reenters the mitotic cycle; the other loses its attachment to the ventricle and becomes a postmitotic premigratory neuroblast (Chenn and McConnell 1995; Guo et al. 1996; Spana and Doe 1996). Lim-1, a gene generated in embryonic stem cells (undifferentiated progenitor cells), is the "head organizer." Mouse embryos homozygous for the null allele (inactivated Lim-1) lack anterior head structures, including the forebrain, although the remaining body axis and neural tube are normally formed (Shawlot and Behringer 1995). Although the earliest expression of Lim-1 is in a small zone of the mammalian epiblast (i.e., dorsal lip of the amphibian gastrula) where the primitive streak forms (Shawlot and Behringer 1995), at a later stage Lim-1 and Zz'ra-3, together with members of another family of organizer genes, islet-1 and islet-2, define subclasses of motor neurons that segregate into columns in the spinal cord (Tsuchida et al. 1994). Motor neurons cannot be generated without islet genes (Pfaff et al. 1996) and Sonic hedgehog (discussed below). Another gene, twist, is equally essential for differentiation of the cranial neural tube; in *twist-mill* mice, the cranial neural folds fail to fuse and there are defects in the head mesoderm and somites (Chen and Behringer 1995).

The gene *Cnot* (*Xnot* in the amphibian), first expressed in Hensen's node, is critical to notochordal identity and hence to induction of the floor plate and further development of the neural tube; a related gene, *goosecoid*, performs a similar programming function for the prechordal mesoderm, inducing the rostral neural tube to form the forebrain (Stein and Kessel 1995). A transition *from goosecoid* to *Cnot* expression may begin while cells are still in the epiblast stage but does not occur after cells assume a mesodermal identity.

Sonic hedgehog (Shh) Family

Sonic hedgehog (Shh) is the name of an early gene of neural induction, the protein product of which is secreted by Hensen's node, the notochord, and floor plate ependymal cells in the ventral midline even before closure of the neural tube (Echelard et al. 1993); the floor plate cells are the first neuroepithelial cells to differentiate. *Hedgehog (hh),* the insect homologue *of Shh,* is a segment polarity gene. *Shh,* one of a family of four *hh* genes in vertebrates, is a regulator of polarity for induction of the ventral CNS and exerts a strong ventralizing influence on dorsal structures; it defines longitudinal columns of cells that are present along the entire neuraxis (Shimamura et al. 1995). *Shh* also programs a strip of posterior and distal mesenchyme on the developing limb bud that is closely associated with the overlying ectoderm (Echelard et al. 1993; Maden et al. 1991; Riddle et al. 1993). The *Shh* protein acts in a concentration-dependent gradient to induce different cell fates across a developing segment of limb bud or neural tissue. *Shh* is unique among the organizer genes in encoding not only a signaling molecule but also a protease required for its own processing (Peifer 1994). Retinoic acid (or its alcohol, retinol or vitamin A) induces *Shh* expression, but excess retinoic acid interferes with rhombomere segmentation in the otic region of r4 and the associated neural crest of r3-r5 by altering the transcriptional activity of *Hox-2.9* and *Krox-20* genes (Maden et al. 1991; Morriss-Kay et al. 1991; Schneider-Maunoury et al. 1993). Retinoic acid is synthesized by both the notochord and the floor plate (Wagner et al. 1990). *Shh* signals from the floor plate induce differentiation of motor neuroblasts. *Shh* is expressed in the ventral part of the forebrain as well as in more posterior regions of the neuraxis, despite the fact that the notochord and floor plate do not extend rostrally beyond the mesencephalic-diencephalic junction. The floor plate is itself induced by the notochord, probably through the synthesis of *Shh* protein and retinoic acid. *Shh* expression activates other important genes in both the CNS and the limb bud, including *Wnt-1* (Echelard et al. 1993) and *Hox* genes (Riddle et al. 1993). Similarly, in insects, *hh* is expressed concomitantly with the segment polarity genes *wg* (homologue of *Wnt-1)* and *engrailed* (homologue of *En-1)* (Lee et al. 1992).

Hox Family and (murine) Krox-20 (human EGR-2)

The primary family of homeobox genes for hindbrain segmentation, known as *Hox,* includes a bHLH transcription factor that encodes a 60-amino-acid homeodomain in the spinal cord and brainstem (Guthrie et al. 1992; Storey et al. 1992). The *Hox* family includes 38 members, which in vertebrates are organized into four gene clusters that are activated during gastrulation. *Hox-2* consists of a cluster of nine genes distributed on four different chromosomes (2, 7, 12, and 17) that specify the anterior limit of each rhombomere: *Hox-2.1* is restricted to the spinal cord; *Hox-2.6* is expressed in the spinal cord and extends rostrally to the boundary of r6/r7; *Hox-2.7* extends further rostrally to specify the boundary of r4/r5; *Hox-2.8* establishes the boundary of r2/r3; and *Hox-2.9* is expressed only in r4 and overlaps the domain *of Hox-1.6,* which includes r4 through r7. Although *Shh* from the floor plate induces initial motor neuron differentiation, *Hox-2* genes preserve their identity in the hindbrain (Kessel 1994). *Hox-2* genes also pattern migratory neural crest cells from r4, *and Hox-1.5* appears to program the formation of mesencephalic neural crest tissue as well as the thymus and parathyroid glands (Chisaka and Capecchi 1991; Hunt et al. 1991).

Another gene, *Krox-20* (mouse gene, same as *EGR-2* in the human), is one of the "zinc fingers" because of zinc-containing histidine and cysteine residues in its transcription factor, it is expressed in alternating rhombomeres, mainly r3 and r5; it is important in neural crest development and also regulates the expression of other genes, particularly those of the *Hox* family (Wilkinson and Krumlauf 1990). Retinoic acid antagonizes the expression of *Hox* genes and thus is considered to be another regulator (Kessel 1993). *Krox-20* (*EGR-2)* suppresses the formation of neural crest tissue. As this tissue forms in the dorsal region of r3 and r5, these neural crest primordia shift rostrally and caudally to join the neural crest forming in the adjacent rhombomeres, so that r3 and r5 appear to have no neural crest contribution.

Pax (Paired) Family

Like *Hox* genes, the family *of paired* homeobox, or *Pax,* genes is also is involved in the establishment of compartments and boundaries that segment the neural tube; in addition, *Pax* genes play a role in dorsal patterning and in establishing neuronal identity in the dorsal half of the neural tube (Chalepakis et al. 1993; Koseki et al. 1993; Stoykova and Gruss 1994). Regional expression *of Pax* genes occurs in response to signals from the notochord and floor plate (Goulding et al. 1993; Koseki et al. 1993). *Pax-2* is expressed in the ventricular zone in two compartments of cells on either side of the sulcus limitans along the entire rhombencephalon and spinal cord; it is also expressed in the ventral half of the optic cup and stalk (Nornes et al. 1990). *Pax-6* is expressed in discrete regions of the forebrain and hindbrain, the eye, and the pituitary and olfactory nasal epithelium (Callaerts et al. 1997; Walther and Gruss 1991). *Pax-1* is expressed in sclerotome cells but only in the presence of an intact notochord (Koseki et al. 1993); it acts as a mediator of notochordal signals for the dorsoventral specification of sclerotomes that will form the ventral parts of vertebrae (Koseki et al. 1993). Signals from the notochord also regulate regionally specific *Pax-3* and *Pax-6* genes in the developing spinal cord (Goulding et al. 1993). These genes continue to be active in the adult CNS in maintaining cell identity and integrity: high levels of *Pax-6* are expressed by cerebellar granule cells, and *Pax-3* transcripts are associated with Bergmann glial cells (Stoykova and Gruss 1994). *Wnt-3* (discussed later), by contrast, is expressed in adult as well as fetal Purkinje cells and is modulated by presynaptic granule cells, presumably under the regulation of *Pax-6*, at the time of neuronal maturation (Salinas et al. 1994). More than one gene may be required for specific cellular lineage. Cerebellar granule cells are maintained not only by *Pax-6* but also by *Zic*, another "zinc finger" gene product (Aruga et al. 1994).

Wnt (Wingless) and En (Engrailed) Families

The *Wnt* family is an important group of genes that program the secretion of cell-signaling or inductive molecules early in differentiation of the nervous system (McMahon 1992). Ten *Wnt* genes have been identified in the mouse embryo; the *Wnt* family is homologous with the segment polarity gene *wingless (wg)* in the fly. Each mammalian *Wnt* gene has a characteristic expression at particular sites in the rostrocaudal axis of the developing neural tube; of equal importance is the dorsoventral polarizing gradient that organizes the brain in the axis perpendicular to the longitudinal axis and exerts a strong "dorsalizing" influence that antagonizes the "ventralizing" induction effect of the notochord and floor plate. In the mouse, *Wnt* expression is strongly expressed in a domain nearly identical to that of the homeobox gene *En-1* (*engrailed* in the larval fly), throughout the midbrain and rostral half of the metencephalon in rl (Joyner and Martin 1987). More caudally, *Wnt-1* expression is confined to the lateral margins of neural plate that later fuse in the dorsal midline with neurulation to become the medulla oblongata and spinal cord. *Wnt-1* is expressed weakly and diffusely rostral to the midbrain neuromere; *Wnt-7*, by contrast, is strongly expressed in the future diencephalon and telencephalon (Parr et al. 1993). The major domain of *Wnt-3* is the myelencephalon, in r3 through r8, where it possesses a strong dorsal polarizing gradient and induces cellular differentiation.

The limits of expression of *En* and *Wnt* genes change with maturation. Neither *En-1* nor *Wnt-1* is active in the mouse embryo before formation of the first somite, but, coinciden-

tal with the condensation of the first mesodermal somite, overlapping expression of *En-1* and *Wnt-1* is detected in the neuroepithelium just rostral to the preotic sulcus. By the three-somite stage, *En-1* and *Wnt-1* domains extend throughout the midbrain neuromere, and many individual cells coexpress the two genes (this is different from what occurs in the fly; however, in that species, a mosaic mixture of cells expressing either *En* or *Wnt* is present in each segment). By the six-somite stage, *Wnt-1* expression is more extensive in the longitudinal axis but is restricted to the dorsal region of the hindbrain and also is stronger dorsally than ventrally in the midbrain. By the 27- through 30-somite stages, *Wnt-1* is almost exclusively confined to the dorsal midline of the midbrain and is no longer detected in ventral regions (McMahon and Bradley 1990; McMahon et al. 1992).

Diencephalic and Telencephalic Gene Families

Several homeotic genes—among them *Wnt-1,Dlx-1, Dlx-2,* and *Nkx-2.2*—are expressed in the developing forebrain, but their functions are incompletely defined (Bulfone et al. 1993; Figdor and Stern 1993; Price et al. 1992; Puelles and Rubenstein 1993; Salinas and Nusse 1992). *Nkx-2.2* also controls the patterning of longitudinal columns of neural cells along the entire neuraxis (Shimamura et al. 1995). Transcriptors of *Cnot* are expressed in the epiphysis and ventral diencephalon at early stages; *goosecoid* is a gene similar to *Cnot* that is expressed only in the prenotochordal mesoderm for forebrain induction (Stein and Kessel 1995). The segmentation established in the hindbrain might also exist in the diencephalon, but the segments appear later and might represent functional units (Figdor and Stern 1993).

Spinal Cord Gene Families

Ironically, the spinal cord remains the only region of the CNS for which no evidence yet exists of an intrinsic segmentation based on compartmental groupings of differentiating neurons (Lim et al.1991). The *Hox-2.1* domain in the spinal cord is an earlier domain of the homeobox gene *Cnot* in the postnodal neural plate caudal to the primordial hindbrain (Stein and Kessel 1995). The apparent segmentation of spinal nerve roots is imposed by surrounding mesodermal structures that form the neural arches of the vertebrae and somites (Sarnat 1992a; Stern et al. 1991; Tosney 1988). The developing neural arches secrete keratan sulfate; this glycosaminoglycan is a strong repellant of axonal growth cones, which prevents the aberrant wandering of developing nerve roots.

DISORDERS OF GENETIC PATTERNING OR NEURAL INDUCTION

Examination of the expression of homozygous mutant genes, or "knockout genes," and the up regulation or overexpression of individual genes can provide a great deal of insight not only into the functions of each of the genes but also into the redundancy of function that allows them to act as substitutes for one another. Researchers have bred and studied many experimental lines of mutant genetic mice with inactivated alleles of specific genes, some of which may relate to human malformations that are not easily explained by classical embryology. Abnormal or defective gene expression is a topic beyond the scope of this chapter.

NEURULATION

The posterior neuropore is not located at the extreme caudal end of the developing neural tube. *Primary neurulation* involves closure of the neural tube at the dorsal midline between the rostral and caudal neuropores and results in formation of the brain and spinal cord to the sacral region. *Secondary neurulation* appears after closure of the caudal neuropore and results in formation of the caudal-most section of spinal cord, the conus medullaris and, in vertebrates with tails, the caudal segments. This part of the spinal cord, as well as other axial tail structures in the human embryo, derives from mesenchymal cells in the tail bud (Lemire 1969; Saraga-Babic et al. 1996). The caudal most segments of the spinal cord develop as a solid rod of neuroepithelial cells that secondarily forms a lumen by ependymal extension of the central canal rather than by closure of a sheet of cells to form a tube. In fishes, the entire spinal cord initially forms as a solid rod of cells rather than as a folded sheet.

Bending of the neural plate to form the neural tube requires both extrinsic and intrinsic mechanical forces (Marin-Padilla 1991; Schoenwolf and Smith 1990). Extrinsic forces are generated in part by the growth of mesodermal tissues flanking the neural plate that will form the somites. Removal of this mesoderm and of the endoderm lateral to the neural plate in the early chick embryo does not prevent neural tube formation but causes the neural tube to be rotated toward the side of the removed tissue (Alvarez and Schoenwolf 1992). Thus, although the mesoderm is important for maintaining the orientation of the neural tube, expansion of the surface epithelium provides the major extrinsic force that bends the neural plate (Alvarez and Schoenwolf 1992; Jacobson 1991). Neural plate cells are motile and attempt to crawl beneath the surface ectoderm along their common boundary, raising neural folds toward the dorsal midline, but the primordial epidermis also offers resistance to neural tube formation (Schoenwolf and Franks 1984). Growth of the embryo as a whole does not appear to be an important factor in neurulation, because neurulation proceeds at the same rate in anamniotes that grow (e.g., birds and mammals) and anamniotes that do not grow (e.g., amphibians) during this period (Jacobson 1991).

Intrinsic forces of primary neurulation begin with the notochordal induction of floor plate differentiation, which establishes the longitudinal axis of the neural plate. The floor plate cells assume the shape of a wedge, narrow at the apex and wide at the base, to accommodate the nucleus, which no longer travels to and fro within the bipolar cytoplasm as it did during mitotic cycling. The wedged shaping of neuroepithelial cells during neurulation may not be as important as was previously thought, except perhaps at certain "hinge points," and not all cells assume this shape (Schoenwolf and Franks 1984; Smith and Schoenwolf 1989). Also, ependymal cells do not completely line the ventricles or central canal of the spinal cord until long after neurulation is complete (Sarnat 1992a, 1992b). Adhesion molecules contribute additional intrinsic factors promoting neurulation. The selective expression of some regulatory genes, such as *Wnt-1*, at the lateral margins of the neural plate during neurulation probably plays an as yet undefined role in the intrinsic curling of the neural plate.

The neural tube closes in the dorsal midline first in the cervical region, with the closure then extending rostrally and caudally so that the anterior neuropore of the human embryo closes at 24 days and the posterior neuropore closes at 28 days, the distances from the cervical region being unequal. This traditional view of a continuous zipper-like closure is an oversimplification. In the mouse embryo, the neural tube closes in the cranial region at four distinct sites, with the closure proceeding bidirectionally or unidirectionally and in general synchrony with somite formation (Golden and Chernoff 1993; Juriloff et al. 1991). An intermittent pattern of anterior neural tube closure involving multiple sites has also been described in human embryos (Busam et al. 1993). In this closure, the principal rostral neuropore closes bidirectionally (O'Rahilly and Muller 1989) to form the lamina terminalis, the primordium of the forebrain (Sarnat 1992a).

Neurulation and the development of the central nervous system pose the question of the fundamental definition of "brain" and its distinction from a "cephalic ganglion." A brain is a rostral, bilobed neural structure with internal architecture of gray and white matter, commissural fibers interconnecting the two halves, and in which the interneuron is the predominant neuron; it regulates the entire body. Ganglia, by contrast, may be rostral or occur anywhere else including the peripheral nervous system, are not bilobed, have no somatotopic internal architecture and no commissural fibers, and interneurons are sparse or absent, the neurons being almost exclusively primary sensory or motor neurons; ganglia subserve restricted segments, not the entire body (Sarnat and Netsky 2002).

NEURAL CREST SEPARATION AND MIGRATION

The neural crest is a tissue of such importance that some authors have even suggested that its status be elevated to that of a "germ layer," equal to the ectoderm, mesoderm, and endoderm. (Hall 2000) Neural crest is the means by which the embryonic neural tube induces many nonneural tissues, including most of the craniofacial structure (Carstens 2004; Hall 1999; Le Douarin and Kalcheim 1999). In addition, neural crest contributes much of the peripheral nervous system, particularly autonomic and somatosensory nerves and ganglia.

Incipient neural crest cells first appear at the lateral margins of the neuroepithelial placode on the day of gastrulation, but these cells are not yet "committed" to a specific fate. As the neural placode bends dorsally on either side to form the neural groove, and then the two sides meet in the dorsal midline and close to form the neural tube, the neural crest cells are those adjacent to the dorsal midline. Shortly thereafter they migrate along prescribed routes throughout the embryo to differentiate after reaching their final destination. They form neural structures of the peripheral nervous system—including neurons of the dorsal root and sympathetic ganglia, Schwann cells of peripheral nerves and chromaffin cells such as those of the adrenal medulla and carotid body. They also form structures of mesodermal origin, including blood vessels and melanocytes or pigment cells, blood vessels and membranous bones including the orbits, cranial vault, and most of the facial skeleton (Carstens 2004; Hall 1999; Le Douarin and Kalcheim 1999; Tan and Morriss-Kay 1985).

Neural crest cells migrate in a somewhat different manner from each part of the embryonic segmental neural tube, the neuromeres. The neural crest may be divided into three groups on this basis (Puelles and Rubenstein 2003). The *prosencephalic neural crest* migrates rostrally into the head as a vertical sheet of cells. The *mesencephalic neural crest,* which arises not only from the mesencephalic neuromere (i.e., future midbrain), but also from the first two hindbrain rhombomeres (neuromeres r1 and r2' or the rostal half of r2), migrates as streams of cells. The *rhombencephalic neural crest,* arising from the hindbrain and spinal cord, migrates as segmental blocks of cells (Bronner-Fraser 1994; Carstens 2004).

Though patterns of genetic expression in the hindbrain probably contribute to the segmental arrangement of neural crest cells, cellular migratory pathways also are guided by attractant and repulsant paracrine molecules secreted by surrounding tissues such as the otic capsule, the somites, and the vertebral neural arches (Jacobson 1991). In addition, neural crest cells possess integrin receptors for interacting with extracellular matrix molecules (Bronner-Fraser 1994). Changes in the distribution of extracellular matrix components during neural crest migration impose migratory guidance limits as well (Sadaghiani et al. 1994).

The neural crest consists of a series of overlapping cell populations that differ in their migratory pathways and fates. The precise origin of neural crest cells is a complex issue, because these cells form so many different mature structures, including some, such as facial bones, that ordinarily would be of mesodermal origin. Why neural crest precursors are so heterogeneous, why neural crest stem cells with multiple potentials exist, and even whether stem cells arising from the neural tube are joined by surrounding cells from the mesodermal germ layer are not as well understood as the migratory pathways of neural crest cells (Selleck et al. 1993). Like other parts of the neural tube, neural crest tissue has a rostrocaudal gradient of differentiation. The fate of neural crest cells is not entirely predetermined; environmental factors may induce differentiation of different cells than ordinarily would have occurred. For example, although early migrating neural crest cells generally form dorsal root ganglion cells, when these early migrating cells are ablated, the late migrating neural crest cells that ordinarily form mesodermal structures will change their fate to become neurons. Furthermore, transplantation of early-migrating neural crest cells does not result in production of neurons under all conditions (Raible and Eisen 1996). Neurotrophic factors (e.g., neurotrophin-3 [NT-3]) also influence the fate of neural crest cells and are essential for survival of sympathetic neuroblasts and innervation of specific organs (El Shamy et al. 1996). NT-3 is the only neurotrophin needed by neurons of the myenteric plexus, but other neural crest derivatives require other factors. Nerve growth factor (NGF) was the first neurotrophin identified and was shown in dorsal root ganglia. Brain-derived neurotrophic factor (BDNF), ciliary neurotrophic factor (CNTF) and glial-derived neurotrophic factor (GNTF) all are associated with neural crest migration or differentiation (Sieber-Blum 1999).

The origin of neural crest is topographically unequal in the neuraxis. The streams of cells arising in the midbrain contributes to formation of the bony orbit, the connective tissue of the eye, the membranous bones of the face, the ciliary ganglion, part of the trigeminal ganglion, and the Schwann cells of nerves (Bronner-Fraser 1994; Le Douarin and Kalcheim 1999; Tan and Morriss-Kay 1985). In the hindbrain, the stream of migratory neural crest cells from r1 and r2 populates the trigeminal ganglion and mandibular arch; cells from r4 form the hyoid arch and the geniculate and vestibular ganglia; and those from r6 populate the third and fourth branchial arches and the associated peripheral ganglia (Bronner-Fraser 1994; Lumsden et al. 1991). Rhombomeres 3 and 5 appear to not generate neural crest cells, but the expression of Krox-20 (human EGR2) only in r3 and r5 causes the neural crest cells of these segments to deviate rostrally and caudally and migrate with cells of adjacent rhombomeres (Bronner-Fraser 1994).

Genetic Programming of Neural Crest

Many genes are essential to the formation of neural crest, but the most important are those having a strong dorsalizing effect in the vertical axis of the neural tube: *ZIC2, BMP4, PAX3.* Ventralizing genes of the vertical axis, such as *Shh,* inhibit neural crest formation, by contrast (Bronner-Fraser 1995). The gene *EGR2* (*Krox-20* in the mouse) is strongly expressed only in rhombomeres r3 and r5 and in the neural crest cells from r5/r6 that migrate caudally around the otic vesicle (Bronner-Fraser 1994). This gene tends to suppress neural crest or cause their precursor cells to migrate to adjacent rhombomeres, rostally and caudally, before migrating into the periphery. *Hox-1.5* and *Hox-2.9* regulate the premigratory and migratory neural crest cells from r4 (Chisaka and Capecchi 1991; Hunt et al. 1991). The gene *SLUG* (*Snail* in invertebrates) seems to be essential for later stages of neural crest differentiation, though it also can be detected in early stages of the neural placode, later regressing in expression and then re-expressed in stronger form. Other genes implicated in neural crest development include *OTX* (*EMX1, 2*), *PHOX*, *DLX*, and *TWIST*. The *PAX* and *MSX* families are of particular importance in craniofacial development associated with prosencephalic and mesencephalic neural crest migration (Bei et al. 2002).

Relation of Neural Crest to CNS Malformations

Many genetically-programmed malformations of the brain are associated with facial dysmorphism that can now be understood in the context of a disturbance of neural crest. Holoprosencephaly is a prime example. The midfacial hypoplasia in many cases of holoprosencephaly was the basis for the DeMyer et al. (1964) frequently quoted statement, "the face predicts the brain." It became apparent that many children with even the most severe alobar form of holoprosencephaly had normal faces, however, and that some children with even the mildest lobar forms of this malformation had severe craniofacial dysgeneses. The reason for this disparity is the extent of the rostrocaudal gradient of expression of the defective gene(s) in holoprosencephaly, which may affect the mesencephalic neural crest in particular. If the gradient extends beyond the diencephalon to cause noncleavage in the dorsal midline of the mesencephalon, neural crest formation or migration is affected and defective development of midline structures of the face, with hypotelorism and absence or hypoplasia of the premaxilla and vomer bones, may result (Sarnat and Flores-Sarnat 2002). This embryonic midbrain involvement is not related to the severity of the forebrain noncleavage. The DeMyer statement was thus further specified as "the face predicts the rostrocaudal gradient of genetic expression that impairs mesencephalic neural crest," providing an explanation as well as a clinical observation. Finally, Carstens (2004) turned the DeMyer statement around in stating, "the brain predicts the face," indicating the primary role of the neural tube in craniofacial development.

Another example of neural crest defects associated with cerebral malformations is the hypertelorism that commonly accompanies agenesis of the corpus callosum. All birds and mammals have their eyes either on the side of the head or directed forward. The natural growth of the orbits is for the eyes to remain the lateral facial structures

that they are in the early fetus. Those animals that have their eyes directed forward (e.g., bears, cats, primates) have an extra bundle of connective tissue, the *intercanthal ligament*, that holds the orbits and periorbital soft tissues together as the face grows. This ligament is in the zone of prosencephalic neural crest origin. The owl provides further confirmation that it arises from neural crest. The owl is the only bird with eyes directed forward. The intercanthal ligament of the owl ossifies, unlike any mammal. The bone formed is membranous bone, which can only originate in neural crest or paraxial mesodermal; since paraxial mesoderm does not form at this rostral level, the presence of membranous bone can only be of neural crest origin.

The importance of the study of craniofacial clefts is that each cleft, indicating an absence of neural crest bone formation, is a marker of the site and timing of the neural crest migration from specific individual neuromeres of the embryonic brain (Carstens 2004).

Relation of Neural Crest to Neurocutaneous Syndromes

Neurocutaneous syndromes are a diverse group of unrelated diseases, some with mendelian inheritance patterns (e.g., tuberous sclerosis complex and neurofibromatosis 1 and 2 as autosomal dominant traits) and others without evident inheritance patterns (e.g., Sturge-Weber syndrome; incontinentia pigmenti). Because the clinical and pathological expression of these diseases is so diverse, it is difficult to generalize about a common embryological origin. Because brain and skin are both of ectodermal origin, and because both tissues are affected in the neurocutaneous syndromes, the traditional view is that these are disorders of ectoderm. This interpretation is probably erroneous for two reasons: (1) organizer genes that program early development are expressed in many tissues and do not respect the traditional germ layers; some of these genes are likely defective in the various neurocutaneous syndromes; (2) neural crest induces not only neural structures of the peripheral nervous system, but also many mesodermal structures of the face, head, and body. A more rational explanation of a common embryology of the neurocutaneous syndromes is that they are all disorders of neural crest. For example, in neurofibromatosis 1, the most frequent, there are disturbances in growth in peripheral nerves (neural crest), melancyte distribution in the dermis (neural crest), a high incidence of pheochromocytoma (neural crest), and an increased incidence of hypertelorism (neural crest). In addition, there are disturbances that are not of neural crest origin, such as the high incidence of optic nerve gliomas, but the *NF-1* gene is also a tumor suppressor gene and may act on nonneural crest tissues. Tuberous sclerosis complex is more problematic in this regard, because there is a cellular dysgenesis that involves almost every organ of the body in addition to failure of tumor suppression function and neural crest abnormalities, such as the angiofibromata of the facial skin ("adenoma sebaceum"). In epidermal nevus syndrome ("linear sebaceous nevus of Jadissohn"), a midline pigmented or depigmented vertical line extends from the forehead onto the nose, clearly a prosencephalic neural crest abnormality of melanocyte differentiation.

This new concept of the embryology of neurocutaneous syndromes deriving from disturbances of neural crest formation or migration may lead to a reclassification of neurocutaneous syndromes as a category of "neuro-cristopathies," with other categories that include aganglionic megacolon (Hirschsprung disease), Waardenburg syndrome, and familial dysautonomia (Riley-Day syndrome) (Sarnat and Flores-Sarnat 2005).

NEUROEPITHELIAL CELL PROLIFERATION AND DIFFERENTIATION

Early cleavages of the fertilized ovum to form the blastula and gastrula involve a simple proliferation of blastomere cells cycling between mitotic (M-phase) and resting (S-phase) states, a process little different from bacterial DNA replication. As the neurectoderm develops in the epiblast at postovulatory week 3 in the human embryo, it becomes organized as pseudostratified columnar epithelium, a sheet of bipolar cells all oriented so that one cytoplasmic process extends to the dorsal (future ventricular) surface and the other process extends to the ventral (future pial) surface. The nucleus of each cell moves to and fro within the cell's cytoplasmic extensions. M-phase occurs at or near the ventricular surface and S-phase occurs at the other surface. The transitional periods between these two states are known as "gap phases," G-l when the nucleus moves distally toward the surface of the brain, and G-2 when it moves proximally toward the ventricular surface (Sauer 1935). During the normal cell cycle, S-phase always follows M-phase; the gap phases allow for adjustments to be made in the replication of DNA in G-l, and the sequence ensures that G-2 cells do not undergo an extra round of S-phase, which would lead to a change in ploidy as the chromosomes segregate in the dividing cell (Nurse 1994). In this way, errors may be corrected before the next mitosis, thus allowing for more plasticity than would the all or none principle of simple cell division. Mitoses continue to occur at the ventricular surface when the neural tube forms with the folding of the neuroepithelial plate. As the brain develops, other sites of mitotic activity include the external granular layer of the cerebellum and the olfactory epithelium, but these are specialized exceptions. A population of quiescent neuroepithelial stem cells in the subventricular region of the mammalian forebrain retains a proliferative potential for gliogenesis and perhaps for neuronogenesis even in the adult (Diener and Bregman 1994).

Disturbances of cellular growth and proliferation characterize several genetic disorders that primarily involve the central nervous system, including Proteus syndrome, tuber-

ous sclerosis, and hemimegalencephaly in multiple syndromes (Cohen 2001; Flores-Sarnat 2002; Flores-Sarnat et al. 2003). In many of these (e.g., tuberous sclerosis, hemimegalencephaly), the primary disturbance is one of cellular lineage, with abnormal individual brain cells expressing mixed glial and neuronal proteins (Curatolo 2003; Flores-Sarnat et al. 2003).

FLOOR PLATE AND EPENDYMA

The floor plate is the first structure of the neuroepithelium to differentiate. This specialized ependyma, a longitudinal column of cells in the midline of the neuroepithelial plate, is induced by the notochord. Like the notochord, the floor plate extends from the caudal end of the neuroepithelium as far rostrally as the midbrain-diencephalic junction; in the diencephalon, the floor plate may transiently form but becomes incorporated into the infundibulum and hence cannot be recognized. Whether a transient floor plate exists briefly in the prosencephalon before "cleavage" into paired telencephalic hemispheres is uncertain, but, even in the absence of a demonstrable corresponding anatomic structure, ventral midline neuroepithelial cells probably serve a similar inductive function. The floor plate exerts a powerful ventralizing influence in the neural tube and, indeed, is a primary organizer of the histological structure of the spinal cord and brainstem (Yamada et al. 1991; Fig. 1.2). Like the notochord but unlike other ependymal cells that differenti-

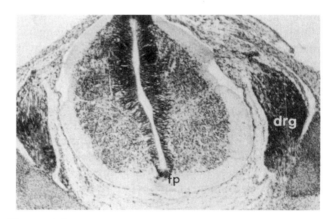

Figure 1.2 Transverse section of fully formed neural tube becoming spinal cord in a 6-week human fetus. The central canal is a large vertical slit whose wall consists largely of undifferentiated neuroepithelium. Dorsal horns and long tracts have not yet formed, but migration of motor neuroblasts is contributing to ventral horn formation. An ependyma is partially differentiated in the region of the roof plate and basal plate but not yet at the alar plate; the floor plate *(fp)* is well formed in the ventral midline. The floor plate is directly induced by the notochord and in turn induces many other structures, including ependyma and motor neurons; it exerts a strong ventralizing effect in the dorsoventral gradient. At this gestational age and earlier, the dorsal root ganglia *(drg)* are large structures lying lateral to the neural tube; they differentiate early from the neural crest after the latter separates from the paramedian dorsal neuroepithelium at the time of dorsal fusion. The dorsal root ganglia show neural crest migration. Hematoxylineosin. *x40.*

ate later, it secretes both retinoic acid and *Sonic hedgehog* glycoprotein. The floor plate induces differentiation of motor neuroblasts, although *Shh* from the notochord may also do this directly.

The adult ependyma is a simple cuboidal epithelial lining of the ventricular system with a function limited to the transport of fluid, ions, and small molecules between the cerebrospinal fluid (CSF) and the cerebral parenchyma. In the fetus, by contrast, the ependyma is a dynamic structure primordial to brain development (Sarnat 1992a, 1992c). A variety of metabolic and structural features distinguish fetal from adult ependyma (Sarnat 1992c).

Structurally, the ependyma differentiates in a precise spatial and temporal sequence in the human fetal CNS, beginning with the floor plate at 3 weeks' gestation and not completely covering the entire surface of the lateral ventricles until 22 weeks' gestation (Sarnat 1992b). The pseudostratified organization represents a continuation of the primitive neuroepithelial structure and gradually becomes thinned to a single layer of cells as the ventricles grow, although the size of the fetal ventricles relative to the mass of the brain is larger than at maturity. Once ependymal cells differentiate, they forever lose their potential for mitotic proliferation, so that the pseudostratified structure allows for the covering of a larger total ventricular surface area as the ependyma becomes a simple epithelium. The postnatal lengthwise growth of the spinal cord is accompanied by progressive narrowing of the central canal and the eventual obliteration of its lumen, because not enough ependymal cells are available to preserve the central canal's tubular shape.

Individual ependymal cells in the fetus have long basal processes that extend radially into the cerebral parenchyma, but these processes do not reach the pial surface in the telencephalon as they do in the brainstem and spinal cord. The processes and their ependymal cell bodies contain cytoskeletal structural proteins such as vimentin, glial fibrillary acid protein (GFAP), and certain cytokeratans; these proteins develop and regress according to a precise schedule, and none of them are expressed by adult ependymal cells. Basal processes are also absent from adult ependymal cells, except for a few small, specialized regions such as the infundibulum and the subcommissural organ. The apical (ventricular) surface of the ependymal cell has microvilli and is ciliated; cilia form early in the differentiation of ependymal cells while the cells are still arranged as a pseudostratified epithelium, and cilia are retained throughout life.

Functionally, the most important difference between fetal and adult ependymal cells is that fetal cells are *secretory* and adult cells are not. The products secreted by fetal cells include (1) glycosaminoglycans and proteoglycans, such as keratan sulfate, that strongly repel axonal growth cones, and (2) other molecules that attract growing axons, such as neton and S-100-beta protein (Kennedy et al. 1994; Sarnat 1992b). The basal processes of ependymal cells intermingle

with developing ascending and descending tracts. One function of the fetal ependyma is to guide the tips of growing axons along their intermediate trajectories (Snow et al. 1990). The influence may be positive or negative: floor plate processes attract and facilitate the passage of commissural fibers but repulse longitudinally growing tracts to prevent aberrant decussation (Bovolenta and Dodd 1990).

Another important function of the fetal ependyma is to arrest mitotic activity of the neuroepithelium. Because nearly all mitoses occur at the ventricular surface, differentiation of an ependyma precludes further cellular proliferation at that site; thus, it is advantageous for ependymal differentiation to be delayed in the fetus as long as possible to allow the requisite number of mitotic cycles to occur and to ensure production of an adequate number of neurons (Sarnat 1992c; Smart 1972).

The ependyma may play a role in transformation of radial glial cells to mature astrocytes, possibly through fetal ependymal secretion of S-100 protein (Sarnat 1992c). Finally, the fetal ependyma, like the adult ependyma, helps to regulate transport of fluid, ions, and small molecules between the CSF and the cerebral parenchyma. Whether the ependyma plays a role in the immune system in the brain is uncertain.

NEURONS

All neurons of a homogeneous population have the same "birthday"—that is, they all differentiate together on the same embryonic day. Examples are the granular cells of layer 3 of the parietal cortex, neurons of various brainstem nuclei, and Purkinje cells of the cerebellum. An exception is the external granule cell of the cerebellum, which proliferates while spreading over the cerebellar cortex from the posterolateral part of the rhombic lip over several days. The external granule cell also is exceptional in being one of only two neurons capable of regeneration; destruction of most (but not all) of the external granule layer by irradiation or by cytotoxic drugs in rodents is followed by cellular proliferation and repopulation of the external granule layer of premigratory neuroblasts (Altman and Anderson 1972; Jones and Gardner 1976; Shimada and Langman 1970). The other neuron capable of regeneration is even more remarkable, because it is fully differentiated; the primary olfactory receptor neuron undergoes a continuous turnover even in adults, a process that is necessary because of its exposed site at the surface of the nasal epithelium and its vulnerability to destruction by upper-respiratory-tract infections. The sensory olfactory neuron is replenished by a population of stem cells at the base of the epithelium that differentiate and establish synaptic contact with target neurons in the mature olfactory bulb (Crews and Hunter 1994).

Among the earliest cells to differentiate within the neural tube after formation of the floor plate are the spinal motor neurons. These are induced by *Shh* gene products secreted by the floor-plate ependyma and the notochord. Differentiation of neurons in the hindbrain occurs first in the even-numbered rhombomeres and then in the odd-numbered segments (Keynes and Lumsden 1990).

How early a neuroepithelial cell is committed to differentiate into a particular type of mature neural cell and, specifically, which type of neuron it is fated to become—questions fundamental to the issue of cerebral plasticity and adaptability of the immature brain to adverse events in fetal life—continue to be highly debated among developmental neurobiologists. Two opposing schools of thought have emerged, each supported by some experimental evidence. The *predetermination hypothesis* presumes that undifferentiated neuroepithelial cells already have different genetic programs, so that their fate is fixed even before all mitotic cycles are completed. The *epigenetic hypothesis* presumes that nongenetic environmental events, such as altered afferent synaptic innervation and the metabolic milieu, may alter the fate of a neuroepithelial cell so that it becomes a different neuron than it would have become under other physiological conditions. In this regard, thalamic differentiation may be more highly programmed than cortical differentiation, and thalamocortical connections may be largely responsible for determining regional cortical specialization, including lamination and cell types (Bayer and Altman 1991). Dorsal and ventral neural tube derivatives can arise from a single precursor of a clone. If an ectopic notochord is homologously transplanted to the region near the roof of the neural tube, where its strong ventralizing influence is mixed with the normal inherent dorsalizing pattern, cells as diverse as dorsal root ganglion neurons and pigment cells of the neural crest, roof-plate ependyma, motor neurons, and floor-plate ependyma can all arise from the same clone (Artinger et al. 1995).

Cell fate has been examined by tagging individual neuroepithelial cells with isotopes, special dyes, or genetic markers introduced into the cell's DNA by retroviruses. Studies using this approach have demonstrated that at the onset of neuronogenesis, there is a heterogeneity of neural progenitor cells within the proliferative ventricular zone (Krushel et al. 1993). A single cell has progeny that differentiate into ependyma, glia, and neurons of several types. Yet separate sets of progenitor cells may give rise to the deep and superficial layers of cortex and may coexist as spatially segregated populations even though their waves of migration are not coincident (Crandall and Herrup 1990). Transplantation of fetal neuroepithelium into ectopic sites in the nervous system or into other embryos of a different gestational age demonstrates that the differentiation of neurons from the transplant may change. Transplanted neurons also selectively eliminate neurites unsuitable for the cortical area to which they are transplanted (O'Leary and Stanfield 1989). Autoradiographic data, by contrast, suggest that the unlaminated cortical plate is not a totally undifferentiated aggregate of identical cells and that lami-

nar specificity is at least partially programmed (Bayer and Altman 1991). Cell cultures of neuroepithelial cells produce uniform populations of maturing neurons or glial cells in some laboratories and mixed populations in others (Lois and Alvarez-Buylla 1993), although the conditions of the culture medium—for example, nutrients, cell density, exposure to cyclicadenosine monophosphate (cAMP)—may influence the phenotypic differentiation of the cells (Juurlink and Hertz 1985). Neurotrophic factors influence whether neural crest cells will develop in vitro as neurons or glia (Sieber-Blum 1999; Silver and Hughes 1974).

GLIAL CELLS

Radial glial cells (Figs. 1.3 and 1.4) are among the earliest neuroepithelial cells to differentiate, and new radial glial cells proliferate mitotically until midgestation (Misson et al. 1988; Schmechel and Rakic 1979). Radial glial cells are identified in the human brain by their coexpression of the cytoskeletal proteins vimentin and GFAP (Roessmann and Gambetti 1986). After the radial glial cells' role in the guidance of migratory neuroblasts and glioblasts is complete, vimentin synthesis ceases, and the long radial process either is retracted or degenerates as the monopolar cell is transformed into a mature multipolar astrocyte that continues to express GFAP (Creutzfeldt 1977). Between 21 and 30 weeks' gestation, fascicles of radial glial fibers become clustered in the intermediate zone of the cerebral hemispheres (Gressens et al. 1992). The transformation of radial glial cells provides the bulk of the population of astrocytes in the deep corticallaminae and in the subcortical white matter at maturity, where as in the superficial cortical layers astrocytes are derived in the second half of gestation from radial migration of subventricular glioblasts and never became radial glia (Cameron and Rakic 1991; Gressens et al. 1992). Cortical radial glial cells transform themselves into astrocytes in vitro as well as in vivo (Culican et al. 1990). During development, there is a close correlation of the perivascular arrangement of astrocytes and the formation of endothelial tight junctions in the blood-brain barrier (Bertossi et al. 1993).

Some radial glial cells may be transformed into oligodendrocytes (Choi et al. 1983), but most oligodendroglia originate from the same pool of subventricular glioblasts that supplies most of the astrocytes (Goldman and Vaysse 1991; Kiernan and Ffrench-Constant 1993; Noll and Miller 1994). Cortical gliogenesis involves a progressively restricted sequence of progenitor cell pools genetically programmed and activated by growth factors and other molecules at the proper time, although astroblasts and oligodendroblasts may be of separate lineages (Kiernan and Ffrench-Constant 1993; Skoff and Knapp 1991). Oligodendrocyte progenitor cells migrate along the optic nerve from the chiasm (Kiernan and Ffrench-Constant 1993). Oligodendrocyte precursors originate from the ventral regions of

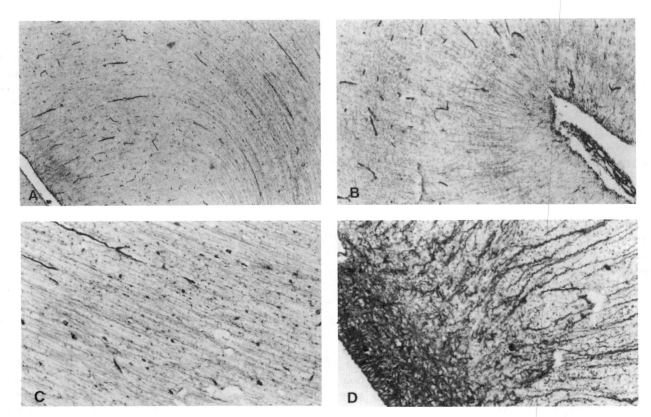

Figure 1.3   (A) Radial glial fibers arch through the subcortical white matter and cerebral cortex of the temporal lobe in a 30-week human fetus. (B) These glial processes extend to the pial surface, where they form end feet with astrocytes of the subpial granular layer. (C) Radial glial fibers in the subcortical white matter (intermediate zone) are seen with migratory neuroblasts and glioblasts gliding along their surface as on a monorail. (D) Radial glial cells in the subventricular zone of the cerebrum. Each cell extends a long process centrifugally, the radial glial fiber. Ependymal cells in the fetus also have basal processes, but these are short and do not guide migratory neuroblasts; immature ependymal cells also express vimentin. Vimentin immunocytochemistry. A: ×40; B–D: ×250.

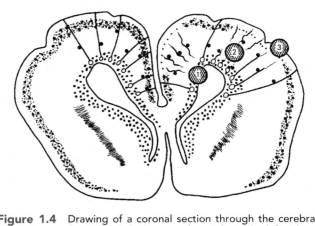

Figure 1.4   Drawing of a coronal section through the cerebral hemispheres of a 25-week fetus or preterm infant. The left side of the figure shows the normal position of radial glial cells in the subventricular zone and their processes spanning the cerebrum; the right side of the figure illustrates three potential sites where acquired lesions could destroy or interrupt the radial glial cell orits process or cause retraction of its end foot from the pial surface. Lesions at these sites arrest migrating neuroblasts and glioblasts and result in heterotopia and abnormal cortical lamination. (Reprinted from Sarnat HB. *Cerebral Dysgenesis: Embryology and Clinical Expression.* New York: Oxford University Press, p. 263, 1992. Copyright 1992, Oxford University Press, Inc. Used with permission.)

the spinal cord (Noll and Miller 1994). Retinoic acid secreted by the floor plate acts as a mitogen for oligodendrocyte precursors but inhibits their maturation in early gestation, thus allowing migration and dispersal of these precursor cells to populate the developing white matter throughout the spinal cord, including the dorsal regions. Later in gestation, basic fibroblast growth factor exerts these same mitogenic and differentiation inhibiting influences, but retinoic acid now abolishes these effects (Noll and Miller 1994). Retinoic acid is thus a regulator of oligodendrocyte development. Extra cellular matrix molecules present in developing white matter tracts at the time of oligodendrocyte progenitor cell migration include laminin and the glycoproteins tenacin and thrombospondin.

Microglia of the CNS are not derived from the neuroepithelium, as are other glial cells; rather, these microglia are intracerebral macrophages of mesodermal origin and generally develop in parallel with the earliest sprouting of the intracerebralvascular system, at about 51 days' gestation. Some microglia may be demonstrated even earlier, at 38 days' gestation (Fujimoto et al. 1989); these early-developing microglia probably are needed to phagocytose the cellular debris of apoptosis. In the developing cerebral cortex, microglia are more numerous, superficial to, and beneath the cortical plate than within it (Fujimoto et al. 1989). Additional microglial cells may enter the brain as transformed amoeboid macrophages from the blood after microcirculation is established, and this process may continue into adult life. Microglia also have anatomic articulations with pericytes—small, undifferentiated cells beneath the basement membrane of capillary endothelial cells of the brain—and pericytes may be the origin of some microglia (Monteiro et al. 1996). The differentiation of human fetal microglia is modulated in vitro by basic fibroblast growth factor (Di Pucchio et al. 1996).

The density of astrocytes in the term neonatal brain is about one sixth that in the normal adult brain and makes it more difficult for the neonatal brain to form dense gliotic "scars" in response to focal lesions. The development of glial cells has long been neglected because of the erroneous view that they serve no purpose except as the glue or the filler substance of the brain, but the complexities and functional importance of glia in the developing fetus, as well as in the mature organism, is being increasingly recognized (Jessen and Richardson 2001).

APOPTOSIS (PROGRAMMED CELL DEATH)

The number of cells generated in the fetal nervous system is 30% to 70% more than the number required at maturity. Surplus cells survive for a finite period, usually days to weeks, and then spontaneously undergo a cascade of degenerative changes and die. This physiological process of programmed cell death, or *apoptosis,* was discovered in 1949 by Hamburger and Levi-Montalcini, who demonstrated its occurrence in the spinal dorsal root ganglion of the chick embryo (Hamburger and Levi-Montalcini 1949). Many investigators subsequently confirmed that apoptosis occurs in all parts of the nervous system and, indeed, that it operates in most organ systems and in all animals, from the simplest worms to humans (Ferrer et al. 1990, 1992; Harris and Mc-Caig 1984; O'Connor and Wyttenback 1974; Okado and Oppenheim 1984). The 120-day half-life of erythrocytes and the continuous turnover of intestinal mucosal cells are examples of apoptosis that continues throughout life. In the fetal nervous system, however, the process is unique in that most differentiated neurons do not regenerate if lost.

Apoptosis differs from cell death by necrosis (due to ischemia, hypoxia, toxins, or infections) in several important morphological details. In neural cell apoptosis, the sequence begins with shrinkage of the nucleus, condensation of the chromatin, and increased electron opacity of the cell, followed by disappearance of the Golgi apparatus, loss of endoplastic reticulum, and disaggregation of polyribosomes; final events are formation of ribosome crystals and breakdown of the nuclear membrane (O'Connor and Wyt-

tenback 1974). Mitochondria are preserved until late in apoptosis, where as they swell and disintegrate early in cellular necrosis. Phagocytic microglial cells remove the debris of apoptotic cells, but lymphocytes and other inflammatory cells do not appear.

Programmed cell death is genetically patterned, as is the case with other early developmental events, but it is more complex than most such events because there does not appear to be any gene or gene combination that initiates the cascade; on the contrary, apoptosis appears to be programmed into every cell but *its expression is blocked* by the genetically-regulated secretion of trophic factors by other cells in the vicinity that preserve metabolic integrity. Nerve growth factor and basic fibroblast growth factor block cell death and preserve the identity of various cell lineages in the nervous system (Diener and Bregman 1994; Gomez-Pinilla et al. 1994; Pittman et al. 1993). Many other trophic factors are also essential for cellular survival. Table 1.2 lists four prominent neurotrophic factors and their specifications for preserving the integrity of various types of neurons.

Not all programmed cell death is an early embryonic event; motor neurons of the cervical spinal cord of the rat continue to show apoptosis in the early postnatal period (Nurcombe et al. 1981). Neural cell apoptosis is a biphasic process; early apoptosis involves undifferentiated or incompletely differentiated neuroepithelial cells, where as late apoptosis involves well-differentiated neurons or glial cells. In one popular analogy, necrosis is compared to "death by murder," where as apoptosis is likened to "death by neglect," because the cell's death is caused not by a toxin but by a deficiency of atrophic factor needed to preserve its integrity.

Apoptosis may be either accelerated or retarded by metabolic "environmental" factors, such as the circulating thyroxine level; fetal hypothyroidism delays apoptosis, and fetal hyperthyroidism enhances it. Neurotoxic excitatory amino acids such as glutamate and aspartate may trigger or accelerate apoptosis (Page et al. 1993). Lactic acidosis, high concentrations of ammonia, electrolyte and calcium imbalances, and many other transient metabolic aberrations may accelerate apoptosis.

Other environmental factors that affect apoptosis involve synaptic relationships. An inverse relationship exists between the rate of apoptosis of spinal motor neurons and synaptogenesis. On the afferent side, neurons that fail to be innervated because of loss of presynaptic neurons degenerate; an example of "transsynaptic degeneration" is what occurs in the lateral geniculate body as a consequence of lesions of the optic nerve. On the efferent side, motor neurons degenerate if they fail to match with target muscle fibers. Removal of a limb bud of a developing embryo results in accelerated loss of motor neurons at the corresponding spinal cord level. The ectopic grafting of a supernumerary limb bud close to a natural limb bud requires innervation by the same pool of motor neurons and causes apoptosis to be retarded or stopped, resulting in an increased number of motor neurons on that side.

TABLE 1.2
NEUROTROPHIN SPECIFICITIES FOR DIFFERENTIATION AND MAINTENANCE OF VARIOUS TYPES OF NEURAL CELLS

Neural Cell	NGF Receptor Trk-A	BDNF Receptor Trk-B	NT-3 Receptor Trk-C (Minor Trk-B)	NT-4/5 Receptor Trk-B
Sympathetic	+++	−	++	−
Parasympathetic	−	−	+	−
Motor				
Lower motor neuron	−	+++	+++	+++
Upper motor neuron (layer 5 pyramidal)	−	−	++	
Sensory				
Small DRG cells	+++	−	+	
Medium DRG cells	−	++	−	
Large DRG cells	−	−	++	
Cochlear ganglion (and organ of Corti)	−	+	+++	
Vestibular ganglion (and labyrinthine neurons)	−	+++	+	
Nodosal ganglion (vagal)	−	++	++	
Nucleus dorsalis (column of Clarke)			++	
Locus coeruleus	−	−	++	
Amygdala			+	
Hippocampus				
CA1, CA2, granular layer of dentate gyrus; calbindin neurons		−	++	
Pyramidal cells; cholinergic neurons	−	++	−	
Cingulate gyrus			++	
Cerebellum	−	+	+++	
Obligodendrocytes	−	−	++	
Schwann cells	−	++	−	
Striated muscle	−	−	++	

Note: − = no expression; + = weak expression; +++ = strong expression; blank spaces indicate incomplete data. BDNF = brain-derived NGF; DRG = dorsal root ganglion; NGF = nerve growth factor; NT-3 = neurotrophin-3; NT-4/5 = neurotrophin-4/5; Trk = tyrosine kinase receptor.

In addition to the well documented apoptosis involving differentiated or maturing neurons and glial cells, some undifferentiated neuroepithelial cells also undergo physiological cell death, but the factors that select these short life cycles are less well understood (Homma et al. 1994). The mechanism may involve activation of the immediate early protooncogene *c-fos*, which is also expressed in regions of cerebral infarction (Gonzales-Martin et al.1992; McLean et al. 1994; Page et al. 1993).

NEUROBLAST MIGRATION

Few, if any, neurons in the mature human brain are ultimately located in the same site where they began their differentiation. Neurons shift position, often migrating over long distances, to form three-dimensional relationships with other neurons with which they must establish synaptic circuitry. The migration of neuroblasts is a precise and orderly process and is intimately associated with specialized fetal glial cells with long processes that serve as guides (Sidman and Rakic 1973; Figs. 1.3 and 1.4). In a few spe-cialized foci, such as the olfactory tract, some neurons may follow axonal guides of others; however, the great majority of neuroblasts slide to their destinations on the outer surface of radial glial fibers. Neurotrophins also play an important role: NT-3 is required for olfactory tract migration and, if defective, results in arrhinencephaly as in holoprosencephaly, though hypoplastic, rudimentary, unmigrated olfactory bulbs may be "fused" to the entorhinal cortex in carefully examined microscopic sections (Sarnat and Flores-Sarnat 2001).

The radial migration of periventricular postmitotic neuroblasts in the cerebrum is regulated in part by the specialized Cajal-Retzius neurons of the initial marginal zone of the early cerebrum, which later becomes the molecular layer or layer 1 of the cerebral cortex when the developing cortical plate from radial migrations forms in the middle of the molecular zone. Cajal-Retzius neurons are mature neurons that form a preplate plexus prior to the first wave of radial migrations. They synthesize GABA and other neurotransmitters, including several calcium-binding proteins such as calmodulin and parvalbumin, and also express several genes that both mediate radial migration and organize the cortical plate; these genes include reelin, LIS1 and DS-CAM. Cajal-Retzius neurons form the first intrinsic cortical circuits, forming synapses with neurons of layer 6 (the first to migrate radially) and later with all cortical layers (Sarnat and Flores-Sarnat 2002). At the end of cerebral development, the Cajal-Retzius neurons become sparse in the molecular zone with growth of the brain but do not disappear; their function in the adult brain is unknown.

In the cerebral hemispheres, the radial glial cell bodies are in the subventricular zone, and their processes extend to the pial surface radially. Groups of postmitotic premigratory neuroblasts migrate together in waves throughout the subcortical white matter (i.e., the intermediate zone) to the surface of the cortical plate; each subsequent "wave of migratory neuroblasts completes its journey superficial to the preceding one, so that the deepest layer of the neocortex is formed by the first migratory wave, and the most superficial neurons in layer 2 are the last to migrate. The inverted arrangement of six-layered neocortex is not the pattern followed in the three-layered paleocortex (hippocampus) or the laminated superior colliculus, however. In these trilaminated cortices, the outermost layer represents the earliest rather than the latest migratory wave. In the cerebellar cortex, Bergmann glial cells in the Purkinje cell layer extend radial processes to the surface and guide the migratory external granule cells to their mature position in the interior of the folia.

In addition to the columnar radial migrations along glial fibers from the subventricular zone to the cortical plate, tangential migration occurs within the intermediate zone (i.e., the future subcortical white matter); a minority of migratory neuroblasts turn to travel perpendicularly to the radial glial fibers for a net effect of tangential dispersion of clonally related cortical neurons (DeDiego et al. 1994; O'Rourke et al. 1992). Time lapse confocal microscopy of living slices of cerebrum demonstrates that these horizontal cell movements are three times faster than radial migrations, suggesting that nonglial substrates such as tangential axons guide this cellular movement (O'Rourke et al. 1992, 1995). The validity of these observations of horizontal migration in the subcortical white matter has been confirmed by other techniques, including retroviral labeling to trace clonal allocation of neuroblasts (Walsh and Cepko 1988) and radioisotope marking of premigratory clones of neuroblasts (O'Rourke et al. 1995). Tangential migrations are not limited to the cerebrum; they also have been documented in the developing optic tectum of the midbrain (Gray and Sanes 1991) and near the surface of the medulla oblongata, where neuroblasts migrate in the subpial region along circumferential axons and perhaps are also guided along the leading processes of other tangentially migrating cells (Ono and Kawamura 1989). Horizontal migrations occur in the developing cerebellar cortex as well (Hager et al. 1995). Even in the spinal cord, longitudinal and tangential migrations serve to disperse and mix different clones and generations of postmitotic neuroblasts (Leber and Sanes 1996).

The signals that mediate neuroblast migration are incompletely understood. The ependyma may play a role in the regulation of radial glia, but this speculation is not well documented. The mechanism of actual migration is uncertain. The neuroblast travels along the radial glial process as if it were a monorail, but the identity of the molecules attracting the migratory neuroblast surface, their location, and the role of adhesive substrates on the radial glial process are unresolved questions. Glycoproteins, including lectin, tenacin, and thrombospondin, may be important in this regard (Bartsch et al. 1992; Lehman et al. 1990; O'Shea et al. 1990). By contrast, S-laminin, a component of the basement membrane, acts as a chemical barrier to cell migration (Porter and Sanes 1995). The plasma membrane of the radial glial cell itself shows a complex dynamic and topographic flow that facilitates cell migration, as is demonstrated in Bergmann glial cell guidance of cerebellar external granule cells (Komuro and Rakic 1995). Genetic programming of neuroblast migration is of primordial importance and regulates many of the other factors that influence this migration (Mochida and Walsh 2004).

Although most neuroblast migration is complete by midgestation, some neuroblasts continue to migrate past this time, perhaps until 34 weeks. In the second half of gestation, most of the post mitotic neuroepithelial cells in the subventricular zone or periventricular "germinal matrix" are glial precursors, and these glioblasts also migrate toward the cerebral cortical surface. After migration is complete, the radial glial cell retracts its process and becomes a mature astrocyte.

Gyri and sulci form in a predictable sequence to enlarge the surface area of the cerebral cortex without concomitantly increasing the volume or mass of the brain (Chi et al. 1977). By 20 weeks' gestation, only the rudimentary primary fissures are formed—the sylvian and calcarine fissures and the early appearance of a Rolandic fissure. The secondary and tertiary gyri develop with further maturation of the cortex and additional radial migration of glioblasts and are fully formed by term. Convolutions of the cerebral cortex thus develop during the phase of glioblast, not neuroblast migration. The forces responsible for gyration of the cerebral cortex are predominantly intracortical rather than subcortical (Richman et al. 1975). They are related more to neurite growth and expansion of the neuropil between cortical plate neurons and to enlargement of the neurons of the cortical plate than to cellular migration.

Neuroblast migration to the cerebral cortex may be divided into three phases, with different genes regulating each and, consequently, mutations of each of these genes resulting in different malformations with arrested migration in different stages. The earliest stage is the initiation of migration from the periventricular region (i.e., the embryonic subventricular zone. The second stage is the centrifugal journey through the subcortical white matter to reach the cortical plate. The third stage is the organization of the cortical plate and lamination of the cortex (Mochida and Walsh 2004; Pinter and Sarnat 2004).

AXONAL PATHFINDING

The outgrowth of a single axon precedes the formation of the multiple dendrites and is one of the first events marking the maturation of neuroblast to neuron, sometimes beginning during the course of neuroblast migration. The tip of the growing axon, termed the *growth cone* by Ramon y Cajal (1909–1911), is neither pointed nor blunt, but rather a constantly changing complex of cytoplasmic fingers, *the filopodia*, enclosed by a membrane that forms veils or webs between the filopodia. Microtubules, filaments, and mitochondria fill the cytoplasm of the filopodia.

Axons must be guided to their destinations, which are often a great distance from the cell body. Three mechanisms are involved in this guidance (Oakley and Tosney 1993; Tessier-Lavigne et al.1988):

1. *Cell-cell interactions.* Molecular signals generated by the target cell induce the growth cone to form a synapse. This mechanism is effective only as the axon approaches to within 1 to 2 mm of the target.
2. *Cell-substrate interactions.* Molecules known as *integrins* bind the cell to an extracellular protein matrix such as fibronectin or laminin. Such substrates serve as adhesive surfaces for growth cones, allowing them to pull themselves along, but might also provide some directional cues as attractants or repellants.
3. *Chemotactic interactions.* Secretory molecules may release powerful attractants or repellants to keep the axon aligned along an intended course of intermediate trajectory; growth cones are exquisitely sensitive to certain chemical sand grow toward or away from these molecules.

An example of a repellant molecule is *keratin sulfate.* This glycosaminoglycan is secreted by many tissues of the fetal body at sites where nerves are not wanted: the epiphyseal plates of growing bones, the epidermis (to prevent nerves from growing through the skin), the notochordal sheath, and the developing neural arches of the vertebrae (to segment and guide nerve roots from the spinal cord) (Oakley and Tosney 1993). The segmental somites are important early guides of neural crest cellular migration and also of axonal projections peripherally (Tosney 1988). Within the CNS, fetalependymal cells synthesize keratan sulfate partly to prevent axons from growing into the ventricles of the brain but also to prevent aberrant decussations of long tracts and wandering of axons toward the wrong targets (Sarnat 1992c). The dorsal median raphe that separates the dorsal columns of the two sides in the dorsal midline of the spinal cord is composed of ependymal roof-plate processes that secrete keratan sulfate at the time when the axons of the dorsal columns are ascending. The raphe repels growth cones that might otherwise decussate (Bovolenta and Dodd 1990; Snow et al. 1990). However, the effects of such repellant molecules are selective. Keratan sulfate secreted by the floor plate and by the dorsal median septum of the midbrain allows the passage of commissural fibers of local interneurons but repulses axons of longitudinal tracts. The floor plate also repulses axons of developing motor neurons, so that they extend into spinal roots only on the same side as the soma (Guthrie and Pini 1995). The commissural axons are actually facilitated in their traversal of the midline septa of ependymal processes by other selective attractant molecules known as *netrins* (Kennedy et al. 1994; Keynes and Cook 1995), but netrins may be bifunctional and may also act as chemorepellants in other sites (e.g., for trochlearaxons) (Colamarino and Tessier-Lavigne 1995; Keynes and Cook 1995). Another family of proteins, the semaphorins/collapsins act mainly as growth-cone repellants both in neural tissue (including the floor plate) and throughout the body in nonneural tissue (Dodd and Schuchardt 1995). Some axons are initially drawn toward the floor plate, perhaps through long-range chemoattraction by a netrin, but then are repelled locally by a semaphorin as they approach the midline and are forced to turn and proceed in another direction. Thus, although the midline septa of ependymal processes act as chemical barriers, they are not the physical barriers to axonal passage that they appear to be in histological sections. Nerve growth factor and S-100 β protein are examples of other growth-cone attractants secreted by ependymal and perhaps other cells of the immature CNS.

The cytoskeleton plays a central role in axonal guidance. The internal organization of actin filaments and microtubules changes rapidly within the growth cone before large scale changes in growth-cone shape are seen, and these changes are evoked by local environmental molecules, which stabilize local changes of cytoskeletal polymers in the growth-cone (Tanaka and Sabry 1995). Although microtubule assembly in the growing axon is required for the axon's extension in forming pathways, drugs that inhibit or disrupt microtubule assembly appear not to impede the process of assembly and grow that the axonal tip, a finding that refutes the hypothesis that the growth cone is the principal site of microtubule assembly (Yu and Baas 1995). Local electrical fields within the neural tissue may play an additional minor role in orienting axons within their trajectories, perhaps by altering receptive properties of the growth-cone membrane to neurotransmitters and molecules that attract or repel (Erskine and McCaig 1995).

Finally, or perhaps first of all, homeobox genes are involved in the regulation of axonal growth as well as earlier stages of development. A gene expressed early in neuronal differentiation, *TOAD-64* (turned-on-after-division, molecular weight 64 kDa), is strongly expressed by its protein transcription product in growth cones and is down regulated after axonal projection is complete; mutations in this gene result in aberrations in axonal out growth in the mouse and also in the simple roundworm *Caenorhabditis elegans*, in which *TOAD-64* is identified as the gene *unc-33*, with an identical nucleotide sequence (Minturn et al. 1995). Overexpression of *Hox-2* reverses axonal pathways from r3 (Kessel 1993). Boundary regions between adjacent domains of regulatory gene expression influence where the first axons will extend (Wilson et al.1993). The establishment of intersegmental connectivity by short axons precedes the development of long ascending and descending tracts (Oppenheim et al. 1988). Initial tract formation is also associated with the selective expression of certain cell adhesion molecules and their regulatory gene transcripts (Chedotal et al. 1995).

MEMBRANE EXCITABILITY

Two features distinguish mature neurons from all other cells: (1) an electrically polarized and excitable membrane and (2) secretory function. Muscle cells have excitable membranes but do not secrete; endocrine and exocrine cells are secretory but have electrically neutral membranes.

The development of electrical polarity of the cell membrane is a maturational feature that marks the transition from neuroblast to neuron. This maturational process depends on the development of ion channels for Na^+, K^+, Cl^-, and Ca^{++} as well as the means for delivering continuous energy production to maintain a resting membrane potential, the Na^+/K^+ adenosine triphosphatase pump (Spitzer 1981). Although the importance of glial cells for ion transport in this regard is incompletely understood, it is thought that astrocytes may play a substantial role in regulation of the cerebral microenvironment in the developing and the mature brain (Walz 1989).

DENDRITIC SPROUTING AND SYNAPTOGENESIS

Dendrites sprout only after the axon of the neuron begins its projection. The branching pattern of dendrites and the formation of spines on these dendritic arborizations upon which synapses form are varied and characteristic for each type of neuron. In the cerebral cortex, synaptogenesis always occurs after migration of the neuron to its mature site is complete, but in the cerebellar cortex, the external granule cells project bipolar axons as "parallel fibers" in the molecular layer and form synapses with Purkinje cell dendrites before migrating to their mature site in the interior of the folium.

Afferent nerve fibers reach the cerebral cortex even before the cortical plate becomes laminated. The first synapses are axodendritic and form both superficial to and deep within the cortical plate, between the Cajal-Retzius cells of the molecular zone and the pyramidal cells of layer 6, the latter representing the earliest wave of radial neuroblast migration from the subventricular zone. However, most of the dendritic arborization and synaptogenesis in the cerebral cortex occurs during the third trimester of gestation and in early infancy, a circumstance that renders this developmental process vulnerable totoxic, hypoxic, ischemic, and metabolic insults in the postnatal period, particularly in preterm neonates.

An excess of synapses is generated, and many of these synapses are later deleted with the retraction of redundant collateral axons. In addition, transitory neurons (e.g., the Cajal-Retzius neurons of the fetal cerebral cortex) form temporary synapses that function for a time and then disappear as the transient neuron undergoes apoptosis.

When an axonal terminal reaches a dendritic spine and cell-cell contact is achieved, a chemical synapse usually forms rapidly. It has been proposed that some "promiscuous" neurons secrete transmitters even before contacting their targets, thus inducing an overabundance of synapses which then undergo additional electrical activity dependent refinement (Haydon and Drapeau 1995). Dendritic spines determine the dynamics of intracellular second-messenger ions such as calcium and very likely provide for synaptic plasticity by establishing compartmentalization of afferent input based on biochemical rather than electrical signals (Koch and Zador 1993). Neurotrophins play an important role in the modulation of synaptogenesis as selective retrograde messengers (Thoenen 1995). Transsynaptic signaling by neurotrophins and neurotransmitters also may influence neuronal architecture such as neurite sprouting and dendritic pruning (Greenough 1984; Lipton and Kater 1989). Prostaglandins and their inducible synthetase enzymes (e.g., cyclooxygenase-2) are expressed by excitatory neurons at postsynaptic sites in the cerebral cortex and hippocampus; they modulate *N*-methyl-D-aspartate (NMDA)-dependent responses such as long-term potentiation and show a spatial and temporal sequence of expression that is demonstrated immunocytochemically in the fetal brain. This expression is highly localized to dendritic spines and reflects functional rather than structural features of synapse formation (Breder et al. 1995; Kaufmann et al. 1996; Lerea and McNamara 1993; Williams et al. 1989). Thus, prostaglandin signaling of cortical development, and synaptogenesis in particular, may be mediated through dendrites, and the same is likely for neurotrophin signaling (Thoenen 1995).

In addition to the axodendritic and axosomatic synapses, a few specialized sites in the developing brain show dendrodendritic contacts, such as those on the spines of olfactory granule cells (Shepherd and Greer 1989).

The electroencephalogram (EEG) is probably the most reliable and accessible noninvasive clinical measure of the functional state of synaptogenesis in the cerebral cortex of the preterm infant. The maturation of EEG patterns involves a precise temporal progression of predictable changes with increasing conceptional age and includes the development of sleep/wake cycles.

BIOSYNTHESIS OF NEUROTRANSMITTERS

The synthesis of secretory products is the function of neurons, and the beginning of this metabolic process denotes the adequacy of the organelles and the maturity of the nerve cell. The number of ribosomes in the cytoplasm of maturing neurons is large if the secretory product is a peptide, such as somatostatin or substance P, or if the product requires the continuous synthesis of protein enzymes of synthesis or degradation, such as those involved in the metabolism of acetylcholine and the monoamines. Nonsecretory neuroblasts have few ribosomes.

Neuropeptides are sometimes synthesized in immature nerve cells but not in mature cells. An example is the peptide substance P, which is present in high concentrations in the cerebellum at 16 to 18 weeks' gestation but is almost undetectable in the cerebellum at term or thereafter; in the second half of gestation, granule cells begin the synthesis of glutamic acid and Purkinje cells produce gamma-aminobutyric acid (GABA) as their neurotransmitters. At this time, the neuropeptides synthesized earlier, in the first half of gestation, probably function more as trophic factors than as synaptic transmitter molecules. Neuropeptide secretory products may coexist with other transmitters, such as acetylcholine and amino acids, in both the fetus and the adult. Cajal-Retzius neurons of the fetal cerebral cortex appear to synthesize both acetylcholine and GABA (Sarnat and Flores-Sarnat 2002).

Neurotransmitters that persist at maturity appear in a predictable sequence during development: serotonin is detected in the fetal brainstem earlier than norepinephrine and dopamine, where as acetylcholine and GABA do not appear until later. Endorphin is found in high concentrations much earlier than substance P, enkephalin, and the hypothalamic hormonal peptides (Lagercrantz 1984). Endogenous glutamate release in the cerebellar cortex produces a dramatic increase in the tonic NMDA receptor channel activity during granule cell migration and synaptogenesis, an effect which suggests that transmitters contribute to the maturational process and are not just end products of maturation (Rossi and Slater 1993).

Equally important to the maturation of secretory capacity of neurons for the biosynthesis of neurotransmitters is the development of specific receptors for each of these molecules on the cell and dendritic membranes of the neurons with which the axons synapse (Rho and Storey 2001; Simeone et al. 2003, 2004).

MYELINATION

The velocity of conduction of a depolarization wave along an axon is important because the transsynaptic propagation of an impulse depends on its temporal summation of generator potentials. Myelination greatly increases the speed of conduction, but myelin is not essential for the integrity or function of many small nerves, such as most of those of the sympathetic nervous system. If a hypothetical axon, whether central or peripheral, conducts 50 impulses per second without myelin and 200 impulses per second with myelin, synaptic block will occur if 100 impulses per second is the critical threshold to release enough quanta of neurotransmitter to trigger the next neuron. For this reason, immature infants without sufficient myelination do not simply move and think more slowly; rather, they have functional synaptic block in many polysynaptic pathways of the brain.

As with other aspects of nervous system development, myelination cycles (i.e., the time of onset and termination of myelination) are specific for each pathway and are precisely time linked. The proximal and distal portions of most pathways myelinate at the same time, but some pathways (e.g., the corticospinal tract) myelinate in rostrocaudal progression. Some cycles are short; the medial longitudinal fasciculus of the brainstem begins myelination at 24 weeks' gestation and completes it at 28 weeks. Others are long; the corticospinal tract begins myelination at about 38 weeks' gestation and is not fully myelinated until 2 years of age. Postnatal myelination is first seen in the forebrain in the thalamus, corona radiata, and posterior limb of the internal capsule at 1 month of age. Myelination is then seen in the optic radiations to the occipital poles at 3 months, the anterior limb of the internal capsule and the radiation to the precentral gyrus at 6 months, the parietal and frontal deep white matter at 8 months, and the white matter of the temporal lobe at 12 months (Brody et al. 1987; Kinney et al. 1988). Myelination in the corpus callosum begins at age 4 months postnatally and finishes in midadolescence. The last pathway of the brain to myelinate is the association bundle connecting the prefrontal cortex with the ipsilateral temporal and parietal lobes, which finally completes its myelination cycle at 32 years of age (Yakovlev and Lecours 1967). These very late cycles require further study and documentation.

Most studies of myelination are based on the staining of postmortem brain tissue with luxol fast blue or other traditional myelin stains (Brody et al. 1987; Gilles 1976; Kinney et al. 1988; Rorke and Riggs 1969; Weidenheim et al. 1992). Newer techniques of histopathological examination use gallocyanin histochemistry, antibodies to myelin basic protein (Bodhireddy et al. 1994; Hasegawa et al. 1992), and special stains that detect myelination more precisely with polarized light or fluorescence microscopy (Miklossy and Van der Loos 1991). In the living patient, T2-weighted magnetic resonance images are a valuable and reliable means of semiquantitatively assessing myelination in the various tracts, fiber bundles, and white matter (Barkovich et al. 1988; Dietrich et al. 1988). When one is comparing studies, care must be taken to ensure that technical conditions in each are the same; for example, results obtained with a 0.5-T magnet will differ from those obtained with a

1.5-T magnet. Although tables of myelination cycles generated by magnetic resonance imaging (MRI) differ somewhat from those based on tissue examination at autopsy in fetuses and infants, the general sequence of myelination of the various tracts correlates well. Conventional Tl- and T2-weighted sequences of MRI show that brain maturation proceeds sequentially, from central to peripheral, from inferior to superior, and from posterior to anterior areas (Barkovich et al. 1988). Compared with conventional MRI, newer techniques of quantitative MRI are potentially more sensitive, less subject to subtle changes in myelination and less open to variable interpretation (Steen et al. 1994).

Early onset of myelination is not always associated with early maturation of myelin (Kinney et al. 1988). On the other hand, an early adult pattern of white matter myelination on MRI has been reported in infants as young as 10 months of age (Dietrich et al. 1988).

Myelination depends both on the normal differentiation and maturation of oligodendroglial cells and on the availability of the lipids needed to form the complex compounds of myelinated membranes. The sequence of proteins and lipids incorporated into myelin may be quantitatively measured by the biochemical study of white matter at autopsy, and the normal sequence of myelination in the human fetus differs from the abnormal sequences in individuals with metabolic diseases involving myelin (Kinney et al. 1994). Like other developmental processes of the nervous system, differentiation of oligodendrocytes from precursor cells and programming of myelin formation are under genetic regulation (Topilko et al. 1994; Yu et al. 1994). The Krox-20 "zinc finger" gene has been identified as playing an important role in the process of myelination by Schwann cells in the peripheral nervous system (Topilko et al. 1994). PMP22/gas3, another gene that programs aprote-olipid protein, encodes an axonally-regulated Schwann cell protein that is incorporated into myelin; this gene is the target of mutations both in a mouse model of defective myelination and in human Charcot-Marie-Tooth disease type la, the most common form of inherited peripheral neuropathy (Lemke 1993). Whether these same genes are active in CNS myelination is not yet known.

In addition to their role in forming myelin sheaths or enveloping unmyelinated axons in both the peripheral and central nervous systems, oligodendrocytes express nerve growth factor and may secrete other molecules that stimulate the growth of axons (Byraven et al. 1994). The number of axons per Schwann cell or per oligodendrocyte becomes reduced with maturation, from as many as 55 to as few as 1 to 4 unmyelinated axons per Schwann cell from midgestation to birth; only rarely does a Schwann cell ensheathe more than one myelinated axon (Hasan et al. 1993).

Myelination as an important parameter of the normal functional maturation of the brain is a clinically measurable index of delayed cerebral maturation (Dambska and Laure-Kamionowska 1990; van der Knaap et al. 1991).

VASCULAR DEVELOPMENT

The development of both the major cerebral arteries and the microvasculature of the brain have an additional influence on cerebral development. Acquired ischemic episodes during fetal life, such as maternal shock, and congenital vascular malformations that alter normal cerebral perfusion may result in abnormal development or in infarcts or hemorrhages before maturation is complete and, at times, resemble genetically determined dysgeneses.

The embryology of the vascular development is complex and was reviewed and illustrated (Sarnat 2004b). The basilar artery initially is a pair of parallel vessels, the longitudinal neural arteries, at the base of the embryonic brain; it then undergoes a true fusion to form the basilar artery. It receives its blood from the internal carotid arteries, with rostrocaudal flow because the plexus that coalesces to form the vertebral arteries occurs at a later stage. The carotid blood is provided to the early fetal basilar artery through a series of transient communicating vessels, mainly the trigeminal, otic, and hypoglossal arteries on each side, and some small and less constant communicators such as the stapedial artery. Because of the pontine flexure, the internal carotid and early basilar arteries lie in parallel and in close proximity, making these transient communicating arteries anatomically feasible. With the straightening of the pontine flexure, the carotid and basilar arteries move farther apart. Occasionally, the transient fetal arteries persist rather than regress, particularly the most rostral or trigeminal artery, and in such cases the carotid circulation also provides most of the blood to half of the brainstem and half of the cerebellum. Persistent fetal cerebral vessels and other congenital vascular malformations of the brain are well described in an article by Pascual-Castroviejo and Pascual-Pascual (2002).

The anterior cerebral artery arises from the first branchial pouch (really, *pharyngeal* pouch, since humans do not have gills at any stage) associated with rhombomere 1, and the middle cerebral artery from the second branchial pouch and rhombomere 2; only later do they fuse with the internal carotid artery on each side. The full circle of Willis, including the anterior and posterior communicating arteries, are the final elements to form.

Most of the microcirculation of the cerebrum is from radial arteriole-like immature fetal vessels that span the cerebral mantle from the subventricular zone to the cortical plate, initially with few collaterals and communications between them, but these increase with advancing gestational age. Vessels in the subventricular zone or "germinal matrix" around the ventricles are mainly thin walled vascular channels, variable in diameter, that are fragile and easily rupture with reperfusion after an episode of systemic hypotension. In the brainstem, the microcirculation arises exclusively from the basilar artery, from a series of 25 to 30 pairs of vessels: the paramedian penetrating and circumferential arteries with short and long branches. The latter course around the brainstem before penetrating the parenchyma to supply the lateral tegmentum. The cerebellum also receives its blood supply from the vertebrobasilar circulation through several vessels: superior, anterior inferior cerebellar, posterior inferior, and middle cerebellar arteries.

Watershed zones are territories between the circulation zones of two major arteries with overlap. In the cerebrum, the major watershed zones are between the anterior and middle cerebral and between the middle and posterior cerebral arteries. In the brainstem, the main watershed zone is in the middle of the tegmentum of the pons and medulla oblongata, and infarcts in this area are usually symmetrical and produce several syndromes that mimic genetic disorders and can cause Möbius syndrome (paralysis of lateral rectus and facial muscles and other cranial neuropathies), central respiratory insufficiency or apnea, dysphagia, ankylosis of the jaw and micrognathia (Sarnat 2004b).

CONCLUSION

Neuroembryology is prerequisite to understanding cerebral dysgeneses because all malformations of the nervous system—focal or widespread, genetic or acquired in utero—are disturbances in one or more of the developmental processes. To explain the pathogenesis of malformations, one must invoke not only descriptive morphogenesis, or "classical" embryology, but also the molecular genetic regulation of programming and induction, the "new" neuroembryology. For pediatric neurologists, neuropsychiatrists, neurosurgeons, neuroradiologists, neuropathologists, and other medical specialists who treat persons with congenital defects of the brain and spinal cord, the foundation that modern neuroembryology provides becomes as practical and indispensable as a knowledge of clinical complications such as hydrocephalus, epilepsy, and cognitive disorders.

REFERENCES

Altman J, Anderson WJ. Experimental reorganization of the cerebellar cortex, I: morphological effects of elimination of all microneurons with prolonged x-irradiation started at birth. J Comp Neurol 146: 355–406, 1972.

Alvarez IS, Schoenwolf GC. Expansion of surface epithelium provides the major extrinsic force for bending of the neural plate. J Exp Zool 261:340–348, 1992.

Artinger KB, Fraser S, Bronner-Fraser M. Dorsal and ventral cell types can arise from common neural tube progenitors. Dev Biol 172: 591–601, 1995.

Aruga J, Yokota N, Hashimoto M, et al. A novel zinc finger protein, zic, is involved in neurogenesis, especially in the cell lineage of cerebellar granule cells. J Neurochem 63:1880–1890, 1994.

Barkovich AJ, Kjos BO, Jackson DE, et al. Normal maturation of the neonatal and infant brain: MR imaging at 1.5 T. Radiology 166: 173–180, 1988.

Bartsch S, Bartsch U, Dorries U, et al. Expression of tenascin in the developing and adult cerebellar cortex. J Neurosci 12:736–749, 1992.

Bayer SA, Altman J. Neocortical Development. New York: Raven, pp. 203–215, 1991.

Bei M, Peters H, Maas RL. The role of PAX and MSX genes in craniofacial development. In: Lin KY, Ogle RC, Jane JA, eds. Craniofacial Surgery. Philadelphia: WB Saunders, 101–112, 2002.

Bertossi M, Roncali L, Nico B, et al. Perivascular astrocytes and endothelium in the development of the blood-brain barrier in the optic tectum of the chick embryo. Anat Embryol (Berl) 188:21–29, 1993.

Bodhireddy SR, Lyman WD, Rashbaum WK, et al. Immunohistochemical detection of myelin basic protein is a sensitive marker of myelination in second trimester human fetal spinal cord. J Neuropathol Exp Neurol 53:144–149, 1994.

Boncinelli E, Somma R, Acampora D, et al. Organization of human homeobox genes. Hum Reprod 3:880–886,1988.

Bottjer DJ. The early evolution of animals. Sci Amer 293:42-47, 2005.

Bovolenta P, Dodd J. Guidance of commissural growth cones at the floor plate in embryonic rat spinal cord. Development 109: 435–447, 1990.

Brand-Saberi B, Ebensperger C, Wilting J, et al. The ventralizing effect of the notochord on somite differentiation in chick embryos. Anat Embryol (Berl) 188:239–245, 1993.

Breder CD, Dewitt D, Kraig RP. Characterization of inducible cyclooxygenase in rat brain. J Comp Neurol 355:296–315, 1995.

Brody BA, Kinney HC, Kloman AS, et al. Sequence of central nervous system myelination in human infancy, I: an autopsy study of myelination. J Neuropathol Exp Neurol 46:283–301, 1987.

Bronner-Fraser M. Neural crest formation and migration in the developing embryo. FASEB J 8:699–706, 1994.

Bronner-Fraser M. Origins and developmental potential of the neural crest. Exp Cell Res 218:405–417, 1995.

Bulfone A, Puelles L, Porteus MH, et al. Spatially restricted expression of Dlx-1 (Tes-1), Gbx-2, and Wnt-3 in the embryonic day 12.5 mouse forebrain defines potential transverse and longitudinal segmental boundaries. J Neurosci 13:3155–3172, 1993.

Busam KJ, Roberts DJ, Golden JA. Clinical teratology counseling and consultation case report: two distinct anterior neural tube defects in a human fetus: evidence for an intermittent pattern of neural tube closure. Teratology 48:399–403, 1993.

Byravan S, Foster LM, Phan T, et al. Murine oligodendroglial cells express nerve growth factor. Proc Natl Acad Sci USA 91:8812–8816, 1994.

Callaerts P, Halider G, Gehring WJ. Pax-6 in development and evolution. Annu Rev Neurosci 20:483–532, 1997.

Cameron RS, Rakic P. Glial cell lineage in the cerebral cortex: a review and synthesis. Glia 4:124–137, 1991.

Carstens M. Neural tube programming and craniofacial cleft formation. Eur J Paediatr Neurol 8: 179–210, 2004.

Chalepakis G, Stoykova A, Wijnholds J, et al. Pax: gene regulators in the developing nervous system. J Neurobiol 24:1367–1384, 1993.

Chedotal A, Pourquie O, Sotelo C. Initial tract formation in the brain of the chick embryo: selective expression of the BEN/SC1/DM-GRASP cell adhesion molecule. Eur J Neurosci 7:198–212, 1995.

Chen Z-F, Behringer RR. Twist is required in head mesenchyme for cranial neural tube morphogenesis. Genes Dev 9:686–699, 1995.

Chenn A, McConnell SK. Cleavage orientation and the asymmetric inheritance of Notch 1 immunoreactivity in mammalian neurogenesis. Cell 82:631–641, 1995.

Chi JG, Dooling EC, Gilles FH. Gyral development of the human brain. Ann Neurol 1:86–93, 1977.

Chisaka O, Capecchi MR. Regionally restricted developmental defects resulting from targeted disruption of the mouse homeobox gene Hox 1.5. Nature 350:473–479, 1991.

Chitnis A, Henrique D, Lewis J, et al. Primary neurogenesis in Xenopus embryos regulated by a homologue of the Drosophila neurogenic gene Delta. Nature 375:761–766, 1995.

Choi BH, Kim RC, Lapham EW. Do radial glia give rise to both astroglial and oligodendroglial cells? Dev Brain Res 8:119–130, 1983.

Cohen MM Jr, Neri G, Weksberg R. Overgrowth Syndromes. New York: Oxford University Press, 2001.

Colamarino SA, Tessier-Lavigne M. The axonal chemoattractant netrin-1 is also a chemorepellant for trochlear motor axons. Cell 81:621–629, 1995.

Crandall JE, Herrup K. Patterns of cell lineage in the cerebral cortex reveal evidence for developmental boundaries. Exp Neurol 109:131–139, 1994.

Creutzfeldt OD. Generality of the functional structure of the neocortex. Naturwissenschaften 64:507–517,1977.

Crews L, Hunter D. Neurogenesis in the olfactory epithelium. Perspect Dev Neurobiol 2:151–161, 1994.

Culican SM, Baumrind NL, Yamamoto M, et al. Cortical radial glia: identification in tissue culture and evidence for their transformation to astrocytes. J Neurosci 10:684–692, 1990.

Curatolo P, ed. *Tuberous Sclerosis Complex: From Basic Science to Clinical Phenotypes.* London, UK: MacKeith Press and International Review of Child Neurology, 2003.

Dambska M, Laure-Kamionowska M. Myelination as a parameter of normal and retarded brain maturation. Brain Dev 12:214–220, 1990.

DeDiego I, Smith-Fernandez A, Fairen A. Cortical cells that migrate beyond area boundaries: characterization of an early neuronal population in the lower intermediate zone of prenatal rats. Eur J Neurosci 6:983–997,1994.

DeMyer W, Zeman W, Palmer CG. The face predicts the brain: diagnostic significance of median facial anomalies for holoprosencephaly (arhinencephaly). Pediatrics 34:256-263, 1964.

De Pomerai D. *From Gene to Animal: An Introduction to the Molecular Biology of Animal Development.* 2nd Ed. Cambridge, UK: Cambridge University Press, 1990.

Dickson ME, Krumlauf R, McMahon AP. Evidence for a mitogenic effect of *Wnt-1* in the developing mammalian central nervous system. Development 120:1453–1471, 1994.

Diener PS, Bregman BS. Neurotrophic factors prevent the death of CNS neurons after spinal cord lesions in newborn rats. Neuroreport 5:1913–1917, 1994.

Dietrich RB, Bradley WG, Zaragoza EJ, et al. MR evaluation of early myelination patterns in normal and developmentally delayed infants. AJNR Am J Neuroradiol 9:69–76, 1988.

Di Pucchio T, Ennas MG, Presta M, et al. Basic fibroblast growth factor modulates in vitro differentiation of human fetal microglia. Neuroreport 7:2813–2817, 1996.

Dodd J, Schuchardt A. Axon guidance: a compelling case for repelling growth cones. Cell 81:471–474, 1995.

Echelard Y, Epstein DJ, St-Jacques B, et al. *Sonic hedgehog,* a member of a family of putative signaling molecules, is implicated in the regulation of CNS polarity. Cell 75:1417–1430, 1993.

ElShamy WM, Linnarsson S, Lee KF, et al. Prenatal and postnatal requirements of NT-3 for sympathetic neuroblast survival and innervation of specific targets. Development 122:491–500, 1996.

Erskine L, McCaig CD. Growth cone neurotransmitter receptor activation modulates electric field-guided nerve growth. Dev Biol 171:330–339, 1995.

Ferrer I, Soriano E, Del Rio JA, et al. Cell death and removal in the cerebral cortex during development. Prog Neurobiol 39:1–43, 1992.

Ferrer I, Serrano T, Soriano E. Naturally occurring cell death in the subicular complex and hippocampus in the rat during development. Neurosci Res 8:60–66, 1990.

Figdor MC, Stern CD. Segmental organization of embryonic diencephalon. Nature 363:630–634, 1993.

Flores-Sarnat L. Hemimegalencephaly. Part 1. Genetic, clinical, and imaging aspects. J Child Neurol 17:373–384, 2002.

Flores-Sarnat L, Sarnat HB, Dávila-Gutiérrez G, Álvarez A. Hemimegalencephaly. Part 2. Neuropathology suggests a disorder of cellular lineage. J Child Neurol 18:776–785, 2003.

Fontain-Perus J. Migration of crest-derived cells from gut: gut influence on spinal cord development. Brain Res Bull 30:251–255, 1993.

Fortini ME, Artavanis-Tsakonas S. *Notch:* neurogenesis is only part of the picture. Cell 75:1245–1247, 1993.

Fujimoto E, Miki A, Mizoguti H. Histochemical study of the differentiation of microglial cells in the developing human cerebral hemispheres. J Anat 166:253–264,1989.

Gilles FH. Myelination in the human brain. Hum Pathol 7:244–248, 1976.

Golden JA, Chernoff GF. Intermittent pattern of neural tube closure in two strains of mice. Teratology 47:73–80, 1993.

Goldman JE, Vaysse PJ. Tracing glial cell lineages in the mammalian forebrain. Glia 4:149–156, 1991.

Gomez-Pinilla F, Lee JW-K, Cotman CW. Distribution of basic fibroblast growth factor in the developing rat brain. Neuroscience 61:911–923, 1994.

Gong Z, Brandhorst BP. Multiple levels of regulation of tubulin gene expression during sea urchin embryogenesis. Dev Biol 130:140–153, 1988.

Gonzalez-Martin C, de Diego I, Crespo D, et al. Transient *c-fos* expression accompanies naturally occurring cell death in the developing interhemispheric cortex of the rat. Brain Res Dev Brain Res 68:83–95, 1992.

Goulding MD, Lumsden A, Gruss P. Signals from the notochord and floor plate regulate the region-specific expression of two *Pax* genes in the developing spinal cord. Development 117:1001–1016, 1993.

Gray GE, Sanes JR. Migratory paths and phenotypic choices of clonally related cells in the avian optic tectum. Neuron 6:211–225, 1991.

Greenough WT. Structural correlates of information storage in the mammalian brain: a review and hypothesis. Trends Neurosci 7:229–233, 1984.

Gressens P, Richelme C, Kadhim HJ, et al. The germinative zone produces the most cortical astrocytes after neuronal migration in the developing mammalian brain. Biol Neonate 61:4–24, 1992.

Guo M, Jan LY, Jan YN. Control of daughter cell fates during asymmetric division: interaction of *Numb* and *Notch.* Neuron 17:27–41, 1996.

Guthrie S, Butcher M, Lumsden A. Patterns of cell division and interkinetic nuclear migration in the chick embryo hindbrain. J Neurobiol 22:742–754, 1991.

Guthrie S, Muchamore I, Kuroiwa A, et al. Neuroectodermal autonomy of *Hox-2.9* expression revealed by rhombomere transpositions. Nature 356:157–159, 1992.

Guthrie S, Pini A. Chemorepulsion of developing motor axons by the floor plate. Neuron 14:1117–1130,1995.

Hager G, Dodt H-U, Zieglgansberger W, et al. Novel forms of neuronal migration in the rat cerebellum. J Neurosci Res 40:207–219, 1995.

Hall BK. The neural crest as a fourth germ layer and vertebrates as quadroblastic not triploblastic. Evol Devel 2:3–5, 2000.

Hall BK. *The Neural Crest in Development and Evolution.* New York: Springer-Verlag, 1999.

Hamburger V, Levi-Montalcini R. Proliferation, differentiation and degeneration in the spinal ganglia of the chick embryo under normal and experimental conditions. J Exp Zool 111:457–502, 1949.

Hardy K, Handyside AH, Winston RML. The human blastocyst: cell number, death and allocation during late preimplantation development in vitro. Development 107:597–604, 1989.

Harris AJ, McCaig CD. Motoneuron death and motor unit size during embryonic development of the rat. J Neurosci 4:13–24, 1984.

Hasan SU, Sarnat HB, Auer RN. Vagal nerve maturation in the fetal lamb: an ultrastructural and morphometric study. Anat Rec 237:527–537, 1993.

Hasegawa M, Houdou S, Mito T, et al. Development of myelination in the human fetal and infant cerebrum: a myelin basic protein immunohistochemical study. Brain Dev 14:1–6, 1992.

Haydon PG, Drapeau P. From contact to connection: early events during synaptogenesis. Trends Neurosci 18:196–201, 1995.

Henrique D, Adam J, Myat A, et al. Expression of *a Delta* homologue in prospective neurons in the chick. Nature 375:787–790, 1995.

Homma S, Yaginuma H, Oppenheim RW. Programmed cell death during the earliest stages of spinal cord development in the chick embryo: a possible means of early phenotypic selection. J Comp Neurol 345:377–395, 1994.

Hunt P, Wilkinson DG, Krumlauf R. Patterning of the vertebrate head: murine *Hox-2* genes mark distinct subpopulations of premigratory and migrating neural crest. Development 112:43–51, 1991.

Jacobson AG. Experimental analyses of the shaping of the neural plate and tube. Amer Zool 31:628–643, 1991.

Jessen KR, Richardson WD, eds. *Glial Cell Development.* 2nd Ed. New York: Oxford University Press, 2001.

Jones MZ, Gardner E. Pathogenesis of methylazoxymethanol-induced lesions in the postnatal mouse cerebellum. J Neuropathol Exp Neurol 35:413–444, 1976.

Joyner AL, Martin GR. *En-1* and *En-2,* two mouse genes with sequence homology to the *Drosophila engrailed* gene: expression during embryogenesis. Genes Dev 1:29–38, 1987.

Juriloff DM, Harris MJ, Tom C, et al. Normal mouse strains differ in the site of initiation of closure of the cranial neural tube. Teratology 44:225–233, 1991.

Juurlink BHJ, Hertz L. Plasticity of astrocytes in primary cultures: an experimental tool and a reason for methodological caution. Dev Neurosci 7:263–277, 1985.

Kaufmann WE, Worley PF, Pegg J, et al. *Cox-2,* a synaptically induced enzyme, is expressed by excitatory neurons at postsynaptic sites in rat cerebral cortex. Proc Natl Acad Sci USA 93:2317–2321, 1996.

Kennedy TE, Serafini T, de la Torre J, et al. Netrins are diffusible chemotropic factors for commissural axons in the embryonic spinal cord. Cell 78:425–435, 1994.

Kessel M. Reversal of axonal pathways from rhombomere 3 correlates with extra *Hox* expression domains. Neuron 10:379–393, 1993.

Kessel M. *Hox* genes and the identity of motor neurons in the hindbrain. J Physiol (Paris) 88:105–109, 1994.

Keynes R, Cook GMW. Axon guidance molecules. Cell 83:161–169, 1995.

Keynes R, Krumlauf R. *Hox* genes and regionalization of the nervous system. Annu Rev Neurosci 17:109–132, 1994.

Keynes R, Lumsden A. Segmentation and the origin of regional diversity in the vertebrate central nervous system. Neuron 4:1–9, 1990.

Kiernan BW, Ffrench-Constant C. Oligodendrocyte precursor (O-2A progenitor cell) migration: a model system for the study of cell migration in the developing central nervous system. Dev Suppl 219–225, 1993.

Kinney HC, Brody BA, Kloman AS, et al. Sequence of central nervous system myelination in human infancy: II: patterns of myelination in autopsied infants. J Neuropathol Exp Neurol 47:217–234, 1988.

Kinney HC, Karthigasan J, Borenshteyn NI, et al. Myelination in the developing human brain: biochemical correlates. Neurochem Res 19:983–996, 1994.

Koch C, Zador A. The function of dendritic spines: devices subserving biochemical rather than electrical compartmentalization. J Neurosci 13:413–422, 1993.

Komuro H, Rakic P. Dynamics of granule cell migration: a confocal microscopic study in acute cerebellar slice preparations. J Neurosci 15:1110–1120, 1995.

Koseki H, Wallin J, Wilting J, et al. A role for *Pax-1* as a mediator of notochordal signals during the dorsoventral specification of vertebrae. Development 119:649–660, 1993.

Krushel LA, Johnston JG, Fishell G, et al. Spatially localized neuronal cell lineages in the developing mammalian forebrain. Neuroscience 53:1035–1047, 1993.

Lagercrantz H. Classical and "new" neurotransmitters during development: some examples from control of respiration. J Dev Physiol 6:195–205, 1984.

Le Douarin N, Kalcheim C. *The Neural Crest.* 2nd Ed. Cambridge, UK: Cambridge University Press, 1999.

Leber SM, Sanes JR. Migratory paths of neurons and glia in the embryonic chick spinal cord. J Neurosci 15:1236–1248, 1995.

Lee JJ, von Kessler DP, Parks S, et al. Secretion and localized transcription suggest a role in positional signaling for products of the segmentation gene *hedgehog.* Cell 71:33–50, 1992.

Lehman S, Kuchler S, Theveniau M, et al. An endogenous lectin and one of its neuronal glycoprotein ligands are involved in contact guidance of neuron migration. Proc Natl Acad Sci USA 87:6455–6459, 1990.

Lemire RJ. Variations in development of the caudal neural tube in human embryos (Horizons XIV–XXI). Teratology 2:361–370, 1969.

Lemke G. The molecular genetics of myelination: an update. Glia 7:263–271, 1993.

Lerea LS, McNamara JO. Ionotropic glutamate receptor subtypes activate *c-fos* transcription by distinct calcium requiring-intracellular signaling pathways. Neuron 10:31–41, 1993.

Lim T-M, Jaques KF, Stern CD, et al. An evaluation of myelomeres and segmentation of the chick embryo spinal cord. Development 113:227–238, 1991.

Lipton SA, Kater SB. Neurotransmitter regulation of neuronal outgrowth, plasticity and survival. Trends Neurosci 12:265–270, 1989.

Lois C, Alvarez-Buylla A. Proliferating subventricular zone cells in the adult mammalian forebrain can differentiate into neurons and glia. Proc Natl Acad Sci USA 90:2074–2077, 1993.

Lumsden A. The cellular basis of segmentation in the developing hindbrain. Trends Neurosci 13:329–335, 1990.

Lumsden A, Sprawson N, Graham A. Segmental origin and migration of neural crest cells in the hindbrain region of the chick embryo. Development 113:1281–1291, 1991.

Maden M, Hunt P, Eriksson U, et al. Retinoic acid-binding protein, rhombomeres and the neural crest. Development 111:35–44, 1991.

Marin-Padilla M. Cephalic axial skeletal-neural dysraphic disorders: embryology and pathology. Can J Neurol Sci 18:153–169, 1991.

McGinnis W, Krumlauf R. Homeobox genes and axial patterning (review). Cell 68:283–302, 1992.

McLean MD, Roy N, Mackenzie AE, et al. Two 5q13 simple tandem repeat loci are in linkage disequilibrium with type 1 spinal muscular atrophy. Hum Mol Genet 3:1951–1956, 1994.

McMahon AP. The *Wnt* family of developmental regulators. Trends Genet 8:236–242, 1992.

McMahon AP, Bradley A. The *Wnt-1 (int-1)* protooncogene is required for development of a large region of the mouse brain. Cell 62:1073–1085, 1990.

McMahon AP, Joyner AL, Bradley A, et al. The midbrain-hindbrain phenotype of *Wnt-1-/Wnt-1-*mice results from stepwise deletion of engrailed-expressing cells by 9.5 days postcoitum. Cell 69:581–595, 1992.

Miklossy J, Van der Loos H. The long-distance effects of brain lesions: visualization of myelinated pathways in the human brain using polarizing and fluorescence microscopy. J Neuropathol Exp Neurol 50:1–15, 1991.

Minturn JE, Fryer HJL, Geschwind DH, et al. *TOAD-64,* a gene expressed early in neuronal differentiation in the rat, is related to *unc-33,* a *C. elegans* gene involved in axon outgrowth. J Neurosci 15:6757–6766, 1995.

Misson J-P, Edwards MA, Yamamoto M, et al. Mitotic cycling of radial glial cells of the fetal murine cerebral wall: a combined autoradiographic and immunohistochemical study. Brain Res 466:183–190, 1988.

Mochida GH, Walsh CA. Genetic basis of developmental malformations of the cerebral cortex. Arch Neurol 61:637–640, 2004.

Monteiro RAF, Rocha E, Marini-Abreu MM. Do microglia arise from pericytes? An ultrastructural and distribution study in the rat cerebellar cortex. J Submicrosc Cytol Pathol 28:457–469, 1996.

Morriss-Kay GM, Murphy P, Hill RE, et al. Effects of retinoic acid on expression of *Hox-2.9* and *Krox-20* and on morphological segmentation in the hindbrain of mouse embryos. EMBO J 10:2985–2995, 1991.

Noll E, Miller RH. Regulation of oligodendrocyte differentiation: a role for retinoic acid in the spinal cord. Development 120:649–660, 1994.

Nornes HO, Dressler GR, Knapik E et al. Spatially and temporally restricted expression of *Pax-2* during murine neurogenesis. Development 109:797–809, 1990.

Nurcombe V, McGrath PA, Bennett MR. Postnatal death of motor neurons during the development of the brachial spinal cord of the rat. Neurosci Lett 27:249–254, 1981.

Nurse P. Ordering S phase and M phase in the cell cycle. Cell 79:547–550, 1994.

Oakley RA, Tosney KW. Contact-mediated mechanisms of motor axon segmentation. J Neurosci 13:3773–3792, 1993.

O'Connor TM, Wyttenbach CR. Cell death in the embryonic chick spinal cord. J Cell Biol 60:448–459, 1974.

Okado N, Oppenheim RW. Cell death of motoneurons in the chick embryo spinal cord. J Neurosci 4:1639–1652, 1984.

O'Leary DDM, Stanfield BB. Selective elimination of axons extended by developing cortical neurons is dependent on regional locale: experiments utilizing fetal cortical transplants. J Neurosci 9:2230–2246, 1989.

Ono K, Kawamura K. Migration of immature neurons along tangentially oriented fibers in the subpial part of the fetal mouse medulla oblongata. Exp Brain Res 78:290–300, 1989.

Oppenheim RWJ, Shneiderman A, Shimizu I, et al. Onset and development of intersegmental projections in the chick embryo spinal cord. J Comp Neurol 275:159–180, 1988.

O'Rahilly R, Muller F. Bidirectional closure of the rostral neuropore in the human embryo. Am J Anatomy 184:259–268, 1989.

O'Rourke NA, Dailey ME, Smith SJ, et al. Diverse migratory pathways in the developing cerebral cortex. Science 258:299–302, 1992.

O'Rourke NA, Sullivan DP, Kaznowski CE, et al. Tangential migration of neurons in the developing cerebral cortex. Development 121:2165–2176, 1995.

O'Shea KS, Rheinheimer JST, Dixit VM. Deposition and role of thrombospondin in the histogenesis of the cerebellar cortex. J Cell Biol 110:1275–1283, 1990.

Page KJ, Saha A, Everitt BJ. Differential activation and survival of basal forebrain neurons following infusions of excitatory amino acids: studies with the immediate early gene *c-fos.* Exp Brain Res 93:412–422, 1993.

Parr B, Shea M, Vassileva G, et al. Mouse *Wnt* genes exhibit discrete domains of expression in the early embryonic CNS and limb buds. Development 119:247–261, 1993.

Pascual-Castroviejo I, Pascual-Pascual SI. Congenital vascular malformations in childhood. Semin Pediatr Neruol 9:254–273, 2002.

Peifer M. The two faces of *hedgehog*. Science 266:1492–1493, 1994.

Pettway Z, Guillory G, Bronner Fraser M. Absence of neural crest cells from the region surrounding implanted notochords in situ. Dev Biol 142:335–345, 1990.

Pfaff SL, Mendelshohn M, Stewart CL, et al. Requirement for *Lim* homeobox gene *Isl-1* in motor neuron generation reveals a motor neuron-dependent step in interneuron differentiation. Cell 84:309–320, 1996.

Pinter JD, Sarnat HB. Neuroembryology. In: Winn HR, ed. *Youman's Neurological Surgery*. 5th Ed. Philadelphia: Saunders, vol. 1, pp. 45–69, 2004.

Pittman RN, Wang S, DiBenedetto AJ, et al. A system for characterizing cellular and molecular events in programmed neuronal cell death. J Neurosci 13:3669–3680, 1993.

Porter BE, Sanes JR. Gated migration: neurons migrate on but not onto substrates containing S-laminin. Dev Biol 167:609–616, 1995.

Pourquie O, Coltey M, Teillet M-A, et al. Control of dorsoventral patterning of somitic derivatives by notochord and floor plate. Proc Natl Acad Sci USA 90:5242–5246, 1993.

Price M, Lazzaro D, Pohl T, et al. Regional expression of the homeobox gene *Nkx-2.2* in the developing mammalian forebrain. Neuron 8:241–255, 1992.

Puelles L, Rubenstein LR. Expression patterns of homeobox and other putative regulatory genes in the embryonic mouse forebrain suggest a neuromeric organization. Trends Neurosci 16:472–479, 1993.

Puelles L, Rubinstein JL. Forebrain gene expression domains and the evolving prosomeric model. Trends Neurosci 26:469-476, 2003.

Raible DW, Eisen JS. Regulative interactions in zebrafish neural crest. Development 122:501–507, 1996.

Ramón y Cajal S. Histologie du systeme nerveux central de l'homme et des vertebres. Paris: Maloine, 1909–1911.

Rho JM, Storey TW. Molecular ontogeny of major neurotransmitter receptor systems in the mammalian central nervous system: norepinephrine, dopamine, serotonin, acetylcholine and glycine. J Child Neurol 16:271–281, 2001.

Richman DP, Stewart RM, Hutchinson JW, et al. Mechanical model of brain convolutional development. Science 189:18–21, 1975.

Riddle RD, Johnson RL, Laufer E, et al. *Sonic hedgehog* mediates the polarizing activity of the ZPA. Cell 75:1401–1416, 1993.

Roessmann U, Gambetti P. Astrocytes in the developing human brain: an immunohistochemical study. Acta Neuropathol (Berl) 70:308–313, 1986.

Rorke LB, Riggs HE. *Myelination of the Brain in the Newborn*. Philadelphia: JB Lippincott, 1969.

Rossi DJ, Slater NT. The developmental onset of NMDA receptor-channel activity during neuronal migration. Neuropharmacology 32:1239–1248, 1993.

Sadaghiani B, Crawford BJ, Vielkind JR. Changes in the distribution of extracellular matrix components during neural crest development in *Xipbophorus spp.* embryos. Can J Zool 72:1340–1353, 1994.

Salinas PC, Nusse R. Regional expression of the *Wnt-3* gene in the developing mouse forebrain in relation to diencephalic neuromeres. Mech Dev 39:151–160, 1992.

Salinas PC, Fletcher C, Copeland NG, et al. Maintenanceof *Wnt-3* expression in Purkinje cells of the mouse cerebellum depends on interactions with granule cells. Development 120:1277–1286, 1994.

Saraga-Babic M, Krolo M, Sapunar D, et al. Differences in origin and fate between the cranial and caudal spinal cord during normal and disturbed human development. Acta Neuropathol (Berl) 91:194–199, 1996.

Sarnat HB. *Cerebral Dysgenesis: Embryology and Clinical Expression*. New York: Oxford University Press, 1992a.

Sarnat HB. Regional differentiation of the human fetal ependyma: immunocytochemical markers. J Neuropathol Exp Neurol 51:58–75, 1992b.

Sarnat HB. Role of human fetal ependyma. Pediatr Neurol 8:163–178, 1992c.

Sarnat HB. CNS malformations: gene locations of known human mutations. Eur J Paediatr Neurol 9: in press, 2005.

Sarnat HB. Regional ependymal upregulation of vimentin in Chiari II malformation, aqueductal stenosis and hyromyelia. Pediatr Devel Pathol 7:48–60, 2004a.

Sarnat HB. Watershed infarcts in the fetal and neonatal brainstem. An etiology of central hypoventilation, dysphagia, Moibius syndrome and micrognathia. Eur J Paediatr Neurol 8:71–87, 2004c.

Sarnat HB, Flores-Sarnat L. Embryology of the neural crest: its inductive role in the neurcutaneous syndromes. J Child Neurol 20: in press, 2005.

Sarnat HB, Benjamin DR, Siebert JR, Kletter GB, Cheyette SR. Agnenesis of the mesencephalon and metencephalon with cerebellar hypoplasia: putative mutation in the *EN2* gene—Report of 2 cases in early infancy. Pediatr Devel Pathol 5:54–68, 2002.

Sarnat HB, Flores-Sarnat L. Neuropathological research strategies in holoprosencephaly. J Child Neurol 16:918–931, 2001.

Sarnat HB, Flores-Sarnat L. Cajal-Retzius and subplate neurons: their role in cortical development. Eur J Paediatr Neurol 6:91–97, 2002.

Sarnat HB, Menkes JH. How to construct a neural tube. J Child Neurol 15:110–124, 2000.

Sarnat HB, Netsky MG. When does a ganglion become a brain? Evolutionary origin of the central nervous system. Sem Pediatr Neurol 9:240–253, 2002.

Sauer FC. Mitosis in the neural tube. J Comp Neurol 62:377–405, 1935.

Schmechel DE, Rakic P. Arrested proliferation of radial glial cells during midgestation in rhesus monkey. Nature 277:303–305, 1979.

Schneider-Maunoury S, Topilko P, Seitanidou T, et al. Disruption of *Krox-20* results in alteration of rhombomeres 3 and 5 in the developing hindbrain. Cell 75:1199–1214, 1993.

Schoenwolf GC, Franks MV. Quantitative analyses of changes in cell shapes during bending of the avian neural plate. Dev Biol 105:257–272, 1984.

Schoenwolf GC, Smith JL. Mechanisms of neurulation: traditional viewpoint and recent advances. Development 109:243–270, 1990.

Seilacher A. Late preCambrian and early Cambrian metazoa: preservational or real extinctions? In: Holland HD, Trendall AF, eds. *Patterns of Change in Earth Evolution*. Berlin: Springer-Verlag, pp. 159–168, 1984.

Selleck MAJ, Scherson TY, Bronner Fraser M. Origins of neural crest cell diversity. Dev Biol 159:1–11, 1993.

Shawlot W, Behringer RR. Requirement for *Lim-1* in head-organizer function. Nature 374:425–430, 1995.

Shelden E, Wadsworth P. Interzonal microtubules are dynamic during spindle elongation. J Cell Sci 97:273–281, 1990.

Shepherd GM, Greer CA. The dendritic spine: adaptations of structure and function for different types of synaptic integrations. In: Lasek R, Black M, eds. *Intrinsic Determinants of Neuronal Form and Function*. New York: A R Liss, pp. 245–314, 1989.

Shimada M, Langman J. Repair of the external granular layer of the hamster cerebellum after prenatal and postnatal administration of methylazoxymethanol. Teratology 3:119–134, 1970.

Shimamura K, Hartigan DJ, Martinez S, et al. Longitudinal organization of the anterior neural plate and neural tube. Development 121:3923–3933, 1995.

Sidman RL, Rakic P. Neuronal migration, with special reference to the developing human brain: a review. Brain Res 62:1–35, 1973.

Sieber-Blum M, ed. *Neurotrophins and the Neural Crest*. Boca Raton, FL: CRC Press, 1999.

Silver J, Hughes AFW. The relationship between morphogenetic cell death and the development of congenital anophthalmia. J Comp Neurol 157:281–302, 1974.

Simeone T, Donevan SD, Rho JM. Molecular biology and ontogeny of γ-aminobutyric acid (GABA) receptors in the mammalian central nervous system. J Child Neurol 18:30–48, 2003.

Simeone T, Sánchez RM, Rho JM. Molecular biology and ontogeny of glutamate receptors in the mammalian central nervous system. J Child Neurol 19:343–360, 2004.

Skoff RP, Knapp PE. Division of astroblasts and oligodendroblasts in postnatal rodent brain: evidence for separate astrocyte and oligodendrocyte lineages. Glia 4:165–174, 1991.

Smart IHM. Proliferative characteristics of the ependymal layer during the early development of the spinal cord in the mouse. J Anat 111:365–380, 1972.

Smith J, Schoenwolf GC. Notochordal induction of cell wedging in the chick neural plate and its role in neural tube formation. J Exp Zool 250:49–62, 1989.

Snow DM, Steindler DA, Silver J. Molecular and cellular characterization of the glial roof plate of the spinal cord and optic tectum: a possible role for a proteoglycan in the development of an axon barrier. Dev Biol 138:359–376, 1990.

Spana EP, Doe CQ. *Numb* antagonizes *Notch* signaling to specify sibling neuron cell fates. Neuron 17:21–26, 1996.

Spemann H, Mangold H. liber Induktion von Embryonalanlagen durch Implantation artfremder Organisatoren. Wilhelm Roux Arch Entwick 100:599–638, 1924.

Spitzer N. Development of membrane properties in vertebrates. Trends Neurosci 4:169–172, 1981.

Steen RG, Gronemeyer SA, Kingsley PB, et al. Precise and accurate measurement of proton Tl in human brain in vivo: validation and preliminary clinical application. J Magn Reson Imaging 4:681–691, 1994.

Stein S, Kessel M. A homeobox gene involved in node, notochord and neural plate formation of chick embryos. Mech Dev 49:37–48, 1995.

Stern CD, Jaques KF, Lim T-M, et al. Segmental lineage restrictions in the chick embryo spinal cord depend on the adjacent somites. Development 113:239–244 1991.

Storey KG, Crossley JM, De Robertis EM, et al. Neural induction and regionalization in the chick embryo. Development 114:729–741, 1992.

Stoykova A, Gruss P. Roles of *Pax*-genes in developing and adult brain as suggested by expression patterns. J Neurosci 14:1395–1412, 1994.

Tajbakhsh S, Buckingham ME. Lineage restriction of the myogenic conversion factor *myf-5* in the brain. Development 121:4077–4083, 1995.

Tan SS, Morriss-Kay GM. The development and distribution of the cranial neural crest in the rat embryo. Cell Tiss Res 240:403–416, 1985.

Tanaka E, Sabry J. Making the connection: cytoskeletal rearrangements during growth cone guidance. Cell 83:171–176, 1995.

Tecott LH, Eberwine JH, Barchas JE, et al. Methodological considerations in the utilization of in situ hybridization. In: Eberwine JH, Valentino KL, Barchas JD, eds. *In Situ Hybridization in Neurobiology: Advances in Methodology.* New York: Oxford University Press, pp. 3–23, 1994.

Tessier-Lavigne M, Placzek M, Lumsden AGS, et al. Chemotropic guidance of developing axons in the mammalian central nervous system. Nature 336:775–778, 1988.

Thoenen H. Neurotrophins and neuronal plasticity. Science 270:593–598, 1995.

Topilko P, Schneider-Maunoury S, Levi G, et al. *Krox-20* controls myelination in the peripheral nervous system. Nature 371:796–799, 1994.

Tosney KW. Somites and axon guidance. Scan Microsc 2:427–442, 1988.

Tsuchida T, Ensini M, Morton SB, et al. Topographic organization of embryonic motor neurons defined by expression of *Lim* homeobox genes. Cell 79:957–970, 1994.

Turner DL, Weintraub H. Expression of *achaete-scute* homolog 3 in *Xenopus* embryos converts ectodermal cells to a neural fate. Genes Dev 8:1434–1447, 1994.

van der Knaap MS, Valk J, Bakker CJ, et al. Myelination as an expression of the functional maturity of the brain. Dev Med Child Neurol 33:849–857, 1991.

Wagner M, Thaller C, Jessell T, et al. Polarizing activity and retinoid synthesis in the floor plate of the neural tube. Nature 345:819–822, 1990.

Walsh C, Cepko CL. Clonally related cortical cells show several migration patterns. Science 241:1342–1345, 1988.

Walther C, Gruss P. *Pax-6*, a murine paired box gene, is expressed in the developing CNS. Development 113:1435–1449, 1991.

Walz W. Role of glial cells in the regulation of the brain microenvironment. Prog Neurobiol 33:309–333, 1989.

Weidenheim KM, Kress Y, Epshteyn I, et al. Early myelination in the human fetal lumbosacral spinal cord: characterization by light and electron microscopy. J Neuropathol Exp Neurol 51:142–149, 1992.

Wilkinson DG, Krumlauf R. Molecular approaches to the segmentation of the hindbrain. Trends Neurosci 13:335–339, 1990.

Williams JH, Errington ML, Lynch MA, et al. Arachidonic acid induces a long-term activity-dependent enhancement of synaptic transmission in the hippocampus. Nature 341:739–742, 1989.

Willmer P. *Invertebrate Relationships: Patterns in Animal Evolution.* Cambridge, UK: Cambridge University Press, 1990.

Wilson SW, Placzek M, Furley AJ. Border disputes: do boundaries play a role in growth-cone guidance? Trends Neurosci 16:316–323, 1993.

Yakovlev PI, Lecours A-R. The myelination cycles of regional maturation of the brain. In: Minkowski A, ed. *Regional Development of the Brain in Early Life.* Philadelphia: FA Davis, pp. 3–70, 1967.

Yamada T, Placzek M, Tanaka H, et al. Control of cell pattern in the developing nervous system: polarizing activity of the floor plate and notochord. Cell 64:635–647, 1991.

Yu W, Baas PW. The growth of the axon is not dependent upon net microtubule assembly at its distal tip. J Neurosci 15:6827–6833, 1995.

Yu W-P, Collarini EJ, Pringle NP, et al. Embryonic expression of myelin genes: evidence for a focal source of oligodendrocyte precursors in the ventricular zone of the neural tube. Neuron 12:1353–1362, 1994.

Zimmerman K, Shih J, Bars J, et al. *XASH-3,* a novel *Xenopus achaetscute* homolog, provides an early marker of planar neural induction and position along the mediolateral axis of the neural plate. Development 119:221–232, 1993.

Normal Childhood Growth and Development of Intellect, Language, Temperament, Emotion, and Social Skills

Marilyn Augustyn, MD

Everything else you grow out of, but you never recover from childhood.
—Beryl Bainbridge

MAJOR THEORIES AND THEORISTS OF CHILD DEVELOPMENT

The changing patterns of abilities and behavior we call "development" present intriguing challenges to clinicians. Children and adolescents are unique because they are changing, and at a greater rate than at any other time in life, which creates a special challenge to clinicians. In this section, we present a brief overview of the major theories of child development and provide principles to guide clinicians. For the various stages of development, we present the classical theory and also describe the clinical manifestations.

One of the forebears of child development, Arnold Gesell, described development as a spiral, with alternating periods of equilibrium and disequilibrium (Gesell and Amatruda 1964). Each transition in the child's progress elicits and requires reciprocal changes in the parents, so that, ideally, parenting has its own developmental course that is coordinated with the child's changing abilities and behaviors.

It is not surprising that such a complex phenomenon fostered several major schools of thought to explain the transitions. In the broadest classifications, the theories can be divided into two frameworks: reactive and structural (Lewis and Volkmar 1990). *Reactive* theorists postulate that the child's mind begins as a *tabula rasa* (i.e., blank slate) and that changes in behavior and development result almost exclusively from environmental events. These theorists believe that abnormal development should be regarded as involving *learned* behaviors and that only through relearning or environmental change can the "symptom" be removed and the behavior modified.

Structural theorists postulate a genetically determined capacity for the development of patterns, or systems, of behavior. The child is seen as interacting with and actively shaping his or her environment. The continuing behavior patterns or stages that emerge are sequential and different from one another; progress is orderly and straightforward, building on the stage before it. Theoretical schools with this perspective are quite diverse and include the psychoanalytic school (Freud) (see Dare 1985), the emotional school (Erikson), the cognitive school (Piaget) (see Hobson 1985), and the attachment school (Mahler). A summary of these theo-

TABLE 2.1

MAJOR STRUCTURAL THEORIES OF CHILD DEVELOPMENT

Age	Psychoanalytic (Freud)	Emotional (Erikson)	Cognitive (Piaget)	Attachment (Mahler)
Newborn	Oral	Trust vs. mistrust	Sensorimotor: Stage I Reflexive	Normal autistic phase
1 month			Sensorimotor: Stage II Primary circular reactions	Normal symbiotic phase
4–5 months			Sensorimotor: Stage III Secondary circular reactions	Peak of symbiosis Beginning of separation and individuation First subphase: Differentiation
7 months				Second subphase: Early practicing phase
9 months			Sensorimotor: Stage IV Coordination of existing scheme	Practicing phase
1 year	Anal	Autonomy vs. shame/doubt	Sensorimotor: Stage V Tertiary circular reactions	
18 months			Sensorimotor: Stage VI Representational period	Third subphase: Rapprochement
2–3 years			Preoperational period	
3–6 years	Oedipal	Initiative vs. guilt		
6–12 years	Latency	Industry vs. inferiority	Concrete operational thought	Object constancy (libidinal)
12–18 years	Genital	Identity vs. identity diffusion	Formal operational thought	Resolution of omnipotence

ries is presented in Table 2.1. Each of these theories provides a different structural lens through which to understand an individual child's development.

The *transactional model*, formulated by Sameroff and colleagues, attempted to reconcile these apparently contradictory views of child development. In this view, both behavioral and biological attributes must be considered in their reciprocal relationships to other characteristics of the child. In this theory, development is conceived of as a fluid, dynamic reciprocal process between biological attributes and environment that can reinforce, modify, or change specific psychological patterns at all age periods—that is, the child affects the environment, and the environment affects the child (Sameroff and Seifer 1983). The transactional model counsels looking at the mutually independent nature of the relationship between a child and his or her environment in order to understand development. The innate characteristics of an individual child (e.g., health, personality, temperament) affect the way a child responds to his or her environment. These patterns of reaction will in turn change certain aspects of the environment (e.g., parental caregiving style). Conversely, the environment has certain qualities (e.g., socioeconomic status, family structure) that have a profound effect on the child. Development must be understood as resulting from the complex interplay of the child and his or her environs. Each modifies and potentiates the other. Together, they weave a complex pattern of development that cannot be under-

stood by examining a single thread of nature or of nurture (Parker et al. 1988).

The process of development is complex and, in spite of much research, still not completely understood. It is helpful when examining human development to apply the preceding above theories as a clarifying, but not conclusive, lens through which to view human behavior and growth. In the following sections, we describe innate characteristics of children that contribute to individual behavioral differences and then explore the stages of human development using the structure of these theories as a framework.

INDIVIDUAL DIFFERENCES THROUGHOUT DEVELOPMENT

Overview of Temperamental Theory

In addition to understanding the theory and sequence of development, it is important to understand individual differences among children. In the early 1900s, it was thought that parents totally shape their children's personalities—in other words, children were born as "lumps of clay" for parents to mold through daily interactions over the course of childhood. Such a theory of personality development, however, does not explain why some children who were born into nurturing families had problems and some who were born into troubled families did well.

Children are intrinsically different from one another, and although parents may love all their children, they respond to each child differently because the children are different. Siblings experience both shared and nonshared aspects of their environment. Research from behavioral genetics suggests that nonshared environmental influences on each child tend to have a greater effect than shared ones. Consequently, parents can respond differently to a persistent, slow-to-warm child—for example, with more frustration or anger—than to a sibling who is more adaptable and less persistent. The folk wisdom is that the person who "invented" temperament was the first parent who had a second child! The dilemma of intrinsic differences between children has led child developmentalists to embrace the concept of innate "temperamental" characteristics that play a role in personality development.

Temperament is often defined as *how* the child behaves, in contrast to *why* the child does what he or she does (motivation) and *what* he or she does (abilities) (Chess and Thomas 1986). The nine characteristics of temperament that were initially described by researchers Stella Chess and Alexander Thomas (1986) in the New York Longitudinal Study are outlined in Table 2.2. This landmark study demonstrated that children are born with a unique combination of temperamental characteristics that describe an individual's particular behavioral style. These characteristics are presumably derived from a combination of genetic, intrauterine, central nervous system, and postnatal environmental factors. Although not fixed, an individual's temperamental style is likely to be consistent over time, especially when the interplay between the individual and the environment is relatively stable.

This is in contrast to *personality* which is commonly defined as what makes one person different from other people, perhaps even unique. This aspect of personality is called *individual differences*. However, personality theorists are just as interested in the *commonalities* among people. The central point is that the major personality traits will vary "with the nature of the adaptive demands created by the social setting, as the profile of animal species varies with the local ecology" ("Normal Personality Development," Kagan, J in *Textbook of Pediatric Neuropsychiatry*, First Edition p. 14).

Specific Temperamental Characteristics

Activity level refers to the motor component of a child's functioning. A child with high activity level is one for whom a parent needs four hands to change a diaper: two to hold the baby down and two to change the diaper. These children are running instead of walking at 1 year of age, and at age 5 years they can sit at the dinner table for only 5 minutes at a time. On the other hand, a child with low activity level moves very little while being dressed or during sleep and, when older, can stay seated through dinner.

Rhythmicity refers to the degree of predictability and rhythm in the timing of biological functions (e.g., sleep, hunger, elimination). A child with predictable rhythms sleeps, eats, and eliminates at roughly the same times each day. Although all newborn infants take a couple of days to adjust to extrauterine life, the child with unpredictable rhythms never seems to develop regular, predictable patterns.

Approach–withdrawal refers to the nature of a child's initial response to new or altered stimuli (e.g., new foods, toys, or people). A child with a positive approach likes new foods and approaches strangers and new surroundings readily. A child with a negative approach–withdrawal

TABLE 2.2
TEMPERAMENTAL CHARACTERISTICS

Characteristic	"Easy"	"Difficult"
Activity level	*Low:* Moves very little while being dressed or sleeping	*High:* Is constantly on the move; four hands needed to change a diaper
Rhythmicity	*Regular:* Eats, sleeps, and eliminates at predictable times	*Irregular:* Is unpredictable from day to day
Approach–withdrawal	*Positive approach:* Approaches strangers easily	*Negative approach:* Does not like new clothes or toys; initially rejects new environments
Adaptability	*Quick:* Easily learns to accept new situations	*Slow:* Has difficult time adjusting to new situations
Threshold of responsiveness	*High:* enjoys being touched and cuddled; is not easily aroused	*Low:* Is easily startled; rejects new textures
Intensity of reaction	*Mild:* Whines but does not cry when angry	*Intense:* Cries loudly and laughs hard
Quality of mood	*Positive:* Generally has a "sunny" disposition	*Negative:* Has serious disposition
Distractibility	*High:* Can be coaxed away from forbidden activities	*Low:* Is not easily drawn away from desired activity
Attention span and persistence	*Long:* Intently concentrates and continues activity despite obstacles	*Short:* Gives up easily; stays briefly on each activity

Source: Adapted from Chess and Thomas 1986.

rejects the first tastes of infant cereal, will not sleep in strange beds, and can be expected to hide behind mother on the first day of school.

Adaptability refers to the ease with which a child's response to new or altered situations can be modified in a desired direction, irrespective of his or her initial response. A highly adaptive child could have been somewhat tentative during the first bath but now enjoys bathing; could have initially rejected new foods but now accepts them well; could have been afraid of certain toy animals at first but now plays with them happily. On the other hand, a child with low adaptability has a difficult time adjusting to new situations, even after multiple exposures. These children have difficulty with transitions; for example, resisting daily dressing and facing the start of each school year or of summer camp with dread.

Threshold of responsiveness refers to the intensity of stimulation that is necessary to evoke a discernible response from a child. Parents of a child with a high threshold of responsiveness do not need to tiptoe around the house during nap times for fear that a sudden noise will awaken their sleeping baby. These children also enjoy being touched and handled and often enjoy roughhousing during play. On the other hand, a child with a low threshold of responsiveness is easily startled, is awakened from sleep by normal household sounds, finds certain articles of clothing unbearable against his or her skin, and refuses to eat foods with certain textures.

Intensity of reaction refers to the energy level or vigor of a child's response (either negative or positive) to stimuli. Intensely reacting children reject foods vigorously, scream when frustrated, and laugh loudly when amused. Children with low intensity of reaction whine but do not cry when angry, and give a brief smile but do not laugh when happy. Some parents of children with low response levels might consider their babies "boring" and have a difficult time establishing an emotional connection because the children offer little or no emotional feedback.

Quality of mood refers to the amount of pleased, joyful, and friendly behavior versus the amount of displeased, crying, and unfriendly behavior. A child with a positive mood is "quick with a smile" or has a "sunny disposition," whereas a child with a negative mood has a serious disposition or frequently acts sullen or cranky. This is not to say that children with negative demeanors never feel pleasure, but rather that they do not express their pleasure openly and with the behaviors typically associated with happiness.

Distractibility refers to the ease with which a child can be diverted from ongoing activity by extraneous peripheral stimuli. Highly distractible children stop crying when their parents sing to them and are alert to sounds and sights in their environment. These children also can be coaxed away from a forbidden activity by being led into something else. Parents who "distract" their children during temper tantrums will be successful with highly distractible children, but not with children who have low distractibility. Children with low distractibility do not seem to hear when they are spoken to if they are involved in their favorite activities.

Attention span and *persistence* refer to the length of time a child will pursue a particular activity and the continued maintenance of the activity in the face of obstacles, respectively. Children with long attention spans and persistence will intently watch toy mobiles over the crib and will stay with tasks like puzzles or blocks for long periods of time. When these children start a temper tantrum, it is difficult to stop it. Children with short attention spans go from one activity to another but, if they have high persistence, will return to the original task. However, if they have low persistence, they have difficulty completing any task.

"Goodness of Fit"

When one is looking at a particular child's behavior, it is possible to see the temperament characteristics of a child emerge and to understand how a child's behavior could affect different parents differently. These characteristics do not in and of themselves cause problems. Rather, it is the "fit" between the child's temperament and the demands and expectations of the parents and other caretakers that can determine whether a struggle will take place. The question is whether the parents and child complement or antagonize each other—in other words, is there a "good fit"?

A classic example of this concept is routinely experienced at dinnertime. There will inevitably be friction between a "10-minute parent" and a "5-minute child," because the parent has the expectation that the child should sit at the table for 10 minutes, but the child can sit there for only 5 minutes. Obviously, if the parent wants the child to stay, he or she will have to fight for the last 5 minutes. On the other hand, a "5-minute parent" with a "5-minute child" has expectations that fit with the child's temperamental capabilities.

If there is a good fit between parent and child, optimal development is likely. On the other hand, if there is a poor fit between parent and child (i.e., parental and caretaker expectations are not consistent with the child's temperament), the ensuing dissonance will result in stress and potential problem behavior. There is a tendency for healthy growth if the fit is good or for disturbed behavior if the fit is poor. Importantly, the notion of goodness of fit is situational. When parents see a consistent style of expression in "good" behavior as well as "bad," they can understand the pattern and see it as a unique feature of their child's temperament.

Children may have a good fit with some, but not all, caregivers or in some, but not all, settings. For example, there may be a good fit with a child in a relaxed home, and he or she is regarded as an "easy" child. Later, upon entering a day care or preschool program, the same child is labeled "difficult" because the expectations and practices in these structured environments can be very different from those in the more relaxed environment the child experiences in the home. The opposite case can also be true. A child thought of as difficult by the parents can be more comfortable—and consequently better behaved—in a structured school environment. Understanding a child's temperamental style will help parents—and, later, teachers—find the appropriate fit.

Temperament in Clinical Practice

Understanding a child's temperament can be a very liberating experience for parents, freeing them from a lot of unproductive parental guilt. For example, parents can be assured that the characteristics of their "colicky" baby are constitutional and not caused by parental inadequacy, or that their intensely reacting child is prone to tantrums unrelated to anything the parents have done. Once parents feel "off the hook," they learn to appreciate the child's unique style and to develop behaviors that complement him or her. A child's basic temperament cannot be changed, but a parent's expectations and behavioral response to the child can be adjusted to create a better fit.

Emotional Regulation and Dysregulation

Another concept useful in understanding the "how" of children's behavior is *emotional regulation,* a process that is intimately connected to temperament (Harris 1995). Emotional regulation is a developmentally acquired process, and various experiences of the child require the child to master this skill (coping), leading to adaptation. Various behaviors, such as out-of-control temper tantrums, social withdrawal, and excessive response to severe pain, can represent failures of emotional regulation, or *dysregulation.* During normal development, there are marked changes in the child's abilities and behavior that allow the child to master new developmental tasks. The failure to *regulate* the emotional input can result in maladaptation or delay. There has been increasing interest in *regulatory disorders* (Diagnostic Classification 0-3, 1997). Regulatory disorders are characterized by the infant or young child's difficulties in regulating behavior and physiological, sensory, attentional, motor, or affective processes, and in organizing a calm, alert, or affectively positive state. The diagnosis of regulatory disorder involves both a sensory, sensory-motor, or processing difficulty and a distinct behavioral pattern indicated by one or more behavioral symptoms.

DEVELOPMENTAL STAGES

It is important to preface a discussion of normal developmental pathways with two caveats. First, the suggestion that development follows a series of discrete stages that proceed in an unvarying order is no longer accepted. The intrinsic variation of each individual is both recognized and respected. Second, at any of the stages following birth, nervous system disease, environmental changes, infections, and so forth can all perturb the normal development discussed. Thus, not only individual variability but also individual

vulnerability from other areas must be considered in assessing the developmental course of any individual child.

Pregnancy

Behavioral development begins long before delivery of the child. Mothers are aware of the pattern a fetus follows: sleep/wake, with certain intermittent periods of increased activity. Ultrasound studies show coordinated movements such as thumb sucking and kicking by 16 weeks; evidence of such movements is that some children are born with blisters on their forearms from the strength of in utero sucking.

There are also developmental stages for parents that begin during pregnancy and continue for the remainder of the child's life (Howard 1990) (Table 2.3). Possibly the largest adjustment, though, takes place when the parents first take the child home from the hospital and recognize the reality of a new life and the issues and responsibilities concomitant with this lifelong commitment. Clinicians can help parents by understanding and discussing this important adjustment.

Early Infancy: "A Small Collection of . . . Reflexes"

Neurobehavior of the Newborn

During the first weeks of life, the physiological organization of infants is not entirely stable. For instance, periodic breathing (i.e., breathing stops and starts) occurs in healthy, full-term infants about 20% of the time during active sleep. Other autonomic functions, including temperature control, skin color, urination, defecation, yawning, gagging, hiccuping, and vomiting, are also variable during the first weeks of life. The normal physiological instability of the newborn is as varied as all aspects of normal development, such as tone. Some infants emit long, lusty squalls; others tend to voice their opinions a bit less noisily but more frequently. There is no average duration to individual crying spells, although there is a tendency toward very abrupt starts and stops. Newborns sleep from 14 to 16 hours per day, or approximately 60% to 70% of the time, and rarely sleep longer than 4.5 hours before waking. In full-term babies, "active" sleep (i.e., rapid eye movement [REM] sleep) occupies 45% to 50% of

TABLE 2.3
PARENTAL DEVELOPMENT DURING PREGNANCY

Stage	Parental Concerns
First trimester: Incorporation	Ambivalence / Anxieties about responsibilities
Second trimester: Differentiation	Recognition of fetus as separate / Fantasies/dreams about child
Third trimester: Separation	Fears about delivery / Concrete preparations

Source: Howard 1990.

TABLE 2.4

DEVELOPMENT OF THE NEWBORN (0–3 MONTHS)

Age	Motor	Communication	Cognition
Birth	Lifts/turns head in prone position Exhibits complete head lag on pull-to-sit motion Hand fisted, flexes arms Is able to track moving object up to 180°	Has mature hearing—prefers human voice frequencies	Has mature vestibular senses Has mature touch, taste, smell—prefers sweet Color vision 20/800
1 month	Lifts head enough to get chin off surface in prone position	Returns parents' gaze	Prefers faces with talking movements
2 months	Lifts head up to 45° in prone position	Coos in response to voices Exhibits social smile	Becomes excited in anticipation of objects Coos in response to voices
3 months	Grasp reflex disappearing; may voluntarily hold/wave a toy Lifts head 90° Makes prereach movements with fingers/toes Is able to sit with support	Chuckles Exhibits vocal-social response	Recognizes taste/smell of mother's breasts Is alert to/consoled by rocking/changes of position

total sleep time, while indeterminate sleep (passing between stages) occupies 10% and "quiet" sleep occupies 35% to 45% of total sleep time.

Colic is often one of the first major developmental obstacles that parents and clinicians encounter. Most basically defined, colic is excessive crying seen in infants who are otherwise well. Usually agreed-on characteristics include the Wessel criteria: unexplained fussiness or crying, child is under age 3 months, lasts (cumulative) more than 3 hours per day, occurs more than 3 days per week, persists longer than 3 weeks. The crying is described as "intense" and lasts for several hours at a time, often on a daily basis, occurring in the late afternoon or evening. Colic starts as a cycle of increased crying and decreased sleep that leads ultimately to neurobehavioral disorganization involving increased tone and reflexes and poor state regulation. The problem affects between 9% and 26% of infants, making it one of the most frequent complaints of parents seeking the help of clinicians in the first year of a child's life (Jenkins et al. 1980). Thus, it is important that clinicians distinguish colic from two other etiologies of crying in this period: normal crying and secondary excessive crying resulting from physical illness.

Normal crying was first studied by Brazelton (1962), who found that in a sample of 80 middle-class infants, crying lasted about 2 hours per day at 2 weeks, increased to a peak of almost 3 hours per day by 6 weeks, and then gradually decreased to about 1 hour per day by 3 months. Thus, when presented with a baby who by history is crying excessively, it is important to recall that the amount of parental concern about crying is not necessarily directly proportional to the degree of crying, since parents can have different thresholds of concern. Likewise, the clinician must evaluate the child for any physical etiology of the crying, including (1) acute disorders, such as infection, intestinal cramping with diarrhea, corneal abrasion, or incarcerated hernia; (2) allergy or lactose intolerance; and (3) external modifiers, such as open diaper pin, occult skin burn, or strangulated finger, toe, or penis.

Neurodevelopment in the Newborn

Infancy is a time of rapid neurological growth and development. During the fetal period, the development of the brain, in terms of volume percentage, proceeds in a caudocranial direction (Tanner 1970). Therefore, at birth, the medulla, pons, and spinal cord are more advanced than the cerebellum. The more advanced development of the former structures is congruent with the newborn's developmental activity, for which complex coordination is not required. The cerebellum, which is least advanced at birth relative to other brain and CNS structures, grows rapidly beginning just before birth and extending through the first year of life. In response to experience, cortical synaptic connections increase during infancy, reaching a maximum of about 50% above the adult mean at age 12 to 24 months and remaining at that level until about age 16 years, at which time they begin to decrease (pruning) to adult levels (Huttenlocher 1979). Some of the motor and sensory milestones of the newborn period are noted in Table 2.4, and the primitive reflexes are listed in Table 2.5.

Examination of Newborn Behavior

Until a generation ago, a newborn was thought to be little more than a warm lump of clay that loosely resembled a miniature human body. Jean Piaget, in *The Origins of Intelligence*, referred to the neonate as a "small collection of somewhat clumsy, unfinished, and isolated reflexes" (Piaget 1952/1985, p. 17). Research and observation of the newborn have shown that the newborn is much more than that. Newborn behavior is commonly classified according

TABLE 2.5
REFLEXES

Reflexes	Appears/Disappears
Postural Reflexes	
Asymmetric tonic neck reflex: When face is turned to one side, arm and leg on that side extend	1 month/4 months
Symmetric tonic neck reflex: When head extends, arms and tongue extend and legs flex; when head is flexed, arms and legs extend	
Primitive Reflexes	
Moro: When head suddenly drops back, arms and fingers first extend, then flex	Extension phase/Startle persists into adult life
Galant: When back is scratched beside the spine, lateral flexion occurs	Birth/6 months
Grasping: When pressure is placed on palm of hand and sole of foot, infant grasps	Birth/6 months
Stepping: When held vertically over a surface, infant touches feet to the surface in an alternating pattern	Birth/2 months
Uncovering: When eyes are covered with cloth, infant fusses and swipes at it	Birth/Becomes voluntary
Leg scraping: When one foot is restrained, infant scrapes that leg with free foot	Birth/Becomes voluntary
Feeding Reflexes	
Rooting and sucking: When the cheek is touched, infant turns head and searches for the nipple; when the nipple touches the lips, infant sucks	Birth/Become differentiated feeding patterns
Cuddling: When held, the infant cuddles up to the chest and grasps at the breast	Birth/Becomes voluntary

to six behavioral states or states of alertness (Nugent 1985) (Table 2.6). The infant's ability to maintain an alert state and to move smoothly from one state to another is an important sign of neurobehavioral integrity (Windmayer and Field, 1980).

The Neonatal Behavioral Assessment Scale (NBAS)
The NBAS was developed by Brazelton to examine newborn behavior in a research setting. A clinical tool, the CLINBAS, has been derived from the NBAS. To conduct the assessment, a graded series of procedures is carried out that involves slowly arousing a sleeping infant and then testing 20 reflexes and 26 behavioral responses over 30 to 40 minutes and rating them on a 9-point scale (Nugent 1985) (see Table 2.7 for specific reflexes and behavioral responses).

TABLE 2.6
NEWBORN BEHAVIORAL STATES

Deep sleep	Breathing/heart rate regular; eyes closed; no spontaneous movement; no rapid eye movement; startles may appear
Light sleep	More modulated motor activity; irregular heart/respiratory rates; rapid eye movements present (often called REM sleep)
Drowsy/Semialert	Eyes may be open or closed; activity levels variable
Alert	Bright look; minimal motor activity
Fussing	Eyes open; considerable motor activity
Active crying	Vocalizations and uncoordinated movement

TABLE 2.7
SUMMARY OF REFLEXES AND BEHAVIORAL RESPONSES ASSESSED ON THE NEONATAL BEHAVIORAL ASSESSMENT SCALE (NBAS)

Item	Task
1	Initial observation of state
2	Habituation to light, rattle, bell, tactile stimulation of the foot
3	Foot reflexes: plantar, Babinski, and ankle clonus
4	Uncovering, undressing, and placing in supine
5	Passive resistance of arms and legs
6	Rooting and sucking
7	Glabella reflex
8	Hand grasp
9	Pull to sit
10	Placing
11	Primary walking
12	Prone position and crawling
13	Galant reflex and tone assessment
14	Spin and nystagmus
15	Defensive movements
16	Asymmetric tonic neck reflex
17	Moro reflex
18	Cuddliness
19	Irritability, crying, and consolability
20	Orientation to animate and inanimate visual stimuli
21	Orientation to animate and inanimate auditory stimuli
22	Signs of stress: Startles
23	Signs of stress: Tremors
24	Signs of stress: Color change
25	Signs of stability: Hand to mouth
26	Signs of stability: Smiles

The NBAS assesses four general categories of infant behavior: habituation, regulation of states of consciousness, motor control, and reflexes. *Habituation* is the capacity of the newborn to cope with environmental stimuli and is assessed by evaluating the decrement of behavioral response to repetitive visual, auditory, or tactile stimuli in the sleeping infant. Infants usually respond to stimuli, for example, with startles that diminish with ongoing presentation of the stimuli. Infants who have difficulty habituating cannot shut out their environments and become aroused or inconsolable with repeated stimulation. This can lead to frustration and anxiety for parents.

Regulation of states of consciousness reflects an infant's ability to maintain an alert, responsive state and to move smoothly from one state to another. Infants with a small range of state, for example, go from sleeping to crying and back to sleep, with little ability to maintain an alert responsive state. Problems with state regulation are also seen with lethargic infants or irritable infants (e.g., those who were exposed to opiates in utero). State control not only reflects neurobehavioral integrity but is a key contributor to parent-infant interactions and parental feelings of competency. An alert, responsive state provides parents with an enhanced opportunity to interact visually and feel connected with their infant. Lethargic infants or those with small ranges of state are difficult to reach, and this leads to some parents becoming disappointed or frustrated. Irritable infants provoke feelings of anger or helplessness because of parents' inability to console them. Some investigators believe that "reading" and understanding the infant's regulation of state is the first developmental task of parenting.

Motor control refers to the smoothness of infants' movements, reflecting the balance between extensor and flexor tone, and the frequency and extent of startles and jitteriness. Smooth movements and minimal startles and jitteriness typically are indicative of a *coordinated* infant, whereas the other extreme raises concerns in the parents about the infant's neurological integrity.

Assessment of *reflexes* provides the neurological context in which to interpret the behavioral findings. Reflexes have most clinical significance in the assessment of neurological integrity when they are absent, asymmetrical, or excessive. The goal of the NBAS and the CLINBAS is to help parents identify specific infant behaviors that enable them to "read" their infants' behavioral cues and therefore respond more contingently.

Bonding and Attachment: The Beginning Stages

The terms *bonding* and *attachment* describe important processes in early infancy by which a unique relationship is established between infant and caregiver (Klaus and Kennel 1982). These two processes can be distinguished by the direction of the parent-child relationship: *bonding* generally refers to the parent's relationship to the infant, whereas *attachment* generally refers to the infant's relationship to the parent. Sensitivity to the importance of early infant relationships generated the preceding research that provided information on the potential detrimental effects that can occur when newborns are separated from their mothers, which was common hospital policy until 25 years ago. Infants with early and extended contact with their mothers were more readily accepted and consoled at 4 months by their mothers. At age 12 months, they showed a significant increase in positive, compared with negative, behaviors in the home (Siegal et al. 1980). Among infants of mothers who were allowed 12 additional hours of contact in the first 2 days of life, there was a significantly lower incidence of child abuse or neglect in the 17 months that the children were followed (O'Connor et al. 1980). However, there has been no scientific research to support a *critical* period of bonding; that is, no evidence that if bonding does not happen in a specified period of time, such as the newborn period, it will not happen.

Later Infancy: "Attachment as a Goal"

Neurodevelopment in Infancy

By 3 months of age, the infant has begun to establish control over physiological processes and states of alertness. Although not mobile, the 3-month-old infant is rapidly developing prerequisites for independent locomotion. Gross motor development in this stage is characterized by increasing control of flexor muscles, especially in the lower back and legs. At the same time, the infant displays increasingly fine control of fingers and hands and inhibition of generalized movements of the opposite extremity, which, along with disappearance of the primitive reflexes, enable him or her to engage in more overtly purposeful movements.

Attachment

The attachment of the infant to primary caregivers begins in the first months of life and continues over time, as noted in the prior discussion. The infant's actual appearance and behavior are major determinants of the attachment process. For example, with an alert infant who reacts readily to parents' faces and responds promptly to consoling maneuvers, parents' positive feelings and sense of competence are enhanced. Conversely, with a drowsy, relatively hypotonic infant who provides less satisfying feedback, parents may feel disappointed when they attempt to gain emotional satisfaction from him or her.

Attachment theory grew out of ethology, developmental psychology, and psychoanalysis to provide a model by which the attachment process could be explained. At the core of attachment theory is the concept of "internal working models," which describe how the infant's sense of self and other unfolds through interactions with a primary caregiver. The motivation for attachment itself, as explained by Bowlby (1958) and Ainsworth (Ainsworth and Bell 1970), is the process of learning: the more the infant seems interested in things, the more he or she wants to see. Since human beings are the most interesting phenomena in his or her environment, the infant becomes most interested in learning more about them. Primary attachment is also based on the baby's biological need to be close to the mother as a means of protection from internal needs (e.g., hunger, cold, pain, and negative feelings) and from dangers in the environment.

Infants respond to their primary attachment figures in a certain pattern. At 3 to 4 months of age, infants smile more quickly at and are consoled more readily by their primary attachment figures than by others. At age 9 months, these infants will cry when their attachment figures leave them, but not when others leave them. At age 12 to 18 months, these infants will use their attachment figures as a secure base to explore new surroundings. They will explore but will return to their attachment figure periodically, for example, frequently burying their head into a parent's lap, a process that can be understood in terms of a "refueling" metaphor.

A commonly used research paradigm to describe attachment relationships was designed by Mary Ainsworth in the 1970s (Ainsworth and Bell 1970). A mother and infant (younger than 24 months of age) are together in a strange environment with age-appropriate toys for the child to explore. A stranger then enters the room, and the infant's response is noted and scored on a scale of behavioral descriptions. The mother then exits from the room, leaving the child with the stranger. The infant's response is then coded. The mother returns, and the child's response to the reunion is observed and scored. The stranger leaves the room, followed by the mother, and the child is left alone. The stranger then returns, followed by the mother. Children are classified on the basis of their response to the strange situation as exhibiting one of the following attachment patterns (Ainsworth and Bell 1970)

- Pattern A: "Anxious/avoidant" attachment (gave the impression of independence and snubbed mother on return; are affect sharing)
- Pattern B: "Secure" attachment (cried on separation, but greeted mother with pleasure on return, seeking to restore proximity and contact after the stress of being away from her)
- Pattern C: "Anxious/resistant" attachment (were ambivalent; anxious initially and at reunion)
- Pattern D: "Disorganized" attachment (had variable, ambiguous response to departure and reunion)

Disorders of primary attachment can have serious implications for a child's future development. Avoidant or anxiously attached children, for example, are often far less able to engage in fantasy play than are securely attached children, and their play often is characterized by irresolvable conflict. Some researchers feel that security of attachment can be an important factor in predicting healthy functioning as far into the future as the teenage years (Karen 1990). Although the quality of attachment can influence the course of development, it should not be considered as a

TABLE 2.8

PHASES IN THE DEVELOPMENT OF ATTACHMENT

Age	Phase
0–3 months	Undiscriminating social responsiveness
3–8 months	Discriminating social responsiveness
7 months–35 months	Active initiative in seeking proximity and contact

fixed attribute in the child's evolving personality, no more than temperament is. Changing life circumstances can alter the quality of attachment, leading to improvement or deterioration, depending on how these changes affect the primary caretakers' availability to the child. The major phases of attachment are summarized in Table 2.8. The general development of the infant is summarized in Table 2.9.

The Toddler Years: Emotional and Adaptive Development to the Forefront

Neurodevelopment in the Toddler Years

Once a child is up on his or her feet and walking, the experiential possibilities (as well as the demands of parenthood!) enter a new and more challenging dimension. Securely attached toddlers usually cope with the developmental tasks of these years with greater ease and competence than do anxiously attached children. For example, they are more cooperative with their mothers and more persistent and enthusiastic in trying to master a developmental task. Securely attached 4-year-old children are often more comfortable with their peers. As 5-year-olds, they are able to problem solve and look at challenges from others' perspectives. At 6 years of age, they are more open-minded and accepting and face fewer behavioral challenges. In this way, a secure early attachment provides a solid foundation by which the child can interact with and learn from the outside world.

The life of a toddler is constantly changing. One new developmental task rapidly builds on the next, and over a course of weeks, children can learn vast amounts of new knowledge. For example, a child at 9 months can be crawling, at 10 1/2 months walking, and by 13 months climbing up stairs "marking time." In terms of fine motor development, toddlers become increasingly capable of refined actions both in their play with other children and when alone, as well as in activities of self-care. Therefore, the toddler is able to string beads easily in play, as well as to become toilet trained and brush his or her teeth. Gross motor development involves balance and coordination skills. The parenting issues that arise with the child's development are primarily those of limit setting, safety, and the parent's physical exhaustion.

TABLE 2.9
DEVELOPMENT OF THE INFANT (3–12 MONTHS)

Age	Gross Motor	Fine Motor	Communication	Cognition
3 months	Rolls over Lifts head 45° in prone position	Makes prereach/pointing motions	Initiates cooing conversation with adults	Interacts differently with different people
4 months	Head midline when pulled to sit Can get chest wall well up from surface in prone position Lifts head 90° in prone position	Bats at objects; may engage in bilateral "hand play"	Laughs and squeals	Associates experiences
5 months	When prone, "swims" with arms/legs	Reaches more with hand closer to object, although both arms activate	Makes raspberries	
6 months	Sits alone When standing supported, will bounce	Obtains objects by raking with both hands equally	Imitates sounds Babbles in one-consonant syllables	Is attached to adults who take care of him or her Looks for falling object at place where it came from
9 months	Crawls Pulls to stand May cruise along furniture	Transfers object from one hand to the other Uses radialized raking motion for reaching small objects	Uses "mama," "dada" specifically	Uncovers object hidden from view
12 months	Most can walk	Uses fine pincer grasp with index finger/thumb	May know one or two words and responds appropriately to several more Understands simple command combined with gesture	Suits actions to object qualities (i.e., explores other ways besides mouthing)

Successful parents are sensitive to their child's changing needs. They are able to be securely bonded to the toddler and yet sensitive to autonomy strivings, wants, and needs while at the same time providing clear and firm guidelines. Parents can encourage this partnership in several ways: by using a tone of voice that conveys conviction; by appealing to the toddler's sense of fairness; by explaining that they, the parents, are the ones in charge of deciding what to do; and by having a sense of humor.

Emotional Development of the Toddler

One of the major emotional milestones of the toddler years is gaining independence, which results largely from attaining mastery motivation. *Mastery motivation* is a psychological force that stimulates a child to attempt independently, in a focused and persistent manner, to solve a problem or to master a skill or task that is at least moderately challenging for him or her (Morgan et al. 1990). Specifically, these mastery skills are obtained in children ages 15 to 36 months and apply to all domains of behavior. There are five domains in which mastery motivation plays out in the emotional life of a toddler: gross motor skills, combinatorial skills, means-end skills, social skills, and symbolic skills. It is this quest for the unknown that drives the toddler to reach the next developmental milestone.

Toddlers fear that their activities can result in the loss of parental love. Thus, a primary motivator for much of the behavior of a toddler is an increase in the love and attention they receive from their primary caretakers. Unfortunately, toddlers lack the cognitive insight to recognize which behaviors result in positive attention and which result in negative attention. Thus, the majority of discipline techniques that are advocated for use with children of this age emphasize the child's innate quest for attention and love. These techniques emphasize the importance of the amount and quality of positive contact between parent and child (called "time-in"). Increasing the amount of parental attention the child receives and teaching parents strategies that encourage positive interactions (i.e., active listening, physical nurturing) are basic tenets of the success of these discipline techniques (Christopherson 1992).

Separation anxiety is another fear experienced by toddlers. It is often distinguished from *stranger anxiety*, which occurs at age 6 to 9 months when the infant has developed a concrete schema of the primary caregiver's face and notes that a stranger's face is now a discrepant one. Separation anxiety and protest, which also begin at approximately 9 months of age and wane at about age 18 months, have two major components. The first occurs when a child is placed in a strange environment without the primary caretaker and realizes that the primary caretaker is gone. The second involves the child's realization that he or she is powerless in the face of the separation—that he or she cannot "get to mother."

The child's and parent's responses to everyday experiences of physical separation, such as bedtime, child care, and parent's vacations or hospitalization, can vary widely. In assessing the developmental progress of the child's internal process of separation, the clinician should anticipate that the child and parent will show mixed feelings about separations. Appropriate management of a physical separation depends on its duration and context as well as on the developmental readiness of both parents and child. If parents are ambivalent about the separation and communicate their feelings to their children, there is greater difficulty in negotiating separation. Parents can help children master separation by introducing the new caretakers over time and having small doses of separation after the initial contact with the new person without *prolonged* separation. By the end of the third year, most children are able to accept the absence of the primary caregiver and to be sufficiently comforted by a secondary figure (e.g., child care provider, friend, other family member). Parents need to prepare themselves and the child and to build a mutual confidence that the experience will be rewarding and the reunion joyous. The process of internal separation does not end in infancy for either parent or child, but it must be negotiated repeatedly throughout the life cycle.

Anger and frustration are prominent emotions in most toddlers, and thus it is not surprising that somewhere between ages 24 and 36 months, most children will have their first (but not their last) temper tantrum. This occurs most frequently at home because of the combination of normal autonomy strivings (children want to do everything themselves) and normal developmental limitations involving gross and fine motor functioning that result in frustrating experiences. Children who are temperamentally intense respond with a high activity level and high persistence and have the longest, loudest tantrums, including throwing themselves on the floor. As language development progresses, most children will begin to verbalize their frustrations instead of acting them out motorically. Though most tantrums diminish by 3 or 4 years of age, parents often need guidance both in understanding the cause of a tantrum and in dealing with the behaviors exhibited.

Gender differences are evident as early as age 12 months. The toddler has already internalized his or her gender, based on how he or she interacts and compares himself or herself with father and mother. The 3-year-old child can reliably state his or her sex and is entering a period of intense gender role practicing. Though there are inherent difficulties in studying the concept of gender identification, research has shown that boys and girls are treated similarly by their parents in the first 3 to 4 years

of life. For example, in areas such as warmth, nurturing, acceptance, restrictiveness, allowing dependency, and allowing aggression, very young boys and girls do not seem to be treated differently by their parents (Maccoby and Jacklin 1980). Boys do seem to receive more physical punishment. This may be a direct result of differential levels of aggression in boys and girls that lead to differing behavior of parents.

Cognition in the Toddler

Children are also exploring in this period the concept of cause and effect. At the end of the sensorimotor period described by Piaget, at 2 years of age, the child has decided that everything happens for a reason and will try to figure out what that reason might be. For Piaget, during the preoperational stage, there are two substages that make the exploration of causality possible: the stage of *symbolic activity and make-believe play* and the stage of *decentration* (discussed later in this chapter). As a result of symbolic activity in play, the child becomes able to reason symbolically rather than motorically as he or she had in infancy. Thus, the child, who as a toddler considered a hairbrush as serving only one purpose, will transform the brush into a phone and a bat and a broom, all within seconds!

The child's reasoning, though, is still limited in two key ways. The first is that the child's judgments are dominated by *his or her perceptions* of events, objects, and experiences. The young child cannot take the perspective of another. This leads to the second limitation, which is that the child can attend only to one perceptual dimension or attribute at a time, to the exclusion of all others. The child's reasoning at this stage is often described as *transductive,* by which is meant events are related not because of any inherent cause-and-effect relationship, but simply on the basis of spatial or temporal contiguity or juxtaposition (Inhelder and Piaget 1958).

Language Development in the Toddler: A Key to the World!

The elaboration of language is one of the most striking developments of the toddler years. Actual language begins when the brain has matured to two thirds of its full extent. (The brain has reached about four fifths of its adult weight by age 3 years [Marshall 1968].) The child progresses in this brief period from speaking 1 to 2 words at 1 year of age to having a vocabulary of as many as 500 words, including first and last names and his or her own sex, by age 2 years, with the largest explosion of new words between ages 18 and 24 months. By age 3 years, the child is speaking sentences that average 3 to 4 words in length. Between the ages of 2 and 4 years, the child has acquired most of the fundamental rules of grammar. The "why" question becomes incessant as the child attempts both to learn the answer to the question and to control the situation with his or her new-found autonomy. This growth occurs equally in expressive and receptive language. By 3 years

TABLE 2.10

DEVELOPMENT IN THE TODDLER YEARS (12–36 MONTHS)

Age	Gross Motor	Fine Motor	Communication	Cognition
12 months	Walks with "tip toddling"	Uses a cup Cooperates briefly in dressing	Uses one to two words Understands gestural commands	Practices independence Begins having temper tantrums Plays peek-a-boo, imitative games
15 months	Runs Pivots Walks backward	Stacks two blocks Does free scribbling Uses spoon	Uses four to six words, simple jargon Understands commands without gestures	Experiences separation anxiety Is self-consoling
18 months	Walks up stairs with rail Throws ball	Makes stroke on paper Can take off most clothes	Uses 10+ words Uses two-word combinations Points to one body part	Is capable of representational play and imitates household tasks
24 months	Jumps with two feet Stands briefly on one foot Kicks ball Walks downstairs two feet/stair "marking time"	Stacks eight blocks Puts on pieces of clothing	Uses 300 words Uses noun-verb sentences 25% of speech intelligible	Tries to figure out how things work Does pretend play
30 months	Jumps forward Stands on one foot for 1 second Pedals tricycle	Pulls on pants	Uses "I"	Can imagine what another child might think/feel
36 months	Alternates feet on stairs Jumps off bottom step	Stacks 10 blocks Copies a circle Copies three-block bridge	Uses 900 words Uses three- to four-word sentences 75% of speech intelligible	Role plays Prefers "gender appropriate" toys Participates in true cooperative play

of age, a child can follow two- or three-step commands and can formulate answers to "what if" questions. The developmental tasks of toddlerhood are summarized in Table 2.10.

THE PRESCHOOL YEARS: "PRACTICING INDEPENDENCE"

Neurodevelopment in the Preschool Years

It is in the span from ages 3 to 6 years that children are transformed from still-dependent toddlers to academically ready 6-year-old children. Motor planning continues to develop, so that complex tasks like "bear walking" can be copied, but posturing and poor balance during such activities are still common. Fine motor planning as well becomes more complex, and children are able to copy and complete a circle by age 3 years, a cross by age 4 years, a box by age 5 years, and a triangle by age 6 years. Language, which grew at logarithmic rates in the previous stage in terms of both reception and expression, begins to be more refined and complex.

Children begin to understand the *semantics* ("meaning") of language as well as *the pragmatics* ("mechanics"). The preschooler still uses language primarily for qualitative description; quantitative language is still to come.

Cognitive Development in the Preschool Years

In terms of cognitive development, the preschooler is increasingly able to understand the subtleties of categories and has firmly entered the *preoperational stage* (i.e., before logical mental operations) described by Piaget. In the second half of the preoperational stage, as Piaget described, there is an *intuitive stage,* from 4 to 7 years of age. In this stage, there is an increased accommodation to reality, with progressive "decentering" from the child's own interests, perception, and point of view. Decentering takes place primarily through socialization, which occurs on entry to school. The child discovers that what one thinks is not necessarily the same as what one's peers think, and so the child learns to take into consideration the points of view of others.

Children's conception of illness causation follows a similar developmental progression, changing from primitive, circular, and egocentric reasoning to more abstract and logical views (Perrin and Gerrity 1981). For example, it is only when a child has mastered concrete operational thought that he or she could be expected to link isolated concrete symptoms to other bodily events and thus understand the relationship between, for example, a cough, runny nose, and fever. This understanding contrasts with that of a child at the preschool level, who can easily think that a broken arm is a result of misbehavior.

Play: Window to a Child's World

Play is an essential occupation of children and becomes an important way for children to test their reasoning as well as to learn and master feelings. The preschooler's play is quite spontaneous, with the child using a wide range of feelings and fantasy themes. Play involves the coordination of the various regulatory systems of the child: neurophysiological-biochemical, cognitive-experiential, and motor-behavioral (Harris 1995). Superheroes often take center stage in this period. Role playing is highly characteristic, with a rich use of dolls, props, and costumes. Much of play at this stage is an attempt to copy adults' behavior and roles, sometimes out of anger, envy, or fear (Lowe 1975). Occasionally, children's play can be an attempt at mastering self-reassurance in stressful situations, such as when the child imitates big and powerful roles such as a parent, doctor, or police officer. In this regard, play can be extremely useful in preparation for a hospitalization or another stressful event such as parental remarriage (Perrin and Gerrity 1981).

Emotional Development of the Preschooler

In the classic psychoanalytic model, the years from 3 to 6 encompass the *oedipal period*, when the child wants the opposite-sex parent all to himself or herself and even thinks of eliminating the same-sex parent. The resolution of these oedipal feelings appears to require some degree of identification with the parent of the same sex and internalization of the good and bad aspects of both parents into the consolidation of the child's individual superego.

Although not a distinctly preschool aspect of development, but one whose roots lie in this period, *moral judgment* is a concept that many theorists have begun to explore in the preschool years. One theorist of moral development, Lawrence Kohlberg, has built on the cognitive stages of Piaget. Kohlberg suggests three major levels of development of moral judgment: *premorality, morality of conventional role conformity*, and *morality of self-accepted moral principles* (Kohlberg 1967). Further work in defining these levels identified two types of reasoning in general, each of which is used to a lesser or greater degree as the child develops. Type A emphasizes *literal* interpretation of the rules, and type B, a more consolidated form, refers to the *larger intent and interpretation of the normative standards* (Colby and Kohlberg 1987). Kohlberg's theory of moral development is summarized in Table 2.11. General preschool development is summarized in Table 2.12.

TABLE 2.11	
KOHLBERG'S STAGES OF MORAL REASONING	
Stage 1	Punishment and obedience orientation (i.e., obedience to parent's superior force)
Stage 2	Naive instrumental relativistic hedonism (i.e., agreement to obey only in return for reward)
Stage 3	Conventional morality: good-boy morality of maintaining good relations/approval of others (i.e., conformity to rules in order to please and gain approval)
Stage 4	Social order: authority maintaining morality (i.e., adherence to the rules for the sake of maintaining social order)
Stage 5	Morality of social contract of individual rights (i.e., reliance on legalistic "social contract")
Stage 6	Morality of individual principles of conscience (i.e., voluntary compliance based on ethical principles)

Middle Childhood: "Crossing the Threshold"

Neurodevelopment in Middle Childhood

Middle childhood represents a period of consolidation, when the pieces of earlier development seem to fit together and function in a smooth, integrated fashion. Gross motor development of children is fairly complete by age 6 years, but the degree of stamina and coordination varies. Children, however, continue to refine their fine motor and perceptual skills. Proficiency in fine motor tasks varies across a wide spectrum, and the child's particular talents and weaknesses become most evident in this stage. This aspect is particularly critical when children enter school and begin having difficulties. Coordinated motor skills that become evident between ages 5 and 12 years include heel-toe walking, performance of rapid, alternating movements, simultaneous sensory stimulation, and performance of crossed commands (e.g., "Put your right hand on your left knee"). Failure to perform one or more of these tasks at certain ages can be associated with the child's difficulty in performing school-related tasks such as reading or writing (McInerny 1995).

Cognitive Development in Middle Childhood

Children's cognitive functioning becomes increasingly complex in middle childhood, and more mature ways of using moral judgment are possible. A child moves from the "law-abiding" morality of the first grader to the more sophisticated perception that rules are necessary to maintain social order. For example, the first grader who needed to focus on the head of the child in front of him to stay in line now becomes the fifth grader who understands that in a fire drill, orderly exit is key to survival. In this period, there is an increased capacity for more complex thought in other cognitive processes in addition to morality.

TABLE 2.12

DEVELOPMENT IN THE PRESCHOOL YEARS

Age	Gross Motor	Fine Motor	Communication	Cognition
3 years	Rides tricycle	Draws circle Draws person with two facial features	Uses prepositions/pronouns Often stutters	Dresses with supervision
4 years	Steers well Hops	Draws square Constructs five-block train Puts clothes on correctly	Understands size concepts Makes novel grammatical errors Enjoys rhyme and wordplay	Understands the rules of social interaction but may not always observe them
5 years	Skips	Draws triangle Copies five-block gate Spreads with knife	Follows three commands	Can compare different objects but still only one feature at a time
6 years	Rides bicycle Walks sideways	Draws Union Jack Copies 10-block steps Ties bow	Understands passive voice Understands double negatives Understands the subjunctive	Understands that dreams are not "real"

Piaget termed this stage the *concrete operations period.* This period, which begins at age 6 to 7 years, has two outstanding characteristics: acquisition of (1) the ability for "reversible operations" (i.e., the child can reason that 6 + 4 = 10 but also that 10 − 6 = 4) and (2) the ability to perceive two or more variables at the same time (i.e., the child can understand "conservation of volume"). An example of the logic involved in the latter is the classic experiment of the two beakers: A child is first asked to make sure that the amount of water in two identical beakers is the same. Water from one of the beakers is then transferred into a tall, thin cylinder, and the child is asked, "Is the amount of water the same?" A child who is in the preoperational stage will say no and then, if asked to explain, the child will say that the taller beaker has more because it is higher. A child in the concrete operations period, having mastered the concept of conservation, will say that the amount of water is the same. Gradually, the thought processes of a child in this stage become increasingly organized into a complex network through which he or she can confront and systematically respond to the surrounding world.

School Entry and the "World Outside"

At 6 years of age, children officially leave the "family circle" and formally enter the world of peers and school. This world becomes the arena for their development and is best summarized by a character from the television show *The Wonder Years* who stated, "Who you are in sixth grade is who the other sixth graders say you are."

It is likewise important to emphasize the pivotal role of sixth grade in a child's development. Most students in sixth grade are 11 years old, physically and emotionally on the brink of puberty. A wide range of body types is evident. The combination of hormonal changes and the tumultuous nature of entering junior high school makes the sixth grade a safety net for the transition between the worlds of childhood and adolescence. Friendships switch rapidly, and these switches of loyalty are experiments in social skills. Children often have an increased body awareness in this stage and thus may present with a steady litany of somatic complaints, especially following stressful experiences. Sexual development begins in this stage, with children exploring how their bodies function. Fears are particularly common in this stage, as a whole new outside world opens up to the child. This is particularly true in school systems where sixth grade marks the passage into junior high school. These range from concrete fears of monsters and ghosts in the earlier years to fears of robbers and child abductors in the later years. Correlated with the child's widening experience of the outside world is the large role played by peer pressure. At the same time, the demands of school and academics loom increasingly larger in a child's world.

Learning and School Failure

All children want to be successful in the academic arena, although their motivation and anxiety level are profoundly influenced by their family expectations. Key elements to success in academics are self-expression and self-esteem, characteristics that are vital to developmental success in middle childhood. In learning, an individual adapts present behavior to the results of previous interactions with the environment. Adequate perception, memory, attention, and motivation are all necessary for learning. Higher cognition is composed of a range of complex "thinking skills." Included in this category of neurodevelopmental function are concept acquisition, problem-solving skill, critical thinking, brainstorming (including creativity), metacognition, and rule recognition and application (Levine 1992).

Children with problems in any of these areas may present with difficulties in learning. Perhaps the single most common problem found in school-age children who come to mental health attention or to pediatric clinics is some form of school learning difficulty, often a reading disability (Rutter 1974). Estimates of the number of children receiving some degree of specialized educational assistance range from 10% to 15% of the school-age population (Mclnerny 1995). School failure has numerous etiologies, including the following:

- Mental retardation
- Learning disability
- Attention-deficit/hyperactivity disorder
- Emotional disturbance
- Chronic illness

The precise definition of *learning disability* is likewise difficult to agree on. Most clinicians agree that a discrepancy of 2 or more years between actual achievement and the child's developmental age constitutes a learning disability, but even this standard is not universally accepted. Others prefer to use a span of greater than 15 points between the verbal and performance portions of a standardized test. Regardless of the criteria used, a learning disability presents significant challenges to a child's sense of success and self-esteem. It is critical to the success of any intervention that the appropriate etiology be sought for school failure. The medical workup for school failure must include a search for the cause of the learning problem(s), including internal factors such as heredity, developmental variations, medical problems (e.g., hypo- or hyperthyroidism, depression, hearing or visual impairment), chromosomal disorders, and prenatal and perinatal insults to the developing CNS, as well as prematurity. External factors include language dysfunction, sociocultural deprivation, prenatal and postnatal toxins, and CNS infections and trauma.

Evaluation of the child must include a thorough physical examination and history. The history must include past and present school performance, as well as pertinent medical history, including any current or past medications. Formal tests that should be part of the evaluation include cognitive testing (e.g., overall IQ score), tests of perception and visual-motor skills (e.g., Bender Visual Motor Gestalt [Bender 1938]), achievement tests (e.g., Wide Range Achievement Test—Revised [Jastak and Wilkinson 1981]), and tests of adaptive behavior (e.g., Vineland Adaptive Behavior Scales [Sparrow et al. 1984]).

Social Development in Middle Childhood

A common phenomenon in middle childhood is *labeling*. Years ago, childhood labels, such as "bully" or "clown," were dismissed as funny and harmless, with their use considered a rite of passage not unlike fraternity hazing. Unfortunately, though, research has shown that labels can become self-fulfilling prophecies. Labeling in its purest form is a natural and necessary human behavior similar to verbal categorization. However, a label impedes a child's development when it closes off other possibilities, and it has the potential to become a self-fulfilling prophecy.

Labeling often intensifies when children begin school; labels such as "bookworm," "class clown," "little princess," "nerd," and "mental" often peg children into slots from which it is difficult to escape. Misleading labels can draw attention away from real problems, which can then go undiagnosed, such as with the child called "shy" who is actually hearing impaired. Parents, teachers, and other involved adults need to help children recognize that the world is full of possibilities and that being "different" is not wrong. The major developmental tasks of middle childhood are summarized in Table 2.13.

Adolescence: "Growing Into Maturity"

Stages in Adolescence

Adolescence, which is felt by many to be the healthiest and yet most challenging phase of development, is often classified into three stages of development: early (12 to 14 years), middle (15 to 17 years), and late (18 years and older). Unlike the earlier phases of development, to which one could easily assign milestones across the four developmental lines (motor, communication, cognition, and social/emotional), adolescence is a period of integration and enhancement of earlier skills. The major domain of growth involves social and psychological development and behavior. Common issues across all stages of adolescence include identity formation, autonomy, achievement, and intimacy. A common definition of the end point of adolescence is the achievement of an adult work role, though in current societies where advanced training can postpone this several years, this definition might be irrelevant.

Physical Development and Neurodevelopment in Adolescence

The onset of adolescence, which more or less coincides with the onset of puberty, is influenced by the physical changes associated with puberty. Puberty starts in girls at about 10 years of age and in boys at about age 12 years (Marshall and Tanner 1969). There has been a downward trend over the past 150 years in the average age at menarche of about 2.3 months per decade, with the most recent average at 12.7 years (Sizonenko 1987) and when stratified by race, 12.16 for African-American girls and 12.88 for White girls (Herman-Giddens et al. 1997). Hence, cognitive or emotional age can be at variance with chronological age during adolescence.

The early adolescent faces new, preemptive challenges when adjusting to the following: (1) the physical changes of puberty, (2) entry into a new social system (namely, high school), and (3) sudden entry into a new role status (i.e., as "teenager"), with all the social challenges that imposes (Hamburg 1974). Obviously, the challenge of each of these areas is formidable in its own right. Additional stress occurs from the superimposition of these challenges at a time when the child's physical being is also rapidly changing (Carnegie Quarterly 1986).

TABLE 2.13
DEVELOPMENT IN MIDDLE CHILDHOOD

Age	Gross Motor	Fine Motor	Communication	Cognition
6 years	Able to broad jump smoothly Hops on one foot	Writes, eats neatly Copies square touching a circle Ties shoe Reverses some letters	Verbalizes emotions Can follow three serial commands Uses dependent clauses	*Preoperational thinking:* Is not yet able to engage in true mental operations, has difficulty keeping more than one aspect of a problem in mind at a time
7 years	Is able to run at least 4 yards Begins to learn complex motor tasks	Draws three interlocking circles Knows right/left	Understands passive voice Articulates clearly	*Concrete operational thinking:* Begins to consider multiple features simultaneously; has internalized mental actions that fit into logical system
8 years	Is more adept at specific sport skills (e.g., batting, kicking)	Draws vertical diamond Cuts with knife		Reasons with increasing exactness or quantitativeness
9 years	Is able to throw a ball overhand at least 6 feet	Draws circle made of eight dots	Masters irregular verbs	Is increasingly able to place things in sequence
10 years	Has more strength Has good eye-hand coordination	Draws cube		
11–12 years	Gender differences in sport skills/interactions apparent Has much-increased strength, endurance, and coordination			*Formal operational thinking:* Is able to consider theoretical possibilities

Cognitive Development in Adolescence

Cognitive development during adolescence is characterized by a widening scope of intellectual activity, increased awareness, and development of a capacity for insight. During adolescence, there is a transition from concrete to abstract thought, the latter defined by Piaget as "formal operations." In the *formal operational period*, the adolescent is able to grasp highly abstract concepts (e.g., infinity) and to reason logically from hypotheses (e.g., generate all possible hypotheses that may apply during a biological experiment) (Inhelder and Piaget 1958). Even with these changes, the egocentrism of middle childhood remains, but in the early adolescent it takes on a new form: the early adolescent is convinced that other people are as obsessed as he or she is with his or her own behavior and appearance. By 15 to 16 years of age, many adolescents have undergone enough reality testing to be able to perceive situations both logically and realistically. It is at this age that the adolescent risk taker starts to be able to weigh choices and visualize consequences more readily. It is after this stage has been accomplished that primary prevention programs that rely on cognitive insight into consequences can be successful.

Socialization in Adolescence

In all cultures, adolescence is a phase of development marked by rites of passage, with the major developmental goal being *socialized* behavior in order to support the continuation of the culture. The process of individuation and separation from family, which plays such a prominent role in the development of an adolescent in Western society, is not universal. In cultures where adolescents are needed to do adult work to support the family, the period of initiation is short, and the identification as adult is based on familial tradition and responsibility. In contrast, in societies where adolescence can be protracted because of prolonged dependence on parents for support—for example, to finance the completion of advanced education—the attaining of adult responsibility can be more philosophical than realistic.

The role of peer relationships in the life of an adolescent cannot be overemphasized. What began in middle childhood as a new arena to test skills becomes an all-encompassing and ruling domain of "peer definition" of self. For early adolescents, the peer group generally consists of members of the same sex. Boys usually belong to a group of friends from childhood, and girls have two or three best friends. These unisexual groups provide a safe haven for early adolescents to test out ideas. In middle adolescence, close peer group relationships are expanded to include heterosexual friendships; this marks the beginning of dating. In late adolescence, individual relationships assume increasing importance, in many cases overriding the peer group. It is often through both the group and individual relationships that adolescents cement and define their gender identity.

Emotional Development of the Adolescent

One cannot ignore the impact of psychological issues—in particular, the role of fluctuating moods and that of risk taking as developmental markers—on the adolescent's development.

Adolescence is a period of development characterized by fluctuating moods and periods of intermittent euphoria and dysphoria. This cycle is a normal part of emotional development in adolescence but can be trying for the individual and the family. Recently several health issues have taken on increased significance in adolescents, specifically their weight. The percentage of overweight adolescents age 12 to 19 years has increased from 5% in 1970 to 14% in 1999. (Centers for Disease Control and Prevention 1999).

The view that risk taking is an integral aspect of adolescent life is supported by statistics. More than half (57%) of adolescents have tried cigarettes by the 12th grade, and 27% of current 12th graders are smokers (Grunbaum et al. 2002). Alcohol is the most commonly used psychoactive substance during adolescence. In 2002, 20% of 8th graders, 35% of 10th graders and 49% of 12th graders admitted to drinking an alcoholic beverage in the 30 days prior to the survey (Johnston et al. 2003). Marijuana is the most commonly used illicit substance; in 2001, 23% of high school students reported using marijuana in the past 30 days (Grunbaum et al. 2002). Sexual activity and identity is a major issue in adolescence. In 2001, 46% of high school students reported that they had been sexually active (Grunbaum et al. 2002). Of the 33% of currently sexually active teenagers in 2001, 58% reported that their partner had used a condom in their last sexual encounter. On a positive note, teenage pregnancy decreased 27% between 1990 and 1999 for girls 15 to 19 years of age (Child Trends 2002).

Risk taking, in essence, defines adolescence and varies throughout the early, middle, and late stages. Much as in the progressive cognitive development of the toddler, early adolescents take risks to test the relation of themselves to their families and peers. Like younger children, they move out from a secure base but require frequent check-ins to reaffirm their place in society. Middle adolescents, who cognitively are now capable of abstract reasoning, are able, often for the first time, to visualize the consequences of their risks, and for that reason preventive education may be successful at this age. Because all teenagers spend most of their time in one of three spheres—school, family, or friends—much information can be gained by evaluating

TABLE 2.14
TASKS OF PSYCHOLOGICAL AND SOCIAL DEVELOPMENT IN ADOLESCENCE

Value system	From self-centered testing of parental values to idealism and identification of individual values, often with rigid concepts of right and wrong
Conceptualization	From concrete thinking to abstract thought
Career plans	From vague and unrealistic goals to specific goals and steps for implementation
Relationships	From unisexual to heterosexual peer group, with individual relationships predominating at conclusion of adolescence
Sexual drives	From curiosity and experimentation to the beginning of adult intimacy and caring
Body image	From adjusting to the physical changes, through "trying on" different self-images, to, eventually, integration of satisfying body image with personality
Independence	From ambivalence about independence to, eventually, integration

Source: Abstracted from Felice 1992.

the adolescent's functioning in each of these areas. It is important to remember that risk taking, at its essence, is often a positive and sustaining characteristic of adolescent development. The tasks of social and psychological development in adolescence are summarized in Table 2.14.

REFERENCES

Adolescent pregnancy: testing prevention strategies. Carnegie Quarterly 31:1–8, 1986.

Ainsworth M, Bell S. Attachment, exploration and separation: illustrated by the behavior of one-year-olds in a strange situation. Child Dev 41:49–67, 1970.

Bender L. *A Visual Motor Gestalt Test and Its Clinical Use* (American Orthopsychiatric Association Res Monogr No 3). New York: American Orthopsychiatric Association, 1938.

Bowlby J. The nature of the child's tie to his mother. Int J Psychoanal 39:350–373, 1958.

Brazelton TB. Crying in infancy. Pediatrics 29:579–588, 1962.

Centers for Disease Control and Prevention (CDC) Wonder Healthy People 2010. Retrieved from http://wonder.cdc.gov/data 2010, 1999.

Chess S, Thomas A. *Temperament in Clinical Practice.* New York: Guilford, 1986.

Child Trends 2002 Facts at a Glance. Retrieved from www.childtrends.org/Files/FAAG 2002.pdf, 2002.

Christopherson ER. Discipline. Pediatr Clin North Am 39:395–411, 1992.

Colby A, Kohlberg L. *The Measurement of Moral Judgment, Vol. 1: Theoretical Foundations and Research Validation.* Cambridge, UK: Cambridge University Press, 1987.

Dare C. Psychoanalytic theories of development. In: Rutter M, Hersov L, eds. *Child and Adolescent Psychiatry: Modern Approaches.* Boston: Blackwell Scientific, pp. 204–215, 1985.

Felice M. Adolescence. In: Levine M, Carey W, Crocker A, eds. *Developmental–Behavioral Pediatrics, 2nd Ed.* Philadelphia: WB Saunders, pp. 65–73, 1992.

Gesell AO, Amatruda CS. *Developmental Diagnosis,* 11th Ed. New York: Paul Hoeber Medical Division, Harper & Row, 1964.

Grunbaum JA, Kann L, Kinchen S, Williams B, Ross JG, Lowry R, Kolbe L. Youth Risk Behavior Surveillance—United States 2001 MMWR; 51(SS-04) 1–64, 2002.

Hamburg B. Early adolescence: a specific and stressful stage of the life cycle. In: Coelho G, Hamburg D, Adams JE, eds. *Coping and Adaptation.* New York: Basic Books, pp. 101–125, 1974.

Harris J. Emotion expression and regulation. In: *Developmental Neuropsychiatry: The Fundamentals.* New York: Oxford University Press, vol I., pp. 203–218, 1995.

Herman-Giddens ME, Slora EJ, Wasserman RC, et al. Secondary sexual characteristics and menses in young girls seen in office practice: a study from the Pediatric Research in Office Setting network. Pediatrics 99:505–512, 1997.

Hobson RP. Piaget: on the ways of knowing in childhood. In: Rutter M, Hersov L, eds. *Child and Adolescent Psychiatry: Modern Approaches.* Boston: Blackwell Scientific, pp. 191–203, 1985.

Howard B. Growing together: a guide to how babies and parents develop. Contemporary Pediatrics, pp. 13–40, April 1990.

Huttenlocher PR. Synaptic density in human frontal cortex—developmental changes and effects of aging. Brain Res 163:195–205, 1979.

Inhelder B, Piaget J. *The Growth of Logical Thinking From Childhood to Adolescence.* New York: Basic Books, 1958.

Jastak S, Wilkinson GS. *The Wide Range Achievement Test—Revised.* Wilmington, DE: Jastak Associates, 1981.

Jenkins S, Bax M, Hart H. Behavior problems in pre-school children. J Child Psychol Psychiatry 21:5–17, 1980.

Johnston LD, O'Malley PM, Bachman JG. *Monitoring the Future National Results on Adolescent Drug Use: Overview of Key Findings, 2002* (National Institutes of Health Publication No. 03-5374). Bethesda, MD: National Institute on Drug Abuse (NIDA), 2003.

Karen R. Becoming attached. *Atlantic Monthly,* pp. 35–70, February 1990.

Klaus MH, Kennel JH. *Parent and Infant Bonding.* St Louis, MO: CV Mosby, 1982.

Kohlberg L. Stage and sequence: the cognitive-developmental approach to socialization. In: Goslin DA, ed. *Handbook of Socialization Theory and Research.* Chicago: Rand-McNally, pp. 347–480, 1967.

Levine M. Neurodevelopmental variation and dysfunction among school children. In: *Developmental–Behavioral Pediatrics.* Levine M, Carey W, Crocker A (eds). Philadelphia: WB Saunders, pp. 477–490, 1992.

Lewis M, Volkmar F. *Clinical Aspects of Child and Adolescent Development.* 3rd Ed. Philadelphia: Lea & Febiger, 1990.

Lowe M. Trends in the development of representational play in infants from one to three years—an observational study. J Child Psychol Psychiatry 16:33–47, 1975.

Maccoby EE, Jacklin CN. Sex differences in aggression: a rejoinder and reprise. Child Dev 51:964–980, 1980.

Marshall WA. *Development of the Brain.* Edinburgh: Oliver & Boyd, 1968.

Marshall WA, Tanner JM. Variations in pattern of pubertal changes in girls. Arch Dis Child 44:291–303, 1969.

Mclnerny T. Children who have difficulty in school: a primary pediatrician's approach. Pediatr Rev 16:325–332, 1995.

Morgan GA, Harmon R, Maslin-Cole C. Mastery motivation: definition and measurement. Early Education and Development 1:318–339, 1990.

Nugent JK. *Using the NBAS With Infants and Their Families.* White Plains, NY: March of Dimes Birth Defects Foundation, 1985.

O'Connor S, Vietze PM, Sherrod KB, et al. Reduced incidence of parenting inadequacy following rooming-in. Pediatrics 66:176–182, 1980.

Parker S, Greer S, Zuckerman B. Double jeopardy: the impact of poverty on early child development. Pediatr Clin North Am 35:1227–1240, 1988.

Perrin E, Gerrity P. There's a demon in your belly: children's understanding of illness. Pediatrics 67:841–849, 1981.

Piaget J. *The Origins of Intelligence in Children* (1952) (translated by Cook M). In: *The Essential Piaget.* Gruber HE, Voneche JJ (eds.) New York: Basic Books, 1985.

Rutter M. Emotional disorder and emotional underachievement. Arch Dis Child 49:249–256, 1974.

Sameroff A, Seifer R. Familial risk and child competence. Child Dev 54:1254–1268, 1983.

Siegal E, Bauman KE, Schaefer ES, et al. Hospital and home support during infancy: impact on maternal attachment, child abuse and neglect, and health care utilization. Pediatrics 66:183–190, 1980.

Sizonenko PC. Normal sexual maturation. Pediatrician 14:191–201, 1987.

Sparrow SS, Balla DA, Cicchetti DV. *Vineland Adaptive Behavior Scales.* Circle Pines, MN: American Guidance Service, 1984.

Tanner JM. Physical growth. In: Mussen PH, ed. *Carmichael's Manual of Child Psychology.* New York: Wiley, 1970.

Thomas A, Chess S, Birch H. *Temperament and Behavior Disorders in Children.* New York: New York University Press, 1968.

Widmayer SM, Field TM. Effects of Brazelton demonstrations on early interactions of preterm infants and their teenage mothers. Infant Behav Dev 3:79–90, 1980.

ZERO TO THREE Diagnostic Classification: Diagnostic Classification of Mental Health and Developmental Task Force. Disorders of Infancy and Early Childhood (DC: 0—3)™. Washington, DC: Zero to Three, 1994.

Clinical Neuropsychiatric Assessment of Children and Adolescents

Paul D. Larsen, MD

Neurology has traditionally claimed the domain of diseases that have a structural or anatomical correlate and can be defined in neuropathological terms. The time-honored clinical pathological correlation has been the gold standard with the utility and validity of the neurological examination and diagnostic tests being measured against the neuropathological examination. Psychiatry grew from medical science's inability to account for mental illnesses that lacked a demonstrable pathological correlate and as a result the mind-brain dichotomy evolved with the mind becoming the providence of psychiatry. The psychiatrist's diagnostic tools became the patient's history and the mental status examination with a combination of symptom complexes used to define disease states. With the tools of functional neuroimaging and genetic-molecular neurobiology, the potential for narrowing the brain-mind divide is ever increasing (Price et al. 2000). The common ground of neuropsychiatry is the remerging of the two disciplines to explain behavior in terms of cortical and subcortical function.

The clinical neuropsychiatric assessment is a blend of the diagnostic strengths of traditional neurology with those of psychiatry. This chapter focuses on assessing children as opposed to adults, comparing and contrasting the adult versus the child examination when appropriate. The emphasis is on how the examination is used for anatomical localization.

The history plus the examination become the diagnostic foundation for determining etiology and the basis for extending the diagnostic process with the tools of appropriate formal neuropsychiatric and neurodiagnostic tests.

ADULT VERSUS CHILD, DIFFERENCES AND COMMON GROUND

To begin with, it is helpful to compare and contrast the differences between the child and the adult brain. One of the immediate and obvious differences is that of growth and development. The term infant's brain weighs about 400 grams, while the adult brain weighs about 1400 grams. The increase in the size of the neurons, the elaboration and proliferation of dendritic and axonal processes and connections, along with myelination accounts for most of this growth. These changes are reflected in the increased metabolic activity and the more widespread activation of the cortex for attention and language tasks in children (Casey 1997; Gaillard 2000). Myelination is reflected by the acquisition of motor and cognitive milestones with the last axonal pathways being myelinated in adolescence and young adulthood.

Understanding these developmental aspects of the brain is important in assessing the child clinically. It is essential to tailor the neuropsychiatric examination to the age and developmental level of the child. It is also essential to interpret the findings in the context of developmental expectations for that age of child. The examination of the newborn is different than the examination of a 3-month-old or 12-month-old infant. If the 12-month-old has the motor and behavior responses of a 3-month-old, then there is significant neurodevelopmental disease. Because of the developmental aspects of brain function, the level of maturity of the brain also affects the expression of disease. An infarction of the left middle cerebral artery in the adult will produce a right hemiparesis. The same infarct in a neonate will present with right-sided focal seizures without any signs of hemiparesis because the motor control of the newborn is predominantly brainstem in nature and lacks cortical modulation. The motor expression of the infarct will not be manifested until at least 4 to 5 months of age. The nature of the infarct has not changed; rather the maturation of the brain has now reached a level where that deficit becomes apparent.

The spectrum of diseases that are seen in children are different than in adults. C. Miller Fisher stated the house officer and student learns neurology "stroke by stroke" (Adams et al. 1997). The incidence of cerebrovascular disease in adults is between 100 to 300/100,000 per year (Chung 2003) compared to 2.7/100,000 per year in children (Broderick et al. 1993). So stroke, although important, is not the mainstay of pediatric neurology practice. Focal lesions, degenerative disease, and the effect of lifestyle and aging are predominant in the adult spectrum of neurological disease while diffuse disease processes, congenital, infectious, and metabolic diseases are predominant in children. Seizure disorders, on the other hand, are a common neurological problem for both adults and children.

Although there are differences between adult and child neuropsychiatry, there is fundamental common ground. The temporal profile of the basic pathological disease processes is the same. The first diagnostic task for both is regional or anatomical localization. The second task is using the temporal profile to identify the disease process. For the child, a third task must be added and that is to take into account neurodevelopment and its affect on the expression of brain function or dysfunction. An emerging fourth task that is impacting both adult and child neurology is the molecular-genetic understanding of disease. The challenge at this level will be to correlate molecular/genetic defects with phenotypic disease realizing that one genotype does not always equal one phenotype.

THE DIAGNOSTIC PROCESS

The first step in approaching the diagnosis in a patient with suspected neuropsychiatric disease is regional or anatomical localization of the lesion. Where in the nervous system is the lesion? Is the lesion focal or diffuse? Both the history and the examination are essential in this process. The second step is to recognize or identify signs or symptoms and laboratory or imaging findings that are specific, demand explanation, and quickly focus attention on a specific diagnosis (Weiner, 1986). For example, in a patient with tremor, ataxia, dystonia, and psychosis, the finding of a Kayser-Fleischer ring leads to the correct diagnosis of Wilson's disease. Similarly, identification of a cherry red spot on funduscopic exam narrows the diagnostic considerations to just a few diseases.

HISTORY

The patient comes to the physician because of a problem—something is wrong and is causing distress, discomfort, or dysfunction. The physician's task is to take the complaint of the patient and work backward to the cause of the problem. To do this, the physician listens to the patient's story, constructs a timeline or temporal profile of the problem, and selects those elements of the story that are essential clues or parts of the puzzle of "What's wrong with me?" The problem or complaint does not occur as an island unto itself but must be considered in the context or the landscape of the patient's past medical history, social history, and family history. Only when the essential elements of the present illness are considered in the context of the patient's overall history can a complete and accurate picture be pieced together, which allows the physician to identify a probable cause (a diagnosis) or generate a list of possible causes (a differential diagnosis). By the time the history portion of the patient encounter is completed, the physician should be well on the way to understanding the patient's problem and formulating a hypothesis, which the physical examination and appropriate diagnostic tests will confirm or negate. The nature of neuropsychiatric problems necessitates a complete and accurate history as a foundation for a diagnosis.

TEMPORAL PROFILE AND NEUROPSYCHIATRIC DISEASE

Constructing a temporal profile of the patient's complaint is essential in arriving at a correct diagnosis. Basic pathologies have certain temporal profiles, and the temporal profile is often the key to the diagnosis. Multiple different pathological processes can cause weakness of the right side of the body from an upper motor lesion. If the temporal profile of the deficit is acute it is most likely a vascular event or stroke, if subacute it could be an infectious or immune process, or if chronic then a neoplastic process. The temporal profile can be conceptualized as a graph (Fig. 3.1). Function can be plotted over time. The patient's baseline function is defined by the patient's past medical history, family and social history, and review of systems. The point of departure from the baseline function is the onset of the chief complaint. The

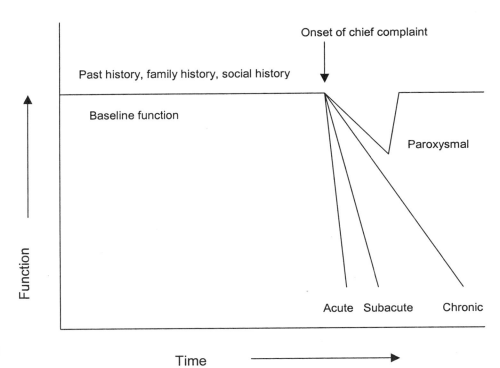

Figure 3.1 Temporal profile of diseases affecting the brain.

signs and symptoms of the chief complaint usually have one of four temporal profiles: acute (seconds, minutes, hours), subacute (hours, days), chronic (days, months), or paroxysmal (episodes of symptoms/signs with return to baseline function). Most diseases of the nervous system are due to one of ten types of pathology. Each one of these pathologies has a usual or typical temporal profile (Benarroch, 1999) (Table 3.1). These pathologies can also be considered in light of their location, whether they affect the nervous system focally or diffusely and whether or not they have a progressive or nonprogressive course (Table 3.2).

CHIEF COMPLAINT AND PRESENT ILLNESS

At the beginning of a patient encounter, the first question that should be asked is "In your own words, what is it that brings you to see me today?" The reply is recorded as the chief complaint. Listen carefully to the story, interrupting only if clarification is needed. Because the patient is a child, it is tempting to skip over the child and obtain the history from the parent. Most of the history will be from the parent, but it is important to circle back to the child

TABLE 3.1
TYPICAL TEMPORAL PROFILE OF PATHOLOGIES AFFECTING THE BRAIN

Acute	Subacute	Chronic	Paroxysmal
Hypoxic	Inflammatory/ Infectious	Congenital	Seizure
Vascular	Immune	Degenerative	Vascular/ Syncope
Trauma	Toxic/Metabolic	Neoplastic	Pain/ Headache

TABLE 3.2
LOCALIZATION AND COURSE OF BASIC BRAIN PATHOLOGIES

Acute

Vascular-focal or diffuse
Hypoxic-diffuse
Trauma-focal or diffuse, progressive

Subacute

Inflammatory/Infectious-focal or diffuse, progressive
Immune-focal or diffuse, progressive
Toxic/Metabolic-diffuse, progressive

Chronic

Congenital-focal or diffuse
Degenerative-diffuse, progressive
Neoplastic-focal, progressive

Paroxysmal

Seizure-focal or diffuse
Vascular/Syncope-diffuse
Pain/Headache-focal or diffuse

and if the child is able, have him or her describe what has happened and what he or she is experiencing. The physician then asks directed questions to fully characterize the chief complaint and present illness. Because the temporal profile is so important for a diagnosis, the physician must be able to reconstruct from the history an accurate and detailed timeline of the symptoms. The physician should seek other characteristics of the symptoms, such as impact on activities of daily living, aggravating and alleviating factors, progression and relationship of symptoms, associated complaints, previous diagnostic studies, and treatments and their effects. Because neuropsychological problems are typically chronic in nature, one important question to ask the parents is "Is there anything that your child used to do that he cannot do now?" This question is helpful in determining if the disease process is static, such as in cerebral palsy, or progressive, such as in one of the neurodegenerative diseases.

PAST MEDICAL HISTORY

For a child, the past medical history starts with a review of the mother's pregnancy, labor, and delivery. It is important to ask if there was any exposure to alcohol, smoking, and drugs during the pregnancy. Complications of the pregnancy and information about fetal movement and results of fetal ultrasound or any diagnostic tests should be noted. Specific questions should be asked about the labor, delivery, and nursery course of the baby. It is not uncommon for parents to attribute the baby's neurodevelopmental problems to a difficult delivery. If the patient did not have any neurological symptoms or signs during the nursery course, but fed well and went home with the mother at the usual time, then the parents can be reassured that the child's problems were not a result of perinatal events (Volpe 2001).

A developmental history should be obtained next. The physician should have a checklist of developmental milestones that either the parent goes through and indicates attainment of milestones or that the physician verbally obtains from the parent. Typically, developmental milestones can be divided into personal-social, language, fine motor, and gross motor skills. Standardized references and tests such as the Denver II or Infant-Toddler Checklist, have been developed and can be used or adapted for screening purposes. The failure of the child to obtain developmental milestones as well as the pattern of developmental delay are important diagnostic clues.

Included in the medical history should be any hospitalizations, surgeries, significant illnesses, trauma (especially head injuries), medications, and allergies. Most of this information can be obtained by having the parent fill out a new patient history form, which the physician reviews with the parent during the visit for any needed clarifications.

TABLE 3.3
FAMILY HISTORY QUESTIONNAIRE

Mother, Father, and Siblings: age, health problems
Is there anyone in the family with the following conditions and what is their relationship with the patient?
Seizures
Mental retardation
Cerebral palsy
Learning problems
Headaches
Fainting
Deafness
Blindness
Muscle disease
Stroke
Ataxia
Tics
Birthmarks (neurocutaneous syndromes)
Degenerative neurological diseases
Depression
Schizophrenia
Attention deficit disorder
Anxiety disorder
Substance abuse and alcoholism
Anyone with the same or similar problem as the patient

FAMILY HISTORY

Because genetic disease has such an important impact on a child's health and can be key to making a diagnosis, this part of the history should be explored in detail. It is important to understand the health and medical problems of the parents and the siblings. The family history is frequently unknown or, due to circumstances such as adoption, can be limited; these limitations should be noted. Constructing a family tree or pedigree chart with ages, medical conditions, and deaths is essential when genetic disease is a possibility for the patient. A review of possible neurological and psychiatric illnesses in the family is particularly important to emphasize. A questionnaire that the parent fills out prior to the clinic visit can facilitate this and be used to further explore diseases that occur in the family (Table 3.3).

SOCIAL HISTORY

The patient's social history should include an understanding of the patient's family constellation and home setting as well as the preschool and school function. This history is the physician's opportunity to gain insight into the child's behavior and adaptation in the important realms of the child's life. Although the parents are the primary source for this information, day care, preschool, school, or special education provider assessments and evaluations are important to obtain and review. The patient's grade level and academic performance should be noted. The results of any formal psychological or psychometric testing should be reviewed. This is the time to review if there are any comorbid psychological problems such as conduct, anxiety, attention, affect, psychotic, or compulsive disorders. Any unusual environmental exposures should be noted and identified.

REVIEW OF SYSTEMS

The review of systems provides the physician with one last chance to make sure that he or she has not missed important elements of the history. It can be done quickly, but should include all major organ systems with the neurological and psychiatric systems review being expanded. It is surprising how often important pieces of information are forgotten or ignored by the family, and this last review will sometimes jog their memory. A checklist can facilitate a rapid but complete review.

NEUROLOGICAL EXAMINATION

As stated previously, the first step in neuropsychiatric problem solving is anatomical or regional diagnosis. The neurological examination is the physician's window to the brain. If the examination is approached in a systematic and logical fashion that is organized in terms of anatomical levels and systems, the physician can establish where in the nervous system the problem is. In a sense, the physician can think of the neuraxis in terms of an "x, y graph" (Larsen 2001) (Fig. 3.2). The vertical location of the lesion on the graph can be determined by examining the cortex (mental status examination and neuropsychological examinations), brainstem (cranial nerve examination), cerebellum (coordination examination), and spinal cord and peripheral nerve (motor and sensory examinations). Because the motor and sensory examinations test the function of crossed descending and ascending tracts that connect the cortex to or from the periphery, these parts of the neurological examination are very helpful, in combination with the other elements of the examination, to determine not only the level of the lesion or disease but also the horizontal (right, left, or midline) location. Cranial nerve and cerebellar findings are also important in determining right versus left location in the neuraxis. Because of cerebral hemisphere dominance and cortical functional location, parts of the mental status examination also help in determining anatomical localization at the cerebral hemisphere level. For example, if the patient has a right hemiparesis plus an expressive aphasia, then the lesion would be localized to the cerebral hemispheres because of the combination of a language deficit plus the motor deficit. If a patient presents with a right hemiparesis plus diplopia from a left third cranial nerve palsy, the only place that the lesion can be located in the neuraxis is at the level of the midbrain, on the left side where the corticospinal tract and the third cranial nerve are in close proximity.

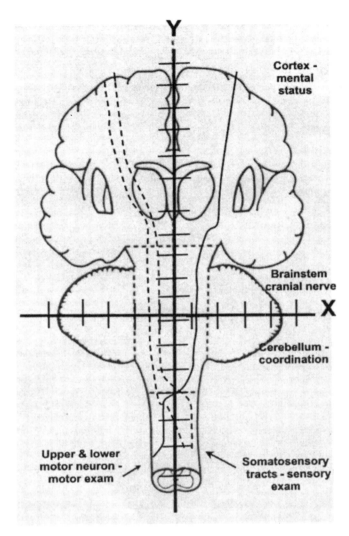

Figure 3.2 Neuraxis and the neurological examination in terms of an "x, y graph."

For children, regional or anatomical localization is the basis of neurological assessment; however, it is not sufficient. The examination and the interpretation of the examination must be couched in the context of neurodevelopmental milestones. As mentioned previously, the assessment of the acquisition of motor and cognitive milestones is an essential part of the neurological examination. Delay in obtaining developmental milestones and abnormal patterns of development are important indicators of underlying neurological disease.

NEUROLOGICAL EXAMINATION IN CHILDREN

Because the infant and child are unable to fully cooperate for the standard neurological examination, the examination must be tailored to their developmental level and temperament (Larsen 2003). The first part of the examination requires the physician to *stop, look, and listen*. More can be learned about the child's neurological status by initial hands-off careful observation than by forcing the child to conform to the physician's set pattern of performing the neurological examination. By watching a baby's spontaneous activity, a great deal can be determined about mental status, cranial nerve function, coordination, and motor status.

The second part of the examination is the hands-on part, which extends and further clarifies the physician's initial observations. For this part of the examination, make it into a game that engages the child's curiosity and imagination. The examination is less threatening and the child is much more cooperative when toys are used and the examination tools are turned into inviting play objects. For example, use a finger puppet for coordination testing and turn the reflex hammer into an imaginary horse when testing deep tendon reflexes.

The third and last part of the examination includes all those things that are the most threatening and unsettling for the child such as undressing the child for a complete body examination, looking at the fundus with an ophthalmoscope, using the otoscope, testing the gag reflex, or measuring the head circumference.

ELEMENTS OF THE MENTAL STATUS EXAMINATION

The purpose of the mental status examination is to examine the function of the cerebral cortex. Because the behavior that is produced by the cortex is dependent on the developmental level of the child, the mental status examination must be directed by age-appropriate expectations. For the newborn, the mental status examination consists mainly of observations of the baby's alertness, sleep-wake changes, temperament, and ability to adapt and react to environmental stimuli (Brazelton 1973). The exam is heavily weighted in reflex behavior. By age 2 to 3 months, a social smile develops and the baby is more socially interactive. At age 6 months, the baby laughs, coos, jabbers, is socially engaging, and is inquisitive. By 12 months of age, the infant has developed stranger anxiety, indicates wants, plays simple games, and has a few meaningful words. As the child becomes verbal, more detailed testing can explore other domains of cortical function. With the preschool and school-aged child, the elements of the traditional psychiatric and neurological mental status examination can be used. Observation of the child's behavior is the main tool of the exam. The mental status examination includes observation of the child's appearance, mood, affect, thought processes, and content. In addition to these areas of behavior, the mental status examination should explore the cognitive domains of attention, executive function, language, memory, and visuospatial function (Guy 2003). These cognitive domains allow functional examination of various regions of the cerebral cortex. Attention and executive function are predominantly frontal lobe functions. Language can be divided into receptive areas in the posterior temporal-inferior parietal lobes and expressive areas in the inferior frontal lobe. The cognitive domain of memory depends on an intact hippocampal-limbic system of the temporal lobes. The parietal lobes are important for visuospatial function. This is an oversimplification of the anatomical location of these cognitive domains, but it provides a working system to organize the clinical approach to the patient and anatomical localization in the cerebral cortex.

Assessment of cortical function is facilitated by the use of standardized tests, which for the infant include the Cattrell Infant Intelligence Test and the Bayley Scales of Infant Development (Table 3.4). For the child 2 to 8 years of age, the McCarthy Scales of Children's Abilities (McCarthy 1972) allows for the assessment of language, memory, and visuospatial skills. Other tests that are helpful in assessing the young child's cognitive function at this age are the Stanford-Binet Intelligence Scale and the Wechsler Preschool and Primary Scale of Intelligence (WPPSI) (Table 3.4). For the child 3 to 12 years of age, the NEPSY allows for testing in the domains of attention-executive function, language, sensorimotor, visuospatial, and memory (Neeper 1998).

These tests require additional evaluation beyond the initial office visit. Table 3.5 provides an outline of the mental status examination of the verbal child, which can be done as part of the initial office visit. It is not a substitute for formal assessment, but it should help the clinician recognize those cognitive domains that will need more extensive assessment.

Frontal Lobe Function

The frontal lobes are important for executive function, judgment, and volition. Dysfunction of the frontal lobes can be seen in many neuropsychiatric conditions including attention deficit disorder, neurotrauma, neoplastic, and neurodegenerative diseases. Functional neuroimaging studies have demonstrated that frontal lobe functions can be tested by specific clinical tests (Sarazin 1998). Conceptualization tests correlate with dorsolateral frontal lobe activity, word generation with medial-frontal, and inhibitory control with orbital-frontal areas. The Frontal Assessment Battery (FAB) is a bedside screening test developed to assess frontal lobe dysfunction (Dubois 2000). Although this battery has not been standardized for children, it has value as a set of six clinical tests that can be done in 10 minutes and can be preformed on older children and adolescents (Table 3.6). Similarities are used to test conceptualization. Mental flexibility and verbal fluency is tested by asking the patient to list in one minute as many words possible that begin with a certain letter. Patients with frontal lobe dysfunction have difficulty with temporal organization and sequencing of motor tasks. Testing this aspect of frontal lobe function can be

TABLE 3.4
NEUROPSYCHOLOGICAL SCREENS AND PSYCHOLOGICAL TESTS FOR INFANTS AND CHILDREN

Instrument	Age Range	Score/Scales	Subtests
Infants and Younger Children			
Prechtl's Neurological Examination (Prechtl 1977) Parmelee's Neurological Examination (Parmelee et al. 1974) Brief Infant Neurobehavioral Optimality Scale (Aylward et al. 1988)	Newborns/Infants		Reflexes Muscle tone Arousal Spontaneous behavior
Neonatal Behavioral Assessment Scale (Brazelton 1973)	Infants		Activity level Visual and auditory orientation Habituation Response to caretakers and environment
Gesell Developmental Schedules (Knobloch et al. 1980)	Infants		Gross and fine motor abilities Adaptive functioning Language development Social interactions
Cattell Infant Intelligence Scale (Cattell 1940)	Infants		Motor Language Cognitive abilities
Bayley Scales of Infant Development (Bayley 1969)	Newborns/Infants (2 months–2$^{1}/_{2}$ years)	Mental Developmental Index (mean = 100, SD = 16)	Shape discrimination Sustained attention Comprehension Memory Naming Problem solving
		Psychomotor Developmental Index (mean = 100, SD = 10)	Purposeful manipulation of objects Imitation Vocalization Gross motor Fine motor
Older Children			
McCarthy Scales of Children's Abilities (McCarthy 1972)	2$^{1}/_{2}$–8$^{1}/_{2}$ years	Verbal Scale (mean = 50, SD = 16)	Pictorial memory Word knowledge Verbal memory Verbal fluency Opposite analogies
		Perceptual Performance Scale (mean = 50, SD = 10)	Block building Puzzle solving Tapping sequence Right-left orientation Draw-a-person Draw-a-child Conceptual grouping
		Quantitative Scale (mean = 50, SD = 10)	Number questions Numerical memory Counting and sorting
		Memory Scale (mean = 50, SD = 10)	Pictorial memory [a] Tapping sequence [b] Verbal memory [a] Numerical memory [c]

(continued)

TABLE 3.4
(continued)

Instrument	Age Range	Score/Scales	Subtests
McCarthy Scales of Children's Abilities (continued)		Motor Scale (mean = 50, SD = 10)	Leg coordination Arm coordination Imitative action Draw-a-design [b] Draw-a-child [h]
		General Cognitive Index [d] (mean = 100, SD = 16)	
Stanford-Binet Intelligence Scale, 4th Ed. (Thorndike et al. 1986)	2 years–23 years, 11 months	Verbal Reasoning (mean = 100, SD = 16)	Vocabulary Comprehension Absurdities Verbal relations
		Abstract/Visual Reasoning (mean = 100, SD = 16)	Pattern analysis Copying Matrices Paper folding and cutting
		Quantitative Reasoning (mean = 100, SD = 16)	Quantitative Number series Equation building
		Short-Term Memory (mean = 100, SD = 16)	Bead memory Memory for sentences Memory for digits Memory for objects
		Test Composite (mean = 100, SD = 16)	
Wechsler Preschool and Primary Scale of Intelligence—Revised (Wechsler 1989)	4 years–7 years, 3 months	Verbal IQ (mean = 100, SD = 15)	Information Vocabulary Arithmetic Similarities Comprehension Sentences
		Performance IQ (mean = 100, SD =15)	Animal house Picture completion Mazes Geometric design Block design
		Full Scale IQ (mean = 100, SD = 15)	
NEPSY (Korkman et al. 1998)	3 years–12 years, 11 months	Attention/Executive Language Sensorimotor Visuospatial Memory	

[a] Also included in the Verbal Scale.
[b] Also included in the Perceptual Performance Scale.
[c] Also included in the Quantitative Scale.
[d] Comprises the 15 subtests from the Verbal, Perceptual Performance, and Quantitative Scales.

done using the Luria technique of having the patient imitate and then demonstrate the fist-palm-edge of hand sequence tests. Proper frontal lobe function allows the child to direct attention and ignore extraneous or competing sensory or environmental stimuli. The Stroop test can be used to determine whether the patient can maintain attention and not be distracted by conflicting sensory cues. The patient is asked to name the color of a printed word rather than saying the color that the word names. In the Frontal Assessment Battery, the same frontal lobe function is tested by asking the patient to do a motor task that is different than what the examiner is doing (Table 3.6). The examiner asks the patient to tap twice when the examiner taps once and to tap once when the examiner taps twice. The patient with frontal lobe dysfunction will be echopractic and will repeat the demonstrated pattern rather than following the directions. Patients

TABLE 3.5
MENTAL STATUS EXAMINATION

Attention/Executive Function

Similarities
Set generation (name all the words you can think of that begin
  with the letter *s*)
Fist-palm-edge motor sequence
Go-No Go test
Working memory: digit span, spell words backward

Language

Naming objects—pen, watch, button, ring, etc
Meaning of these words: money, flower, summer, book, and so on
Repeat "no ifs, ands or buts"
Following commands
Show a picture and make up a story
Read an age-appropriate paragraph, observe for accuracy and
  fluency
Ask questions about the paragraph content, check comprehension
Write a sentence (dictated and spontaneous), check for spelling
  and grammar

Memory

List of three words—recall in 5 minutes
Question recent and remote events

Visuospatial

Copy a design (simple to complex depending on age)
Draw a person (count body parts, see and draw a man reference)
Draw a clock—draw certain time if age appropriate
Name fingers
Tell right-left and mirror right-left (age appropriate)

with orbital-frontal lobe dysfunction have difficulty controlling impulsiveness and inhibiting inappropriate responses. The Go–No Go test assesses this aspect of frontal lobe function. The patient is asked to tap when the examiner taps once and not to tap when the examiner taps twice. The Go–No Go test has been studied in children and it has been demonstrated that the same underlying prefrontal circuitry is activated in children as in adults (Casey 1997). The last subtest of the Frontal Assessment Battery tests environmental autonomy. Patients with prefrontal lobe dysfunction cannot inhibit their motor response to environmental cues. Testing for environmental autonomy is done by instructing the patient not to grasp the examiner's hand and then placing a hand in the patients outstretched hand. Normally the patient should be able to inhibit the impulse to grab the examiner's hand.

Another area of assessment for frontal lobe function is testing working memory, which evaluates the child's ability to maintain and focus attention. Digit span, spelling words backward, and naming the months of the year backward are good screening tests for working memory.

Language Function

In the classical construct of language there are two nodes: the receptive node in the posterior superior gyrus of the dominant hemisphere (Wernicke's area) and the expressive node in the inferior frontal gyrus (Broca's area). The nodes are connected by the arcuate fasciculus. Language is certainly more complex than this simple paradigm, but this model allows the clinician to organize an approach to the child. Children with language disorders can have difficulty with phonology, morphology, syntax, semantics, and pragmatics (Crosley 1999).

The child initially develops recognition of spoken words (phonology and morphology) and attaches meaning to words (semantics). This is a function of Wernicke's area and the adjacent association cortex in the superior temporal-inferior parietal area. Children with developmental receptive dysphasias are often uncomfortable in verbal settings and have difficulty with hearing words correctly and understanding their meaning. They are most comfortable in nonverbal settings and prefer visual and tactile interaction. Assessment of receptive language must take into account age-appropriate expectations. The 12- to 18-month-old should know the meaning of "no," "come here," and be able to point to body parts. By 24 months the child should obey simple commands and be able to point to many named objects. By 3 to 4 years the child should be able to name objects by their actions and understand prepositions. Important speech and language milestones are outlined in Table 3.7. Comprehension and inner vocabulary can be tested for age-appropriate levels by using a screening test such as the Weinberg Symbol Language and Communication Battery (SLCB) (Table 3.8, item 1) (Weinberg 1998, 2001).

Expressive language skills are slower to develop than receptive language skills. In a child who has language delay, expressive language is typically more affected than receptive language. It is not uncommon to have children comprehend more than they express. An infant first develops babbling, then nonspecific "da-da" or "ma-ma." At age 10 to 12 months the infant will develop one to two specific words. A vocabulary growth spurt occurs at age 18 to 24 months, and two-word sentences are used by 2 years of age (Rescorla 1997). By age 3 to 4 years the child uses three-word to four-word sentences and past and future verb tenses (Table 3.7).

Assessment of expressive language begins with listening to the child's spontaneous speech. The child can be encouraged to talk by showing colorful action pictures and asking the child questions about the picture. More formal assessment of expressive language can be accomplished by asking the child to repeat words and name colors, shapes, numbers, and letters. The hallmark of expressive dysphasia is nonfluency, grammatical errors, and articulation problems. The older child should be able to use correct grammar including pronouns, possessives, prepositions, and

TABLE 3.6

FRONTAL ASSESSMENT BATTERY (FAB)

1. Similarities (conceptualization)
   "In what way are they alike?"
   A banana and an orange (in the event of total failure: "they are not alike" or partial failure: "both have peel," help the patient by saying, "both a banana and an orange are . . ." but credit 0 for the item; do not help the patient for the following items).
   A table and a chair
   A tulip, a rose, and a daisy
   Score (only category responses [fruits, furniture, flowers] are considered correct)

Three correct:	3
Two correct:	2
One correct:	1
None correct:	0

2. Lexical fluency (mental flexibility)
   "Say as many words as you can, beginning with the letter S, any words except surnames or proper nouns."
   If the patient gives no response during the first 5 seconds, say, "for instance, snake." If the patient pauses 10 seconds, stimulate him by saying, "any word beginning with the letter S. The time allowed is 60 seconds.
   Score (word repetitions or variations [shoe, shoemaker], surnames, or proper nouns are not counted as correct responses)

More than nine words:	3
Six to nine words:	2
Three to five words:	1
Less than three words:	0

3. Motor series (programming)
   "Look carefully at what I'm doing."
   The examiner, seated in front of the patient performs alone three times with his left hand the series of Luria "fist-edge-palm." "Now, with your right hand do the same series, first with me, then alone." The examiner performs the series three times with the patient, then says to him or her, "Now, do it on your own."
   Score

Patient performs six correct consecutive series alone:	3
Patient performs at least three correct consecutive series alone:	2
Patient fails alone, but performs three correct consecutive series with the examiner:	1
Patient cannot perform three correct consecutive series even with the examiner:	0

4. Conflicting instructions (sensitivity to interference)
   "Tap twice when I tap once."
   To be sure that the patient has understood the instruction, a series of three trials is run: 1-1-1. "Tap once when I tap twice." To be sure that the patient has understood the instruction, a series of three trials is run: 2-2-2. The examiner performs the following series: 1-1-2-1-2-2-2-1-1-2.
   Score

No error:	3
One or two errors:	2
More than two errors:	1
Patient taps like the examiner at least four consecutive times:	0

5. Go–No Go (inhibitory control)
   "Tap once when I tap once."
   To be sure that the patient has understood the instruction, a series of three trials is run: 1-1-1. "Do not tap when I tap twice." To be sure that the patient has understood the instruction, a series of three trials is run: 2-2-2. The examiner performs the following series: 1-1-2-1-2-2-2-1-1-2.
   Score

No error:	3
One or two errors:	2
More than two errors:	1
Patient taps like the examiner at least four consecutive times:	0

6. Prehension behavior (environmental autonomy)
   "Do not take my hands."
   The examiner is seated in front of the patient. Place the patient's hands palm up on his or her knees. Without saying anything or looking at the patient, the examiner brings his or her hands close to the patient's hands and touches the palms of both the patient's hands, to see if he or she will spontaneously take them. If the patient takes the hands, the examiner will try again after asking him or her, "Now, do not take my hands."
   Score

Patient does not take the examiner's hands:	3
Patient hesitates and asks what he or she has to do:	2
Patient takes the hands without hesitation:	1
Patient takes the examiner's hand even after he or she has been told not to do so:	0

Source: Reprinted from Dubois et al. The FAB: a frontal assessment battery at bedside. Neurology 55:1621–1626, 2000. Used with permission.

TABLE 3.7
IMPORTANT SPEECH AND LANGUAGE MILESTONES

Receptive Language	Age	Expressive Language
Turns to sound of bell	6 months	Cries, laughs, babbles
Waves bye-bye	9 months	Imitates sounds and makes dental sounds during play (e.g., "da-da")
Knows meaning of "no" and "don't touch"	12 months	Uses 1–2 words (e.g., "da-da" "mama" "bye")
Responds to "come here"	15 months	Uses jargon (speech-like babbling during play)
Points to nose, eyes, hair	18 months	Uses 8–10 words (one third are nouns); puts two words together (e.g., "more cookie"), repeats requests
Points to a few named objects	24 months	Asks one- to two-word questions (e.g., "Where kitty?")
Obeys simple commands		
Repeats two numbers	30 months	Uses "I" "you" "me"
Can identify by name "What barks?" and "What blows?"		Names objects
		Uses three-word simple sentences
Responds to prepositions "on" and "under"	3 years	Masters consonants *b, p, m*
Responds to prepositions "in," "out," "behind," "in front of"	4 years	Speaks in three- to four-word sentences
		Uses future and past tenses
		Masters consonants *d, t, g, k*
Can repeat a seven-word sentence	6.5 years	Masters *th* sound
		Uses six- to seven-word sentences
		Says numbers up to 30s

Source: Reprinted from Olson WH, Brumback RA, Gascon GG, et al. *Handbook of Symptoms-Oriented Neurology.* 2nd Ed. St. Louis, MO: Mosby-Year Book, p. 347, 1994, Copyright 1994, Mosby-Year Book. Used with permission.

correct sentence structure (syntax). Children with expressive dysphasia will have trouble repeating words or sentences. For example, a child who has an expressive dysphasia would have trouble repeating the phrase, "no ifs, ands, or buts." This is also seen in conductive dysphasia. The child with conductive dysphasia from a lesion of the arcuate fasciculus has adequate comprehension (i.e., Wernicke's area is intact) and spontaneous speech (i.e., Broca's area is spared), but the child cannot repeat what is said.

Another important aspect of language that should be assessed in the older child is written language, including both reading comprehension and written expression. Comprehension of written language is assessed by having the child read age-appropriate material and checking for both accuracy and fluency. The young child with dyslexia will have problems with phonology and decoding the word, but comprehension will be intact. Another hallmark of dyslexia is that reading fluency is always impaired so that the child's reading is slow and laborious. Dyslexics also have difficulty with spelling. Early identifiable risk factors for dyslexia include delay in speaking, difficulties in pronunciation, insensitivity to rhyme, and inability to learn the names and sounds of the letters (Shaywitz 2003). Screening tests for reading readiness, phonemic recall, and spelling ability, which are associated with reading ability as well as tests for reading accuracy and comprehension, are outlined in the Weinberg SLCB, subtests 2 to 4 (Table 3.8). Another informal way of assessing the child's reading ability is to have a collection of children's books in the office from the first

grade to high school level. The child can then be tested for age-appropriate reading accuracy, fluency, and comprehension. Formal reading assessment tools include the Woodcock-Johnson III, the Woodcock Reading Mastery Test, and the Gray Oral Reading Tests.

Prosody is the affective and emotional quality of language. Much of the meaning of language is embodied in the way or manner that something is said (pragmatics). Intonation, inflexion, rate, volume, and emphasis of speech, as well as facial expression and body gesturing, are all a part of the meaning of language. An example of this would be the changing of a statement into a question by adding an inflexion at the end or the use of sarcasm to mean just the opposite of what is said. A simple declarative statement such as "I'm going to school now" can convey a state of being sad, happy, or angry about going to school. The prosody of language is a function of the nondominant cerebral hemisphere with the same anatomical nodal organization of reception and expression as semantic language in the dominant hemisphere. The anatomical location for the receptive node of prosody is the posterior part of the nondominant superior temporal gyrus analogous to Wernicke's area in the opposite hemisphere. Likewise, expressive prosody is located in the posterior region of the nondominant inferior frontal gyrus analogous to Broca's area. The receptive and expressive prosody nodes are connected by a fasciculus. The disorders of prosody (aprosody or dysprosody) are clinically categorized in the same way as left hemisphere aphasias (receptive, expressive, and conductive).

TABLE 3.8

SELECTED TESTS FROM WEINBERG SYMBOL LANGUAGE AND COMMUNICATION BATTERY (SLCB)

1. Reading Readiness

This section of the test asks the child age 3 to 6 years to name the classic symbols: colors, shapes, numbers, and letters. A child unable to name the symbols should be presented with a multiple-choice format using three choices. If the child is unable to select the proper choice, then assume that the symbol has not been stored.

    a. **Color naming.** "What color is this?" Show the child red, blue, green, yellow, and brown. Children ages 3 to 4.5 years should be able to name colors.

    b. **Geometric shapes.** "What shape is this?" Show the child a square, triangle, diamond, cross, and star. Children ages 3.5 to 6 years should be able to name geometric shapes.

    c. **Number discrimination.** "What number is this?" Show the child a 1, 3, 6, 7, and 9. If the child is unable to name the number, offer three possible responses for the child to choose from. Children ages 4 to 5 years should be able to name numbers.

    d. **Number naming.** "What number is this?" Show the child a 1, 3, 6, 7, 9, 25, and 50. Children ages 5 to 6 years should be able to name numbers.

    e. **Letter discrimination.** "What letter is this?" Show the child the uppercase A, B, C, D, and E. If the child is unable to name the letter, offer three possible responses for the child to choose from. Children ages 4 to 5 should be able to discriminate letters.

    f. **Letter naming.** "What letters are these?" Show the child lowercase a, b, c, d, h, j, k, m, n, p, u, w, x, y, and z. Children ages 5 to 6 years should be able to name letters.

2. Reading Comprehension

(Spelling words A: Backward words spelling test). This test relates directly to reading comprehension.

    a. "Spell the word **dog**." "Spell **dog** backward." "What does that new word spell?" Children ages 6 to 7 years should correctly spell and label the backward word (**god**) and should understand first-grade reading material.

    b. "Spell the word **was**." "Spell **was** backward." "What does that new word spell?" Children ages 7 to 8 years should correctly spell and label the backward word (**saw**) and should understand second-grade reading material.

    c. "Spell the word **tip**, like the **tip** of my finger." "Spell **tip** backward." "What does that new word spell?" Children ages 7.5 to 8.5 years should correctly spell and label the backward word (**pit**) and should understand third-grade reading material.

    d. "Spell the word **not**. Like, 'I will **not** go.'" "Spell **not** backward." "What does that new word spell?" Children ages 9 to 10 years should correctly spell and label the backward word (**ton**) and should understand fourth-grade reading material.

    e. "Spell the word **live**." "Spell **live** backward." "What does that new word spell?" Children ages 9.5 to 10.5 years should correctly spell and label the backward word (**evil**) and should understand fifth-grade reading material.

"Spell the word **dial**. Like, 'dial a telephone number.'" "Spell **dial** backward." "What does that new word spell?" Children ages 9.5 to 11 years should correctly spell and label the backward word (**laid**) and should understand fifth-grade to sixth-grade reading material. A child able to do **live/evil** and **dial/laid** is literate.

3. Phonemic Recall and Sequencing of Graphemes

(Spelling words B). "Now, these are more difficult words. Some may be fifth-grade words, but do the best you can. Spell them as well as you can." Children who are able to spell the fifth-grade words are considered to be literate for spelling.

a. **First-grade words**	(ages 6–7 years):	it, cat, look, stop, spot
b. **Second-grade words**	(ages 7–7.5 years):	hit, hot, hat, hut
	(ages 7.5–8 years):	work, talk, girl, went
c. **Third-grade words**	(ages 8–9.5 years):	should, could, phone, house
d. **Fourth-grade words**	(ages 9–10.5 years):	monkey, elephant, receive, friend
e. **Fifth-grade words**	(ages 10–11.5 years):	purchase, ethics, delicate, delicious

4. Word Storage

(Inner vocabulary) Ask the child to define one or more age-appropriate words. If the child is unable to do so, offer three verbal choices. If the child is unable to choose the correct definition, offer three pictorial choices. If the child is still unable to do this task, then offer one or more words appropriate for a younger age group. If the child is unable to offer a definition, then offer three verbal choices. If the child is unable to choose the correct definition, offer three pictorial choices.

a. **Ages 6 to 8 years:**	baby, name, green, second
b. **Ages 8 to 10 years:**	visit, spring, money, thought
c. **Ages 10 to 12 years:**	grasp, moist, stride, browse, coward
d. **Ages 12 to 14 years:**	freight, obsolete, drought, absorb, occupation
e. **Ages 14 to 16 years:**	fortuitous, vaguely, judicious, vocation, absurd
f. **Ages greater than 16 years:**	serendipity, foment, impecunious, litigious

(continued)

TABLE 3.8
(continued)

5. Gilmore Oral Reading Test—Form C: Accuracy (Gilmore and Gilmore 1968).

"I want you to read for me. Some of the words may be difficult. That's okay; just do the best you can. I am going to ask you some questions after you have read the stories." Start by having the child reading aloud at a grade level below the child's estimated ability. When possible, find the grade level at which the child makes no errors (base) and at which he or she makes four or fewer errors (ceiling). Stop after the fifth error at a grade level. Record the number of errors made for each test grade level. Types of errors are substitutions, omissions, blanks, mispronunciations, and skipping around on the page.

6. Gilmore Oral Reading Test—Form C: Comprehension (Gilmore and Gilmore 1968).

Using the child's ceiling paragraph, read the questions to the child. For each question that the child cannot answer, present a multiple choice using three choices, with one being correct.

Source: Modified from Coffey CE, Brumback RA. *Textbook of Pediatric Neuropsychiatry.* Washington, D.C., London: American Psychiatric Press, Inc. 1998. Used with permission.

Prosody develops early in infancy and is fully established for communication by the late toddler and early preschool years (Weinberg, 1998, 2001). A child who has problems with receptive or expressive prosody is significantly impaired in social and contextual interactions. Such a child can understand the meaning of words and say them correctly, but without normal prosody the child is bewildered and frustrated with social language.

The examiner can learn the most about the child's prosody by watching spontaneous verbal and gestural interactions. The examiner should note if the child understands the emotional and contextual aspects of language and if the gestures and language prosody are appropriate for the occasion. Formal screening can be divided into tests for gestural prosody and verbal prosody (Weinberg 1998, 2001). For gestural prosody, use cards or the examiner's own face and ask the child to identify the expression of happy, sad, or angry (Fig. 3.3). Then ask the child to demonstrate facial expressions of these same emotions. Verbal prosody is tested by having the child listen to the examiner say a sentence in a happy, sad, or angry fashion and then asking the child to identify the correct emotion. The child can then demonstrate the ability to express these same emotions in a sentence. While testing verbal prosody, the examiner and child should not be able to see each other's facial expression.

Memory

Memory can be subdivided into episodic and semantic memory (Tulving 1972). Episodic memory is the ability to recall personal experiences including time, place, persons, and objects. Semantic memory is knowledge of facts without a personal reference such as general knowledge of world events or rules of arithmetic. Both types of memory depend on an intact hippocampus for consolidation.

Insight into the child's memory function is obtained throughout the mental status examination as well as the history part of the evaluation by observing responses to questions asked during the course of the office visit. A specific screening test for recent memory is to give the child a list of three things to remember, and then later in the examination ask the child to recall the list. If the child can't recall all of the objects, then progressive prompting should be used to see how much help the child needs to be able to recall the objects. Another way of testing recent memory is to give the child a list of words to be memorized and then later in the examination have the child pick out the memorized words from a longer list of words. The same testing can be done for nonverbal recent memory by showing the child several pictures to remember and then later in the examination having the child identify the memorized pictures from a larger assortment of pictures. Episodic memory can be tested by asking the child to recall recent personal events or activities as well as important personal historical events. Semantic memory can be tested by asking the child to recall presidents of the United States, events of history, or other age-appropriate world knowledge.

Parietal Lobe Function and Visuospatial Processing

The parietal lobes are important for somatosensory perception and visuospatial organization. The nondominant parietal lobe is particularly important for visuospatial tasks. Testing for parietal lobe function can be subdivided into tests for cortical discriminatory somatosensory function, sensory neglect, visuospatial tasks of constructional praxis, and a constellation of tests used to examine the function of the dominant inferior parietal area for evidence of the developmental Gerstmann syndrome.

Cortical discriminatory somatosensory function is tested in several ways. Having the child identify numbers that are written on the palm of the hand with eyes closed tests for graphesthesia. Having the child name objects that are placed in the hand with the child's eyes closed tests stereognosis. Tactile direction movement is a sensitive test

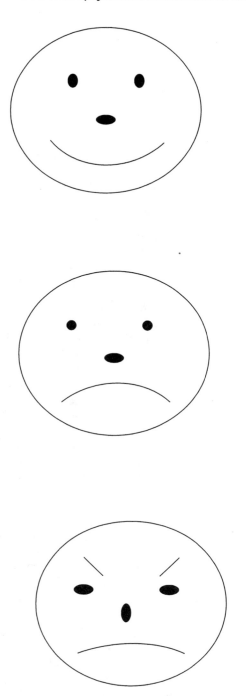

Figure 3.3   Faces for testing gestural prosody.

parietal lesion. This is sensory neglect. Subtle neglect can be detected by testing double simultaneous stimulation. The child is tested by touching homologous parts of the body on one side, the other side, or both sides at once with the child's eyes closed and asking the child to identify right, left, or both. If the child neglects one side on double simultaneous stimulation (extinction or simultanagnoisa), this indicates dysfunction of the contralateral posterior parietal lobe. This test can also be done with visual stimuli.

Constructional praxis is tested by asking a child to draw a person, a clock, or geometric figures. By 5 years of age, a child should be able to draw a person, and by age 7 to 8 years, the child should be able to draw a clock. Difficulty with these visuospatial tasks can be seen in nondominant inferior parietal lobe dysfunction.

The dominant inferior parietal lobe is important for symbol sequencing such as in counting, number processing, letter writing, and spatial orientation such as in right-left orientation. By age 6 to 8 years, the child should be able to identify right and left on herself or himself, and by age 8 to 9 years, the child should be able to identify right and left on others and the environment. Children with dominant inferior parietal lobe dysfunction will have elements of the developmental Gerstmann syndrome, such as right-left confusion, finger agnosia, dyscalculia, and dysgraphia. It is interesting that finger naming (finger gnosia) is a predictor of arithmetic abilities in children (Fayol 1998).

CRANIAL NERVE EXAMINATION

The cranial nerve (CN) examination allows the physician to "view" the neuraxis from the level of the olfactory and optic tracts to the caudal extent of the medulla. The 12 cranial nerves can be divided into four anatomical levels: CN 1 and 2-telencephalon, CN 3 and 4-midbrain, CN 5 through 8-pons, and CN 9 through 12-medulla. Cranial nerve findings when combined with long tract findings (corticospinal and somatosensory) are important for localizing lesions in the brainstem.

The cranial nerve examination in children must be adapted to the age and cooperation of the child (Larsen 2003). Most of the exam can be completed by specifically observing the function of each of the cranial nerves during the patient's spontaneous behavior and play. Cranial nerves 3, 4, and 6 are tested as the child tracks and follows a colorful toy. Observing smiling, crying, and spontaneous facial expression and blinking indicate CN 7 function. The child turning to soft noises or clicks of a toy is an initial screening for hearing (certainly more detailed audiometric screening of hearing must be done if there is any question of language delay or hearing loss). Listening to the child's vocalizations, then watching chewing and swallowing, reflects CN 5, 9, and 10 function. For the older child, repeating "lahpahkah," tests CN 12, 7, and 10.

of cortical discriminatory function (Casey 2000). First, explain and demonstrate to the child that the examiner is going to ask the child to report which direction the skin is stroked with a pointed object, either up or down, to the right or left. A young child can point to the direction of movement rather than say the direction. The examiner then applies a stimulus of at least 2 to 3 cms length on the right and left sides of the body with the child's eyes closed.

Children with a parietal lobe lesion neglect space on the side opposite of the lesion, especially with a nondominant

TABLE 3.9
CRANIAL NERVE EXAMINATION ADAPTED FOR CHILDREN

Cranial Nerve (CN)	Sensory/Motor	Standard Test	Adaption for Infants and Children
CN 1	Sensory	Identify nonnoxious odor	Use small container of lemon, orange, vanilla. Ask if child can smell something with eyes closed.
CN 2	Sensory	Snellen or Rosenbaum chart	Does infant regard small objects. Is the object held too close to the eyes? Use E or animal pictures Snellen chart.
		Visual fields	Child focuses on object in front of him while another object is introduced form the side into his field of vision.
		Funduscopic exam	Check for symmetric red reflexes. Have child focus on colorful object as fundus is examined.
CN 3, 4, and 6	Motor	Six cardinal positions of gaze	For neonate, rotate head in horizontal and vertical planes and observe conjugate eye rotation in opposite direction. For infant and child, use face, finger puppet, doll, or colorful object for the child to tract and follow.
CN 5	Motor	Jaw movement	Watch baby suck, older infant chew and open mouth.
CN 5	Sensory	Corneal and facial sensation	Blink and grimace to corneal reflex. Nasal tickle also tests ophthalmologic division of CN5. Observe reaction to tickle of regions of the face.
CN 7	Motor	Muscles of facial expression	Infant: Watch cry, smile, grimace. Child: Blow kisses, blow on tissue, response to tickle, say "pah-pah-pah."
CN 8	Sensory	Soft click, softly spoken words, each ear	Infant: Turns to voice, click or novel sounds. Test both right and left ear.
CN 9 and 10	Motor/Sensory	Say "ah," gag	Infant: Watch suck and swallow, sound of cry and vocalizations, gag reflex—save until end of the exam. Child: Watch swallow, say "kah-kah-kah," listen for hypernasalized sound to vocalizations, gag reflex.
CN 11	Motor	Turn head against resistance, shrug shoulders	Infant: Turn head and watch for sternocleidomastoid muscle action to resist the turning. Child: Touch chin on shoulder, shrug shoulders.
CN 12	Motor	Side to side and in-out tongue movements	Lick lips, wiggle tongue side to side, try to touch tongue to nose, say "lah-lah-lah."

Observations of spontaneous cranial nerve function should be combined with examination maneuvers directed to assess specific cranial nerve function. Table 3.9 lists the cranial nerves and suggestions for examination adaptations for children.

COORDINATION

The principle area of the brain that is examined by the coordination examination is the cerebellum. The cerebellum is important for motor learning and timing of motor activity. Recent research indicates that it is a sensory coordinator, integrating and processing sensory input that is essential for feedback and feed-forward control of motor movements (Bower 2003). It fine-tunes the force of agonist and antagonist muscle activity simultaneously and sequentially across multiple joints to produce smooth flowing, goal-directed movements. Its integration and timing function also extend beyond the motor control realm to include a role in cognition. At the present time, the cerebellum is examined in terms of motor coordination. To test the cerebellum, the motor and somatosensory systems have to be sufficiently developed and intact because the cerebellum has a primarily supportive function for these systems. For the newborn, the coordination examination is not even a part of the neurological examination. At age 3 to 6 months, the infant has developed the ability to start to reach for objects and grasp objects. At this point most of the tasks that are tested in the infant are gross motor skills. In the 6 to 12 months age range, the fine motor skills start to emerge and as the repertoire increases, the need for cerebellar input also increases. As the baby develops a fine pincer grasp at 10 to 12 months of age and is manipulating small objects, fine motor testing takes on the familiar characteristics of coordination testing. As an infant develops the ability to sit,

---

TABLE 3.10
COORDINATION EXAMINATION ADAPTED FOR CHILDREN

Appendicular coordination
  Pick up small object such as a Cheerio or raisin. Observe for pincer grasp development.
  Take small object and place in a small container.
  Reach for and grasp the end of a measuring tape.
  Touch nose or eyes of a finger puppet.
  Stack blocks (15-month-old: tower of 2, 18-month old: 4–6 blocks, 30-month old: 6–8 blocks, 3-year old: 3 block bridge).
  Drawing/copying geometric shapes (age appropriate): line, circle, triangle, square
Midline or gait coordination
  Sitting: able to stabilize trunk
  Standing: stable station, broad based as toddler, narrower as older child
  Stoop and recover: 12–14 month old
  Toddlers gait: 10–18 months
  Stand on one foot: 3-year-old
  Hop on one foot: 4-year-old
  Tandem walk: 6-year-old

---

stand, and then walk, the immaturity of the cerebellar system is demonstrated in the unsteadiness of the toddler's gait and motor movements. With time and maturation, the gait and movements become more coordinated. The station narrows and the gait becomes more steady. At 3 to 4 years of age, the child is able to balance on one foot. At age 6 years, the child can narrow the station to the point of being able to tandem walk.

Cerebellar dysfunction results in the decomposition of movements and the undershooting and overshooting of goal-directed movements (dysmetria). Decomposition of movements and dysmetria are the main elements of ataxia. Ataxias can be divided into gait ataxia and appendicular ataxias (ataxia of an extremity). Gait ataxia is usually caused by disease of the midline cerebellar structures (vestibulocerebellum and spinocerebellum), whereas appendicular ataxia is caused by the ipsilateral cerebellar hemisphere (cerebrocerebellum). Suggestions for adapting the coordination examination to children are given in Table 3.10.

SOMATOSENSORY EXAMINATION

The somatosensory examination is the most subjective portion of the neurological examination and perhaps the hardest to perform in children. A child who is verbal, can follow instructions, and can report sensation accurately is tested in the same manner as an adult. A younger child can only be tested for the presence or absence of sensation. The child should be able to localize where he or she is touched. Also, children should have an affective response to noxious or painful stimuli such as pinprick. Obviously, once a painful stimulus is used, the child's cooperation will diminish and

the potential to continue the examination will be limited. For children, the sensory examination is most important when there is a possible spinal cord, nerve root, or peripheral nerve lesion. When a child is old enough to follow directions and stand with eyes closed, testing needs to be performed to determine the ability to maintain balance. A positive Romberg sign is present when the child can maintain balance with their eyes open but loses balance when eyes are closed. If the child loses balance only with eyes closed, that is a proprioceptive problem and an important indicator of dorsal column-medial lemniscus system disease. If the child has poor balance with eyes open or closed, that is a cerebellar problem and not a sensory problem.

MOTOR EXAMINATION

The motor examination includes observing muscle bulk and palpating of the muscles when appropriate; assessing tone, strength, deep tendon reflexes; and noting any pathological reflexes. For infants and children, attainment of motor milestones and the assessment of primitive and postural reflexes should be added to these standard elements of the motor examination.

Inspection of the child's muscle bulk is the beginning of the motor examination. Any atrophy or asymmetry should be noted. Atrophy is pronounced in neuromuscular disease, while it is less noticeable in diseases of the upper motor neuron. The distribution of the atrophy is also important. A lesion of the brachial plexus, such as an Erb's palsy, will have a characteristic distribution of atrophy and weakness, while a disease like spinal muscular atrophy will give diffuse weakness. When weakness is present, the muscle should be palpated for tenderness, consistency, or contractures.

Muscle tone is the resistance of the muscle to stretch. Two types of tone are assessed clinically: postural and phasic (Fenichel 2001). Postural tone is the bias or tension maintained by the muscle to resist gravity. The examiner can assess it by applying a sustained low amplitude stretch of the muscle with passive range of motion. Phasic tone is assessed by applying a high amplitude quick stretch of the muscle with a resulting brief phasic contraction of the muscle. Testing deep tendon reflexes (DTRs) refers to the clinical method of assessing phasic tone.

Tone assessment is important in determining the intact function of the upper motor neuron (connections from the motor cortex to the anterior horn cell) as well as the lower motor neuron unit (anterior horn cell, nerve, and muscle). Diseases of the upper motor neuron typically cause increased postural and phasic tone (spasticity and hyperreflexia), whereas diseases of the lower motor unit cause decreased postural and phasic tone (hypotonia and hyporeflexia). In infants and young children, an upper motor neuron lesion can cause cerebral or central hypotonia. Postural tone is diminished, but phasic tone is preserved or even increased. Cerebral hypotonia is seen with congenital

TABLE 3.11
TONE, REFLEXES, AND STRENGTH IN CENTRAL VERSUS PERIPHERAL NERVOUS SYSTEM DISEASE

	Postural Tone	Phasic Tone	Pathological Reflexes	Weakness
Spasticity: UMN	Increased	Increased	Present	Variable
Cerebral hypotonia: UMN	Decreased	Increased or normal	Present	Variable
Peripheral hypotonia: LMN	Decreased	Decreased	Absent	Invariable

brain malformations, chromosome disorders, metabolic diseases, and as a type of cerebral palsy. When hypotonia is cerebral in origin, additional neurological findings are usually present, such as pathological reflexes, persistent primitive reflexes, cognitive impairment, and other signs of central nervous system dysfunction. Table 3.11 summarizes the tone changes and other findings in central versus peripheral nervous disease.

Strength testing can be a challenge in children who cannot follow directions or who are uncooperative. In the child who can follow directions, strength testing is the same as in the adult examination. For the infant, strength can be tested by putting the baby through maneuvers that require muscle strength to oppose gravity (Table 3.12). For the hypotonic infant, it is important to determine if the child can increase tone and demonstrate strength when irritated and crying. The infant with cerebral hypotonia will be able to reinforce tone and strength when angry or upset, but the infant with peripheral hypotonia will not. This is an important diagnostic clue in determining the cause of hypotonia (Table 3.11). For the older, uncooperative child, strength testing

can be observed when getting out of a chair, getting up off the ground, walking, running, squatting, and rising. The examiner can have the child do a push up or use the wheelbarrow maneuver to assess shoulder girdle strength.

For the infant, an important part of the motor examination is the testing for primitive reflexes and postural reflexes. Neurodevelopmentally, primitive reflexes, such as the Moro, Galant, root, suck, and grasp (Table 3.13), should be present in the newborn and their absence is pathologic. The primitive reflexes normally diminish over the next 4 to 6 months. The postural reflexes, such as the positive support reflex, Landau, lateral propping, and parachute (Table 3.13), emerge at 3 to 8 months of age. Postural reflexes are essential for postural stability and without them the child will be unable to sit independently or walk. Persistence of primitive reflexes and the lack of development of the postural reflexes are the hallmark of an upper motor neuron abnormality in the infant.

Other reflexes to test for in the motor examination are pathological reflexes. An upgoing great toe on noxious plantar stimulation is normal during the first year of life be-

TABLE 3.12
ASSESSING STRENGTH IN AN INFANT

Head Control

The newborn should be able to lift the head to upright position at least for a few seconds while sitting. By 3 months, there may be some wobbling of the head but most of the time the head is held upright with good control.

Traction

While pulling the newborn to sitting from the supine position, the head will lag behind the trunk but not in full extension. By 3 months, there may be slight head lag. By 6 months, the head leads the trunk when the baby is pulled to the sitting position. The baby then sits with a straight back and good head control.

Ventral Suspension

With the newborn suspended in the prone position, the head should stay in the same plane as the back and the extremities would be a semiflexed position. By 3 months, the baby's back should be straight, the head extended and looking forward.

Vertical Suspension

The examiner should be able to hold the baby in the vertical position without the baby slipping through his hands because of shoulder girdle weakness. By 3 months, the baby should be able to support some weight on his or her feet.

Prone Position

The newborn should be able to turn the head side to side and the extremities should be in flexion. By 3 months, the baby should lift the head 45 to 90 degrees off the mat, support weight on the forearms. By 6 months, the chest should be off the mat and weight is on the hands.

TABLE 3.13
PRIMITIVE AND POSTURAL REFLEXES

Primitive Reflexes

Moro: With sudden downward movement of a supine baby, the arms will fully extend and abduct and then return to midline.
Root, suck: When the cheek is gently stroked toward the lips, the baby should open his or her month and turns toward the stimulus. Suck should be strong with a coordinated stripping action of the tongue.
Galant (trunk incurvation): With the baby in ventral suspension, stroking the skin on one side of the lower back will cause the trunk and hips to swing toward the side of the stimulus.
Grasp: The baby should have a strong grasp with the fingers or toes when pressure is applied to the palm of the hand or ball of the foot.

Postural Reflexes

Positive support: When held in the vertical position with feet touching a surface, the infant will extend the legs and attempt to support his or her weight.
Landau: With the infant held in ventral suspension, the head and legs will extend.
Lateral propping: In the sitting position, the infant will extend the appropriate arm and hand to prevent falling.
Parachute: When the infant is turned upside down and suspended in the air, the arms extend forward and the hands spread out in order to catch him or her. This is the last of the postural reflexes to appear.

cause of the incomplete myelination of the corticospinal tracts during this time. After 1 year of age, extension of the great toe (or Babinski sign) is abnormal and is a sign of corticospinal tract disease. When a child is old enough to cooperate, he or she should be tested for pronantor drift. The patient extends the arms in front with the palms up and eyes closed. The examiner watches for any pronation and downward drift of either arm. Any pronantor drift indicates corticospinal tract disease. This sign is a sensitive indicator of corticospinal tract disease and has the same clinical significance as a Babinski sign.

Attainment of motor milestones is an important part of the motor examination (Larsen 2003). The development of motor control proceeds in a head to toe fashion and reflects the progressive myelination of the corticospinal tracts. The baby first develops head then trunk control (able to sit) and finally develops motor control of the lower extremities to be able to walk. Delay in obtaining motor milestones can indicate the presence of neurological disease. The infant less than 1 year of age does not have a hand preference and uses both hands equally well. Early handedness is an indication of a motor deficit of the nonpreferred hand. Significant motor milestones are listed in Table 3.14, along with the age at which they typically are obtained.

For many of the children that are assessed for neuropsychiatric problems, the findings on the standard motor examination will be normal yet they are often noted to be awkward or clumsy. These children will frequently have subtle neurological findings such as mirror movements, associated or overflow movements, and impaired fluency and accuracy of repetitive movements (Denckla 1985). In assessing subtle neurological findings, it is important to remember the neurodevelopmental aspect of when these findings should disappear (Table 3.15). These subtle motor neurological findings do not have the same anatomical localization power as the classic motor examination findings. Nevertheless, they have value in

indicating that the motor control in these children is not totally normal and these findings can be associated with such conditions as attention deficit disorder and learning disorders. Other unusual movements that should be searched for include tics, repetitive self-stimulation movements.such as hand flapping, twirling, rocking, choreiform movements, and pseudochoreiform movements (pseudochoreiform movements are seen in hyperactive children and can be difficult to distinguish from true chorea).

GAIT

Assessing the child's gait is an essential part of the neurological examination. As infants develop, they will start to support weight on their legs at 3 to 4 months, get in and out of the sitting position at 7 to 9 months, cruise at 10 to 12 months, and walk by 12 to 16 months. As infants start to walk, the station is wide based and the arms are held up in front in the high guard position as if they are ready to catch themselves. Gradually, over the next few months, the position of the arms is lowered to the midguard, then low-

TABLE 3.14
MOTOR MILESTONES

Milestone	Age Accomplished
Rollover	2–4 months
Sitting without support	5–7 months
Crawling	6–8 months
Getting to sitting	8–9 months
Creeping	8–10 months
Cruising	9–11 months
Walking	12–16 months
Running	14–18 months
Hop on one foot	3–4 years

TABLE 3.15
SUBTLE NEUROLOGICAL SIGNS

Sign or Finding	Age
Can't hop on one leg 5 times	4 years
Can't hop on one leg 25 times	6 years
Can't balance on one leg for 10 seconds	5 years
Can't balance on one leg for 30 seconds	8 years
Persistence of feet-to-hands overflow (hands mirror position of feet) on toe walking	6 years
Persistence of feet-to-hands overflow on heel walking	7 years
Persistence of mirror movements of any simple repetitive movement (such as hand or foot patting)	7 years
Persistence of feet-to-hands overflow with walking on sides of feet	9 years
Persistence of mirror movements with complex movement of repetitive hand patting front to back	10 years
Persistence of mirror movements with the thumb opposing each finger sequentially	13 years

Source: Modified from Denckla MB. Revised Neurological Examination for Subtle Signs (1985). Psychoparmacology Bull 21:773–800, 1985. Used with permission.

guard position. By 18 months, the arms are held down by the side and the normal associated swing of the arms is present with walking. For the older child, maneuvers to stress the gait can be used such as toe, heel, hop, and tandem walking. Although there are multiple types of abnormal gaits, most children with neuropathological gaits will fit in one of seven basic types (Table 3.16). Each of these pathological gaits can be recognized by the distribution and pattern of the gait abnormality (Larsen 2001).

GENERAL PHYSICAL EXAMINATION: IMPORTANT ASPECTS

Growth parameters are important in assessing the child with neuropsychiatric problems. Height, weight, and head circumference should be measured and plotted on standardized growth curves. Obtaining previous measurements is helpful so that growth trends can be analyzed. Excessive somatic growth is seen in the overgrowth syndromes, such as Sotos, Weaver, or Beckwith–Wiedemann Syndromes (Jones 1997). Short stature is associated with numerous syndromes and chromosomal abnormalities. Head circumference is an essential part of the neurological evaluation of the infant and child. The measurement is obtained by measuring the head around the greatest circumference, which is from the frontal prominence around the most prominent part of the occiput. The most accurate measurements are obtained with a plastic or steel tape rather than a paper tape because the paper tape can stretch. A head that is less than the 2nd percentile is microcephalic and correlates with a brain that is abnormally small (micrencephaly). A head circumference greater than the 98th percentile is macrocephaly or macrocrania and can be caused by abnormal collections of blood (subdural hematomas), obstructed CSF pathways (hydrocephalus), or a larger than normal brain (megalencephaly). Head shape is determined by growth of the cranial bones, which occurs

perpendicular to the cranial sutures. A misshapen head can be caused by craniosynostosis (premature closure of the sutures) or by a positional deformity. The most common type of misshapen head is a positional deformity with flattening of the occiput (usually the right side) with a compensatory prominence of the ipsilateral forehead (plagiocephaly). This deformation is caused by the baby being placed on the back to sleep and the head being turned to one side as the preferred position. The abnormal head shape of craniosynostosis is determined by which suture is prematurely closed and the compensatory growth that occurs in sutures that remain open. Synostosis of the sagittal suture causes scaphocephaly (the most common form of craniosynostosis) and is usually an isolated finding, while synostosis of the coronal suture causes brachycephaly and is often associated with an underlying syndrome, such as Apert, Crouzon, Pfeiffer, or Saethre–Chotzen syndromes (Jones, 1997). Synostosis of the metopic suture results in trigonocephaly, which can be an isolated finding or can be associated with brain malformations and cognitive and behavior abnormalities.

A child should be carefully examined for any dysmorphic features that may have an associated brain malformation. This is especially true of the face. There is the adage that *the face predicts the defective brain* (DeMyer 2004). This is especially true for defects in the parts of the face that are embryologically derived from the frontonasal process. The frontonasal process produces the forehead, upper eyelids, nose, and the medial third of the upper lip. Dysmorphic findings in these facial structures should prompt evaluation of an associated brain malformation. Not only should the face be carefully analyzed for dysmorphic features, but there should be inspection of the rest of the body including the hands and feet for anomalies. A constellation of dysmorphic features can be the key for making a syndrome diagnosis with brain involvement (Jones 1997).

The eye examination of a child with neuropsychiatric problems should not be neglected. Observation of pupillary

TABLE 3.16
PATHOLOGICAL GAITS

Hemiplegic	Diplegic
The patient has unilateral weakness and spasticity with the upper extremity held in flexion and the lower extremity in extension. The foot is in extension so the leg is "too long," therefore the patient will have to circumduct or swing the leg around to step forward. This type of gait is seen with a UMN lesion.	The patient has spasticity in the lower extremities greater than the upper extremities. The hips and knees are flexed and adducted with the ankles extended and internally rotated. When the patient walks, both lower extremities are circumducted and the upper extremities are held in a middle or low guard position. This type of gait is usually seen with bilateral periventricular lesions. The legs are more affected than the arms because the corticospinal tract axons that are going to the legs are closest to the ventricles.
Neuropathic	**Myopathic**
This type of gait is most often seen in peripheral nerve disease where the distal lower extremity is most affected. Because the foot dorsiflexors are weak, the patient uses a high stepping gait in an attempt to avoid dragging the toe on the ground.	With muscular diseases, the proximal pelvic girdle muscles are usually the weakest. Because of this, such patients will not be able to stabilize the pelvis as they lift their leg to step forward, so the pelvis will tilt toward the non–weight-bearing leg, which results in a waddle type of gait.
Parkinsonian	**Choreiform**
This type of gait is seen with rigidity and hypokinesia from basal ganglia disease. The patient's posture is stooped forward. Gait initiation is slow, and steps are small and shuffling. Turning is en bloc like a statue.	This is a hyperkinetic gait seen with certain types of basal ganglia disorders. There is intrusion of irregular, jerky, involuntary movements in both the upper and lower extremities.
Ataxic	
The patient's gait is wide based with truncal instability and irregular lurching steps, which results in lateral veering and if severe, falling. This type of gait is seen in midline cerebellar disease. It can also be seen with severe lose of proprioception (sensory ataxia).	

Source: Modified from Larsen PD, Stensaas SS. *NeuroLogic: an Anatomical Approach to the Neurological Examination* [online]. http://medstat.med.utah.edu/neurologicexam, 2001. Used with permission.

reactivity, ocular alignment, conjugate eye movements, and visual acuity is a part of the cranial nerve examination. Added to these observations should be a funduscopic examination. The appearance of the optic nerve, optic disc margin, vessels, and retinal background should be noted.

Because the skin and the brain share a common embryological origin, cutaneous lesions can lead to the diagnosis of one of the neurocutaneous disorders. As a part of the neurological evaluation there must be a careful head-to-toe skin search. The most common lesions that have neurological significance include the hypopigmented lesions and facial angiofibromas of tuberous sclerosis, café au lait spots and axillary freckling of neurofibromatosis I, and the forehead and upper eyelid port-wine nevus of Sturge–Weber syndrome.

In the context of a child who is developmentally delayed or who has lost neurodevelopmental milestones, it is important to exam the abdomen for visceromegaly. Enlargement of the liver and the spleen occurs in the storage diseases such as Gaucher, Tay–Sachs, or Hurler syndrome. The spine should be inspected for scoliosis and the lumbarsacral region should be inspected for cutaneous lesions, masses, unusual hair patterns, and cutaneous dimples and tracts. These clinical findings can be an indication of an underlying defect of the lower spinal cord and nerve roots.

PATTERNS OF ABNORMAL NEURODEVELOPMENT

There are certain basic patterns of abnormal neurodevelopment that the clinician should be familiar with and readily recognize in children who present with neuropsychiatric problems (Table 3.17). A delay in language acquisition should first be evaluated with a formal hearing evaluation. In the infant this can be done using evoked otoacoustic emissions or with auditory brainstem evoked responses, but in the child who can cooperate, it should be done with audiometric testing. The pattern of failure to develop meaningful language associated with impaired social interaction and stereotypical behavior is seen with infantile autism. In a child who looses receptive language abilities after a period of normal language development, the diagnosis of acquired epileptiform aphasia should be considered. Most of these children will have a history of having seizures, and the electroencephalogram (EEG) is important in confirming the diagnosis (Tuchman 1997).

A delay in the acquisition of motor milestones can be seen in multiple disorders of the nervous system, but there are patterns of motor abnormalities that help make a diagnosis. The motor abnormalities of cerebral palsy are static,

TABLE 3.17
PATTERNS OF ABNORMAL NEURODEVELOPMENT

Abnormality	Condition
Isolated language delay	Neurosensory hearing loss
Language deficits plus behavior abnormalities	Autism
Loss of language plus seizures	Acquired epileptic aphasia
Static motor deficits with persistent primitive reflexes, lack of postural reflexes and may have other associated neurological deficits	Cerebral palsy (types include quadriplegia, diplegia, hemiplegia, hypotonic, choreoathetoid, and cerebellar)
Loss of motor milestones	Neurodegenerative
Hypotonic infant without associated CNS deficits	Neuromuscular disease
Motor delay with symmetric delay in language and social skills, may have mild hypotonia	Mental retardation

nonprogressive, and usually fit the pattern of an upper motor neuron lesion or, less frequently, a lesion of the basal ganglia or cerebellum (Table 3.17). There can be associated findings such as epilepsy, mental retardation, or neurobehavioral problems depending on the severity of the prenatal event that caused the brain injury. One of the hallmarks of cerebral palsy is the persistence of the primitive reflexes and the failure to develop the postural reflexes. In making the diagnosis of cerebral palsy it is important to establish that the motor deficits are static and nonprogressive. If there is loss of developmental milestones, then the pattern is not that of cerebral palsy but of a neurodegenerative disease or a progressive lesion of the brain. The pattern of hypotonia with preserved cognitive function can be seen in neuromuscular diseases. Global developmental delay that is symmetric in all areas of development and without pathological motor findings except for perhaps mild hypotonia is often the pattern of mental retardation.

EXTENSION OF THE EXAMINATION: DIAGNOSTIC TESTING

The choice of the appropriate diagnostic tests is based on the differential diagnosis that is generated by the history and physical examination of the patient. As a general rule, diagnostic testing has its highest yield in a child who has severe mental retardation, focal neurological deficits, or findings on physical examination that suggest a specific disease entity. The main diagnostic tests that are considered include imaging the brain for structural abnormalities (magnetic resonance imaging, cranial tomography, head ultrasound in the neonate), tests for brain and nerve function (electroencephalography, evoked potentials, electromyography and nerve conduction studies, positron-emission tomography, single-photon emission computed tomography, and functional magnetic resonance imaging), cytogenetic studies (particularly in the setting of the dysmorphic child), and

metabolic studies (inborn errors of metabolism). Other diagnostic tests to be considered are tests of neurodevelopment, intelligence, language, behavior, and other specific cortical skills and functions. These neuropsychological tests are discussed in the following chapter.

NEUROIMAGING

For the neonate, head ultrasound can be done at the cribside in the newborn intensive care unit and is valuable in assessing midline structures and ventricular anatomy. The periventricular brain parenchyma can be visualized, but ultrasound is inadequate for assessing cortical and posterior fossa anatomy.

Head cranial tomography (CT) is most valuable in the acute emergency setting when the patient is being assessed for increased intracranial pressure, mass effect, and hemorrhage. CT is also the modality of choice when assessing bone and looking for intracranial calcifications as seen in congenital infections.

Head magnetic resonance imaging (MRI) has become the imaging modality of choice in most diagnostic settings where imaging the brain is important. The images are obtained in three different planes and with different acquisition parameters that help identify pathology. Cortical anatomy and the ability to identify brain malformations are much greater with MRI than with CT. For evaluation of posterior fossa abnormalities, malformations, tumors, and imaging for seizures and headaches, MRI has replaced CT.

FUNCTIONAL STUDIES

The traditional mainstay study for assessing neuronal function has been electroencephalography (EEG). The EEG is a summation of dendritic synaptic potentials recorded from various locations on the scalp and therefore reflects underlying brain cortical activity. It has some localization power, but because the electrodes are recording at a distance from the surface of the brain and the waveforms are a summation of neuronal activity, the precision of localization is approximate. EEG is most helpful in the diagnosis, classification, and management of seizure disorders. It is not, however, a substitute for a detailed and accurate history since most paroxysmal events, such as seizures, are diagnosed by history and not by laboratory studies. The EEG can also be helpful in assessing altered states of consciousness and encephalopathic states. Some EEG findings are specific for certain diseases, but most EEG findings are nonspecific as far as etiology. A routine EEG has limited value in assessing psychiatric illness. It may help in the assessment of the child who has possible seizures, intermittent explosive disorder, or organic disorders (Johnson 1996). When a paroxysmal event is frequent but it is difficult to determine whether or not the event is seizure, then video EEG monitoring can be helpful.

Evoked potentials, both visual and auditory, have value when assessing the central pathways of these special senses in the appropriate clinical setting. Visual evoked potentials are useful in inflammatory and demyelinating diseases affecting the optic nerve, tract, and radiations. Auditory evoked potentials can identify and localize lesions in the auditory pathways from the auditory nerve to the level of the inferior colliculus. In the infant who is too young for audiometric testing, auditory evoked potentials is an indirect way of assessing hearing by assessing the brainstem auditory pathways.

Electromyography (EMG) and nerve conduction studies are used to assess the peripheral nervous system. In neuropsychiatry, these tests are mainly used in the setting of diseases that can affect the brain and nerve or muscle. The dystrophies and mitochondrial diseases that affect the brain and muscle can have neuropsychiatric manifestations. Nerve conduction studies are useful in establishing the presence of myelination abnormalities in diseases such as the leukodystrophies and axonal abnormalities in diseases such as Friedreich's Ataxia.

Positron-emission tomography (PET) scanning with the tracer 2-deoxy-2[^{18}F]fluoro-D-glucose combines the structural definition of computed tomography with the measurement of glucose utilization which indicates metabolic activity. PET scanning has been used to study the maturation of cerebral function and is clinically useful in epilepsy surgery, neurooncology, and as a research tool. At this point in time, its application in neuropsychiatry is limited except as a research tool. Single-photon emission computed tomography (SPECT) scans use changes in regional blood flow as an indirect measure of localized cerebral function.

Functional magnetic resonance imaging (fMRI) combines the anatomical definition of MRI with changes in regional blood flow. This change in blood flow serves as an indicator of neuronal activation by specific tasks that activate that particular region(s) of the brain. fMRI has become the major research tool for localization of cerebral function

in behavioral and cognitive neuroscience in both adults and children. It has opened the door to understanding normal and abnormal function in the brain in vivo. Its role in clinical practice has yet to be established, but its promise is exciting to consider. Magnetic resonance spectroscopy (MRS) is used to measure the level of biochemical substances in the brain, such as creatine and N-acetyl-aspartate. It is being used in the setting of hypoxic brain injury, traumatic brain injury, and metabolic diseases especially where levels of lactate may be elevated in the brain (Wycliffe 1999).

CYTOGENETIC STUDIES

More genes are expressed in the brain than in any other organ of the body. Genetic syndromes and chromosomal defects are often associated with neurological dysfunction. Cytogenetic studies that are useful in child neuropsychiatry include high-resolution chromosome studies, DNA studies for trinucleotide repeat diseases such as fragile X, myotonic dystrophy, and spinocerebellar atrophies, fluorescence in situ hybridization (FISH) of subtelomeric deletions, for syndromes such as Prader–Willi, Angelman, and Williams, and testing for mutation in the X-linked gene causing Rett syndrome (methyl-CpG-binding protein 2- MECP2). Even in the child who has global developmental delay without dysmorphic features, cytogenetic studies can have a diagnostic yield (see Table 3.18).

TABLE 3.18
DIAGNOSTIC YIELD OF TESTS IN CHILDREN WITH GLOBAL DEVELOPMENTAL DELAYS

Test	Diagnostic yield, %
Neuroimaging	
MRI scan, nonenhanced	55.3
CT scan	39.0
Genetic studies	
Routine cytogenetic studies	3.7
Subtelomeric deletion	6.6
Fragile X screen	2.6
MECP2	Unknown
Metabolic testing[a]	$\approx$**1**
Thyroid screen (serum TSH, T4)	Near 0 if UNS; $\approx$4 if no UNS
Serum lead level	**Unknown**
EEG (routine)	$\approx$1

[a]Metabolic testing usually consists of urine organic acids, serum amino acids, serum lactate, ammonia level, and a capillary blood gas.
TSH = thyroid stimulating hormone; T4 = thyroxine; UNS = universal newborn screening
Source: Reprinted from Shevell et al. Practice parameter: evaluation of the child with global developmental delay. Neurology 60:367–380, 2003. Used with permission.

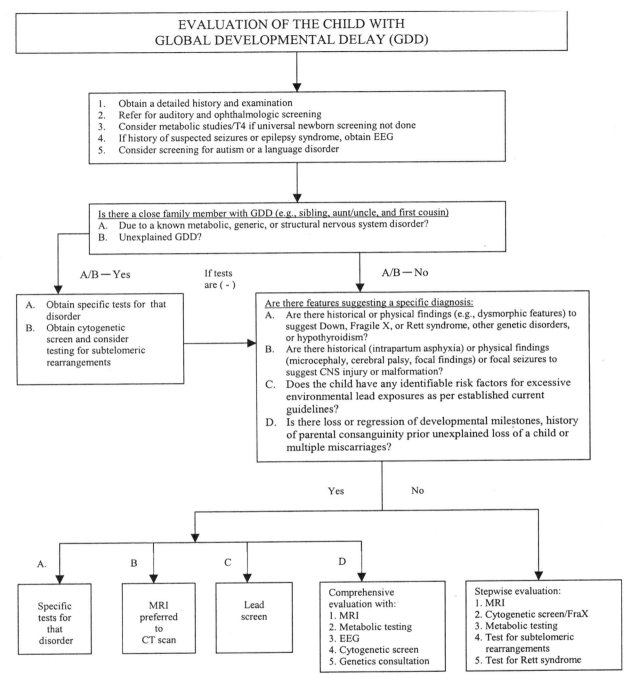

Figure 3.4 Algorithm for the evaluation of the child with developmental delay. (Reprinted from Shevell et al. Practice parameter: Evaluation of the child with global developmental delay. Neurology 60:367–380, 2003. Used with permission.)

METABOLIC STUDIES

Multiple identifiable inborn errors of metabolism effect the developing brain. These diseases should be considered when there is a loss of developmental milestones. These studies also have their place (although the yield is low; see Table 3.18) in the child without an explanation for his or her developmental delay when neuroimaging and cytoge-

netic screening have been nondiagnostic. Because the phenotypes of the metabolic diseases are so variable, multiple metabolic pathways are usually screened simultaneously unless the clinical presentation and findings are specific enough to suggest a certain disease (Table 3.19).

One of the most common evaluations that face the clinician in neurology is the child with global developmental delay. A practice parameter has been developed for the

TABLE 3.19

METABOLIC SCREENING

Serum amino acids: amino acidopathies
Urine organic acids: organic acidurias
Serum lactate and pyruvate: deficits in intermediary metabolism and respiratory chain
Serum ammonia: urea cycle defects
Thyroid function studies: hypothyroidism
Plasma acylcarnitine profile: fatty acid oxidation defects
Plasma very long chain fatty acids: peroxisomal defects
Leukocyte lysosomal enzyme profile: lysosomal storage diseases

evaluation of the child with global developmental delay (Shevell et al. 2003). Figure 3.4 is an algorithm that provides a useful guide in this situation and reflects the thought pattern that is generally used in evaluating most children with neurodevelopmental disease. Table 3.18 provides perspective as to the frequency these tests provide a diagnosis in the child with global developmental delay.

CONCLUSION

This chapter provides the clinician with an overview of the clinical neuropsychiatric assessment of children. The essential elements of that evaluation are an understanding of the temporal profile of the child's disease as well as regional or anatomical localization. A complete accurate history and the neurological examination are the clinician's window to the brain, and they have not been replaced by laboratory or diagnostic tests. For neuropsychiatric problems, an expanded mental status evaluation is particularly important. The elements of the mental status examination allow for examination of the cerebral cortex and the behaviors that are associated with cortical function. The bedside neuropsychiatric examination is not a substitute for formal neuropsychological testing, but rather it should establish the formulation of the physician's diagnostic concerns, which will then direct and provide focus for the more detailed evaluation of neuropsychological testing as well as selection of the appropriate neuroimaging, neurophysiologic, and diagnostic laboratory studies. The neuropsychiatric evaluation of the child must include an understanding of neurodevelopment and how neurodevelopment influences the examination process, expectations, and diagnostic interpretation.

REFERENCES

Adams, RD, Victor M, Ropper AH. Cerebrovascular diseases. In: *Principles of Neurology.* 6th Ed. New York: McGraw-Hill, pp. 777–873, 1997.
Aylward GP. Infant and early childhood assessment. In: Tramontana MG, Hooper SR, eds. *Assessment Issues in Child Neuropsychology.* New York: Plenum, pp. 225–248, 1988.
Bayley N. *Bayley Scales of Infant Development.* New York: The Psychological Corporation, 1969.
Benarroch EE, Westmoreland BF, Daube JR Reagan TJ, Sandok BA. *Medical Neurosciences.* 4th Ed. Philadelphia: Lippincott Williams & Wilkins, 1999.
Bower JM, Parsons LM. Rethinking the "lesser brain." Sci Am, 289:50–57, 2003.
Brazelton TB. *Neonatal Behavioral Assessment Scale. Clinics in Developmental Medicine No. 50.* London: Spastics International Medical Publications/William Heinemann Medical Books; Philadelphia: J. B. Lippincott, 1973.
Broderick J, Talbot T, Prenger E, Leach A, Brott T. Stroke in children within a major metropolitan area: the surprising importance of intracerebral hemorrhage. J Child Neurol 8:250–255, 1993.
Casey KL. The somatosensory system. In: Gilman S, ed. *Clinical Examination of the Nervous System.* New York: McGraw-Hill, pp. 175–212, 1999.
Casey BJ, Trainor RJ, Orendi JL, Schubert AB, Nystrom LE, Giedd JN, Castellanos FX, Haxby JV, Noll DC, Cohen JD, Forman SD, Dahl RE, Rapoport JL. A developmental functional MRI study of prefrontal activation during performance of a go-no-go task. J Cognitive Neuroscience 9:835–847, 1997.
Cattell RB. *Cattell Infant Intelligence Scale.* New York: The Psychological Corporation, 1940.
Chung CS, Caplan LR. Neurovascular disorders. In: Goetz CG, ed. *Textbook of Neurology.* 2nd Ed. Philadelphia: WB Saunders, 2003.
Crosley CJ. Speech and language disorders. In: *Pediatric Neurology: Principles and Practice.* 3rd Ed. Swaiman KF, Ashwal S, eds. Minneapolis, MN: Mosby, pp. 568–575, 1999.
DeMyer WE. *Technique of the Neurological Examination.* 5th Ed. New York: McGraw-Hill, 2004.
Denckla MB. Revised neurological examination for subtle signs (1985). *Psychopharmacol Bull* 21:773–800, 1985.
Dubois B, Slachevsky A, Litvan I, Pillon B. The FAB: a frontal assessment battery at bedside. Neurology 55:1621–1626, 2000.
Fayol M, Barrouillet P, Marinthe C. Predicting arithmetical achievement from neuropsychological performance: a longitudinal study. Cognition 68:B63–B70, 1998.
Fenichel GM. The hypotonic infant. In: *Clinical Pediatric Neurology.* 4th Ed. Philadelphia: WB Saunders, pp. 149–170, 2001.
Gaillard WD, Hertz-Pannier L, Mott SH, Barnett AS, LeBihan D, Theodore WH. Functional anatomy of cognitive development: fMRI of verbal fluency in children and adults. Neurology 54:180–185, 2000.
Gilmore JV, Gilmore EC. *Gilmore Oral Reading Test-Form C.* New York: Harcourt, Brace Jovanovich, 1968.
Guy SK, Cummings JL. The mental status exam. In: Feinberg TE, Farah MJ, eds. *Behavioral Neurology and Neuropsychology.* 2nd Ed. New York: McGraw-Hill, pp. 23–32, 2003.
Johnson CJ, Larsen PD, Altman C. Electroencephalography in inpatient child psychiatry and its impact on management. Scientific Proceedings of Annual Meeting. American Academy of Child and Adolescent Psychiatry 12:127, 1996.
Jones KL. *Smith's Recognizable Patterns of Human Malformation.* 5th Ed. Philadelphia: WB Saunders, 1997.
Knobloch H, Stevens F, Malone AF. *Manual of Developmental Diagnosis.* Hegerstown, MD: Harper & Row, 1980.
Korkman, M, Kirk U, Kemp S. *NEPSY Manual: A Developmental Neuropsychological Assessment.* San Antonio, TX: The Psychological Corporation, 1998.
Larsen PD, Stensaas SS. NeuroLogic: an anatomical approach to the neurological examination [online]. Retrieved from http://medstat.med.utah.edu/neurologicexam, 2001.
Larsen PD, Stensaas SS. PediNeuroLogic exam: a neurodevelopmental approach [online]. Retrieved from http://medstat.med.utah.edu/pedineurologicexam/home_exam.html, 2003.
McCarthy DA. *Manual for the McCarthy Scales of Children's Abilities.* San Antonio, TX: The Psychological Corporation, 1972.
Neeper R, Huntzinger R, Gascon GG. Examination I: special techniques for the infant and young child. In: Coffey CE, Brumback RA, eds. *Textbook of Pediatric Neuropsychiatry.* Washington, D.C., London: American Psychiatric Press, pp. 153–170, 1998.
Parmelee AH, Michaelis R, Kopp CB, et al. Newborn neurological examination. UCLA Infant Studies Project Report 1974.

Prechtl HFR. The Neurological Examination of the Full-Term Newborn Infant. 2nd Ed. (Clinics in Developmental Medicine No. 63). London: Spastics International Medical Publications/William Heinemann; Philadelphia: Lippincott, 1977.

Price BH, Adams RD, Coyle JT. Neurology and psychiatry: closing the great divide. Neurology 54:8–14, 2000.

Rescorla L, Mirak J. Normal language development. Seminars in Pediat Neurol 4:70–77, 1997.

Sarazin M, Pillon B, Giannakopoulos P, Rancurel G, Samson Y, Dubois B. Clinicometabolic dissociation of cognitive functions and social behavior in frontal lobe lesions. Neurology 51:142–148, 1998.

Shaywitz S. *Overcoming Dyslexia.* New York: Knopf, 2003.

Shevell M, Ashwal S, Donley D, Flint J, Gingold M, Hirtz D, Majnemer A, Noetzel M, Sheth RD. Practice parameter: evaluation of the child with global developmental delay. Neurology 60:367–380, 2003.

Thorndike, RI, Hagen EP, Sattler JM. *Guide for Administering and Scoring the Stanford-Binet Intelligence Scale.* 4th Ed. Chicago: Riverside, 1986.

Tuchman RF. Acquired epileptiform aphasia. Semin Pediat Neurol 4:93–101, 1997.

Tulving E. Episodic and semantic memory. In: Tulving E, Donaldson W, eds. *Organization of Memory.* New York: Academic Press, 1972.

Volpe JJ. Hypoxic-ischemic encephalopathy: clinical aspects. In: *Neurology of the Newborn.* 4th Ed. Philadelphia: WB Saunders, pp. 331–394. 2001.

Wechsler D. Manual for the Wechsler Preschool and Primary Scale of Intelligence—Revised. San Antonio, TX: The Psychological Corporation, 1989.

Weinberg WA, Harper CR, Brumback RA. Examination II: clinical evaluation of cognitive/behavioral function. In: Coffey CE, Brumback RA, eds. *Textbook of Pediatric Neuropsychiatry.* Washington, DC, London: American Psychiatric Press, pp. 171–220, 1998.

Weinberg WA, Harper CR, Brumback RA. *Attention, Behavior, and Learning Problems in Children: Protocols for Diagnosis and Treatment.* Hamilton, Ontario, Canada: BC Decker, 2001.

Weiner HL. Case 25-1986. Case records of the Massachusetts General Hospital. NEJM 314:1689–1699, 1986.

Wycliffe ND, Thompson JR, McLeary M, Hoshouser B, Ashwal S. Pediatric neuroimaging. In: Swaiman KF, Ashwal S, eds. *Pediatric Neurology: Principles and Practice.* 3rd Ed. St. Louis, MO: Mosby, pp. 122–141, 1999.

Neuropsychological and Psychoeducational Testing

Renée Lajiness-O'Neill, PhD   *Isabelle Beaulieu, PhD*

Pediatric neuropsychology has seen significant advances over the past several decades, surfacing as one of the areas of unrivaled growth in psychology and psychiatry. Pediatric neuropsychology emerged concurrent with adult neuropsychology when the primary populations serviced were children with traumatic injuries and learning disorders from various etiologies. Historically, children were examined as if they were merely downward extensions of adults (Reitan and Herring 1985). Advances in the cognitive neurosciences, particularly developmental neuropsychiatry, as well as in technologies that have improved mortality have assisted in widening the breadth of populations serviced by pediatric neuropsychology as is evident with the autistic spectrum disorders (Happe and Frith 1996; Ozonoff et al. 2004), genetic and metabolic syndromes (Diamond et al. 1997; Lajiness-O'Neill and Beaulieu 2002; Phillips et al. 2004), and low birth weight (Taylor et al. 2004). An increasing awareness of the utility of a child's cognitive and behavioral phenotype to aid in diagnosis as well as the use of his or her strengths and weaknesses to guide intervention efforts has become apparent (Volkmar et al. 2004). The first comprehensive compendium strictly devoted to the measures and methods used in the neuropsychological assessment of children including the compilation of normative data has been published (Baron 2004), an analog to the well-known compendium by Lezak (1995).

More recently, a substantially greater reliance on developmental theory has impacted test construction and the approach to the assessment of children (Gottlieb 2001; Rourke et al. 2002a). Nonetheless, the general approach remains consistent with what is seen in adult assessment with three core components necessary. The assessment begins with an examination of the *clinical presentation* or *presenting problem*. This information is often obtained from multiple informants such as the referral source, a parent or legal guardian, and in some cases from the child depending on his or her age. Presenting complaints from the child are sometimes limited by his or her developmental level of functioning, conceptual capacity and self-awareness, and limitations stemming directly from the difficulties for which the child was referred for evaluation (e.g., mutism, brain damage). Consistency and contradictions in the nature and severity of presenting problems described by various informants must be considered. Also, the pervasiveness of the problems—that is, their persistence across setting—should be closely assessed. This information will be useful with regard to understanding the role that certain environmental contingencies may play in supporting or alleviating problem behaviors. Determination of the timeline during which problems have been present is important in helping to identify etiological factors (e.g., developmentally based, acute reaction to stressors, acute or graded onset).

For children, the presenting complaints are typically related to development, learning, or behavior from a known or suspected etiology. Unlike adult referral questions that are often interested in examining a more specific complaint such as memory, as is seen in dementia, referrals for children are often prompted by academic or learning difficulties given that school is a child's occupation, and this is the functional area most often impacted. Unfortunately, the reasons for "learning difficulties" are extremely varied and can result from developmental (e.g., developmental delay), medical (e.g., epilepsy), or acquired (e.g., head injury) etiologies. As such, it is important to recognize that a suspected "learning disorder" is always justification for the neuropsychological examination of a child. Obviously, children with medical illnesses known to negatively impact the central nervous system also benefit substantially from a comprehensive neuropsychological assessment. Behavioral or social concerns are frequently encountered referral questions, and neuropsychological testing can help to illuminate markers that will aid in diagnosis. For example, impaired sustained attention and executive deficits (e.g., poor impulse control, decreased working memory, etc.) are typically encountered in children with attention-deficit/hyperactivity disorder (Roth and Saykin 2004). Likewise, nonverbal learning disability is often noted in children with Asperger syndrome (Stein et al. 2004), although the ability to discriminate Asperger syndrome from high-functioning autism (HFA) continues to be an area of much debate (Ghaziuddin and Mountain-Kimchi 2004).

The second component consists of a comprehensive review of the relevant *history*. This involves obtaining information about the child's developmental history including prenatal, intrapartum, and postnatal events, developmental milestones, medical and psychiatric history including relevant family history, academic history, and longstanding functioning in social, emotional, and adaptive domains. The majority of this information will have to be obtained from a parent or guardian and through a review of the medical and school records. It is also important to interview children and adolescents regarding social and emotional issues as their developmental level of function allows. After sufficient appraisal of the presenting problems and the relevant historical data, the pediatric neuropsychologist develops hypotheses about the possible etiology, pattern of strengths and weaknesses, and the possible severity of neuropsychological deficits that are reasonable to expect.

Research within pediatric neuropsychology and the neurosciences as it relates to brain-behavior relationships aids the clinician in the development of his or her hypotheses regarding a child's expected areas of impairment. Traditional areas of practice and research such as traumatic brain injury have provided a strong foundation for the field, with more recent clinical practice and research in traumatic brain injury focusing on factors affecting outcome, such as age at injury and the presence of family support (Ewing-Cobbs et al. 2003; Wade et al. 2003). While lesion "localization" was an objective in pediatric neuropsychology during its inception in traditional areas of practice, current practice does not constrain itself by attempting to suggest a focal region of disruption as there is a clear appreciation that the central nervous system is a complex array of vast neural networks and systems that work in concert to execute all aspects of complex cognition and behavior (Booth et al. 2004; Sporns et al. 2004). Pediatric neuropsychology has become increasingly interested in attempting to understand the cognitive and behavioral phenotypes of the multitude of developmental neuropsychiatric disorders to aid in diagnosis and guide treatment efforts as well as to increase our understanding of the neurobiological basis of these disorders. Predictable cognitive and behavioral phenotypes are also evident in acquired disorders such as those form teratogen exposure, whether from a drug of abuse (e.g., alcohol) (Connor et al. 2000) or environmental toxin (e.g., lead) (Canfield et al. 2004).

The final component is the *neuropsychological examination* itself. This involves the utilization of a variety of technical procedures. Selection of procedures depends, in part, on the nature of the referral question. It also depends on the child's age and on his or her physical and mental capacities. The specific tests used in a neuropsychological examination will vary according to the neurophysiologist's own preferences. Despite these variations, the comprehensive neuropsychological examination will attempt to measure, at least in a molar fashion, all domains of neuropsychological functions believed to be of importance for supporting the child's abilities to successfully interact in his or her environment. Making decisions as to which tests are most appropriate under what circumstances requires substantial sophistication and training. Such training includes an understanding of the psychometric characteristics of the procedures themselves and of their validity and reliability in the context in which they are being considered. A number of excellent books and reviews of psychological and neuropsychological tests are used in the context of neuropsychology available (Baron 2004; Lezak 1995; Spreen and Strauss 1998). A detailed listing of those measures more commonly used is reviewed in this chapter.

The development of pediatric measures has appropriately evolved from being atheoretical in its approach to being significantly more grounded in developmental and neuroscience theory (Korkman 1999). Early batteries such as the Halstead-Reitan Test Battery for Children (Reitan and Wolfson 1985) and the Luria-Nebraska Test Battery for Children (Golden 1987) further advised a fixed battery approach. That is, all subtests of a well-defined battery were administered in a generally fixed manner. As pediatric neuropsychology began to embrace a more diverse referral base that included preschool-aged children and those with complex neurodevelopmental and medical conditions, more flexibility has been necessary to garner the appropriate data.

As stated, comprehensive neuropsychological evaluation requires sufficient coverage of the full domain of neuropsychological functions believed to be important for supporting developmentally "normal" behavior. Although neuropsychological domains are not entirely or even mostly independent constructs, they do have some level of functional independence from each other, and neuropsychological tests are commonly labeled based on the primary domain that the test putatively measures (e.g., memory, speech and language, executive, etc.). Although clinicians can vary substantially in the specific tests included in their neuropsychological test batteries (e.g., Wechsler Intelligence Scale for Children-IV versus Stanford-Binet Intelligence Scale, 5th Edition), there is substantial agreement about which neuropsychological constructs or domains of functioning should be measured to obtain a comprehensive assessment. Domains to be considered include intellectual, academic achievement, speech and language, visuospatial and perceptual-motor, memory and learning, and attention and executive functioning. In addition, assessment of basic sensory and motor functions is typically included because of their established importance for diagnosing and lateralizing brain dysfunction as well as their importance for understanding the potential contribution of impaired performance on "cognitive tasks" that have a sensorimotor component as well. In general, for pediatric neuropsychological assessment, a broad-based comprehensive examination is necessary to provide the clinician with multiple data points from which to make inferences. The data will provide the clinician with a profile or pattern of strengths and weaknesses from which to generate diagnoses as well as compensatory, remedial, therapeutic, and rehabilitation recommendations. Other tests, called "sign tests," should be included. These are tasks on which poor performance is generally seen as pathognomonic for a specific neuropsychological syndrome (e.g., presence of clearly aphasic speech). Multiple tests that assess abilities believed to be normally distributed (i.e., distributed along bell curve) in the general population (e.g., IQ, memory) should be administered. These tests lend themselves most readily to interpretation based on the child's level of performance relative to normative expectation. Behavioral, social, and emotional adjustment are also evaluated in the comprehensive neuropsychological examination.

Often, in addition to assessment of children's performance across multiple domains (e.g., reading skill), further, "process"-oriented assessment is performed in an attempt to better understand the qualitative aspects of performance of the child and its relationship to specific and overall functioning (Kaplan 1990). Testing of limits is also often conducted as well to discern a child's maximum capability. For example, after a child's reading abilities have been identified as poor, it may be useful to eliminate time demands to discern if processing speed has negatively impacted performance.

NORMAL AND ABNORMAL DEVELOPMENTAL ISSUES

The nature and extent of the neuropsychological examination are, in large part, determined by the developmental level of the child. Many pediatric neuropsychologists develop expertise in the assessment of school-aged children

from approximately 5 years of age to adulthood. However, clinicians interested in the mental retardation syndromes, pervasive developmental disorders, and developmental delay must develop expertise that extends to as young as 2 years of age. Extensive knowledge of normal childhood development is a unique aspect of the pediatric neuropsychologists' repertoire of skills. Likewise, a strong appreciation of the extremely wide range of normal variability is critical. The issue of reliability is an often-encountered problem in testing young children. Nonetheless, this is typically addressed through the examination of core abilities with multiple measures as well as with serial testing so that patterns of strengths and weaknesses can be monitored closely. Since the mid-1990s, a number of measures and batteries used to assess neurocognitive and developmental levels of functioning in children and toddlers with developmental neuropsychiatric disorders have been developed, such as the Differential Ability Scale (DAS), NEPSY, and Mullen Scales of Early Learning (Elliott 1990; Korkman et al. 1997; Mullen 1995). This has been fueled by an increasing awareness that distinct cognitive and behavioral profiles exist even in children with mental retardation syndromes, and this is often with islets of abilities that can aid in the eventual diagnosis and treatment planning. Moreover, these distinct profiles are likely to lead to subsequent markers for disorders and the identification of potential etiological variables.

In general, the etiology of neuropathology in infants and children is substantially different from that in adults. For example, children are far more likely to be referred for evaluation because of difficulties stemming from congenital or developmental rather than acquired conditions. More specifically, as noted, learning and attentional problems are often encountered referral questions. If a child is referred for an acquired condition, the primary etiology and contributing factors are often different than that noted in the adult population. For example, intracranial neoplasms identified in children are much more often found to be subtentorial compared with tumors found in adults (Spreen et al. 1995). The primary risk for strokes in children occurs during the prenatal period (Schoenberg et al. 1978), and the neurocognitive outcome is typically more variable given multiple developmental factors (Sreenan et al. 2000; Stiles et al. 2003). Children with traumatic brain injuries are most likely to occur from falls, whereas in adults traumatic brain injuries most commonly occur in the context of motor vehicle accidents (Annegers et al. 1980). In adults, neurological injury affects the cognitive-behavioral substrate (the brain) after the individual has acquired and mastered skills. In children, however, brain damage often has a cascading effect on later developing cognitive and neurobehavioral functions, with a particular impact on prefrontal and executive functions (Eslinger and Biddle 2000).

Although prediction from infants' and young children's test performance to later ability level is possible at the extremes of the ability distribution, there has been generally poor success with predicting later skill levels from test scores obtained in infancy among those infants who were not unusually delayed or gifted (Aylward et al. 1987; Bornstein and Sigman 1987; Gibbs 1990). Nonetheless, distinguishing a global developmental delay (GDD) from a specific delay in development (e.g., mixed receptive and expressive language disorder) can be an important question answered by neuropsychological testing, which will subsequently guide immediate therapeutic efforts. The distinction between GDD and mental retardation is often a perplexing one for clinicians examining children of toddler age, and it frequently surfaces as a comorbid issue in children within the autistic spectrum. As stated in the Practice Parameters set forth by the American Academy of Neurology (Shevell et al. 2003), the diagnosis of GDD typically is reserved for younger children (i.e., younger than 5 years) who exhibit age-specific deficits in learning and adaptation (i.e., two standard deviations or more below the mean on an age-appropriate norm referenced test), for which the etiology is heterogenous and the degree of improvement following intervention is yet to be determined. In general, a diagnosis of mental retardation should rarely be made prior to age 5 when the assessment of intellectual abilities is much less valid and reliable.

An equally difficult distinction to make is between children with pervasive developmental disorder not otherwise specified and those with significant developmental language disorders. Neuropsychological testing can often illuminate many of the distinguishing features with standardized tools such as the Autism Diagnostic Interview-Revised (ADI-R: Lord et al. 1994) or the Autism Diagnostic Observation Schedule (ADOS: WPS Edition; Lord et al. 1999) in conjunction with traditional neuropsychological measures. In concert, these tools can improve diagnostic specificity as well as provide the clinician with a pattern of cognitive and behavioral strengths and weaknesses from which to generate remedial interventions.

Issues typically assessed in school-aged children are related to academic or learning, and behavioral difficulties, although the etiologies are vast. As noted, the etiology may be congenital, ideopathic, or acquired (e.g., epilepsy or traumatic brain injury), and the neuropsychological assessment will help to define cognitive deficits that may negatively impact academic functioning. For example, delayed processing speed in a child with a brain injury may suggest the need to extend or eliminate time demands to maximize the child's performance. With the advances made in modern medicine in improving infant mortality, school-aged children with histories of low birth weight are becoming an increasingly prevalent diagnostic group assessed by pediatric neuropsychology (Doyle and Casalaz; Victorian Infant Collaborative Study Group 2001; Taylor et al. 2004). Children with low birth weight (LBW) often encounter long-term neurocognitive and behavioral difficulties secondary to the known medical complications that are linearly related to the degree of LBW, such as

intraventricular hemorrhage, hydrocephalus, cerebral palsy, and retinopathy of prematurity.

NEUROPSYCHOLOGY IN THE PEDIATRIC NEUROPSYCHIATRIC SETTING

Neuropsychological evaluation has a substantial role to play in pediatric neuropsychiatry. Research in child psychopathology has demonstrated that many of the disorders of childhood that were previously only presumed to result, in large part, from dysfunctional brain systems have been found, in fact, to be related to aberrant patterns of connectivity within the central nervous system (e.g., learning disorders [Bigler et al. 1998; Hiemenz and Hynd 2000], attention-deficit/hyperactivity disorder [ADHD] [Hale et al. 2000]). Several of the DSM-IV childhood behavior disorders (e.g., conduct disorder, oppositional defiant disorder, ADHD) are associated with a high prevalence of comorbid learning problems, and for this reason the use of neuropsychological assessment in these patient groups is commonly indicated. Likewise, children with Tourette's frequently encounter comorbid attentional, learning, and emotional difficulties, and neuropsychological testing can be useful in distinguishing an attentional disorder from anxiety.

The role of pediatric neuropsychology in the assessment of children with suspected or known genetic disorders that present with comorbid psychiatric illness is also becoming increasingly prevalent. Genomic disorders such as velocardiofacial syndrome (VCFS)(22q11.2 deletion syndrome), William syndrome, Prader-Willi syndrome, and Angelman syndrome present with characteristic physical, cognitive, and behavioral features (Lajiness-O'Neill et al. 2005; Nichols et al. 2004). For example, the rate of schizophrenia, bipolar disorder, and possibly obsessive compulsive disorder has been reported to be as high as 30% in individuals with 22q11.2 deletion syndrome, significantly higher than the general population (Eliez et al. 2001). As discussed by Finegan (1998), behavioral phenotypes will play a critical role in (1) delineating syndromes, (2) illuminating intrasyndrome variability, (3) spawning theory development, and (4) understanding brain-behavior relationships and the genetic bases of behavior.

Children with teratogen exposure often present to the pediatric neuropsychologist due to significant behavioral and learning difficulties. For example, children who have chronic and significant lead exposure experience a predictable pattern of difficulties that includes substantial dysregulation and features of attention-deficit/hyperactivity disorder, aggression, and learning disorders (Ris 2003; Trask and Kosofsky 2000). Without a thorough assessment, these children are often missed or misdiagnosed, with an emphasis placed on the manifest behavior (oppositional defiant disorder, conduct disorder) and without a clear understanding of the precipitant.

NEUROPSYCHOLOGY IN THE PEDIATRIC MEDICAL REHABILITATION SETTING

Historically, both neuropsychiatry and neuropsychology have been involved in the assessment and treatment of children with medical disorders that have a direct impact on central nervous system functioning such as hydrocephalus, brain injury, tumors, and epilepsy (Yeates et al. 1999). A sizable empirical knowledge base has developed demonstrating that medical disorders secondarily affecting the central nervous system (e.g., craniofacial) or primarily affecting nonbrain organ systems can, under certain conditions, have neuropsychological sequelae as well. Examples include research relating cardiac, renal, pulmonary, and immune disorders to neuropsychological deficits (Fennell 1999; Pulsifer and Aylward 1999). Of course, behavioral adjustment to certain medical procedures and conditions can be difficult even in the absence of neuropsychological sequelae. Loss of cognitive functioning, however, can make emotional and behavioral adjustment even more difficult.

Neuropsychologists, because of their background in both clinical psychology and neuropsychology, have special skills to offer pediatric medical patients and their families. The neuropsychologist can assist in behavioral management, family treatment, and consultation to the child's other treatment providers. Children with behavioral difficulties stemming from neurological disorders may present with poor compliance behaviors, emotional lability, or general adjustment difficulties. Illness, recovery from injury, and certain treatments are difficult for cognitively intact children to manage. This set of circumstances becomes even more overwhelming for the child who may be experiencing confusion or frustration because cognitive (including perceptual, language, and conceptual) processes have become impaired. The neuropsychologist can be particularly useful in both assisting the child with behavioral adjustment and in making recommendations to physicians, parents, and teachers about intervention strategies.

NEUROPSYCHOLOGY IN THE SCHOOL SETTING

Outpatient pediatric practices include referral of a large number of children whose difficulties are recognized primarily within the classroom setting. Difficulties prompting referrals include behavioral, emotional, and academic problems. Diagnosis and treatment planning can be substantially aided by comprehensive neuropsychological assessment. A complex issue that frequently surfaces in the academic setting is that of the distinction between attention-deficit/hyperactivity disorder (ADHD) and learning disability. Children are often perceived or diagnosed as having (ADHD) when learning disability is the primary source of their inattention and distractibility. Nonetheless, it is also important to recognize that many individuals with ADHD also have comorbid learning disorders, with rates as high as 10% to 25% reported (American Psychiatric Association: Diagnostic and Statistical Manual of Mental Disorders-IV, 1994). Likewise, primary language disorders can significantly interfere with the acquisition of reading while sensorimotor deficits may negatively impact graphomotor and written language abilities. Provision of data on the child's cognitive strengths and weaknesses can allow more realistic, positive, and useful strategies to be developed for use in the classroom.

Emotional and interpersonal adjustment difficulties are commonly seen in combination with cognitive deficits. The neuropsychological assessment can help to distinguish a primary anxiety or mood disorder from an attentional or learning disorder. Neuropsychological evaluation may help the treatment provider and family members understand why a child is having a difficult time interpersonally. Clinicians and researchers have begun to identify additional forms of learning disorders such as nonverbal learning disability (NLD) (Rourke 1995) that may serve as a marker for other developmental (e.g., Asperger syndrome) and psychiatric conditions for which interpersonal difficulties is a crucial feature. Children with NLD display a predictable pattern of cognitive strengths and weaknesses that are purported to underlie their social deficits. More specifically, children with NLD exhibit deficits in sensorimotor, visuospatial, perceptual motor functioning, nonverbal memory, and novel problem solving with a concomitant weakness in mathematics. The constellation of deficits is purported to contribute to the child's inability to accurately interpret the subtle nuances in social exchanges, which interferes with appropriate reciprocity in relationships and subsequently cascades into significant interpersonal deficits.

EXAMINATION OF BRAIN-BEHAVIOR RELATIONSHIPS

Domains of Neuropsychological Functioning

General Intelligence/Developmental Assessments

Intelligence, most commonly represented by IQ tests, is an area of broad coverage that should be included in the neuropsychological examination of children. Intelligence measures are widely used across disciplines, specialties, and settings. They provide an assessment of cognitive abilities and intellectual potential that can be used to compare a child's relative standing with that of his or her same age peers and corresponding demographic factors. They have been found most useful in predicting academic success. However, they also offer clinicians important information on a child's pattern of cognitive strengths and weaknesses. For example, certain tests will provide information on verbal compared to visual-spatial intellectual skills, attention and working memory abilities, and processing speed, as well as information processing styles. However, certain limitations exist that must be taken into consideration when choosing to administer an intelligence test. For example, IQ subtest scores are thought to provide limited information as to domain-specific abilities, to be relatively insensitive to brain dysfunction including mild cognitive impairment (Peavy et al. 2001), and to have limited value and reliability in identifying students with learning disabilities based on the IQ-academic achievement discrepancy model (Stuebing et al. 2002; Vellutino et al. 2000).

Since the late twentieth century, several tests have been designed to assess intellectual potential in children (Table 4.1). The well-known Wechsler series of intelligence tests typically assess verbal and nonverbal intellectual abilities, processing speed, and working memory performances. These tests are designed to measure intellectual potential in toddlers (i.e., WPPSI-III), children and adolescents (i.e., WISC-IV), and adults (i.e., WAIS-III). An abbreviated version also exists that can be used in children and adults (i.e., WASI). Other widely used measures of intellectual potential include, but are not limited to, tests that assess both verbal and visual-spatial intellectual abilities in the context of fluid versus crystallized forms of intelligence (e.g., SB-5), tests that co-norm results of cognitive ability and academic achievement (e.g., DAS and WJ-III-Tests of Cognitive Abilities), tests of nonverbal intelligence where language influences are reduced to a minimum (e.g., TONI-3 and Leiter-R), and tests assessing intelligence through sequential versus simultaneous mental processing styles (e.g., K-ABC-II). The choice of which test to select depends on the individual's age, cultural aspects (e.g., familiarity with the English language), reason for referral, presence of specific or global delays in development, report of functional impairments (e.g., impaired hearing or vision), and nature and severity of psychopathology.

In light of recent advances in the early detection of neurodevelopmental disorder, pediatric neuropsychologists are more than ever asked to provide developmental assessment of toddlers and preschoolers. These assessments are often requested when an underlying neurodevelopmental

TABLE 4.1
SELECTED TESTS OF INTELLIGENCE AND ACADEMIC ACHIEVEMENT

Test	Age/Grade Range
Intelligence	
Cattell Infant Intelligence Scale	3–30 months
Detroit Test of Learning Aptitude–4 (DTLA-4)	6–17 years
Differential Ability Scale (DAS)	2½–17 years
Kaufman Assessment Battery for Children–II (K-ABC-II)	3–18 years
Leiter International Performance Scale, Revised (Leiter–R)	2–20 years
Miller Assessment for Preschoolers	2¾–5 years
Slosson Intelligence Test, Revised 3 (SIT R3) for Children and Adults	4–65 years
Stanford-Binet Intelligence Scale, 5th Ed. (SB-5)	2–85 years
Test of Nonverbal Intelligence, 3rd Ed. (TONI-3)	6–89 years
Wechsler Adult Intelligence Scale, 3rd Ed. (WAIS-III)	6–89 years
Wechsler Intelligence Scale for Children–IV (WISC-IV)	6–16 years
Wechsler Preschool and Primary Scale of Intelligence, 3rd Ed. (WPPSI-III)	2½–7¼ years
Woodcock Johnson III (WJ-III) Tests of Cognitive Abilities	2–90+ years
Academic Achievement	
Kaufman Test of Educational Achievement–II (K-TEA-II)	4½–25 years
Peabody Individual Achievement Test, Revised (PIAT-R)	5–18 years
Wechsler Individual Achievement Test, 2nd Ed. (WIAT-II)	4–85 years
Wide Range Achievement Test, 3rd Ed. (WRAT-3)	5–75 years
Woodcock Johnson Tests of Achievement, 3rd Ed. (WJ-III)	2–90 years
Specific Academic Areas	
Boder Test of Reading-Spelling Patterns	6–24 years
Gray Oral Reading Test, 4th Ed. (GORT-4)	6–18 years
Nelson-Denny Reading Test	Grades 9–16
Test of Early Mathematics Ability, 3rd Ed. (TEMA-3)	3–8 years
Test of Early Reading Ability, 3rd Ed. (TERA-3)	3½–8½ years
Test of Early Written Language, 2nd Ed. (TEWL-2)	3–10 years
Test of Mathematical Abilities, 2nd Ed. (TOMA-2)	8–18 years
Test of Reading Comprehension, 3rd Ed. (TORC-3)	7–17 years
Test of Written Expression (TOWE)	6½–14 years
Test of Written Language, 3rd Ed. (TOWL-3)	7½–17 years

Dashes in age/grade ranges indicate "through."

TABLE 4.2
SELECTED TESTS OF DEVELOPMENTAL AND ADAPTIVE FUNCTIONING

Test	Age Range
Adaptive Behavior Assessment System, 2nd Ed. (ABAS 2nd Ed.)	0–89 years
Adaptive Behavior Inventory	6–18 years
Adaptive Behavior Scale–School, 2nd Ed. (ABS-S:2)	3–21 years
Batelle Developmental Inventory, 2nd Ed. (BDI-2)	0–8 years
Bayley Scales of Infant Development, 3rd Ed. (BSID-3)	0–3½ years
Child Development Inventory (CDI)	0–6 years
Denver Developmental Screening Test-II (DDST-II)	0–6 years
Developmental Profile II (DP-II)	0–7 years
Mullen Scales of Early Learning	0–68 months
Scales of Independent Behavior-Revised (SIB-R)	Infancy to 80+ years
Vineland Adaptive Behavior Scales	Birth to 18 years

Dashes in age ranges indicate "through."

disorder is suspected early on, when delays are noted in specific areas (e.g., motor, language, or socialization development), to determine a child's need for early intervention and treatment, and to determine a child's readiness for school. A number of tests were constructed based on developmental models and use developmentally appropriate tasks (Tables 4.2 and 4.3). For example, the BSID–3 is a measure of early motor and cognitive development that can be used with infants and toddlers and is adjustable to account for prematurity. This test yields index scores that can be translated into age equivalents to determine a child's developmental level of functioning. Other tests such as the Mullen Scales of Early Development and NEPSY provide information on a range of abilities such as motor development, expressive and receptive language skills, visuospatial skills, memory, and executive functions. During the toddler and early childhood years, tests such as the Bracken Basic Concept Scale-Revised (Bracken 1998) measures basic concept acquisition and receptive language skills to determine a child's readiness for school by assessing preliteracy skills. However, caution is suggested in interpreting the results generated from these measures as they are not designed to

be used as predictors of eventual long-term cognitive deficits. Instead, an impaired performance on these measures would lead to recommendations that would include the need for follow-up neuropsychological evaluations of those identified as developmentally delayed or at-risk, as well as recommendations toward appropriate medical, psychological and academic interventions.

Academic Achievement

Children who are perceived as struggling academically should be referred for a comprehensive psychoeducational or neuropsychological evaluation. Deficits in acquiring general academic skills (reading, spelling, mathematics) in the first few years of elementary school set the child up for having difficulties in the later grades, when these skills must be efficiently used to acquire new knowledge and to keep up with the classroom curriculum. In addition to information that is typically obtained through a psychoeducational evaluation usually provided by a school psychologist, neuropsychological assessments are helpful in ruling out other factors that might be contributing to a child's academic difficulties beyond learning disabilities, such as problems with executive functioning abilities and behavioral regulation, language processing difficulties, sensorimotor problems, and emotional factors. In light of federal guidelines, the model used to determine a child's eligibility for educational services is that of a discrepancy between intellectual abilities and academic achievement. Over the years, many concerns have been raised about the use of the IQ-achievement discrepancy model as the basis for identifying and providing services to children with learning disabilities. Efforts have been made to pass a bill for which response to intervention would be used to identify students with learning disabilities.

Reading
Many students with a reading disorder or dyslexia have difficulty with one or more aspects of the reading process

TABLE 4.3
SELECTED NEUROPSYCHOLOGICAL TEST BATTERIES

Test	Age Range
Halstead-Reitan Neuropsychological Test Battery for Children	9–14 years
Luria-Nebraska Neuropsychological Test Battery for Children	8–12 years
NEPSY: A Developmental Neuropsychological Assessment	3–12 years
Reitan-Indiana Neuropsychological Test Battery for Children	5–8 years

Dashes in age ranges indicate "through."

that cannot be accounted for by intellectual limitations, functional impairments, or inadequate schooling. Some students have difficulty decoding words; others have problems acquiring a sight vocabulary or accessing words rapidly; still others have difficulty comprehending (Catts et al 2002). Dyslexia may also be categorized depending on a child's primary deficits: problems with phonetic processing (dysphonetic dyslexia), problems with orthographic retrieval (dyseidetic dyslexia), or a combination of both (dysphonetic/dyseidetic dyslexia) (Boder and Jarrico 1982). Nonetheless, it is important to recognize that attempts at subtyping are purely descriptive as no valid subtypes have been delineated. As Pennington (2002) noted, reading disorders are a form of language disorder, and two primary processes have been found to be critical for efficient reading: phonological decoding and rapid naming. As such, reading diagnostic tests are typically designed to assess phonological processing such as word attack skills and rapid automatized naming as well as sight word reading, reading rate, fluency, and reading comprehension (Table 4.1).

Problems with reading are often observed when a child is asked to read single words orally. Although tests for oral reading of sight words are widely used to determine word recognition and decoding skills, they are not sufficient for planning intervention. They typically yield information about expected age and grade-level performance, but they provide limited information as to the etiology of these difficulties, such as problems with phonological processing, rapid access to sight words, and so on. To assist in evaluating phonological processing abilities, clinicians will administer tasks that examine many aspects of phonological processing, such as a child's ability to transform sounds into graphemes, apply phonic rules to decode nonwords, substitute syllables in words, detect initial or final sounds of words, categorize sounds, or segment words by syllable and phoneme. Several studies have found that students with dyslexia and related reading disabilities struggle with phonological processing (Habib 2000; McCandliss and Noble 2003; Temple 2002).

As noted, rapid access of words from one's lexicon or naming is considered to be a critical skill for efficient reading. Tests that assess this skill may require the subject to rapidly name letters, numbers, or objects with specific characteristics, under time constraints. Therefore, the subject must first process the information visually, followed by forming a semantic representation, accessing a corresponding phonological word and recognizing the sequence of articulated phonemes (Denckla and Rudel 1976). Another aspect of reading that is often identified as problematic is a child's reading comprehension skills. Tests that assess literal and inferential reading comprehension typically require that a student read brief or lengthy passages or stories, silently or out loud, and then answer questions. Certain children, such as those within the autistic spectrum, are often noted to exhibit another form of reading disorder called hyperlexia syndrome, in which superior ability for reading is noted with poor reading comprehension (Grigorenko et al. 2002).

Writing

Several aspects of writing should be examined when a disorder of written expression or dysgraphia is suspected (Sandler et al. 1992). Therefore, the use of tests that diagnose deficits in legibility, fluency, spelling, written grammar, and thought expression are frequently used (Table 4.1). In a significant portion of children, the written language disturbance is associated with reading difficulties, developmental language disorders, or developmental motor coordination disorders. Visuomotor integration or copying ability as well as fine motor problems should first be ruled out as contributing factors (see Sensorimotor Functions), as these difficulties can interfere with a student's ability to convey ideas in writing. Spelling skills are typically assessed through dictation. However, in children with severe graphomotor problems, tests for which the student identifies the correct word can be administered (e.g., Peabody Individual Achievement Test—Revised). Third, written grammar should be assessed to determine if writing problems are secondary to the student's oral language or unique to the written domain. Certain measures also test for proofing, punctuation, and spelling (e.g., WJ-III). Finally, the ability to express ideas through a written modality should be assessed to evaluate organization, cohesion, and sense of audience, as well as other skills discussed earlier. Often, problems related to spelling, vocabulary, and grammar interfere with written discourse. However, some students have particular difficulty generating and organizing their ideas. Some have difficulty adjusting their language to meet the needs of the reader. Tests assessing this dimension of written language usually require the child to write a story about a picture or write sentences to complete short paragraphs. Results are analyzed for vocabulary, cohesion, organization, level of abstraction, and thematic maturity, as well as for contextual spelling and grammar. When working with younger children, tests such as the TEWL-2 focus on a child's ability to copy, spell words, write sentences from dictation, and write simple messages, notes, and other types of discourse expected of the developing writer.

Mathematics

Certain students have a specific learning disability that affects primarily the acquisition of arithmetic skills (Shalev and Gross-Tsur 2001). This type of learning disability is referred to as a mathematics disorder or dyscalculia. Although dyscalculia typically refers to children who exhibit significant difficulty with computations or difficulty with problem-solving abilities, other students with visual-spatial difficulties can display problems understanding quantitative and measurement concepts or aligning numbers properly to perform calculations. Tests measuring aspects such as calculations, mathematical fluency through rote memorization of basic calculations, and the ability to apply mathematical concepts through story problems are helpful in determining the presence of this type of learning disability (Table 4.1). However, the presence of comorbid learning disabilities should be examined as those with reading disorders may have adequate understanding of concepts and computation abilities but struggle with understanding story problems.

Sensorimotor Functions

Sensorimotor functions have traditionally been considered markers of normal development and provide the clinician with information regarding lateralized dysfunction (Thelen 1995). Prior to generating an interpretation based on observations and test results of more complex integrative skills, primary sensory processes must be intact. Therefore, determining a child's visual and auditory acuity through documentation of recent screens, as well as observations during testing, is crucial. Moreover, the assessment of complex sensory integrative functions (e.g., visual, auditory, and tactile) are assessed by examining sensory suppressions (extinction) in response to bilateral sensory stimulation. Neurological soft signs are a useful component of a neuropsychological assessment. They can provide insight into the presence and severity of neurological compromise, provide information as to areas of cerebral dysfunction, and document developmental as opposed to acquired brain dysfunction. For example, rapid alternating and fine finger movements as well as evidence of dysmetria are examined. Handedness is generally established by the time a child is starting elementary school and provides information as to lateralization of cognitive functions. Dominance may be determined by using tests and inventories of hand, eye, and foot preference in a number of activities or by observing hand preference in tasks such as writing. Bilateral fine motor speed, dexterity, and strength are typically assessed through tasks in which the child is asked to manipulate small objects, accomplish simple finger movements in a rapid fashion, and grip an apparatus. Deficits in tactile and kinesthetic information processing may also be measured. Deficits in these areas may lead to difficulty in tasks that rely heavily on motor control such as graphomotor activities, manual coordination, and eye-hand coordination (Levine 1987; Luria 1973). A number of children who are described as clumsy or uncoordinated and who are otherwise neurologically intact may be apraxic or dyspraxic. In other words, they struggle with movement representation and performance of sequential movements to accomplish an action (Luria 1973). Asking a child to pantomime acts such as brushing his or her hair, hammering a nail, and waving good-bye may assess this condition. An informal screen of other aspects of motor functioning such as oculomotor and oral motor functions is also frequently conducted to discern their relative contribution to a child's difficulties.

Visuospatial, Visuoconstructional, and Visuoperceptual Functions

Deficits in this cognitive domain can lead to academic difficulties and reluctance of a student to engage in tasks that rely heavily on perceptual and spatial abilities, such as

mathematics, drawing, and handwriting. In more severe cases, it can affect a child's ability to process social cues and nonverbal communication and lead to emotional distress and stress in social settings (Dimitrovsky et al. 1998; Ross et al. 2000; Rourke et al. 2002b; Wooden et al. 2001). Many tests exist that measure different aspects of visual-spatial abilities from basic perceptual processes to basic drawing abilities, visuospatial orientation, figure-ground discrimination, visuospatial reasoning, and so on (Table 4.4). Children may be asked to draw a picture as a way of initiating testing while assessing perceptual-motor skills, emotional status, and developmental maturity. One of the most widely used measures of developmental visuomotor ability is the Beery-Buktenica Developmental Test of Visual-Motor Integration (Beery et al. 2004), which involves the reproduction of increasingly complex shapes. For school-aged children, the Rey Complex Figure Test is another popular visuomotor test that provides information on a child's ability to plan and execute a complex design. To assess visuoconstructional praxis and provide information about other aspects of visual-spatial and executive functioning abilities, clock drawing may be used in children (Cohen et al. 2000). In children with suspected fine motor deficits, motor-free tests that measure visuospatial abilities are useful.

Speech and Language

Speech refers to the mechanics of oral communication while language refers to the ability to communicate information. Children who display early language impairments are at greater risk of developing academic difficulties (Rapin 1998). Difficulties in communication, either in receptive or expressive language functions, may be developmental or acquired. A number of screening measures ex-

TABLE 4.4
SELECTED TESTS OF SENSORIMOTOR, PERCEPTUAL, AND CONSTRUCTIONAL FUNCTIONS

Test	Age Range
Bender Visual-Motor Gestalt Test, 2nd Ed.	4 years–adulthood
Benton Visual Retention Test, 5th Ed.	8 years–adulthood
Developmental Test of Visual-Motor Integration, 5th Ed. (Beery VM1-5)	2–18 years
Developmental Test of Visual Perception, 2nd Ed. (DTVP-2)	4–10 years
Grooved Pegboard	4 years–adulthood
Judgment of Line Orientation (JOLO)	7 years–adulthood
Perceptual-Motor Assessment for Children	4–16 years
Purdue Pegboard Test	5 years–adulthood
Test of Visual Motor Integration	4–17 years
Test of Visual-Perceptual Skills (Nonmotor), Revised	4–12 years
Wide Range Assessment of Visual Motor Abilities	3–17 years

Dashes in age ranges indicate "through."

TABLE 4.5	
SELECTED TESTS OF LANGUAGE FUNCTIONS	
Test	**Age/Grade Range**
Aphasia Screening Test	5–8 and 9–14 years
Beery Picture Vocabulary Test	2–12 years
Boston Naming Test	6 years–adulthood
Clinical Evaluation of Language Functions, 4th Ed. (CELF-4)	K–grade 12
Comprehensive Receptive and Expressive Vocabulary Test, Second Edition (CREVT-2)	4–17 years
Comprehensive Test of Phonological Processing (CTOPP)	5–24 years
Controlled Oral Word Association Test (COWAT)	6 years–adulthood
Expressive One-Word Picture VocabularyTest, 2000 Ed. (EOWPVT-2000)	2–18 years
Lindamood Auditory ConceptualizationTest, 3rd Ed. (LAC-3)	5–18 years
Multilingual Aphasia Examination, 3rd Ed. (MAE-3)	6–adulthood
Peabody Picture Vocabulary Test, 3rd Ed. (PPVT-III)	2½–90+ years
Test of Early Language Development, 3rd Ed. (TELD-3)	2–7 years
Test of Language Development, Primary and Intermediate (TOLD-P:3 and TOLD-I:3)	4–8 years and 8–12 years
Test of Word Finding, 2nd Ed. (TEF-2)	4–12 years
Token Test	3 years–adulthood
Western Aphasia Battery	13 years–adulthood

Dashes in age/grade ranges indicate "through."

ist that assess several aspects of expressive and receptive language skills such as articulation, phonological processing, naming, verbal fluency, repetition, reading, spelling (oral and written), written expression, and comprehension of instructions (Table 4.5). Difficulties with phonological processing, naming, reading, spelling, and writing skills were previously discussed (see Academic Achievement). Other aspects of language that are frequently assessed are receptive and expressive language skills.

Receptive Language

To ascertain whether a child has a disturbance in auditory receptive language, he or she may be required to demonstrate an understanding of spoken words, but with demands on verbal responding reduced. For example, the child may be given a set of pictures and asked to identify the one that corresponds with words spoken by the examiner (e.g., "Point to rectangle"). Certain tests that are considered to be a measure of the child's vocabulary can also be used as a screening measure for verbal intelligence. Some children understand single words but have difficulty understanding more complex language. Certain tests are designed to assess receptive language components such as comprehension of oral language, figurative language, and other types of discourse. Listening skills may also be assessed by asking a child to follow commands when grammatical and syntactical complexity is increased. Children who struggle with behavior regulation, with holding on to verbal information, or with sequencing oral instructions may display poorer performances on these tasks. Memory is essential for comprehension, and some children have

difficulty retaining what they have heard because of deficits in auditory memory. Therefore, they may struggle in school not because they are unable to complete assignments, but because they cannot remember a series of oral directions. Failure to understand spoken language may result in problems with social communication and academic difficulties.

Expressive Language

Children who have a history of delays or difficulty with expressive language skills tend to struggle academically in areas such as reading as well as oral and written expression (Lewis et al. 2000; Rescorla 2002). Expressive language deficits may also interfere with impairments in arithmetic skills (Manor et al. 2001). Measures used to assess basic expressive language skills focus on a child's ability to name objects and pictures. More complex expressive language skills involve other aspects of language, such as word definition and the ability to formulate and express ideas and thoughts orally. These skills are assessed by asking children to explain how to make or do something, to tell a story, or to give directions. Finally, pragmatics, or social language use, is evaluated. Pragmatics, which is in some respects the most important aspect of language, involves the ability to use language for various functions, to meet the needs of listeners in various contexts, and to use nonverbal communication appropriately. Disturbances in any of the previously discussed areas of language can interfere with pragmatics. These individuals may have adequate phonology, vocabulary, and syntax but do not use language appropriately for communication. They may not use good listening behaviors; for example, they may not look at the speaker, or they may not wait for the speaker to finish a sentence. Others cannot maintain a conversation or focus on a topic. Generally, pragmatic problems can be observed throughout the evaluation during informal conversations and by noting eye contact, turn taking, requests for clarification, and the ability to convey ideas clearly.

Attention and Concentration

Neuropsychologists are often recruited to determine whether a child has attentional problems or attention deficit/hyperactivity disorder (ADHD), as a neuropsychological evaluation can assist in ruling out whether attentional problems may be secondary to other factors, such as learning disabilities or emotional disturbances. Disrupted attentional processes can be responsible for performance deficits on other tests that examine cognitive abilities such as memory, problem solving, visual-spatial processing, and so forth. The comprehensive neuropsychological battery will include tests, some computer-based, that assist in isolating deficits in attentional processes from deficiencies in other cognitive domains (Table 4.6). Depending on the type and severity of attentional problems, different treatment approaches may be recommended in both home and school settings.

Attention and concentration are thought to be composed of several different components that may be assessed through tests. For example, selective/focused attention refers to an individual's level of vigilance in monitoring information in the presence of distracting stimuli. Tests that measure this type of attentional skills assess an individual's ability to stay focused despite the presence of distractors. For example, a child could be asked to scan a page with different stimuli and cross out target stimuli. Divided attention refers to an individual's ability to attend to more than one task at a time. This type of attention refers to one's ability to multitask and appears to have the most effect on daily experiences. Tests that would measure this attentional skill

would, for example, require the child to perform two types of tasks at the same time, such as remembering three letters for a brief period of time while counting backward out loud. Sustained attention refers to one's ability to maintain vigilance and performance over time, in the context of a continuous or repetitive activity. The two latter types of attention are particularly affected in children with ADHD, as they tend to struggle on tests for which sustained attention over an extended period of time is required. Finally, alternating attention is used in describing an individual's ability to mentally shift his or her attention from one task to another. Tests that measure this type of attention will typically examine a child's tendency to perseverate in their response pattern despite instructions or redirection during testing. Children with an autistic spectrum disorder tend to struggle with this aspect of attention (Baron 2004).

Tests that examine brief auditory attentional capacity or a child's ability to hold on to as much information as possible are referred to as span tests. For example, on such tests a child may be instructed to repeat a series of letters, numbers, or words in a specific order, or repeat a sequence of hand movements. In adults, an average span has traditionally been of $7 +/-2$ bits of information (Miller 1956). Children will increase their ability to hold on to information with cerebral maturation and reach adult level performance around age 9 (Rudel and Denckla 1974). Children who struggle with these tasks are often described as forgetful and as struggling with following multistep instructions.

Memory and Learning

Problems with memory are often cited as reasons for referrals for a neuropsychological evaluation in almost all age groups. Many children and adolescents struggle with remembering instructions and with learning information, hindering their academic success. Although memory deficits or amnestic disorders exist in children, they are quite rare and are most often secondary to cerebral insult such as epilepsy, anoxia, brain tumors, or head injuries (Vargha-Khadem et al. 2003; Williams and Sharp 1999). Memory or learning problems most often reflect difficulties with other cognitive functions such as attentional processes, executive functioning, and language or visuospatial processing. Most child memory batteries or tests will use downward extensions of tasks used in adult memory batteries and assess a child's ability to encode and consolidate information, as well as retrieve or recognize the information after a short and long delay (Table 4.7). Memory tasks have been developed for children as young as 3. They typically involve tasks that assess verbal and nonverbal memory processes, or both simultaneously. Verbal memory can be examined by asking a child to repeat stories, sentences, lists of words, or words that have been paired with other words, and so on. Nonverbal memory tasks may involve remembering faces, locations, and designs or pictures, for example. The child's performance across separate memory

TABLE 4.6

SELECTED TESTS OF ATTENTION, CONCENTRATION, AND MENTAL PROCESSING SPEED

Test	Age Range
Auditory Continuous Performance Test	6–11 years
Conners Continuous Performance Test, Second Edition (CCPT-II)	4 years–adulthood
D2 Test of Attention	9–59 years
Gordon Diagnostic System	4–16 years
Symbol Digit Modality Test	8 years–adulthood
Test of Everyday Attention for Children (TEA-Ch)	6–16 years
Test of Variables of Attention	4–80 years
Trail Making Test	9 years–adulthood

Dashes in age ranges indicate "through."

TABLE 4.7
SELECTED TESTS OF MEMORY

Test	Age Range
Benton Revised Visual Retention Test	8 years–adulthood
California Verbal Learning Test, Children's Version (CVLT-C)	5–16 years
Children's Memory Scale (CMS)	5–16 years
Rey Complex Figure Test and Recognition Trial (RCFT)	6–89 years
Rivermead Behavioural Memory Test	5 years–adulthood
Test of Memory and Learning (TOMAL)	5–19 years
Wechsler Memory Scale, 3rd Ed. (WMS-III)	16–89 years
Wide Range Assessment of Memory and Learning, 2nd Ed. (WRAML-2)	5–90 years

Dashes in age ranges indicate "through."

TABLE 4.8
SELECTED MEASURES OF EXECUTIVE FUNCTIONS

Test	Age Range
Behavioral Assessment of the Dysexecutive Syndrome for Children (BADS-C)	8–16 years
Behavioral Rating Inventory of Executive Functioning (BRIEF)	5–18 years
Children's Category Test	5–16 years
Delis-Kaplan Executive Function System (D-KEFS)	8–89 years
Raven's Progressive Matrices	5 years–adulthood
Stroop Color and Word Test: Children's Version	5–14 years
Tower of London, Drexel University	7–60 years
Wisconsin Card Sorting Test	6½ years–adulthood

Dashes in age ranges indicate "through."

tests will provide the clinician with a reliable pattern of strengths and weaknesses (e.g., visual versus verbal learning) that assist in the elaboration of educational strategies.

Executive Functions

Executive functions refer to a wide variety of complex cognitive processes and behaviors. For example, complex problem solving and reasoning, working memory, mental flexibility, inhibition, initiation, planning, and organization all fall under the umbrella of executive functions (Denckla 1989; Welsh et al. 1991). Executive dysfunction is a core aspect of the difficulties encountered by many children, and these deficits may be developmental in nature (i.e., ADHD, autism, Tourette's syndrome) or acquired (e.g., traumatic brain injury). Executive dysfunction may manifest as problems with attention, impulse control, perseveration, apathy, or emotional dysregulation (Gioia et al. 2002). Students with learning disabilities tend to display executive functioning difficulties such as problems with initiation, inhibition, and set shifting (Hooper et al. 2002). Tests have been developed to assess executive functioning in children starting at a very young age (Table 4.8). When executive functions are of concern, it is also important to obtain information about the student's behavior in natural contexts, since highly structured test situations do not always reveal the problems. Observations by parents, teachers, and the student themselves are helpful in noting whether assistance and accommodations are needed.

Personality and Psychosocial Functioning

The evaluation of psychological, social, and behavioral factors is an important part of the neuropsychological evaluation (Table 4.9). It provides information about a child's emotional and behavioral level of functioning across settings, as well as information about his or her coping abilities when faced with difficulties. Although formal projective personality measures can be administered (ex. CAT, Rorschach Test), the assessment of a child's emotional and

psychological level of functioning relies heavily on information obtained from parents and teachers. Attention and concentration difficulties, problems with impulse control, mood disturbances, social difficulties, and other behavioral or emotional problems may be assessed through a variety of subjective paper-and-pencil questionnaires completed by the parent, teacher, and the child. This information is useful for interpreting performance on cognitive tests, as deficits may be accounted for by developmental psychopathology (for example, ADHD) or exacerbated by the onset of emotional distress (such as depression).

INTERPRETATION OF THE EXAMINATION

Validity of Test Scores

Interpretation within the neuropsychological assessment is not performed in a vacuum. There are multiple potential explanations for a child's poor performance on any test. The first point to consider in determining the validity of obtained test scores is the child's level of cooperation and effort. Test scores, unlike radiographs or other medical procedures, require the child's cooperation before they can be considered a true reflection of that child's capabilities. When a child does not cooperate with the test procedures, the confidence with which statements can be made about the child's abilities across various domains of neuropsychological functioning is lessened. The conclusion that a child may not be performing up to his or her true ability level is based in part on an experienced clinician's and technician's observation of level of effort allocated toward the test procedures. More recently, formal measures have been developed that are used exclusively to determine whether an adolescent has provided their best effort or if less than optimal effort has been

TABLE 4.9
SELECTED MEASURES OF PSYCHOSOCIAL AND PERSONALITY FUNCTIONING

Test	Age/Grade Range
Achenbach System of Empirically Based Assessment (ASEBA Child Behavior Checklist)	6–18 years
Behavior Rating Profile, 2nd Ed. (BRP-2)	6–18 years
Brown Attention-Deficit Disorder Scales	12 years–adulthood
Children's Apperception Test (CAT)	3–10 years
Children's Depression Inventory (CDI)	6–17 years
Conners' Rating Scales-Revised (CRS-R)	3–17 years
Devereux Scales of Mental Disorders	5–18 years
Minnesota Multiphasic Personality Inventory—Adolescents (MMPI-A)	14–17 years
Multidimensional Self-Concept Scale	Grades 5–12
Personality Inventory for Children, 2nd Ed. (PIC-2)	5–19 years
Revised Children's Manifest Anxiety Scale (RCMAS)	6–19 years
Reynold's Adolescent Depression Scale, 2nd Ed. (RADS-2)	11–20 years
Rorschach Inkblot Test	8 years–adulthood

Dashes in age/grade ranges indicate "through."

extended during memory testing (Green et al. 1996). This type of testing has been found to be particularly useful in forensic examination. Validity is also examined in the profiles completed by a child's parent to discern if a parent is endorsing symptoms in a child to a degree that are in excess of what would likely be expected in most children and may suggest a plea for help.

BRAIN-BEHAVIOR RELATIONSHIPS

Methods of Inference

If the test data are judged to be a valid and reliable measure of the child's abilities, then multiple methods of inference are used to interpret the neuropsychological data. Historically, the major methods of inference have been level of performance, pattern of performance, pathognomonic signs, right-left patterns, and test-retest performance patterns. As brain-behavior relationships have become more fully illuminated other axes including cortical-subcortical, anterior-posterior, orbitomedial and dorsolateral, and dorsal-ventral stream patterns of performance have become important aspects of the method of inference. Figure 4.1 provides a partial example of a method of inference that a neuropsychologist would employ in the interpretation of the test data. The conclusions drawn from the aforementioned inferential method will be subsequently integrated with information obtained regarding the presenting concerns and historical data in formulating the case with regard to potential diagnoses, brain-behavior relationships, and strengths and weaknesses. The future of pediatric neuropsychological assessment is, however, entering an era in which the etiological yield is likely to be the most fruitful

when conducted in conjunction with neuroimaging and there is a more substantial appreciation of the variance in performance and outcome based on environmental contingencies (see Table 4.10).

Level of Performance

Drawing conclusions about functions based on a child's norm-referenced performance level on a test is a common method of inference used by both psychologists (e.g., IQ score) and nonpsychologists (e.g., values of laboratory tests). For example, standardized IQ tests typically provide scores ranging from around 50 to approximately 150. Individuals who take an IQ test can be compared with the population with regard to their standing in the distribution. Someone with an IQ of 110 is in the upper 25th percentile of the general population, whereas someone with an IQ of 85 is at the lower 15th percentile. Neither of these IQ scores implies normality or abnormality, but they do position an individual with regard to his or her competitive level in a number of respects. Knowing that a person is consistently above or below average and the degree of difference from the average of the population are significant elements in proper educational and occupational placement.

The risk of considering level of performance in isolation from other data is that performance level does not provide adequate information about whether or not the obtained scores are normal or abnormal for any given child. An individual with lifelong cognitive abilities in the superior range who now has average intelligence is certainly not normal. In addition to the individual's having lost mental skills to the level of average, it may be the case that those losses have occurred in areas sufficiently specific to preclude behavior consistent with that typifying

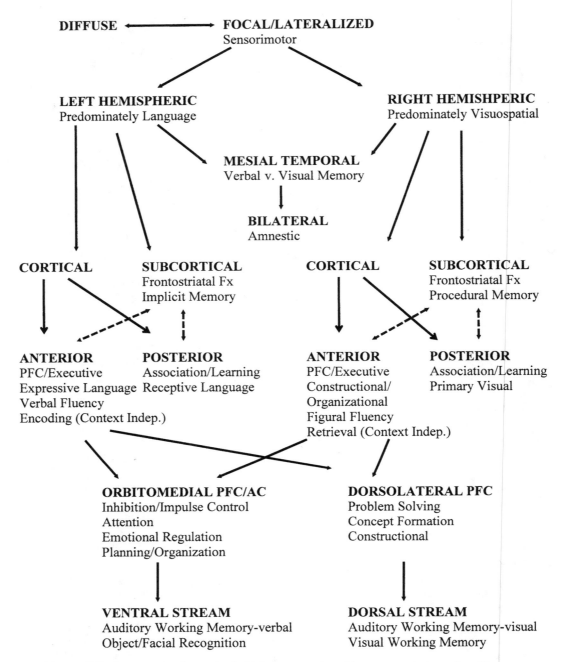

Figure 4.1 An example of a method of inference employed in neuropsychology. Cognitive constructs listed are intended to be merely examples of abilities known or suspected to be representative of the specific brain region or system. *Note:* Brain regions: PFC, prefrontal cortex; AC, anterior cingulate.

the broad range of individuals with lifelong average cognitive abilities. The frustrations experienced by such a child who has lost intellectual abilities are difficult to appreciate and are simply not elucidated by obtaining an IQ score of 95 to 105. Thus, an "average" IQ considered alone can be quite misleading by suggesting that all is well, when, in fact, dramatic changes may have occurred.

Similarly, even subtle changes in motor functioning (from superior to average), though not likely to be apparent in a variety of clinical evaluations, may make a substantial difference in a child's athletic prowess, thereby affecting the child's self-concept and perceptions by his or her peers. Certainly, brief neuropsychological screenings run a substantial risk of missing these kinds of difficulties.

Level of performance encourages the utilization of tests with adequate normative data, and this method of inference is appropriate to a broad range of neuropsychological tests. Test reports that fail to provide information on level

TABLE 4.10
SUMMARY OF THE NEUROSCIENCE OF PSYCHOPATHOLOGIES

| | Etiology | | Brain Findings | | | |
	Genes	Environment	Neurochemical	Structural	Functional	Neuropsychology
Motivation						
Depression	5-HT transporter?	Loss, stress	Cortisol, NE, 5HT	FL, BG	HPA, Amyg, PFC, ACG	Dysregulated stress response
Anxiety	5-HT transporter	Threat, Stress	NE, 5-HT GABA, CCK	—	Amyg, PFC	Conditioned fear response
PTSD	?	Trauma	Cortisol, Opiates	HC	Amyg, OFC, ACG	Conditioned fear response?
Bipolar disorder	18p, q: 21q	Stress	DA, NE, GABA	WM, Cortex	PFC	Overactive approach system
Action Selection						
Attention-deficit/hyperactivity disorder	DRD4: DAT1	FAS, CHI	DA	PFC, BG, CC	PFC, BG	Executive inhibition
Conduct disorder	MAOA, TPH	Harsh parenting abuse	5-HT	PFC	PFC, Amyg,	Inhibition, low autonomic arousal
Tourette's syndrome	4q, 8p	Strep infection	DA	BG	BG, OFC, ACG	Inhibition?
Obsessive-compulsive disorder	5-HT transporter?	Strep infection	DA	BG	OFC, CN, ACG	Inhibition?
Schizophrenia	6p, 8p, 22q, 15q	OCs, viral infection	DA, GABA, glutamate, Ach	Ventricles, TL, Thal	PFC	Low IQ, WM, LTM
Language and Cognition						
Autism	7q, 15q	Extreme neglect?	5-HT	Large brain	P300, OFC, FG	EF, ToM, praxis, emotional processing?
Down syndrome	Trisomy 21	—	Ach?	Small brain, HC, cerebellum, PFC	—	Verbal STM, syntax, LTM
Fragile X syndrome	FMRI	—	—	Large brain	—	Pragmatic language, EF
Williams syndrome	7p microdeletion	—	—	Small brain	—	Spatial deficit, language strengths
Dyslexia	1p, 2p, 6p, 15q, 18p	?	—	Language cortex	—	Phonological

Note: Neurotransmitters: NE, norepinephrine; 5-HT, serotonin; DA, dopamine; Ach, acetylcholine; GABA, gamma-aminobutyric acid; CCK, cholecystokinin. *Brain regions:* FL, frontal lobes; BG, basal ganglia; HPA, hypothalamic-pituitary-adrenal axis; Amyg, amygadala; ACG, anterior cingulate gyrus; PFC, prefrontal cortex; OFC, orbitofrontal cortex; WM, white matter; HC, hippocampus; CN, caudate nucleus; TL, temporal lobes; Thal, thalamus; FG, fusiform gyrus; CC, Corpus callosum. *Other:* DRD-4, dopamine receptor 4; DAT1, dopamine transporter 1; TPH, tryptophan hydroxylase; MAOA, monoamine oxidase A; FAS, fetal alcohol syndrome; CHI, closed head injury; Strep, streptococcus; OCs, obstetrical complications; ToM, theory of mind; WM, working memory; LTM, long-term memory; STM, short-term memory; EF, executive function; FMRI, fragile X mental retardation gene 1; P300, a component of the evoked response.
Source: Reprinted with permission from Pennington, BR. *The Development of Psychopathology. Nature and Nurture.* New York: The Guilford Press, 2002.

of performance are hardly ever fully informative; test reports that rely exclusively on the child's position relative to a normative sample leave out significant amounts of information that may be pertinent to the child's day-to-day performance.

Pattern of Performance
Pattern analysis has the advantage of encouraging utilization of a wide range of psychological tests covering broad domains of functioning. Identifying and interpreting "unusual" patterns of performance within and across tests re-

quires knowledge about the base rates for specific patterns and the relationship of specific patterns to neurological or developmental syndromes.

The most common pattern referred to is the split between scores on verbal versus performance subtests of the Wechsler intelligence scales, since such splits have been associated with various types of neurological impairment. However, verbal-performance differences on the Wechsler scales do not necessarily reflect neurological impairment in children, much less necessarily indicate lateralized brain damage to the left or right hemisphere (Boll and Barth 1981; Chadwick and Rutter 1983). Despite this, many clinical reports continue to allude to left and right brain differences in children based on these data without neurological criteria to support such conclusions. Drawing inferences based on the amount of variability in performance among the Wechsler subscales, a process often referred to as "scatter analysis," is also invoked as a way of deriving information from these scales. Unfortunately, no scientifically valid data of a criterion-based nature have been produced to suggest that specific relationships among subtests have a particular reference either to presence or absence or to location of brain damage. Nonetheless, the degree of spread or IQ discrepancy in a profile will be critical in the interpretation in some forms of developmental and learning disorders. For example, Figure 4.2 reveals data of a child with an NLD who was subsequently diagnosed with Asperger syndrome. In this case, superior verbal intellectual abilities relative to low average visuospatial intellectual skills have resulted in the regression to an average overall IQ, and an exclusive reliance on any IQ in isolation will not help one to appreciate the degree to which the child is struggling. Moreover, his generally low average visuospatial IQ does not fully illuminate his rather profound constructional and organizational deficit (Fig. 4.3). Qualitative interpretation of the vocabulary responses (Fig. 4.2) further reveals a classic feature of language in Asperger syndrome: the tendency to be pedantic. It is important to note that NLD is an academic distinction that may or may not be evident in Asperger syndrome, though it is frequently observed.

A more valid and reliable form of analysis occurs when one examines and compares the pattern of performance across a variety of different types of tests covering a broad range of neuropsychological domains. In other words, a child who displays a relative strength on tests of language but a substantial weakness in motor functioning provides information with regard to the child's areas of needed emphasis and required intervention, independent of whether or not these relative strengths and weaknesses relate in a specific way to underlying brain damage, normally occurring individual differences, or poorly understood (in terms of brain substrate) neuropsychological syndromes (e.g., hyperlexia).

Children whose pattern of performance across multiple tests is substantially different from the normative pattern (e.g., substantial differences between performance on IQ tests and performance on achievement tests) may have learning difficulties requiring further assessment. At times, the pattern is puzzling for families and school personnel. For example, many children with autism with hyperlexia and hypergraphia as depicted in Figure 4.4 are frequently believed to be "bright" given their often early and rather exquisitely developed sight reading abilities until more complex reading demands are required. Pattern analysis is helpful for raising questions, answering questions, identifying areas of strength toward which learning strategies can be targeted, and identifying areas of deficit for which remediation may be attempted. Relative strengths and weaknesses can also help explain a child's preferences for a variety of tasks and activities that might otherwise be attributed to personality variables. Recognizing that

Male, Age 10	
COGNITIVE/ACADEMIC PROFILE: NONVERBAL LEARNING DISABILITY (Mean = 100; S.D. = 15) CLINICAL DIAGNOSIS: ASPERGER SYNDROME	
Verbal IQ = 127	Reading SS = 105
Performance IQ = 85	Spelling SS = 81
Full Scale IQ = 104	Arithmetic SS = 62
Vocabulary Sample:	
Umbrella: An object used to keep—to displace rain over a taut surface—or to keep a section of an area dry. *Bicycle:* A two wheeled transportation unit powered by the legs.	

Figure 4.2 Selected cognitive data from a 10-year-old boy with nonverbal learning disability and Asperger syndrome. Note his verbal greater than performance intellectual pattern and preserved sight reading, but significantly impaired mathematics performance. Spelling is below average partially due to orthographic errors. Further note examples of his rather pedantic vocabulary.

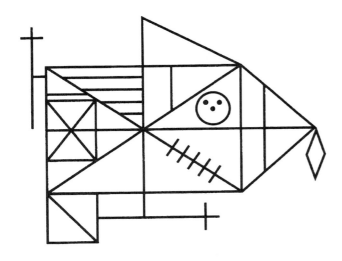

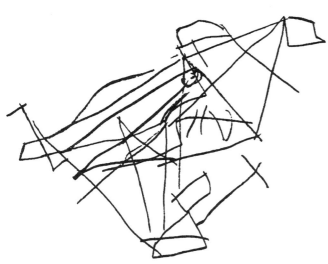

Figure 4.3 Top figure: Rey complex figure stimulus. Bottom figure: The copy of the Rey complex figure by the 10-year-old boy with nonverbal learning disability and Asperger syndrome. Note his severe visuoconstructional skills combined with his superior verbal intellectual skills. Further note the lack of sensitivity of performance IQ, which is low average, to reveal the profound nature of his visuoconstructional impairment.

personality and ability interact in determining preferences helps lead to a more holistic understanding of the child's behavior and, it is hoped, to a more informed base from which to plan intervention strategies.

Right-Left Patterns/Anterior-Posterior/ Orbitomedial-Dorsolateral/ Subcortical-Cortical/Dorsal-Ventral

A comparison of the efficiency of sensory and motor functions on the two sides of the body (right-left patterns) provides important data that contribute to neuropsychological interpretation. Systematically obtained and consistently identified deficits on one side of the body are

likely to have a neurological origin (central or peripheral) and are unlikely to be influenced by environmental, motivational, academic background, or emotional factors as scores on "level of performance" tests can be. Lateralized sensory-motor deficits (e.g., right-sided manual weakness, speed, and coordination), when related to cortical lesion, will commonly co-occur with deficits in cognitive processes (e.g., language deficits in this example). As noted, it is now possible to consider additional axes of potential disruption, such as cortical-subcortical, anterior-posterior, orbitomedial and dorsolateral, and dorsal-ventral stream patterns, in the formulation of the assessment (Fig. 4.1). Research has suggested that some developmental disorders likely, in fact, represent disruptions in specific neural networks (e.g., William syndrome, dorsal stream) (Atkinson et al., 2003).

Test-Retest Performance Patterns

Test-retest analysis is particularly useful in assessing children. The child's performance on a battery of tests at an initial time is compared with his or her performance on retesting at a second time, usually 12 months or more after the initial testing. A child may perform poorly on one or another test because a real deficit is present, a temporary developmental lag is occurring, or certain nonneurological events (e.g., poor motivation) are at work. By retesting the child after a period of time, observations are made with regard to the stability of certain performance strengths and weaknesses.

Another important reason for use of test-retest comparisons is that in the developing child at risk given a history of early injury (e.g., prenatal/intrapartum stroke or traumatic brain injury in early childhood), initial testing may not reveal pronounced deficits. However, as the child develops there is frequently a cascading effect on more complex cognitive, particularly executive functions, as life demands increase.

CONCLUSION

Neuropsychological testing represents only one of the three components of the neuropsychological evaluation. The neuropsychological test results are considered in the context of a comprehensive understanding of the presenting complaints and the child's life history to include developmental history, medical history, and longstanding functioning across behavioral, social, emotional, and cognitive domains. Selection of tests to include in the neuropsychological examination of the child will vary among neuropsychologists. However, substantial agreement exists indicating that the comprehensive child neuropsychological test battery will include tests and procedures that cover the following domains:

- Intellectual or developmental level of functioning
- Academic achievement
- Sensorimotor functions
- Visuospatial and perceptual-motor functions

Male, Age 11	
COGNITIVE/ACADEMIC PROFILE: HYPERLEXIA AND HYPERGRAPHIA (Mean = 100; S.D. = 15) CLINICAL DIAGNOSIS: AUTISTIC DISORDER	
Intellectual	*Academic*
Verbal IQ = 53 Performance IQ = 57 Full Scale IQ = 65	Sight Reading SS = 100 Spelling SS = 116 Arithmetic SS = 108
Speech and Language	Oral Reading (Mean = 10; S.D. =3) Rate SS = 8
PPVT-III SS (Receptive Vocabulary) = 59 EOWPVT SS (Expressive Vocabulary) = 64	Accuracy SS = 11 Comprehension SS = 4 Oral Reading Quotient = 82

Figure 4.4 Selected cognitive data from an 11-year-old boy with autism who displays mental retardation with hyperlexia and hypergraphia. Note his preserved sight reading and spelling despite mental impairment and significantly impaired expressive and receptive vocabulary. Further note his significantly impaired reading comprehension despite preserved sight reading, reading rate, and accuracy.

- Speech and language functions
- Memory and learning
- Attention and executive functions
- Behavioral and emotional adjustment

Neuropsychological interpretation involves drawing conclusions based on the use of multiple levels of inference considered in the context of the child's pertinent developmental and medical history as well as what is known about the natural history of certain pathological conditions.

In the hands of a skilled child neuropsychologist, a neuropsychological evaluation (conducted in 2 to 5 hours) can be a useful diagnostic and treatment-relevant assessment tool that is also cost-effective. The information obtained from a comprehensive neuropsychological evaluation is unique, and in many cases pivotal to the diagnosis, and detailed enough to be useful in the development of psychological, medical, and educational interventions.

REFERENCES

Academic Therapy Publications: Expressive One-Word Picture Vocabulary Test, 2000 Ed. (2000). Austin, TX: Pro-Ed.

Achenbach TM & Rescorla LA (2001). *Achenbach System of Empirically Based Assessment.* Burlington, VT: ASEBA.

Adams W & Sheslow D (1995). *Wide Range Assessment of Visual Motor Abilities.* San Antonio, TX: The Psychological Corporation.

Adams W & Sheslow D (2003). *Wide Range Assessment of Memory and Learning,* 2nd ed. San Antonio, TX: The Psychological Corporation.

Alpern G, Boll T, & Shearer M (2000). *Developmental Profile II Manual.* Los Angeles: Western Psychological Services.

American Psychiatric Association. (1994). *Diagnostic and Statistical Manual of Mental Disorders,* 4th ed. Washington, DC: Author.

Annegers JF, Grabow JD, Kurland LT, and Laws ER Jr. (1980). The incidence, causes, and secular trends of head trauma in Olmstead County, Minnesota, 1935–1974. Neurology 30:912–919.

Atkinson J, Braddick O, Anker S, Curran W, Andrew R, Wattam-Bell J, Braddick F (2003). Neurobiological models of visuospatial cognition in children with Williams syndrome: measures of dorsal-stream and frontal function. *Developmental Neuropsychology* 23:139–172.

Aylward GP, Gustafson N, Verhulst SJ, et al. (1987). Consistency in the diagnosis of cognitive, motor, and neurologic function over the first three years. *J Pediatr Psych* 12:77–98.

Baron IS (2004). *Neuropsychological Evaluation of the Child.* New York: Oxford University Press.

Bayley N (1993). *Bayley Scales of Infant Development,* 2nd ed. San Antonio, TX: The Psychological Corporation.

Beery KE, Buktenica NA, & Beery NA (2004). *Developmental Test of Visual-Motor Integration,* 5th ed. Austin, TX: Pro-Ed.

Beery KE & Taheri CM (1992). *Beery Picture Vocabulary Test and Beery Picture Vocabulary Screening Series.* Odessa, FL: Psychological Assessment Resources.

Bellak L & Bellak S (1974). *Children's Apperception Test.* Los Angeles, CA: Western Psychological Services.

Bender L (2003). *Bender Visual Motor Gestalt Test.* San Antonio, TX: The Psychological Corporation.

Benton AL (1991). *Revised Visual Retention Test,* 4th ed. San Antonio, TX: The Psychological Corporation.

Benton AL & Hamsher K deS (1989). *Multilingual Aphasia Examination,* 2nd ed. Iowa City, IA: AJA Associates.

Benton AL, Hamsher K deS, & Rey GJ (1994). *Multilingual Aphasia Examination,* 3rd ed. Iowa City, IA: AJA Associates.

Benton AL, Hamsher K deS, Varney NR, et al. (1983). *Contributions to Neuropsychological Assessment.* New York: Oxford University Press.

Benton-Sivan A (1992). *Benton Visual Retention Test* 5th ed. San Antonio, TX: The Psychological Corporation.

Bigler ED, Lajiness-O'Neill R, & Howes NL (1998). Technology in the assessment of learning disability. *J Learn Disabil* 31:67–82.

Boder E & Jarrico S (1982). *Boder Test of Reading-Spelling Pattern Test: A diagnostic screening test for subtypes of reading disability.* San Antonio, TX: The Psychological Corporation.

Boll TJ (1993). *The Children's Category Test.* San Antonio, TX: The Psychological Corporation.

Boll TJ & Barth JB (1981). Neuropsychology of brain damage in children In: Filskov SB, Boll TJ, eds. *Handbook of Clinical Neuropsychology.* New York: Wiley, pp. 418–452.

Booth JR, Burman DD, Meyer JR, et al. (2004). Brain-behavior correlation in children depends on the neurocognitive network. Human Brain Mapping 23:99–108.

Bornstein MH & Sigman MD (1986). Continuity in mental development from infancy. Child Development 57:251–274.

Bracken BA (1992). *Multidimensional Self-Concept Scale.* Austin, TX: Pro-Ed.

Bracken B. (1998). *The Braken Basic Concept Scale-Revised.* San Antonio, TX: The Psychological Corporation.

Brickenkamp R & Zillmer E (1998). *d2 Test of Attention.* Seattle, WA: Hogrefe & Huber.

Brown L & Hammill DD (1990). *Behavior Rating Profile 2nd ed. (BRP-2).* Austin, TX: Pro-Ed.

Brown L & Leigh JE (1986). *Adaptive Behavior Inventory.* Austin, TX: Pro-Ed.

Brown L, Sherbenou RJ, & Johnsen SK (1997). *Test of Nonverbal Intelligence (TONI-3).* Austin, TX: Pro-Ed.

Brown TE (1996). *Brown Attention-Deficit Disorder Scales.* San Antonio, TX: The Psychological Corporation.

Brown VL, Cronin ME, & McEntire E (1994). *Test of Mathematical Abilities,* 2nd Ed. Austin, TX: Pro-Ed.

Brown VL, Hammill DD, & Wiederholt JL (1995). *Test of Reading Comprehension,* 3rd Ed. Austin, TX: Pro-Ed.

Bruininks RH, Woodcock RW, Weatherman RF, et al. (1996). *Scales of Independent Behavior-Revised.* Itasca, IL: Riverside.

Butcher JN, Williams CL, Graham JR, et al. (1992). *Minnesota Multiphasic Personality Inventory for Adolescents (MMPI-A): Manual for Administration, Scoring, and Interpretation.* Minneapolis, MN: University of Minnesota Press.

Canfield RL, Gendle MH, & Cory-Slechta DA (2004). Impaired neuropsychological functioning in lead-exposed children. Dev Neuropsychol 26:513–540.

Cattell P (1992). *Cattell Infant Intelligence Scale.* San Antonio, TX: The Psychological Corporation.

Catts HW, Gillispie M, Leonard LB, et al. (2002). The role of speed of processing, rapid naming, and phonological awareness in reading achievement. J Learn Disab 35:509–524.

Chadwick O & Rutter M (1983). Neuropsychological assessment. In: Rutter M, ed. *Developmental Neuropsychiatry.* New York: The Guilford Press, pp. 181–212.

Cohen M (1997). San Antonio, TX: Psychological Corporation.

Cohen MJ, Ricci CA, Kibby MY, & Edmonds JE (2000). Developmental progression of clock face drawing in children. Child Neuropsychol 6:64–76.

Conners CK (1985). *The Conners' Rating Scales.* Austin, TX: Pro-Ed.

Conners KC (2000). *Conners Continuous Performance Test.* San Antonio, TX: The Psychological Corporation.

Connor PD, Sampson PD, Bookstein FL, et al. (2000). Direct and indirect effects of prenatal alcohol damage on executive function. Dev Neuropsychol 18:331–354.

Delis DD, Kaplan E, & Kramer JH (2001). *Delis-Kaplan Executive Function System.* San Antonio, TX: Psychological Corporation.

Delis DC, Kramer JH, Kaplan E, & Ober BA California Verbal Learning Test-Second Edition (CVLT II). (1994). San Antonio, TX: The Psychological Corporation.

Denckla MB (1989). Executive function, the overlap zone between attention deficit hyperactivity disorder and learning disabilities. International Pediatr 4:155–160.

Denckla MB & Rudel RG (1976). Rapid "automatized" naming (R.A.N.): dyslexia differentiated from other learning disabilities. Neuropsychologia 14:471–479.

Diamond A, Prevor MB, Callender G, & Druin DP (1997). Prefrontal cortex cognitive deficits in children treated early and continuously for PKU. Monogr Soc Res Child Dev 62:i–v, 1–208.

Dimitrovsky I, Spector H, Levy-Shiff R, & Vakil E (1998). Interpretation of facial expressions of affect in children with learning disabilities with verbal or nonverbal deficits. J Learn Disabil 31:286–292, 312.

DiSimoni F (1978). *Token Test for Children: Manual.* Allen, TX: DLM Teaching Resources, 1978.

Doyle LW, Casalaz D, Victorian Infant Collaborative Study Group (2001). Outcome at 14 years of extremely low birth weight infants: a regional study. Arch Dis Child Fetal Neonatal Ed 85: F159–164.

Dunn LM & Dunn LM (1997). *Peabody Picture Vocabulary Test,* 3rd ed. Circle Pines, MN: American Guidance Service.

Eliez S, Antonarakis SE, Morris MA, Dahoun SP, & Reiss AL (2001). Parental origin of the deletion 22q11.2 and brain development in velocardiofacial syndrome: a preliminary study. Arch Gen Psychiatry 58:64–68.

Elliot CD (1990). *Differential Ability Scales.* San Antonio, TX: The Psychological Corporation.

Emslie H, Wilson C, Burden B, et al. (2004). *Behavioral Assessment of the Dysexecutive Syndrome for Children (BADS-C).* Lutz, FL: Psychological Assessment Resources.

Eslinger PJ & Biddle KR (2000). Adolescent neuropsychological development after early right prefrontal cortex damage. Dev Neuropsychol 18: 297–329.

Ewing-Cobbs L, Barnes MA, & Fletcher JM (2003). Early brain injury in children: development and reorganization of cognitive function. Dev Neuropsychol 24:669–704.

Exner JE (1982). *The Rorschach: A Comprehensive System,* Vols. 1–3. New York: Wiley.

Fennell EB (2000). Neuropsychological effects of end-stage renal disease. In: Yeates KO, Ris MD, & Taylor HG, eds. *Pediatric Neuropsychology: Research, Theory and Practice.* New York: The Guilford Press, pp. 366–380.

Finegan JA (1998). Study of behavioral phenotypes: goals and methodological considerations. Am J Med Genet 28:148–155.

Frankenburg WK, Dodds JB, Archer P, et al. (1992). The Denver II: a major revision and restandardization of the Denver Developmental Screening Test. Pediatrics 89:91–97.

Gardner M (1991). *Test of Visual-Perceptual Skills (Nonmotor), Revised.* North Tonawanda, NY: Multi-Health Systems.

German DJ (1989). National College of Education *Test of Word Finding-Second Edition.* Austin, TX: Pro-Ed.

Ghaziuddin M & Mountain-Kimchi K (2004). Defining the intellectual profile of Asperger Syndrome: comparison with high-functioning autism. J Autism Dev Disord 34:279–284.

Gibbs ED (1990). Assessment of infant mental ability: conventional tests and issues of prediction. In: Gibbs ED, Teti DM, eds. *Interdisciplinary Assessment of Infants: A Guide for Early Intervention Professionals.* Baltimore: Paul H Brookes, pp. 77–89.

Ginsburg HP & Baroody AJ (2003). *Test of Early Mathematics Ability,* 3rd Ed. Austin, TX: Pro-Ed.

Gioia GA, Isquith PK, Guy SC, & Kenworthy L (2000). *Behavior Rating Inventory of Executive Function.* Lutz, FL: Psychological Assessment Resources.

Goia GA, Isquith PK, Kenworthy L, & Barton RM (2002). Profiles of everyday executive function in acquired and developmental disorders. Neuropsychol Dev Cogn C Child Neuropsychol 8(2):121–137.

Golden CJ (1987). *Luria-Nebraska Neuropsychological Battery: Children's Revision.* Los Angeles, CA: Western Psychological Services.

Golden CJ, Freshwater SM, & Golden Z (2002). *Stroop Color and Word Test: Childrens Version.* Wood Dale, IL: Stoelting.

Gordon M (1983). *The Gordon Diagnostic System.* DeWitt, NY: Gordon Systems.

Gottlieb G (2001). The relevance of developmental-psychobiological metatheory to developmental neuropsychology. Dev Neuropsychol 19:1–9.

Green W, Allen LM III, & Astner K (1996). *The Word Memory Test: A user's guide to the oral and computer-administered forms. US Version 1.1.* Durham, NC: CogniSyst.

Greenberg L, Leark RA, Dupuy TR, et al. (1996). Tests of Variables of Attention (TOVA/TOVA-A): Clinical Guide. Los Alamitos, CA: Lutz, FL: Psychological Assessment Resources, Inc. Universal Attention Disorders.

Grigorenko EL, Klin A, Pauls DL, et al. (2002). A descriptive study of hyperlexia in a clinically referred sample of children with developmental delays. J Autism and Dev Disorders, 32:3–12.

Habib M (2000). The neurological basis of developmental dyslexia: an overview and working hypothesis. Brain 123: 2373–2399.

Hale TS, Hariri AR, & McCracken JT (2000). Attention-deficit/hyperactivity disorder: perspectives from neuroimaging. Ment Retard Dev Disabil Res Rev 6:214–219.

Halstead WC & Wepman JM (1959). The Halstead-Wepman Aphasia Screening Test. J Speech Hear Disord 14:9–15.

Hammill DD (1998). *Detroit Tests of Learning Aptitude 3.* Austin, TX: Pro-Ed.

Hammill DD & Larsen SC (1996). *Test of Written Language-Third Edition.* Austin, TX: Pro-Ed.

Hammill DD & Newcomer PL. (1999). *Test of Language Development-Intermediate: Third Edition (DLD-I3).* Austin, TX: Pro-Ed.

Hammill DD, Pearson NA, & Voress JK (1993). *Developmental Test of Visual Perception.* Austin, TX: Pro-Ed.

Hammill DD, Pearson NA, & Voress JK (1996). *Test of Visual Motor Integration.* Austin, TX: Pro-Ed.

Happe F & Frith U (1996). *The neuropsychology of autism.* Brain 119:1377–1400.

Harrison P & Oakland T (2003). *Adaptive Behavior Assessment System—second edition.* San Antonio, TX: The Psychological Corporation.

Heaton RK, Chelune GJ, Talley J, et al. (1993). *Wisconsin Card Sorting Test Manual.* Odessa, FL: Psychological Assessment Resources.

Hiemenz JR & Hynd GW (2000). Sulcal/gyral pattern of morphology of the perisylvian language region in developmental dyslexia. Brain Lang 74:113–133.

Hooper SR, Swartz CW, Wakely MB, et al. (2002). Executive functions in elementary school children with and without problems in written expression. J Learn Disab 35:57–68.

Hresko WP, Herron SR, & Peak PK (1996). *Test of Early Written Language, 2nd Ed. (TEWL-2).* Austin, TX: Pro-Ed.

Hresko WP, Reid DK, & Hammill DD (1991). *Test of Early Language Development,* 3rd ed. Austin, TX: Pro-Ed.

Ireton H (1992). *Child Development Inventory.* Minneapolis, MN: Behavior Science Systems.

Kaplan E (1990). The process approach to neuropsychological assessment of psychiatric patients. J Neuropsychiatry Clin Neurosci 2:72–87.

Kaplan EF, Goodglass H, & Weintraub S (1983). *Boston Naming Test,* 2nd ed. Philadelphia: Lea & Febiger.

Kaufman AS & Kaufman NL (2003). *Kaufman Test of Educational Achievement,* 2nd ed. (K-TEA-II). Circle Pines, MN: American Guidance Service.

Kaufman AS & Kaufman NL (2004). *KABC-II: Kaufman Assessment Battery for Children,* 2nd ed. Circle Pines, MN: American Guidance Service.

Keith RW (1994). *Auditory Continuous Performance Test.* San Antonio, TX: The Psychological Corporation.

Kertesz A (1982). *Western Aphasia Battery.* San Antonio, TX: The Psychological Corporation.

Korkman M (1999). Applying Luria's diagnostic principles in the neuropsychological assessment of children. Neuropsychol Rev 9:89–105.

Korkman M, Kirk U, & Kemp S (1998). *NEPSY: A Developmental Neuropsychological Assessment.* San Antonio, TX: The Psychological Corporation.

Kovacs M (1992). *Children's Depression Inventory (CDI).* Lutz, FL: Psychological Assessment Resources.

Lajiness-O'Neill R & Beaulieu I (2002). Neuropsychological findings in two children diagnosed with hamartoses: evidence of a NLD phenotypic profile. Neuropsychol Dev Cogn C Child Neuropsychol 8:27–40.

Lajiness-O'Neill RR, Beaulieu I, Titus JB, Asamoah A, Bigler ED, Bawle EV, & Pollack R (2005). Memory and learning in children with 22q11.2 deletion syndrome: evidence for ventral and dorsal stream disruption? Neuropsychol Dev Cogn Child Neuropsychol C 11:55–71.

Lambert NM, Nihira K, & Leland H (1993). *AAMR Adaptive Behavior Scale-School,* 2nd ed. (ABS-S:2). Washington, DC: American Association on Mental Retardation.

Levine MD (1987). *Developmental Variation and Learning Disorders.* Cambridge, MA: Educators Publishing Service.

Lewis BA, Freebairn LA, & Taylor HG (2000). Follow-up of children with early expressive phonology disorders. J Learn Disab 33:433–444.

Lezak MD (1995). *Neuropsychological Assessment,* 3rd ed. New York: Oxford University Press.

Lindamood PC & Lindamood P (2004). *Lindamood Auditory Conceptualization Test (LAC-3).* Circle Pines, MN: American Guidance Service.

Lord C, Rutter M, DiLavore PC, & Risi S (1999). *Autism Diagnostic Observation Schedule.* Los Angeles: Western Psychological Services.

Lord C, Rutter M, & Le Couteur A (1994). Autism Diagnostic Interview-Revised: a revised version of a diagnostic interview for caregivers of individuals with possible pervasive developmental disorders. J Autism Dev Disord 24:659–685.

Luria AR (1973). *The Working Brain: An Introduction to Neuropsychology* (B. Haigh, Trans.). London: Penguin.

Manly T, Robertson IH, Anderson V, & Nimmo-Smith I (1999). *Test of Everyday Attention for Children (TEA-Ch).* Bury St Edmunds, UK: Thames Valley Test.

Manor O, Shalev RE, Joseph A, & Gross-Tsur V (2001). Arithmetic skills in kindergarten children with developmental language disorders. Euro J Paediatr Neurol 5:71–77.

Markwardt FC (1998). *Peabody Individual Achievement Test-Revised (PIAT-R).* Circle Pines, MN: American Guidance Service.

Mather N & Woodcock RW (1989). *Woodcock-Johnson Tests of Achievement.* Allen, TX: DLM Teaching Resources.

Matthews CG & Klove H (1964). *Instruction Manual for the Adult Neuropsychology Test Battery.* Odessa, FL: Psychological Assessment Resources.

McCandliss BD & Noble KG (2003). The development of reading impairment: a cognitive neuroscience model. Ment Retard and Dev Disabil Res Rev 9:196–204.

McGhee R, Bryant BR, Larsen SC, et al. (1995). *Test of Written Expression.* Austin, TX: Pro-Ed.

Meyers JE & Meyers K (1996). *Rey Complex Figure Test and Recognition Trial (RCFT).* Lutz, FL: Psychological Assessment Resources.

Miller GA (1956). The magical number seven, plus or minus two: Some limits on our capacity for processing information. Psychological Review 63:81–97.

Miller LJ (1982). *Miller Assessment for Preschoolers.* San Antonio, TX: The Psychological Corporation.

Mullen EM (1995). *Mullen Scales of Early Learning.* Circle Pines, MN: American Guidance Service.

Naglieri JA, LeBuffe PA, & Pfeiffer SI (1994). *Devereux Scales of Mental Disorders.* San Antonio, TX: The Psychological Corporation.

Newborg J, Stock JR, & Wnek L (1984). *Battelle Developmental Inventory.* Allen, TX: DLM Teaching Resources.

Newcomer PL & Hammill DD (1988). *Test of Language Development-Primary,* 3rd ed. (TOLD-P3). Austin, TX: Pro-Ed.

Nichols S, Jones W, Roman MJ, et al. (2004). Mechanisms of verbal memory impairment in four neurodevelopmental disorders. Brain Lang 88:180–189.

Ozonoff S, Cook I, Coon H, et al. (2004). Performance on Cambridge Neuropsychological Test Automated Battery subtests sensitive to frontal lobe function in people with autistic disorder: evidence from the Collaborative Programs of Excellence in Autism network. J Autism Dev Disord 34:139–150.

Peavy GM, Salmon DP, Bear I, et al. (2001). Detection of mild cognitive deficits in Parkinson's disease patients with the WAIS-R NI. J Int Neuropsych Soc 7:535–543.

Pennington BR (2002). *The Development of Psychopathology. Nature and nurture.* New York: The Guilford Press.

Phillips CE, Jarrold C, Baddeley AD, et al. (2004). Comprehension of spatial language terms in Williams syndrome evidence for an interaction between domains of strength and weakness. Cortex 40:85–101.

Pulsifer MB & Aylward EH (1999). *Human Immunodeficiency Virus.* In: Yeates KO, Ris DH, & Taylor MD, eds. *Pediatric Neuropsychology: Research, Theory and Practice.* New York: The Guilford Press, pp. 381–404.

Rapin I (1998). Understanding childhood language disorders. Curr Opin in Pediatr 10:561–566.

Raven JC, Court JH, & Raven J (1986). *Manual for Raven's Progressive Matrices and Vocabulary Scales, Section 2: Coloured Progressive Matrices* (with U.S. norms). London: Lewis.

Reid DK, Hresko WP, & Hammill DD (2001). *Test of Early Reading Ability,* 3rd ed. Austin, TX: Pro-Ed.

Reitan RM & Herring, S. (1985). A short screening device for identification of cerebral dysfunction in children. J Clin Psychol 41:643–650.

Reitan RM & Wolfson D (1985). *The Halstead-Reitan Neuropsychological Test Battery.* Tucson, AZ: Neuropsychology Press.

Rescorla L (2002). Language and reading outcomes to age 9 in late-talking toddlers. J Speech Lang Hear Res 45:360–371.

Reynolds CR & Bigler ED (1994). *Test of Memory and Learning.* Austin, TX: Pro-Ed.

Reynolds CR & Richmond BO (1997). *Revised Children's Manifest Anxiety Scale (RCMAS).* Los Angeles, CA: Western Psychological Services.

Reynolds WM (2004). *Reynolds Adolescent Depression Scale,* 2nd ed. (RADS-2). Lutz, FL: Psychological Assessment Resources.

Ris MD (2003). Causal inference in lead research: introduction to the special section on the neurobehavioral effects of environmental lead. Neuropsychol Dev Cogn C Child Neuropsychol 9:1–9.

Roid GH & Miller LJ (1997). *Leiter International Performance Scale-Revised.* Los Angeles: Western Psychological Services.

Ross J, Zinn A, & McCauley E (2000). Neurodevelopmental and psychosocial aspects of Turner syndrome. Ment Retard Dev Disabil Res Rev 6:135–141.

Roth RM & Saykin AJ (2004). Executive dysfunction in attention-deficit/hyperactivity disorder cognitive and neuroimaging findings. Psychiatr Clin North Am 27:83–96.

Rourke BP (1995). *Syndrome of Nonverbal Learning Disabilities. Neurodevelopmental manifestations.* New York: The Guilford Press.

Rourke BP, Ahmad SA, Collins DW, et al. (2002a). Child clinical/pediatric neuropsychology: some recent advances. Ann Rev Psychol 53:309–339.

Rourke BP, van der Vlut H, & Rourke SB (2002b). *Practice of Child-Clinical Neuropsychology.* Lisse, Netherlands: Swets & Zeitlinger.

Rudel R & Denckla MB (1974). Relationship of forward and backward digit repetition to neurological impairment in children with learning disabilities. Neuropsychologia 12:109–118.

Sandler AD, Watson TE, Footo M, et al. (1992). Neurodevelopmental study of writing disorders in middle childhood. J Dev Behav Pediatr 13:17–23.

Schoenberg BS, Mellinger JF, Schoenberg DG (1978). Cerebrovascular disease in infants and children: a study of incidence, clinical features, and survival. Neurology 28:763–768.

Sreenan C, Bhargava R, & Robertson CM (2000). Cerebral infarction in the term newborn: clinical presentation and long-term outcome. J Pediatr 137:351–355.

Semel EM, Wiig EH, & Secord WA (2003). *Clinical Evaluation of Language Fundamentals.* San Antonio, TX: The Psychological Corporation.

Shalev RS & Gross-Tsur V (2001). Developmental dyscalculia. Pediatr Neurol 24:337–342.

Shevell M, Ashwal S, Donley D, et al. (2003). Practice parameter: Evaluation of the child with global developmental delay. Neurol 60:367–380.

Slosson RL, Nicholson CL, & Hibpshman T (1991). *Slosson Intelligence Test-Revised 3 (SITR3) for Children and Adults.* North Tonawanda, NY: Multi-Health Systems.

Smith A (1982). *Symbol Digit Modalities Test: Manual.* Los Angeles: Western Psychological Services.

Sparrow SS, Balla DA, & Cicchetti DV (1984). *Vineland Adaptive Behavior Scales.* Circle Pines, MN: American Guidance Service.

Sporns O, Chialvo DR, Kaiser M, & Hilgetag CC (2004). Organization, development and function of complex brain networks. Trends Cogn Neurosci 8:418–425.

Spreen O, Risser AH, & Edgell D (1995). *Developmental Neuropsychology.* New York: Oxford University Press.

Spreen O & Strauss E (1998). *A Compendium of Neuropsychological Tests,* 2nd ed. New York: Oxford University Press.

Stein MT, Klin A, & Miller K. (2004). When Asperger's syndrome and a nonverbal learning disability look alike. J Dev Behav Pediatr 25:S59–S64.

Stiles J, Moses P, Roe K, et al. (2003). Alternative brain organization after prenatal cerebral injury: convergent fMRI and cognitive data. J Int Neuropsychol Soc 9:604–622.

Stuebing KK, Fletcher JM, LeDoux JM, et al. (2002). Validity of IQ discrepancy classifications of reading disability: A meta-analysis. Amer Ed Res J 30:469–518.

Taylor HG, Minich NM, Klein N, & Hack M (2004). Longitudinal Outcomes of very low birthweight: neuropsychological findings. J Int Neuropsychol Soc 10:149–163.

Temple E (2002). Brain mechanisms in normal and dyslexic readers. Curr Opin Neurobiol 12:178–183.

Thelen E (1995). Motor development: A new synthesis. Am Psychol 50:79–95.

Thorndike RL, Hagen EP, & Sattler JM (2003). *Guide for Administering and Scoring the Stanford-Binet Intelligence Scale,* 4th ed. Chicago: Riverside.

Tiffin J (1968). *Purdue Pegboard Examiner's Manual.* Rosemont, IL: London House.

Trask C, Kosofsky BE (2000). Developmental considerations of neurotoxic exposure. Neurol Clin 18:541–562.

Vargha-Khadem F, Salmond CH, Watkins KE, et al. (2003). Developmental amnesia: effect of age at injury. Proc Natl Acad Sci USA 100:10055–10060.

Vellutino FR, Scanlon DM, & Lyon GR (2000). Differentiating between difficult-to-remediate and readily remediated poor readers: more evidence against the IQ-achievement discrepancy definition and reading disability. J Learn Dis 33:223–238.

Volkmar FR, Lord C, Bailey A, et al. (2004). Autism and pervasive developmental disorders. J Child Psychol Psychiatry 45:135–170.

Wade SL, Taylor HG, Drotar D, et al. (2003). Parent-adolescent interactions after traumatic brain injury: the relationship to family adaptation and adolescent adjustment. J Head Trauma Rehabil 18:164–176.

Wagner R, Torgesen JK, & Rushotte C (1999). *Comprehensive Test of Phonological Processing.* Austin, TX.: Pro-Ed.

Wallace G, Hammill DD (1994). *Comprehensive Receptive and Expressive Vocabulary Test,* 2nd ed. Austin, TX: Pro-Ed.

Wechsler D. (1997a). *Wechsler Adult Intelligence Scale,* 3rd ed. San Antonio, TX: Harcourt Assessment.

Wechsler D (1997b). *Wechsler Memory Scale Revised.* San Antonio, TX: The Psychological Corporation.

Wechsler D (2001). *Wechsler Individual Achievement Test.* San Antonio, TX: The Psychological Corporation.

Wechsler D (2002). *Manual for the Wechsler Preschool and Primary Scale of Intelligence,* 3rd ed. San Antonio, TX: Psychological Corporation.

Wechsler D (2003). *Manual for the Wechsler Intelligence Scale for Children,* 4th ed. San Antonio, TX: The Psychological Corporation.

Welsh MC, Pennington BF, & Groisser DB (1991). A normative-developmental study of executive function: A window on prefrontal function in children. Developmental Neuropsychology 7:131–49.

Wiederholt JL & Bryant BR (2001). *Gray Oral Reading Test-Third Edition.* Austin, TX: Pro-Ed.

Wilkinson GS (1993). *Wide Range Achievement Test Revised.* Wilmington, DE: Jastak Associates.

Williams J & Sharp GB (2000). *Epilepsy.* In: Yeates KO, Ris MD, & Taylor HG, eds. *Pediatric Neuropsychology: Research, Theory and Practice.* New York: The Guilford Press, p8. 47–73.

Wilson B, Cockburn J, & Baddeley A (1991). *Rivermead Behavioural Memory Test.* Los Angeles: Western Psychological Services.

Wirt RD, Lachar D, Klinedinst JK, et al. (2001). *Multidimensional Description of Child Personality: A Manual for the Personality Inventory for Children-Revised.* Los Angeles: Western Psychological Services.

Woodcock RW, McGrew KS, & Mather N (2001). *Woodcock-Johnson Tests of Cognitive Abilities (WJ-III).* Allen, TX: DLM Teaching Resources.

Wooden M, Wang PP, Aleman D, et al. (2001). Neuropsychological profile of children and adolescents with the 22q11.2 microdeletion. Genetic Medicine 3:34–39.

Yeates KO, Ris MD, & Taylor HG (1999). *Pediatric Neuropsychology: Research, Theory and Practice.* New York: The Guilford Press.

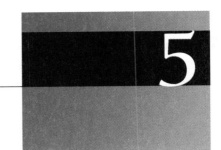

Anatomic Imaging of the Developing Human Brain

Jay N. Giedd, MD

Many neuropsychiatric disorders of childhood may reflect subtle deviations in the normal development of the brain. Adult psychiatric illnesses, such as schizophrenia, are also increasingly being viewed from a neurodevelopmental perspective (Bloom 1993; Weinberger 1995).

Understanding of the relationship between abnormal brain development and developmental neuropsychiatric disorders has been challenged by nature's efforts to protect this most vital organ. Wrapped in a tough leathery membrane, immersed in fluid, and completed encased by bone, the brain's protective system has long served to thwart environmental insults, but it has also posed considerable obstacles for those studying the brain. Fortunately, advances in neuroimaging technology now provide an unprecedented opportunity to examine in vivo brain structure and function.

To meaningfully assess pathologic deviations it is imperative to first characterize the normal pathways of brain development. Postmortem data are of limited availability since the mortality rate is low for this age group and autopsies are infrequently performed. For example, only 13 of 483 "normal" brains in the Yakovlev Brain Collection in Washington, D.C., are from subjects aged 3 to 18 years. The use of ionizing radiation for in vivo imaging techniques, such as conventional radiography, computerized tomography (CT), or positron emission tomography, render them unsuitable for the study of normal pediatric populations.

Magnetic resonance imaging (MRI) provides many advantages for in vivo imaging studies. In addition to absence of ionizing radiation, MRI offers the capability to acquire images in any plane of view; provides excellent spatial resolution and the ability to discriminate gray matter, white matter, and cerebrospinal fluid; has the flexibility to assess a variety of tissue characteristics (as opposed to relying solely on patency to radiographs); and can be used to visualize structures (temporal lobes, frontal lobes, posterior fossa) often obscured by interference from bone on CT scans. The lack of ionizing radiation with MRI also allows sequential exams, which is very desirable for developmental studies. These factors make MRI the imaging modality of choice for most pediatric neuroimaging studies.

In this chapter, which focuses on normal brain development from ages 4 to 18 years, we discuss methodologic issues relevant to pediatric neuroimaging, review previous imaging studies of normal development with emphasis on the National Institute of Mental Health (NIMH) Pediatric Brain MRI project, and conclude with a discussion of developmental changes in brain anatomy as they relate to the study of pediatric neuropsychiatry.

METHODOLOGICAL CONSIDERATIONS

Subject Selection

Clinically Referred Versus Community Recruited Subjects

The common practice of deriving normative measures from children referred for clinical reasons whose scans were subsequently read as "normal" is problematic on at least two counts. First, children referred for clinical scans are overrepresented in clinical groups, such as attention-deficit/hyperactivity disorder (ADHD). Second, a small but perhaps meaningful number of healthy children may have scans read as abnormal and excluding these subjects confounds comparisons to clinical groups. Recruitment of healthy subjects directly from the community provides a more appropriate sample to assess normal development.

Psychiatric History

Abnormalities of brain structure have been observed in a number of pediatric neuropsychiatric illnesses, including autism (Brambilla et al. 2003), ADHD (Giedd et al. 2001), childhood-onset schizophrenia (Giedd et al. 1999; Gogtay et al. 2004; Keller et al. 2003; Sporn et al. 2003), dyslexia (Duara et al. 1991; Eckert and Leonard 2000; Eckert et al. 2003; Hynd and Semrud-Clikeman 1989; Hynd et al. 1990; Larsen et al. 1990; Rae et al. 2002; Rumsey et al. 1986), eating disorders (Laessle et al. 1989), obsessive compulsive disorder (Giedd et al. 1996), Sydenham's chorea (Giedd et al. 1995), and Tourette's syndrome (Peterson et al. 1993, 1994, 2000). It is evident that a normative sample must be carefully screened to rule out these conditions. Likewise, affective disorders (Coffey et al. 1993) and substance abuse (Cascella et al. 1991; Lishman 1990) have been associated with structural anomalies in adults and should be considered as potential confounds in pediatric samples as well.

Intelligence

Studies have found small but statistically significant relationships between brain size and intelligence (Andreasen et al. 1993; Reiss et al. 1996; Willerman et al. 1991). Although in the most robust of these findings IQ accounts for only 17% of the variance (Andreasen et al. 1993), this parameter should be considered in any group comparison. Education and socioeconomic status have been reported to influence brain size as well, although the interdependence with factors such as nutrition, prenatal care, and IQ is not clear.

Handedness

Beginning with Geschwind, several investigators have noted a relationship between handedness and structural or symmetry measures of the brain (Geschwind 1978; Kertesz et al. 1992; Witelson 1989). Handedness should not be viewed as strictly left or right, but as a continuum (Coffey et al. 1992) and quantified as such. Patient and control groups must be matched for handedness since symmetry differences are often key features in discriminating groups such as ADHD (Giedd et al. 2001), dyslexia (Hynd 1990, et al. Larsen et al. 1990), or Tourette's disorder (Peterson et al. 1993, 1994, 2000).

Body Size

The relationship between brain size and body size in humans is surprisingly poor (Harvey and Krebs 1990). In contrast to the relative stability of brain weight after childhood, body weight varies widely among individuals and can vary substantially within individuals from time to time. Height is also a poor indicator of brain size as can be implied by contrasting the notable increases in height from ages 4 to 18 years with the lack of corresponding increase in brain size. This general trend for the young to have disproportionately large head-to-height ratios compared to adults, termed neonatogony, is widely observed throughout the mammalian species.

Image Acquisition

General Considerations

MRI can provide excellent resolution between gray matter, white matter, and cerebrospinal fluid (CSF). This capacity is critical for quantitative anatomical studies since such contrasts define the boundaries of most brain structures. Generally, resolution can be purchased with the currency of time; that is, improvements in image quality must be weighed against patient discomfort from prolonged time in the scanner. Most children can tolerate scan times between 45 minutes and 1 hour.

The discomforts associated with getting an MRI scan are potential feelings of claustrophobia from being placed in the tunnel-like barrel of the scanner, the loud noise generated by rapid heating and cooling of gradient coils, and the need to remain relatively still during the approximately 10-minute intervals of image acquisition.

Although sedation is not an ethical option in acquiring scans of healthy children, several nonpharmacological steps may be taken to minimize these discomforts in a pediatric population. Allowing the child to become familiar and comfortable with the staff conducting the scan, scanning in the evening to promote the natural falling asleep, allowing the child to bring in a favorite blanket or stuffed animal, and assuring the children that they may stop the procedure at any time can all increase the chances of acquiring adequate scans and make the experience more enjoyable for the child.

Slice thickness is an important parameter in MRI scans. Greater slice thickness results in larger partial voluming effects and in less spatial resolution, especially critical for small but clinically pertinent subcortical structures.

The use of multichannel versus single-channel scanning protocols is another factor to consider in image acquisition. Multichannel scanning protocols provide nearly simultaneously acquired spatially registered image sets that highlight different tissue characteristics. The most common multichannel scanning protocol is one that combines a sequence best for identifying tissue pathology and white matter lesions (T2-weighted) with one that provides optimal discrimination between brain tissue and CSF (proton density weighted). The advantage of multichannel acquisition is that by combining information from the image sets, automated computer programs can maximally discriminate gray matter, white matter, and CSF (Rajapakse et al. 1996).

The disadvantage to multichannel images is that they characteristically have greater slice thickness (5 mm or greater). The most common single-channel sequences yield T1-weighted images, which are well suited for providing anatomical detail.

Functional MRI

Functional MRI takes advantage of the fact that oxygenated hemoglobin has different magnetic properties than deoxygenated hemoglobin. This difference provides a natural contrast agent that can be detected by a properly configured MR scanner. As neuronal activity increases metabolic demands trigger an increase of blood flow to that area. By comparing blood flow while the subject performs an experimental task with blood flow during a passive control condition, images of brain activity can be generated. Both spatial (1 mm) and temporal (5 to 7 seconds, limited by blood flow characteristics) resolution far surpass the capabilities of Positron Emission Tomography (PET). The potential to study dynamic activity of the brain in real time without the use of ionizing radiation offers great promise for pediatric studies (Casey 1995, 1996).

Image Analysis

General Considerations

Validation of MR image analysis techniques is hindered by lack of an absolute gold standard. Postmortem data, even if more abundant, are less than ideal on several counts. When removed from the intracranial cavity and the cerebrospinal fluid in which it is immersed, the brain collapses on its own weight, distorting in vivo morphology. Fixation and drying processes affect different brain structures to different degrees with gray matter and white matter shrinking at separate rates. Also, age itself is a confound, since younger brains have higher water content and are differentially affected by fixation processes.

Studies using models that mimic the shape and tissue characteristics of the human brain can be useful, but valid models are difficult to construct. The standard for validation of automated measures for the quantification of many structures remains a comparison to results obtained from manual tracing by expert human raters.

MR image data are in the form of pixels (picture elements) or their three-dimensional counterpart voxels (volume elements). Each of these elements may have only one intensity value. At the time of image acquisition, these values may range from 1 to 65,536 (2^{16}). However, to reduce the memory requirements for computation, most image analysis systems restrict this intensity value range to 256 (2^8). A general goal of structural image analysis is to classify each voxel in the image data set according to tissue characteristic (e.g., gray matter, white matter, CSF, vasculature), as well as to assign it to the structure or region in which it belongs.

Sample Size/Longitudinal Study Design

The enormous normal variability in size of brain structures calls for large samples and longitudinal study designs to characterize the heterochronous developmental changes of the pediatric population. Fortunately, the feasibility of longitudinal studies is supported by the relative stability of morphologic measures from scans acquired at 2- to 4-week intervals (Giedd et al. 1995). This stability indicates that quantitative differences in longitudinal scans are reflections of genuine changes in brain structure and not from variability related to the scan acquisition itself.

DETERMINATES OF BRAIN SIZE

Human brain development, like central nervous system development in all vertebrates, takes place by an overproduction and then selective elimination of cells. The size of a given brain structure is determined by the size, number, and packing density of its constituent cells. The majority of dynamic brain development takes place in utero; however, changes in brain structure and function continue throughout the life span (see Fig. 5.1).

Brain cells are of two general types: neurons and glial cells. Although neuronal number peaks during gestation (Rabinowicz 1986), neuronal size changes with age (Blinkov and Glezer 1968) as axonal thickness, dendritic number, and number of synaptic connections undergo cyclic changes throughout development (Thatcher 1992). Environmental factors influence which synaptic connections and neurons thrive and remain viable. For instance, in children with cataracts who do not receive treatment prior to age 1, irreversible cortical blindness occurs (Lewis et al. 1986).

Synaptic pruning of neurons is an important aspect in the functional development of the brain but may have little impact on overall structure size. Estimates from research on the primary visual cortex of the macaque monkey indicate that a total loss of all boutons would result in only a 1% to 2% decrease in volume (Bourgeois and Rakic 1993). However, synaptic pruning may have an effect on the thickness of the parent axon or dendritic branches.

The other main class of CNS cells is made up of the glial cells, which unlike neurons continue to actively proliferate and die postnatally. Glial cells outnumber neurons by ratios ranging from 1.7 to 10 (Brizzee et al. 1964). Myelination by a subclass of glial cells, oligodendrocytes, is an important determinant of increases in structure size during childhood and adolescence. Ultimate structure size is determined by this dynamic interplay between glial cells and decreasing numbers but increases in size of neurons.

Another parameter to consider in structure size is packing density, which is influenced by degree of vascularity, extracellular volume, and hydration. Genetics, hormones, growth factors, nutrients in the developing nervous system, diet, infections, toxins, trauma, stress, or degree of enriched

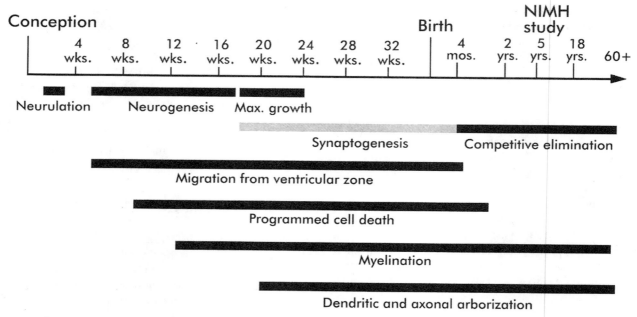

Figure 5.1 Time course of critical events in the determination of human brain morphometry.

environment (Diamond et al. 1964; Jacobson 1991) all have a role in determining structure size and the complexity of these factors and their interactions should be considered in any interpretation of the clinical significance of gross structural volume.

SUMMARY OF PREVIOUS STUDIES

More than 1,000 studies have been reported regarding brain MRI in fetuses or infants. However, only a handful of brain MRI studies have assessed healthy children from the ages of 4 to 18 years. In one study (Jernigan et al. 1991) of 23 males and 16 females, ages 8 to 35 years, both cortical and subcortical gray matter decreased with age, and cerebrospinal fluid (CSF) volumes increased with age. Another study of 88 clinically referred subjects, ages 3 months to 30 years, also found age-related decreases in gray matter, as well as increases in cortical white matter, but no changes in CSF volume (Pfefferbaum et al. 1994).

Postmortem studies or PET studies of this age group are equally rare. A postmortem study including subjects aged 3, 5, 11, and 13 years indicated developmental changes in synaptic density, neuronal density, and dendritic arborization occurring at least up until adolescence (Huttenlocher 1990). PET studies also indicate dynamic changes throughout development with cerebral metabolic rates rising rapidly during the first years of life, maintaining higher-than-adult levels throughout childhood, and declining to adult levels during adolescence (Chugani et al. 1987).

NATIONAL INSTITUTE OF MENTAL HEALTH PEDIATRIC NEUROIMAGING PROJECT

The child psychiatry branch of the NIMH is conducting an ongoing brain imaging project to assess the hypothesis that many of the most severe neuropsychiatric disorders of childhood-onset are associated with deviations from normal brain development, the anatomical substrates of which may be detectable by MRI. The study includes twin and nontwin healthy controls and subjects from a variety of diagnostic groups. Longitudinal scans are acquired at approximately 2-year intervals.

The healthy control subjects are recruited from the community and undergo screening including physical and neurological exams, clinical interviews and family history assessment, and an extensive neuropsychologic battery. Approximately one in six initial contacts are accepted for the study. For this chapter, only nontwin healthy subjects are used and only one subject from each family. The resulting sample is 329 scans from 95 boys and 66 girls (longitudinal scans acquired at approximately 2-year intervals) across ages 4 to 20 years.

Once the images are acquired, they are analyzed by a variety of automated and manual tracing techniques through collaboration with several imaging centers throughout the world. Further details of the testing and screening of this sample and the methods of image analysis are published elsewhere (Chung et al. 2001; Giedd et al. 1999; Zijdenbos et al. 1994).

Brain Maturational Changes During Childhood and Adolescence

Total Cerebral Volume

In the longitudinal NIMH sample, the total cerebral volume of children and adolescents remained relatively stable across ages 4 to 20 years (Fig. 5.2). This is consistent with our previous cross-sectional studies (Giedd et al. 1996) and postmortem studies indicating the brain is approximately 95% of its adult size by age 5 years (Dekaban 1977; Dekaban and Sadowsky 1978). However, the finding is counterintuitive to anyone who has tried putting an adult's hat on a 5-year-old and watched it fall down over the child's eyes. Indeed, head circumference does increase from age 4 to 18 years (approximately, 2.0 inches in boys and 1.9 inches in girls) (Nellhaus 1968), but this is accounted for by an increase in skull thickness (Shapiro and Janzen 1960) and less so by an increase in ventricular volume. Although total cerebral volume remains relatively constant, various subcomponents of the brain do undergo significant age-related changes (see Fig. 5.2).

Male brains were approximately 12% larger on average than those of females. This difference was statistically significant, even when controlling for height and weight. Of course, gross size of structures may not reflect sexually dimorphic differences in neuronal connectivity or receptor density. Given the myriad of parameters influencing brain size, size alone should not be interpreted as imparting any sort of functional advantage or disadvantage.

Ventricles

In the NIMH sample, lateral ventricular volume increased robustly with age (see Fig. 5.2), a fact not widely appreciated for children and adolescents. This pattern is noteworthy in light of the fact that increased ventricular volumes, or ventricular-to-brain ratios, are associated in a nonspecific fashion with a broad range of neuropsychiatric conditions. That this phenomenon is a normally occurring event in healthy adolescents adds to the complexity of interpreting changes in ventricular volume in patient populations.

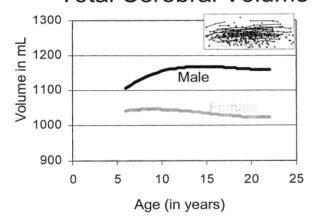

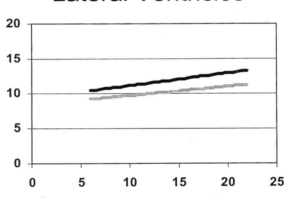

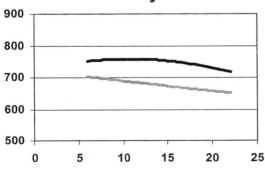

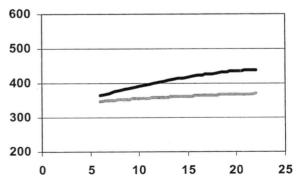

Figure 5.2 Changes in volume of the total cerebral, lateral ventricles, total gray matter, and total white matter derived from 329 scans of 95 boys and 66 girls (longitudinal scans acquired at approximately 2-year intervals) across ages 4 to 20 years.

Frontal White Matter

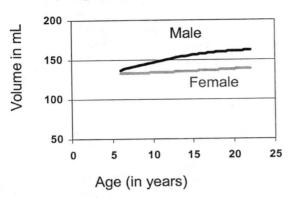

Temporal White Matter

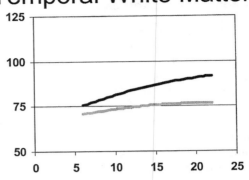

Parietal White Matter

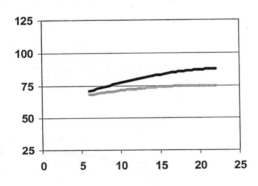

Corpus Callosum

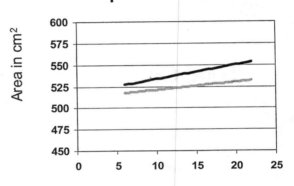

Figure 5.3 White matter volume changes in the frontal lobes, temporal lobes, parietal lobes, and the midsagittal cross-ectional area of the corpus callosum from 329 scans of 95 boys and 66 girls (longitudinal scans acquired at approximately 2-year intervals) across ages 4 to 20 years.

White Matter

Regional Volumes of White Matter

On MRI scans, white matter indicates myelinated axons. Throughout childhood and adolescence the amount of white matter in the brain generally increases (see Fig. 5.2). The white matter increases are roughly linear and the slope of increase is approximately the same in the frontal, temporal, and parietal lobes (Fig. 5.3).

Corpus Callosum

The corpus callosum is the most prominent white matter structure consisting of approximately 200 million myelinated fibers, most of which connect homologous areas of the left and right cortex. The midsagittal cross-sectional area of the corpus callosum is easily visualized on MRI scans, which along with its clinical interest has made it a frequent target of investigations. The organization of the corpus callosum is roughly topographic with anterior segments containing fibers from the anterior cortical regions, middle segments containing fibers from the middle cortical regions, and so on. Several studies have indicated that development of the corpus callosum continues to progress throughout adolescence (Allen et al. 1991; Cowell et al. 1992; Pujol et al. 1993; Rauch and Jenkins 1994), and anomalous corpus callosal morphology has been reported in several disorders manifesting in childhood (Bigelow et al. 1983; Giedd et al. 1994; Hynd et al.1990, 1991; Njiokiktjien 1991; Peterson et al. 1994; Parashos et al. 1995; Rosenthal and Bigelow 1972). Effects of sex have been widely debated with some authors finding gender-related differences (Clarke et al. 1989; Cowell et al. 1992; de Lacoste 1986; Holloway and de Lacoste 1986), while many have not (Bell and Variend 1985; Byne et al. 1988; Oppenheim et al. 1987; Weis et al. 1988, 1989; Witelson 1985a, 1985b). In the NIMH sample, total midsagittal corpus callosum area increased robustly from ages 4 to 18 years, but there were no significant gender effects (see Fig. 5.3).

The functions of the corpus callosum can generally be thought of as integrating the activities of the left and right cerebral hemispheres and include unifying sensory fields (Berlucchi 1981; Shanks et al. 1975), facilitating memory storage and retrieval (Zaidel and Sperry 1974), allocating attention and arousal (Levy 1985), and enhancing language and auditory functions (Cook 1986). The relationship between improved capacities for these functions during childhood and adolescence and the noted morphologic changes is intriguing. Creativity and intelligence have been linked to efficiency of interhemispheric integration (Bogen and Bogan 1969), and interhemispheric integration becomes more critical as task difficulty increases (Hellige et al. 1979; Levy and Trevarthen 1981).

Gray Matter

Cortical Gray Matter

Unlike white matter increases, which tend to be mostly linear, cortical gray matter volume tends to follow an "inverted U" developmental course with different peak volumes in different lobes (Fig. 5.4). For example, frontal lobe gray matter reaches its maximal thickness at 11 years in girls and 12.1 years in boys. Temporal lobe cortical gray matter peaks at 16.7 years in girls and 16.2 years in boys. Parietal lobe cortical gray matter peaks at 10.2 years in girls and 11.8 years in boys (Giedd et al. 1999).

The thickening and thinning of gray matter is thought to reflect changes in the size and complexity of neurons, not a change in the actual number. The increasing size may reflect a process called arborization as the cells grows extra branches, twigs, and roots, growing bushier and making a greater number of connections to other cells. The decreasing amount of gray matter may reflect the process of pruning where certain connections are eliminated.

The forces guiding these processes of arborization and pruning are not well understood. Genetics, nutrition, toxins, bacteria, viruses, hormones, and many other factors have been shown to have an effect. One hypothesis for the pruning phase is the "use it or lose it" principle in which those connections that are used well survive and flourish, whereas those connections that are not used will wither and die. If

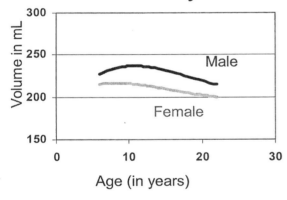

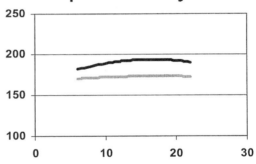

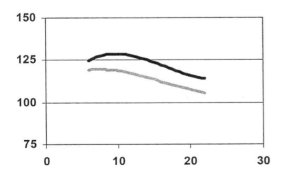

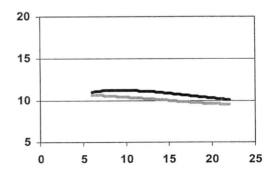

Figure 5.4 Gray matter volume changes in the frontal lobes, temporal lobes, parietal lobes, and caudate nucleus from 329 scans of 95 boys and 66 girls (longitudinal scans acquired at approximately 2-year intervals) across ages 4 to 20 years.

this hypothesis is correct, the activities of the child or teen may have a powerful influence on the ultimate physical structure of the brain.

To examine cortical gray matter development with greater regional specificity we examined the change in gray matter density on a voxel-by-voxel basis in a group of 13 subjects who had each been scanned four times at approximately 2-year intervals (Gogtay et al. 2004). An animation of these changes is available at www.loni.ucla.edu/~thompson/DEVEL/dynamic.html.

As gray matter volume reaches its maximum at about the time of puberty, a reduction in cortical gray matter volume is interpreted as maturation, in the sense that is becoming closer to the adult state. Cortical gray matter loss occurs earliest in the primary sensorimotor areas and latest in the dorsolateral prefrontal cortex (DLPFC) and superior temporal gyrus. The general pattern is for those regions subserving primary functions, such as motor and sensory systems, to mature earliest and the higher order association areas, which integrate those primary functions to mature later. For instance, in the temporal lobes the latest part to mature is the superior temporal gyrus/sulcas, which serves as a heteromodal association site integrating memory, audiovisual input, and object recognition functions (along with prefrontal and inferior parietal cortices) (Calvert 2001; Martin and Chao 2001; Mesulam 1998).

Subcortical Gray Matter

Basal Ganglia

The basal ganglia consist of the caudate, putamen, globus pallidus, subthalamic nucleus, and substantia nigra. Of these only the first three are readily quantifiable by MRI. In addition to their central role in control of movement and muscle tone, basal ganglia structures are also involved in circuits mediating higher cognitive functions, attention, and affective states.

Caudate volumes decreased significantly from ages 4 to 20 years (see Fig. 5.4). Caudate nucleus volume differences have been reported for several pediatric neuropsychiatric disorders such as ADHD (Castellanos et al. 1996; Giedd et al. 1994; Hynd et al. 1993), early onset schizophrenia (Chakos et al. 1994; Frazier et al. 1996; Keshavan et al. 1994), Sydenham's chorea (Giedd et al. 1995), and Tourette's syndrome (Peterson 1993, 2000; Singer et al. 1993).

Amygdala and Hippocampus

The temporal lobes, amygdala, and hippocampus are integral players in the arenas of emotion, language, and memory (Nolte 1993). Human capacity for these functions changes markedly between the ages of 4 and 18 years (Diener et al. 1985; Jerslid 1963; Wechsler 1974), although the relationship between the development of these capacities and morphological changes in the structures subserving these functions is poorly understood.

The amygdala and hippocampus have not been quantified for the longitudinal sample. In a previous report from a cross-sectional sample subset of the NIMH sample, amygdala volume increased significantly only in males and hippocampal volume increased significantly with age only in females (Giedd et al. 1996). This pattern of gender-specific maturational volumetric changes is consistent with nonhuman primate studies indicating that the amygdala contains high numbers of androgen receptors (Clark et al. 1988) and a smaller number of estrogen receptors (Sholl and Kim 1989), while the hippocampus contains higher amounts of estrogen receptors (Morse et al. 1986).

Influence of estrogen on the hippocampus is further supported by both rodent and human studies. Gonadectomized female rats have lower density of dendritic spines and decreased fiber outgrowth in the hippocampus, which can be alleviated with hormone replacement (Gould et al. 1990; Morse et al. 1986). In humans, women with gonadal hypoplasia have smaller hippocampi (Murphy et al. 1993). A MRI study of 20 young adults also showed proportionately larger hippocampal volumes in females (Filipek et al. 1994).

Further support for these findings is provided by a postmortem study of hippocampal volume in 164 psychiatrically normal individuals, ages newborn to 76 years, which revealed ongoing myelination in the subicular and presubicular regions of the hippocampus throughout adolescence and into adulthood (Benes et al. 1994). A sexually dimorphic effect was also noted in this postmortem study, with females showing a greater degree of myelin staining from 6 to 29 years, but with no significant differences thereafter.

RELATIONSHIP BETWEEN BRAIN STRUCTURE AND BEHAVIOR

Because even the simplest of tasks eventually involves the majority of brain systems, it is not surprising that straightforward relationships between volumes of a single structure and performance on a particular cognitive task are not usually found. The diversity of afferent and efferent connections to the many distinct nuclei of most structures as well as the intricacy of their various neurochemical systems further complicates functional correlates of gross volume size.

Despite this complexity, relationships between memory function and hippocampal size have been noted. For instance, food-storing species of birds have larger hippocampi than related nonfood-storing species (Krebs et al. 1989; Sherry et al. 1989). This relationship has been found in mammals as well, particularly for voles. Male voles of the polygamous species travel far and wide in search of mates. They perform better than their female counterparts on laboratory measures of spatial ability and have significantly larger hippocampi (Sherry et al. 1992). Conversely, in the monogamous vole species, which do not show male-female differences in spatial ability, no sexual dimorphism of hippocampal size is seen (Jacobs et al. 1990). In humans also, correlations between memory for stories and left hippocampal volume have been noted (Goldberg et al. 1994; Lencz et al. 1992).

A sizable literature has addressed cognitive ability/brain structure relationships in patients with dementia. However, literature regarding healthy subjects has been sparse, and results have been conflicting (Coffey 1994).

CONCLUSION

Although total cerebral volume approaches adult sizes at a young age (5 to 8 years), developmental changes in various subcomponents of the brain across childhood and adolescence are striking. Indeed, examination of maturational changes in several regions throughout the brain indicates a dynamic balance achieved between growth and regression throughout childhood and adolescence. In particular, changes are noted in basal ganglia structures, the lateral ventricles, the amygdala, and the hippocampus. It is of note that structures undergoing the most robust developmental changes are by and large the same structures implicated in neuropsychiatric disorders of childhood onset (Castellanos et al. 1994; Frazier et al. 1996; Hynd et al. 1990, 1991, 1993; Semrud-Clikeman et al. 1994; Singer et al. 1993).

REFERENCES

Allen LS, Richey MF, Chai YM, Gorski RA. Sex differences in the corpus callosum of the living human being. *J Neurosci* 1991;11:933–942.

Andreasen NC, Flaum M, Swayze V, 2nd, et al. Intelligence and brain structure in normal individuals. *Am J Psychiatry* 1993;150:130–134.

Bell AD, Variend S. Failure to demonstrate sexual dimorphism of the corpus callosum in childhood. *J Anat* 1985;143:143–147.

Benes FM, Turtle M, Khan Y, Farol P. Myelination of a key relay zone in the hippocampal formation occurs in the human brain during childhood, adolescence, and adulthood. *Arch Gen Psychiatry.* 1994;51:477–484.

Berlucchi G. Interhemispheric asymmetries in visual discrimination: a neurophysiological hypothesis. *Doc Opthal Proc Ser* 1981;30:87–93.

Bigelow LH, Nasrallah HA, Rauscher FP. Corpus callosum thickness in chronic schizophrenia. *Br J Psychiatry* 1983;142:284–287.

Blinkov SM, Glezer II. *The human brain in figures and tables. A quantitative handbook.* New York: Plenum Press; 1968.

Bloom FE. Advancing a neurodevelopmental origin for schizophrenia. *Arch Gen Psychiatry* 1993;50:224–227.

Bogen JE, Bogen GM. The other side of the brain. *Bull Los Ang Neurol Soc* 1969;34:73–220.

Bourgeois JP, Rakic P. Changes of synaptic density in the primary visual cortex of the macaque monkey from fetal to adult stage. *J Neurosci* 1993;13:2801–2820.

Brambilla P, Hardan A, di Nemi SU, Perez J, Soares JC, Barale F. Brain anatomy and development in autism: review of structural MRI studies. *Brain Res Bull* 2003;61:557–569.

Brizzee KR, Vogt J, Kharetehko X. Postnatal changes in glia neuron index with a comparison of methods of cell enumeration in the white rat. *Prog Brain Res* 1964;4:136–149.

Byne W, Bleier R, Houston L. Variations in human corpus callosum do not predict gender: a study using magnetic resonance imaging. *Behav Neurosci* 1988;102:222–227.

Calvert GA. Crossmodal processing in the human brain: insights from functional neuroimaging studies. *Cereb Cortex* 2001;11:1110–1123.

Cascella NG, Pearlson G, Wong DF. Effects of substance abuse on ventricular and sulcal measures assessed by computed tomography. *Br J Psychiatry* 1991;159:217–221.

Casey BJ, Cohen JD, Jezzard P, et al. Activation of prefrontal cortex in children during a non-spatial working memory task with functional MRI. *Neuroimage* 1995;2:221–229.

Casey BJ, Cohen JD, Noll DC, Schneider W, Giedd JN, Rapoport JL. Functional magnetic resonance imaging: studies of cognition. In: Bigler ED, ed. *The handbook of human brain function: neuroimaging.* New York: Plenum Press; 1996.

Castellanos FX, Giedd JN, Eckburg P, et al. Quantitative morphology of the caudate nucleus in attention deficit hyperactivity disorder. *Am J Psychiatry* 1994;151(12):1791–1796.

Castellanos FX, Giedd JN, Marsh WL, et al. Quantitative brain magnetic resonance imaging in attention-deficit hyperactivity disorder. *Arch Gen Psychiatry* 1996;53:607–616.

Chakos MH, Lieberman JA, Bilder RM, et al. Increase in caudate nuclei volumes of first-episode schizophrenic patients taking antipsychotic drugs. *Am J Psychiatry* 1994;151:1430–1436.

Chugani HT, Phelps ME, Mazziotta JC. Positron emission tomography study of human brain functional development. *Ann Neurol* 1987; 22:487–497.

Chung MK, Worsley KJ, Paus T, et al. A unified statistical approach to deformation-based morphometry. *Neuroimage* 2001;14:595–606.

Clark AS, MacLusky NJ, Goldman-Rakic PS. Androgen binding and metabolism in the cerebral cortex of the deveoping rhesus monkey. *Endocrinology* 1988;123:932–940.

Clarke S, Kraftsik R, Van Der Loos H, Innocenti GM. Forms and measures of adult and developing human corpus callosum: is there sexual dimorphism? *J Comparative Neurology* 1989;280:213–230.

Coffey CE. Anatomic imaging of the aging human brain: computed tomography and magnetic resonance imaging. In: Coffey CE, Cummings JL, eds. *The American Psychiatric Press textbook of geriatric neuropsychiatry.* Washington, DC: American Psychiatric Press; 1994:160–194.

Coffey CE, Wilkinson WE, Parashos IA, et al. Quantitative cerebral anatomy of the aging brain: a cross sectional study using magnetic resonance imaging. *Neurology* 1992;42:527–536.

Coffey CE, Wilkinson WE, Weiner RD, et al. Quantitative cerebral anatomy in depression. A controlled magnetic resonance imaging study. *Arch Gen Psychiatry* 1993;50:7–16.

Cook ND. *The brain code. Mechanisms of information transfer and the role of the corpus callosum.* London: Methuen; 1986.

Cowell PE, Allen LS, Zalatimo NS, Denenberg VH. A developmental study of sex and age interactions in the human corpus callosum. *Dev Brain Res* 1992;66:187–192.

de Lacoste MC, Holloway RL, Woodward DJ. Sex differences in the fetal human corpus callosum. *Hum Neurobiol* 1986;5:93–96.

Dekaban AS, Sadowsky D. Changes in brain weight during the span of human life: relation of brain weights to body heights and body weights. *Ann Neurol* 1978;4:345–356.

Dekaban AS. Tables of cranial and orbital measurements, cranial volume, and derived indexes in males and females from 7 days to 20 years of age. *Ann Neurol* 1977;2:485–491.

Diamond MC, Krech D, Rosenzweig MR. The effects of an enriched enviroment on the histology of the rat cerebral cortex. *J Comp Neur* 1964;123:111–120.

Diener E, Sandvik E, Larsen RF. Age and sex effects for affect intensity. *Developmental Psychology* 1985;21:542–546.

Duara R, Kushch A, Gross-Glenn K, et al. Neuroanatomic differences between dyslexic and normal readers on magnetic resonance imaging scans. *Arch Neurol* 1991;48:410–416.

Eckert MA, Leonard CM, Richards TL, Aylward EH, Thomson J, Berninger VW. Anatomical correlates of dyslexia: frontal and cerebellar findings. *Brain* 2003;126:482–494.

Eckert MA, Leonard CM. Structural imaging in dyslexia: the planum temporale. *Ment Retard Dev Disabil Res Rev* 2000;6:198–206.

Filipek PA, Richelme C, Kennedy DN, Caviness VS, Jr. The young adult human brain: an MRI-based morphometric analysis. *Cereb Cortex* 1994;4:344–360.

Frazier JA, Giedd JN, Hamburger SD, et al. Brain anatomic magnetic resonance imaging in childhood onset schizophrenia. *Arch Gen Psychiatry* 1996;53:617–624.

Geschwind N. Anatomical asymmetry as the basis for cerebral dominance. *Fed Proc* 1978;37:2263–2266.

Giedd JN, Blumenthal J, Jeffries NO, et al. Brain development during childhood and adolescence: a longitudinal MRI study. *Nat Neurosci* 1999;2:861–863.

Giedd JN, Blumenthal J, Molloy E, Castellanos FX. Brain imaging of attention deficit/hyperactivity disorder. *Ann NY Acad Sci* 2001; 931:33–49.

Giedd JN, Castellanos FX, Casey BJ, et al. Quantitative morphology of the corpus callosum in attention deficit hyperactivity disorder. *Am J Psychiatry* 1994;151:665–669.

Giedd JN, Jeffries NO, Blumenthal J, et al. Childhood onset schizophrenia: progressive brain changes during adolescence. *Biol Psychiatry* 1999.

Giedd JN, Kozuch P, Kaysen D, et al. Reliability of cerebral measures in repeated examinations with magnetic resonance imaging. *Psychiatry Res* 1995;61:113–119.

Giedd JN, Rapoport JL, Kruesi MJ, et al. Sydenham's chorea: magnetic resonance imaging of the basal ganglia. *Neurology* 1995; 45:2199–2202.

Giedd JN, Rapoport JL, Leonard HL, Richter D, Swedo SE. Acute basal ganglia enlargement and obsessive compulsive symptoms in an adolescent boy. *J Amer Acad Child Adol Psychiat* 1996;35:913–915.

Giedd JN, Snell JW, Lange N, et al. Quantitative magnetic resonance imaging of human brain development: ages 4–18. *Cereb Cortex* 1996;6:551–560.

Giedd JN, Vaituzis AC, Hamburger SD, et al. Quantitative MRI of the temporal lobe, amygdala, and hippocampus in normal human development: ages 4–18 years. *J Comp Neurol* 1996;366:223–230.

Gogtay N, Giedd JN, Lusk L, et al. Dynamic mapping of human cortical development during childhood through early adulthood. *Proc Natl Acad Sci USA* 2004;101:8174–8179.

Gogtay N, Sporn A, Clasen LS, et al. Comparison of progressive cortical gray matter loss in childhood-onset schizophrenia with that in childhood-onset atypical psychoses. *Arch Gen Psychiatry* 2004;61: 17–22.

Goldberg TE, Torrey EF, Berman KF, Weinberger DR. Relations between neuropsychological performance and brain morphological and physiological measures in monozygotic twins discordant for schizophrenia. *Psychiatry Res* 1994;55:51–61.

Gould E, Woolley CS, Frankfurt M, McEwen BS. Gonadal steroids regulate dendritic spine density in hippocampal pyramidal cells in adulthood. *J Neurosci* 1990;10:1286–1291.

Harvey PH, Krebs JR. Comparing brains. *Science* 1990;249:140–146.

Hellige JB, Cox JP, Litvac L. Information processing in the hemispheres: selective hemisphere activation and capacity limitations. *J Exp Psychol Gen* 1979;108:251–259.

Holloway RL, de Lacoste MC. Sexual dimorphism in the human corpus callosum: an extension and replication study. *Hum Neurobiol* 1986;5:87–91.

Huttenlocher PR. Morphometric study of human cerebral cortex development. *Neuropsychologia* 1990;28:517–527.

Hynd GW, Hern KL, Novey ES, Eliopulos D, Marshall R, Gonzalez JJ. Attention deficit hyperactivity disorder (ADHD) and asymmetry of the caudate nucleus. *J Child Neurology* 1993;8:339–347.

Hynd GW, Semrud-Clikeman M, Lorys AR, Novey ES, Eliopulos D, Lyytinen H. Corpus callosum morphology in attention deficit-hyperactivity disorder: morphometric analysis of MRI. *J Learn Disabil* 1991;24:141–146.

Hynd GW, Semrud-Clikeman M, Lorys AR, Novey ES, Eliopulos D. Brain morphology in developmental dyslexia and attention deficit disorder/hyperactivity. *Arch Neurol* 1990;47:919–926.

Hynd GW, Semrud-Clikeman M. Dyslexia and brain morphology. *Psychol Bull* 1989;106:447–482.

Jacobs LF, Gaulin SJ, Sherry DF, Hoffman GE. Evolution of spatial cognition: sex-specific patterns of spatial behavior predict hippocampal size. *Proc Natl Acad Sci USA* 1990;87:6349–6352.

Jacobson M. *Developmental neurobiology.* New York: Plenum Press; 1991.

Jernigan TL, Trauner DA, Hesselink JR, Tallal PA. Maturation of human cerebrum observed in vivo during adolescence. *Brain* 1991; 114:2037–2049.

Jerslid AT. *The psychology of adolescence.* 2nd ed. New York: Macmillan; 1963.

Keller A, Castellanos FX, Vaituzis AC, Jeffries NO, Giedd JN, Rapoport JL. Progressive loss of cerebellar volume in childhood-onset schizophrenia. *Am J Psychiatry* 2003;160:128–133.

Kertesz A, Polk M, Black SE, Howell J. Anatomical asymmetries and functional laterality. *Brain* 1992;115:589–605.

Keshavan MS, Bagwell WW, Haas GL, Sweeney JA, Schooler NR, Pettegrew JW. Changes in caudate volume with neuroleptic treatment. *Lancet* 1994;344:1434.

Krebs JR, Sherry DF, Healy SD, Perry VH, Vaccarino AL. Hippocampal specialization of food-storing birds. *Proc Natl Acad Sci USA* 1989;86:1388–1392.

Laessle RG, Krieg JC, Fichter MM. Cerebral atrophy and vigilance performance in patients with anorexia nervosa and bulimia nervosa. *Neuropsychobiology* 1989;21:187–191.

Larsen JP, Hoien T, Lundberg I, Odegaard H. MRI evaluation of the size and symmetry of the planum temporale in adolescents with developmental dyslexia. *Brain Lang* 1990;39:289–301.

Lencz T, McCarthy G, Bronen RA, et al. Quantitative magnetic resonance imaging in temporal lobe epilepsy: relationship to neuropathology and neuropsychological function. *Ann Neurol* 1992;31:629–637.

Levy J, Trevarthen C. Color-matching, color naming and color memory in split brain patients. *Neuropsychol* 1981;19:523–541.

Levy J. Interhemispheric collaboration: single mindedness in the asymmetric brain. In: Best CT, ed. *Hemisphere function and collaboration in the child.* New York: Academic Press; 1985:11–32.

Lewis TL, Maurer D, Brent HP. Effects on pereceptual development of visual deprivation during infancy. *Brit J Ophthalmol* 1986; 70:214–220.

Lishman WA. Alcohol and the brain. *Brit J Psychiatry* 1990;156: 635–644.

Martin A, Chao LL. Semantic memory and the brain: structure and processes. *Curr Opin Neurobiol* 2001;11:194–201.

Mesulam MM. From sensation to cognition. *Brain* 1998;121: 1013–1052.

Morse JK, Scheff SW, DeKosky ST. Gonadal steroids influence axonal sprouting in the hippocampal dentate gyrus: a sexually dimorphic response. *Exp Neurol* 1986;94:649–658.

Murphy DGM, DeCarli CD, Daly E, et al. X chromosome effects on female brain: a magnetic resonance imaging study of Turner's Syndrome. *Lancet* 1993;342:1197–1200.

Nellhaus G. Head circumference: girls and boys 2–18 years. *Pediatrics* 1968;41:106.

Njiokiktjien C. *Pediatric behavioral neurology, vol. 3: the child's corpus callosum.* Amsterdam: Suyi Publications; 1991.

Nolte J. Olfactory and Limbic Systems. In: Farrell R, ed. *The human brain: an introduction to its functional anatomy.* 3rd ed. St. Louis, MO: Mosby-Year Book; 1993:397–413.

Oppenheim JS, Benjamin AB, Lee CP, Nass R, Gazzianga MS. No sex-related differences in human corpus callosum based on magnetic resonance imagery. *Ann Neurol* 1987;21:604–606.

Parashos IA, Wilkinson WE, Coffey CE. Magnetic resonance imaging of the corpus callosum: predictors of size in normal adults. *J Neuropsychiatry* 1995;7:35–41.

Peterson B, Riddle MA, Cohen DJ, et al. Reduced basal ganglia volumes in Tourette's syndrome using three-dimensional reconstruction techniques from resonance images. *Neurology* 1993; 43:941–949.

Peterson BS, Leckman JF, Duncan JS, Wetzles R, Riddle MA. Corpus callosum morphology from magnetic resonance images in Tourette's syndrome. *Psychiatry Res: Neuroimaging* 1994;55:85–99.

Peterson BS, Staib L, Scahill L, Zhang H, Anderson C, Leckman JF, Cohen DJ, Gore JC, Albert J, Webster R. Regional brain and ventricular volumes in Tourette syndrome. *Arch Gen Psychiatry.*

Pfefferbaum A, Mathalon DH, Sullivan EV, Rawles JM, Zipursky RB, Lim KO. A quantitative magnetic resonance imaging study of changes in brain morphology from infancy to late adulthood. *Arch Neurol* 1994;51:874–887.

Pujol J, Vendrell P, Junque C, Marti-Vilalta JL, Capdevila A. When does human brain development end? Evidence of corpus callosum growth up to adulthood. *Ann Neurology* 1993;34:71–75.

Rabinowicz T. The differentiated maturation of the cerebral cortex. In: Falkner F, Tanner JM, eds. *Human growth, vol. 2.* New York: Plenum Press; 1986:385–410.

Rae C, Harasty JA, Dzendrowskyj TE, et al. Cerebellar morphology in developmental dyslexia. *Neuropsychologia* 2002;40:1285–1292.

Rajapakse JC, DeCarli C, McLaughlin A, et al. Cerebral magnetic resonance image segmentation using data fusion. *J Comput Assist Tomogr* 1996;20:206–218.

Rauch RA, Jinkins JR. Analysis of cross-sectional area measurements of the corpus callosum adjusted for brain size in male and female subjects from childhood to adulthood. *Behav Brain Res* 1994;64: 65–78.

Reiss AL, Abrams MT, Singer HS, Ross JL, Denckla MB. Brain development, gender and IQ in children. A volumetric imaging study. *Brain* 1996;119:1763–1774.

Rosenthal R, Bigelow L. Quantitative brain measurements in chronic schizophrenia. *Brit J Psychiatry* 1972;121:259–264.

Rumsey JM, Dorwart R, Vermess M, Denckla MB, Kruesi MJP, Rapoport JL. Magnetic resonance imaging of brain anatomy in severe developmental dyslexia. *Arch Neurol* 1986;43:1045–1046.

Semrud-Clikeman M, Filipek PA, Biederman J, et al. Attention-deficit hyperactivity disorder: magnetic resonance imaging morphometric analysis of the corpus callosum. *J Am Acad Child Adolesc Psychiatry* 1994;33:875–881.

Shanks MF, Rockel AJ, Powel TPS. The commissural fiber connections of the primary somatic sensory cortex. *Brain Res* 1975;98:166–171.

Shapiro R, Janzen AH. *The normal skull.* New York: Paul B. Hoeber; 1960.

Sherry DF, Jacobs LF, Gaulin SJ. Spatial memory and adaptive specialization of the hippocampus [see comments]. *Trends Neurosci* 1992;15:298–303.

Sherry DF, Vaccarino AL, Buckenham K, Herz RS. The hippocampal complex of food-storing birds. *Brain Behav Evol* 1989;34:308–317.

Sholl SA, Kim KL. Estrogen receptors in the rhesus monkey brain during fetal development. *Dev Brain Res* 1989;50: 189–196.

Singer HS, Reiss AL, Brown JE, et al. Volumetric MRI changes in basal ganglia of children with Tourette's syndrome. *Neurology* 1993;43:950–956.

Sporn AL, Greenstein DK, Gogtay N, et al. Progressive brain volume loss during adolescence in childhood-onset schizophrenia. *Am J Psychiatry* 2003;160:2181–2189.

Thatcher RW. Cyclic cortical reorganization during early childhood. *Brain Cogn* 1992;20:24–50.

Wechsler D. *Wechsler intelligence scale for children–revised.* New York: The Psychological Corporation; 1974.

Weinberger DR. From neuropathology to neurodevelopment. *Lancet.* 1995;346:552–557.

Weis S, Weber G, Wenger E, Kimbacher M. The controversy about sexual dimorphism of the human corpus callosum. *Int J Neurosci* 1989;47:169–173.

Weis S, Weber G, Wenger E, Kimbacher M. The human corpus callosum and the controversy about sexual dimorphism. *Psychobiol* 1988;16:411–415.

Willerman L, Schultz R, Rutledge JN, Bigler ED. In vivo brain size and intelligence. *Intelligence* 1991;15:223–228.

Witelson SF. Hand and Sex Differences in the Isthmus and Genu of the Human Corpus Callsoum. *Brain* 1989;112:799–835.

Witelson SF. On hemisphere specialization and cerebral plasticity from birth. In: Best CT, ed. *Hemisphere function and collaboration in the child.* Orlando: Academic Press; 1985a:33–85.

Witelson SF. The brain connection: the corpus callosum is larger in left-handers. *Science* 1985b;229:665–668.

Zaidel D, Sperry RW. Memory impairment after commissurotomy in man. *Brain.* 1974;97:263–272.

Zijdenbos AP, Dawant BM, Margolin RA. Automatic detection of intracranial contours in MR images. *Comput Med Imaging Graph* 1994;18:11–23.

Functional Imaging of the Developing Human Brain

Harry T. Chugani, MD   Csaba Juhász, MD PhD

Functional neuroimaging modalities include primarily positron emission tomography (PET) and single photon emission computed tomography (SPECT). Through PET and SPECT applications, a variety of physiological and biochemical processes in the brain can now be imaged quantitatively and noninvasively. Functional magnetic resonance imaging (fMRI) techniques and applications have become widely used in adults because of their ready availability, although clinical applications in children remain limited. After briefly reviewing some clinically relevant fMRI applications, this chapter discusses the impact of PET and SPECT technologies and findings on pediatric neuropsychiatric disorders and indicates some potential future applications in this rapidly evolving field.

FUNCTIONAL MAGNETIC RESONANCE IMAGING

Functional MRI (fMRI) is a noninvasive technique that is able to map activity of neural networks that underlie various (normal and abnormal) cerebral functions. fMRI is clinically feasible because it can be performed by using a regular 1.5 T clinical MRI scanner. The most commonly used technique is the blood oxygen level-dependent (BOLD) echo planar imaging, which is based on a delayed (few seconds after stimulus onset) change in oxy/deoxy-hemoglobin ratio following regional brain activation. Application of fMRI in children is particularly advantageous since it does not involve radiation exposure. However, there are important physiologic and anatomic differences between pediatric and adult fMRI studies, affecting the acquisition, analysis, and interpretation of pediatric fMRI data (Gaillard et al. 2001). The main disadvantage of this technique is its sensitivity to motion artifacts. Since most activation tests require patient cooperation, only older, more cooperative children can be studied with fMRI. Sedation of children is not typically used because it interferes with most activation paradigms. For young children or children with cognitive impairment, it is often difficult or impossible to achieve sufficient cooperation to perform a task while limiting motion. Conditioning and personal interactions can improve compliance, and motion reduction techniques can diminish artifacts due to head motion. Application of fMRI is most successful in children of 7 to 8 years of age or older, and normal children at these ages appear to have similar activation maps as adults (Gaillard et al. 2001, 2003).

Functional MRI is increasingly being used to determine language dominance noninvasively, but currently there is no universally accepted clinical indication for fMRI in children (International League Against Epilepsy Commission Report 2000). Language activation fMRI studies can be useful to localize eloquent cortical areas before resective brain (e.g., epilepsy) surgery, and they also provide novel data on development of language dominance in the human brain. Initial studies on children older than 8 years of age demonstrated that normal patterns of verbal fluency are established by this age, but the general extent of speech-related activation is larger than that in normal adults (Gaillard et al. 2000). Also, while hemispheric language dominance is largely established by 7 to 8 years of age (Lee et al. 1999), the degree of lateralization increases as children approach adulthood (Holland et al. 2001). In addition to language functions, other cognitive functions investigated by fMRI in children have included working memory, spatial memory, reading visual recognition, as well as motor and sensory tasks (reviewed by Gaillard et al. 2001). fMRI was reported to be comparable in accuracy to the carotid Amobarbital (Amytal) test for cerebral lateralization of language functions (Yetkin et al. 1998) and can provide clinically useful localizing information for sensory and motor function. In patients with intractable epilepsy, fMRI alone or combined with other techniques such as transcranial magnetic stimulation can demonstrate reorganization of motor function preoperatively (Macdonell et al. 1999), thus predicting motor outcome following resection. More recently, combination of fMRI and diffusion tensor imaging (DTI)-based tractography has been explored to analyze motor connectivity in vivo (Guye et al. 2003). Another potential clinical application of fMRI can be to localize actively spiking epileptic foci. This, however, is feasible only in patients with frequent seizures or in those in status epilepticus. In patients with motor seizures or impaired cooperation during seizures, movement artifacts preclude meaningful data acquisition, while fMRI signals arising from an area close to air cavities can be poor (Lazeyras et al. 2000). Localization of interictal epileptiform activity using EEG-triggered fMRI is more feasible (Krakow et al. 1999), although resective epilepsy surgery generally cannot purely rely on functional data derived from interictal epileptiform activity.

In summary, fMRI holds the promise of being a safe, powerful clinical tool for noninvasive mapping of various brain functions in older children with intractable epilepsy.

PET AND SPECT METHODOLOGY

The development of PET technology has allowed the imaging and quantification of local chemical functions in various body organs to be carried out noninvasively in humans (Phelps et al. 1975; Ter-Pogossian et al. 1975; Ter-Pogossian 1995). This technique utilizes detectors that are capable of detecting the paired photons (each with energy of 511 KeV) that travel in opposite directions (coincidence detection) and are released as a result of positron-electron annihilations. Quantification of the biochemical or physiological process being imaged can be achieved with tracer kinetic mathematical models that describe the in vivo behavior of the PET probe, which is labeled with a positron-emitting isotope. In general, the isotopes used in PET have short half-lives (Table 6.1) and are produced onsite with a cyclotron. Use of PET tracers in children has allowed the measurement of local cerebral metabolic rates for glucose

TABLE 6.1
POSITRON-EMITTING ISOTOPES

Isotopes	Half-Life (min)	Energy (MeV)[a]
^{18}F	109.7	0.6–1
^{11}C	20.4	0.96
^{13}N	9.9	1.19
^{15}O	2.1	1.72
^{82}Rb	1.2	3.36

[a]Maximal energy.

utilization, cerebral blood flow, oxygen utilization, protein synthesis, and neurotransmitter function.

SPECT is also a noninvasive functional imaging technique, but it uses simpler and less expensive equipment than does PET. SPECT provides tomographic imaging through the use of either a single rapidly rotating gamma camera or multiple gamma cameras to detect and reconstruct gamma-ray emissions (Ell et al. 1987). Because of the longer half-life of SPECT isotopes compared with the isotopes used in PET, and the readily available equipment, SPECT is suited for even the smallest hospitals and clinics. The isotopes can be obtained commercially and can be stored onsite. However, the spatial resolution of SPECT images is about half of that achieved with PET, a distinction that is particularly relevant in pediatric studies. Furthermore, SPECT techniques are semiquantitative at best, compared with PET, which is fully quantitative.

In brain studies, SPECT has been used primarily to provide an index of cerebral blood flow. Radioactive probes developed for this purpose have included xenon, iodamines, technetium-99m hexamethyl propylene amine oxime (99mTc-HMPAO), and technetium-99m-ethyl cysteinate dimer (ECD). Scanning of the brain can be initiated at leisure after the brain uptake phase because the trapped agent remains relatively stable for at least 1 hour, and the isotopes used in SPECT have rather long half-lives (e.g., ^{123}I has a half-life of 13 hours). These properties are particularly favorable for studies in children (Iivanainen et al. 1990).

NORMAL BRAIN DEVELOPMENT

Developmental studies using PET with the tracer 2-deoxy-2[^{18}F]fluoro-d-glucose (FDG) have shown that the pattern of brain glucose utilization in the human infant evolves during the first year of life from a simple neonatal pattern to one that qualitatively resembles an adult pattern. Beyond the first year, the brain continues to manifest metabolic maturational changes that persist well into the second decade of life (Chugani and Phelps 1986, Chugani et al. 1987b).

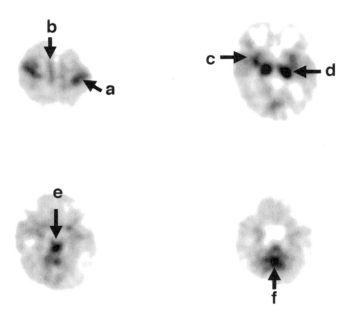

Figure 6.1 PET images from a human newborn showing the pattern of brain glucose metabolism. Although there is relatively low glucose metabolism in most of the cerebral and cerebellar cortex, a number of brain regions appear to be metabolically active including (a) sensorimotor cortex, (b) cingulate cortex, (c) striatum, (d) thalamus, (e) brainstem, and (f) cerebellar vermis. The auditory cortex is also relatively active in newborns.

ONTOGENY OF BRAIN GLUCOSE UTILIZATION

The pattern of glucose utilization in the newborn brain is markedly different from that in the adult brain. In the newborn, glucose metabolic activity is most prominent in primary sensory and motor cortex, thalamus, brainstem, and cerebellar vermis (Chugani 1994; Chugani and Phelps 1986; Chugani et al. 1987b; Kinnala et al. 1996). More recent studies with high-resolution PET scanners have suggested that the cingulate cortex, amygdala, hippocampus,

striatum, and auditory cortex may also show relatively prominent activity in the newborn period (Fig. 6.1) (Chugani 1999). The limited number of brain regions displaying metabolic activity could be related to the relatively limited behavioral repertoire of newborns (Table 6.2). For example, reaching movements in newborns are relatively poor and imprecise (von Hofsten 1982) because of inadequate visual-motor integration. Intrinsic brainstem reflex behaviors, such as the Moro, root, and grasp responses, are present transiently in newborns and are gradually suppressed with further brain maturation (Andre-Thomas and Saint-Anne Dargassies 1960).

Between ages 2 and 4 months, glucose utilization increases in several cortical regions, including parietal, temporal, and primary visual cortex, as well as in the basal ganglia and cerebellar hemispheres (Chugani 1994; Chugani and Phelps 1986; Chugani et al. 1987b; Kinnala et al. 1996). The frontal cortex, however, remains relatively dormant in terms of glucose consumption (Fig. 6.2). Coinciding with these changes in glucose metabolism is the emergence of a number of behaviors, such as improved visual-spatial and visual-sensorimotor integration (Bronson 1974) and the disappearance or reorganization of neonatal brainstem reflex behaviors (Table 6.2) (Andre-Thomas and Saint-Anne Dargassies 1960; Parmelee and Sigman 1983). The cortical maturation is evident also on the electroencephalogram (EEG), which undergoes dramatic changes during this period as a result of increasing cortical influence (Kellaway 1979).

The frontal cortex is the last cortical region to undergo a maturational rise in glucose consumption. Even within the frontal lobe, there is a rank order of metabolic maturation, with the lateral and inferior portions of the frontal cortex becoming active between ages 6 and 8 months (Fig. 6.3), and the dorsal and medial frontal regions showing increased glucose utilization between ages 8 and 12 months (Fig. 6.4). These maturational changes in frontal lobe coincide with the appearance of more cognitively related

TABLE 6.2
RELATIONSHIP BETWEEN LOCAL CEREBRAL GLUCOSE METABOLISM AND BEHAVIORAL LANDMARKS IN THE FIRST YEAR OF LIFE

Age	Glucose Metabolic Pattern	Behavior
≤ 1 month	Active sensorimotor cortical and subcortical regions, midbrain, brainstem, paleocerebellum	Predominantly, subcortical and primitive sensorimotor level of function; intrinsic brainstem reflexes
2–4 months	Increasing glucose metabolic activity in basal ganglia, cerebral cortex (except frontal and association regions), and cerebellar hemispheres	Suppression of intrinsic subcortical reflexes; visual-sensorimotor integration. *Electroencephalogram:* disappearance of neonatal patterns (trace alternans, frontal sharp transients, frontal rhythmic delta); appearance of sleep spindles and precursor of alpha rhythm
8–12 months	Increasing glucose metabolic activity in frontal and association cortices	Cognitive or hypothesis-forming development; stranger anxiety; more meaningful interaction with surroundings

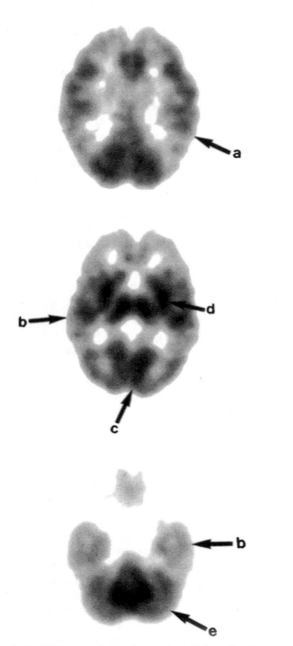

Figure 6.2 PET images from a 3-month-old infant showing maturational increases of glucose metabolism in *(a)* parietal cortex, *(b)* temporal cortex, *(c)* occipital cortex, *(d)* striatum, and *(e)* cerebellar cortex. Note the persistently low metabolic activity in frontal cortex.

behaviors, such as stranger anxiety (Kagan 1972), and improved performance on the delayed response task (Table 6.2) (Goldman-Rakic 1984; Fuster 1997). Neuroanatomic studies have shown that toward the end of the first postnatal year, dendritic fields expand (Schade and van Groenigen 1961) and capillary density increases (Diemer 1968) in the frontal cortex. A pattern of glucose utilization not unlike that seen in adults is present by

approximately 1 year of age (Chugani 1994; Chugani and Phelps 1986; Chugani et al. 1987b), although a few brain structures (e.g., in the thalamus) undergo further maturation as late as beyond 6 years of age (Van Bogaert et al. 1998).

Glucose Metabolic Rates

Measurement of absolute rates of glucose utilization during development indicates that the brain is far from mature at 1 year of age. The cerebral cortex undergoes a dynamic course of metabolic maturation that persists until ages 16 to 18 years (Chugani 1994; H. T. Chugani 1999; Chugani and Phelps 1986; Chugani et al. 1987b). Initially, there is a rise in the rates of glucose utilization from birth to about age 4 years, at which time the amount of glucose used in the child's cerebral cortex is more than twice that used in the adult's cerebral cortex (Fig. 6.5). From ages 4 to 10 years, these high rates of glucose consumption are maintained, and only after age 10 years is there a gradual decline of glucose metabolic rates, with rates reaching adult values by age 16 to 18 years. Similar changes, but of lesser magnitude, are observed in basal ganglia and thalamus, whereas the brainstem and cerebellum do not show significant changes of glucose metabolic rates over the course of postnatal development.

Significance of Brain Glucose Metabolic Changes

The important maturational changes just described could be determined only following the development of PET technology. Similar studies using SPECT have confirmed some of the observations described with PET (Chiron et al. 1992; Rubinstein et al. 1989; Tokumaru et al. 1999), but the poor spatial resolution of SPECT precludes its being useful in the study of maturation in small brain regions such as the amygdala and hippocampus.

Functional brain imaging has shown that in the first year of life, the ontogeny of glucose metabolism follows a phylogenetic order, with functional maturation of older anatomic structures preceding that of newer areas. In addition, the ranking of structures in terms of the degree to which maturational increases in glucose metabolic rates exceed adult values follows a phylogenetic order; with the greatest changes observed in cerebral cortex, followed by basal ganglia and thalamus, and, lastly, cerebellum and brainstem. Although a general relationship between the maturational sequence of regional glucose metabolism and the behavioral maturation of the infant has been shown, further studies are required to explore this anatomic-behavioral relationship that forms the basis for the development of complex neuroanatomic networks that mediate human behavior.

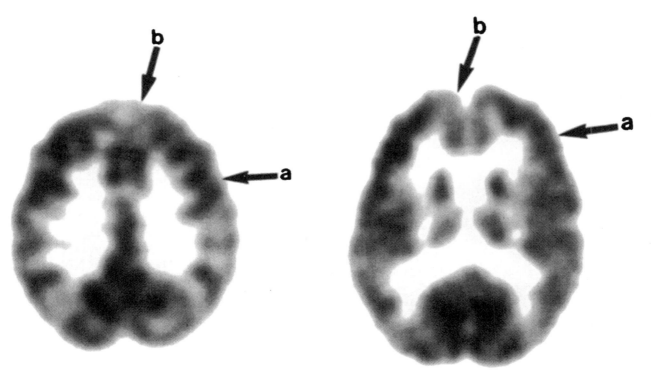

Figure 6.3 PET images from an 8-month-old infant showing the pattern of brain glucose metabolism. Note that glucose metabolic maturation in lateral frontal cortex *(a)* precedes that in dorsal mesial frontal cortex *(b)*.

The dynamic profile of glucose metabolic rates in cerebral cortex as a function of age (Fig. 6.5) matches that of synaptic proliferation and dendritic pruning in the postnatal period. We believe that the ascending portion of the implied curve in Figure 6.5, representing a period of rapid increase in glucose metabolic rates, corresponds to the period of rapid overproduction of synapses and nerve terminals that is known to occur in the human brain. The "plateau" period, during which glucose metabolic rates exceed adult values, corresponds to the period of increased cerebral energy demand that is a result of transient exuberant connectivity. Finally, the descending portion of the curve, representing the

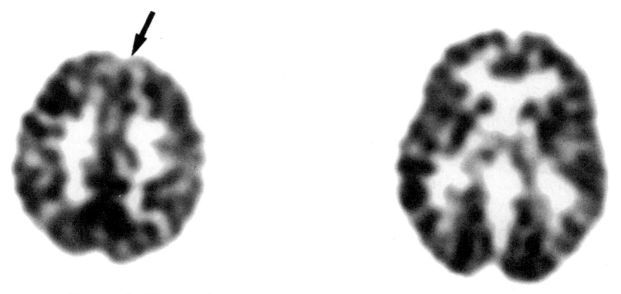

Figure 6.4 PET images from a 10-month-old infant showing the pattern of brain glucose metabolism. An adult pattern of glucose metabolism is almost present, except for in the most rostral portion of the mesial prefrontal cortex *(arrow)*.

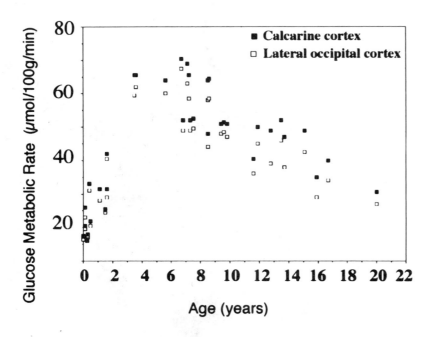

Figure 6.5 Absolute values of local cerebral glucose metabolic rates (LCMRglc) in cortical (lateral occipital and calcarine) brain regions plotted as a function of age in individual healthy infants and children.

developmental decline in the rates of glucose utilization, corresponds to the period of selective elimination, or "pruning," of excessive connectivity and marks the time when developmental plasticity markedly diminishes in humans. This interpretation is supported by our studies in the cat (Chugani et al. 1991) and the rhesus monkey (Jacobs et al. 1995). Furthermore, there is an abundance of data to suggest that in humans, developmental brain plasticity begins to decline at about the time of puberty (Awaya 1978; Curtiss 1981; Lenneberg 1967; Newport and Supalla 1990; Schwartz et al. 1987; Vaegan and Taylor 1979).

EPILEPSY

Both PET and SPECT are used clinically to define epileptogenic brain regions in children with medically refractory epilepsy who are being evaluated for possible surgical treatment. These functional neuroimaging tools are particularly useful in epileptic patients who show no evidence of structural abnormalities on MRI and in whom, therefore, EEG localization is the sole guide for the localization of epileptic foci. With these patients, *interictal* PET with FDG and other tracers is a powerful tool for determining functional disturbances in the cortex associated with epilepsy. When PET is not available, *ictal* SPECT can provide localization of seizure onset. In patients with a single epileptic focus and seizures that are frequent and last at least a minute or so, ictal SPECT may be sufficient. However, when multiple foci, large epileptogenic regions, or brief and infrequent seizures are present, ictal SPECT is of limited value. In addition, interictal SPECT is not nearly as sensitive as PET in delineating epileptogenic zones. Ictal PET, on the other hand, is not practical with these patients, since PET isotopes have a short half-life (e.g.,

108 minutes for ^{18}F and 20 minutes for ^{11}C). The routine use of functional neuroimaging in presurgical evaluation has reduced the necessity for chronic invasive EEG monitoring in many children undergoing epilepsy surgery (reviewed by Zupanc 1997).

Partial Epilepsy

In patients with refractory temporal lobe epilepsy, interictal FDG-PET scans reveal decreased glucose utilization of the affected temporal lobe in about 85% of cases. These areas of hypometabolism correspond anatomically to pathological and depth-electrode EEG localization of epileptogenicity (Henry et al. 1993). It is important to monitor the EEG during the PET tracer uptake period, since an active focal epileptiform discharge present on the EEG can be associated with local *hypermetabolism*, even on the interictal PET scan. In such instances, the relative hypometabolism on the contralateral (normal) side could be mistakenly interpreted as an interictal epileptic focus; an interpretation that would lead to false lateralization of the focus (Chugani et al. 1993a). Advances in analysis techniques of MRI have eliminated the need for functional imaging or invasive EEG monitoring in the majority of patients with temporal lobe epilepsy. FDG-PET rarely provides additional clinical information when hippocampal atrophy is present on the MRI (Gaillard et al. 1995) and is increasingly reserved for those cases in which the MRI fails to provide the necessary localization.

In seizures of extra-temporal lobe origin, particularly frontal lobe epilepsy, FDG-PET was initially less sensitive in detecting focal areas of abnormal metabolism than in temporal lobe epilepsy. Recently developed high-resolution PET scanners, however, are able to show hypometabolic

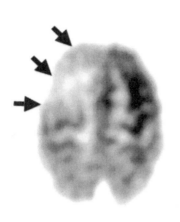

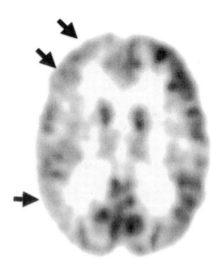

Figure 6.6 PET scan from a 14-year-old girl with uncontrolled seizures and no evidence of focal abnormalities on MRI. Decreased glucose metabolism is clearly seen in the right front cortex *(arrows)*, also extending posteriorly with milder hypometabolism in the parietal region. Intracranial EEG showed right frontal seizure onset.

cortical regions in the majority of children with intractable frontal lobe epilepsy (da Silva et al. 1997a) (Fig. 6.6). A different strategy has been to use PET with various tracers other than FDG. For example, PET studies of the central benzodiazepine receptor with the antagonist ^{11}C-labeled flumazenil (FMZ) have shown that adult patients with partial epilepsy have significantly reduced binding in the epileptic focus (Savic et al. 1988). Subsequent studies with detailed intracranial EEG comparisons showed that FMZ-PET was more sensitive than FDG-PET in delineating cortex with seizure onset and frequent interictal spiking in children with intractable epilepsy of extratemporal origin (Muzik et al. 2000).

Frontal lobe seizures that begin in the neonatal period or in early infancy typically are associated with an underlying structural lesion detected by MRI. However, when the MRI is normal, PET with FDG almost always shows the area of seizure onset, with the result that early surgical treatment is possible. The area of metabolic abnormality correlates with the extent of microdysgenesis (Chugani et al. 1988), but the extent of decreased FMZ binding appears to be more accurate to delineate the epileptogenic zone to be resected to achieve seizure-free surgical outcome (Juhasz et al. 2001a).

Interictal SPECT studies are generally less sensitive than ictal SPECT studies in localizing the epileptic focus in children, but have some clinical utility. The typical interictal SPECT scan is either normal or shows one or more areas of decreased perfusion. For example, in one 99mTc-HMPAO-SPECT study of 14 children with frequent seizures (Heiskala et al. 1993), the typical finding in 11 patients with partial secondary generalized seizures was a single hypoperfused area involving the cerebral cortex. The 3 children with Lennox-Gastaut syndrome had multiple areas of hypoperfusion and a worse clinical outcome. In this study, SPECT was more sensitive than EEG, CT, or MRI in detecting abnormalities. Similar sensitivity of interictal SPECT was found in another study of 14 children with intractable temporal lobe epilepsy (Cross et al. 1997).

However, most studies using SPECT interictally have found a sensitivity of no more than 50% (Harvey et al. 1993).

Ictal SPECT is more sensitive than interictal studies in detecting the epileptic focus in both temporal lobe and extra-temporal lobe epilepsy. A well-circumscribed area of increased perfusion is the most common finding (Fig. 6.7), and in patients whose ictal EEGs are nonlocalizing, the SPECT localization is particularly useful in surgical planning (Marks et al. 1992). Harvey and coworkers (1993) found that ictal, but not interictal, studies were informative in 14 of 15 children with temporal lobe epilepsy, with ictal SPECT findings corresponding well with ictal EEG, MRI,

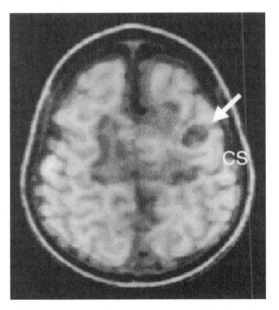

Figure 6.7 Ictal SPECT focus in a 2.5-year-old girl with seizures of left frontal origin. The red area represents the region with highest blood flow increase. Coregistration with high-resolution MRI demonstrated that the focus (arrow) was just in front of the precentral gyrus (CS = central sulcus). Seizure onset on intracranial EEG monitoring colocalized with the SPECT focus. (For color detail, see color insert.)

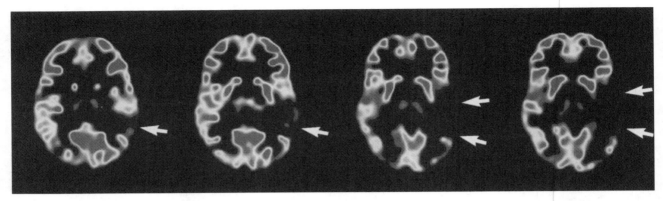

Figure 6.8 PET scan of an infant with medically refractory infantile spasms and with normal MRI. The focus of decreased glucose utilization in the left temporal lobe *(arrows)* corresponded to the interictal and ictal epileptiform activity on the EEG.

and pathology. Even in patients with focal cortical dysplasias seen on the MRI but a nonlocalizing EEG, ictal 99mTc-HMPAO-SPECT can prove to be invaluable in providing the necessary localizing data to proceed to surgical resection (Kuzniecky et al. 1993). Sensitivity and spatial accuracy of ictal SPECT findings can be enhanced by using subtraction ictal SPECT coregistered to MRI (SISCOM) (Vera et al. 1999); that is, the interictal SPECT images are subtracted from the ictal images and the results displayed on coregistered MR images. In 40 children with epilepsy, SISCOM showed localized hyperperfusion in agreement with the seizure onset zone in 95% of the cases. Importantly, previously not appreciated MRI abnormalities (such as areas of subtle cortical dysplasia) can be identified in some cases (Chiron et al. 1999b). One study compared the value of ictal SPECT to localize the ictal onset as defined by intracranial EEG in children with epilepsy and found that the area with highest ictal perfusion increase colocalized with the onset area in 12 of 15 children, while it was consistent with early propagation in the remaining 3 (Kaminska et al. 2003). False localization was due to rapid seizure propagation or subclinical seizure onset. In addition, the majority (70%) of children with favorable outcome of resective epilepsy surgery had their SPECT focus colocalized with the resected area.

Some investigators claim that *postictal* SPECT is more sensitive than interictal SPECT in identifying the epileptogenic cortex. Rowe and coworkers (1989) found increased uptake mainly in the anteromesial temporal region in 83% of patients during the first several minutes after the seizure. The mesial temporal hyperperfusion was often accompanied by hypoperfusion in the lateral temporal cortex and other areas of the ipsilateral cortex corresponding to both degree and extent of postictal slow-wave activity on the EEG. This postictal hypoperfusion can last up to 20 minutes. The unilateral seizure focus was localized correctly in 31 of 45 patients as a result of postictal SPECT (Rowe et al. 1991). Studies have demonstrated that postictal SPECT localization of epileptic foci can also be improved by subtraction of interictal studies, and then coregistering with MRI (O'Brien et al. 1999).

Infantile Spasms

Infantile spasms are seizures that typically have their onset at between 3 and 8 months of age and are characterized by brief jerks of the neck, trunk, or extremities resulting in flexion, extension, or a combination of the two. Depending on whether an underlying condition has been identified or not, the spasms are classified as *symptomatic* or *cryptogenic*. A third group, the *idiopathic* group, is distinctly rare and is characterized by rapid response to treatment, benign course, and favorable outcome (Dulac and Plouin 1994).

Glucose metabolism PET studies in children with intractable cryptogenic infantile spasms have shown unifocal (Fig. 6.8) and, more commonly, multifocal (Fig. 6.9) cortical areas of hypometabolism interictally. Less commonly, increased focal glucose utilization can be seen if the study is performed ictally or in the presence of an actively

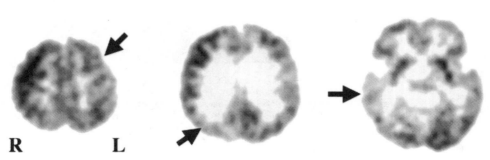

R   L

Figure 6.9 PET images from an infant with medically refractory infantile spasms showing multifocal cortical hypometabolism *(arrows)*. Although MRI showed normal results, PET showed foci of decreased glucose utilization in the left frontal and in the right parietal cortex as well as in the right temporal region.

discharging focus on the EEG. The EEG localization of focal ictal or interictal abnormalities corresponds well to the PET focus in most cases (Chugani et al. 1990, 1993b). However, when hypsarrhythmia is present on the EEG, focal electrographic abnormalities either preceding or following the presence of hypsarrhythmia correlate best with the location of PET cortical abnormalities. When available, therefore, EEGs performed before the onset of spasms must be reexamined in conjunction with the PET study.

The discovery of these focal cortical metabolic abnormalities on PET has allowed some infants with refractory spasms to be treated with cortical resection. Thus, when a single region of abnormal glucose metabolism is present, and there is good correlation between the region localized with PET and the focus identified on the EEG, surgical removal of the epileptogenic region results not only in seizure control but also in complete or partial reversal of the associated developmental delay. Neuropathological examination of the resected tissue typically reveals cortical dysplasia (Chugani et al. 1990, 1993b; Vinters et al. 1992).

Unfortunately, about 65% of infants with cryptogenic infantile spasms show more than one area of cortical hypometabolism on the PET scan (Chugani and Conti 1996) and are therefore not ideal candidates for cortical resection (Fig. 6.9). Within this group is a subgroup of infants with bilateral temporal hypometabolism and a typical clinical phenotype, comprising about 10% of all infants with cryptogenic infantile spasms. The clinical features include severe developmental delay (particularly in the language domain) and autism (Chugani et al. 1996).

The high sensitivity of PET in detecting focal cortical abnormalities allows most infants diagnosed with cryptogenic infantile spasms to have their spasms reclassified into the "symptomatic" category. In a study of 140 infants with infantile spasms, 97 had infantile spasms that were initially classified as cryptogenic before the application of PET in evaluation of etiology (Chugani and Conti 1996). With PET, unifocal cortical metabolic abnormalities were uncovered in 30 and multifocal abnormalities in 62 of these infants. Whereas these findings were confirmed to represent cortical dysplasia in many of the infants with unifocal abnormalities, because the infants underwent cortical resection (Chugani et al. 1990, 1993b), pathological studies were not available for the infants with multifocal abnormalities. It is likely that these lesions represent cortical dysplasia or ischemic insults. Importantly, only 5 of the 97 infants in this study continued to be classified as having cryptogenic infantile spasms after the benefit of a PET study. It is now recommended that all infants with intractable cryptogenic infantile spasms undergo an evaluation with PET. In some cases, PET reveals bilateral symmetric or generalized cortical (with or without associated cerebellar) hypometabolism (Fig. 6.10). This pattern suggests an underlying genetic/metabolic condition, rather than cortical dysplasia, and strongly discourages pursuing of presurgical evaluation but may prompt more detailed metabolic and genetic studies.

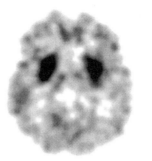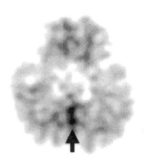

Figure 6.10 Generalized cortical hypometabolism in a 6-month-old child with infantile spasms. Note the prominent basal ganglia and cerebellar vermis (arrow) as a result of diffuse cortical cerebral and cerebellar hypometabolism. In such cases, a genetic or metabolic condition can be suspected and presurgical evaluation is typically not pursued.

Another important finding with PET in patients with infantile spasms is evidence of complex cortical-subcortical interactions believed to be important in the secondary generalization of focal cortical discharges to result in the infantile spasms. PET studies have shown that, regardless of the type or extent of cortical abnormality, prominent glucose metabolism in lenticular nuclei and brainstem is a common feature in infantile spasms (Chugani et al. 1992). It is postulated that the infantile spasms result primarily from focal or diffuse cortical abnormalities interacting with brainstem and lenticular nuclei and that this type of generalization accounts for the bilateral motor involvement and relative symmetry of the majority of infantile spasms even in the presence of a discrete focal lesion (Chugani et al 1992; reviewed in Juhasz et al. 2001b).

Investigators using SPECT technology have also found focal areas of cortical hypoperfusion in patients with infantile spasms (Dulac et al. 1987). Furthermore, one study found that the mean cerebral blood flow decreased just after corticosteroid treatment (Chiron et al. 1993). Correlation of focal hypoperfusion with behavior of the infants showed that parietal-occipital SPECT foci are often associated with visual inattention at the time when the infants present with infantile spasms and with long-term cognitive compromise (Jambaque et al. 1993). Both visual inattention and cognitive delay have been reversed with successful focal cortical resection. In a study of 40 children with West syndrome, localized cortical perfusion abnormalities were seen in 24 patients (60%), supporting that focal cortical lesions play an important role in the development of West syndrome (Haginoya et al. 2000). However, the existence of cortical dysfunction as defined by SPECT did not seem to predict seizure prognosis or developmental outcome in that study.

Other Epilepsy Syndromes

Both PET and SPECT have been used in the study of various other epilepsy syndromes occurring in infants and children. *Lennox-Gastaut syndrome* in children has diverse etiologies but manifests three common features: a slow spike-wave pattern (1 to 2.5 Hz) on the EEG, some degree of intellectual impairment, and the presence of multiple seizure types, including tonic seizures (Blume et al. 1973). Studies with FDG-PET have provided a new classification of Lennox-Gastaut syndrome based on metabolic anatomy. Four metabolic subtypes have been identified: (1) unilateral focal, (2) unilateral diffuse, (3) bilateral diffuse hypometabolism, and (4) normal patterns (Chugani et al. 1987a; Iinuma et al. 1987; Theodore et al. 1987). These glucose metabolic patterns can be useful in determining the type of surgical intervention indicated for those patients with uncontrolled seizures. Surprisingly, there were no differences in glucose metabolic rates between PET studies performed during continuous slow spike-wave activity and studies in which there was minimal epileptiform activity on the EEG (Chugani et al. 1987a).

Sturge-Weber syndrome is a sporadic neurocutaneous syndrome characterized by facial capillary nevus (port-wine stain) in the distribution of one or more divisions of the fifth cranial nerve and ipsilateral leptomeningeal angiomatosis. Neurological consequences include intracerebral calcification, epilepsy, hemiparesis, hemianopia, and glaucoma (reviewed in Sujansky and Conradi 1995). In children with Sturge-Weber syndrome, FDG-PET typically reveals hypometabolism ipsilateral to the facial nevus and thus allows the degree and extent of hemispheric involvement to be determined (Chugani and Dietrich 1992; Chugani et al. 1989). In addition, the rate of hemispheric deterioration can he determined by quantifying the degree of hypometabolism in sequential PET studies. PET has been useful both in guiding the extent of focal cortical resection (i.e., correlating better with intraoperative electrocorticography than CT or MRI) and in assessing candidacy for early hemispherectomy in patients with Sturge-Weber syndrome. Paradoxically, children with mild but extensive glucose hypometabolism (confined to one hemisphere) often have worse cognitive outcome than children with early and severe unilateral hypometabolism (Lee et al. 2001); this finding suggests that early and rapid demise of the affected hemisphere could be beneficial in allowing unaffected areas to take over lost functions. In contrast, when the affected areas show slow deterioration, seizures tend to persist and plasticity is not optimal; such patients should be good candidates for resective surgery in our efforts to prevent cognitive decline. Interestingly, an unusual pattern of ipsilateral hypermetabolism (Fig. 6.11) can be seen instead of hypometabolism in young infants with Sturge-Weber syndrome studied in the interictal state (Chugani et al. 1989). The cause of this transient increased glucose utilization is yet to be clarified. SPECT studies demonstrated presence of regional hyperperfusion even before the occurrence of clinical seizures (Pinton et al. 1997). After 1 year of age, the pattern of hypoperfusion is typically seen on SPECT; and this corresponds topographically to the CT scan abnormality in Sturge-Weber syndrome (Chiron et al. 1989).

Hemimegalencephaly is a brain malformation characterized by congenital hypertrophy of one cerebral hemisphere with ipsilateral ventriculomegaly. The larger hemisphere is the more abnormal one and is highly epileptogenic, often requiring hemispherectomy for alleviation of the seizures (Vigevano et al. 1989). PET scanning of glucose metabolism in infants and children with hemimegalencephaly reveals the expected, severe interictal hypometabolism of the affected hemisphere and, more important, allows the functional integrity of the better hemisphere to be evaluated. In a study of eight children with hemimegalencephaly, seven of whom underwent hemispherectomy, a general correlation was found between the degree of metabolic involvement of the less-affected hemisphere and overall prognosis (Rintahaka et al. 1993). Another study, using SPECT in two children with hemimegalencephaly, showed a similar pattern of decreased perfusion in the malformed hemisphere (Konkol et al. 1990), despite the patients having very different EEG findings.

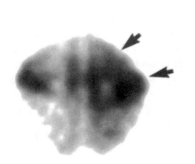 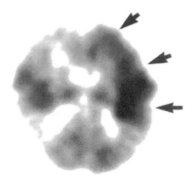 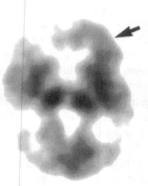

Figure 6.11   Interictal glucose metabolism PET scan from a 2-month-old infant with seizures and Sturge-Weber syndrome. The left facial port-wine stain, left-sided epileptogenicity on the EEG, right hemiparesis, and subsequent development of left cerebral calcifications were all consistent with an abnormal left cerebral hemisphere. However, note the increased interictal glucose metabolism *(arrows)* in left frontal, parietal and superior temporal cortex, which is in contrast to the right hemisphere, in which there is a normal pattern of glucose metabolism for age (cf. Figure 6.1).

Tuberous sclerosis complex (TSC) is a neurocutaneous disorder, characterized by tumor growths that involve multiple organs, including brain, retina, kidney, heart, and skin. It is inherited as an autosomal dominant trait with a high degree of penetrance and a high spontaneous mutation rate. Approximately 70 to 90% of patients with TSC have seizures, which are attributed to the presence of brain cortical malformations, which typically are evident as areas of cortical hypometabolism on interictal FDG-PET. These hypometabolic areas often extend beyond the structural lesions visible on MRI. However, FDG-PET is not able to identify which of the multiple tubers are epileptogenic and, therefore, is not useful to guide surgical resection in TSC patients with medically intractable seizures. A relatively new PET tracer, α-[^{11}C]methyl-L-tryptophan (AMT) has proven to be helpful in this respect. AMT, which has been developed as a tracer for serotonin synthesis with PET (Diksic et al. 1990), is an analogue of tryptophan, the precursor for serotonin biosynthesis. The properties of AMT make it a suitable tracer substance for the PET measurement of serotonin biosynthesis in vivo in humans (Chugani et al. 1998b; Muzik et al. 1997)(see Autism on page 121). Alternatively, increased AMT uptake can occur due to activation of the alternative kynurenine pathway, producing important neurotoxic and convulsant metabolites, such as quinolinic acid (reviewed by Stone 2001).

AMT PET can identify a single tuber or a small subset of epileptogenic tubers with increased uptake in approximately two thirds of the cases, while nonepileptogenic tubers show decreased AMT uptake (Asano et al. 2000; Chugani et al. 1998a; Fedi et al. 2003) (Fig. 6.12). Thus, AMT PET is a powerful imaging tool to guide intracranial electrode placement for resective epilepsy surgery in children with TSC. More recent studies have also shown AMT PET to be a promising imaging method to localize epileptic foci in children with extratemporal epilepsy not associated with TSC. In such cases, AMT PET can identify epileptogenic cortex as an area of increased uptake even if FDG-PET and MRI show ambiguous results, and appears to be most sensitive in epilepsies associated with malformations of cortical development (Juhasz et al. 2003). Increased cortical AMT uptake can also identify nonresected epileptic cortex after failed resective epilepsy surgery (Juhasz et al. 2004)(Fig. 6. 13).

DISORDERS OF COGNITIVE DEVELOPMENT

Structural neuroimaging with CT and MRI has been of limited value in the evaluation of children with cognitive disorders. For example, anatomic abnormalities are rarely evident with CT or MRI in children with learning disabilities (such as developmental dyslexia). Yet, most learning disabilities are believed to be neurobiologically based (Filipek 1995; Pennington 1995; Weinberg et al. 1995). Furthermore, the

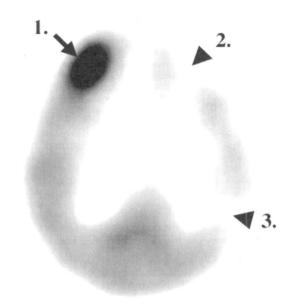

Figure 6.12 α-[^{11}C]Methyl-L-tryptophan (AMT) PET identifies an epileptogenic tuber by showing increased uptake in a child with tuberous sclerosis and intractable epilepsy. Out of the three tubers (1. right frontal; 2. left frontal; 3. left parietal) shown on this plane, only the right frontal one showed increased AMT uptake, while the other two had decreased uptake. Ictal EEG confirmed that the right frontal region was epileptogenic.

various types of learning disorder probably have their abnormal function in different brain regions and circuits, and functional neuroimaging could be suitable in detecting these neuroanatomic substrates. With this strategy in mind, Zametkin and colleagues (1990) evaluated adults with

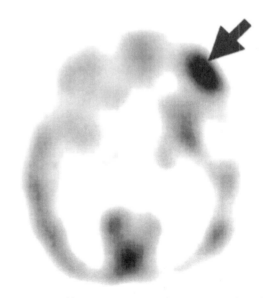

Figure 6.13 α-[^{11}C]Methyl-L-tryptophan (AMT) PET can identify nonresected epileptic regions following a failed cortical resection in some patients. This 8-year-old boy had undergone a left superior frontal, parietal, and temporal resection but continued to have seizures. AMT PET showed an area of increased uptake in the left inferior frontal cortex (arrow), which was corroborated as a residual seizure focus by ictal intracranial EEG.

childhood-onset hyperactivity using FDG-PET and found about 8% reduction of global cerebral glucose metabolic rates in the patients compared with control subjects, with the largest degree of reduction in premotor and superior prefrontal cortical regions bilaterally. These studies suggested that functional neuroimaging with PET and SPECT could be powerful tools for the evaluation of various disorders of cognitive development, including the learning disabilities.

When performed in the resting state, PET and SPECT studies indicate brain regions of abnormal function. In contrast, when obtained during the performance of a specific task by the subject, a PET scan of ^{15}O-labeled water will show patterns of cerebral blood flow that indicate the circuits activated by the task and whether they are functioning abnormally (Posner and Raichle 1994). The advantage of PET activation studies, compared with SPECT activation studies, is that the half-life of ^{15}O is about 2 minutes, allowing multiple tasks to be performed within a session. In contrast, SPECT allows only a single activation paradigm to be studied. Task activation of neuronal circuits can also be achieved with echoplanar MRI technique (functional MRI, discussed earlier). Since absolute cooperation of the subject is required in activation studies, these methods are generally not suitable in young children.

Developmental Dyslexia

Both resting FDG-PET studies and PET/SPECT activation studies have been performed in patients with developmental dyslexia. Resting FDG-PET studies in dyslexic subjects have revealed several patterns of abnormal glucose metabolism, including bilateral hypometabolism of temporal and parietal cortex (Fig. 6.14), bilateral temporal hypometabolism, and unilateral left temporal hypometabolism (Chugani, un-

published data). These findings are in agreement with neuropsychological data indicating heterogeneity in patients with developmental dyslexia. Activation studies with SPECT in adults who were dyslexic as children have demonstrated deficient Wernicke's area activation and excessive temporoparietal activation during a spelling task, findings that suggest a trait anomaly of the left hemisphere (Flowers et al. 1991). Subsequent PET studies using ^{15}O-labeled water in dyslexic adults showed a failure to activate the left temporoparietal cortex during a rhyme detection task, and reduced activation/unusual deactivation in mid- and posterior temporal cortex bilaterally and in inferior parietal cortex, predominantly on the left side, during both pronunciation and decision making (Rumsey et al. 1992, 1997). More recent PET studies have also revealed abnormal cerebellar activation (Nicolson et al. 1999) and functional disconnection of the left angular gyrus from other parts of the reading network in adults with persistent developmental dyslexia (Horwitz et al. 1998). Subsequent fMRI studies support the notion that impaired activation of key regions for language perception and auditory attention in dyslexic subjects could account for persistent deficits in phonological awareness and reading tasks (Ruff et al. 2003).

Developmental Dysphasia

Two groups of children with developmental language disabilities (expressive dysphasia and expressive-receptive dysphasia) and a group of children with attention-deficit/hyperactivity disorder (ADHD) were evaluated with SPECT in the resting condition, during the performance of a simple auditory task, and during performance of an auditory phonemic discrimination task. Unlike the expressive and ADHD groups, the expressive-receptive group showed

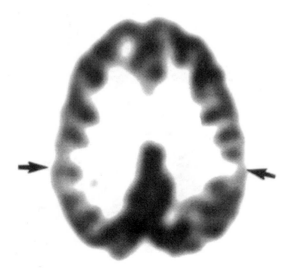
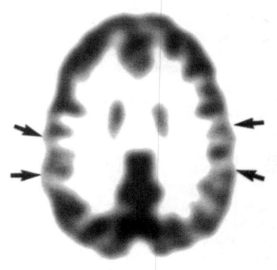

Figure 6.14 PET images from an adolescent boy with developmental dyslexia showing cerebral glucose metabolism. Note the bilateral parietal cortex hypometabolism (arrows). The MR images did not show any abnormalities.

an absence of left-hemispheric activation during the phonemic discrimination task. In addition, neither of the two language disability groups showed the left inferior parietal activation seen in the children with ADHD (Tzourio et al. 1994). A subsequent study added to these findings by demonstrating a lack of increase of rCBF in the left hemisphere (in Broca's area) but increased rCBF in the right hemisphere (in the region homologous to Broca's area) during a dichotic listening task given to boys with expressive dysphasia (Chiron et al. 1999a). The resting physiological asymmetry was reversed in favor of the right hemisphere in all areas except Broca's area. These findings illustrate how functional imaging can demonstrate abnormal lateralization and localization of language functions in the brain.

Learning Disability in Turner's Syndrome

Turner's syndrome is one of the most common of the human chromosomal aneuploidies, with an incidence of about 1 in 2,500 live female births. Both the severity and the type of cognitive impairment are highly variable among individuals with Turner's syndrome and cannot easily be accounted for by genotypic differences associated with chromosomal karyotype. The cognitive impairments often involve visuospatial and mathematical difficulties. Structural neuroimaging with MRI and CT scanning, and even neuropathological studies, have failed to identify any consistent abnormality to account for the cognitive difficulties in Turner's syndrome. On the other hand, PET investigations have shown a consistent pattern of bilateral occipital and parietal hypometabolism in adults with Turner's syndrome (Clark et al. 1990). A study of children with Turner's syndrome showed similar results, with the additional findings of temporal lobe hypometabolism in some subjects and a general correlation between the neuropsychological profile and the metabolic pattern (Elliott et al. 1996). This has been confirmed by subsequent quantitative PET studies of cerebral glucose metabolism, which have also revealed, in addition to focal hypometabolism in associative cortical areas, a generalized cerebral hypermetabolism in patients with Turner's syndrome, probably reflecting abnormal neuronal packing (Murphy et al. 1997). These studies suggest that the X chromosome is likely to be involved in development of cortical association areas in the brain.

Autism

Functional neuroimaging has been used in attempts to identify the neuroanatomic substrates involved in autism. In one study, elevated glucose metabolic rates were found in multiple brain regions of 10 autistic adults, but there was considerable overlap with control subjects, and no common regional abnormality could be identified in the autistic subjects (Rumsey et al. 1985). Further analysis of these data using correlation coefficients, a method that allows the strength of functional association between brain regions to be measured, revealed abnormal correlations between frontal and parietal regions and between the neostriatum and thalamus (Horwitz et al. 1988). In a study involving 18 autistic children, neither the rates nor the regional distribution of brain glucose metabolism was different from that in control subjects (De Volder et al. 1987). Similarly, Siegel et al. (1992) compared autistic adults and normal controls mixed for gender and found no difference in global cerebral glucose metabolism. In another study involving autistic children, some of whom had seizures and other coexisting conditions, MRI revealed evidence of neuronal migration anomalies in 3 of 13 children, and PET showed evidence of abnormalities in 5; however, no common or uniform abnormality could be demonstrated (Schifter et al. 1994). In contrast, Haznedar et al. (1997) performed MRI and glucose PET scans on high-functioning autistic patients and reported that the right anterior cingulate was significantly smaller in relative volume and was metabolically less active in the autistic patients compared to the normal subjects. The data from SPECT studies on autism have also been hard to interpret. One study found global hypoperfusion as well as hypoperfusion in the right lateral temporal lobe and right, left, and midfrontal lobes in four autistic adults compared with control subjects (George et al. 1992). Another study found no regional perfusion abnormalities in 21 autistic children evaluated with SPECT (Zilbovicius et al 1992). In a subsequent longitudinal study, the same group studied five autistic children (three males, two females) at the age of 3 to 4 years and again 3 years later, in comparison to two age-matched groups of nonautistic children (five children ages 3 to 4 years and seven children aged 6 to 12 years) with normal development (Zilbovicius et al 1995). The investigators reported frontal hypoperfusion in the autistic children at ages 3 to 4 years, but not at the ages of 6 to 7 years, suggesting a delayed frontal maturation in childhood autism. Another SPECT study showed hypoperfusion in the temporoparietal region in six autistic patients between 9 and 21 years of age, but further clinical information on these subjects was not provided (Mountz et al. 1995).

Studies investigating alterations in neurotransmitters, hormones, and their metabolites in the blood, cerebrospinal fluid (CSF), and urine of autistic patients have provided some evidence for the potential involvement of several neurotransmitters in autism (for review, see Anderson 1994). Furthermore, given that there is evidence for dysfunction in widely distributed brain regions in autism, the monoamine neurotransmitters are interesting candidates to be examined due to their widespread modulatory role in the brain. To this purpose, functional imaging has been used to examine in autism the role of two monoamine transmitters, dopamine (Ernst et al. 1997) and serotonin (Chugani et al. 1997, 1999).

Ernst et al. (1997) studied 14 medication-free autistic children with [^{18}F]-labeled fluorodopa (F-DOPA) using PET. F-DOPA is a precursor of dopamine, which is taken up, metabolized, and stored by dopaminergic terminals.

These authors reported a 39% reduction of the dopaminergic activity in the anterior medial prefrontal cortex in the autistic group, but no significant differences in any of the other regions measured. It was therefore suggested that decreased dopaminergic function in prefrontal cortex could contribute to the cognitive impairment seen in autism.

Although there is evidence for the potential involvement of several other neurotransmitters in autism, the most consistent findings involve serotonin. Pharmacological treatments that decrease serotonergic neurotransmission, such as tryptophan depletion, have been reported to result in an exacerbation of symptoms in autistic subjects (McDougle et al. 1996b). Conversely, administration of serotonin reuptake inhibitors appears to result in improvement of compulsive symptoms, repetitive movements, and social difficulties in autistic adults (Cook et al. 1992; Gordon et al. 1993; McDougle et al. 1996a).

Chugani et al. (1997) used AMT PET scanning (see also the earlier section on tuberous sclerosis) to study healthy, seizure-free children with autism (seven males and one female, ages 4 to 11 years) and their healthy nonautistic siblings (four males and one female, ages 8 to 14 years). Gross asymmetries of AMT standard uptake value (SUV) in frontal cortex, thalamus, and cerebellum were visualized in seven autistic boys (Fig. 6.15), but not in the one autistic girl studied or in four of the five siblings. Decreased AMT accumulation was seen in the left frontal cortex and thalamus in five of seven autistic boys. This was accompanied by an elevated AMT accumulation in the right cerebellum, in the region of the cerebellar dentate nucleus. In the remaining two autistic boys, AMT accumulation was decreased in the *right* frontal cortex and thalamus and elevated in the left dentate nucleus. The overall difference in asymmetry scores between the autistic boys and their siblings was found to be statistically significant, and regional asymmetry scores in the frontal cortex and thalamus were also found to differ significantly. The specificity of these abnormalities to serotonin synthesis was apparent when comparing the AMT scans to the FDG-PET and MRI scans, both of which were normal. Chugani et al. (1999) also measured whole brain serotonin synthesis capacity in autistic and nonautistic children at different ages using AMT and PET. Global brain values for serotonin synthesis capacity were obtained for 30 healthy, seizure-free autistic children (24 males and 6 females, ages 2 to 15 years),

eight of their healthy nonautistic siblings (six males and two females, ages 2 to 14 years), and 16 epileptic children without autism (nine males and seven females, ages 3 months to 13 years). For nonautistic children, serotonin synthesis capacity was greater than 200% of adult values until the age of about 5 years and then declined toward adult values. Serotonin synthesis capacity values declined at an earlier age in girls than in boys. In autistic children, serotonin synthesis capacity increased between the ages of 2 years and 15 years to values 1.5 times of the adult normal values and showed no gender difference. The data indicated a period of high brain serotonin synthesis capacity during childhood, and that this developmental process is disrupted in autistic children.

Landau-Kleffner Syndrome (Acquired Epileptic Aphasia)

Landau-Kleffner syndrome, or acquired epileptic aphasia, is characterized by progressive language loss after the acquisition of normal language function. The associated epilepsy is usually relatively mild (Landau and Kleffner 1957). During slow-wave sleep, continuous spike-and-wave discharges can be seen in some patients, but the presence of this electroencephalographic pattern is not required to make the diagnosis. Typically, the CT and MRI scans in Landau-Kleffner syndrome are normal. An FDG-PET study performed during sleep in three children with Landau-Kleffner syndrome showed metabolic disturbances consisting of hypermetabolism or hypometabolism in the temporal lobes and were right-sided, left-sided, or bilateral (Maquet et al. 1990). In children with Landau-Kleffner syndrome and continuous spike-and-wave discharges during sleep, PET scans have shown bilaterally increased temporal lobe glucose metabolism in the sleep state compared with the awake state, suggesting that the temporal lobes could be involved in the generation of continuous spike-and-wave discharges during slow-wave sleep (Rintahaka et al. 1995). The role of temporal lobe dysfunction in the pathophysiology of this condition has been also supported by a subsequent FDG-PET study of 17 children with Landau-Kleffner syndrome, demonstrating bilateral temporal lobe hypometabolism in 15 of them, although several other cortical regions also displayed hypometabolism in a subset of the patients (da Silva et al. 1997b).

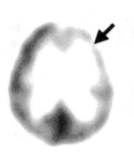 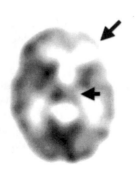 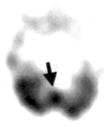

Figure 6.15 Focal abnormalities of tryptophan metabolism in an autistic boy, demonstrated by α-[^{11}C]methyl-L-tryptophan (AMT) PET. The figure shows a typical pattern of decreased AMT uptake in the left frontal cortex and thalamus, and an increased uptake in the cerebellum, in the region of the dentate nucleus (arrows).

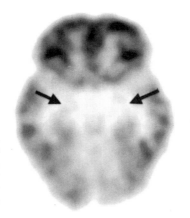 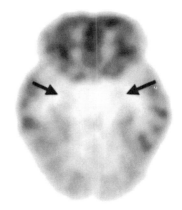

Figure 6.16 FDG-PET scan of a 6.5-year-old child who was adopted from an Eastern European orphanage. Note the severe hypometabolism in the region of hippocampus and amygdala bilaterally (arrows). An objective group analysis using SPM revealed further hypometabolic areas in the orbital frontal and infralimbic prefrontal cortex, the lateral temporal cortex, and the brainstem (Chugani et al. 2001).

Children With Early Severe Socioemotional Deprivation

Previous studies conducted in orphans adopted from Eastern European orphanages have found a variety of physical, cognitive, and social disturbances in such children (Ames 1997; Rutter 1998). The behavioral abnormalities reported in these children are similar to those seen in early socially deprived nonhuman primates (Suomi 1997). The impact of early social deprivation on human brain function has been studied recently using functional neuroimaging. In one study, FDG-PET scans in 10 postinstitutionalized Romanian orphans (ages 7.1 to 11.3 years) revealed decreases of brain glucose metabolism in mostly limbic structures, including the medial temporal region (amygdala and head of hippocampus), orbital frontal and infralimbic prefrontal cortex, the lateral temporal cortex, and the brainstem (Chugani et al. 2001) (Fig. 6.16). These brain regions form networks that have been shown to be activated by stress and damaged with prolonged stress (Lopez et al. 1999). Findings from these imaging studies suggest that the chronic stress endured by children from severe socioemotional deprivation during infancy can result in altered development of limbic structures and that altered functional connections in these circuits could represent the mechanism underlying persistent behavioral disturbances. Although preliminary, such functional neuroimaging studies provide an unprecedented opportunity to further understand the biological basis of early social deprivation and could prove useful to monitor therapeutic attempts in the future.

PERINATAL HYPOXIC-ISCHEMIC BRAIN INJURY

The earliest PET studies performed in the pediatric population involved newborns with perinatal asphyxia. These studies provided a new perspective on the mechanisms of neonatal brain injury and established the feasibility of PET studies on sick neonates.

In preterm infants with intraventricular hemorrhage, FDG-PET studies found that the area of metabolic abnormality (hypometabolism) extended beyond the regions that had been noted to be anatomically abnormal with CT (Doyle et al. 1983). Subsequently, measurements of local cerebral blood flow with PET in preterm infants with intraventricular and intracerebral hemorrhage demonstrated that in addition to a paucity of cerebral blood flow in the area of hemorrhagic involvement, there was markedly reduced blood flow throughout the affected cerebral hemisphere (Volpe et al. 1983). It therefore appeared that in these premature infants, intracerebral hemorrhage was but one manifestation of a large ischemic infarct. In *full-term* asphyxiated neonates, PET showed that the most consistent abnormality of cerebral blood flow was a relative hypoperfusion to the parasagittal regions of the brain (Volpe et al. 1985). In a further study, the same investigators found that cerebral blood flow rates of less than 10 ml/100 g/minute in newborns are compatible with normal neurological development (Altman et al. 1988). A subsequent study of children suspected of having hypoxic-ischemic brain injury found that children who were developing normally had the expected maturational increases of brain glucose uptake, whereas children who were developing abnormally tended to show persistently low glucose metabolism (Suhonen-Polvi et al. 1993). Similar observations have been made with SPECT, which showed hypoperfusion of all parts of the brain except the basal ganglia, brainstem, and sensorimotor cortex in neurologically affected infants (Konishi et al. 1994). A correlational study of PET findings with neurological outcome in term infants with hypoxic-ischemic encephalopathy found that total cerebral glucose metabolism rates measured during the first 3 weeks after birth was predictive of neurological sequelae, which were still present at 2 years of age (Thorngren-Jerneck et al. 2001).

Spastic Diplegia

Spastic diplegia is the typical motor manifestation in children with static encephalopathy associated with premature birth. The expected neuropathology, referred to

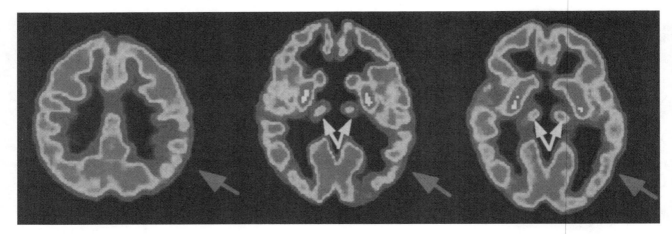

Figure 6.17 PET images from a 4-year-old child with spastic diplegic cerebral palsy associated with premature birth who was evaluated for delayed language skills. MRI revealed irregular contour to the walls of the lateral ventricles and high signal intensity in the periventricular white matter but no abnormalities in the cortex. PET revealed moderate hypometabolism in the left parietal and temporal cortex *(large arrows)*. In addition, there may be mild thalamic hypometabolism bilaterally *(small arrows)*.

as *periventricular leukomalacia,* in these children is readily identified on MRI scanning and represents ischemic lesions in the watershed region peculiar to the premature infant (Volpe 1995). These lesions are limited to white matter tracts dorsal and lateral to the lateral ventricles, seen most frequently near the foramen of Monro and the occipital horn. Cognitive difficulties are common in children with spastic diplegia, with an incidence of up to 20 to 40% in some follow-up studies of low-birth-weight infants (Blennow et al. 1986; Lefebvre et al. 1988). These cognitive problems are poorly predicted by MRI studies (e.g., Feldman et al 1990). Functional neuroimaging studies in children with spastic diplegia associated with premature birth have demonstrated focal areas of SPECT hypoperfusion (Denays et al. 1989) or PET hypometabolism (Kerrigan et al. 1991) in the parietal-occipital cortex adjacent to ultrasound or CT/MRI lesions representing periventricular leukomalacia. These findings suggest that the hypoperfusion and hypometabolism are the result of disrupted white matter tracts to and from the cortex (Fig. 6.17). Focal cortical volume loss was subsequently demonstrated in these children using MRI volumetry (Inder et al. 1999), thus confirming the functional neuroimaging studies. The clinical significance (and possible predictive value) of these focal cortical functional lesions with respect to the cognitive difficulties so frequently encountered in these children is currently being examined.

Choreoathetoid/Dystonic Form of Cerebral Palsy

In the full-term infant who has suffered from perinatal asphyxia, a static encephalopathy associated with chorea, athetosis, or dystonia can be seen. The neuropathological correlate of this disorder is usually gliosis and dysmyelina-

tion of the thalamus and basal ganglia, particularly the striatum (Volpe 1995). FDG-PET studies in a number of such children have shown either absent or markedly depressed glucose metabolism in the thalamus and lenticular nuclei, with relative sparing of the caudate nucleus (Kerrigan et al. 1991). The cerebral cortex is also relatively spared (Fig. 6.18), a finding that is consistent with the clinical observation that most of these children have relative preservation of cognitive function compared with their severe motor impairment. FDG-PET can be used in this group of children to evaluate their cognitive potential as a guide to early intervention.

CEREBROVASCULAR DISEASE

Functional neuroimaging is often helpful in the study of pediatric cerebrovascular disease, providing an assessment of the extent of functional involvement, which generally involves an area exceeding in size the anatomically affected area. In a series of 15 infants and children presenting with cerebrovascular disorders, SPECT showed focal hypoperfusion in all patients, with three patients also being shown to have adjacent hyperemia. Interestingly, two of the patients showed no abnormalities on repeated CT scans (Shahar et al. 1990). In patients with sickle cell disease, PET studies have shown increased regional cerebral blood flow and blood volume, but no differences in oxygen extraction or consumption, compared with control subjects (Herold et al. 1986). A subsequent FDG-PET study of 49 children with sickle cell disease showed abnormalities in glucose metabolism that were much more extensive and often bilateral when MRI abnormalities were lacking or subtle (Powars et al. 1999). PET was particularly sensitive in detecting focal abnormalities in children with no overt

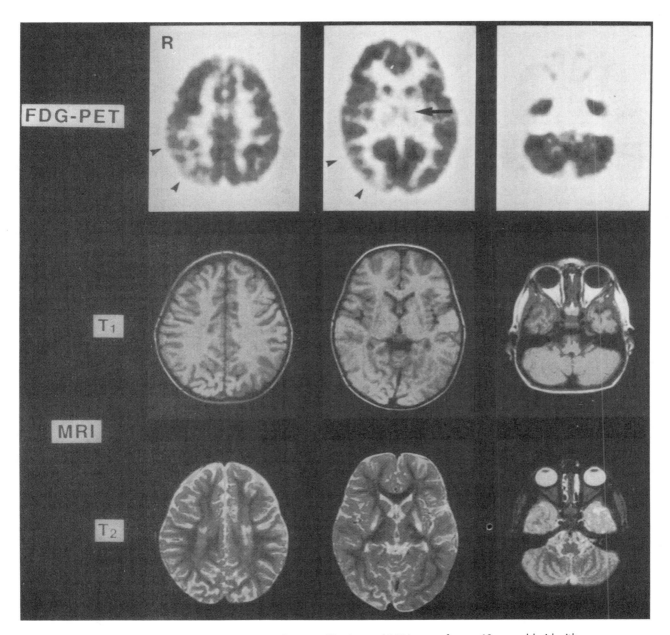

Figure 6.18 PET images showing glucose utilization and MR images from a 10-year-old girl with choreoathetoid cerebral palsy associated with abruptio placentae and birth asphyxia at term. The MR images show increased T2 signal intensity in the periventricular white matter, thalamus, and lenticular nuclei. The PET images show bilateral hypometabolism in the thalamus and lenticular nuclei *(arrow)*; the cerebral cortex is relatively normal except for hypometabolism in the right parietotemporal region *(arrowheads)*.

neurological symptoms. Thus, PET can be a sensitive and objective clinical tool to monitor response to therapeutic interventions in children with sickle cell anemia.

MOVEMENT DISORDERS

Most of the functional neuroimaging studies performed in this category have been on adults with disorders such as parkinsonism, Huntington's disease, and dystonia. For these and other dyskinesias in adults, PET studies using ^{18}F-labeled 6-fluorodopa to measure presynaptic dopaminergic function have been particularly useful (see, e.g., Turjanski et al. 1993). But use of PET with FDG or other PET ligands—for example, [^{11}C]raclopride, which labels the dopamine D_2 receptors (Brooks et al. 1992), and [^{11}C]-l-deprenyl, which labels monoamine oxidase B (Fowler et al. 1993)—has also provided useful information. Only a few studies have been performed in children, and these also have yielded interesting findings.

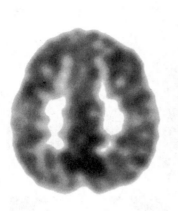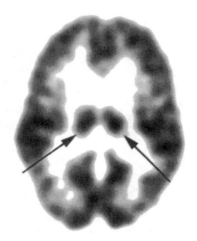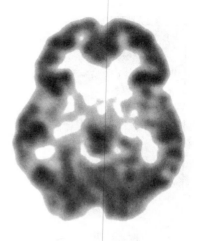

Figure 6.19 PET images from a 16-year-old girl with Huntington's disease showing glucose metabolism. Note the absence of metabolic activity in the caudate and lenticular nuclei. The thalami appear normal *(arrows)*.

Huntington's Disease in Children

Abnormal basal ganglia metabolism is seen in children with juvenile Huntington's disease, in whom the caudate and lenticular nuclei show markedly decreased glucose utilization (Fig. 6.19) (De Volder et al. 1988a). This finding is interesting because it is similar to what is found in adult Huntington's disease (Kuhl et al. 1982), yet the clinical presentations are quite different between the two forms. The juvenile form is characterized by intellectual decline, rigidity, seizures, and behavioral difficulties, whereas the adult form has as major manifestations chorea and dementia. Another study, however, found that the metabolic pattern in a child with juvenile Huntington's disease consisted of hypometabolism in the posterior nuclei of the thalamus (Matthews et al. 1989), a pattern that has not been seen in the adult form of the disease.

Tourette's Syndrome

In the few children with Tourette's syndrome who have been studied with FDG-PET, no consistent abnormalities have been found. However, a perfusion SPECT study reported subcortical asymmetries in Tourette's syndrome patients due to reduced right basal ganglia perfusion (Klieger 1997). Several studies evaluated various aspects of dopaminergic transmission, since it is believed that disturbances in the dopaminergic system contribute to the pathophysiology of Tourette's syndrome. Such studies reported elevated striatal dopamine transporter levels (Krause et al. 2002) and also abnormal presynaptic DOPA decarboxylase activity (Ernst et al. 1999). Another study also demonstrated increased dopamine release in the striatum of Tourette's syndrome patients (Singer et al. 2002). Preliminary imaging data using AMT PET (discussed previously) appear to support the role of abnormal serotonergic neurotransmission in the pathophysiology of Tourette's syndrome and some of its comorbid conditions, such as ADHD and obsessive-compulsive disorder (Ho et al. 2003).

NEURODEGENERATIVE DISORDERS

Some neurodegenerative disorders of childhood are characterized by relatively specific findings on CT or MRI scanning. For example, in Hallervorden-Spatz disease, a disorder of abnormal iron metabolism in brain, the MRI shows hypointense areas in the basal ganglia and substantia nigra (see Rouault 2001 for review). However, structural neuroimaging in many childhood neurodegenerative disorders reveals nonspecific abnormalities such as progressive cerebral atrophy and is of limited value in these cases. In such disorders, imaging of glucose metabolism or a variety of biochemical processes with PET or SPECT can provide more specific findings and yield important insight into the pathophysiology of these disorders.

Mitochondrial Encephalopathies

The combined use of PET and magnetic resonance spectroscopy (MRS) can be useful in the evaluation of children with disorders involving mitochondrial function. In one such study, FDG-PET in children with defects of oxidative phosphorylation and lactic acidosis showed a massive increase in glycolysis, believed to be a result of compensatory efforts to meet energy requirements of the brain. Elevated lactate in the brain was confirmed with MRS. An increase in glycolysis was not seen in children with normal respiratory chain activity and lactic acidosis due to stress and exercise (Duncan et al. 1995). An earlier study on subjects with mitochondrial diseases evaluated both oxygen and glucose utilization with PET and found that patients with brain disease in addition to muscle disease had a lower ratio of oxygen-to-glucose consumption in the brain, a finding

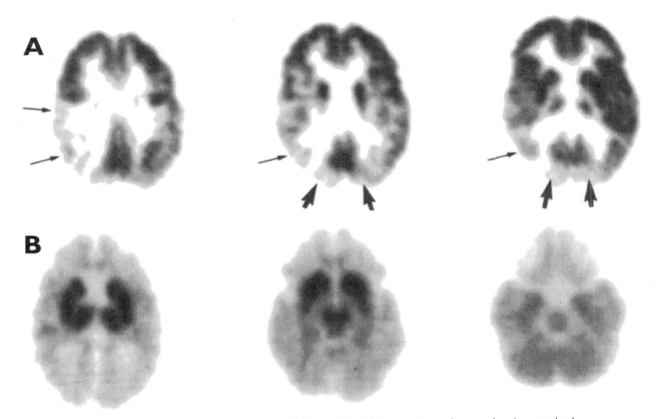

Figure 6.20 PET images from two children with Spielmeyer-Vogt disease showing cerebral glucose metabolism. **(A)** Early in the course, there is hypometabolism in the occipital cortex *(thick arrows);* as the disease progresses, hypometabolism is seen in other posterior cortical regions and may be asymmetric, as shown in the images from this child, with occipital, right parietal, and posterior temporal cortex hypometabolism *(thin arrows).* **(B)** Diffuse and severe cortical hypometabolism is seen in the late stages of the disease. Note the relative preservation of glucose metabolism in the basal ganglia, thalamus, brainstem, and mesial temporal structures.

which suggests that there is aerobic glycolysis to lactate and possibly other intermediate metabolites (Frackowiak et al. 1988). Elevated brain lactate level is indeed an important diagnostic finding in mitochondrial diseases and, since it can indicate functional involvement irrespective of structural MRI abnormalities, MRS can be a useful complementary tool to monitor disease progression or treatment efficacy (Castillo et al. 1995; Pavlakis et al. 1998). SPECT has also been used to evaluate children with mitochondrial disorders. SPECT is less useful than PET in this context but does show focal areas of decreased perfusion believed to be related to stroke events (Fujii et al. 1995).

Neuronal Ceroid Lipofuscinoses

The neuronal ceroid lipofuscinoses are a group of autosomal recessive diseases that are characterized, in general, by seizures, developmental regression, and progressive visual impairment. The juvenile form (CLN-3) is also known as Spielmeyer-Vogt (or Batten) disease. FDG-PET studies in children with Spielmeyer-Vogt disease evaluated early in the course of the disease have revealed decreased glucose

metabolism in the calcarine cortex (Philippart et al. 1994) (Fig. 6.20). In contrast, late infantile neuronal ceroid lipofuscinosis (CLN-2; Jansky-Bielschowsky disease, with curvilinear inclusions) is characterized by rapid degeneration with generalized cortical and subcortical hypometabolism (Philippart et al. 1997). As the juvenile form of the disease progresses, a rostral spread of glucose hypometabolism to other cortical areas is observed. We have not seen this pattern of abnormality in any other childhood or adult neurodegenerative processes, and, therefore, PET may be of diagnostic value in Spielmeyer-Vogt disease. In addition, the rate of disease progression can be monitored with PET.

RETT SYNDROME

The few studies that have been performed with PET in children with Rett syndrome have shown conflicting results. One study found reduced rates of oxygen metabolism and oxygen extraction fraction, particularly in frontal cortex (Yoshikawa et al. 1991), but another study found slightly increased glucose metabolism in frontal cortex and hypometabolism in occipital cortex (Naidu et al. 1988). In addition, PET with [^{18}F]-6-fluorodopa and [^{11}C]-raclopride have been used to study dopaminergic function in young patients with Rett syndrome (Dunn et al. 2002). MRI scans of these patients showed significant volume reductions of the basal ganglia (caudate heads and thalami), which was corroborated by reduced fluorodopa uptake in the caudate and putamen. In contrast, dopamine D_2 receptor binding was increased significantly by almost 10% in both of these structures, suggesting a mild presynaptic deficit of nigrostriatal activity in Rett syndrome.

Canavan's Disease

Canavan's disease is an autosomal recessive hereditary leukodystrophy due to deficiency of the enzyme aspartoacylase, which is the primary enzyme involved in the catabolic metabolism of N-acetylaspartate (NAA). Structural imaging studies typically show severe nonspecific white matter abnormalities compatible with demyelination. Proton MRS studies can be useful to support the presumed diagnosis of Canavan's disease by showing increased levels of NAA as compared to choline and creatine in the affected brain regions (Wittsack et al. 1996).

Subacute Sclerosing Panencephalitis

In a single child with the rapidly progressive form of subacute sclerosing panencephalitis (SSPE), the absolute rates of glucose metabolism were markedly decreased in cortical gray matter structures but normal in caudate and lenticular nuclei. In contrast, cerebral glucose metabolic rates were normal in another child who appeared to have slow progression of the disease (Yanai et al. 1987). There is one study suggesting that abnormal patterns of cerebral glucose metabolism can return to normal in patients with SSPE following treatment with human interferon beta. A case was reported in which the patient prior to such treatment was shown to have symmetric hypometabolism in the thalamus, cerebellum, and cortex (except primary motor region) and hypermetabolism in the lenticular nuclei. After treatment, which was associated with some clinical improvement, glucose metabolic rates returned to normal in the cerebral cortex. However, the bilateral focal necrosis present in the putamen as shown on CT and MRI scans indicated disease progression. Persistent hypermetabolism was evident in the caudate and in the spared superoposterior portion of the putamen (Huber et al. 1989). The findings from this study are somewhat difficult to interpret, but further studies have not been performed.

Alternating Hemiplegia of Childhood

Between attacks, FDG-PET studies in patients with alternating hemiplegia have shown normal findings (Mikati and Fischman 1995). However, an 11-year-old boy with alternating hemiplegia studied with $C^{15}O_2$ and PET during an acute episode of right hemiplegia was found to have slightly increased perfusion in the insula, putamen, and claustrum in the left hemisphere (Tada et al. 1989). Although this finding has been interpreted as suggesting a vascular etiology, this is not necessarily the explanation, because cerebral blood flow is tightly coupled to cerebral metabolism, and, therefore, intrinsic neuronal perturbations could also result in blood flow alterations. A more recent PET study of cerebral tryptophan metabolism in children with alternating hemiplegia performed during or shortly after an attack showed increased serotonin synthesis capacity in the frontoparietal cortex, lateral and medial temporal structures, striatum, and thalamus when compared to controls, and subjects with alternating hemiplegia studied interictally. In addition, larger estimated lifetime attack numbers were associated with delay in communication and daily living skills. These studies suggest that attacks in alternating hemiplegia are associated with increased regional serotonergic activity, and that frequent attacks can have an effect on neurodevelopment, thus supporting the notion that alternating hemiplegia of childhood can be a progressive disorder (Pfund et al. 2002).

Other Childhood Neurodegenerative Disorders

Glutaricaciduria type I (Ozand and Gascon 1991a, 1991b) is an autosomal recessive disorder in the oxidative pathway of lysine, hydroxylysine, and tryptophan that is caused by a defect of the enzyme glutaryl-CoA dehydrogenase. The clinical presentation of individuals with this disorder is heterogeneous, with intermittent metabolic acidosis or extrapyramidal signs. FDG-PET shows a dramatic pattern of absent metabolic activity in the striatum bilaterally and diffuse cortical hypometabolism (Fig. 6.21). These findings suggest that although the brain is diffusely affected in this metabolic disorder, the striatum is particularly vulnerable to damage (Awaad et al. 1996).

In another inborn error of metabolism, adenylosuccinase deficiency, in which there is a deficiency in the synthesis of purine nucleotides, psychomotor retardation with autism is a prominent clinical feature (Jaeken and Van den Berghe 1984). PET scanning in this disorder has shown a consistent pattern of markedly diminished glucose metabolism in all gray matter structures except the cerebellum. The hypometabolism was most pronounced in the frontal lobes (De Volder et at. 1988b). The typical pattern of glucose metabolism on FDG-PET in patients with Wilson's disease is hypometabolism of the lenticular nuclei (Hawkins et al. 1987). When patients with Wilson's disease have been studied with PET and [^{11}C]raclopride, reduced uptake is seen in the striatum; after treatment with d-penicillamine, [^{11}C]raclopride uptake shows improvement, and this suggests that the defect in striatal neurons is reversible (Schwarz et al. 1994). Wilson's disease is an

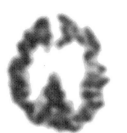 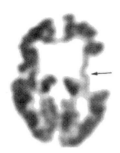 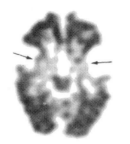 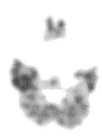

Figure 6.21 PET images from a 3-year-old boy with glutaricaciduria type I. Note the virtual absence of glucose metabolism in the basal ganglia and the open opercula (*arrows*) with severe frontotemporal atrophy.

example of a disorder in which the effectiveness of therapy can be monitored with PET, which provides unique information not otherwise obtainable.

CONCLUSION

This chapter has shown how functional neuroimaging with PET, SPECT, proton MRS, and fMRI modalities continue to emerge as important tools in the diagnosis, monitoring, and eventual treatment of a variety of neuropsychiatric disorders in infants and children. In some cases, such as infantile spasms, functional imaging has led directly to new treatment options previously not considered. In other instances, properly selected functional imaging methods can provide specific diagnostic markers (such as increased NAA on proton MRS in Canavan's disease). In most cases, anatomic and functional neuroimaging provide complementary data and should be carefully used together for optimum management. Studies over the past few years have provided several examples of how application of new PET and SPECT tracers have gained clinical importance (e.g., those for imaging benzodiazepine and dopamine receptors, or serotonergic neurotransmission). With both SPECT and PET, the synthesis of even newer tracers designed to evaluate various biochemical processes in the brain is proceeding at a rapid pace. These tracers are being applied to pediatric neuropsychiatric disorders to yield a wealth of new and specific information related to pathophysiology and therapeutic guidance. Imaging specific biochemical functions can also lead to identification of various patterns of abnormal brain function. This sub-classification allows more accurate genotyping in future genetic studies aimed to clarify the genetic background of pediatric neuropsychiatric disorders.

REFERENCES

Altman Dl, Powers WJ, Perlman JM, et al. Cerebral blood flow requirement for brain viability in newborn infants is lower than in adults. Ann Neurol 24:218–226, 1988.

Ames, EW. The development of Romanian orphanage children adopted into Canada. Final report to Human Resources Development, Canada, 1997.

Anderson, GM. Studies on the neurochemistry of autism. In: Bauman ML, Kemper TL, eds. *The Neurobiology of Autism*. Baltimore: Johns Hopkins University Press, pp. 227–242, 1994.

Andre-Thomas CY, Saint-Anne Dargassies S. *The Neurological Examination of the Infant*. London: Medical Advisory Committee of the National Spastics Society, 1960.

Asano E, Chugani DC, Muzik O, et al. Multimodality imaging for improved detection of epileptogenic foci in tuberous sclerosis complex. Neurology 54:1976–1984, 2000.

Awaad Y, Shamoto H, Chugani HT. Hemidystonia improved by baclofen and PET scan findings in a patient with glutaric aciduria Type 1. J Child Neurol 11:167–169, 1996.

Awaya S. Stimulus vision deprivation amblyopia in humans. In: Reinecke RD, ed. *Strabismus*. New York: Grune & Stratton, pp. 31–44, 1978.

Blennow G, Pleven H, Lindroth M, et al. Long-term follow-up of ventilator-treated low birthweight infants, II: neurological and psychological outcome at 6–7 years. Acta Paediatrica Scandinavica 75:827–831, 1986.

Blume WT, David RB, Gomez MR. Generalized sharp and slow wave complexes: associated clinical features and long-term follow-up. Brain 96:289–306, 1973.

Bronson G. The postnatal growth of visual capacity. Child Dev 45:873–890, 1974.

Brooks DJ, Ibanez V Sawle GV et al. Striatal D-2 receptor status in patients with Parkinson's disease, striatonigral degeneration, and progressive supranuclear palsy, measured with 11-C-raclopride and positron emission tomography. Ann Neurol 31:184–192, 1992.

Castillo M, Kwock L, Green C. MELAS syndrome: imaging and proton MR spectroscopic findings. AJNR Am J Neuroradiol 16:233–239, 1995.

Chiron C, Dulac O, Bulteau C, et al. Study of regional cerebral blood flow in West syndrome. Epilepsia 34:707–715, 1993.

Chiron C, Pinton F, Masure MC, Duvelleroy-Hommet C, Leon F, Billard C. Hemispheric specialization using SPECT and stimulation tasks in children with dysphasia and dystrophia. Dev Med Child Neurol 41:512–520, 1999a.

Chiron C, Raynaud C, Maziere B, et al. Changes in regional cerebral blood flow during brain maturation in children and adolescents. J Nucl Med 33:696–703, 1992.

Chiron C, Raynaud C, Tzourio N, et al. Regional cerebral blood flow by SPECT imaging in Sturge-Weber disease: an aid for diagnosis. J Neurol Neurosurg Psychiatry 52:1402–1409, 1989.

Chiron C, Vera P, Kaminska A, et al. Single-photon emission computed tomography: ictal perfusion in childhood epilepsies. Brain Dev 21:444–446, 1999b.

Chugani DC, Chugani HT, Muzik O, et al. Imaging epileptogenic tubers in children with tuberous sclerosis complex using α-[^{11}C] methyl-L-tryptophan positron emission tomography. Ann Neurol 44:858–866, 1998a.

Chugani DC, Muzik O, Behen ME, et al. Developmental changes in brain serotonin synthesis capacity in autistic and non-autistic children. Ann Neurol 45:287–295, 1999.

Chugani DC, Muzik O, Chakraborty PK, et al. Human brain serotonin synthesis capacity measured in vivo with alpha-[C-11] methyl-L-tryptophan. Synapse 28:33–43, 1998b.

Chugani DC, Muzik O, Rothermel R, et al. Altered serotonin synthesis in the dentatothalamo-cortical pathway in autistic boys. Ann Neurol 14:666–669, 1997.

Chugani HT, Hovda D, Villablanca J, et al. Metabolic maturation of the brain: a study of local cerebral glucose utilization in the cat. J Cereb Blood Flow Metab 11:35–47, 1991.

Chugani HT. Development of regional brain glucose metabolism in relation to behavior and plasticity. In: Dawson G, Fischer KW, eds. *Human Behavior and the Developing Brain.* New York: Guilford, pp. 153–175, 1994.

Chugani HT. Metabolic imaging: a window on brain development and plasticity. The Neuroscientist 5:29–40, 1999.

Chugani HT, Behen ME, Muzik O, Juhász C, Nagy F, Chugani DC. Local brain functional activity following early deprivation: a study of post-institutionalized Romanian orphans. Neuroimage 14:1290–1301, 2001.

Chugani HT, Conti J. Etiological classification of infantile spasms in 140 cases: role of positron emission tomography. J Child Neurol 11:44–48, 1996.

Chugani HT, da Silva E, Chugani DC. Infantile spasms, III: prognostic implications of bitemporal hypometabolism on positron emission tomography. Ann Neurol 39:643–649, 1996.

Chugani HT, Dietrich RB. Sturge-Weber syndrome: recent developments in neuroimaging and surgical considerations. In: Fukuyama Y, Suzuki Y, Kamoshita S, and Caesar P, eds. *Fetal and Perinatal Neurology,* Basel: Karger, pp. 187–196, 1992.

Chugani HT, Mazziotta JC, Engel JJ, et al. The Lennox-Gastaut syndrome: metabolic subtypes determined by 2-deoxy-2[18-F] fluoro-d-glucose positron emission tomography. Ann Neurol 21:4–13, 1987a.

Chugani HT, Mazziotta JC, Phelps ME. Sturge-Weber syndrome: a study of cerebral glucose utilization with positron emission tomography J Pediatr 114:244–253, 1989.

Chugani HT, Phelps ME. Maturational changes in cerebral function in infants determined by 18-FDG positron emission tomography. Science 231:840–843, 1986.

Chugani HT, Phelps ME, Mazziotta JC. Positron emission tomography study of human brain functional development. Ann Neurol 22:487–497, 1987b.

Chugani HT, Shewmon D, Khanna S, et al. Interictal and postictal focal hypermetabolism on positron emission tomography. Pediatr Neurol 9:10–15, 1993a.

Chugani HT, Shewmon D, Peacock W, et al. Surgical treatment of intractable neonatal-onset seizures: the role of positron emission tomography. Neurology 38:1178–1188, 1988.

Chugani HT, Shewmon D, Sankar R, et al. Infantile spasms, II: lenticular nuclei and brainstem activation on positron emission tomography. Ann Neurol 31:212–219, 1992.

Chugani HT, Shewmon D, Shields W et al. Surgery for intractable infantile spasms: neuroimaging perspectives. Epilepsia 34:764–771, 1993b.

Chugani HT, Shields W, Shewmon D, et al. Infantile spasms, I: PET identifies focal cortical dysgenesis in cryptogenic cases for surgical treatment. Ann Neurol 27:406–413, 1990.

Clark C, Klonoff H, Hayden M. Regional cerebral glucose metabolism in Turner syndrome. Can J Neurol Sci 17:140–144, 1990.

Cook EH, Rowlett R, Jaselskis C, et al. Fluoxetine treatment of children and adults with autistic disorder and mental retardation. J American Academy of Child and Adolescent Psychiatry 31:739–745, 1992.

Cross JH, Gordon I, Connelly A, et al. Interictal 99T c(m) HMPAO SPECT and ^{1}H MRS in children with temporal lobe epilepsy. Epilepsia 38:338–345, 1997.

Curtiss S. Feral children. In: Wortis J, ed. *Mental Retardation and Developmental Disabilities XII.* NewYork: Brunner/Mazel, pp. 129–161, 1981.

da Silva EA, Chugani DC, Muzik O, Chugani HT. Identification of frontal lobe epileptic foci in children using positron emission tomography. Epilepsia 38:1198–1208, 1997a.

da Silva EA, Chugani DC, Muzik O, Chugani HT. Landau-Kleffner syndrome: metabolic abnormalities in temporal lobe are a common feature. J Child Neurol 12:489–495, 1997b.

Denays R, Van Pachterbeke T, Tondeur M, et al. Brain single photon emission computed tomography in neonates. J Nucl Med 30:1337–1341, 1989.

De Volder A, Bol A, Michel C, et al. Brain glucose metabolism in children with the autistic syndrome: positron tomography analysis. Brain Dev 9:581–587, 1987.

De Volder AG, Bol A, Michel C, et al. Brain glucose utilization in childhood Huntington's disease studied with positron emission tomography (PET). Brain Dev 10:47–50, 1988a.

De Volder AG, Jaeken J, Van Den Berghe G, et al. Regional brain glucose utilization in adenylosuccinase-deficient patients measured by positron emission tomography. Pediatr Res 24:238–242, 1988b.

Diemer K. Capillarisation and oxygen supply of the brain. In: Lubbers DW, Luft UC, Thews G, et al., eds. *Oxygen Transport in Blood and Tissue.* Stuttgart: Thieme, pp. 118–123, 1968.

Diksic M, Nagahiro S, Sourkes TL et al. A new method to measure brain serotonin synthesis in vivo. I. Theory and basic data for a biological model. J Cereb Blood Flow Metab 9:1–12, 1990.

Doyle LW, Nahmias C, Firnau G, et al. Regional cerebral glucose metabolism of newborn infants measured by positron emission tomography Dev Med Child Neurol 25:143–151, 1983.

Dulac O, Chiron C, Jambaque I, et al. infantile spasms. Progress in Clinical Neuroscience 2:97–109, 1987.

Dulac O, Plouin P. Cryptogenic/idiopathic West syndrome. In: Dulac O, Chugani HT, Bernardina BD, eds. *Infantile Spasms and West Syndrome.* London: WB Saunders, pp. 232–243, 1994.

Duncan DB, Herholz K, Kugel H, et al. Positron emission tomography and magnetic resonance spectroscopy of cerebral glycolysis in children with congenital lactic acidosis. Ann Neurol 37:351–358, 1995.

Dunn HG, Stoessl AJ, Ho HH, et al. Rett syndrome: investigation of nine patients, including PET scan. Can J Neurol Sci 29:345–357, 2002.

Ell PJ, Jarritt PH, Costa DC, et al. Functional imaging of the brain. Semin Nucl Med 17:214–229, 1987.

Elliott TK, Watkins JM, Messa C, et al. Positron emission tomography and neuropsychological correlations in Turner syndrome. Developmental Neuropsychology 12:365–386, 1996.

Ernst M, Zametkin A, Matochik J, et al. Low medial prefrontal dopaminergic activity in autistic children. The Lancet 350:638, 1997.

Ernst M, Zametkin AJ, Jons PH, Matochik JA, Pascualvaca D, Cohen RM. High presynaptic dopaminergic activity in children with Tourette's disorder. J Am Acad Child Adolesc Psychiatry 38:86–94, 1999.

Fedi M, Reutens DC, Andermann F, et al. Alpha-[^{11}C]-methyl-L-tryptophan PET identifies the epileptogenic tuber and correlates with interictal spike frequency. Epilepsy Res 52:203–213, 2003.

Feldman HM, Scher MS, Kemp SS. Neurodevelopmental outcome of children with evidence of periventricular leukomalacia on late MRI. Pediatr Neurol 6:296–302, 1990.

Filipek P. Neurobiologic correlates of developmental dyslexia: how do dyslexics' brains differ from those of normal readers? J Child Neurol 10 (suppl 1):62–69, 1995.

Flowers LD, Wood FB, Naylor CE. Regional cerebral blood flow correlates of language processing in reading disability. Arch Neurol 48:637–43, 1991.

Fowler JS, Volkow ND, Logan J, et al. Monoamine oxidase B (MAO B) inhibitor therapy in Parkinson's disease: the degree and reversibility of human brain MAO B inhibition by Ro 19 6327. Neurology 43:1984–1992, 1993.

Frackowiak RSJ, Herold S, Petty RKH, et al. The cerebral metabolism of glucose and oxygen measured with positron tomography in patients with mitochondrial diseases. Brain 111:1009–1024, 1988.

Fujii T, Okuno T, Ito M, et al. 123I-IMP SPECT findings in mitochondrial encephalomyopathies. Brain Dev 17:89–94, 1995.

Fuster JM. *The Prefrontal Cortex: Anatomy, Physiology, and Neuropsychology of the Frontal Lobe.* 3rd Ed. Philadelphia: Lippincott-Raven, pp. 177–178, 1997.

Gaillard WD, Bhatia S, Bookheimer SY, Fazilat S, Sato S, Theodore WH. FDG-PET and volumetric MRI in the evaluation of patients with partial epilepsy. Neurology 45:123–126, 1995.

Gaillard WD, Grandin CB, Xu B. Developmental aspects of pediatric fMRI: considerations for image acquisition, analysis, and interpretation. Neuroimage 13:239–249, 2001.

Gaillard WD, Hertz-Pannier L, Mott SH, Barnett AS, LeBihan D, Theodore WH. Functional anatomy of cognitive development: fMRI of verbal fluency in children and adults. Neurology 54:180–185, 2000.

Gaillard WD, Sachs BC, Whitnah JR, Ahmad Z, Balsamo LM, Petrella JR, Braniecki SH, McKinney CM, Hunter K, Xu B, Grandin CB. Developmental aspects of language processing: fMRI of verbal fluency in children and adults. Hum Brain Mapp 18:176–185, 2003.

George MS, Costa DC, Kouris K, et al. Cerebral blood flow abnormalities in adults with infantile autism. J Nerv Ment Dis 180:413–417, 1992.

Goldman-Rakic PS. The frontal lobes: uncharted provinces of the brain. Trends Neurosci 7:425–429, 1984.

Gordon CT, State RC, Nelson JE, et al. A double-blind comparison of clomipramine, desipramine and placebo in the treatment of autistic disorder. Arch Gen Psych 50:441–447, 1993.

Guye M, Parker GJ, Symms M, et al. Combined functional MRI and tractography to demonstrate the connectivity of the human primary motor cortex in vivo. Neuroimage 19:1349–1360, 2003.

Haginoya K, Kon K, Yokoyama H. The perfusion defect seen with SPECT in West syndrome is not correlated with seizure prognosis or developmental outcome. Brain Dev 22:16–23, 2000.

Harvey AS, Bowe JM, Hopkins IJ, et al. Ictal 99mTc-HMPAO single photon emission computed tomography in children with temporal lobe epilepsy. Epilepsia 34:869–877, 1993.

Hawkins RA, Mazziotta JC, Phelps ME. Wilson's disease studied with FDG and positron emission tomography. Neurology 37:1707–1711, 1987.

Haznedar M, Buchsbaum M., Metzger M, et al. Anterior cingulate gyrus volume and glucose metabolism in autistic disorder. Am J Psych 154:1047–1050, 1997.

Heiskala H, Launes J, Pihko H, et al. Brain perfusion SPECT in children with frequent fits. Brain Dev 15:214–218, 1993.

Henry TR, Chugani HT, Abou-Khalil BW et al. Positron emission tomography. In: Surgical Treatment of the Epilepsies. 2nd Ed. New York: Raven, pp. 211–243, 1993.

Herold S, Brozovic M, Path FRC, et al. Measurement of regional cerebral blood flow, blood volume and oxygen metabolism in patients with sickle cell disease using positron emission tomography. Stroke 17:692–698, 1986.

Ho A, Juhasz C, Chugani HT, Behen ME. PET scanning of tryptophan metabolism in Tourette syndrome (TS). Neurology Suppl 1:A211, 2003.

Holland SK, Plante E, Weber Byars A, Strawsburg RH, Schmithorst VJ, Ball WS Jr. Normal fMRI brain activation patterns in children performing a verb generation task. Neuroimage 14:837–843, 2001.

Horwitz B, Rumsey JM, Donohue BC. Functional connectivity of the angular gyrus in normal reading and dyslexia. Proc Natl Acad Sci USA 95:8939–8944, 1998.

Horwitz B, Rumsey JM, Grady CL, et al. The cerebral metabolic landscape in autism: intercorrelations of regional glucose utilization. Arch Neurol 45:749–755, 1988.

Huber M, Herholz K, Pawlik G, et al. Cerebral glucose metabolism in the course of subacute sclerosing panencephalitis. Arch Neurol 46:97–100, 1989.

Iinuma K, Yanai K, Yanagisa T, et al. Cerebral glucose metabolism in five patients with Lennox-Gastaut syndrome. Pediatr Neurol 3:12–14, 1987.

Iivanainen M, Launes J, Pihko H, et al. Single-photon emission computed tomography of brain perfusion: analysis of 60 paediatric cases. Dev Med Child Neurol 32:63–68, 1990.

ILAE Commission Report. Commission on diagnostic strategies. Recommendations for functional neuroimaging of persons with epilepsy. Epilepsia 41:1350–1356, 2000.

Inder TE, Huppi PS, Warfield S, et al. Periventricular white matter injury in the premature infant is followed by reduced cerebral cortical gray matter volume at term. Ann Neurol 46:755–760, 1999.

Jacobs B, Chugani HT, Allada V et al. Developmental changes in brain metabolism in sedated rhesus macaques and velvet monkeys revealed by positron emission tomography. Cereb Cortex 3:222–233, 1995.

Jaeken J, Van den Berghe G. An infantile autistic syndrome characterized by the presence of succinyl purines in body fluids. Lancet 2:1058–1061, 1984.

Jambaque I, Chiron C, Dulac O, et al. Visual inattention in West syndrome: a neuropsychological and neurofunctional imaging study. Epilepsia 34:692–700, 1993.

Juhász C, Chugani DC, Muzik O, et al. Relationship of flumazenil and glucose PET abnormalities to neocortical epilepsy surgery outcome. Neurology 56:1650–1658, 2001a.

Juhász C, Chugani DC, Muzik O, Shah A, Asano E, Mangner T, Chakraborty PK, Sood S, Chugani HT. Alpha-methyl-L-tryptophan PET detects epileptogenic cortex in children with intractable epilepsy. Neurology 60:960–968, 2003.

Juhász C, Chugani DC, Padhye UN, et al. Evaluation with α [11C]methyl-L-tryptophan PET for reoperation after failed epilepsy surgery. Epilepsia 45:124–130, 2004.

Juhász C, Chugani HT, Muzik O, Chugani DC. Neuroradiological assessment of brain structure and function and its implication in the pathogenesis of West syndrome. Brain Dev 23:488–495, 2001b.

Kagan J. Do infants think? Sci Am 226:74–82, 1972.

Kaminska A, Chiron C, Ville D, et al. Ictal SPECT in children with epilepsy: comparison with intracranial EEG and relation to postsurgical outcome. Brain 126:248–260, 2003.

Kellaway P. An orderly approach to visual analysis: parameters of the normal EEG in adults and children. In: Klass DW, Daly DD, eds. Current Practice of Clinical Electroencephalography. New York: Raven, pp. 69–147, 1979.

Kerrigan J, Chugani HT, Phelps M. Regional cerebral glucose metabolism in clinical subtypes of cerebral palsy. Pediatr Neurol 7:415–425, 1991.

Kinnala A, Suhonen-Polvi H, Aarimaa T, et al. Cerebral metabolic rate for glucose during the first six months of life: an FDG positron emission tomography study. Arch Dis Child Fetal Neonatal Ed 74:F153–157, 1996.

Klieger PS, Fett KA, Dimitsopulos T, Karlan R. Asymmetry of basal ganglia perfusion in Tourette's syndrome shown by technetium-99m-HMPAO SPECT. J Nucl Med 38:188–191, 1997.

Konishi Y, Kuriyama M, Mori I, et al. Assessment of local cerebral blood flow in neonates with N-isopropyl-P-[123-I]iodoamphetamine and single photon emission computed tomography. Brain Dev 16:450–453, 1994.

Konkol RJ, Maister BH, Wells RG, et al. Hemimegalencephaly: clinical, EEG, neuroimaging, and IMPSPECT correlation. Pediatr Neurol 6:414–418, 1990.

Krakow K, Woermann FG, Symms MR, et. al. EEG-triggered functional MRI of interictal epileptiform activity in patients with partial seizures. Brain 122:1679–1688, 1999.

Krause KH, Dresel S, Krause J, Kung HF, Tatsch K, Lochmuller H. Elevated striatal dopamine transporter in a drug naive patient with Tourette syndrome and attention deficit/hyperactivity disorder: positive effect of methylphenidate. J Neurol 249:1116–1118, 2002.

Kuhl DE, Phelps ME, Markham CH, et al. Cerebral metabolism and atropy in Huntington's disease determined by 18-FDG and computed tomographic scan. Ann Neurol 12:425–434, 1982.

Kuzniecky R, Mountz JM, Wheatley G, et al. Ictal single-photon emission computed tomography demonstrates localized epileptogenesis in cortical dysplasia. Ann Neurol 34:627–631, 1993.

Landau WM, Kleffner FR. Syndrome of acquired aphasia with convulsive disorder in children. Neurology 7:27–531, 1957.

Lazeyras F, Blanke O, Perrig S, Zimine I, Golay X, Delavelle J, Michel CM, de Tribolet N, Villemure JG, Seeck M. EEG-triggered functional MRI in patients with pharmacoresistant epilepsy. J Magn Reson Imaging 12:177–185, 2000.

Lee BC, Kuppusamy K, Grueneich R, El-Ghazzawy O, Gordon RE, Lin W, Haacke EM. Hemispheric language dominance in children demonstrated by functional magnetic resonance imaging. J Child Neurol 14:78–82, 1999.

Lee JS, Asano E, Muzik O, et al. Sturge-Weber syndrome: correlation between clinical course and FDG PET findings. Neurology 57:189–195, 2001.

Lefebvre F, Bard H, Veilleux A, et al. Outcome at school age of children with birth-weights of 1,000 grams or less. Dev Med Child Neurol 30:170–180, 1988.

Lenneberg E. Biological Foundations of Language. New York: Wiley, 1967.

Lopez, JF, Akil, H, and Watson SJ. Role of biological and psychological factors in early development and their impact on adult life. Biol Psychiatry 46:1461–1471, 1999.

Macdonell RA, Jackson GD, Curatolo JM, et al. Motor cortex localization using functional MRI and transcranial magnetic stimulation. Neurology 53:1462–1467, 1999.

Maquet P, Hirsch E, Dive D, et al. Cerebral glucose utilization during sleep in Landau-Kleffner syndrome: a PET study. Epilepsia 31:778–783, 1990.

Marks DA, Katz A, Hoffer P, et al. Localization of extratemporal epileptic foci during ictal single photon emission computed tomography. Ann Neurol 31:250–255, 1992.

Matthews PM, Evans AC, Andermann F, et al. Regional cerebral glucose metabolism differs in adult and rigid juvenile forms of Huntington disease. Pediatr Neurol 5:353–356, 1989.

McDougle CJ, Naylor ST, Cohen DJ, et al. A double-blind, placebo-controlled study of fluvoxamine in adults with autistic disorder. Arch Gen Psych 53:1001–1008, 1996a.

McDougle CJ, Naylor ST, Cohen DJ, et al. Effects of tryptophan depletion in drug-free adults with autistic disorder. Arch of Gen Psych 53:993–1000, 1996b.

Mikati M, Fischman AJ. Positron emission tomography in children with alternating hemiplegia of childhood. In: Andermann F, Aicardi J, Vigevano F, eds. Alternating Hemiplegia of Childhood (International Review of Child Neurology Series). New York: Raven, pp. 109–114, 1995.

Mountz JM, Tolbert LC, Lill DW, et al. Functional deficits in autistic disorder: characterization by technetium-99m HMPAO and SPECT. J Nucl Med 36:1156–1162, 1995.

Murphy DG, Mentis MJ, Pietrini P, et al. A PET study of Turner's syndrome: effects of sex steroids and the X chromosome on brain. Biol Psychiatry 41:285–298, 1997.

Muzik O, Chugani DC, Chakraborty PK, et al. Analysis of [C-11] alpha-methyl-tryptophan kinetics for the estimation of serotonin synthesis rate in vivo. J Cerebr Blood Flow Metab 17:659–669, 1997.

Muzik O, da Silva E, Juhász C, et al. Intracranial EEG vs. flumazenil and glucose PET in children with extratemporal lobe epilepsy. Neurology 54:171–179, 2000.

Naidu S, Wong DF, Sanche RP, et al. Rett syndrome: positron emission tomography metabolic-clinical correlates (abstract). Ann Neurol 24:305, 1988.

Newport EL, Supalla T. Maturational constraints on language learning. Cognitive Science 14:11–28, 1990.

Nicolson RI, Fawcett AJ, Berry EL, Jenkins IH, Dean P, Brooks DJ. Association of abnormal cerebellar activation with motor learning difficulties in dyslexic adults. Lancet 353:1662–1667, 1999.

O'Brien TJ, So EL, Mullan BP, et al. Subtraction SPECT co-registered to MRI improves postictal SPECT localization of seizure foci. Neurology 52:137–146, 1999.

Ozand PT, Gascon GG. Organic acidurias: a review, Part 1. J Child Neurol 6:196–219, 1991a.

Ozand PT, Gascon GG. Organic acidurias: a review, Part 2. J Child Neurol 6:288–303, 1991b.

Parmelee AH, Sigman MD. Perinatal brain development and behavior. In: Haith MM, Campos JJ, eds. Handbook of Child Psychology. 4th Ed. Vol 2. Infancy and Developmental Psychobiology. New York: Wiley, pp 95–155, 1983.

Pavlakis SG, Kingsley PB, Kaplan GP, Stacpoole PW, O'Shea M, Lustbader D. Magnetic resonance spectroscopy: use in monitoring MELAS treatment. Arch Neurol 55:849–852, 1998.

Pennington BF. Genetics of learning disabilities. J Child Neurol 10 (suppl 1):69–77, 1995.

Pfund Z, Chugani DC, Muzik O, et al. Alpha [¹¹C] methyl-L-typtophan positron emission tomography in patients with alternating hemiplegia of childhood. J Child Neurol 17:253–260, 2002.

Phelps ME, Hoffman EJ, Mullani NA, et al. Application of annihilation coincidence detection to transaxial reconstruction tomography. J Nucl Med 16:210–224, 1975.

Philippart M, da Silva E, Chugani HT. The value of positron emission tomography in the diagnosis and monitoring of late infantile and juvenile lipopigment storage disorders (so-called Batten or neuronal ceroid lipofuscinoses). Neuropediatrics 28:74–76, 1997.

Philippart M, Messa C, Chugani HT. Spielmeyer-Vogt (Batten, Spielmeyer-Sjogren) disease: distinctive patterns of cerebral glucose utilization. Brain 117:1085–1092, 1994.

Pinton F, Chiron C, Enjolras O, Motte J, Syrota A, Dulac O. Early single photon emission computed tomography in Sturge-Weber syndrome. J Neurol Neurosurg Psychiatry 63:616–621, 1997.

Posner MI, Raichle ME. Images of Mind. New York: Scientific American Library, 1994.

Powars DR, Conti PS, Wong WY. Cerebral vasculopathy in sickle cell anemia: diagnostic contribution of positron emission tomography. Blood 93:71–79, 1999.

Rintahaka P, Chugani HT, Messa C, et al. Hemimegalencephaly: evaluation with positron emission tomography. Pediatr Neurol 9:21–28, 1993.

Rintahaka P, Chugani HT, Sankar R. Landau-Kleffner syndrome with continuous spikes and waves during slow-wave sleep. J Child Neurol 10:127–133, 1995.

Rouault TA. Systemic iron metabolism: a review and implications for brain iron metabolism. Pediatr Neurol 25:130–137, 2001.

Rowe CC, Berkovic SF, Austin MC, et al. Patterns of postictal blood flow in temporal lobe epilepsy: qualitative and quantitative analysis. Neurology 41:1096–1103, 1991.

Rowe CC, Berkovic SF, Sia STB, et al. Localization of epileptic foci with postictal single photon emission computed tomography. Ann Neurol 26:660–668, 1989.

Rubinstein M, Denays R, Ham HR, et al. Functional imaging of brain maturation in humans using iodine-123 iodoamphetamine and SPECT. J Nucl Med 30:1982–1985, 1989.

Ruff S, Marie N, Celsis P, Cardebat D, Demonet JF. Neural substrates of impaired categorical perception of phonemes in adult dyslexics: an fMRI study. Brain Cogn 53:331–334, 2003.

Rumsey JM, Andraeson P, Zametkin AJ, et al. Failure to activate the left temporoparietal cortex in dyslexia. Arch Neurol 49:527–534, 1992.

Rumsey JM, Duara R, Grady C, et al, Brain metabolism in autism: resting cerebral glucose utilization rates as measured with positron emission tomography. Arch Gen Psychiatry 42:448–455, 1985.

Rumsey JM, Nace K, Donohue B, Wise D, Maisog JM, Andreason P. A positron emission tomographic study of impaired word recognition and phonological processing in dyslexic men. Arch Neurol 54:562–573, 1997.

Rutter, M. Developmental catch-up, and deficit, following adoption after severe global early privation. English and Romanian Adoptees (ERA) Study Team. J Child Psychol Psychiatry 39:465–476, 1998.

Savic I, Persson A, Roland P, et al. In vivo demonstration of benzodiazepine receptor binding in human epileptic foci. Lancet 2:863–866, 1988.

Schade JP, van Groenigen WB. Structural organization of the human cerebral cortex. Acta Anat (Basel) 47:74–111, 1961.

Schifter T, Hoffman JM, Hatten HP, et al. Neuroimaging in infantile autism. J Child Neurol 9:155–161, 1994.

Schwartz TL, Linberg JV, Tillman W et al. Monocular depth and vernier acuities: a comparison of binocular and uniocular subjects (abstract). Invest Ophthalmol Vis Sci 28 (suppl):304, 1987.

Schwarz J, Antonini A, Kraft E, et al. Treatment with D-penicillamine improves dopamine D-2-receptor binding and T-2-signal intensity in de novo Wilson's disease. Neurology 44:1079–1082, 1994.

Shahar E, Gilday DL, et al. Pediatric cerebrovascular disease: alterations of regional cerebral blood flow detected by TC 99m-HMPAO SPECT. Arch Neurol 47:578–584, 1990.

Siegel BV, Jr., Asarnow R, Tanguay P, et al. Regional cerebral glucose metabolism and attention in adults with a history of childhood autism. J Neuropsychiatry Clin Neurosci 4:406–414, 1992.

Singer HS, Szymanski S, Giuliano J, Yokio F, Dogan S, Brasic J, Zhou Y, Grace A, Wong DF. Elevated intrasynaptic dopamine release in Tourette's syndrome measured by PET. Am J Psychiatry 159:1329–1336, 2002.

Stone TW. Kynurenines in the CNS: from endogenous obscurity to therapeutic importance. Prog Neurobiol 64:185–218, 2001.

Suhonen-Polvi H, Kero P, Korvenranta H, et al. Repeated fluoro-deoxyglucose positron emission tomography of the brain in infants with suspected hypoxic-ischaemic brain injury. Eur J Nucl Med 20:759–765, 1993.

Sujansky E, Conradi S. Sturge-Weber syndrome: age of onset of seizures and glaucoma and the prognosis for affected children. J Child Neurol 10:49–58, 1995.

Suomi, SJ. Early determinants of behavior: evidence from primate studies. Br Med Bull 53:170–184, 1997.

Tada H, Miyake S, Yamada M, et al. A patient with alternating hemiplegia in childhood. No 1b Hattatsu 21:283–288, 1989.

Ter-Pogossian MM. Positron emission tomography. In: Wagner HN, Szabo Z, Buchanan JW, eds. Principles of Nuclear Medicine. London: WB Saunders, pp. 342–346, 1995.

Ter-Pogossian MM, Phelps ME, Hoffman EJ, et al. A positron emission transaxial tomograph for nuclear imaging (PETT). Radiology 114:89–98, 1975.

Theodore WH, Rose D, Patronas N, et al. Cerebral glucose metabolism in the Lennox-Gastaut syndrome. Ann Neurol 21:14–21, 1987.

Thorngren-Jerneck K, Ohlsson T, Sandell A, et al. Cerebral glucose metabolism measured by positron emission tomography in term newborn infants with hypoxic ischemic encephalopathy. Pediatr Res 49:495–501, 2001.

Tokumaru AM, Barkovich AJ, O'uchi T, Matsuo T, Kusano S. The evolution of cerebral blood flow in the developing brain: evaluation with iodine-123 iodoamphetamine SPECT and correlation with MR imaging. AJNR Am J Neuroradiol 20:845–852, 1999.

Turjanski N, Bhatia K, Burn DJ, et al. Comparison of striatal 18F-dopa uptake in adult-onset dystonia-parkinsonism, Parkinson's disease, and dopa-responsive dystonia. Neurology 43:1563–1568, 1993.

Tzourio N, Heim A, Zilbovicius M, et al. Abnormal regional CBF response in left hemisphere of dysphasic children during a language task. Pediatr Neurol 10:20–26, 1994.

Vaegan, Taylor D. Critical period for deprivation amblyopia in children. Tran Ophthalmol Soc UK 99:432–439, 1979.

Van Bogaert P, Wikler D, Damhaut P, Szliwowski HB, Goldman S. Regional changes in glucose metabolism during brain development from the age of 6 years. Neuroimage 8:62–68, 1998.

Vera P, Kaminska A, Cieuta C, et al. Use of subtraction ictal SPECT co-registered to MRI for optimizing the localization of seizure foci in children. J Nucl Med 40:786–792, 1999.

Vigevano F, Bertini E, Boldrini R, et al. Hemimegalencephaly and intractable epilepsy: benefits of hemispherectomy. Epilepsia 30:833–834, 1989.

Vinters HV Fisher RS, Cornford ME, et al. Morphological substrates of infantile spasms: studies based on surgically resected cerebral tissue. Childs Nerv Syst 8:8–17, 1992.

Volpe JJ. *Neurology of the Newborn.* 3rd Ed. Philadelphia: WB Saunders, pp, 403–430, 1995.

Volpe JJ, Herscovitch P, Perlman JM, et al. Positron emission tomography in the asphyxiated term newborn: parasagittal impairment of cerebral blood flow. Ann Neurol 17:287–296, 1985.

Volpe JJ, Herscovitch P, Perlman JM, et al. Positron emission tomography in the newborn: extensive impairment of regional cerebral blood flow with intraventricular hemorrhage and hemorrhagic intracerebral involvement. Pediatrics 72:589–601, 1983.

von Hofsten C. Eye-hand coordination in the newborn. Developmental Psychology 18:450–461, 1982.

Weinberg WA, Harper CR, Brumback RA. Neuroanatomic substrate of developmental specific learning disabilities and select behavioral syndromes. J Child Neurol 10 (suppl 1):78–80, 1995.

Wittsack HJ, Kugel H, Roth B, Heindel W. Quantitative measurements with localized ^{1}H MR spectroscopy in children with Canavan's disease. J Magn Reson Imaging 6:889–993, 1996.

Yanai K, Ilinuma K, Tada K, et al. Regional cerebral metabolic rate for glucose in subacute sclerosing panencephalitis. Eur J Pediatr 146:288–289, 1987.

Yetkin FZ, Swanson S, Fischer M, et al. Functional MR of frontal lobe activation: comparison with Wada language results. AJNR Am J Neuroradiol 19:1095–1098, 1998.

Yoshikawa H, Fueki N, Suzuki H, et al. Cerebral blood flow and oxygen metabolism in Rett syndrome. J Child Neurol 6:237–242, 1991.

Zametkin AJ, Nordahl TE, Gross M, et al. Cerebral glucose metabolism in adults with hyperactivity of childhood onset. N Engl J Med 323:1361–1461, 1990.

Zilbovicius M, Garreau B, Samson Y, et al. (1995). Delayed maturation of the frontal cortex in childhood autism. Am J Psychiatry 152:248–252, 1995.

Zilbovicius M, Garreau B, Tzourio N, et al. Regional cerebral blood flow in childhood autism: a SPECT study. Am J Psychiatry 149:924–930, 1992.

Zupanc ML. Neuroimaging in the evaluation of children and adolescents with intractable epilepsy: II. Neuroimaging and pediatric epilepsy surgery. Pediatr Neurol 17:111–121, 1997.

Clinical Electrophysiology of the Developing Human Brain

Leslie J. Carver, PhD

Martha Ann Bell, PhD

The electroencephalogram (EEG) and event-related potentials (ERPs) are two brain imaging methodologies that provide functional information about the developing brain. Both EEG and ERPs represent electrical activity recorded from the scalp, with the assumption that the origin of these electrical signals is in the brain itself. Although once thought to be the product of action potentials, there now is general agreement among researchers that the scalp signal is the summation of postsynaptic potentials (Nelson & Monk, 2001). The EEG signal is spontaneous but context-related, with the signal generated during quiet rest being different from that generated during mental activity. The ERP signal is event specific, with onset aligned to a temporarily locked event. This means that both the EEG and ERP signals have temporal resolution on the order of milliseconds. Thus, postsynaptic changes immediately are reflected in the EEG and ERP, making these methodologies outstanding for tracking rapid shifts in brain functioning. Furthermore, these brain electrical signals are robust and the techniques by which they are obtained are somewhat easy, noninvasive, and relatively inexpensive. These characteristics make the EEG and ERP methods some of the more favorable ones for studying brain development in infants and children and for relating brain development to changes in behavior (Casey & de Hann, 2002; de Haan & Thomas, 2002; Taylor & Baldeweg, 2002).

In this chapter we highlight the value of EEG/ERP for the study of typical and atypical brain/behavior relations in infancy and childhood. We begin with an overview of the basic methodology associated with EEG and ERP techniques. Next, we describe research studies that have used the EEG in examining individual differences in social and emotional behaviors. The focus of this section is on studies examining behavioral inhibition or extreme shyness. In the final section, we describe studies that have been conducted using ERPs to measure the neural correlates of cognitive and social behavior in typically developing and atypical populations. Our review in this section focuses on studies of face processing, one method that has proven especially useful in studies of development.

ELECTROENCEPHALOGRAM (EEG) AND EVENT-RELATED POTENTIALS (ERP) METHODOLOGY

The EEG and ERP signals represent the electrical potential between two scalp electrodes. In reality, however, researchers utilize multiple electrodes in EEG/ERP studies. For ease and speed in application with pediatric populations, electrodes are available in configurations that contain multiple electrodes. Typically, one of two methods is used for electrode application. A Lycra stretch cap that can be custom made to different head sizes and number of electrodes is available for use with infants and children as well as adults (Fig. 7.1). After the EEG cap is placed on the head, recommended procedures regarding EEG data collection

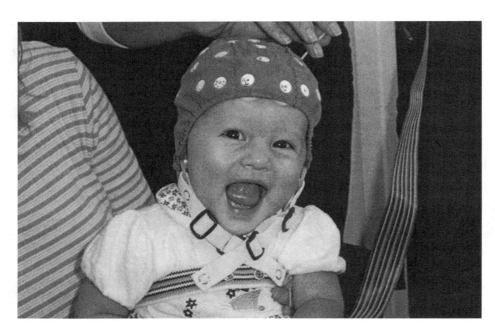

Figure 7.1 Infant wearing EEG/ERP electrodes.

with infants and young children should be followed (EEG: Pivik et al., 1993; ERP: Picton et al., 2000). Specifically, a small amount of abrasive gel is placed into each electrode-recording site and the scalp gently rubbed. This prepares the scalp by gently removing any dry skin that may interfere with EEG recordings. Following this, conductive gel is placed in each site.

A second method of electrode application is the geodesic net system (Electrical Geodesics, Inc.; Tucker, 1993). This system provides a large number of electrodes that are distributed evenly across the scalp. This system of electrode placement has the advantage of being very easy to apply even to young infants. In addition, the geodesic system uses high-impedance amplifiers that do not require scalp abrasion to improve the connection between electrode and scalp. The use of these amplifiers is somewhat controversial, although studies are beginning to emerge that show similar findings between this system and the Lycra cap system (Johnson et al., 2001).

A standard set of electrode placements referred to as the International 10–20 system has been used by most researchers (Jasper, 1958). For a number of reasons, the validity of this electrode application has been challenged over the years. Of greatest relevance for this summary are problems with application of the 10–20 system to infants and young children. The Jasper system relies for placement of electrodes on a ratio of distances between anterior and posterior sites. It is unclear whether this same ratio exists across development or whether different regions of the brain mature at different rates, leading to differences in the relation between anterior and posterior growth. However, several researchers have examined this problem, primarily through autopsy (Blume, Buza, & Okazaki, 1974) and radiograph (Hellstrom, Karlsson, & Mussbichler, 1963), and have found that the 10–20 system does an adequate job in defining placement of electrodes across key cortical regions. However electrodes are distributed across the scalp, it is important to note that electrical activity is volume conducted at different rates through different materials (e.g., scalp, meninges, brain, cerebrospinal fluid). Thus, the scalp distribution of electrical activity only provides an approximation of the location of the source of the activity. High-density recordings likely increase the accuracy of these estimates; however, electrophysioloical methods remain significantly less accurate for estimating the location of activity as they do the time course of that activity.

EEG Data Reduction and Measures

The methods for recording "clinical" EEG and "quantitative" EEG are identical. Clinical EEG records are analog tracings that focus on the time domain. These clinical EEG records are inspected by visual analysis and yield valuable information regarding neuropathology in infants and children, as well as gestational age/maturation level of premature infants. Quantitative EEG is a digital record that is converted from the time domain to the frequency domain using fast Fourier transform. This is accomplished to assess mathematical changes in brain electrical activity and corresponding psychological functions. Quantitative techniques can also be used to assess developmental changes in the EEG during infancy and childhood. This chapter focuses on quantitative EEG.

Theoretically, the EEG signal is composed of multiple sine waves cycling at different frequencies. The Fourier transform decomposes the EEG into these different sine waves and estimates the spectral power (in mean square microvolts) at each frequency. The result is information regarding the contribution of each individual frequency to the entire EEG spectrum at a particular electrode site. Power is thought to reflect the excitability of groups of neurons. Increasing power values across age are considered indicative of brain development (Bell, 1998; Marshall, Bar-Haim, & Fox, 2002). The power data are normalized because EEG power data are usually positively skewed. The most common normalization for EEG data is the natural log (Davidson, Jackson, & Larson, 2000).

Power values are usually totaled across frequency bins to form measures of power in a specific frequency band. *Alpha* activity, so named by Berger (1929) because it was the first EEG rhythm he discussed, cycles at 8 to 13 Hz and is the predominant frequency band for adults. Activation of brain areas underlying specific scalp electrodes is assumed when alpha power values at those electrode sites are lower during stimulus processing than they were during resting baseline (Bell & Fox, 2003; Davidson, Chapman, Chapman, & Henriques, 1990). Similarly, activation of brain areas underlying specific electrodes also is assumed when alpha power values at those electrode sites are lower during rest than are alpha power values at corresponding electrodes sites on the opposite hemisphere (Davidson et al., 2000).

Interest in the normal developmental course of the EEG began with Berger's (Berger, 1932) report of EEG differences among infants, young children, and adults. This work immediately generated longitudinal studies of EEG development during infancy and childhood (Henry, 1944; Lindsley, 1939; Smith, 1938a, 1938b). These pioneering researchers used visual inspection of EEG records to describe the appearance of a 3–5 Hz rhythm over the occipital area at 3 months of age that increased to a frequency of 6 to 7 Hz by 12 months of age. More recently, researchers have noted, based on these earlier studies, that by the second half of the first year of life the majority of infant EEG activity can be found in the 3 to 12 Hz band (Fox & Davidson, 1987, 1988). Furthermore, there appears to be a peak in EEG activity at 6 to 9 Hz during this same time period (Bell, 1998; Johnson et al., 2001; Molfese, 1989; Molfese, Wetzel, & Gill, 1993; Sato, Kochiyama, Yoshikawa, & Matsumura, 2001). This period of rapid EEG development during the first year of life continues into early childhood and is then followed by a more gradual change in EEG. In longitudinal studies of EEG development during childhood, frequencies of 9 to 10 Hz at occipital locations have been reported by 8 years of age (Bell, 1998; Lindsley, 1939; Smith, 1938b; see Bell, 1998, for a detailed review of the ontogeny of EEG during infancy and childhood). Thus, the pediatric EEG signal has different frequency, as well as amplitude, characteristics relative to the adult EEG signal (Fig. 7.2). Researchers must take care to examine frequency components that are appropriate for infant and child populations.

ERP Data Reduction and Measures

As with EEG, ERP data are scored for artifact before data analysis is conducted. Some ERP data-collection programs include algorithms for detecting data that include eyeblinks, motor artifact, and environmental noise. Other researchers choose to manually inspect data, as is frequently

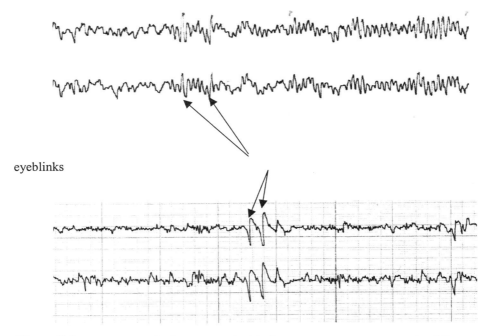

Figure 7.2 Comparison of infant (top) and adult (bottom) EEG tracings. Note the differences in frequency and amplitude. Eyeblinks (arrows) are labeled in each tracing.

done in EEG recording. Regardless of which method is used, researchers should inspect averaged data from each individual subject for artifact.

After artifact detection, data from the raw EEG recording are averaged over some number of trials that are defined by the onset of some temporally-locked event (e.g., the presentation of a stimulus). In this way, the background EEG is removed over trials, and ERP components emerge. Several components are usually observed in developmental ERP research. A complete review of the components elicited in most ERP studies is beyond the scope of this chapter. We describe the components typically elicited and analyzed in visual ERP paradigms used with children, as this is the type of study we describe in a later section of the chapter. The reader should be aware that a number of other components are elicited in studies using auditory stimuli and in studies conducted with adults (see Fig. 7.3).

Visual ERP studies conducted with infant and child populations typically elicit characteristic ERP components. Characteristic ERP patterns seen in visual ERP studies with infants are shown in Figure 7.4. Among the first of these to be identified and the one that seems to be most pervasive in the developmental literature is the Nc component. This component was first identified by Courchesne (Courchesne, 1978; Courchesne, Ganz, & Norcia, 1981). The Nc component is a middle latency (peaking at about 500 msec after stimulus presentation) negative component. The scalp distribution of the Nc was first described as involving

frontal and central midline electrodes. Since the development of high-density recording methods, it has become clear that the Nc is broadly distributed over the frontal scalp. The Nc is thought to be related to the infant's attentional response to a salient stimulus (Courchesne, 1978; Courchesne et al., 1981; de Haan & Nelson, 1997, 1999; Nelson, 1994; Nelson & Collins, 1991). The more salient the infant finds the stimulus, the larger the amplitude of the Nc that is elicited. Thus, if an infant sees a novel object, and has a novelty preference, the amplitude of the Nc will be larger than that elicited by a familiar stimulus. However, if the familiar stimulus is highly salient (e.g., a picture of the infant's mother), the Nc can be larger to the familiar stimulus. In addition, early in development, the Nc can respond to the frequency with which a familiar stimulus is presented, so that the Nc is larger to a infrequently presented familiar stimulus than to a more frequently presented familiar stimulus (Nelson & Collins, 1990, 1991). The Nc component is typically elicited in young children and can be seen until at least 7 years of age (Courchesne, 1978). It is not typically seen in adults.

Other ERP components elicited in many developmental studies are also seen in adults. Early components thought to reflect sensory processing are elicited over occipital scalp locations and are similar in morphology to early sensory components seen in adults (Courchesne, 1978). These components are typically labeled in relation to their polarity and peak latency (e.g., P250) or by their polarity and

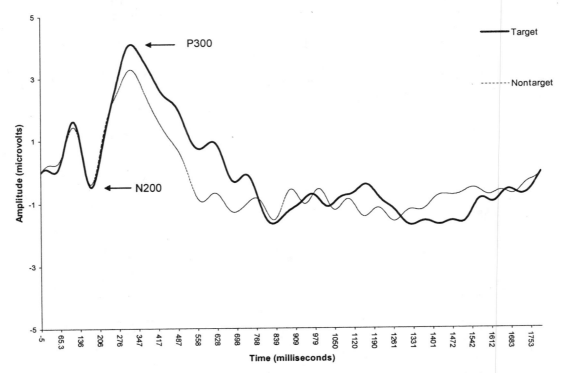

Figure 7.3 Adult ERP waveform recorded at a posterior electrode site in a target/nontarget paradigm. The top arrow indicates the P300, which is larger in response to the target stimulus. The second arrow indicates the early sensory component, N200.

(a)

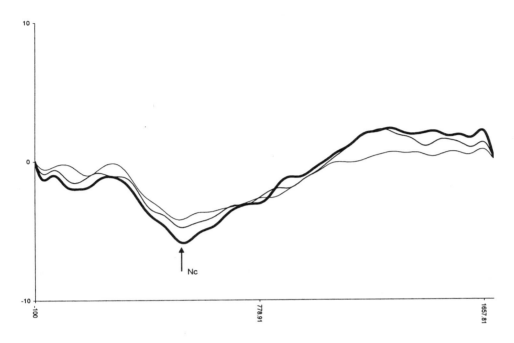

(b)

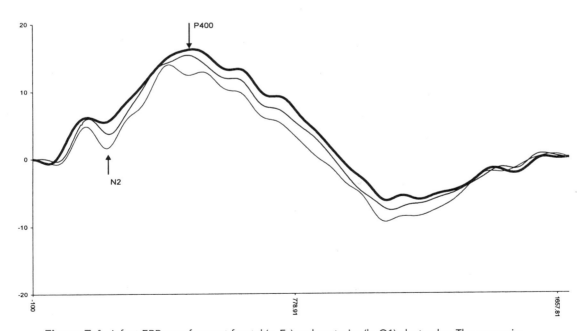

Figure 7.4 Infant ERP waveforms at frontal (a, Fz) and posterior (b, O1) electrodes. The arrows indicate the Nc component (in [a]), the P500 component (positive peak in [b]), and the early sensory component N200 (in [b]). The Nc and P500 components are larger to a highly salient stimulus (in this case, a negative facial expression).

ordinal position (e.g., the second negative component would be referred to as N2). A large amplitude positive component (P500) has been observed over occipital scalp locations. This component has been described primarily in studies of face recognition, although it has also been elicited in studies of object recognition. The function of this component is not entirely clear; however, it appears to have some face-specific response characteristics, making it a potential candidate for a precursor to the face-specific component observed in adults (de Haan, Pascalis, & Johnson, 2002). Finally, slow-wave activity (activity that does not resolve in a clear peak) has been observed in studies of memory (Nelson & Collins, 1990, 1991). This slow-wave activity occurs late in the recording epoch, and its polarity may be related to memory updating, novelty detection, or recognition.

A final component that is important for the discussion of face processing is the N170. This is an early component that peaks over posterior parietal electrode sites and is sensitive to aspects of face processing (Bentin, Allison, Puce, Perez, & McCarthy, 1996). The N170 is larger in response to faces than other classes of stimuli and is sensitive to the orientation in which faces are displayed. The N170 is larger in amplitude and slower in latency for inverted faces than for upright faces. It is not clear whether the N170 can be identified in developmental studies. De Haan and colleagues (de Haan et al., 2002) suggested that early developmental precursors to the N170 are apparent in the P400 and the negative peak that immediately precedes it.

Typical dependent measures in ERP studies include the peak amplitude of the component and its latency, as well as the area underneath the curve formed by the component, and the average amplitude of the component. Principle components analysis (PCA) and independent components analysis (ICA) have also been used in some studies in attempts to isolate multiple underlying neural sources that could contribute to activity recorded at the scalp (Grice et al., 2001).

In ERP studies, the stimuli typically belong to two or several categories or conditions and are analyzed across these conditions, leads (i.e., activity at different electrode sites), and any grouping variables. Data from clinical populations are typically compared to that from a control group, although the choice of control group needs to be made with great care. For example, in studies of children with developmental delay, controls might typically be matched on mental age. However, there are significant maturational changes in children that could preclude the choice of a much younger control group. In such cases, it is often helpful to test a group of children who have developmental delay of a different etiology and thus are matched on both maturation and level of cognitive functioning.

Limitations of EEG/ERP

EEG and ERP are among the more favorable brain imaging methods for use with infants and children; however,

these methodologies have some drawbacks. Although the EEG and ERP signals have outstanding temporal resolution, they have poor spatial resolution. There are at least three reasons for this shortcoming (Davidson et al., 2000). First, even with multiple electrodes, there are gaps between electrodes on the scalp. This prohibits a complete electrical mapping of the scalp. Second, the skull behaves like a low-pass filter and distorts the underlying brain electrical activity over a large area of the scalp. Finally, scalp potentials are likely generated by multiple groupings of cortical and subcortical generators spread across a relative wide area. Thus, an electrode is likely detecting electrical activity generated from nonlocal groups of neurons.

The accuracy of algorithms devised to localize electrical activity in the brain from scalp surface recordings is a source of debate (Dien, Spencer, & Donchin, 2003; Mosher, Leahy, & Lewis, 1999; Picton et al., 2000). These considerations are amplified in studies with infants, primarily due to challenges in electrode application, testing parameters, and physical differences between infants and adults (Johnson et al., 2001). These differences include myelination of certain brain areas and dendritic arborization (Greenough, Black, & Wallace, 1987; Greenough & Volkmar, 1973), and differences between adults and children in factors that affect the transmission of electrical signals, such as differences in skull and meninges thickness, and open fontanels in infancy. Our limited understanding of neural development in humans compounds the problem of accurate localization of source activity in the young infant. Johnson and colleagues (2001) reported that reasonable source localization can be estimated in about half of infant subjects. Thus, improvements in methods for both analyzing source information and recording brain electrical activity are needed before we can accurately estimate the source of such ERP activity in infants.

Another drawback is that the EEG is prone to distortion because of motor movement. Artifact may result from such gross motor activity as waving of the arms and legs or from motor activity as fine as a blink or a slight eye movement. Although adult research participants are generally cooperative when requested to sit without moving, young children often have great difficulty in refraining from gross motor movements. Researchers must ensure that their expectations for the behavior of young children in EEG and ERP paradigms are developmentally appropriate.

CLINICAL APPLICATIONS OF EEG STUDIES

EEG methodology has proven very useful in studies of cognitive and socioemotional development. We have highlighted the use of the EEG in research on cognitive development elsewhere (Bell & Wolfe, 2004). Here we focus on the use of the EEG in research on socioemotional development and specifically examine EEG correlates of behavioral inhibition. Behavioral inhibition is a childhood temperament profile of great interest to developmentalists because of its association with later developing anxiety disorders (Biederman et al., 2001; Kagan, 1997; Ollendick & Hirshfeld-Becker, 2002; Schwartz, Wright, Shin, Kagan, & Rauch, 2003). In this selective overview, we describe the development of behavioral inhibition, briefly discuss the neural circuitry hypothesized to be involved in behavioral inhibition, and then detail EEG correlates of behavioral inhibition in children. Although the EEG cannot be used as a diagnostic tool for behavioral inhibition, its inclusion in research projects may help provide a convergent piece of evidence toward the goal of understanding the biological underpinnings of behavioral inhibition.

Development of Behavioral Inhibition

Temperament refers to relatively enduring individual differences in affective moods and behaviors observed during infancy and early childhood. Current theories of temperament consider these individual differences to have a biological basis and most likely a genetic basis as well (Kagan, 1998; Rothbart & Bates, 1998; Schmidt, Polak, & Spooner, 2001). Much of the work on individual differences in temperament can be delineated along the behavioral dimensions of approach and withdrawal (Fox, 1994; Schmidt & Fox, 1999). Thus, behavioral inhibition, more specifically "inhibition to the unfamiliar" (Kagan, 1994, 1999), is a temperament profile that describes children who tend to withdraw from unfamiliar people, objects, and situations, whereas uninhibited children tend to approach under these circumstances.

The term "behavioral inhibition" is most often associated with the work of Jerome Kagan and his colleagues at Harvard, who have reported that behavioral inhibition is associated not only with behavioral withdrawal but also with negative affect (Garcia-Coll, Kagan, & Reznick, 1984) and physiological arousal (Kagan, Reznick, & Snidman, 1987). In longitudinal studies from infancy to adulthood, Kagan and colleagues have focused on individuals who are at the extremes of approach and withdrawal profiles because these were the groups of children who displayed the most consistent behavior across laboratory tasks, although this consistency was not acute (Kagan, 1999; Kagan, Reznick, Snidman, Gibbons, & Johnson, 1988). Others also have noted that behavioral inhibition can be moderately stable throughout childhood for some individuals (Fox, Henderson, Rubin, Calkins, & Schmidt, 2001; Scarpa, Raine, Venables, & Mednick, 1995).

Although temperament profiles are considered to be rather enduring individual differences in affective moods and behaviors, it is probably *not* the case that specific, microscopic behaviors are permanent. Kagan (1998) holds that infants are born with a particular temperamental profile that undergoes change as a result of experiences with parents, teachers, and peers. Because of all these changes, the actual descriptive names of temperament profiles in in-

fancy should differ from those used to describe older children. Thus, it appears that the most notable temperament profile in infancy is distress or irritability (Kagan, 1998; Rothbart, Derryberry, & Posner, 1994), whereas the most notable temperament profile in childhood is shyness or, more aptly, fearfulness (Kagan, 1998). These different temperament profiles at different times in development may be related to the development of behavioral inhibition.

In Kagan's work, as well as the work of others, infant predictors of inhibited and uninhibited behaviors in childhood center on motor and affective reactivity to sensory stimuli (Calkins, Fox, & Marshall, 1996; Fox et al., 2001; Kagan, 1997; Kagan & Snidman, 1991). Highly reactive infants have been shown to display high motor activity and high negative affect to visual, auditory, and olfactory stimuli at 4 months of age. Low-reactive infants remained motorically inactive and display little affect to sensory stimuli at 4 months. During the toddler period (ages 14 and 21 months), many (but not all) of these high-reactive infants exhibited fearful behavior to unfamiliar people, objects, and situations. The low-reactive group typically exhibited minimal fear (e.g., Kagan, 1997). By age 4, members of the original high-reactive group were less likely to talk and smile to an unfamiliar adult than were members of the low-reactive group. With unfamiliar peers, the original high-reactive group were avoidant and quiet (Kagan, 1998).

This temperament profile was not rigidly stable, however. Only a small percentage of the original high-reactive and low-reactive infant groups exhibited consistent inhibited or uninhibited profiles across each age and at each assessment period (Fox et al., 2001; Kagan, 1998). Maternal behavior (Schmidt et al., 2001) and possibly day care experience (Fox et al., 2001) have been implicated in the instability of the behavioral inhibition temperament profile. Thus, it appears that experience may be able to dampen, or perhaps even enhance, original temperament quality (Kagan, 1998).

Of most interest to developmentalists is the evidence that individuals with stable behavioral inhibition profiles across childhood are at risk for social anxiety disorder (Biederman et al., 2001; Schwartz et al., 2003). Social anxiety disorder is the most common anxiety disorder in adolescence and adulthood. It is the third most common of all neuropsychiatric disorders, following major depression and alcohol dependency (Ollendick & Hirshfeld-Becker, 2002). Most models of social anxiety hypothesize interactions between biological and psychological variables, as well as genetic influences. Children with behavioral inhibition from the original Kagan studies had parents with higher rates of social phobia than the parents of the uninhibited children (Rosenbaum et al., 1991). Similarly, in another parent-child sample, behavioral inhibition was associated with social anxiety among children whose parents had panic disorder. Furthermore, behavioral inhibition predicted childhood social anxiety beyond what could be predicted from parent panic disorders (Biederman et al., 2001). Kagan has emphasized, however, that most children with behavioral inhibition will not develop an anxiety disorder. It is more likely that behavioral inhibition in childhood will be associated with introverted, or shy, adult personality (Kagan, 1998).

Neurological Basis for Behavioral Inhibition

Many developmentalists propose that individual differences in behavioral inhibition may reflect variation in excitability of the limbic system, specifically the amygdala and its neural circuitry (Kagan, 1997, 1998; Marshall & Stevenson-Hinde, 2001) or perhaps even dysregulation of this neural circuitry (Schmidt & Fox, 1999, 2002; Schmidt et al., 2001). In particular, the central nucleus of the amygdala is associated with fear (LeDoux, 1996; Nader & LeDoux, 1999), the most distinguished temperament profile in childhood (Kagan, 1998). As noted previously, fearfulness is the primary behavioral component of behavioral inhibition in childhood, and this has led Kagan and others to propose that behavioral inhibition is associated with the functioning of the amygdala and associated circuitry (Davidson & Rickman, 1999; Kagan, 1997, 1998; Schmidt & Fox, 1999, 2002). Indeed, recent fMRI evidence lends support to this hypothesis. Young adults who had been categorized as having behavioral inhibition when toddlers exhibited greater amygdalar responses to novel versus familiar faces compared with young adults categorized as uninhibited as toddlers (Schwartz et al., 2003).

Data from animal studies have been used to suggest that the frontal cortex is also an integral part of the fear system (see Schmidt & Fox, 2002, and Schmidt et al., 2001, for overviews of the neural circuitry of the fear system). In humans, the frontal cortex is associated with emotion expression, regulation, and associated processes (Davidson, 1992, 1995; Fox, 1991, 1994). Functional connections have been demonstrated between the frontal cortex and the amygdala, and this is of importance for any model of behavioral inhibition. Communication between these two brain areas may be important for regulating withdrawal responses to aversive stimuli and approach responses to appetitive stimuli (Davidson & Rickman, 1999; Marshall & Stevenson-Hinde, 2001).

Both Fox (1991, 1994) and Davidson (1992, 1995) have proposed two basic circuits involving the frontal cortex and associated affects and motivations. The approach system focuses on positive emotions that are implicated in pregoal attainments. This system involves reduced negative affect and active social approach and is associated with left hemisphere frontal functioning. The withdrawal system involves negative emotions that are implicated in aversive situations. This system has reduced positive affect and active social withdrawal and is associated with right hemisphere frontal functioning (Davidson & Rickman, 1999).

These two affect/motivation circuits have major implications for EEG work in studies of behavioral inhibition. One could readily hypothesize that behavioral inhibition would be associated with functioning of the right frontal cortex relative to the left frontal cortex. As previously noted, EEG methodology is especially suited for research with infants and children (Casey & de Hann, 2002; Taylor & Baldeweg, 2002). Thus, the EEG is an excellent research tool for examination of the biology/physiology associated with behavioral inhibition.

Frontal EEG and Behavioral Inhibition

A difference in EEG power values between left and right frontal EEG scalp electrodes is assumed to reflect relative differences in neuronal activity between the left and right hemispheres of the frontal cortex. Evidence presented by Davidson and colleagues (Davidson, 1992, 1995; Davidson & Rickman, 1999; Davidson, Schaffer, & Saron, 1985) indicates that within a normal adult population differences in tonic or baseline EEG alpha (8–13 Hz) hemispheric activation are associated with affective style. EEG alpha values are inversely related to cortical involvement. Thus, lower power values in a hemisphere (or region) reflect greater cortical activation of that hemisphere (or region) relative to the other hemisphere (Davidson et al., 2000; Lindsley & Wicke, 1974). For example, adults rating themselves high on the Beck Depression Inventory exhibit greater right frontal activation (i.e., lower EEG alpha values) during a resting baseline condition than adults rating themselves low on the inventory. Likewise, adults who are clinically depressed also exhibit right frontal activation during baseline (Henriques & Davidson, 1990). Conversely, left frontal activation is associated with higher positive affect on self-report measures (Sutton & Davidson, 1997; Tomarken, Davidson, Wheeler, & Doss, 1992).

In the adult EEG literature, Davidson has reported that asymmetries in frontal cortical functioning also are associated with variations in emotional behavior during tasks designed to evoke different emotion responses (Davidson, 1992, 1994, 1995; Davidson et al., 1990). Specifically, greater levels of left frontal activation relative to right frontal activation are associated with positive affect or approach behaviors. Greater levels of right frontal activation, relative to left frontal, are associated with negative affect or withdrawal behaviors.

Developmental evidence seems to suggest that electrocortical differences in affective style or temperament can be evident as early as the first year of life. The EEG power values used for infants are at developmentally appropriate lower frequency (i.e., 6–9 Hz) than the traditional 8 to 13 Hz adult alpha levels and may reflect similar processes as the adult alpha frequency band (Marshall et al., 2002). Fox and colleagues have shown that infants who cry at maternal separation are more likely to exhibit right frontal EEG activation during rest or baseline (Bell & Fox, 1994; Davidson & Fox, 1989; Fox, Bell, & Jones, 1992; Fox, Calkins, & Bell, 1994; Fox & Davidson, 1987). Dawson (Dawson, 1994a, 1994b; Dawson, Panagiotides, Grofer Klinger, & Hill, 1992) has reported that type and intensity of emotional expression during emotion-eliciting tasks is related to specific patterns of left and right hemisphere frontal EEG activation in infants. Infants exhibited frontal activation relative to baseline during a brief maternal separation. Furthermore, during emotion-eliciting situations, infants exhibited right frontal activation during sad, or withdrawal, situations and left frontal activation during more positive, or approach, situations. Others have reported similar EEG findings with infant populations (Buss et al., 2003; Davidson & Fox, 1982). All this infant emotion reactivity research has implications for EEG work on behavioral inhibition.

Using Kagan's methodology to select infants who may later on be high or low on behavioral inhibition, Fox has reported that infants who display negative affect and high motor activity at age 4 months exhibit right frontal EEG activation at age 9 months and inhibited behavior at age 14 months (Calkins et al., 1996). Infants who exhibited a pattern of stable right frontal activation across the 9- and 14-month time period were more likely to be inhibited at both age 14 and 24 months relative to those infants who exhibited a pattern of stable left frontal EEG activation (Fox et al., 1994). Schmidt has speculated that infants may have a temperamental bias toward the emergence of behavioral inhibition in very early childhood. These bias features appear early in the first year of life and remain stable during the first 2 years of life (Schmidt et al., 2001). The frontal EEG indicators of this temperament bias may be indexing individual differences in forebrain and limbic sensitivity (Schmidt & Fox, 2002).

For many infants, these individual differences in affective style and EEG activation persist throughout the preschool years and early school age years. Fox has reported that when these same infants were 4 years old, those who displayed a high level of behavioral inhibition during play groups with three unfamiliar peers exhibited greater relative right frontal EEG activation during baseline rest compared with children displaying less behavioral inhibition behaviors (Fox et al., 2001; Henderson, Fox, & Rubin, 2001; Henderson, Marshall, Fox, & Rubin, 2004). It is of note, however, that not all behavioral inhibition toddlers exhibited behavioral inhibition behaviors at age 4 years (Fox et al., 2001), much like the data reported by Kagan and colleagues (see Kagan, 1998, for a review of this work). Schmidt reported that by age 7 years, these children who displayed high levels of behavioral inhibition at the preschool years exhibited an increase in right, but not left, frontal EEG activity during a self-presentation task as the task became more demanding (Schmidt, Fox, Schulkin, & Gold, 1999). The self-presentation task was used with the school-age children because issues of self-evaluation appear to be at the crux of many social anxieties (Schmidt & Fox, 1999).

Davidson and colleagues have reported similar EEG data for children at age 3 years (Davidson & Rickman, 1999; Finman, Davidson, Colton, Straus, & Kagan, 1989). Children were exposed to a play session during which mild stressors were presented (e.g., talking robot, adult stranger). Play sessions were experienced with an unfamiliar same-gender peer. Later the children who exhibited the most behavioral inhibition behaviors and those exhibiting the least behavioral inhibition behaviors returned for EEG baseline recordings. The group of 3-year-old children with the highest levels of behavioral inhibition had relatively more right than left frontal EEG activity, whereas the children with the lowest levels of behavioral inhibition had relatively more left than right activity. EEG power was calculated on a slightly higher frequency band than that used in the Fox studies. Power was formulated for 7 to 11 Hz.

Returning at age 9 years for more behavioral testing and then at age 10 years for EEG recordings, these children mimicked the behavioral inhibition-EEG data at age 3 years (Davidson & Rickman, 1999). Comparison of the 3-year-old data with the 9- to 10-year-old data revealed no stability in either behavioral inhibition or EEG hemispheric activation for the entire group of children. Much like the previously noted reports of Fox and Kagan, however, there was a smaller group of children who exhibited greater relative right frontal EEG activity at both ages, and these were the children who exhibited behavioral inhibition behaviors at both ages. One possible explanation for this apparent lack of behavioral stability in behavioral inhibition is that the laboratory measures were not analogous, each being based on developmentally appropriate tasks (Davidson & Rickman, 1999). It is also the case that individual differences in EEG activation patterns and behavioral inhibition behaviors are influenced by maturational patterns of brain development (Davidson & Rickman, 1999).

In summary, these EEG studies indicate an association between behavioral inhibition and frontal EEG activation from infancy through the middle childhood years. These associations lend some credence to the hypothesis that behavioral inhibition can be linked to the dysregulation of some components of the fear system involving the frontal cortex and the amygdala (Schmidt et al., 2001). Thus, although these data provide evidence of a biological predisposition to behavioral inhibition in some children, there is also evidence that many children do not exhibit stability in behavioral inhibition-EEG associations (Davidson & Rickman, 1999; Fox et al., 2001). Likewise, there is the suggestion that there are environmental contributions to behavioral inhibition as well (Fox et al., 2001). The interested reader is directed to the writings of Schmidt (Schmidt et al., 2001) for a discussion of possible environmental correlates of childhood shyness or behavioral inhibition.

CLINICAL APPLICATIONS OF ERP STUDIES

ERPs have been used to test a variety of types of function in populations with developmental disorders. Because they are noninvasive, EEG and ERP can be used to understand a number of aspects of brain development and function in populations that might otherwise be difficult to test. We will describe studies that focused on measuring brain function related to social behavior in children with typical development, autism, Williams syndrome, and developmental delay. We will describe a paradigm that has proven highly useful in studying these populations, as well as children with typical development.

Typical Development

Faces have long proved a powerful stimulus for use in ERP studies with infants and very young children. Because participants of this age cannot make verbal or motor responses, researchers depend on their attention to salient stimuli, which are then varied on some parameter (e.g., familiarity). Because infants like to look at faces from very early in development, they are more likely to reliably attend to presentations of face stimuli than almost any other type of stimulus. Thus, faces have been used to measure infants' ability to learn about faces through familiarization (Nelson, 1994, 1998, 2001). They have also been used in studies designed to elicit and differentiate ERP activity related to encoding, novelty detection, and memory updating in infancy (Nelson & Collins, 1991). Faces have also been used to measure infants' emotion recognition ability (Nelson, 1993; Nelson & de Haan, 1996; Nelson & Horowitz, 1983).

In most previous studies, infants typically viewed faces that, prior to the experiment, were entirely novel to them. Infants were typically familiarized with one face or emotional expression, and subsequent ERP activity was measured to that face or expression in contrast with a novel (unfamiliarized) face or expression. De Haan and Nelson (1997, 1999) devised a novel but elegant method by which infants' ERP responses to an already familiar stimulus could be compared to their responses to a new, novel stimulus. A digital image was taken of the infants' mother, and was shown paired with an unfamiliar face. De Haan and Nelson (1997) systematically varied the degree to which the unfamiliar face resembled the mother's face. In 6-month-olds, the similarity between the mother's face and the stranger's face affected infants' ERP responses to the mother's face. Thus, the context in which the familiar face was seen had an impact on how that face was processed.

In a second study, de Haan and Nelson (1999) compared ERP response to the mother's face versus a stranger's face to their responses to a very familiar object (a favorite toy brought to the lab from home) versus an unfamiliar toy (a toy provided by the lab and confirmed by the mother to be unfamiliar to the infant). This study revealed differences in the laterality of the Nc component for faces versus objects where faces elicited a greater Nc over the right hemisphere than the left. (Objects were bilaterally distributed across the scalp hemispheres.) These data provided evidence of the lateralization of face processing mechanisms as distinct from general familiarity mechanisms.

A number of labs have adapted the mother's face recognition paradigm for use with both typically developing infants and children, and children with developmental disabilities. Carver and colleagues (2002) tested 13-month-old to 4-year-old typically developing children using the mother's face paradigm. The results indicated age-related changes in the differences between the amplitude of the Nc component to the mother's face and the stranger's face. Further analysis revealed that this correlation occurred primarily because the infants' Nc to the mother's face decreased over time, whereas the Nc to the stranger's face remained fairly constant. Based on the ages over which this change occurred, the authors suggested that the effect may be due to changes in the relative salience of the mother's face as infants emerge from the stage of attachment. Studies are currently under way to test this hypothesis.

Autism

One of the key areas of impairment in autism is in social development. Children with autism fail to attend preferentially to faces as do other children, and adults with autism show impairments in face recognition tasks and unusual patterns of brain activity in response to faces. Thus, face recognition tasks provide an important avenue from which to explore the brain basis of the social impairments in autism. Dawson and colleagues (Dawson et al., 2002) tested 3- and 4-year-olds with typical development, developmental delay, and autism spectrum disorders using the mother's face paradigm and the very familiar object paradigm (de Haan & Nelson, 1997, 1999). The researchers noted that 3- and 4-year-olds with autism showed ERP patterns that were similar to those elicited for children with typical development in responses to very familiar versus unfamiliar objects. Children in both groups showed differences in the amplitude of the P500 component. The amplitude was larger for the unfamiliar object than for the very familiar object. Children with typical development also showed a difference in the amplitude of the Nc component to familiar and unfamiliar objects. The Nc effect was similar in children with autism, although it did not reach statistical significance (Dawson et al., 2002). A very different pattern was observed for faces. Children with typical development showed differences between responses to the mother's face and a stranger's face for the Nc component, the P500 component, and the slow wave component. Children with autism showed no differences between the ERP response to the mother's face and the stranger's face for any of these components. Interestingly, children with developmental delay showed a third pattern, in which ERP activity differentiated the familiar from the novel stimulus for both faces and objects, but only in the slow-wave activity. The authors interpreted these results as indicating that children with typical development and developmental delay both were able to differentiate both social (faces) and nonsocial (objects) stimuli, although the components in which this differentiation occurred varied between these populations. Children with autism, in contrast, showed differential ERP activity only to objects, suggesting a specified impairment in the processing of social information. In future studies, the mother's face paradigm could be used longitudinally to examine the long-term effects of autism on face processing.

ERPs have also been used in a study of face processing in adults with autism (McPartland, Dawson, Webb, Panagiotides, & Carver, 2004). In this experiment, high-functioning individuals with autism where tested using standardized behavioral measures of face recognition ability, and ERPs to faces were tested using a paradigm described by Bentin and colleagues (1996). High-functioning volunteers with autism and typical control volunteers saw random presentations of upright and inverted pictures of unfamiliar faces and furniture. People with autism failed to show the usual inversion effect in the N170 (slower and larger amplitude to inverted faces). The N170 was also not lateralized to the right hemisphere in the patients with autism, whereas it was in the typical controls. Finally, slower latency of the N170 component over the left hemisphere predicted better performance on the face recognition task for people with autism, whereas faster N170 over the right hemisphere predicted better performance for typical controls. These data suggest that individuals with autism use a different brain system for processing faces than do controls. In addition, the results suggest that the extent to which such compensatory strategies are developed may relate to the severity of the face recognition impairment in autism.

Williams Syndrome

Williams syndrome is a rare genetic disorder that, in many ways, seems to be the polar opposite of autism. Patients with Williams syndrome are hypersocial where patients with autism are asocial. Patients with Williams syndrome also show a pattern of severe impairment in spatial cognitive abilities with less impairment in verbal abilities. This pattern is the opposite of that typically seen in autism, where most patients show severe impairments in verbal abilities and less severe spatial cognitive deficits. In one area, however, patients from these seemingly disparate disorders are strikingly similar. Patients with autism and Williams syndrome show similar behavioral profiles in face recognition tasks. Both groups fail to show an inversion effect, in which inverted faces are recognized less well than upright faces. ERPs to faces have also been used to test patients with Williams syndrome. In one study, ERPs of individuals with Williams syndrome, autism, and typical controls were compared in a face processing task (Grice et al., 2001). Both of the patient groups showed different ERP patterns than did controls. Patients with autism showed an increased amplitude to inverted faces (which is a typical pattern) but did not show differential latency of the

activation. Patients with Williams syndrome showed a latency difference, but not an amplitude difference between inverted and upright faces. Thus, ERPs proved helpful in differentiating the underlying neurophysiology between autism and Williams syndrome, despite similar or identical behavioral profiles.

Other Populations

In addition to studies of children with autism, ERP methods can be used with any number of other populations. Pollak and colleagues (Pollak, Cicchetti, Klorman, & Brumaghim, 1997) measured ERP responses to facial expressions of emotion in children who had or had not been physically abused. Children who had suffered abuse showed enhanced ERP activity to negative facial expressions, especially to angry expressions. The authors interpreted these results as indicating that the children's perception of emotions differed as a function of their abuse history. These results may prove important in future studies of children who have experienced any number of different environments (e.g., children raised by caregivers with major depression) and point to a potential aspect of brain plasticity that might be involved in their behavioral profiles.

CONCLUSION

EEG and ERP studies have proven useful for investigating a number of aspects of development in typically developing children as well and in clinical populations. The results of these studies have provided important insights into the nature of the differences found in these populations, as well as providing information from which hypotheses about their brain bases can be generated. EEG has proven useful in our understanding of the brain basis of behavioral inhibition, in both its normative variance and clinical application. Electrophysiological methods can, in the future, provide even more information about both normal and atypical development. ERP methods would be even more powerful if used in conjunction with other methods. For example, functional imaging methods provide high-resolution spatial information. ERPs used in conjuction with imaging could provide important information about both the spatial and temporal characteristics of brain activity. ERP and EEG methods could also be combined to gain converging information from their relative strengths. Finally, electrophysiological methods should be used in conjunction with behavioral observations to provide the strongest possible estimate of the neural correlates of behavioral change.

REFERENCES

Bell, M. A. (1998). The ontogeny of the EEG during infancy and childhood: Implications for cognitive development. In B. Garreau

(Ed.), *Neuroimaging in child neuropsychiatric disorders*. Berlin: Springer-Verlag.

Bell, M. A., & Fox, N. A. (1994). Brain development over the first year of life: Relations between electroencephalographic frequency & coherence and cognitive & affective behaviors. In G. Dawson & K. W. Fischer (Eds.), *Human behavior and the developing brain*. New York: Guilford Press.

Bell, M. A., & Fox, N. A. (2003). Cognition and affective style: Individual differences in brain electrical activity during spatial and verbal tasks. *Brain and Cognition, 53*, 441–451.

Bell, M. A. & Wolfe, C. D. (in press). The use of the electroencephalogram in research on cognitive development. In L. A. Schmidt & S. J. Segalowitz (Eds.), *Developmental psychophysiology*. New York: Cambridge University Press.

Bentin, S., Allison, T., Puce, A., Perez, E., & McCarthy, G. (1996). Electrophysiological studies of face perception in humans. *Journal of Cognitive Neuroscience, 8*, 551–565.

Berger, H. (1929). On the electroencephalogram of man. I. *Archiv for Psychiatric and Nervenkrankheiten, 87*, 527–570.

Berger, H. (1932). On the electroencephalogram of man. V. *Archiv for Psychiatric and Nervenkrankheiten, 98*, 231–254.

Biederman, J., Hirshfeld-Becker, D. R., Rosenbaum, J. F., Herot, C., Friedman, D., Snidman, N., Kagan, J., & Faraone, S. V. (2001). Further evidence of association between behavioral inhibition and social anxiety in children. *American Journal of Psychiatry, 158*, 1673–1679.

Blume, W.R., Buza, R.C., & Okazaki, H. (1974). Anatomic correlates of the ten-twenty electrode placement system in infants. *Electroencephalography and Clinical Neurophysiology, 36*, 303–307.

Buss, K. A., Schumacher, J. R. M., Dolski, I., Kalin, N. H., Goldsmith, H. H., & Davidson, R. J. (2003). Right frontal brain activity, cortisol, and withdrawal behavior in 6-month-old infants. *Behavioral Neuroscience, 117*, 11–20.

Calkins, S. D., Fox, N. A., & Marshall, T. R. (1996). Behavioral and physiological antecedents of inhibited and uninhibited behavior. *Child Development, 67*, 523–540.

Carver, L. J., Dawson, G., Panagiotides, H., Meltzoff, A. N., McPartland, J., Gray, J., & Munson, J. (2002). Age-related differences in neural correlates of face recognition during the toddler and preschool years. *Developmental Psychobiology, 42*, 148–159.

Casey, B. J., & de Hann, M. (2002). Introduction: new methods in developmental science. *Developmental Science, 5*, 265–267.

Courchesne, E. (1978). Neurophysiological correlates of cognitive development: Changes in long-latency event-related potentials from childhood to adulthood. *Electroencephalography Clinical Neurophysiology 45*, 468–482.

Courchesne, E., Ganz, L., & Norcia, A. M. (1981). Event-related brain potentials to human faces in infants. *Child Development, 52*, 804–811.

Davidson, R. J. (1992). Anterior cerebral asymmetry and the nature of emotion. *Brain and Cognition, 20*, 125–151.

Davidson, R. J. (1994). Temperament, affective style, and frontal lobe asymmetry. In G. Dawson & K. W. Fischer (Eds.), *Human behavior and the developing brain* (pp. 518–536). New York: Guilford Press.

Davidson, R. J. (1995). Cerebral asymmetry, emotion, and affective style. In R. J. Davidson & K. Hugdahl (Eds.), *Brain asymmetry* (pp. 361–387). Cambridge, MA: MIT Press.

Davidson, R. J., Chapman, J. P., Chapman, L. J., & Henriques, J. B. (1990). Asymmetrical brain electrical activity discriminates between psychometrically-matched verbal and spatial cognitive tasks. *Psychophysiology, 27*, 528–543.

Davidson, R. J., & Fox, N. A. (1982). Asymmetrical brain activity discriminates between positive versus negative affective stimuli in human infants. *Science, 218*, 1235–1237.

Davidson, R. J., & Fox, N. A. (1989). Frontal brain asymmetry predicts infants' response to maternal separation. *Journal of Abnormal Psychology, 98*, 127–131.

Davidson, R. J., Jackson, D. C., & Larson, C. L. (2000). Human electroencephalography. In J. T. Cacioppo & L. G. Tassinary & G. G. Berntson (Eds.), *Handbook of psychophysiology (2nd Edition)* (pp. 27–52). Cambridge, UK: Cambridge University Press.

Davidson, R. J., & Rickman, M. (1999). Behavioral inhibition and the emotional circuitry of the brain: Stability and plasticity during the early childhood years. In L. A. Schmidt & J. Schulkin (Eds.), *Extreme fear, shyness, and social phobia: Origins, biological mechanisms, and clinical outcomes* (pp. 67–87). New York: Oxford University Press.

Davidson, R. J., Schaffer, C. E., & Saron, C. (1985). Effects of lateralized stimulus presentations on the self-report of emotion and EEG asymmetry in depressed and non-depressed subjects. *Psychophysiology, 22*, 353–364.

Dawson, G. (1994a). Development of emotional expression and emotion regulation in infancy: Contributions of the frontal lobe. In G. Dawson & K. W. Fischer (Eds.), *Human behavior and the developing brain* (pp. 346–379). New York: Guilford Press.

Dawson, G. (1994b). Frontal electroencephalographic correlates of individual differences in emotion expression in infants: A brain systems perspective on emotion. In N. A. Fox (Ed.), *The development of emotion regulation: Biological and behavioral considerations.* (Vol. 59, 2–3, Serial No. 240, pp. 135–151).

Dawson, G., Carver, L. J., Meltzoff, A. N., Panagiotides, H., McPartland, J., & Webb, S. J. (2002). Neural correlates of face and object recognition in young children with autism spectrum disorder, developmental delay, and typical development. *Child Development, 73*, 700–717.

Dawson, G., Panagiotides, H., Grofer Klinger, L., & Hill, D. (1992). The role of frontal lobe functioning in the development of self-regulatory behavior in infancy. *Brain and Cognition, 20*, 152–175.

de Haan, M., & Nelson, C. A. (1997). Recognition of the mother's face by six-month-old infants: A neurobehavioral study. *Child Development, 68*, 187–210.

de Haan, M., & Nelson, C. A. (1999). Brain activity differentiates face and object processing in 6-month-old infants. *Developmental Psychology, 35*, 1113–1121.

de Haan, M., Pascalis, O., & Johnson, M. H. (2002). Specialization of neural mechanisms underlying face recognition in human infants. *Journal of Cognitive Neuroscience, 14*, 199–209.

de Haan, M., & Thomas, K. M. (2002). Application of ERP and fMRI techniques to developmental science. *Developmental Science, 5*, 335–343.

Dien, J., Spencer, K. M., & Donchin, E. (2003). Localization of the event-related potential novelty response as defined by principal components analysis. *Cognitive Brain Research, 17*, 637–650.

Finman, R., Davidson, R. J., Colton, M. B., Straus, A. M., & Kagan, J. (1989). Psychophysiological correlates of inhibition to the unfamiliar in children. *Psychophysiology, 26*, S24.

Fox, N. A. (1991). If it's not left, it's right: Electroencephalograph asymmetry and the development of emotion. *American Psychologist, 46*, 863–872.

Fox, N. A. (1994). Dynamic cerebral processes underlying emotion regulation. In N. A. Fox (Ed.), *The development of emotion regulation: Biological and behavioral considerations. Monographs of the Society for Research in Child Development* (Vol. 59, 2–3, Serial No. 240).

Fox, N. A., Bell, M. A., & Jones, N. A. (1992). Individual differences in response to stress and cerebral asymmetry. *Developmental Neuropsychology, 7*, 161–184.

Fox, N. A., Calkins, S. D., & Bell, M. A. (1994). Neural plasticity and development in the first two years of life: Evidence from cognitive and socio-emotional domains of research. *Development and Psychopathology, 6*, 677–698.

Fox, N. A., & Davidson, R. J. (1987). EEG asymmetry in ten month old infants in response to approach of a stranger and maternal separation. *Developmental Psychology, 23*, 233–240.

Fox, N. A., & Davidson, R. J. (1988). Patterns of brain electrical activity during the expression of discrete emotions in ten month old infants. *Developmental Psychology, 24*, 230–236.

Fox, N. A., Henderson, H. A., Rubin, K. H., Calkins, S. D., & Schmidt, L. A. (2001). Continuity and discontinuity of behavioral inhibition and exuberance: Psychophysiological and behavioral influences across the first four years of life. *Child Development, 72*, 1–21.

Garcia-Coll, C., Kagan, J., & Reznick, J. S. (1984). Behavioral inhibition in young children. *Child Development, 55*, 1005–1019.

Greenough, W. T., Black, J., & Wallace, C. (1987). Effects of experience on brain development. *Child Development, 58*, 540–559.

Greenough, W. T., & Volkmar, F. R. (1973). Pattern of dendritic branching in the occipital cortex of rats reared in complex environments. *Experimental Neurology, 40*, 491–504.

Grice, S. J., Spratling, M. W., Karmiloff-Smith, A., Halit, H., Csibra, G., de Haan, M., & Johnson, M. H. (2001). Disordered visual processing an oscillatory brain activity in autism and Williams Syndrome. *Neuroreport, 12,* 2697–2700.

Hellstrom, B., Karlsson, B., & Mussbichler, H. (1963). Electrode placement in EEG of infants and its anatomical relationshipstudied radiographically. *Electroencephalography and Clinical Neurophysiology, 15,* 115–117.

Henderson, H. A., Fox, N. A., & Rubin, K. H. (2001). Temperamental contributions to social behavior: The moderating roles of frontal EEG asymmetry and gender. *Journal of the American Academy of Child and Adolescent Psychiatry, 40,* 68–74.

Henderson, H. A., Marshall, P. J., Fox, N. A., & Rubin, K. H. (2004). Psychophysiological and behavioral evidence for varying forms oand functions of nonsocial behavior in preschoolers. *Child Development, 75,* 251–263.

Henriques, J. B., & Davidson, R. J. (1990). Regional brain electrical asymmetries discriminate between previously depressed and healthy control subjects. *Journal of Abnormal Psychology, 99,* 22–31.

Henry, J. R. (1944). Electroencephalograms of normal children. *Monographs of the Society for Research in Child Development, 9, (3 Serial No 39).*

Jasper, H. H. (1958). The ten-twenty electrode system of the International Federation. *Electroencephalography Clinical Neurophysiology, 10,* 371–375.

Johnson, M. H., de Haan, M., Oliver, A., Smith, W., Hatzakis, H., Tucker, L. A., & Csibra, G. (2001). Recording and analyzing high-density event-related potentials with infants using the geodesic sensor net. *Developmental Neuropsychology, 19,* 295–323.

Kagan, J. (1994). *Galen's prophecy: Temperament in human nature.* New York: Basic Books.

Kagan, J. (1997). Temperament and the reactions to unfamiliarity. *Child Development, 68,* 139–143.

Kagan, J. (1998). Biology and the child. In N. Eisenburg (Ed.), *Handbook of child psychology: Vol. 3. Social, emotional, and personality development* (pp. 177–235). New York: Wiley.

Kagan, J. (1999). The concept of behavioral inhibition. In A. Schmidt & J. Schulkin (Eds.), *Extreme fear, shyness, and social phobia: Origins, biological mechanisms, and clinical outcomes* (pp. 3–13). New York: Oxford University Press.

Kagan, J., Reznick, J. S., & Snidman, N. (1987). The physiology and psychology of behavioral inhibition in children. *Child Development, 58,* 1459–1473.

Kagan, J., Reznick, J. S., Snidman, N., Gibbons, J., & Johnson, M. O. (1988). Childhood derivatives of inhibition and lack of inhibition to the unfamiliar. *Child Development, 59,* 1580–1589.

Kagan, J., & Snidman, N. (1991). Temperamental factors in human development. *American Psychologist, 46,* 856–862.

LeDoux, J. E. (1996). *The emotional brain.* New York: Simon & Schuster.

Lindsley, D. B. (1939). A longitudinal study of the occipital alpha rhythm in normal children: Frequency and amplitude standards. *Journal of Genetic Psychology, 55,* 197–213.

Lindsley, D. B., & Wicke, J. D. (1974). The EEG: Autonomous electrical activity in man and animals. In R. Thompson & M. N. Patterson (Eds.), *Bioelectrical recording techniques* (pp. 3–83). New York: Academic Press.

Marshall, P. J., Bar-Haim, Y., & Fox, N. A. (2002). Development of the EEG from 5 months of 4 years of age. *Clinical Neurophysiology, 113,* 1199–1208.

Marshall, P. J., & Stevenson-Hinde, J. (2001). Behavioral inhibition: Physiological correlates. In W. R. Crozier & L. F. Alden (Eds.), *International handbook of social anxiety: Concepts, research and intervention relating to the self and shyness* (pp. 53–76). New York: Wiley.

McPartland, J., Dawson, G., Webb, S. J., Panagiotides, H., & Carver, L. J. (2004). Event-related brain potentials reveal anomalies in temporal processing of faces in autism. *Journal of Child Psychology and Psychiatry and Allied Disciplines.*

Molfese, D. (1989). Electrophysiological correlates of word meanings in 14-month-old human infants. *Developmental Neuropsychology, 5,* 79–103.

Molfese, D., Wetzel, W. F., & Gill, L. A. (1993). Known versus unknown word discriminations in 12-month-old infants: Electrophysiological correlates. *Developmental Neuropsychology, 9,* 241–258.

Mosher, J. C., Leahy, R. M., & Lewis, P. S. (1999). EEG and MEG: Forward solutions for inverse methods. *IEEE Transactions on Biomedical Engineering, 46,* 245–299.

Nader, K., & LeDoux, J. (1999). The neural circuits that underlie fear. In L. A. Schmidt & J. Schulkin (Eds.), *Extreme fear, shyness, and social phobia: Origins, biological mechanisms, and clinical outcomes* (pp. 119–139). New York: Oxford University Press.

Nelson, C. A. (1993). The recognition of facial expression in infancy: Behavioral and electrophysiological evidence. In D. Boysson-Bardies (Ed.), *Developmental neurocognition: Speech and face processing in the first year of life* (pp. 187–198). Dordrecht, Netherla: Kluwer Academic.

Nelson, C. A. (1994). Neural correlates of recognition memory in the first postnatal year. In G. Dawson & D. M. Fisher (Eds.), *Human behavior and the developing brain.* New York: Guilford Press.

Nelson, C. A. (1998). The nature of early memory. *Preventive Medicine, 27,* 172–179.

Nelson, C. A. (2001). The development and neural bases of face recognition. *Infant and Child Development, 10,* 3–18.

Nelson, C. A., & Collins, P. F. (1990). The lateralization of language comprehension using event-related potentials. *Brain and Cognition, 14,* 92–112.

Nelson, C. A., & Collins, P. F. (1991). Event-related potential and looking-time analysis of infants' responses to familiar and novel events: Implications for visual recognition memory. *Developmental Psychology, 27,* 50–58.

Nelson, C. A., & de Haan, M. (1996). Neural correlates of infants' visual responsiveness to facial expressions of emotion. *Developmental Psychobiology, 29,* 577–595.

Nelson, C. A., & Horowitz, F. D. (1983). The perception of facial expressions and stimulus motion by two- and five-month-old infants using holographic stimuli. *Child Development, 54,* 868–877.

Nelson, C. A., & Monk, C. S. (2001). The use of the event-related potentials in the study of cognitive development. In C. A. Nelson & M. Luciana (Eds.), *Handbook of developmental cognitive neuroscience* (pp. 125–136). Cambridge, MA: MIT Press.

Ollendick, T. H., & Hirshfeld-Becker, D. R. (2002). The developmental psychopathology of social anxiety disorder. *Biological Psychiatry, 51,* 44–58.

Picton, T. W., Bentin, S., Berg, P., Donchin, E., Hillyard, S. A., Johnson Jr., R., Miller, G. A., Ritter, W., Ruchkin, D. S., Rugg, M. D., & Taylor, M. J. (2000). Guidelines for using human event-related potentials to study cognition: Recording standards and publication criteria. *Psychophysiology, 37,* 127–152.

Pivik, R. T., Broughton, R. J., Coppola, R., Davidson, R. J., Fox, N. A., & Nuwer, M. R. (1993). Guidelines for the recording and quantitative analysis of electroencephalographic activity in research contexts. *Psychophysiology, 30,* 547–558.

Pollak, S. D., Cicchetti, D., Klorman, R., & Brumaghim, J. (1997). Cognitive brain event-related potentials and emotion processing in maltreated children. *Child Development, 68,* 773–787.

Rosenbaum, J. F., Beiderman, J., Hirshfeld, D. R., Boldus, E. A., Faraone, S. V., Kagan, J., Snidman, N., & Reznick, J. S. (1991). Further evidence of an association between behavioral inhibition and anxiety disorders: Results from a family study of children from a non-clinical sample. *Journal of Psychiatry Research, 25,* 49–65.

Rothbart, M. K., & Bates, J. C. (1998). Temperament. In N. Eisenburg (Ed.), *Handbook of child psychology: Vol. 3. Social, emotional, and personality development* (pp. 105–176). New York: Wiley.

Rothbart, M. K., Derryberry, D., & Posner, M. I. (1994). A psychobiological approach to the development of temperament. In J. E. Bates & T. D. Wachs (Eds.), *Temperament: Individual differences at the interface of biology and behavior* (pp. 83–116). Washington, DC: APA.

Sato, W., Kochiyama, T., Yoshikawa, S., & Matsumura, M. (2001). Emotional expression boosts early visual processing of the face: ERP recording and its decomposition by independent component analysis. *Neuroreport, 12,* 709–714.

Scarpa, A., Raine, A., Venables, P. H., & Mednick S.A., (1995). The stability of inhibited/uninhibited temperament from ages 3–11 years in Mauritian children. *Journal of Abnormal Child Psychology, 23,* 607–618.

Schmidt, L. A., & Fox, N. A. (1999). Conceptual, biological and behavioral distinctions among different categories of shy children. In

L. A. Schmidt & J. Schulkin (Eds.), *Extreme fear, shyness, and social phobia: Origins, biological mechanisms, and clinical outcomes* (pp. 47–66). New York: Oxford University Press.

Schmidt, L. A., & Fox, N. A. (2002). Individual differences in childhood shyness: Origins, malleability, and developmental course. In D. Cervone & W. Mischel (Eds.), *Advances in personality science* (pp. 83–105). New York: Guilford Press.

Schmidt, L. A., Fox, N. A., Schulkin, J., & Gold, P. W. (1999). Behavioral and psychophysiological correlates of self-presentation in temperamentally shy children. *Developmental Psychobiology, 35*, 119–135.

Schmidt, L. A., Polak, C. P., & Spooner, A. L. (2001). Biological and environmental contributions to childhood shyness: A diathesis-stress model. In W. R. Crozier & L. F. Alden (Eds.), *International handbook of social anxiety: Concepts, research and intervention relating to the self and shyness* (pp. 29–51). New York: Wiley.

Schwartz, C. E., Wright, C. I., Shin, L. M., Kagan, J., & Rauch, S. L. (2003). Inhibited and uninhibited infants "grown up": Adult amygdalar response to novelty. *Science, 300*, 1952–1953.

Smith, J. R. (1938a). The electroencephalogram during normal infancy and childhood: I. Rhythmic activities present in the neonate and their subsequent development. *Journal of Genetic Psychology, 53*, 431–453.

Smith, J. R. (1938b). The electroencephalogram during normal infancy and childhood: II. The nature and growth of the alpha waves. *Journal of Genetic Psychology, 53*, 455–469.

Sutton, S. K., & Davidson, R. J. (1997). Prefrontal brain asymmetry: A biological substrate of the behavioral approach and inhibition systems. *Psychological Science, 8*, 204–210.

Taylor, M. J., & Baldeweg, T. (2002). Application of EEG, ERP, and intracranial recordings to the investigation of cognitive functions in children. *Developmental Science, 5*, 318–334.

Tomarken, A.J., Davidson, R. J., Wheeler, R. E., & Doss, R. (1992). Individual differences in anterior brain asymmetry and fundamental dimensions of emotion. *Journal of Personality and Social Psychology, 62*, 676–687.

Tucker, D. M. (1993). Spatial sampling of head electrical fields: The geodesic sensor net. *Electroencephalography and Clinical Neurophysiology, 87*, 154–163.

Neuropsychiatric Aspects of Psychiatric and Behavioral Disorders of Children and Adolescents

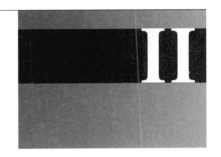

Mental Retardation

8

Suzanne T. P. V. Sundheim, MD   *Ruth M. Myers, MD*
Kytja K.S. Voeller, MD

Mental retardation syndromes should be of great interest to those who study normal development and psychopathology. In the last decade molecular biological techniques and the stimulus of the Human Genome Project have made it possible to identify many of the genes that are involved in these disorders. Simultaneously, research in neuroscience has provided clues as to the role of these genes during brain development and in postnatal brain function. Studies in cognitive neuroscience, particularly in the area of neuroimaging, have made it possible to study the differences in information processing in individuals with a specific mental retardation syndrome compared to unaffected persons. In some cases, it has been possible to demonstrate an association between the genotype and cognitive function; as for example in the performance of individuals with fragile X on tasks demanding prefrontal executive resources. Moreover, it has become apparent that certain psychiatric disorders are strongly associated with certain mental retardation syndromes, such as the link between schizophrenia and velocardiofacial syndrome or Prader-Willi syndrome, or the fascinating association of Prader-Willi syndrome and obsessive-compulsive disorder. Although there remains much that needs to be learned about the precise mechanisms by which the genetic perturbations result in the neuropsychiatric phenotype, the mental retardation syndromes provide the neuropsychiatrist with a remarkable opportunity to understand how the neurobiological underpinnings of these disorders affect cognitive and emotional behaviors. In this chapter we have attempted to provide the reader with an overview of the genetics, cognitive, neurological and psychiatric features (and, where relevant, medical disorders), of several well-studied mental retardation syndromes.

CURRENT DEFINITIONS OF MENTAL RETARDATION

Mental retardation is the term used to describe the condition of individuals with intellectual impairment and compromised adaptive behavior with onset prior to 18 years of age (in some situations, age 21 years). Three formal definitions of mental retardation are currently recognized. The *Diagnostic and Statistical Manual of Mental Disorders*, 4th Edition (DSM-IV) (1) definition (Table 8.1) establishes an IQ of approximately 70 as a cutoff-point. If, for example, an individual has an IQ of 75 but has adaptive functioning with impairment in two or more skill areas of onset prior to age 18 years, the criteria for mental retardation are met. This represents a change from the 1987 definition in DSM-III-R (2), which neither recognized that the classification was continuous nor attempted to integrate IQ and adaptive functioning. In the American Association on Mental Retardation (AAMR) definition, mental retardation is viewed not as an absolute trait, but rather as an interaction between the individual and the environment (3). The AAMR approach is multidimensional, involving a systematic, three-step evaluation of psychological/emotional, physical/health/etiological, and environmental factors, focusing on an individual's specific deficits and providing adaptive supports to optimize functioning. The International Classification of Diseases, 10th Revised Edition (ICD-10) (4) provides a description of each condition rather than a symptom menu as in DSM-IV. It clearly describes the same three qualitative features that are critical to the diagnosis of mental retardation in DSM-IV. Like the DSM-IV nosology, ICD-10 defines levels of mental retardation in terms of measured IQ level.

Individual Differences in Profile and Changes Across the Life Cycle

Individuals with mental retardation have specific strengths and weaknesses in both cognitive and adaptive areas: one person might have strong spatial abilities but impaired language, whereas another might be independent in self-care skills and home management but have poor functional math skills and require help in money management. A thoughtful, multidimensional neuropsychiatric evaluation

TABLE 8.1

DSM-IV DIAGNOSTIC CRITERIA FOR MENTAL RETARDATION

a. Significantly subaverage intellectual functioning: an IQ of approximately 70 or below on an individually administered IQ test (for infants, a clinical judgment of significantly subaverage intellectual functioning).
b. Concurrent deficits or impairments in present adaptive functioning (i.e., the person's effectiveness in meeting the standards expected for his or her age by his or her cultural group) in at least two of the following areas: communication, self-care, home living, social/interpersonal skills, use of community resources, self-direction, functional academic skills, work, leisure, health, and safety.
c. The onset is before age 18 years.

Diagnostic Code	Degree of Severity of MR	IQ Level
317	Mild	50–55 to approximately 70
318.0	Moderate	35–40 to 50–55
318.1	Severe	20–25 to 35–40
318.2	Profound	Below 20 or 25
319	Severity unspecified	When there is strong presumption of MR but the person's intelligence is untestable by standard tests

Source: Reprinted from American Psychiatric Association: *Diagnostic and Statistical Manual of Mental Disorders,* 4th Edition. Washington, DC, American Psychiatric Association, 1994. Copyright 1994, American Psychiatric Association. Used with permission.

mental retardation functions. An adequate evaluation should include a systematic review of the patient's developmental, medical, and family history, as well as cognitive function, daily living skills, and capacity for autonomous function. Temperament, social, emotional, psychosexual, and moral functioning also need to be explored. Moreover, these cognitive and behavioral profiles do not necessarily remain static, but may change across the life cycle in both a syndrome-specific and individual manner. For example, children with fragile X syndrome may reach a cognitive plateau in adolescence, whereas those with Williams syndrome start out with delayed language but then go on to develop a remarkably rich vocabulary. Each child's personal strengths and life experiences, physical health, and their family and educational environment will also affect how this basic pattern is manifested.

COGNITIVE AND ADAPTIVE MEASURES

Measurement of Intelligence

Intellectual functioning is measured by standardized tests that yield an intelligence quotient (IQ). Intelligence tests were originally developed to predict academic success and measure general intelligence. However, they do not necessarily provide much information about performance in real-world situations.

Assessment of Adaptive Functioning

Adaptive functioning refers to an individual's ability to perform tasks of daily living compared to others of the same age and cultural group. It provides a real-life, practical measure of performance and a second source of information about areas of competence and deficit. Without an assessment of adaptive functioning, the diagnosis of mental retardation is only provisional. What constitutes a significant impairment in adaptive behavior has not yet been tightly defined. The Vineland Adaptive Behavior Scales (VABS) (5) and the AAMR Adaptive Behavior Scales (6–8), are commonly used instruments. The VABS is restricted to four domains—communication, daily living skills, socialization, and motor skills—not the entire spectrum of adaptive behaviors, and is of limited use in longitudinal studies because of the fluctuation of means and standard deviations across age groups (9).

Epidemiology

From a purely statistical point of view, mental retardation is defined by an arbitrary cut-off of two standard deviations below the mean on a continuum of intelligence test scores. In the Wechsler tests, which have a mean of 100 and a standard deviation of 15, the cutoff is 70. On the Stanford-Binet, with a mean of 100 and a standard deviation of 16, the cutoff is 68. When adaptive functioning criteria are considered, the prevalence drops to the 1 to 1.5% range (1, 10, 11). Depending on the specific criteria that are used to determine special education services, 0.3 to 2.5% of school-aged children are defined as being mentally retarded.

Approximately 85% of the mentally retarded population fall into the range of mild mental retardation, 10% have moderate, 3 to 4% to have severe, and 1 to 2% have profound mental retardation (1). Medical complications and mortality increase with severity of mental retardation, and contribute to the discrepancy between expected and identified prevalence rates.

Psychiatric Assessment

Individuals with mental retardation are at high risk for psychiatric disorders. The term *dual diagnosis* is used for individuals with mental retardation and comorbid mental health disorders. Depending on the types of population sampling strategies used, between 10 and 40% meet the criteria for a dual diagnosis. (12)

Psychiatrists are often consulted to address an isolated behavioral symptom, such as self-injurious behavior, aggression, or destructiveness. These symptoms may arise from any number of different interacting neurobiological and environmental factors. Two pitfalls in the diagnosis of patients with mental retardation are especially worth mentioning. *Diagnostic overshadowing* refers to using the diagnosis of mental retardation as an explanation for the symptoms instead of applying more standard diagnostic approaches. As a result, a symptom that would be diagnosed and treated in an individual of normal intelligence is instead diagnosed and treated differently when it is associated with mental retardation. (13–15). *Diagnostic presumption* is a term coined by Sundheim to describe the phenomenon of assuming that a specific psychiatric diagnosis applies to an individual with mental retardation purely on the basis of its frequent association with the syndrome instead of systematically exploring the full range of other diagnostic possibilities. For example, assuming that a 20-year-old individual with Down syndrome who has increasing difficulty with day-to-day functioning is demented, rather than exploring the possibility of a depressive disorder.

Patients with mental retardation often have difficulty verbalizing the reasons for their distress. Otitis, dental pain, urinary tract infection, migraine headaches, or gastritis may lead to irritability, aggressive, or self-injurious behavior. Thus, in many cases it may be necessary to refer the patient for a medical evaluation. Medical conditions, such as hypothyroidism and epilepsy, are often associated with mental retardation syndromes and appropriate treatment may improve function. Adequate neuropsychiatric assessments of patients with mental retardation are optimally served in the context of a team of other physicians, educators, and behavioral specialists (16). In light of the emerging syndromal subtypes and their association with different psychiatric and behavioral manifestations, genetic evaluation is an essential part of diagnostic evaluation and treatment planning.

Although most people with developmental disabilities are able to communicate using words, it may be necessary to modify the interview to work around the linguistic limitations of the patient. Nonverbal individuals develop ways of expressing themselves (sometimes the strategy used is troublesome enough to be the reason for the referral!). Information must be obtained from parents, caregivers, and teachers about past and present functioning. When possible, direct, systematic observation of the individual in his home or daytime environment can be extremely helpful for understanding the circumstances involved in problematic behaviors and the development of effective interventions.

Even for a patient who has difficulty communicating in words, the mental status examination remains critical. The nonverbal person may be able to utilize sign language, respond to yes-no questions, or use a picture book to facilitate the interview. Subjective experience may be cautiously inferred from facial expression and body language.

GENETIC AND NEUROPSYCHIATRIC ASPECTS OF CERTAIN MENTAL RETARDATION SYNDROMES

In the following sections, six common, well-studied genetic mental retardation syndromes are reviewed, with the goal of exploring the diversity of medical and neuropsychiatric features associated with mental retardation.

Fragile X Syndrome

Epidemiology/Phenotype

Fragile X syndrome, the most common form of inherited mental retardation, affects approximately 1 in 1,200 males and 1 in 2,500 females. Males with fragile X are more severely involved than females and have some phenotypic features which become more apparent with age—an elongated face, large mandible, long ears, head circumference > 50th percentile, hyperextensible metacarpophalangeal joints, soft skin over the dorsum of the hands, a hallucal crease, and enlarged testicles (not noted in children under age 8 years). There is usually a family history of mental retardation (17–20). However, these phenotypic features are variable and do not reliably identify affected individuals. They should not be used as the only basis for deciding to conduct molecular DNA testing.

Genetics

In 1969, Lubs described a secondary constriction on the long arm of the X chromosome and noted the relationship between this anomaly and X-linked mental retardation (21). However, this "fragile site" as it was called, is apparent only when a folate-deficient culture medium is used and it was not until the early 1980s that the critical role of folate was appreciated (22). The fragile X mental retardation gene (*FMR1*) is located at Xq27.3 (23). Fragile X syndrome results from a large expansion (>200 repeats) of an unstable CGG trinucleotide in the 5' untranslated region of the FMR1 gene (24). In unaffected individuals, this repeat is less than 50. A "transmitting" (carrier) male who is normal in appearance, has CGG repeats in the range of 50 to 200 (termed a "premutation") which are transmitted to his daughters with little change in size. However, the daughter's children (both males and females) inherit CGG repeats that are significantly longer (ranging from 200 to over

1,000). This coincides with the appearance of the clinical phenotype (25). This large CGG repeat results in hypermethylation of the promoter region with transcriptional suppression of the *FMR1* gene, in turn shutting down the production of fragile X mental retardation protein (FMRP). FMRP is widely expressed in neurons (26), with highest levels of expression in the cholinergic cells in the nucleus basalis and the hippocampus (27–29). FMRP is involved in synaptic plasticity, and plays a role both in fetal brain development and learning in the mature brain (30). Although neurogenesis and neuronal migration are relatively normal, there is disruption of the later "pruning" phase. During normal brain development, the numerous, small synapses distributed along long, thin dendritic spines undergo a transition during pruning to fewer, larger synapses on broader and shorter spines. The immature pattern is retained in brains of individuals with fragile X as well as of knockout mice lacking the *FMR1* gene (31–34).

An intriguing finding is that there is a high level of FMRP expression in the magnocellular layers of the lateral geniculate nucleus in normal humans and monkeys, whereas a loss of the normal laminar structure of the lateral geniculate was noted in a male with fragile X. Clear evidence of magnocellular pathway pathology in fragile X was demonstrated by motion-perception deficits without impairment of function of the parvocellular pathway. The magnocellular pathway feeds into the dorsal visual stream/parietal lobe system which integrates visuospatial and motor processing, an area of significant weakness in individuals with fragile X (35).

Medical and Neurological Disorders

About 28% of carrier females have premature ovarian failure, probably the result of decreased follicle number and function, (36) with a risk of osteoporosis (37). Males with premutations (CGG repeats <200) were long believed to be unaffected. However, neuroimaging studies have revealed clear differences in gray and white matter volumes were relative to controls (38). Approximately a third of male premutation carriers over the age of 50 develop fragile X-associated tremor/ataxia syndrome (FXTAS), characterized by cerebellar ataxia, intention tremor, cognitive decline, peripheral neuropathy, lower-limb proximal muscle weakness, and autonomic dysfunction (39, 40). Female premutation carriers may develop a more subtle presentation but are not demented (41, 42). Diffuse eosinophilic intranuclear inclusions are found in both neurons and astrocytes and MRI studies have revealed atrophic changes (43, 44). Thus, when reviewing family history in a child in which fragile X is considered a diagnostic possibility, it is helpful to explore late-onset progressive motor dysfunction in older relatives.

Dysregulation of hypothylamic/pituitary/adrenal axis and neuroendocrine functions can be seen, with a blunted response to thyrotropin releasing hormone (45). The exaggerated hormonal response to stress and elevated glucocor-

ticoid hormones under basal conditions described in fragile X is relevant because of the difficulties affected individuals manifest in managing stress and anxiety. Hessl et al. conducted an in-home evaluation of a large group of children with fragile X full mutation and their unaffected siblings. Children with fragile X (in particular the boys), had higher levels of salivary cortisol and increased cortisol was significantly associated with behavior problems. Lauterborn also demonstrated an exaggerated response to stress in FMR1 knock-out mice compared to wild-type mice (46).

Neurocognitive Profile

Intellectual ability in fragile X ranges from frank mental retardation in males to bright normal intelligence in females. In a study of 144 families neurocognitive status was significantly correlated with the amount of FMRP present. However, the genetic variance accounted for less than half of the total variance in full scale IQ (47).

There is evidence of a decline in IQ in fragile X which becomes apparent during early puberty (48–56). Young boys with the full mutation typically have IQs in the borderline-to-mild mental retardation range, whereas the IQs of adult males fell in the moderate-to-severe range (57, 58). The decline in IQ is correlated with the methylation status of *FMR1* (with a resulting decrease in FMRP) (56, 59–61). Even male premutation carriers have significant deficits in executive function and memory compared to controls (62).

Although the cognitive profile of women with full expression of fragile X syndrome is similar to that of males (58, 63–68), there are significant enough differences to warrant treating them separately in the following discussion.

Males with the Full Fragile X Mutation

Language

Although language is a relative strength in boys with fragile X, their linguistic age ends up being roughly equivalent to that of a 4-year-old (69, 70). In fact, fragile X should be a diagnostic consideration in any preschool child with delayed language (71). Receptive language lags behind expressive language (72). Adolescent and adult males with fragile X have a characteristic rapid, perseverative, jocular, tangential, "cluttered," and echolalic speech (64, 73–76). It may be a way of managing social anxiety (77) or allowing more time to process verbal information.

Psychiatric and Behavioral Features in Males

Fragile X has been reported to be associated with a broad range of psychiatric disorders. Schizotypal features are prominent enough to warrant molecular testing even in males with relatively normal IQs (78). In adults, dysthymia, abusive verbal behaviors, and antisocial personality disorder behaviors have been reported (79). Self-injurious behaviors, usually restricted to hand- or finger-biting, occur in 58% of boys with fragile X (80). These behaviors appear before age 3 years and are triggered by changes in routine or when the child is asked to perform a difficult task. Selective mutism (81), social phobia (82), Tourette syndrome, and OCD have been reported (83, 84). Hagerman (65) suggests that complex stereotypies are only vaguely differentiated from motor tics and that the bursts of pressured speech represent complex vocal tics, which increase with anxiety.

Hyperactivity is common in fragile X syndrome, and although prominent in early childhood (69, 85), it is also present in adolescents and adults in somewhat diminished form (58, 86–89). There is a high level of sensitivity to sensory stimuli, often labeled "tactile defensiveness" which can be quite impairing (90). Young males with fragile X have deficits in prepulse inhibition (an indicator of impaired sensory gating in rodents), which is strongly associated with intellectual deficits, impaired attention and adaptive skills as well as autistic behaviors (91). Curiously, FMR1 knock-out mice show enhanced prepulse inhibition which would suggest a different compensatory mechanism in that species.

In the 1980s, a series of papers appeared that drew attention to the similarities between fragile X syndrome and autistic disorder (69, 73, 92–98). The atypical social interactions, stereotypies, hypersensitivity and bizarre responses to sound and other sensory stimuli, self-injurious behaviors, smelling of nonfood objects are all strongly reminiscent of autism spectrum disorders. Moreover, depending on the sample, up to 16% of males with autism manifest the fragile site (99). Autism is more prevalent in males (6.5%) than in females with fragile X (4%) (65).

Current information suggests that individuals with fragile X and autistic-spectrum behaviors represent a distinct subgroup. Autistic behaviors were significant predictors of slower development (100, 101), greater cognitive, adaptive, and social impairment (102), and increased age-related cognitive decline (60). Autistic behaviors occur more frequently in individuals with the full mutation (103), although Bailey et al. were unable to demonstrate a relationship between autistic behavior and the level of FMRP expression (100). On the other hand, children without autistic features and higher levels of FMRP expression features also demonstrated higher levels of adaptive behaviors (104).

The diagnosis of autistic disorder in individuals with fragile X must be approached cautiously because many of the "autistic" behaviors are qualitatively quite different. The social indifference that is the hallmark of autism is not seen in boys with fragile X: they are aware of the feelings of others and capable of reciprocal interactions, and their social skills improve with maturation (95, 105, 106). Men with fragile X are more likely to achieve adaptive functional levels commensurate with IQ than those with nonspecific mental retardation or autism (107). Males with fragile X syndrome are shy, socially awkward, anxious, and have a characteristic approach-withdrawal interactive style with an invariant set of mannerisms (108, 109). They have

peculiar greeting behaviors (such as looking away and making repetitive, out-of-context comments while also putting out a hand to shake) (92, 93, 110, 111, Cohen, 1991 #2395;Hatton, 2002 #5108;Merenstein, 1996 #7757;Wolff, 1989 #12464;). This "go away closer" quality is quite perplexing to those who are interacting with them. In social contexts their speech is more perseverative and less echolalic than observed in autism (112). These stereotypical utterances may serve to increase processing time (105, 113).

The neurobiological factors underlying gaze avoidance in fragile X also appear different from those involved in autistic disorder. Gaze avoidance in autistic disorder has been attributed to attentional factors or an inability to integrate eye contact into social interactions (94, 105). Individuals with autism appear to be indifferent and unaware of gaze but do not find it aversive, whereas individuals with fragile X are highly aware of gaze but disturbed by it (93). As discussed below, individuals with fragile X appear to have atypical activation neural activation patterns in regions subserving face and gaze-processing.

Females With the Fragile X Gene

Although once believed to be unaffected, fragile X carriers also manifest the somatic and neurobehavioral features of the disorder, albeit in attenuated form (114–116). The IQ of female fragile X carriers typically falls in the normal to mildly mentally retarded range, and there is a gradient of severity, with those with the full FMR1 mutation having greater cognitive deficits than those with the premutation. Women with the premutation did not differ from sibling controls (117). The verbal IQ is higher than the performance IQ. Subtests that are usually impaired include the Arithmetic, Digit Span, Block Design, and Object Assembly subtests (55). Short-term memory deficits, visual memory deficits, and impaired prefrontal executive function are typically seen (118–121). Girls with fragile X are often diagnosed as learning disabled. The typical academic profile of women with fragile X is characterized by relative strengths in reading and spelling and weakness in arithmetic (122).

Despite their relative strength in language, and even in the presence of average- to above-average intelligence, women with fragile X manifest deficiencies in expressive language and have conceptual disorganization with unusual thought content. This is accompanied by deficits in the expression and modulation of affect. Stereotypes are often observed. Compared to controls, they are more prone to schizophrenia-spectrum diagnoses, in particular schizotypy (115, 123). They are also more likely to have a diagnosis of avoidant disorder, mood disorder, as well as greater impairment in social interactions than controls (124–126). Mood disorders occur in 40% of the women with the premutation and are three times more common than in the control groups. Women with fragile X are shy, socially anxious and avoidant (127). They are often quite disorganized, inattentive, distractible, and impulsive (121, 125, 126, 128, 129).

Keysor and colleagues (130) noted a heightened level of baseline physiological arousal in 12- to 22-year-old girls with the full mutation. The length of the CGG repeat (therefore a lower level of FMRP) and inheritance of the gene from the mothers are associated with increased severity of psychiatric symptoms (75, 123, 125, 131). The cognitive and neuropsychiatric profile presented by women with fragile X is similar to that of nonverbal learning disability (125).

Neuroimaging Studies

In some ways, brains of children with fragile X are not different from brains in normally developing children. There is no significant difference in total cerebral volume in fragile X and it remains relatively stable after the age of 5 years. As in normal subjects, males have larger total cerebral volumes than females, with larger gray matter volumes in the male accounting for the difference, and there is the normal pattern of a decrease in gray matter volume with age, with an increase in white matter volume (132–134). However, there is evidence of disruption of the frontal and parietal white matter pathways in females with fragile X compared to controls (135).

Interestingly, the age-related decrease in gray matter volumes in boys with fragile X is slower than that in affected girls (136). In normal populations, total cerebral volume (specifically prefrontal and subcortical gray matter) explain 20% of the variance in IQ (134, 137). However, although there was a highly significant difference in IQ scores between fragile X males and females (mean full scale IQ 85 ± 18 for females versus 54 ± 15 for males), there was no evidence of a relationship between gray matter volumes and IQ, even after correcting for total brain volume difference. The volume of the lateral ventricles is increased and is also correlated with IQ. An atypical pattern of hemispheric asymmetry was noted, with larger right-sided cortical gray matter volumes (132)

Significant regional morphometric differences between individuals with fragile X and normal individuals have been noted in several studies. The cerebellar vermis is smaller in fragile X (males more so than in females) compared to both normal controls and other subjects with developmental disabilities. This reduction in size appears be due to a failure of normal brain growth rather than atrophy (138, 139). The growth impairment is particularly prominent in cerebellar lobules VI and VII and correlates with lower IQ (140) as well as increased stereotypy (126). An age-related increase in hippocampal volume is observed in the fragile X group by some investigators (136, 141) but not by others (118). Interestingly, FMRP is highly expressed in both the cerebellum and hippocampus and further research is required to understand this differential effect (26, 29). A decrease in size of the superior temporal gyrus, also age-related, has been reported (136). Subcortical structures have been reported to be enlarged, possibly as a result of increased dendritic density (142). Enlargement of the thalamus was also observed in females.

The caudate nucleus is enlarged in males and is correlated with methylation status and IQ (143), in contrast to the decrease in size observed in normally-developing children (144).

Although previously thought to be unaffected, adult males with premutations also manifest significant reduction in grey and white matter voxel densities across a broad range of cerebral structures. These reductions were correlated with increased CGG repeat size and decreased percent of FMRP positive lymphocytes (38).

Functional neuroimaging studies, largely restricted to females with fragile X, are particularly instructive as they not only provide valuable information about the recruitment of prefrontal cortex in the performance of difficult tasks, but also demonstrate that women with fragile X have particular difficulty with this process compared to controls. Highly relevant to these studies is the concept of *deactivation* (that is the control or baseline condition minus the cognitive task condition, which is the opposite of activation, cognitive task condition minus baseline). Deactivation may be viewed as the suspension or inhibition of ongoing background neuronal activity in specific brain regions during the performance of tasks requiring increased cognitive activity (145). A number of studies have demonstrated that women with fragile X differ from control groups not only in activation patterns but also in their inability to deactivate or turn off this ongoing background activity and impairment in performance is correlated with diminished FMRP levels. Thus, anomalous activation and inactivation MRI patterns were noted in fragile X females and controls while they performed a STROOP interference task (146). In an arithmetic task with two levels of difficulty, women with fragile X showed less activation and did not increase activation in response to greater task difficulty in contrast to the controls. FMRP expression was positively correlated with activation of a number of frontoparietal structures. (147).

In an fMRI Go–No Go study, the accuracy and reaction time of females with fragile X did not differ significantly from that of the controls, despite a lower mean IQ score. However, FMRP expression was positively correlated with activation in a number of areas, including the hippocampus, cerebellum, and frontostriatal regions. Controls manifested an *increased* level of activation in prefrontal ventromedial cortex area during the baseline "Go" task compared to the "No Go" task. A markedly different pattern was noted in the women with fragile X (148).

In an fMRI study examining visuospatial working memory in females with fragile X (149), similar anomalies in the activation and deactivation patterns were noted in comparison to controls. Although they were able to perform the simple version in a manner similar to the controls, on the difficult task, the performance of the fragile X females deteriorated significantly and they activated a number of prefrontal areas, suggesting that they were unable to recruit neural areas in a coherent manner on the more difficult task. The lack of FMRP may impair the transcriptional machinery required for rapid protein synthesis of protein in synapses, which underlies learning. In a study of visual memory encoding (150), girls with fragile X showed significantly less activation in the hippocampus and the basal forebrain.

In a study examining accuracy in identifying the direction of facial gaze, females with fragile X syndrome were less accurate and did not manifest enhanced left superior temporal sulcus, or the differential activation in the fusiform gyrus in response to forward faces relative to angled faces, as was seen in controls (151). This study provides a somewhat different perspective on the issue of gaze aversion in individuals with fragile X. It would suggest that there is an underlying impairment in the neural systems for processing faces and direction of gaze.

Management

One of the "take home" messages in this section about fragile X is that when a child comes for psychiatric evaluation and treatment, it is unusual to have just one affected individual in the family. It is likely that management of the child will need to take into consideration the neurocognitive status of the parents. It is also apparent that there is a broad range of variability in the cognitive and neuropsychiatric features so that a careful assessment of the child is indicated. This assessment should include evaluation of the child's temperament, ability to interact in social situations, and function in school.

Individual assessment of temperament, and functional analysis with subsequent parent counseling and environmental modification is an important first step that can help delay the use of medications very early in life (152–154). A careful initial evaluation will provide the basis for a treatment plan, which may include appropriate psychopharmacology. In some cases, sensorimotor integration therapy may be helpful in managing the high arousal level (155), and cognitive behavioral therapy may be useful in selected cases (81, 156–158, Sundheim, unpublished data). Assisting the parents in finding an appropriate school setting and anticipating the type of educational difficulties that the child is likely to encounter (poor grasp of arithmetic and difficulty making inferences) will be beneficial. Providing structured, supportive settings for learning socially appropriate behaviors is helpful. Parents benefit from counseling regarding the longterm outcome and assistance in locating vocational training opportunities tailored to their child's abilities. Some patients will require considerable structure and support to function adequately, whereas others will be able to manage with relative independence.

Future Avenues in Treatment

Learning and memory are regulated by a delicate balance between the creation functional and stable synapses and the elimination of redundant synapses. There is a considerable body of research which supports the role of long term

potentiation (LTP) in establishing and maintaining such functional synaptic connections, whereas long term depression (LTD) is one of the processes involved in the pruning of non-functional connections. There are several different pathways leading to LTD. One pathway involves the activation of group 1 metabotropic glutamate receptors (Gp1 mGluRs) by mGluR agonists which in turn results in the translation of preexisting mRNA in the postsynaptic neuron leading to a rapid increase in dendritic protein synthesis (158a), as well as the rapid (and, importantly, irreversible) loss of both AMPA and NMDA receptors from synapses, a putative antecedent of synaptic elimination (158b). Importantly, the activation of Gp1 mGluRs also stimulates the synaptic synthesis of FMRP. One might expect that in fragile X syndrome, the absence of FMRP at the synapse would result in a decrease in protein-synthesis dependent LTD. Surprisingly, in the *Fmr1* knockout mouse model, LTD is *enhanced* rather than diminished (158c). This finding makes sense in the context of research that shows that FMRP is a translational repressor—part of the RNA-induced silencing complex (RISC) that mediates the degradation of mRNAs and stops transcription (158d). These findings have led Bear et al. to propose that the neuropsychiatric profile of fragile X is the result of a failure of FMRP to silence synthesis of specific proteins at an appropriate developmental stage with an ensuing pathological exaggeration of LTD (158e). Thus, at a time when the developing brain should be generating and strengthening synaptic connections, the fragile X brain is slowing and eliminating synaptic connections with a predictable and devastating impact on learning and memory. Anatomically, the anomalous long, thin dendritic spines seen in fragile X brains would fit with this model. This opens an exciting therapeutic possibility, namely that Gp1 mGluR antagonists may serve to treat or mitigate the symptoms observed in fragile X. These agents (one of which is lithium) have been used in mouse and drosophila models of fragile X and have materially decreased the pathological behaviors seen in these mutant animals (158f; 158g). These mGluR antagonists are being actively investigated because of their role in the treatment of other neuropsychiatric disorders—anxiety, addictive and bipolar disorders. The challenge here will be to select an appropriate time window as LTD induced by mGluR functions differently at different phases of development (158h). Moreover, the mechanisms of LTP and LTD vary depending on brain region and function.

Down Syndrome

Down syndrome (DS)(trisomy 21) is the most common genetic mental retardation syndrome, occurring in 1 in 660 live births (159). Very young mothers and those over age 40 years are at increased risk of having a child with DS (the risk increases to 1 per 50 live births over age 40).

The individual with DS is short and has a small, brachycephalic head. Atypical facial features include hypotelorism, midface hypoplasia, epicanthal folds, uptilted palpebral fissures, small ears, an enlarged tongue, and a high-arched palate. Hands are broad with short fingers and an incurved fifth finger. They are hypotonic, with hyperextensible joints. DS is associated with serious congenital anomalies of the heart and gut, both congenital and acquired thyroid disease, and a 19-fold increase in risk of acute leukemia (160, 161). Children with DS are at increased risk for celiac disease (162). Epilepsy occurs in about 8% of children with DS; with close to a third having infantile spasms of infancy (163, 164).

Genetics
Trisomy (three copies of chromosome 21) occurs in 95% of individuals with DS. About 5% have a translocation (165, 166). Two to 4% of cases are mosaics (167). The DS critical region has been mapped to a 5 Mb area on chromosome 21(168–172). Some genes are overexpressed, such as C21orf2, synaptojanin, and the Minibrain (Mng) gene (183, 184, 185). Others are unchanged, and some, such as HACS1, a signaling pathway mediator, are underexpressed. As a result, there is a dysregulation and "misexpression" in the balance of protein products (173–185). Many of the dysregulated genes play important roles in neuronal function and connectivity. At 19 gestational weeks samples of fetal cortex from patients with DS revealed significant reduction in proteins associated with synaptogenesis and dendritic tree arborization (186). Examination of DS fetal brains also reveals marked reduction of protein products associated with genes on other chromosomes (179).

Neuroanatomical Aspects
Brain weight is reduced to about 76% of normal, although in some studies, the cerebellum and brain stem are disproportionately small (187–189). The convolutional pattern is simple, with a narrow superior temporal gyrus and gaping insula. Frontal cortex, anterior corpus callosum, and limbic structures (uncus, amygdala, hippocampus, and parahippocampal gyrus) are disproportionately reduced in volume, with relative sparing of the parietal cortex (190, 191). The amount of gray matter is proportional to the volume of the cerebrum (192). However, thalamus, putamen and globus pallidus, but not caudate are increased in size compared to normal controls (190, 192, 193).

Brain Development
Given the fact that several of the genes essential for normal brain development are disrupted in DS, one would expect to see anomalies in the earliest stages of brain development. Surprisingly, evidence of abnormal brain growth is apparent, albeit relatively subtly, only around the 22nd gestational week (194, 195). Despite the fact that in the DS mouse, there is evidence that the normal sequence of neuronal migration is disrupted (196) the DS brain is not particularly aberrant at birth. Dendritic differ-

entiation in infants with DS at 2½ months is similar to that of controls (197), but there is a 20–50% decrease in neuronal density with maturation (189, 195, 198, 199). Myelination is delayed, particularly fibers linking frontal and temporal cortices as well as U-fibers, and particularly in infants who had congenital heart lesions (200). Deceleration in brain growth and emergence of the characteristic foreshortening of the DS brain becomes apparent by 6 months of age (195).

The dendritic and synaptic structure within the DS brain is quite anomalous (200). Dendritic arborization is curtailed and there is a decline in the number of dendritic spines with age (201, 202). In a mouse model of DS, dendritic spines and synaptic boutons are markedly enlarged with abnormal internal membranes. There are shifts in the pattern of spine density and inhibitory inputs (203).

Neurocognitive Profile
Forty-five years ago, the developmental picture for children with DS was bleak, and institutionalization was recommended. Today, it is not uncommon for individuals with DS to be married, live and work independently, raise children, and even attend college (204). Several young persons have been able to pursue careers as television actors. In 1976 the average IQ of persons with trisomy 21 was 52, and the average for the mosaic DS subject was 67. It is now recognized that the IQ can extend into the normal range (205). A trend to higher academic achievement scores from 1986 to 2000 has also been documented (206).

This shift toward higher functional ability reflects two major factors: First, birth defects and medical conditions are now treated early and effectively. Second, the discouraging prognoses have been replaced by much more positive attitudes, now infant stimulation programs and educational mainstreaming are the norm (189).

Children with DS are at risk for decreased visual acuity as well as hearing impairment, secondary to anomalies of the external auditory canal, and otitis media (207, 208). These preventable sensory impairments interfere with normal development and the child benefits immensely from early evaluation and treatment.

Children with DS typically manifest relatively rapid acquisition of skill in early childhood (albeit at a slower rate than normally developing peers), but the developmental pattern is asynchronous and skills are not consolidated, so that a plateau occurs at different points in different cognitive domains (209).

Overall, children with DS are weak in language and have somewhat greater strengths in processing visuospatial information. They acquire language at a slower rate than their normally developing peers (210). Adolescents with DS continue to manifest impoverished vocabulary and grammar, word meanings, appropriate contextual use, and syntax (211, 212). Working memory is impaired in these children and is associated with acquisition of receptive vocabulary. As a group, children with DS have a better understanding of word meanings than their grasp of grammar and syntax and their comprehension is better than expression (213–216). Their narratives are wordy and complex and lack cohesion (217). A well-designed longitudinal study has shown that teenagers continue to acquire receptive vocabulary (albeit at about half the rate of normal peers), but comprehension of grammar begins to plateau in early adolescence (218). Comprehension at the initial evaluation and the rate of growth in comprehension provided the best predictors of expressive language (219).

Despite the expressive language delays, children with DS use gestural communication effectively and to the same extent as peers matched for mental age, although like other areas of development, they acquire gestures at a slower rate than normally developing children (205, 220, 221).

Visuospatial function is a relative strength in children with DS. Performance on visuospatial tasks continues to improve in adolescence, whereas several aspects of language acquisition either plateau or decline (218). Compared to children with Williams syndrome, children with DS perform better on visuospatial short-term memory tasks, even though they are impaired in auditory working memory (222). The deficits in working memory (due to limited storage capacity) and grammar would suggest that prefrontal functions are mainly compromised (223). Children with Williams syndrome have great difficulty with global processing, whereas those with DS grasp the gestalt more readily than the details (i.e., they see the "forest" but not the "trees") (212, 224).

Social-Emotional Development

Children with DS are described as having pleasant, easygoing personalities. However, there are two developmental features of young children with DS which may hinder social interactions with parents and social development. First, children with DS appear to make little effort to learn new skills, and fail to consolidate and use skills already acquired (225, 226). Their decreased engagement in a task may reflect attentional and intentional deficits (227). Infants with DS appear to have difficulty shifting attention from one target to another (228) and persisting in continuous goal-directed exploratory behavior (227). These attentional features may reflect an early manifestation of prefrontal dysfunction in infants with DS. Children with DS respond empathetically to facial emotional signals and gestures of distress but in tasks which involved processing of more abstract information about emotional states of others, their performance began to plateau at age 4 years (229, 230). This is somewhat unexpected, given the apparent sociability of these children and their relative strengths processing visuospatial information (212). Nonetheless, children with DS have considerable awareness of their social environment. Preverbal children with DS vary gestural patterns depending on social context. Patterns of visual checking also vary with the social context (more social checking occurs with a peer).

Symbolic play does not appear to be particularly delayed in children with DS (231). Although they may engage in more play acts than their normally developing peers, they are less likely to request objects or assistance (231, 232).

Academic

Children with DS can decode single words but have difficulty comprehending what they have read (233). They have difficulty grasping mathematical concepts, lack a well-developed number concept and have difficulty applying their mathematical knowledge to novel problems (205, 234).

Brain Function in DS

Functional neuroimaging studies on healthy, non-demented adults with DS have demonstrated elevated global cerebral glucose metabolism (235), particularly in inferior temporal/entorhinal cortex (236), and functional disruption of neural circuits involved in attentional processing (237). Several studies have described age-related decreases in regional gray matter of temporal lobe structures in nondemented adults with Down's syndrome. Amygdala and hippocampal volumes were positively correlated with memory measures (193, 238). Neuroimaging studies in nondemented adults with DS indicate that there are progressive changes in the structure and function of various areas of the brain before the appearance of clinical evidence of dementia.

Neuropsychiatric Disorders

The overall incidence of psychiatric disorders in children, adolescents, and adults with DS is around 20% (239–244). The pattern of psychiatric disorders shifts with age. Externalizing behaviors—ADHD, oppositional defiant disorder, conduct disorder, and aggression—are prominent in the school age child. Adolescents and young adults manifest more internalizing behaviors—withdrawal, shyness, impaired self-confidence. Depression is very common in older adolescents and adults with DS and should be considered before attributing a functional decline to dementia (245–248). It can lead to potentially lethal suicidal behavior (249). Obsessional slowness has been reported in individuals with DS who can spend hours performing daily routines (250). Anorexia nervosa is not unusual in DS (251–254) and has been reported in association with obsessive-compulsive disorder and depression (255). Other anxiety disorders, phobias, autistic disorder, stereotypy, and self-injurious behaviors are relatively rare. Dementia of the Alzheimer's type appears as early as age 40 and 77% receive the diagnosis after the age of 60 years.

Management

The neuropsychiatric management of patients with DS depends in part on the age of the patient. Counseling the parents of young children with DS can provide support while they struggle with any of the early medical complications. They need encouragement to provide early social and developmental stimulation. Wishart recommends that parents and teachers focus on consolidation of existing skills and on dealing with the child's tendency to avoid challenging tasks (which may compromise performance on cognitive assessments) (226). There are multiple treatable etiologies for neuropsychiatric symptoms in DS patients that are unrelated to dementia (e.g., hypothyroidism).

Williams Syndrome

Williams syndrome (WS) occurs in 1 per 25,000 to 1 per 50,000 live births. Individuals with WS are short (256) have a characteristic "elfin" facial appearance—a depressed nasal bridge with anteverted nares, medial eyebrow flare, stellate irides, small, low-set ears with prominent lobes, thick lips with a wide mouth, and curly hair. The voice is low-pitched, hoarse, and metallic (257–261). There is an exaggerated lumbar lordosis with flexion at the knees and hips (262, 263). Infants with WS are often of low birth weight and gain weight slowly. They are constipated, irritable, and overreactive to noises (264). Hypercalcemia, usually mild, occurs in the neonatal period and resolves spontaneously by age 2 years (265).

Neurological examination reveals esotropia (266), hypotonia, cerebellar signs and corticospinal tract signs as well as a higher incidence of left-handedness than in the general population (211).

Recurrent otitis media occurs in over 60% of children with WS (267), with the associated risk of a conductive hearing loss. Decreased visual acuity and strabismus occur frequently (268). Serious cardiac and vascular problems are associated with WS. In one series, 59% of children and adults with WS had a structural heart defect (supravalvular aortic stenosis, pulmonic artery stenosis, coarctation of the aorta, and cardiomyopathy) or vascular disease (vasospasm and stenoses resulting in stroke) (269). The vascular problems are the result of a deficiency of elastin in vessel walls (270). Thus, individuals with WS are at high risk for cerebral infarction at a young age (271). Hypertension occurs in about 50% of individuals with WS, likely secondary to the generalized arteriopathy discussed above, and increases the risk of stroke (274).

Genetics

The WS critical region is composed of some 30 genes at 7q11.23. Over 99% of the DNA sequence of human chromosome 7 has now been identified and the orthologous sequences on mouse chromosome 5G have also been mapped with high accuracy (275). Identifying the genes responsible for WS challenges conventional mapping techniques because of the high density of repetitive sequences and the large (~300 kb) duplicated DNA sequences, which are nearly identical and vary from individual to individual (276). These result from the misalignment and crossing over of these low-copy repeat sequences which flank the WS critical region, and lead to chromosomal instability. Identifying the genes responsible for the cognitive and behavioral features of WS phenotype has been particularly challenging. A number of different reports describing rare individuals with small deletions and only some of the somatic and cognitive phenotypic features characteristic of WS have appeared but definitive information is not yet available (277–279).

Many of the vascular features of WS results from haploinsufficiency of the elastin gene (ELN) (280–285). The decreased production of elastin alters the structure and mechanical properties of arterial walls (286). LIM kinase-1 has been considered a candidate gene for the cognitive deficits seen in WS (279, 285, 287, 288). It is a component of an intracellular signaling pathway, which regulates neuronal cytoskeleton, synapses and apoptosis through formation of actin fibers (289–291). LIM kinase-1 is expressed in fetal development, including neuronal differentiation of hippocampal progenitor cells (292, 293). It is also involved in hippocampal long-term potentiation (LTP), which is critical to memory formation (294). LIM kinase-1 knockout mice exhibit significant abnormalities in spine morphology, synaptic function, including hippocampal long-term potentiation and show altered fear response and spatial learning (295, 296).

Other candidate genes include those in the general transcriptions factor family, which are widely expressed throughout the brain during fetal brain development (297) and maybe related to mental retardation (279). Syntaxin 1A (STIX) and the gene for the human homologue of the *Drosophila* gene "frizzled", *FZD9*, were considered potential candidates but some patients with the classical WS phenotype have small deletions which spare these loci (298–302).

Neurocognitive Profile

The IQ of most individuals with WS falls in the mild to moderate range of mental retardation (mean of 55; range 40 to 90) and remains stable across the lifespan (303, 304). Thus, the clinician can expect to encounter considerable variability in cognitive functioning among patients with WS.

There are several fascinating aspects of the neurocognitive profile of WS. As these children develop, an uneven cognitive profile emerges, characterized by relative strength in language, impaired visuospatial abilities, and a strong drive to engage in social interactions. In the preschool years, expressive language, and motor skills are often delayed. By school-age, the child with WS appears fluent and articulate, if not "verbose and pseudo-mature" (305). By the time that they are adolescents, children with WS have large, sophisticated vocabularies, consisting of unusual words. To give the flavor of these remarkable linguistic abilities of some individuals with WS, the following quote (the response of one of Dr. Bellugi's patients when asked what he would want other people to know about WS) is cited:

> It is what you're born with, it is what you have to accept,
> and it is something that you go on day to day, year to year,
> month to month with. And no matter how people treat

people with Williams syndrome, you always have to stand tall and ignore the things that are said because they are, they don't understand the things that we go through every day that we wake up. We should be treated the same way somebody else should be treated. Even when times are bad we still try to shine a light upon other people, and to give that sense of glow to our friends . . . You have to accept things you cannot change. (306).

The language in WS has been a focus of considerable interest for linguists, as it is relevant to theories of the neural representations of language. Despite the relatively strong vocabulary of individuals with WS (albeit below that of controls) the way they organize their lexical information differs from that of normally developing individuals. (307–311). They use unusual low-frequency words both in spontaneous speech and when performing verbal semantic fluency tasks (e.g., words such as "brontosaurus" and "yak") (211). Words are also used by individuals with WS in unusual ways; for example, "I have to evacuate the glass," a phrase uttered by a girl with WS as she emptied a glass of water (210, p. 13). The WS profile has been the subject of considerable controversy. Bellugi maintains that individuals with WS have intact morphosyntactic rule and grammar systems and a deviant lexicosemantic system (307, 312), whereas others believe that the morphosyntactic abilities are in fact impaired (313). Clahsen has reported that individuals with WS performed as well as controls when inflecting regular forms but had difficulty on irregular forms, applying regular inflection forms to the irregular verbs; (for example, *ring→ringed* (314). Based on the assumption that regular inflections are computationally-based and irregular inflections are lexically-based and stored in longterm memory, the investigators concluded that these children understand the rule-based systems of language (and thus are quite good in terms of managing regular syntax) but have difficulty with the items requiring access to the associative memory (lexical) system, required for manipulation of irregular forms. Cross-linguistic studies have tended to support this view (309).

Working memory is a relative strength in WS (mean digit span 4.6), (222, 309). Subjects with WS who had good working memory showed particular strength in producing irregular grammatical forms. Working memory was also associated with use of low-frequency words, suggesting that children with WS rely on phonological working memory to a much greater degree than normal children in the process of learning language. It would also explain their deficits in manipulating irregular syntax (315).

In comparison to relative strength in working memory which persists into adulthood, most individuals with WS have deficient episodic memory, particularly in the visuospatial domain, which becomes increasingly impaired as they age (222, 305, 307, 316–318).

Performance on visuospatial, graphomotor, and constructional tasks are significantly impaired in individuals with WS (312, 319–321). Children with WS have difficulty

integrating visual features into a global configuration—they see "the trees" rather than "the forest" (210, 211, 224). Drawings lack coherence and spatial orientation, perspective or depth, consisting of parts of objects scattered across the page. These deficits are not secondary to either fine motor or vision impairment per se (268, 322). Rather, the deficit involves the integration of visuospatial information and motor programming, thus implicating the dorsal parietal and frontoparietal functions (323).

Although verbal mediation can be used to compensate for these deficits, language describing spatial relationships is also impaired in individuals with WS (210, 324). They have difficulty understanding terms describing spatial relationships, in contrast to their relative strength in other conceptual areas (325).

Some individuals with WS have been reported to have a higher frequency of perfect pitch (1 per 20) compared to the general population (1 per 10,000) (326, 327).

Hypersociability

The hypersociability of individuals with WS is a distinctive attribute. Babies with WS will stare intensely at faces for long periods of time (328). They tolerate brief separations from their mothers with few manifestations of distress (329). Older children with WS approach strangers in a fearless manner and engage them in conversation, a trait which is particularly concerning to mothers of adolescent girls (277, 329).

In story-telling tasks, children with WS demonstrated a remarkable ability to engage their audience. They changed their voices and used exaggerated prosody to enhance the story, provided interpretations of the mental states of the characters in the stories, and employed "audience hookers" (e.g., "Guess what happened next?" "What do you know?" and "Lo and behold, the frog was gone!"). These devices were utilized to a much greater extent than normal controls. Similar behaviors were noted in the course of a semistructured interview (329).

The performance of persons with WS on Theory of Mind tasks (i.e., the ability to make inferences about another individual's perspectives and motivations) is again uneven. Older children and young adults with WS were able to make appropriate inferences about the intention of others at a level comparable to that seen in normally developing controls. They were able to deal with more difficult tasks, such as the interpretation of sarcasm, and 44% passed second-order knowledge questions, but some had difficulty discriminating lies from jokes (330).

However, despite their apparent sociability, children and adults with WS are not very successful in developing and keeping friendships (331). They typically relate to adults better than to peers (329, 332).

Although some aspects of the WS profile resemble that of individuals with nonverbal learning disorder or right-hemisphere dysfunction, individuals with WS are more attuned to the emotional state of others and more able to describe their own emotions in detail. They lack the prosodic flatness that is often seen in persons with right hemisphere dysfunction. Their performance on the Facial Recognition and Noncanonical Views tasks (i.e., a test in which one is given views of an object in different lighting and from different vantage points) is surprisingly proficient. However, the strategies they use are different than those employed by controls, suggesting that facial processing follows an abnormal course of development (311, 333, 334).

Academic Achievement

Children with WS remain in special education classes throughout their educational exposure (335, 336). Although they perform as well as controls (matched for reading and verbal mental age) on most phonological awareness tasks and are able to link a word's orthographic form to its phonological representations, they do not necessarily associate the word with its meaning (337, 338). Thus, in some ways they are hyperlexic—they may perform better in single word reading than would be predicted by IQ, but their comprehension is poor (339, 340). Writing and arithmetic are areas of weakness, which persist into adulthood (210, 341).

Neuropsychiatric Disorders

Children with WS are rated by parents and teachers as being fussy, fearful, anxious, shy, distractible, and hyperactive (342–347). One interesting aspect of the attention problem is "sticky fixation"—difficulty disengaging and shifting attention from one target to another. This may reflect dysfunction in the dorsal (parietal) pathway (323). Sticking fixation is seen in normally developing infants aged 3 to 5 months, but not after 6 months. In the child with WS, it may persist until the age of 5 to 6 years. These children also have particularly difficulty modulating incoming stimuli and regulating their levels of arousal. This is particularly true with regard to loud noises which provoke great distress—crying, rocking, and self-injurious behaviors (267, 348). As many as 95% have hyperacusis, which tends to improve with age (263). Clinically significant anxiety, obsessions, and phobias often persist into adulthood (349, 350). Depressive symptoms tend to increase with age (351).

Difficulty initiating and sustaining sleep, associated with frequent nocturnal arousals and difficulty settling back to sleep is a common problem. Parents often need to soothe the child who cannot otherwise settle down to sleep. The arousals may be related to periodic limb movements (352).

Brain Structure and Function

The brain in WS is small (800 to 1000 grams; MRI morphometric studies reveal a reduction of 13% in total brain volume compared to controls). There is relative preservation of cerebellar volume: lobules VI-VII and VIII-X are enlarged and the posterior vermis is significantly larger, after controlling for the reduction in the size of the WS brain

(353). Brainstem tissue volume is reduced by 20%. In general, there is relative sparing of frontal regions and a selective reduction in posterior areas of the WS brain (188, 190, 211, 354–356). In an MRI study using much thinner slices and better resolution, this observation was only partially replicated: decreased occipital gray matter volume, particularly on the right and increased parietal gray matter volume was noted (300). Schmitt et al. described the distinctive shape of the WS brain, characterized by less of a curve in the corpus callosum as well as in the angulation of the anterior/posterior areas relative to frontal areas in the sagittal plane which may reflect the decrease in the ratio of frontal to parietaloccipital volumes (357).

There is a disproportional reduction of cerebral white matter with relative sparing of gray matter (300). In particular, gray matter in the superior temporal gyrus (STG) volumes in subjects with WMS were proportionally larger compared to controls. The corpus callosum is noted to be decreased in size, particularly in the isthmus and splenium (358, 359). However, women with WS were noted to have decreased gray matter volumes bilaterally in the superior, not the inferior parietal lobule (360). This finding would implicate specific involvement of dorsodorsal stream which control "on line" motor behaviors. Lesions in this area result in optic ataxia (361), and would be consistent with the deficits in visuomotor integration observed in individuals with WS. Corroborating information from functional neuroimaging studies have demonstrated that the parietal segment of the dorsal stream is hypoactivated in WS (362).

Anomalous patterns of cortical gyrification have been noted. Increased gyrification was noted most prominently in the left frontal and right parietal and occipital areas (363). Shortening of the central sulcus with relative hypoplasia of the occipitoparietal regions has been observed. The cytoarchitecture of cortical forebrain areas is relatively normal (354).

During face perception tasks, WS subjects show a pattern of activation of the fusiform gyrus that is similar to controls (364). However, in an ERP study of face processing, individuals with WS demonstrated an abnormally small negativity at 100 msec (N100) and an abnormally large negativity at 200 msec (N200) to both upright and inverted faces. The small N100/large N200 ERP may represent an electrophysiologic marker for abnormal face perception in WS (334).

These structural and functional neuroimaging studies provide further evidence for the anomalous anatomical features of the WS brain. However, at this point in time, the genes in the WS critical region that result in these aberrant morphological features have not been identified. The aberrant gyrification patterns, reduction of gray matter in the parietal lobe, and the relative decrease in white matter suggest that brain development is affected at different points in time and by different mechanisms across development. The relationship between the structural and functional anomalies in the dorsodorsal parietal region provides a pathophysiological basis for the visuospatial deficits seen in WS.

Management

The management of persons with WS starts with a detailed assessment of intellectual and functional ability. The high rate of medical complications associated with WS, particularly with aging, requires close collaboration with other physicians.

Young children with WS are often particularly handicapped by a combination of visuospatial deficits, deficient expressive language, hyperacusis, severe ADHD, and an array of anxieties, phobias, and a lower threshold for arousal. Tomc suggests that parents should be counseled regarding these difficult temperamental characteristics and supported in their attempts to deal with a difficult child who "should be easy"; (that is, they appear friendly and outgoing) (365). ADHD may respond to treatment with psychostimulants (366). Sensory integration techniques aimed at helping the child to modulate arousal level and hypersensitivity to environmental stimuli (particularly auditory stimuli) may be helpful. The use of auditory filters has been suggested (348). It is helpful for the parents, teachers, and mental health professionals to understand the developmental trajectory of children with WS—namely, that as they mature they may develop relative strengths in the area of expressive language but continue to have severe intellectual and academic deficiencies. The school-age child will require selection of an appropriate class placement and learning disability support.

The remarkable language skills of persons with WS and their engaging way of relating may lead caretakers into erroneously assuming that the individual's functional ability is comparable to their linguistic skill. In fact, the individual with WS has a simplistic understanding of the functional aspects of day-to-day living (e.g., the purpose of going to the bank is to get money). They continue to struggle with fine motor skill deficits (they need help in tying shoelaces), visuospatial deficits, and difficulty with social relationships. Most adults with WS live a solitary existence; are restless, anxious, and fearful; and continue to be troubled by hyperacusis. Fewer than 5% are employed in the general work force. Most live and work in sheltered environments (335, 367).

Turner Syndrome

Epidemiology

Turner Syndrome (TS) is the most common sex chromosome abnormality in females, occurring in 1 in 1,500 to 2,500 live born females (368, 369). Two to three percent of all females conceived have an XO karyotype. Only 1 to 1.5% survive to term (370).

Characteristic features include short stature, low posterior hairline, lymphedema of the hands and feet, anomalous ears, and a narrow maxilla. A webbed neck and increased chest diameter ("shield chest"), are strong predictors of aortic and pulmonary venous anomalies (371). Gonadal dysgenesis, apparent in the 20-week fetus, results in ovarian failure which can occur either before puberty or later. Most (85 to 95%) of the girls with monosomy (45X)

and 60% of mosaic TS fail to enter puberty spontaneously (372). Women with TS are at high risk for osteoporosis and other medical complications associated with estrogen deficiency. Spontaneous pregnancy is rare and the rate of fetal wastage and birth defects is very high (373, 374).

Serious medical problems in TS include cardiac anomalies (17 to 45%), prominently coarctation of the aorta and bicuspid aortic valve (375), aortic dissection (373), hypertension (in 7 to 17% of children and 24 to 40% of adults) (375), and congenital renal anomalies (25 to 43%) (373, 376–378). A mild conductive hearing loss (as a result of chronic otitis) occurs in over 50% of girls with TS. A progressive sensorineural hearing loss may also occur (379–381). Impaired glucose tolerance, insulin resistance with Type 2 diabetes mellitus, (382), hyperlipidemia, ulcerative colitis, Crohn's disease, and autoimmune thyroid disease are frequently associated with TS (383). Growth failure secondary to a primary bone defect, and possibly a relative growth hormone deficiency result in slow growth in childhood. The height of adults with TS falls two standard deviations below the mean (373).

Genetic Features

TS is characterized by the absence of part or all of the second X chromosome (in some cases, absence of part of the Y chromosome). Approximately half of the girls with TS have monosomy X- (45, XO), which is associated with the most severe anomalies (373, 384). In 70%, the single X chromosome is of maternal origin.

Two copies of the X chromosome are required for normal development of the female (385). Early in the normal embryonic development of females, one X chromosome in each cell is transcriptionally silenced (or "inactivated"), with the exception of the genes in the pseudoautosomal region 1 (PAR-1), located in a 2.6 Mb region—Xp11.2–p22.1—at the distal end of the short arm. (In males, the short arm of the Y chromosome contributes a similar set of genes from PAR-1). Thus, deletion of one copy of PAR-1 genes can result in the TS phenotype (380, 386). Genes associated with ovarian failure, high-arched palate, and autoimmune thyroid disease have also been mapped to this region (386).

The X-inactivation site (XIST) is located at Xq11.2–q21 on the long arm of the X chromosome. It is required for the transcriptional silencing of the second copy of the genes on the X chromosome, except for those in PAR-1. Inactivation typically involves any faulty genes. Genes (specifically paternal genes) are initially silenced well before cellular differentiation, later reactivated, and then randomly silenced again (387). Deletion of the XIST site, which occurs in some cases of small ring chromosomes in TS, may be associated with severe anomalies or retardation (388–390).

Imprinting, that is, whether the X chromosome comes from the father (X^+) or mother (X^m), may also result in different cognitive and behavioral phenotypes.

Somewhat different genetic patterns are associated with different TS phenotypes. Seven to 18% of individuals with

TS have an isochromosome (46,Xi(Xq), that is, two identical chromosome arms due to duplication of one arm and loss of the other arm. This genotype is linked to increased risk of deafness and autoimmune disorders. Mosaicism (45, X/46, XX) occurs in 10% and is associated with a milder neurocognitive phenotype, less growth impairment, and less ovarian dysfunction (391). Approximately 2% of women with TS have 46,XXp- and 46,XXq- genotypes with variable phenotypes. Ring chromosome, 46,Xr(X), sometimes associated with a severe phenotype, occurs in 6 to 10% of TS subjects (388–390). In about 7% of TS cases, Y chromosome material is present as a result of deletion of the Y chromosome (45,X/46,XY) as demonstrated by polymerase chain reaction (392, 393). There is a significantly increased risk for gonadoblastoma; virilization is inconsistently present (392, 393).

Neurocognitive Profile

The TS cognitive profile is characterized by average-range verbal skills and impaired visuospatial/motor/perceptual skills, visual memory, prefrontal executive function and processing social-emotional interactions (394–408).

A study was undertaken comparing the neurocognitive performance of women with TS to those with premature ovarian failure (409). Both groups had early estrogen deficiency and both had received estrogen replacement therapy (410). The performance of the women with premature ovarian failure did not differ from that of normal controls; whereas the women with TS manifested the characteristic visuospatial perceptual skills deficit, suggesting that the cognitive deficits in TS are the result of anomalous brain development rather than estrogen deficiency. In a study in which adolescent girls with TS were randomly assigned to placebo and androgen (oxandrolone) treatment groups for two years, there was a small but significant improvement in working memory in the treatment group (411).

In the academic sphere, reading skills in TS are relatively intact. Individuals with TS are able to read irregular words, and manifest strength in phonological awareness and comprehension (412). Despite the strength in phonologic awareness, they are impaired in nonword reading, which is an unusual pattern and may be a manifestation of executive function deficits (394).

Poor performance in the area of arithmetic, especially numerical ability, mental calculation, geometry, and reasoning are characteristic of the TS population (403, 413–415) and is apparent in kindergarten and shows little improvement. They perform poorly on tasks involving cognitive estimation and rapid enumeration of small quantities which depends in part on storing a specific configuration in memory and calculation ability (400, 414, 416).

Girls with TS have difficulty with facial affect recognition, particularly identifying fearful facial expressions. Their deficit is as impaired as that seen in patients with bilateral amygdalectomies (397, 417, 418). Similar impairment was noted in a study in which they were asked to identify mental state from images of the upper face ("reading the mind in the eyes") (419). Some studies evaluating their ability to detect small shifts in gaze have indicated impairment as well (420).

The TS neurocognitive/behavioral profile (in 70% of females with TS)— verbal ability superior to visuospatial ability, motor impairment, prefrontal executive function deficit, relative strength in language-based academic tasks compared to weakness in arithmetic coupled with difficulty in the social-emotional sphere— bears a strong resemblance to nonverbal learning disability (421).

There is considerable variability in individuals, and the degree of impairment on task performance depends, in part, on the complexity of the task and the cognitive load that is placed on frontal-executive system resources (407, 408). In addition, the specific pattern of affected genes may determine the neurocognitive profile, although more data will be required before firm conclusions can be drawn. The genes related to the TS neurocognitive profile have been mapped to the PAR-1 region (380). Overall, TS subjects with monosomy perform more poorly than mosaic TS subjects, who may perform within the range of controls on some verbal tasks. Both the mosaic and monosomic TS groups are significantly impaired on visuospatial and memory tasks compared to controls, suggesting specific impairment of association neocortex (422). Imprinting may contribute to the TS cognitive phenotype. Skuse found the women with 45,X^p to have superior verbal and executive function and better social adjustment (423). Moreover, 40% of the subjects with 45,X^m had been in special education settings in comparison to only 16% of the subjects with 45,X^p. Autistic disorder in TS occurs in association with the 45,X^m phenotype more frequently than would be expected in the general population (424). Severe social problems, significant obsessive features, aggression, impulsivity, and attention problems have been reported in patients with small ring X chromosomes (425).

Psychiatric and Behavioral Aspects

The social difficulties of girls with TS require sensitive handling. As children, they are at risk for being teased and marginalized by peers because of their unusual appearance, short stature, and poor motor skills (381, 426, 427). They have few friends and are often socially isolated (427). Their impaired social skills, which arise in part because of difficulties processing emotional signals, may also result from their decreased emotional arousal and restricted emotional facial expressions, and need to be addressed in their management (428–430). Not surprisingly, girls with TS have serious deficits in self-esteem (369, 427, 431, 432).

Inattention, hyperactivity, and impulsivity are often severe enough to meet formal criteria for ADHD, and impair academic performance and social interactions. When compared to their sisters who do not have TS, affected girls had higher ratings of social, attention or thought problems on the Child Behavior Checklist (126). Anxiety has been reported but is not consistently found (428, 433).

Neuroimaging Studies

Total brain volume of individuals with TS does not differ from that of controls (434). However, as might be predicted from the neurocognitive profile, neuroimaging studies demonstrate abnormal structure and function in areas subserving visuospatial and executive functions. The structural anomalies in the TS brain are prominently in the occipito-parieto-temporal regions. These include regional decreases in tissue volumes in the parietal areas, particularly the superior parietal and postcentral gyri (435), as well as occipital white matter (with some imprinting effects) (436), and reduced size of the genu of the corpus callosum (408). Anomalies of the right intraparietal sulcus have been reported (407). Reiss noted increased proportions of white and gray matter in the right posterior area (434). White matter pathways in the temporal lobe, the gray-white interface of superior temporal sulcus, and the inferior interparietal region are disrupted (406–408). Full-Scale IQ scores showed a significant positive correlation with postcentral tissue volume (435).

Anomalous structural and functional features of the superior temporal gyrus, which plays a crucial role in the processing of social-emotional signals, have been noted. Gray matter volumes in this area are larger than observed in controls (an effect particularly obvious in the 45,X^m suggesting that neuronal pruning is differentially regulated in some way) (437). In a sample limited to 7- to 12-year-old girls with XO monosomy, (not on estrogen replacement, thus, eliminating issues of age or hormonal effect), an increase in temporal lobe gray matter was noted (394). Magnetic resonance spectroscopy findings were also consistent with a possible failure of normal neuronal pruning, which may also be reflected in the disturbed gyrification and sulcation that is prominent in the superior temporal sulci (407). The size of temporal gyri was correlated negatively with performance on auditory rhyme and semantic fluency (394).

The amygdala, a structure implicated in the recognition of fearful facial expression (438) is significantly larger in TS females than normal XX females and interestingly, even larger than in 46, XY males (417). It is a sexually dimorphic structure: normal 46,XY males have significantly increased amygdala volumes in comparison to normal 46,XX females, so that the finding of the larger amygdala in TS females is a distinct anomaly. The amygdala is tightly interconnected with orbitofrontal cortex and forms one of the functional neural units involved in emotion-processing. The finding that the orbitofrontal cortex is larger in TS females than in normal XX females or XY males provides a possible explanation for the deficits that TS women manifest in the processing of facial emotional displays, particularly in the recognition of fearful emotional expressions. Good et al. suggest that the amygdala and orbitofrontal cortex constitute a functional unit which is specifically affected in TS.

Although hormonal factors are a possible explanation, Good et al. did not note any clear relationship between ovarian function and neuroimaging or neuropsychological findings. Enlargement of the left amygdala was also noted in a study involving younger subjects suggesting that rather than any hormonal effects, it is X-linked genes gene dosage effects that influence amygdala development (439).

Decreased hippocampal gray matter volume is associated with memory deficits on neuropsychological testing in TS (434, 436, 439, 440). Smaller volumes of the caudate, lenticular, and thalamic nuclei were noted in women with TS (441). Some studies have noted abnormalities in the cerebellum and brainstem, but the findings are inconsistent and may be explained by different technical methods (406, 408, 436, 442–445).

Functional neuroimaging studies have demonstrated that women with TS not only fail to activate the cortical areas employed by normally developing individuals during the performance of certain specific cognitive tasks, but also fail to employ frontal resources when required to deal with increased task difficulty (406, 407, 444, 445). For example, subjects with TS activated the same frontal-parietal network as normal controls when performing simple computational tasks, but decreased activation in these areas when they were required to perform exact calculation of large numbers, (406, 444). They performed more poorly than controls on both the easy and hard versions (1-back and 2-back) of a visuospatial working memory task, and, unlike controls increased activation bilaterally in the supramarginal gyrus during the 1-back task, and during the 2-back task decreased supramarginal gyrus activation as well as dorsolateral prefrontal cortex, and caudate (446). Thus, cognitive function in TS appears to result from dysfunction of posterior association cortices, possibly as the result disturbance of neuronal pruning as well dysfunctional connectivity as a result of disruption of the underlying white matter pathways.

Management

The array of cognitive and executive function deficits presents a formidable challenge for the treating psychiatrist. The problems surrounding social competence and sexuality in combination with numerous medical disorders make the girls and women with TS particular vulnerable to emotional problems. The medical problems associated with TS continue throughout the life span. Parents of young children need guidance in understanding the cognitive and psychosocial implications of the diagnosis and making reasonable choices with regard to growth hormone and estrogen replacement. The psychiatrist will play an important role in helping the girl with TS who is approaching puberty understand the implications of ovarian dysfunction and the absence of pubertal development and child-bearing potential as well as working through the risks and benefits of estrogen replacement therapy. In addition, assisting the girl with TS in dealing with the difficulty in reading social cues and developing effective coping strategies is beneficial.

Prader-Willi Syndrome

Epidemiology

The prevalence of PWS has been estimated as falling between 1 per 10,000 and 1 per 52,000 (447–450). There is no specific racial preponderance. Boys and girls are equally affected, except for one particular genetic subtype, uniparental disomy, in which there is a male predominance (451).

Physical and Behavioral Phenoytypic Features

Persons with PWS are typically short, obese, with small hands and feet, delicately, tapering fingers, a narrow bifrontal diameter, full cheeks and almond-shaped eyes. About 75% of patients are hypopigmented relative to other members of the family (452–454). Ocular hypopigmentation has been found in about half of patients with PWS and is often associated with strabismus and nystagmus (455). The physical and behavioral features of PWS change with maturation. Even before they are born, mothers report diminished fetal activity (456). Newborns are small, profoundly hypotonic, have hypoactive reflexes, severe feeding problems, failure to thrive, and may have apnea. During the first year of life, the feeding problems resolve. Initially pleasant and rather docile in the second to third years of life, the PWS child develops rampant food-seeking behaviors which leads to gross obesity around 6 years of age (457, 458). Anger, aggression, and obsessive-compulsive behaviors also emerge during the preschool years.

Thus, when making a diagnosis of PWS, the child's age must be taken into consideration. The following criteria for genetic testing, DNA methylation analysis, which take the age-related shift in the phenotypic profile into account were proposed by Gunay-Aygun in 2001 (459). In the birth to 2-year old age range children presenting with hypotonia and poor suck in the neonatal period should be tested. Similarly, in the 2- to 6-year range a child with this neonatal history, hypotonia, and global developmental delay should undergo testing. Those in the 6- to 12-year range with this neonatal and developmental history, coupled with excessive eating with central obesity are candidates. Adolescents and adults with this history, mild mental retardation, excessive eating with central obesity, hypothalamic hypogonadism, and/or the typical PWS obsessive-compulsive behaviors and temper outbursts should be screened (459). The parent-specific DNA methylation imprint is present in the PW critical region in over 99% of patients with PWS. Once the diagnosis is confirmed by methylation analysis, the specific type of mutation is identified.

Genetic Features

The PW critical region is on chromosome 15q11–q13 encompasses 4 million base pairs containing 50 to 100 genes/transcripts, some of which are highly relevant to the neuropsychiatric features. There are several different genetic subtypes of PWS. The most common (70% of cases) involves an interstitial deletion (absence of the paternal genes), 25% have maternal disomy (that is, two copies of the maternal gene, and none from the father), and 2 to 3% have a mutation of the imprinting center or other anomalies of the imprinting process. There is evidence that suggests that maternal disomy results from the "correction" of a trisomy 15 state.

There are some differences in the somatic and cognitive/behavioral phenotypes depending on the particular genetic subtype. The typical phenotype is seen in children with paternal deletions. Individuals with mosaic trisomy 15 have the most severe phenotype, whereas those with maternal uniparental disomy have a milder phenotype (460). The oculocutaneous albinism II (OCA2) gene (formerly the P gene) is located at 15q 11.2–12 and is deleted in most patients with paternal deletions. These children are hypopigmented relative to other members of their families. Less than half of those with uniparental disomy are hypopigmented (451, 452, 454). Highly relevant to the psychiatric manifestations of PWS is the fact that the genes encoding the alpha (5), beta (3), and gamma (3) subunits of the gamma-aminobutyric acid type-A (GABA(A)) receptor lie within the PWS critical region (461–465). There are rare cases of patients with the PWS phenotype who on genetic testing have a chromosome 15 deletion and imprinting defect typical of Angelman's syndrome (a genetic disorder which involves the same region of 15q as PWS but disomic individuals have two copies of the maternal chromosome) (466).

A number of genes which regulate various aspects of brain development have been mapped to the PW critical region (in the mouse orthologous genes are located on mouse chromosome 7C). Although a number of genes have been identified in this region the molecular features of PWS have not as yet been fully identified. One of the genes is the small nuclear ribonucleoprotein particles (snRPN) gene, which is maternally imprinted. Mutations of this gene might affect RNA-splicing (467). Magel2 is specifically expressed in developing hypothalamus. Other genes, such as the highly conserved genes NIPA 1 and NIPA 2, which may function as transporters or receptors, have also been identified. The precise role of these genes has yet to be identified. Loss of expression of small nucleolar RNAs, involved in various aspects of RNA-processing, has been suggested to be an important factor in the PWS phenotype (468).

Neurocognitive Profile

Individuals with PWS have intelligence quotients ranging from average to severe mental retardation. In a population-based study the IQ distribution was normal, but shifted downward by about 40 points (469). Typically there are relative strengths in visuospatial ability and relative weakness in the verbal sphere, although not all persons follow this pattern (470, 471). PWS children may perform as well as peers of normal intelligence on word searches and outperform them on puzzles (472).

Speech and language deficits are prominent. In the preschool child, oral motor and articulation difficulties are primarily affected (473–475). Kleppe et al. reported that in their sample of children with PWS, 88.9% fell below the 6th percentile on tests of receptive language (474). This may be related to the behavioral problems that are characteristic of PWS children, as receptive language delays contribute to oppositional, angry, aggressive outbursts and academic frustration (469, 476). Developmental language disorder also contributes to impaired reading comprehension. It is thus of interest that Burd and Kerbeshian described such a hyperlexic adult with PWS with an IQ of 75 who was able to read fluently but with poor comprehension (477). It is common, however, for the academic performance of children with PWS to fall considerably below the level of their measured intelligence. Whittington et al. attributed it to placement in restrictive educational environments because of behavior problems (469).

Cognitive and behavioral profiles appear to be related primarily to the particular genetic subtype (478). Subjects with uniparental disomy had better verbal abilities but impaired coding ability, compared to the deletion group. Some subjects in the deletion group had strong visuospatial skills. Cassidy compared 37 individuals with paternal deletion to 17 individuals with uniparental disomy and noted that the group with uniparental disomy had less skill with jigsaw puzzles, and had a more normal pain threshold and less skin picking (453). Butler et al. (479) examined PWS subjects with large deletions (500 kb or more), those with smaller deletions, and those with uniparental disomy. Large deletions were associated with lower adaptive behavior scores, and more academic difficulty compared to the smaller deletions. Those with the large deletions also manifested more OCD behaviors than subjects with disomy 15. Butler et al. noted that four recently identified genes are deleted in the large not the small deletion and that these genes are implicated in OCD behaviors. Somewhat different conclusions were reached by another group, who conducted a telephone survey using the Autism Screening Questionnaire (ASQ) and the Vineland Adaptive Behavior Scales. These investigators found that subjects with maternal uniparental disomy manifested more autistic symptomatology (480).

Psychiatric and Behavioral Aspects

The toddler with PWS is often friendly, charming, well-intentioned and generous. However, during the preschool years, there is a dramatic change in behavior. The child develops incessant food-seeking behavior, aggressive rages and tantrums, becomes stubborn and perseverative, and has repetitive skin-picking, and obsessive-compulsive behaviors. Children with PWS tend to be rigid and inflexible in their thinking. These behaviors reach a peak in adolescence and

young adulthood, and start to decline in intensity around age 30 years (481–484). A variety of psychiatric disorders have been described in patients with PWS—obsessive-compulsive disorders, conduct disorder, depression, bipolar disorder, ADHD, psychosis, and self-injurious behavior.

Obsessive-compulsive symptoms are prominent in patients with PWS and include hoarding, ordering and arranging, repetitive concerns, and symmetry (485, 486). Anger and irritability are extremely common, occurring in 84.8% of subjects with PWS. Nearly half (42.1%) meet DSM-III-R criteria for conduct disorder in childhood (486).

Depression is also noted in some patients with PWS. In one study 16.4% had a history of depressed mood for more than 2 weeks (486). More boys than girls appeared to be affected (481). Attempted suicide was reported in 4.9% (486). ADHD is seen in pre-adolescents (487). Anxiety disorder or panic attacks/panic disorder occur rarely (in less than 10% of subjects with PWS) (486).

Psychosis has also been described in patients with PWS. In a longterm study, 6 of 59 patients with PWS experienced a psychotic episode during adolescence (488). The presenting features included agitation of sudden onset, abnormal beliefs, and auditory hallucinations and severe affective disorder (488–492). Virtually all of these cases of psychosis occurred in patients with maternal uniparental disomy and were not associated with paternal deletions.

Self-injurious behavior (repetitive skin-picking and hair pulling) is a common problem and a source of constant stress for parents (80, 493, 494). The sores heal very slowly and sometimes not at all because of repetitive injury. Rectal digging is a variant of this behavior and has been misdiagnosed as inflammatory bowel disease (495). It has been suggested that picking behaviors may be an attempt to increase sensory input, or may represent a behavior in the OCD spectrum (486, 496–498).

Gamma amino butyric acid (GABA) is a widely distributed inhibitory neurotransmitter which plays an important role in neuropsychiatric function. GABA(A) receptors are ligand-operated chloride channels assembled from five subunits, which mediate fast inhibitory neurotransmission (499). The physiological and pharmacological properties of these receptors are related to the particular combination of receptors. This permits flexibility in signal transduction and allosteric modulation, enabling neuronal networks to detect pre- and postsynaptic signals, and select and stabilize response patterns. This changing pattern of sensitivity in receptors enables the synapse to respond differentially to the same type of stimulus and thus permits remarkable response modulation (500, 501). Different brain regions are associated with specific GABA(A) receptor subunit configurations, suggesting that there are functional differences depending on the combination of receptor subunits in that region (499, 502).

There is a remarkable structural heterogeneity in the GABA (A) receptor family. Twenty-one GABA(A) receptor subunits have been identified at this point, distributed among 8 different subunit "families." (502–506). Genes encoding the alpha (5), beta (3) and gamma (3) subunits of the gamma-aminobutyric acid type-A, GABA (A), receptor have been mapped to the PWS critical region. Given the crucial role of GABA (A) in receptors in brain development and neuronal signaling, one would expect that the absence of these subunits of the GABA (A) receptor would have a profound effect on neuronal connectivity, cognition, and behavior. These subunit types are concentrated in the neostriatum, lateral geniculate nucleus, amygdala, hypothalamus, and hippocampus in a rat brain— all regions shown to be involved in the regulation of social behaviors, mood, autonomic regulation, memory, and motor behaviors (499, 507–510).

Although GABA is viewed as an inhibitory neurotransmitter in the adult brain, it is expressed in the fetal brain and plays a crucial role in brain development (511–514). During the early phases of fetal brain development, GABA (A) receptor subunits regulate cell proliferation in neocortex (515, 516) and hippocampus (517). As brain development progresses, they play a role in the regulation of neuronal migration (518), as well as synaptogenesis (519–521). Thus, GABA (A) is an important regulator of neuronal plasticity (522).

In the adult brain, the finely-tuned GABAergic activity in hippocampal inhibitory interneurons contributes to synaptic plasticity and thus to learning and memory (523, 524). The GABA (A5) subunit is expressed abundantly in the hippocampus and only minimally in other areas of the brain. A number of studies have demonstrated that in the GABA (A5) knock-out mouse in which GABA (A5) activity is decreased, performance on hippocampus-dependent learning tasks, particularly those involving visuospatial memory, is enhanced (525, 526). Similarly, when the alpha 5 subunit binds inverse agonists (that is, agents which shifts the equilibrium of the receptor toward its inactive state), enhanced memory is observed with improved spatial learning (527, 528).

What are the observed effects of the deletion of these GABA (A) receptors in PWS? Plasma GABA levels are much higher than normal in individuals with PWS and Angelman's syndromes (in which the same area is deleted) but not in obese or mentally retarded control subjects, possibly because of increased release of presynaptic GABA as a compensation for the decrease in GABA-A receptor units (529). However, since not all GABA receptor types map to the region of the deletion, the remaining GABA receptors are exposed to much higher neurotransmitter levels than is normal. Given the important role that GABA (A) plays in early brain development, neuronal connectivity and neuronal transmission may be affected. Certainly, many of the behaviors seen in PWS—aggression, arousal, impaired motor function, decreased response to pain, and impaired satiety mechanisms—could be attributed to this sequence of problems. Moreover, given the role of GABAergic interneurons in binding and synchronizing the neuronal activity of various cortical networks and, on a cognitive level,

conscious experience, GABA has been postulated to play a role in the development of psychosis (530–532).

Overeating and food-seeking behaviors in patients with PWS result in severe obesity and all the secondary medical problems that are associated with obesity (including cardiovascular disease, obstructive sleep apnea, diabetes, and degenerative joint changes). The behavioral problems associated with food-seeking pose formidable challenges for parents in their day-to-day management of these children. Behavioral problems are positively correlated with body mass index (482, 483). There is little question that persons with PWS can ingest enormous quantities of food when left to their own devices. In one study, subjects with PWS ate steadily for an hour and consumed more than three times as much food as did normal controls (1,292 vs. 369 calories) (533). Satiety was reached only when subjects became markedly hyperglycemic (534). Moreover, individuals with PWS, even underweight infants, have proportionately more body fat than controls, as measured by skin fold thickness (535). Abnormal fat metabolism is, in part, related to growth hormone deficiency (536). Although it appears likely that the overeating is related to hypothalamic dysfunction, the precise pathophysiological mechanism has yet to be identified. An fMRI study demonstrated that hypothalamic activation in PWS subjects in response to a glucose load occurred only after a 24-minute delay, in contrast to healthy lean subjects who showed this activation in 10 minutes, and obese subjects in 15 minutes. The activation of other areas (prefrontal cortex, insula, ventral basal ganglia) which regulate hunger and satiety was also delayed (537). Considerable attention has been focused on ghrelin, a peptide expressed in the stomach and hypothalamus that stimulates both growth hormone and prolactin secretion. In normal individuals, increased plasma ghrelin concentrations are associated with increased subjective ratings of hunger. Individuals with PWS have markedly elevated ghrelin levels compared to other obese patients (538–540). However, two short-duration studies failed to demonstrate that lowering ghrelin levels effectively inhibited food-seeking behavior (540, 541).

Other evidence of hypothalamic dysfunction is suggested by extremely high fevers in young infants with PWS, deficient growth hormone production (542), decreased size of the adrenal glands (543), and decreased bone mass density probably as a result of high bone turnover and in males appeared to be related to lower levels of sex steroids (544). The posterior hypothalamus is involved in the regulation of wakefulness and REM sleep (545–547), and dysfunction in this area may underlie the sleep disturbance frequently noted in PWS.

Management

Treatment of persons with PWS requires broad behavioral, medical and neuropsychiatric approaches. Interventions should include control of weight including restriction to foods in all environments (548), management of sleep apnea, if present, exercise (549, 550), hormone replacement, and psychopharmacological treatment of self-injurious behaviors, and psychiatric issues.

Receptive language impairment can have a negative impact on social interaction. Taking time to understand what the individual understands in a given conversation is essential. Furthermore, the use of visually-based communication (for example, gestures and visual cues), the more effective, successful, and helps the person with PWS with a greater sense of being understood and self-control.

Limiting access to food in all environments, as well as exposure to food-related stimuli (e.g., viewing pictures of food, working in food preparation, having access to leftovers and garbage) is the foundation of effective weight management. Foods should be prepared by others in limited portions, and in most households it is necessary to lock cupboards and the refrigerator. Limiting access to food is much more effective than any other approach. (533, 551, 552). Hormonal replacement with growth hormone improves growth, body composition (decrease in fat mass and increase in lean body mass), physical strength (including respiratory muscles), agility, bone density and fat utilization in children with PWS, as well as improvement in depressive symptoms and behavior (487, 553–556), although there are also reports of adverse events associated with growth hormone therapy (487, 553).

Velocardiofacial Syndrome

Epidemiology
Velocardiofacial syndrome (VCFS), originally described by Shprintzen, is a genetic syndrome found once in every 2,000–4,000 live births (557, 558, 559).

Physical Features
The VCFS phenotype is extremely variable. Some affected children have major cardiac defects and thymus aplasia, so severe as to be fatal, whereas others may have only subtle craniofacial dysmorphic features. Patients are often of short stature. There is a typical facial appearance—narrow palpebral fissures, prominent tubular nose, narrow alae nasi, low-set, dysplastic ears, and retrognathia. Cardiovascular malformations include anomalies of the aortic arch, pulmonary arteries, defects of the infundibular septum, and malformations of the semilunar valves (560). These congenital heart defects require surgical repair in early childhood (561). Renal anomalies may also occur (561). Cleft palate and velopalatal insufficiency result in feeding problems in infancy, and speech and articulation problems later in childhood (562–564). Absent or hypoplastic adenoids and laryngotracheal anomalies and laryngeal stenosis also contribute to communication problems (561). Congenital ear anomalies result in middle ear infection in almost 50% of children with VCFS, with a secondary conductive hearing loss. About 11% of individuals with VCFS also have a sensorineural hearing loss (562). Hypocalcemia or immune disturbances may occur (561). Although VCFS is associated with a high rate of birth defects and dysmorphic features, one third of individuals with VCFS do not have such anomalies (565). Thus, the absence of these congenital anomalies is not a reason for not performing genetic testing (565–567).

Genetic Aspects
VCFS results from a microdeletion at 22q11.2. Most deletions are de novo, sporadic deletions. There is considerable phenotypic overlap between VCFS, DiGeorge syndrome, and conotruncal anomaly face syndrome, all of which involve deletion of the same region of 22q11.2. In DiGeorge syndrome a developmental anomaly of the derivatives of the 3rd and 4th pharyngeal pouches is associated with the absence or hypoplasia of thymus and parathyroid glands. Conotruncal heart defects include truncus arteriosus, transposition of the great arteries, double outlet of the right ventricle, and tetralogy of Fallot. These three syndromes are sometimes grouped under the acronym CATCH-22 (for Cardiac defects, Abnormal facies, Thymic hypoplasia, Cleft palate, and Hypocalcemia) (568).

The genetic anomaly in VCFS is complex and there are a variety of deletions in the 22q11 region that result in the VCFS phenotype. A large (3 Mb) deletion is found in about 87% of the cases, whereas 8% have a smaller (1.5 Mb) deletion within that region, 4% have other deletions, and a small percentage have unique deletions (569). After examination of patients with more restricted deletions, the critical region has been narrowed to a 250 kb area at the proximal end of the larger deletion (570). In some cases, microduplication of the del(22)(q11.2q11.2) results in a similar phenotype (571).

The 22q11 region is highly susceptible to chromosomal rearrangements, which has been attributed to a set of common chromosomal breakpoints, called low copy repeats (569, 572, 573). Low copy repeats are rich in palindromic AT repetitive sequences, which may result in a hairpin turn of the chromosomal material, facilitating more frequent chromosomal rearrangement (573–575). These exchanges of chromosomal material occur during meiosis I and seem to happen more frequently than in deletions on other chromosomes, suggesting a difference in the meiotic behavior of chromosome 22 (576). This has made it hard to pinpoint the mechanism by which haploinsufficiency results in the VCFS phenotype. Even monozygotic twins do not always have the same phenotypic presentation (577).

A number of genes in the VCFS region are expressed in the brain during early development, although some are not unique to developing brain (578). Genes of the latter type include the goosecoid-like homeobox gene (579, 580), Tbx1, a gene encoding transcription factors involved in developmental processes (578), ubiquitin fusion degradation 1-like (UFD1L) gene (581), and PIK4CA, a member of the phosphatidylinositol 4-kinase family (582).

Some genes in the VCFS deleted region have been implicated in psychiatric disorders (schizophrenia and bipolar disorder), which occur in very high frequency in VCFS. However, controversy remains considerable and none of these genes have been demonstrated to be involved in the psychiatric symptoms in all populations. These include the proline dehydrogenase (PRODH) gene (583), the NoGo (RTNF4) gene, a glycosylphosphatidylinositol-linked protein, which inhibits axonal growth, is involved in myelination, and is also a factor in hippocampal neuronal plasticity during development (584, 585). The claudin gene (CLDN5), is involved in myelinization (586).

An important gene in this area is the catecholamine-O-methyltransferase (COMT) gene that codes for the COMT enzymes, which inactivates catecholamines. There are two polymorphisms, the val and met forms, resulting from a G-to-A transition at codon 158 (thus, a valine-to-methionine substitution). Individuals, who have two copies of the met allele, have a three to fourfold reduction in COMT activity, with a marked increase in catecholamines.

Neurological Features and Neurocognitive Profile

Some patients are microcephalic and have severe cognitive dysfunction. Spina bifida and hydrocephalus have been described in VCFS (587). Unprovoked seizures are more frequent in VCFS than in the general population, and are not explained by any associated medical problems (588). Children with VCFS are hypotonic and delayed in acquiring motor milestones, and have poor coordination (589). IQs range from profound mental retardation to the average range. About half of the patients have an IQ below 70. The typical VCFS patient is mildly mentally retarded—mean IQ of 70, (range 46 to 100) (590).

Language development is often significantly impaired and severe articulation difficulties are prominent. The situation is made more complicated by the global developmental delay often seen in these children, as well as the craniofacial anomalies (cleft palate or nasopharyngeal insufficiency which results in hypernasality and audible nasal air emission). Hearing deficits also contribute to the slow language acquisition of these children. However, a number of studies comparing children with VCFS to other groups with similar birth defects and developmental delays have suggested that the delay in language is not simply the result of these physical anomalies or developmental problems (591–593).

One study examined 27 subjects with VCFS (6 to 19 years of age) matched to a group of children with idiopathic developmental delay, and for certain tasks, typically developing children. The parental origin of the deletion was confirmed in 21 of these subjects. The assessment, which included the *Clinical Evaluation of Language Fundamentals–III*, revealed that Receptive Language scores were significantly lower than Expressive Language scores in the VCFS group. In contrast, the reverse pattern was seen in the developmentally delayed group. The mean full scale IQ was 69.4 (range 40–105) (those with maternally-derived deletions had a mean full-scale IQ of 64.4 ± 23.7; range 46 to 81) whereas those with a deletion of paternal origin had a full-scale IQ score of 76.2 ± 18.56 (range 40–105). The VCFS children in which the deletion was of maternal origin scored significantly lower in receptive language than those whose deletion was paternally derived; a trend in the same direction was also noted in expressive language. These findings are also intriguing because of the possibility that there is an imprinting effect, namely that the parental origin of the deletion affects the phenotype. The authors, noting the lack of congruence with the findings reported by others (594, 595), suggested that their findings might be related to the specific test instruments used, or to the increasing demands for abstract reasoning with age. They suggested that their findings are consistent with the volume reduction noted in cortical language area on morphometric MRIs (596, 597).

Despite the early language deficits and uniformly poor cognitive profile in the young child with VCFS (598), the cognitive profile in older children and adolescents is characterized by low-normal to borderline-range Full-Scale IQ with a Verbal IQ in the range of 80 and a Performance IQ of about 70. The gap between the Verbal Comprehension and Perceptual Organization indices is even greater. In about 90% of individuals with VCFS, reading and spelling achievement scores (high 80s) are higher than arithmetic achievement scores (low 80s) (594). Moss et al. point out that this is an unusual pattern as one usually sees poor academic performance on language-based tasks in children with early language impairment (594).

Gross and fine motor skills are impaired. Visuospatial skills, visual attention, and visual-spatial memory are deficient and affected individuals have difficulty grasping new and complex information (599). Adults with VCFS have a cognitive profile characterized by deficits in visual working memory, visual recognition, attention, certain aspects of social cognition, and frontal executive deficits, a profile resembling that seen in nonverbal learning disability particularly in view of the deficits in social-emotional behaviors (600, 601). Moreover, patients who were hemizygous for COMT-met performed better on executive function tasks (set-shifting, verbal fluency, attention, and working memory tasks) than did those who were hemizygous for the val allele (602).

Psychiatric Aspects

High rates of attention deficit hyperactivity disorder (ADHD), aggression (603), anxiety disorders (specifically obsessive-compulsive disorder and separation anxiety disorder), mood disorder, in particular, bipolar disorder, schizotypal features, and schizophrenia have been noted in persons with VCFS (604).

ADHD (both with and without hyperactivity) has been reported in 35 to 50% of children with VCFS (the higher prevalence occurring in those children whose first degree relatives also had ADHD). There was no apparent relationship to dysmorphic features, perinatal problems, or developmental delay (603). Based on the pattern of errors on the

Attention Network Test, Sobin et al. concluded that the attentional disturbances in the VCFS group are consistent with executive function deficits (605, 606).

Behavioral disorders typically emerge in prodromal form in the preschool years. Several studies involving different populations of youngsters with VCFS have described them as having difficulty with attention/concentration, and atypical thinking (607). They are also withdrawn and retiring (589, 607), and compared to children with learning disabilities, less aggressive (589, 608). However, these internalizing, withdrawn behaviors do not appear to be related to craniofacial abnormalities. Compared to a matched control group of children with craniofacial abnormalities, VCFS children had significantly higher scores on the internalizing scale of the Achenbach Child Behavior Checklist and Teacher Rating Scale, as well as significantly higher scores on the thought problems, attention problems, and social problems scales (609).

Bipolar disorder has been reported to occur more frequently in persons with VCFS. Based on a study involving a structured interview, review of records, and a clinical interview by two research psychiatrists, Papolos et al. concluded that 64% of an unselected series of children and adults with VCFS (age range 5 to 34 years) met DSM-III-R diagnostic criteria for bipolar disorder (610). Moreover, they suggested that homozygosity for the COMT-met allele could predispose to the ultra-ultra or ultradian cycling form of bipolar disorder (611). Mean age of onset was 12 years standard deviation = 3 years. None of the patients in this series met diagnostic criteria for schizophrenia, and only four had psychotic symptoms which emerged in their 20s or 30s. However, approaching the association from the other direction—namely, genotyping patients with bipolar disorder, Lachman et al. were unable to find any association between bipolar disorder and the COMT-met polymorphism (612).

Approximately one third of individuals with VCFS also have Obsessive-Compulsive disorder (OCD). Gothelf noted that 32.6% of their subjects met diagnostic criteria for OCD using the YBOCs (613). The disorder appeared relatively early and responded to fluoxetine. The symptoms included contamination concerns, somatic preoccupations, hoarding, repetitive questions and cleaning. Comorbid ADHD was present in 37.2% of the subjects in this series. Psychosis was present in 16.2%.

Difficulty in the realm of social-emotional functioning is quite prominent in older children and adults with VCFS, ranging from disorders in the autistic spectrum (590) to a cognitive/behavioral phenotype reminiscent of nonverbal learning disorder characterized by delayed motor development, Verbal IQ> Performance IQ, coupled with academic deficits in arithmetic, impaired visuospatial skills, and social withdrawal and anxiety (589). Some, (55%), of children with VCFS fit into this diagnostic category. Language is often more impaired than is typical in most children with nonverbal learning disorder. In one study it was noted that even in persons with VCFS who were of normal intelligence, there

was often a behavioral profile resembling prefrontal dysfunction, characterized by apathy and difficulty with initiation (590).

Individuals with a 22q11 deletion are at particularly high risk for schizophrenia— as many as 25% may develop schizophrenia—a rate substantially higher than that of the general population (0.025%) (614, 615). In fact, only the offspring of two parents with schizophrenia are at higher risk (616). Bassett et al. compared a group of patients with the 22q11.2 deletion to a sample of patients with familial schizophrenia. The groups did not differ in age of onset, positive/negative schizophrenic symptom scores, severity of anxiety-depression or cognitive symptoms. The subjects with VCFS had more problems with impulse control, uncooperativeness, and hostility. These symptoms were not secondary to mania. The conclusion was that the schizophrenic phenotype in VCFS is essentially indistinguishable from other forms of schizophrenia. However, there were significant differences in that 75% of the VCFS group had either congenital cardiac defects and/or palatal defects, whereas none of the comparison subjects had a congenital birth defect. A family history of psychosis was present in only one of the 16 patients with VCFS (6.3%) (a result of the high rate of spontaneous deletion in VCFS) compared to 82.6% in the comparison group (565). Although the *absence* of dysmorphic features cannot be used to eliminate the possibility of a 22q11 deletion (617, 618), the *presence* of dysmorphic features, cardiac abnormalities, or mental retardation would make the diagnosis of VCFS well worth considering. In short, at this point in time, a careful review of developmental, medical and family history in a person with schizophrenia may be helpful in determining whether genetic testing for VCFS is indicated.

A relatively dense genetic map of single nucleotide polymorphisms in the entire 1.5 Mb schizophrenia critical region on 22q11 was extensively studied by Liu et al. (619, 620). They identified two subregions in this area suggesting that the 22q11 microdeletion schizophrenia phenotype might be a contiguous gene syndrome. In the proximal ~ 30 kb segment the only two genes identified at that time were PRODH2 and DGCR6 and this region appeared to be associated more closely with childhood and early onset schizophrenia. In the distal subregion, measuring 80 kb, a number of genes were identified and appear to contribute to schizophrenia independently of the timing of onset. In addition, numerous other genes have been suggested as possibly involved in schizophrenia, but none have as yet been consistently shown to be related.

Neuroimaging studies
An overall reduction in total cerebral volume in patients with VCFS has been reported (621, 622). This is not surprising, given the prevalence of microcephaly in the VCFS population. In the study by Èliez et al. there was even greater (9%) reduction in volume when the deletion was on the paternal chromosome (621). In adults with both

with both schizophrenia and VCFS the reduction in total cerebral volume is quite striking. A significant reduction in cerebellar volume (particularly the vermis) compared to controls has been noted in most studies (621–624). Eliez also noted a reduction in the size of the pons and in vermal lobules VI–VII (621). Lynch reported an adult with VCFS with evidence of cerebellar atrophy of unknown origin (625). Decreases in frontal and temporal lobe volumes have also been noted, although this does not reach statistical significance when corrected for multiple comparisons (626).

A spectrum of neuromigrational abnormalities has been described in VCFS ranging from lissencephaly to abnormal gyrification (627, 628). Regional anomalies, such as widening of the sylvian fissure have been reported (629). Midline abnormalities such as cavum septum pellucidum are more frequent in persons with VCFS than in controls (622, 623, 626, 630). Anomalies of the septum pellucidum have been reported in subjects with VCFS with and without schizophrenia. However, anomalies of the septum pellucidum are found in subjects with schizophrenia without the 22q11 deletion, particularly in schizophrenia of childhood onset (631, 632) and may reflect the close embryological and functional relationship of the septum pellucidum to limbic structures (633). (In individuals with schizophrenia, an enlarged cavum septum pellucidum has been associated with reduced volumes of the parahippocampal gyrus) (634). The finding of other midline anomalies in the VCFS population suggests that there may be a specific disturbance in the formation of midline structures (635).

A number of studies have reported decreased white matter volumes, particularly in the frontal area, and particularly in those with schizophrenia and the VCFS deletion.

White matter hyperintensities and cysts in the vicinity of the frontal horns have been noted (624, 626). Van Amelsvoort compared patients with VCFS without schizophrenia to those with schizophrenia and to a group of IQ-matched controls who did not meet criteria for psychiatric disorders or conditions that might affect the brain. The group with schizophrenia and VCFS had a significant generalized reduction in total brain volume and total white matter (626). A diffusion tensor imaging study revealed disruption of white matter connectivity in fronto-temporal-parietal pathways (636). Deep frontal white matter was reduced significantly (by about 23%) in VCFS subjects compared to controls (637). Kates et al. noted that it was not clear if this was related to a disturbance in myelination or simply reflected delayed myelination.

The reduced volumes in the frontal area have been associated with increased volumes of the caudate nucleus (left > right) (638). Kates et al. reported increased volume of the right caudate nucleus in the VCFS group (637). In that study, the VCFS group did not show the association between the right caudate and right frontal region which was present in the controls, providing anatomical support for the frontostrial dysfunction that is clinically noted in the VCFS population.

Shashi et al. noted that total area of the corpus callosum was significantly increased in the group with VCFS, in particular the isthmus (which includes interhemispheric fibers from posterior parietal and superior temporal cortex) (639). In the NIMH study of very early onset schizophrenia, increased ventricular volume and increased midbody area of the corpus callosum was noted in the subjects with VCFS when compared to persons with non-VCFS childhood-onset schizophrenia and healthy controls (640).

Relatively few functional imaging studies have been performed on patients with VCFS. Eliez et al. studied children with VCFS and controls as they performed a mathematical computation task and noted increased activation of the left supramarginal gyrus in children with VCFS compared to controls which correlated with increased task difficulty (621, 641).

Management

Children with VCFS pose a challenge to the neurologists and psychiatrists who are caring for them. In early childhood, children with VCFS often require multiple surgical procedures for congenital heart lesions and/or palatal defects. In addition to the emotional problems often experienced by children who have been subjected to multiple surgical procedures and hospitalizations at an early age, they also have multiple neurodevelopmental problems. Thus, early identification and treatment of any hearing and speech problems, as well as language impairment requires sophisticated evaluations. Proactively identifying and helping the child, the child's parents and teachers to work with the social-emotional problems that are typically associated with VCFS is extremely helpful. Being aware of the significant psychiatric morbidity that this diagnosis is associated with can hopefully mitigate some of these problems.

Children with VCFS are likely to be functioning below the average range and supporting the parents and assisting in finding appropriate educational settings will be highly beneficial. Children with VCFS often have strong aptitudes for music and computers. Educational interventions which use music and computers often meet with greater success in reading and math and socially with improvements noted in self-esteem, motivation, and confidence (642, 643). Success is also facilitated when information is presented in small increments that can be successfully mastered.

Clinicians should be aware of the increased risk of bipolar disorder, schizophrenia, and obsessive-compulsive disorder in this population. There are several genes which map to the VCFS critical region which potentially play a role in bipolar disorder. One of these genes, PIC4CA, is involved in the synthesis of phosphatidylinositol 4,5-bisphosphate, a phosphoinositide that regulates signal transduction and synaptic vesicle function. Some patients with bipolar disorder show an atypical response to lithium, which is a noncompetitive inhibitor in this metabolic pathway. There is a suggestion that this gene may be involved in bipolar disorder and schizophrenia (582).

Patients with VCFS who have the COMT-met polymorphism (with reduced levels of COMT and high levels of catecholamines) may be at high risk for mania, particularly if treated with psychostimulants. In the case of psychiatric symptoms that are refractory to more standard psychological treatment, the possibility that the deletion of the COMT gene results in high levels of circulating catecholamines should be considered. The use of alpha-methyl-tyrosine, a competitive inhibitor of tyrosine hydroxylase, which lowers the concentration of homovanillic acid, and in turn decreases endogenous levels of catecholamines, has been reported to improve function and have minimal side effects (644). O'Hanlon described a case in which seizures and hallucinations were controlled with improved cognitive function (645). Selective serotonin reuptake inhibitors for OCD have been useful in this population (613). Given the possibility that COMT levels are decreased, and therefore the inactivation of catecholamines is compromised, concern has been expressed regarding the use of psychostimulants, the fear being possibly precipitating or exacerbating mood disorder or psychotic symptoms. One small-n, 4-week study reported that treatment with low-dose (0.3mg/kg) methylphenidate resulted in significant behavioral improvement in patients with VCFS, without any evidence of increased cognitive dysfunction and only mild side effects (646). However, given the fact that the dose level was relatively low, the treatment of short duration, and the COMT genotype of the subjects unknown, the results of this study should be taken with caution. Gothelf et al. have suggested that some patients with VCFS and schizophrenia respond poorly to standard neuroleptics (although two of the four responded to clozapine) (567).

Conclusion

In this chapter we have reviewed the neuropsychiatric features of some of the common mental retardation syndromes, and the importance of making a diagnosis not only on the basis of IQ but also in terms of adaptive functioning. Given the variability in neuropsychiatric presentation in mental retardation syndromes as well as the variability in individuals who carry the same diagnosis, it is important to be aware of the characteristic neuropsychiatric features associated with these syndromes while at the same time having a diagnostic approach that is sensitive to this variability. Although the relationships between the genetic factors and neurobehavioral profile are still incompletely delineated, there is a burgeoning research literature that will make it possible to understand more clearly the pathophysiology of these syndromes and ultimately provide a rational approach to management. At this point, neuropsychiatric diagnosis and management should include a detailed history and examination that takes into account the medical and neuropsychiatric features associated with these syndromes

but is flexible enough to evaluate the psychosocial and medical issues of each patient on an individual basis.

REFERENCES

1. American Psychiatric Association. *Diagnostic and Statistical Manual of Mental Disorders*, 4th Ed. Washington, D.C.: American Psychiatric Association, 1994.
2. American Psychiatric Association. *Statistical Manual of Mental Disorders*, 3rd Ed., *revised.* Washington, D.C.: American Psychiatric Association, 1987.
3. American Association on Mental Retardation. *Mental Retardation: Definition, Classification and Systems of Support.* Washington, D.C.: American Association on Mental Retardation, 1992.
4. World Health Organization. *The ICD-10 Classification of Mental and Behavioural Disorders: Clinical Descriptions and Diagnostic Guidelines.* Geneva: World Health Organization, 1992.
5. Sparrow, SS, Balla DA, Cichetti DV. *Vineland Adaptive Behavior Scales.* Circle Pines MN: American Guidance Service, 1984.
6. Lambert, N, Nihira K, Leland H. *AAMR Adaptive BehaviorScales—School.* Austin, TX: Pro-Ed, 1993.
7. Nihira, K, Foster R, Shellaus M, et al. *Manual for Aamd Adaptive Behavior Scale.* Austin, TX: Pro-Ed, 1974.
8. Nihira, K, Leland H, Lambert N. *AAMR Adaptive Behavior Scales—Residential and Community.* Austin, TX: Pro-Ed, 1993.
9. Silverstein, AB. Nonstandard standard scores on the vineland adaptive behavior scales: A cautionary note. Am J Ment Defic 1986;91:1–4.
10. Baroff, GS. *Developmental Disabilities: Psychological Aspects.* Austin, Tx: Pro-Ed, 1991.
11. McLaren, J, Bryson SE. Review of recent epidemiological studies in mental retardation: Prevalence, associated disorders, and etiology. Am J Ment Retard 1987;92:243–254.
12. Reiss, S. Prevalence of dual diagnosis in community-based day programs in the Chicago metropolitan area. Am J Ment Retard 1990;94:578–585.
13. Reiss, S, Szyszko J. Diagnostic overshadowing and professional experience with mentally retarded persons. Am J Ment Defic 1983;87:396–402.
14. Reiss, S, Levitan GW, Szyszko J. Emotional disturbance and mental retardation: Diagnostic overshadowing. Am J Ment Defic 1982;86:567–574.
15. Weisz, JR. Effects of the "mentally retarded" label on adult judgments about child failure. J Abnorm Psychol 1981;90:371–374.
16. Reiss, S. Psychopathology in mental retardation. In Bouras, N, ed. *Mental Health in Mental Retardation: Recent Advances and Practices.* Cambridge: Cambridge University Press, 1994:67–78.
17. Butler, MG, Allen GA, Haynes JL, et al. Anthropometric comparison of mentally retarded males with and without the fragile x syndrome. Am J Med Genet 1991;38:260–268.
18. Hagerman, PJ. Clinical features of the fragile x syndrome. In Hagerman, PJ and McBogg, P, eds. *The Fragile X Syndrome: Diagnosis, Biochemistry, and Intervention.* Dillan, CO: Spectra, 1983: 17–53.
19. Partington, MW. The fragile x syndrome II: Preliminary data on growth and development in males. Am J Med Genet 1984;17: 175–194.
20. Lachiewicz, AM, Dawson DV, Spiridigliozzi GA. Physical characteristics of young boys with fragile x syndrome: Reasons for difficulties in making a diagnosis in young males. Am J Med Genet 2000;92:229–236.
21. Lubs, HA. A marker x chromosome. Am J Hum Genet 1969;21: 231–244.
22. Glover, TW. Fudr induction of the x chromosome fragile site: Evidence for the mechanism of folic acid and thymidine inhibition. Am J Hum Genet 1981;33:234–242.
23. Verkerk, AJ, Pieretti M, Sutcliffe JS, et al. Identification of a gene (fmr-1) containing a cgg repeat coincident with a breakpoint cluster region exhibiting length variation in fragile x syndrome. Cell 1991;65:905–914.
24. Yu, S, Pritchard M, Kremer E, et al. Fragile x genotype characterized by an unstable region of DNA. Science 1991;252:1179–1181.

25. Oberle, I, Rousseau F, Heitz D, et al. Instability of a 550-base pair DNA segment and abnormal methylation in fragile x syndrome. Science 1991;252:1097–1102.
26. Devys, D, Lutz Y, Rouyer N, et al. The fmr-1 protein is cytoplasmic, most abundant in neurons and appears normal in carriers of a fragile x premutation. Nat Genet 1993;4:335–340.
27. Abitbol, M, Menini C, Delezoide AL, et al. Nucleus basalis magnocellularis and hippocampus are the major sites of fmr-1 expression in the human fetal brain. Nat Genet 1993;4:147–153.
28. Hinds, HL, Ashley CT, Sutcliffe JS, et al. Tissue specific expression of fmr-1 provides evidence for a functional role in fragile x syndrome. Nat Genet 1993;3:36–43.
29. Tamanini, F, Willemsen R, van Unen L, et al. Differential expression of fmr1, fxr1 and fxr2 proteins in human brain and testis. Hum Mol Genet 1997;6:1315–1322.
30. Weiler, IJ, Irwin SA, Klintsova AY, et al. Fragile x mental retardation protein is translated near synapses in response to neurotransmitter activation. Proc Natl Acad Sci USA 1997;94:5395–5400.
31. Irwin, SA, Galvez R, Greenough WT. Dendritic spine structural anomalies in fragile-x mental retardation syndrome. Cereb Cortex 2000;10:1038–1044.
32. Galvez, R, Gopal AR, Greenough WT. Somatosensory cortical barrel dendritic abnormalities in a mouse model of the fragile x mental retardation syndrome. Brain Res 2003;971:83–89.
33. Hinton, VJ, Brown WT, Wisniewski K, et al. Analysis of neocortex in three males with the fragile x syndrome. Am J Med Genet 1991;41:289–294.
34. Rudelli, RD, Brown WT, Wisniewski K, et al. Adult fragile x syndrome. Clinico-neuropathologic findings. Acta Neuropathol (Berl) 1985;67:289–295.
35. Kogan, CS, Boutet I, Cornish K, et al. Differential impact of the fmr1 gene on visual processing in fragile x syndrome. Brain 2004;127:591–601.
36. Welt, CK, Smith PC, Taylor AE. Evidence of early ovarian aging in fragile x premutation carriers. J Clin Endocrinol Metab 2004;89:4569–4574.
37. Hundscheid, RD, Smits AP, Thomas CM, et al. Female carriers of fragile x premutations have no increased risk for additional diseases other than premature ovarian failure. Am J Med Genet A 2003;117:6–9.
38. Moore, CJ, Daly EM, Tassone F, et al. The effect of pre-mutation of x chromosome cgg trinucleotide repeats on brain anatomy. Brain 2004;127:2672–2681.
39. Jacquemont, S, Hagerman RJ, Leehey MA, et al. Penetrance of the fragile x-associated tremor/ataxia syndrome in a premutation carrier population. JAMA 2004;291:460–469.
40. Rogers, C, Partington MW, Turner GM. Tremor, ataxia and dementia in older men may indicate a carrier of the fragile x syndrome. Clin Genet 2003;64:54–56.
41. Hagerman, RJ, Leavitt BR, Farzin F, et al. Fragile-x-associated tremor/ataxia syndrome (fxtas) in females with the fmr1 premutation. Am J Hum Genet 2004;74:1051–1056.
42. Zuhlke, C, Budnik A, Gehlken U, et al. Fmr1 premutation as a rare cause of late onset ataxia:Evidence for fxtas in female carriers. J Neurol 2004;251:1418–1419.
43. Hagerman, PJ, Greco CM, Hagerman RJ. A cerebellar tremor/ataxia syndrome among fragile x premutation carriers. Cytogenet Genome Res 2003;100:206–212.
44. Hagerman, PJ, Hagerman RJ. Fragile x-associated tremor/ataxia syndrome (fxtas). Ment Retard Dev Disabil Res Rev 2004;10:25–30.
45. Bregman, JD, Leckman JF, Ort SI. Thyroid function in fragile-x syndrome males. Yale J Biol Med 1990;63:293–299.
46. Lauterborn, JC. Stress induced changes in cortical and hypothalamic c-fos expression are altered in fragile x mutant mice. Brain Res Mol Brain Res 2004;131:101–109.
47. Loesch, DZ, Bui QM, Grigsby J, et al. Effect of the fragile x status categories and the fragile x mental retardation protein levels on executive functioning in males and females with fragile x. Neuropsychology 2003;17:646–657.
48. Fisch, GS, Simensen R, Arinami T, et al. Longitudinal changes in iq among fragile x females: A preliminary multicenter analysis. Am J Med Genet 1994;51:353–357.
49. Fisch, GS, Carpenter N, Holden JJ, et al. Longitudinal changes in cognitive and adaptive behavior in fragile x females: A prospective multicenter analysis. Am J Med Genet 1999;83:308–312.
50. Fisch, GS, Carpenter NJ, Holden JJ, et al. Longitudinal assessment of adaptive and maladaptive behaviors in fragile x males: Growth, development, and profiles. Am J Med Genet 1999; 83:257–263.
51. Fisch, GS, Carpenter NJ, Simensen R, et al. Longitudinal changes in cognitive-behavioral levels in three children with fraxe. Am J Med Genet 1999;84:291–292.
52. Hodapp, RM, Dykens EM, Hagerman RJ, et al. Developmental implications of changing trajectories of iq in males with fragile x syndrome. J Am Acad Child Adolesc Psychiatry 1990;29:214–219.
53. Hodapp, RM, Dykens EM, Ort SI, et al. Changing patterns of intellectual strengths and weaknesses in males with fragile x syndrome. J Autism Dev Disord 1991;21:503–516.
54. Lachiewicz, AM, Gullion CM, Spiridigliozzi GA, et al. Declining iqs of young males with the fragile x syndrome. Am J Ment Retard 1987;92:272–278.
55. Miezejeski, CM, Jenkins EC, Hill AL, et al. A profile of cognitive deficit in females from fragile x families. Neuropsychologia 1986;24:405–409.
56. Wright-Talamante, C, Cheema A, Riddle JE, et al. A controlled study of longitudinal iq changes in females and males with fragile x syndrome. Am J Med Genet 1996;64:350–355.
57. Opitz, JM, Sutherland GR. Conference report: International workshop on the fragile x and x-linked mental retardation. Am J Med Genet 1984;17:5–94.
58. Hagerman, PJ. Learning disabilities and attentional problems in boys with the fragile x syndrome. Am J Dis Child 1985;139:674–678.
59. Fisch, GS, Carpenter N, Howard-Peebles PN, et al. Lack of association between mutation size and cognitive/behavior deficits in fragile x males: A brief report. Am J Med Genet 1996;64:362–364.
60. Fisch, GS, Simensen RJ, Schroer RJ. Longitudinal changes in cognitive and adaptive behavior scores in children and adolescents with the fragile x mutation or autism. J Autism Dev Disord 2002;32:107–114.
61. Hagerman, RJ, Hull CE, Safanda JF, et al. High functioning fragile x males: Demonstration of an unmethylated fully expanded fmr-1 mutation associated with protein expression. Am J Med Genet 1994;51:298–308.
62. Moore, CJ, Daly EM, Schmitz N, et al. A neuropsychological investigation of male premutation carriers of fragile x syndrome. Neuropsychologia 2004;42:1934–1947.
63. Abrams, MT, Reiss AL, Freund LS, et al. Molecular-neurobehavioral associations in females with the fragile x full mutation. Am J Med Genet 1994;51:317–327.
64. Freund, LS, Reiss AL. Cognitive profiles associated with the fra(x) syndrome in males and females. Am J Med Genet 1991;38:542–547.
65. Hagerman, RJ. Physical and Behavioral Phenotype. In Fragile X Syndrome: Diagnosis, Treatment, and Research. Hagerman, RJ and Cronister, AC, eds. 2nd ed. Baltimore: Johns Hopkins University Press, 1996b:283–331.
66. Loesch, DZ, Hay DA, Sutherland GR, et al. Phenotypic variation in male-transmitted fragile x: Genetic inferences. Am J Med Genet 1987;27:401–17.
67. Kemper, MB, Hagerman RJ, Ahmad RS, et al. Cognitive profiles and the spectrum of clinical manifestations in heterozygous fra (x) females. Am J Med Genet 1986;23:139–156.
68. Schapiro, MB, Murphy DG, Hagerman RJ, et al. Adult fragile x syndrome: Neuropsychology, brain anatomy, and metabolism. Am J Med Genet 1995;60:480–93.
69. Borghgraef, M, Fryns JP, Dielkens A, et al. Fragile (x) syndrome: A study of the psychological profile in 23 prepubertal patients. Clin Genet 1987;32:179–186.
70. Fisch, GS, Holden JJ, Carpenter NJ, et al. Age-related language characteristics of children and adolescents with fragile x syndrome. Am J Med Genet 1999;83:253–256.
71. Mazzocco, MM, Myers GF, Hamner JL, et al. The prevalence of the fmr1 and fmr2 mutations among preschool children with language delay. J Pediatr 1998;132:795–801.

72. Roberts, JE, Mirrett P, Burchinal M. Receptive and expressive communication development of young males with fragile x syndrome. Am J Ment Retard 2001;106:216–230.
73. Hanson, DM, Jackson AW, 3rd, Hagerman RJ. Speech disturbances (cluttering) in mildly impaired males with the martinbell/fragile x syndrome. Am J Med Genet 1986;23:195–206.
74. Howard-Peebles, PN, Stoddard GR, Mims MG. Familial x-linked mental retardation, verbal disability, and marker x chromosomes. Am J Hum Genet 1979;31:214–222.
75. Reiss, AL, Freund L, Vinogradov S, et al. Parental inheritance and psychological disability in fragile x females. Am J Hum Genet 1989;45:697–705.
76. Newell, K, Sanborn B, Hagerman R. Speech and language dysfunction in the fragile x syndrome. In Hagerman, RJ and McBogg, P, eds. *The Fragile X Syndrome: Diagnosis, Biochemistry, and Intervention.* Dillan, Co: Spectra 1983:175–200.
77. Sudhalter, V, Belser RC. Conversational characteristics of children with fragile x syndrome: Tangential language. Am J Ment Retard 2001;106:389–400.
78. Merenstein, SA, Shyu V, Sobesky WE, et al. Fragile x syndrome in a normal iq male with learning and emotional problems. J Am Acad Child Adolesc Psychiatry 1994;33:1316–1321.
79. Dorn, MB, Mazzocco MM, Hagerman RJ. Behavioral and psychiatric disorders in adult male carriers of fragile x. J Am Acad Child Adolesc Psychiatry 1994;33:256–264.
80. Symons, FJ, Clark RD, Hatton DD, et al. Self-injurious behavior in young boys with fragile x syndrome. Am J Med Genet 2003;118A:115–121.
81. Hagerman, RJ, Hills J, Scharfenaker S, et al. Fragile x syndrome and selective mutism. Am J Med Genet 1999;83:313–317.
82. Coupland, NJ. Social phobia: Etiology, neurobiology, and treatment. J Clin Psychiatry 2001;62 Suppl 1:25–35.
83. Hagerman, RJ. Fragile-x chromosome and learning disability. J Am Acad Child Adolesc Psychiatry 1987;26:938.
84. Kerbeshian, J, Burd L, Martsolf JT. Fragile x syndrome associated with tourette symptomatology in a male with moderate mental retardation and autism. J Dev Behav Pediatr 1984;5:201–203.
85. Largo, RH, Schinzel A. Developmental and behavioural disturbances in 13 boys with fragile x syndrome. Eur J Pediatr 1985;143:269–275.
86. Einfeld, S, Tonge B, Turner G. Longitudinal course of behavioral and emotional problems in fragile x syndrome. Am J Med Genet 1999;87:436–439.
87. Fryns, JP. The fragile x syndrome. A study of 83 families. Clin Genet 1984;26:497–528.
88. Fryns, JP. X-linked mental retardation. Prog Clin Biol Res 1985;177:309–319.
89. Mattei, JF, Mattei MG, Aumeras C, et al. X-linked mental retardation with the fragile x. A study of 15 families. Hum Genet 1981;59:281–289.
90. Rogers, SJ, Hepburn S, Wehner E. Parent reports of sensory symptoms in toddlers with autism and those with other developmental disorders. J Autism Dev Disord 2003;33:631–642.
91. Frankland, PW, Wang Y, Rosner B, et al. Sensorimotor gating abnormalities in young males with fragile x syndrome and fmr1-knockout mice. Mol Psychiatry 2004;9:417–425.
92. Cohen, IL, Fisch GS, Sudhalter V, et al. Social gaze, social avoidance, and repetitive behavior in fragile x males: A controlled study. Am J Ment Retard 1988;92:436–446.
93. Cohen, IL, Vietze PM, Sudhalter V, et al. Parent-child dyadic gaze patterns in fragile x males and in non-fragile x males with autistic disorder. J Child Psychol Psychiatry 1989;30:845–856.
94. Cohen, IL, Vietze PM, Sudhalter V, et al. Effects of age and communication level on eye contact in fragile x males and non-fragile x autistic males. Am J Med Genet 1991;38:498–502.
95. Hatton, DD, Hooper SR, Bailey DB, et al. Problem behavior in boys with fragile x syndrome. Am J Med Genet 2002;108:105–116.
96. Hagerman, PJ. An analysis of autism in fifty males with fragile x syndrome. Am J Med Genet 1986;23:195–206.
97. Levitas, A, Hagerman RJ, Braden M, et al. Autism and the fragile x syndrome. J Dev Behav Pediatr 1983;4:151–158.
98. Wolf-Schein, EG, Sudhalter V, Cohen IL, et al. Speech-language and the fragile x syndrome: Initial findings. Asha 1987;29:35–38.
99. Smalley, SL, Asarnow RF, Spence MA. Autism and genetics. A decade of research. Arch Gen Psychiatry 1988;45:953–961.
100. Bailey, DB, Jr., Hatton DD, Skinner M, et al. Autistic behavior, fmr1 protein, and developmental trajectories in young males with fragile x syndrome. J Autism Dev Disord 2001;31:165–174.
101. Philofsky, A, Hepburn SL, Hayes A, et al. Linguistic and cognitive functioning and autism symptoms in young children with fragile x syndrome. Am J Ment Retard 2004;109:208–218.
102. Kau, AS, Tierney E, Bukelis I, et al. Social behavior profile in young males with fragile x syndrome: Characteristics and specificity. Am J Med Genet 2004;126A:9–17.
103. Cohen, IL, Nolin SL, Sudhalter V, et al. Mosaicism for the fmr1 gene influences adaptive skills development in fragile x-affected males. Am J Med Genet 1996;64:365–369.
104. Hatton, DD, Wheeler AC, Skinner ML, et al. Adaptive behavior in children with fragile x syndrome. Am J Ment Retard 2003;108:373–390.
105. Turk, J. The fragile x syndrome: Recent developments. Curr Opin Psy 1992;5:677–682.
106. Reiss, AL, Freund L. Fragile x syndrome, DSM-III-R, and autism. J Am Acad Child Adolesc Psychiatry 1990;29:885–891.
107. Dykens, E, Leckman J, Paul R, et al. Cognitive, behavioral, and adaptive functioning in fragile x and non-fragile x retarded men. J Autism Dev Disord 1988;18:41–52.
108. Bregman, JD, Leckman JF, Ort S. Fragile x syndrome: Genetic predisposition to psychopathology. J Autism Dev Disord 1988;18:343–354.
109. Wolff, PH, Gardner J, Paccla J, et al. The greeting behavior of fragile x males. Am J Ment Retard 1989;93:406–411.
110. Cohen, RM, Semple WE, Gross M, et al. Functional localization of sustained attention: Comparison to sensory stimulation in the absence of instruction. Neuropsychiatry, Neuropsychology, and Behavioral Neurology 1988;1:3–20.
111. Cohen, NJ, Davine M, Meloche-Kelly M. Prevalence of unsuspected language disorders in a child psychiatric population. J Am Acad Child Adolesc Psychiatry 1989;28:107–111.
112. Sudhalter, V, Cohen IL, Silverman W, et al. Conversational analyses of males with fragile x, down syndrome, and autism: Comparison of the emergence of deviant language. Am J Ment Retard 1990;94:431–441.
113. Ferrier, LJ, Bashir AS, Meryash DL, et al. Conversational skills of individuals with fragile-x syndrome: A comparison with autism and down syndrome. Dev Med Child Neurol 1991;33:776–788.
114. Loesch, DZ, Hay DA, Mulley J. Transmitting males and carrier females in fragile x—revisited. Am J Med Genet 1994;51:392–399.
115. Reiss, AL, Hagerman RJ, Vinogradov S, et al. Psychiatric disability in female carriers of the fragile x chromosome. Arch Gen Psychiatry 1988;45:25–30.
116. McConkie-Rosell, A, Lachiewicz AM, Spiridigliozzi GA, et al. Evidence that methylation of the fmr-1 locus is responsible for variable phenotypic expression of the fragile x syndrome. Am J Hum Genet 1993;53:800–809.
117. Franke, P, Leboyer M, Hardt J, et al. Neuropsychological profiles of fmr-1 premutation and full-mutation carrier females. Psychiatry Res 1999;87:223–231.
118. Jakala, P, Hanninen T, Ryynanen M, et al. Fragile-x: Neuropsychological test performance, cgg triplet repeat lengths, and hippocampal volumes. J Clin Invest 1997;100:331–338.
119. Borghgraef, M, Umans S, Steyaert J, et al. New findings in the behavioral profile of young frax females. Am J Med Genet 1996;64:346–349.
120. Mazzocco, MM, Hagerman RJ, Cronister-Silverman A, et al. Specific frontal lobe deficits among women with the fragile x gene. J Am Acad Child Adolesc Psychiatry 1992;31:1141–1148.
121. Hagerman, RJ, Sobesky WE. Psychopathology in fragile x syndrome. Am J Orthopsychiatry 1989;59:142–152.
122. Riddle, JE, Cheema A, Sobesky WE, et al. Phenotypic involvement in females with the fmr1 gene mutation. Am J Ment Retard 1998;102:590–601.
123. Sobesky, WE, Hull CE, Hagerman RJ. Symptoms of schizotypal personality disorder in fragile x women. J Am Acad Child Adolesc Psychiatry 1994;33:247–255.
124. Freund, LS, Reiss AL, Hagerman R, et al. Chromosome fragility and psychopathology in obligate female carriers of the fragile x chromosome. Arch Gen Psychiatry 1992;49:54–60.

125. Freund, LS, Reiss AL, Abrams MT. Psychiatric disorders associated with fragile x in the young female. Pediatrics 1993;91: 321–329.

126. Mazzocco, MM, Baumgardner T, Freund LS, et al. Social functioning among girls with fragile x or turner syndrome and their sisters. J Autism Dev Disord 1998;28:509–517.

127. Lachiewicz, AM, Dawson DV. Behavior problems of young girls with fragile x syndrome: Factor scores on the conners' parent's questionnaire. Am J Med Genet 1994;51:364–369.

128. Hagerman, RJ, Jackson C, Amiri K, et al. Girls with fragile x syndrome: Physical and neurocognitive status and outcome. Pediatrics 1992;89:395–400.

129. Borghgraef, M, Fryns JP, van den Berghe H. The female and the fragile x syndrome: Data on clinical and psychological findings in 7 fra(x) carriers. Clin Genet 1990;37:341–346.

130. Keysor, CS, Mazzocco MM, McLeod DR, et al. Physiological arousal in females with fragile x or turner syndrome. Dev Psychobiol 2002;41:133–146.

131. Franke, P, Maier W, Hautzinger M, et al. Fragile-x carrier females: Evidence for a distinct psychopathological phenotype? Am J Med Genet 1996;64:334–339.

132. Eliez, S, Blasey CM, Freund LS, et al. Brain anatomy, gender and iq in children and adolescents with fragile x syndrome. Brain 2001;124:1610–1634.

133. Giedd, JN, Snell JW, Lange N, et al. Quantitative magnetic resonance imaging of human brain development: Ages 4–18. Cereb Cortex 1996;6:551–560.

134. Reiss, AL, Abrams MT, Singer HS, et al. Brain development, gender and iq in children. A volumetric imaging study. Brain 1996; 119:1763–1774.

135. Barnea-Goraly, N, Eliez S, Hedeus M, et al. White matter tract alterations in fragile x syndrome: Preliminary evidence from diffusion tensor imaging. Am J Med Genet 2003;118B:81–88.

136. Reiss, AL, Lee J, Freund L. Neuroanatomy of fragile x syndrome: The temporal lobe. Neurology 1994;44:1317–1324.

137. Andreasen, NC, Flaum M, Swayze V, 2nd, et al. Intelligence and brain structure in normal individuals. Am J Psychiatry 1993;150: 130–134.

138. Reiss, AL, Aylward E, Freund LS, et al. Neuroanatomy of fragile x syndrome: The posterior fossa. Ann Neurol 1991;29:26–32.

139. Reiss, AL, Freund L, Tseng JE, et al. Neuroanatomy in fragile x females: The posterior fossa. Am J Hum Genet 1991;49: 279–288.

140. Mostofsky, SH, Mazzocco MMM, Aakalu G, et al. Decreased cerebellar posterior vermis size in fragile x syndrome. Correlation with neurocognitive performance. Neurology 1998;50:121–130.

141. Kates, WR, Abrams MT, Kaufmann WE, et al. Reliability and validity of mri measurement of the amygdala and hippocampus in children with fragile x syndrome. Psychiatry Res 1997;75:31–48.

142. Comery, TA, Harris JB, Willems PJ, et al. Abnormal dendritic spines in fragile x knockout mice: Maturation and pruning deficits. Proc Natl Acad Sci U S A 1997;94:5401–5404.

143. Reiss, AL, Abrams MT, Greenlaw R, et al. Neurodevelopmental effects of the fmr-1 full mutation in humans. Nat Med 1995;1: 159–167.

144. Castellanos, FX, Giedd JN, Marsh WL, et al. Quantitative brain magnetic resonance imaging in attention-deficit hyperactivity disorder. Arch Gen Psychiatry 1996;53:607–616.

145. Raichle, ME, MacLeod AM, Snyder AZ, et al. A default mode of brain function. Proc Natl Acad Sci U S A 2001;98:676–682.

146. Tamm, L, Menon V, Johnston CK, et al. Fmri study of cognitive interference processing in females with fragile x syndrome. J Cogn Neurosci 2002;14:160–171.

147. Rivera, SM, Menon V, White CD, et al. Functional brain activation during arithmetic processing in females with fragile x syndrome is related to fmr1 protein expression. Hum Brain Map 2002;16:206–218.

148. Menon, V, Leroux J, White CD, et al. Frontostriatal deficits in fragile x syndrome: Relation to fmr1 gene expression. Proc Natl Acad Sci U S A 2004;101:3615–3620.

149. Kwon, H, Menon V, Eliez S, et al. Functional neuroanatomy of visuospatial working memory in fragile x syndrome: Relation to behavioral and molecular measures. Am J Psychiatry 2001;158: 1040–1051.

150. Greicius, MD, Boyett-Anderson JM, Menon V, et al. Reduced basal forebrain and hippocampal activation during memory encoding in girls with fragile x syndrome. Neuroreport 2004;15: 1579–1583.

151. Garrett, AS, Menon V, MacKenzie K, et al. Here's looking at you, kid: Neural systems underlying face and gaze processing in fragile x syndrome. Arch Gen Psychiatry 2004;61:281–288.

152. Hatton, DD, Bailey DB, Jr., Hargett-Beck MQ, et al. Behavioral style of young boys with fragile x syndrome. Dev Med Child Neurol 1999;41:625–632.

153. van Lieshout, CF, De Meyer RE, Curfs LM, et al. Family contexts, parental behaviour, and personality profiles of children and adolescents with prader-willi, fragile-x, or williams syndrome. J Child Psychol Psychiatry 1998;39:699–710.

154. von Gontard, A, Backes M, Laufersweiler-Plass C, et al. Psychopathology and familial stress - comparison of boys with fragile x syndrome and spinal muscular atrophy. J Child Psychol Psychiatry 2002;43:949–957.

155. Hagerman, PJ. Psychopathology in fragile x syndrome. Am J Orthopsychiatry 1989;59:142–152.

156. Berry-Kravis, E, Potanos K. Psychopharmacology in fragile x syndrome—present and future. Ment Retard Dev Disabil Res Rev 2004;10:42–48.

157. Hagerman, PJ. Medical follow-up and pharmacotherapy. In Hagerman, RJ and Cronister, AC, eds. *Fragile X Syndrome: Diagnosis, Treatment, and Research*, 2nd Ed. Baltimore; MD: Johns Hopkins University Press, 1996:283–331.

158. Linden, MG, Tassone F, Gane LW, et al. Compound heterozygous female with fragile x syndrome. Am J Med Genet 1999; 83:318–321.

158a. Huber, KM, Roder JC, Bear MF. Chemical induction of mGluR5- and protein synthesis—dependent long-term depression in hippocampal area CA1. J Neurophysiol 2001;86:321–325.

158b. Snyder, EM, Philpot BD, Huber KM, et al. Internalization of ionotropic glutamate receptors in response to mGluR activation. Nat Neurosci 2001;4:1079–1085.

158c. Huber, KM, Gallagher SM, Warren ST, et al. Altered synaptic plasticity in a mouse model of fragile X mental retardation. Proc Natl Acad Sci USA 2002;99:7746–7750.

158d. Caudy, AA, Myers M, Hannon GJ, et al. Fragile X-related protein and VIG associate with the RNA interference machinery. Genes Dev 2002;16:2491-2496.

158e. Bear, MF, Huber KM, Warren ST. The mGluR theory of fragile X mental retardation. Trends Neurosci 2004;27:370–377.

158f. McBride, SM, Choi CH, Wang Y, et al. Pharmacological rescue of synaptic plasticity, courtship behavior, and mushroom body defects in a Drosophila model of fragile X syndrome. Neuron 2005; 45:753–764.

158g. Yan, QJ, Rammal M, Tranfaglia M, et al. Suppression of two major Fragile X Syndrome mouse model phenotypes by the mGluR5 antagonist MPEP. Neuropharmacology 2005; (e publication ahead of print).

158h. Nosyreva, ED, Huber KM. Developmental switch in synaptic mechanisms of hippocampal metabotropic glutamate receptor-dependent long-term depression. J Neurosci 2005;25:2992–3001.

159. Jones, KL. *Smith's Recognizable Patterns of Human Malformations*, 4th Ed. Philadelphia: WB Saunders, 1988.

160. van Trotsenburg, AS, Vulsma T, van Santen HM, et al. Lower neonatal screening thyroxine concentrations in down syndrome newborns. J Clin Endocrinol Metab 2003;88:1512–1515.

161. Goldacre, MJ, Wotton CJ, Seagroatt V, et al. Cancers and immune related diseases associated with down's syndrome: A record linkage study. Arch Dis Child 2004;89:1014–1017.

162. Cogulu, O, Ozkinay F, Gunduz C, et al. Celiac disease in children with down syndrome: Importance of follow-up and serologic screening. Pediatr Int 2003;45:395–399.

163. Goldberg-Stern, H, Strawsburg RH, Patterson B, et al. Seizure frequency and characteristics in children with down syndrome. Brain Dev 2001;23:375–378.

164. Pueschel, SM, Louis S, McKnight P. Seizure disorders in down syndrome. Arch Neurol 1991;48:318–320.

165. Thuline, HC, Pueschel SM. Cytogenetics in down syndrome. In: Pueschel, SM and Rynders, JE, eds. *Down syndrome Advances in*

Biomedicine and the Behavioral Sciences. Cambridge: Ware Press, 1982: p. 133.

166. Hook, EG. Epidemiology of down syndrome. In: Pueschel, SM and Rynders, JE, eds. *Down syndrome advances in biomedicine and the behavioral sciences*. Cambridge: Ware Press, 1982: p. 11.

167. Mikkelsen, M. Down syndrome: Cytogenetical epidemiology. Hereditas 1977;86:45–50.

168. Delabar, JM, Theophile D, Rahmani Z, et al. Molecular mapping of twenty-four features of down syndrome on chromosome 21. Eur J Hum Genet 1993;1:114–124.

169. Korenberg, JR, Chen XN, Schipper R, et al. Down syndrome phenotypes: The consequences of chromosomal imbalance. Proc Natl Acad Sci U S A 1994;91:4997–5001.

170. McCormick, MK, Schinzel A, Petersen MB, et al. Molecular genetic approach to the characterization of the "down syndrome region" of chromosome 21. Genomics 1989;5:325–331.

171. Rahmani, Z, Blouin JL, Creau-Goldberg N, et al. Critical role of the d21s55 region on chromosome 21 in the pathogenesis of down syndrome. Proc Natl Acad Sci U S A 1989;86:5958–5962.

172. Korenberg, JR. Toward a molecular understanding of down syndrome. Prog Clin Biol Res 1993;384:87–115.

173. Engidawork, E, Lubec G. Protein expression in down syndrome brain. amino acids 2001;21:331–361.

174. Barbiero, L, Benussi L, Ghidoni R, et al. Bace-2 is overexpressed in down's syndrome. Exp Neurol 2003;182:335–345.

175. Lubec, G, Bajo M, Cheon MS, et al. Increased expression of human reduced folate carrier in fetal down syndrome brain. J Neural Transm Suppl 2003;95–103.

176. Engidawork, E, Gulesserian T, Fountoulakis M, et al. Aberrant protein expression in cerebral cortex of fetus with down syndrome. Neuroscience 2003;122:145–154.

177. Cheon, MS, Kim SH, Ovod V, et al. Protein levels of genes encoded on chromosome 21 in fetal down syndrome brain: Challenging the gene dosage effect hypothesis (Part III). Amino Acids 2003;24:127–134.

178. Ferrando-Miguel, R, Cheon MS, Lubec G. Protein levels of genes encoded on chromosome 21 in fetal down syndrome brain (Part V): Overexpression of phosphatidyl-inositol-glycan class p protein (dscr5). Amino Acids 2004;26:255–261.

179. de Haan, JB, Susil B, Pritchard M, et al. An altered antioxidant balance occurs in down syndrome fetal organs: Implications for the "gene dosage effect" hypothesis. J Neural Transm Suppl 2003;67–83.

180. Olson, LE, Richtsmeier JT, Leszl J, et al. A chromosome 21 critical region does not cause specific down syndrome phenotypes. Science 2004;306:687–690.

181. Shim, KS, Ferrando-Miguel R, Lubec G. Aberrant protein expression of transcription factors bach1 and erg, both encoded on chromosome 21, in brains of patients with down syndrome and alzheimer's disease. J Neural Transm Suppl 2003;39–49.

182. Cheon, MS, Shim KS, Kim SH, et al. Protein levels of genes encoded on chromosome 21 in fetal down syndrome brain: Challenging the gene dosage effect hypothesis (Part IV). Amino Acids 2003;25:41–47.

183. Cheon, MS, Kim SH, Yaspo ML, et al. Protein levels of genes encoded on chromosome 21 in fetal down syndrome brain: Challenging the gene dosage effect hypothesis (Part I). Amino Acids 2003;24:111–117.

184. Engidawork, E, Baiic N, Fountoulakis M, et al. Beta-amyloid precursor protein, ets-2 and collagen alpha 1 (vi) chain precursor, encoded on chromosome 21, are not overexpressed in fetal down syndrome: Further evidence against gene dosage effect. J Neural Transm Suppl 2001;335–346.

185. Greber-Platzer, S, Schatzmann-Turhani D, Cairns N, et al. Expression of the transcription factor ets2 in brain of patients with down syndrome—evidence against the overexpression-gene dosage hypothesis. J Neural Transm Suppl 1999;57:269–281.

186. Weitzdoerfer, R, Dierssen M, Fountoulakis M, et al. Fetal life in down syndrome starts with normal neuronal density but impaired dendritic spines and synaptosomal structure. J Neural Transm Suppl 2001;59–70.

187. Crome, L, Cowie V, Slater E. A statistical note on cerebeller and brain-stem weight in mongolism. J Ment Defic Res 1966;10:69–72.

188. Jernigan, TL, Bellugi U. Anomalous brain morphology on magnetic resonance images in williams syndrome and down syndrome. Arch Neurol 1990;47:529–533.

189. Wisniewski, KE. Down syndrome children often have brain with maturation delay, retardation of growth, and cortical dysgenesis. Am J Med Genet Suppl 1990;7:274–281.

190. Jernigan, TL, Bellugi U, Sowell E, et al. Cerebral morphologic distinctions between williams and down syndromes. Arch Neurol 1993;50:186–191.

191. Wang, PP, Doherty S, Hesselink JR, et al. Callosal morphology concurs with neurobehavioral and neuropathological findings in two neurodevelopmental disorders. Arch Neurol 1992;49:407–411.

192. Jernigan, T, Bellugi, M. Neuroanatomical distinctions between williams and down syndromes. In Broman, S and Grafman, J, eds. *Atypical Cognitive Deficits in Developmental Disorders: Implications for Brain Function*. Hillsdale, NJ: Lawrence Gilbaum, 1994:57–66.

193. Aylward, EH, Li Q, Honeycutt NA, et al. Mri volumes of the hippocampus and amygdala in adults with down's syndrome with and without dementia. Am J Psychiatry 1999;156:564–568.

194. Brooksbank, BW, Walker D, Balazs R, et al. Neuronal maturation in the foetal brain in down's syndrome. Early Hum Dev 1989;18:237–246.

195. Schmidt-Sidor, B, Wisniewski KE, Shepard TH, et al. Brain growth in down syndrome subjects 15 to 22 weeks of gestational age and birth to 60 months. Clin Neuropath 1990;9:181–190.

196. Cheng, A, Haydar TF, Yarowsky PJ, et al. Concurrent generation of subplate and cortical plate neurons in developing trisomy 16 mouse cortex. Dev Neurosci 2004;26:255–265.

197. Vuksic, M, Petanjek Z, Rasin MR, et al. Perinatal growth of prefrontal layer iii pyramids in down syndrome. Pediatr Neurol 2002;27:36–38.

198. Ross, MH, Galaburda AM, Kemper TL. Down's syndrome: Is there a decreased population of neurons? Neurology 1984;34:909–916.

199. Wisniewski, KE, Laure-Kamionowska M, Connell F, et al. Neuronal density and synaptogenesis in the postnatal stage of brain maturation in down syndrome. In: Epstein, CJ, ed. *The Neurobiology of Down Syndrome*. New York: Raven Press, 1986:29–44.

200. Wisniewski, KE, Schmidt-Sidor B. Postnatal delay of myelin formation in brains from down syndrome infants and children. Clin Neuropathol 1989;8:55–62.

201. Scott, BS, Becker LE, Petit TL. Neurobiology of down's syndrome. Prog Neurobiol 1983;21:199–237.

202. Takashima, S, Becker LE, Armstrong DL, et al. Abnormal neuronal development in the visual cortex of the human fetus and infant with down's syndrome. A quantitative and qualitative golgi study. Brain Res 1981;225:1–21.

203. Belichenko, PV, Masliah E, Kleschevnikov AM, et al. Synaptic structural abnormalities in the ts65dn mouse model of down syndrome. J Comp Neurol 2004;480:281–298.

204. Hamill, LB. Going to college: The experiences of a young woman with down syndrome. Ment Retard 2003;41:340–353.

205. Wisniewski, HM, Miezejeshi, CM and Hill, AL. Neurological and psychological status of individuals with down syndrome. In Nadel, L, ed. *The Psychobiology of Down Syndrome: Issues in the Biology of Language and Cognition*. Cambridge: MIT Press, 1988: 315–345.

206. Turner, S, Alborz A. Academic attainments of children with down's syndrome: A longitudinal study. Br J Educ Psychol 2003; 73:563–583.

207. John, FM, Bromham NR, Woodhouse JM, et al. Spatial vision deficits in infants and children with down syndrome. Invest Ophthalmol Vis Sci 2004;45:1566–1572.

208. Kanamori, G, Witter M, Brown J, et al. Otolaryngologic manifestations of down syndrome. Otolaryngol Clin North Am 2000;33:1285–1292.

209. Hodapp, RM, Evans DW, Gray FL. Intellectual development in children with down syndrome. In: Rondal, JA, Perera, J and Nadel, L, eds. *Down Syndrome: A Review of Current Knowledge*. London: Whurr, 1999: 124–132.

210. Bellugi, U, Lichtenberger L, Jones W, et al. I. The neurocognitive profile of williams syndrome: A complex pattern of strengths and weaknesses. J Cogn Neurosci 2000;12 Suppl 1:7–29.

211. Bellugi, U, Bihrle A, Jernigan T, et al. Neuropsychological, neurological, and neuroanatomical profile of williams syndrome. Am J Med Genet Suppl 1990;6:115–125.

212. Wang, PP, Bellugi U. Williams syndrome, down syndrome, and cognitive neuroscience. Am J Dis Child 1993;147:1246–1251.

213. Miller, JF. Profiles of language development in children with down syndrome. In: Miller, JF, Leahy, M and Leavitt, LA, eds. *Improving the Communication of People with Down Syndrome.* Baltimore, M.D.: Paul Brookes Publishing Co. Inc., 1999:11–39.

214. Chapman, RS, Schwartz SE, Bird EK. Language skills of children and adolescents with down syndrome: I. Comprehension. J Speech Hear Res 1991;34:1106–1120.

215. Chapman, RS, Seung HK, Schwartz SE, et al. Language skills of children and adolescents with down syndrome: Ii. Production deficits. J Speech Lang Hear Res 1998;41:861–873.

216. Fowler, AE. Language abilities in children with down syndrome: Evidence for a specific syntactic delay. In: Cicchetti, D and Beeghly, M, ed. *Children with Down Syndrome: A Developmental Perspective.* New York: Cambridge University Press, 1990:302–328.

217. Boudreau, DM, Chapman RS. The relationship between event representation and linguistic skill in narratives of children and adolescents with down syndrome. J Speech Lang Hear Res 2000; 43:1146–1159.

218. Laws, G, Gunn D. Phonological memory as a predictor of language comprehension in down syndrome: A five-year follow-up study. J Child Psychol Psychiatry 2004;45:326–337.

219. Chapman, RS, Hesketh LJ, Kistler DJ. Predicting longitudinal change in language production and comprehension in individuals with down syndrome: Hierarchical linear modeling. J Speech Lang Hear Res 2002;45:902–915.

220. Smith, L, von Tetzchner S, Michelsen B. The emergence of language skills in young children with down syndrome. In Nadel, L, ed. *The Psychobiology of Down Syndrome: Issues in the Biology of Language and Cognition.* Cambridge: MIT Press, 1988:145–165.

221. Iverson, JM, Longobardi E, Caselli MC. Relationship between gestures and words in children with down's syndrome and typically developing children in the early stages of communicative development. Int J Lang Commun Disord 2003;38:179–197.

222. Wang, PP, Bellugi U. Evidence from two genetic syndromes for a dissociation between verbal and visual-spatial short-term memory. J Clin Exp Neuropsychol 1994;16:317–322.

223. Jarrold, C, Baddeley AD, Hewes AK. Verbal short-term memory deficits in down syndrome: A consequence of problems in rehearsal? J Child Psychol Psychiatry 2000;41:233–244.

224. Bihrle, AM, Bellugi U, Delis D, et al. Seeing either the forest or the trees: Dissociation in visuospatial processing. Brain Cogn 1989;11:37–49.

225. Wishart, JG. Early learning in infants and young children with down syndrome. In Nadel, L, ed. *The Psychobiology of Down Syndrome: Issues in the Biology of Language and Cognition.* Cambridge: MIT Press, 1988:7–50.

226. Wishart, JG. The development of learning difficulties in children with down's syndrome. J Intellect Disabil Res 1993;37:389–403.

227. Ruskin, EM, Mundy P, Kasari C, et al. Object mastery motivation of children with down syndrome. Am J Ment Retard 1994;98:499–509.

228. Legerstee, M, Bowman TG. The development of responses to people and a toy in infants with down syndrome. Infant Behav Dev 1989;12:465–477.

229. Kasari, C, Freeman SF, Hughes MA. Emotion recognition by children with down syndrome. Ment Retard 2001;106:59–72.

230. Wishart, JG, Pitcairn TK. Recognition of identity and expression in faces by children with down syndrome. Am J Ment Retard 2000;105:466–479.

231. Mundy, P, Sigman M, Kasari C, et al. Nonverbal communication skills in down syndrome children. Child Dev 1988;59:235–249.

232. Franco, F, Wishart JG. Use of pointing and other gestures by young children with down syndrome. Am J Ment Retard 1995;100:160–182.

233. Byrne, A, MacDonald J, Buckley S. Reading, language and memory skills: A comparative longitudinal study of children with down syndrome and their mainstream peers. Br J Educ Psychol 2002;72:513–529.

234. Gelman, R, Cohen M. Qualitative differences in the way down syndrome and normal children solve a novel counting problem. In Nadel, L, ed. *The Psychobiology of Down Syndrome: Issues in the Biology of Language and Cognition.* Cambridge: MIT Press, 1988: 51–99.

235. Schwartz, M, Duara R, Haxby J, et al. Down's syndrome in adults: Brain metabolism. Science 1983;221:781–783.

236. Haier, RJ, Alkire MT, White NS, et al. Temporal cortex hypermetabolism in down syndrome prior to the onset of dementia. Neurology 2003;61:1673–1679.

237. Schapiro, MB, Grady CL, Kumar A, et al. Regional cerebral glucose metabolism is normal in young adults with down syndrome. J Cereb Blood Flow Metab 1990;10:199–206.

238. Krasuski, JS, Alexander GE, Horwitz B, et al. Relation of medial temporal lobe volumes to age and memory function in nondemented adults with down's syndrome: Implications for the prodromal phase of alzheimer's disease. Am J Psychiatry 2002; 159: 74–81.

239. Clark, D, Wilson GN. Behavioral assessment of children with down syndrome using the reiss psychopathology scale. Am J Med Genet 2003;118A:210–216.

240. Gath, A, Gumley D. Behaviour problems in retarded children with special reference to down's syndrome. Br J Psychiatry 1986; 149:156–161.

241. Lund, J. Psychiatric aspects of down's syndrome. Acta Psychiatr Scand 1988;78:369–374.

242. Menolascino, FJ. Psychiatric aspects of mongolism. Am J Ment Defic 1965;69:653–660.

243. Menolascino, FJ. Down's syndrome: Clinical and psychiatric findings in an institutionalized sample. Psychiatric Approaches of Mental Retardation 1970;191–204.

244. Myers, BA, Pueschel SM. Psychiatric disorders in persons with down syndrome. J Nerv Ment Dis 1991;179:609–613.

245. Cooper, SA, Collacott RA. Clinical features and diagnostic criteria of depression in down's syndrome. Br J Psychiatry 1994;165: 399–403.

246. Dykens, EM, Shah B, Sagun J, et al. Maladaptive behaviour in children and adolescents with down's syndrome. J Intellect Disabil Res 2002;46:484–492.

247. Nicham, R, Weitzdorfer R, Hauser E, et al. Spectrum of cognitive, behavioural and emotional problems in children and young adults with down syndrome. J Neural Transm Suppl 2003; 173–191.

248. Pary, RJ, Loschen EL, Tomkowiak SB. Mood disorders and down syndrome. Semin Clin Neuropsychiatry 1996;1:148–153.

249. Hurley, AD. Two cases of suicide attempt by patients with down's syndrome. Psychiatr Serv 1998;49:1618–1619.

250. Charlot, L, Fox S, Friedlander R. Obsessional slowness in down's syndrome. J Intellect Disabil Res 2002;46:517–524.

251. Cottrell, DJ, Crisp AH. Anorexia nervosa in down's syndrome—a case report. Br J Psychiatry 1984;145:195–196.

252. Fox, R, Karan OC, Rotatori AF. Regression including anorexia nervosa in a down's syndrome adult: A seven year follow up. J Behav Ther Exp Psychiatry 1981;12:351–354.

253. Heal, M, O'Hara J. The music therapy of an anorectic mentally handicapped adult. Br J Med Psychol 1993;66:33–41.

254. Holt, GM, Bouras N, Watson JP. Down's syndrome and eating disorders. A case study. Br J Psychiatry 1988;152:847–848.

255. Raitasuo, S, Virtanen H, Raitasuo J. Anorexia nervosa, major depression, and obsessive-compulsive disorder in a down's syndrome patient. Int J Eat Disord 1998;23:107–109.

256. Pankau, R, Partsch CJ, Gosch A, et al. Statural growth in williams-beuren syndrome. Eur J Pediatr 1992;151:751–755.

257. Beuren, A. Supravalvular aortic stenosis: A complex syndrome with and without mental retardation. Birth Defects 1972;8:45–56.

258. Holmstrom, G, Almond G, Temple K, et al. The iris in williams syndrome. Arch Dis Child 1990;65:987–989.

259. Jones, KL, Smith DW. The williams elfin facies syndrome. A new perspective. J Pediatr 1975;86:718–723.

260. Smith, DW. Recognizable patterns of human malformation. Genetic, embryologic and clinical aspects. Third edition. Major Probl Clin Pediatr 1982;7:1–653.

261. Winter, M, Pankau R, Amm M, et al. The spectrum of ocular features in the williams-beuren syndrome. Clin Genet 1996;49: 28–31.

262. Metcalfe, K. Williams syndrome: An update on clinical and molecular aspects. Arch Dis Child 1999;81:198–200.
263. Donnai, D, Karmiloff-Smith A. Williams syndrome: From genotype through to the cognitive phenotype. Am J Med Genet 2000; 97:164–171.
264. Martin, ND, Snodgrass GJ, Cohen RD. Idiopathic infantile hypercalcaemia—a continuing enigma. Arch Dis Child 1984;59: 605–613.
265. Bzduch, V. Hypercalcemic phase of williams syndrome. J Pediatr 1993;123:496.
266. Kapp, ME, Noorden GK, Jenkins R. Strabismus in williams syndrome. Am J Ophthalmol 1995;119:355–360.
267. Klein, AJ, Armstrong BL, Greer MK, et al. Hyperacusis and otitis media in individuals with williams syndrome. J Speech Hear Disord 1990;55:339–344.
268. Atkinson, J, Anker S, Braddick O, et al. Visual and visuospatial development in young children with williams syndrome. Dev Med Child Neurol 2001;43:330–337.
269. Eronen, M, Peippo M, Hiippala A, et al. Cardiovascular manifestations in 75 patients with williams syndrome. J Med Genet 2002;39:554–558.
270. Brooke, BS, Bayes-Genis A, Li DY. New insights into elastin and vascular disease. Trends Cardiovasc Med 2003;13:176–181.
271. Ardinger, RH, Jr., Goertz KK, Mattioli LF. Cerebrovascular stenoses with cerebral infarction in a child with williams syndrome. Am J Med Genet 1994;51:200–202.
272. Soper, R, Chaloupka JC, Fayad PB, et al. Ischemic stroke and intracranial multifocal cerebral arteriopathy in williams syndrome. J Pediatr 1995;126:945–948.
273. Wollack, JB, Kaifer M, LaMonte MP, et al. Stroke in williams syndrome. Stroke 1996;27:143–146.
274. Rose, C, Wessel A, Pankau R, et al. Anomalies of the abdominal aorta in williams-beuren syndrome—another cause of arterial hypertension. Eur J Pediatr 2001;160:655–658.
275. DeSilva, U, Elnitski L, Idol JR, et al. Generation and comparative analysis of approximately 3.3 mb of mouse genomic sequence orthologous to the region of human chromosome 7q11.23 implicated in williams syndrome. Genome Res 2002;12:3–15.
276. Hillier, LW, Fulton RS, Fulton LA, et al. The DNA sequence of human chromosome 7. Nature 2003;424:157–164.
277. Doyle, TF, Bellugi U, Korenberg JR, et al. "everybody in the world is my friend" hypersociability in young children with williams syndrome. Am J Med Genet 2004;124A:263–273.
278. Hirota, H, Matsuoka R, Chen XN, et al. Williams syndrome deficits in visual spatial processing linked to gtf2ird1 and gtf2i on chromosome 7q11.23. Genet Med 2003;5:311–321.
279. Morris, CA, Mervis CB, Hobart HH, et al. Gtf2i hemizygosity implicated in mental retardation in williams syndrome: Genotype-phenotype analysis of five families with deletions in the williams syndrome region. Am J Med Genet 2003;123A:45–59.
280. Ewart, AK, Morris CA, Atkinson D, et al. Hemizygosity at the elastin locus in a developmental disorder. Williams syndrome. Nature Genet 1993;5:11–16.
281. Lowery, MC, Morris CA, Ewart A, et al. Strong correlation of elastin deletions, detected by fish, with williams syndrome: Evaluation of 235 patients. Am J Hum Genet 1995;57:49–53.
282. Ewart, AK, Jin W, Atkinson D, et al. Supravalvular aortic stenosis associated with a deletion disrupting the elastin gene. J Clin Invest 1994;93:1071–1077.
283. Morris, CA, Thomas IT, Greenberg F. Williams syndrome: Autosomal dominant inheritance. Am J Med Genet 1993;47: 478–481.
284. Osborne, LR, Martindale D, Scherer SW, et al. Identification of genes from a 500-kb region at 7q11.23 that is commonly deleted in williams syndrome patients. Genomics 1996;36:328–336.
285. Wu, YQ, Sutton VR, Nickerson E, et al. Delineation of the common critical region in williams syndrome and clinical correlation of growth, heart defects, ethnicity, and parental origin. Am J Med Genet 1998;78:82–89.
286. Farnham, JM, Camp NJ, Neuhausen SL, et al. Confirmation of chromosome 7q11 locus for predisposition to intracranial aneurysm. Hum Genet 2004;114:250–255.
287. Frangiskakis, JM, Ewart AK, Morris CA, et al. Lim-kinase1 hemizygosity implicated in impaired visuospatial constructive cognition. Cell 1996;86:59–69.
288. Hoogenraad, CC, Akhmanova A, Galjart N, et al. Limk1 and clip-115: Linking cytoskeletal defects to williams syndrome. Bioessays 2004;26:141–150.
289. Tomiyoshi, G, Horita Y, Nishita M, et al. Caspase-mediated cleavage and activation of lim-kinase 1 and its role in apoptotic membrane blebbing. Genes Cells 2004;9:591–600.
290. Yang, E, Kim H, Lee J, et al. Overexpression of lim kinase 1 renders resistance to apoptosis in pc12 cells by inhibition of caspase activation. Cell Mol Neurobiol 2004;24:181–192.
291. Tojima, T, Ito E. Signal transduction cascades underlying de novo protein synthesis required for neuronal morphogenesis in differentiating neurons. Prog Neurobiol 2004;72:183–193.
292. Foletta, VC, Moussi N, Sarmiere PD, et al. Lim kinase 1, a key regulator of actin dynamics, is widely expressed in embryonic and adult tissues. Exp Cell Res 2004;294:392–405.
293. Yang, EJ, Yoon JH, Min do S, et al. Lim kinase 1 activates camp-responsive element-binding protein during the neuronal differentiation of immortalized hippocampal progenitor cells. J Biol Chem 2004;279:8903–8910.
294. Meng, Y, Zhang Y, Tregoubov V, et al. Regulation of spine morphology and synaptic function by limk and the actin cytoskeleton. Rev Neurosci 2003;14:233–240.
295. Meng, Y, Zhang Y, Tregoubov V, et al. Abnormal spine morphology and enhanced ltp in limk-1 knockout mice. Neuron 2002; 35:121–133.
296. Sarmiere, PD, Bamburg JR. Head, neck, and spines: A role for limk-1 in the hippocampus. Neuron 2002;35:3–5.
297. Bayes, M, Magano LF, Rivera N, et al. Mutational mechanisms of williams-beuren syndrome deletions. Am J Hum Genet 2003;73: 131–151.
298. Botta, A, Novelli G, Mari A, et al. Detection of an atypical 7q11.23 deletion in williams syndrome patients which does not include the stx1a and fzd3 genes. J Med Genet 1999;36: 478–480.
299. Huang, HC, Klein PS. The frizzled family: Receptors for multiple signal transduction pathways. Genome Biol 2004;5:234.
300. Reiss, AL, Eliez S, Schmitt JE, et al. Iv. Neuroanatomy of williams syndrome: A high-resolution mri study. J Cogn Neurosci 2000; 12 Suppl 1:65–73.
301. Wang, YK, Samos CH, Peoples R, et al. A novel human homologue of the drosophila frizzled wnt receptor gene binds wingless protein and is in the williams syndrome deletion at 7q11.23. Hum Mol Genet 1997;6:465–472.
302. Korenberg, JR, Chen XN, Hirota H, et al. Vi. Genome structure and cognitive map of williams syndrome. J Cogn Neurosci 2000; 12 Suppl 1:89–107.
303. Bellugi, U, Klima ES, Wang PP. Cognitive and neural development: Clues from genetically based syndromes. In: Magnussen, D, ed. *The Life-Span Development of Individuals: Behavioral, Neurobiological, and Psychosocial Perspectives.* New York, NY: The Nobel Symposium. Cambridge University Press, 1996:223–243.
304. Searcy, YM, Lincoln AJ, Rose FE, et al. The relationship between age and iq in adults with williams syndrome. Am J Ment Retard 2004;109:231–236.
305. Udwin, O, Yule W. A cognitive and behavioural phenotype in williams syndrome. J Clin Exp Neuropsychol 1991;13:232–244.
306. St. George M, Bellugi U. Preface. J Cogn Neurosci 2000;12:1–6.
307. Bellugi, U, Wang P, Jernigan T. Williams syndrome: An unusual neuropsychological profile. In: Broman, SH and Grafman, J, ed. *Atypical cognitive deficits in developmental disorders implications for brain function.* Hillsdale, NJ: Erlbaum Press, 1994:23–56.
308. Grant, J, Karmiloff-Smith A, Gathercole SA, et al. Phonological short-term memory and its relationship to language in william syndrome. Cognitive Neuropsychiatry 1997;2:81–99.
309. Pleh, C, Lukacs A, Racsmany M. Morphological patterns in hungarian children with williams syndrome and the rule debates. Brain Lang 2003;86:377–383.
310. Jarrold, C, Baddeley AD, Hewes AK. Verbal and nonverbal abilities in the williams syndrome phenotype: Evidence for diverging developmental trajectories. J Child Psychol Psychiatry 1998;39: 511–523.
311. Karmiloff-Smith, A. Development itself is the key to understanding developmental disorders. Trends Cogn Sci 1998;2:389–398.
312. Bellugi, U, Bihrle A, Neville H. Language, cognition, and brain organization in a neurodevelopmental disorder, in developmen-

tal behavioral neuroscience. Minnesota Symposia on Child Psychology 1992;24:201–232.

313. Karmiloff-Smith, A, Grant J, Berthoud I, et al. Language and williams syndrome: How intact is "intact"? Child Dev 1997;68: 246–262.

314. Clahsen, H, Almazan M. Syntax and morphology in williams syndrome. Cognition 1998;68:167–198.

315. Robinson, BF, Mervis CB, Robinson BW. The roles of verbal short-term memory and working memory in the acquisition of grammar by children with williams syndrome. Dev Neuropsychol 2003;23:13–31.

316. Devenny, DA, Krinsky-McHale SJ, Kittler PM, et al. Age-associated memory changes in adults with williams syndrome. Dev Neuropsychol 2004;26:691–706.

317. Vicari, S, Brizzolara D, Carlesimo GA, et al. Memory abilities in children with williams syndrome. Cortex 1996;32:503–514.

318. Vicari, S. Memory development and intellectual disabilities. Acta Paediatr Suppl 2004;93:60–63–64.

319. Crisco, JJ, Dobbs JM, Mulhern RK. Cognitive processing of children with williams syndrome. Dev Med Child Neurol 1988; 30:650–656.

320. Farran, EK, Jarrold C. Visuospatial cognition in williams syndrome: Reviewing and accounting for the strengths and weaknesses in performance. Dev Neuropsychol 2003;23:173–200.

321. Wang, PP, Doherty S, Rourke SB, et al. Unique profile of visuo-perceptual skills in a genetic syndrome. Brain Cogn 1995;29:54–65.

322. Anker, S, Atkinson J. Visual acuity measures in a sample of william syndrome. Perception 1997;26:763–768.

323. Atkinson, J, Braddick O, Anker S, et al. Neurobiological models of visuospatial cognition in children with williams syndrome: Measures of dorsal-stream and frontal function. Dev Neuropsychol 2003;23:139–172.

324. Landau, B, Zukowski A. Objects, motions, and paths: Spatial language in children with williams syndrome. Dev Neuropsychol 2003;23:105–137.

325. Phillips, CE, Jarrold C, Baddeley AD, et al. Comprehension of spatial language terms in williams syndrome: Evidence for an interaction between domains of strength and weakness. Cortex 2004;40:85–101.

326. Hopyan, T, Dennis M, Weksberg R, et al. Music skills and the expressive interpretation of music in children with williams-beuren syndrome: Pitch, rhythm, melodic imagery, phrasing, and musical affect. Neuropsychol Dev Cogn Sect C Child Neuropsychol 2001;7:42–53.

327. Sacks, O. Musical ability. Science 1995;268:621–622.

328. Mervis, CB, Morris CA, Klein-Tasman BP, et al. Attentional characteristics of infants and toddlers with williams syndrome during triadic interactions. Dev Neuropsychol 2003;23:243–268.

329. Jones, W, Bellugi U, Lai Z, et al. Ii. Hypersociability in williams syndrome. J Cogn Neurosci 2000;12 Suppl 1:30–46.

330. Sullivan, K, Winner E, Tager-Flusberg H. Can adolescents with williams syndrome tell the difference between lies and jokes? Dev Neuropsychol 2003;23:85–103.

331. Laws, G, Bishop D. Pragmatic language impairment and social deficits in williams syndrome: A comparison with down's syndrome and specific language impairment. Int J Lang Commun Disord 2004;39:45–64.

332. Bellugi, U, Adolphs R, Cassady C, et al. Towards the neural basis for hypersociability in a genetic syndrome. Neuroreport 1999;10:1653–1657.

333. Deruelle, C, Mancini J, Livet MO, et al. Configural and local processing of faces in children with williams syndrome. Brain Cogn 1999;41:276–298.

334. Mills, DL, Alvarez TD, St George M, et al. Iii. Electrophysiological studies of face processing in williams syndrome. J Cogn Neurosci 2000;12 Suppl 1:47–64.

335. Udwin, O. A survey of adults with williams syndrome and idiopathic infantile hypercalcaemia. Dev Med Child Neurol 1990; 32:129–141.

336. Udwin, O, Davies M, Howlin P. A longitudinal study of cognitive abilities and educational attainment in williams syndrome. Dev Med Child Neurol 1996;38:1020–1029.

337. Menghini, D, Verucci L, Vicari S. Reading and phonological awareness in williams syndrome. Neuropsychology 2004;18:29–37.

338. Majerus, S, Barisnikov K, Vuillemin I, et al. An investigation of verbal short-term memory and phonological processing in four children with williams syndrome. Neurocase 2003;9: 390–401.

339. Howlin, P, Davies M, Udwin O. Cognitive functioning in adults with williams syndrome. J Child Psychol Psychiatry 1998;39: 183–189.

340. Laing, E, Hulme C, Grant J, et al. Learning to read in williams syndrome: Looking beneath the surface of atypical reading development. J Child Psychol Psychiatry 2001;42:729–739.

341. MacDonald, GW, Roy DL. Williams syndrome: A neuropsychological profile. J Clin Exp Neuropsychol 1988;10:125–131.

342. Arnold, R, Yule W, Martin N. The psychological characteristics of infantile hypercalcaemia: A preliminary investigation. Dev Med Child Neurol 1985;27:49–59.

343. Greer, MK, Brown FR, 3rd, Pai GS, et al. Cognitive, adaptive, and behavioral characteristics of williams syndrome. Am J Med Genet 1997;74:521–525.

344. Klein-Tasman, BP, Mervis CB. Distinctive personality characteristics of 8-, 9-, and 10-year-olds with williams syndrome. Dev Neuropsychol 2003;23:269–290.

345. Udwin, O, Yule W, Martin N. Cognitive abilities and behavioural characteristics of children with idiopathic infantile hypercalcaemia. J Child Psychol Psychiatry 1987;28:297–309.

346. von Arnim, G, Engel P. Mental retardation related to hypercalcaemia. Dev Med Child Neurol 1964;6:366–377.

347. Einfeld, SL, Tonge BJ, Florio T. Behavioral and emotional disturbance in individuals with williams syndrome. Am J Ment Retard 1997;102:45–53.

348. O'Reilly, MF, Lacey C, Lancioni GE. Assessment of the influence of background noise on escape-maintained problem behavior and pain behavior in a child with williams syndrome. J Appl Behav Anal 2000;33:511–514.

349. Davies, M, Udwin O, Howlin P. Adults with williams syndrome. Preliminary study of social, emotional and behavioural difficulties. Br J Psychiatry 1998;172:273–276.

350. Dykens, EM. Anxiety, fears, and phobias in persons with williams syndrome. Dev Neuropsychol 2003;23:291–316.

351. Gosch, A, Pankau R. Personality characteristics and behaviour problems in individuals of different ages with williams syndrome. Dev Med Child Neurol 1997;39:527–533.

352. Arens, R, Wright B, Elliott J, et al. Periodic limb movement in sleep in children with williams syndrome. J Pediatr 1998; 133: 670–674.

353. Schmitt, JE, Eliez S, Warsofsky IS, et al. Enlarged cerebellar vermis in williams syndrome. J Psychiatr Res 2001;35: 225–229.

354. Galaburda, AM, Bellugi U. V. Multi-level analysis of cortical neuroanatomy in williams syndrome. J Cogn Neurosci 2000;12 Suppl 1:74–88.

355. Wang, PP, Hesselink JR, Jernigan TL, et al. Specific neurobehavioral profile of williams' syndrome is associated with neocerebellar hemispheric preservation. Neurology 1992;42: 1999–2002.

356. Jernigan, TL, Tallal P. Late childhood changes in the brain morphology observable with mri. Developmental Medicine and Child Neurology 1990;32:379–385.

357. Schmitt, JE, Eliez S, Bellugi U, et al. Analysis of cerebral shape in williams syndrome. Arch Neurol 2001;58:283–287.

358. Schmitt, JE, Eliez S, Warsofsky IS, et al. Corpus callosum morphology of williams syndrome: Relation to genetics and behavior. Dev Med Child Neurol 2001;43:155–159.

359. Tomaiuolo, F, Di Paola M, Caravale B, et al. Morphology and morphometry of the corpus callosum in williams syndrome: A t1-weighted mri study. Neuroreport 2002;13:2281–2284.

360. Eckert, MA, Hu D, Eliez S, et al. Evidence for superior parietal impairment in williams syndrome. Neurology 2005;64:152–153.

361. Rizzolatti, G, Matelli M. Two different streams form the dorsal visual system: Anatomy and functions. Exp Brain Res 2003; 153: 146–157.

362. Meyer-Lindenberg, A, Kohn P, Mervis CB, et al. Neural basis of genetically determined visuospatial construction deficit in williams syndrome. Neuron 2004;43:623–631.

363. Schmitt, JE, Watts K, Eliez S, et al. Increased gyrification in williams syndrome: Evidence using 3d mri methods. Dev Med Child Neurol 2002;44:292–295.

364. Schultz, RT, Grelotti DJ, Pober B. Genetics of childhood disorders: Xxvi. Williams syndrome and brain-behavior relationships. J Am Acad Child Adolesc Psychiatry 2001;40:606–609.

365. Tomc, SA, Williamson NK, Pauli RM. Temperament in williams syndrome. Am J Med Genet 1990;36:345–352.

366. Power, TJ, Blum NJ, Jones SM, et al. Brief report: Response to methylphenidate in two children with williams syndrome. J Autism Dev Disord 1997;27:79–87.

367. Davies, M, Howlin P, Udwin O. Independence and adaptive behavior in adults with williams syndrome. Am J Med Genet 1997; 70:188–195.

368. Saenger, P. Turner's syndrome. N Engl J Med 1996;335: 1749–1754.

369. Ross, J, Zinn A, McCauley E. Neurodevelopmental and psychosocial aspects of turner syndrome. Ment Retard Dev Disabil Res Rev 2000;6:135–141.

370. Cockwell, A, MacKenzie M, Youings S, et al. A cytogenetic and molecular study of a series of 45,x fetuses and their parents. J Med Genet 1991;28:151–155.

371. Ho, VB, Bakalov VK, Cooley M, et al. Major vascular anomalies in turner syndrome: Prevalence and magnetic resonance angiographic features. Circulation 2004;110:1694–1700.

372. Reynaud, K, Cortvrindt R, Verlinde F, et al. Number of ovarian follicles in human fetuses with the 45,x karyotype. Fertil Steril 2004;81:1112–1119.

373. Elsheikh, M, Dunger DB, Conway GS, et al. Turner's syndrome in adulthood. Endocr Rev 2002;23:120–140.

374. Tarani, L, Lampariello S, Raguso G, et al. Pregnancy in patients with turner's syndrome: Six new cases and review of literature. Gynecol Endocrinol 1998;12:83–87.

375. Sybert, VP. Cardiovascular malformations and complications in turner syndrome. Pediatrics 1998;101:E11.

376. Lippe, B, Geffner ME, Dietrich RB, et al. Renal malformations in patients with turner syndrome: Imaging in 141 patients. Pediatrics 1988;82:852–856.

377. Flynn, MT, Ekstrom L, De Arce M, et al. Prevalence of renal malformation in turner syndrome. Pediatr Nephrol 1996;10: 498–500.

378. Frias, JL, Davenport ML. Health supervision for children with turner syndrome. Pediatrics 2003;111:692–702.

379. Hultcrantz, M. Ear and hearing problems in turner's syndrome. Acta Otolaryngol 2003;123:253–257.

380. Ross, JL, Roeltgen D, Kushner H, et al. The turner syndrome-associated neurocognitive phenotype maps to distal xp. Am J Hum Genet 2000;67:672–681.

381. Saenger, P, Wikland KA, Conway GS, et al. Recommendations for the diagnosis and management of turner syndrome. J Clin Endocrinol Metab 2001;86:3061–3069.

382. Bakalov, VK, Cooley MM, Quon MJ, et al. Impaired insulin secretion in the turner metabolic syndrome. J Clin Endocrinol Metab 2004;89:3516–3520.

383. Chiovato, L, Larizza D, Bendinelli G, et al. Autoimmune hypothyroidism and hyperthyroidism in patients with turner's syndrome. Eur J Endocrinol 1996;134:568–575.

384. Sybert, VP, McCauley E. Turner's syndrome. N Engl J Med 2004; 351:1227–1238.

385. Bailey, JA, Carrel L, Chakravarti A, et al. Molecular evidence for a relationship between line-1 elements and x chromosome inactivation: The lyon repeat hypothesis. Proc Natl Acad Sci U S A 2000;97:6634–6639.

386. Zinn, AR, Tonk VS, Chen Z, et al. Evidence for a turner syndrome locus or loci at xp11.2–p22.1. Am J Hum Genet 1998;63: 1757–1766.

387. Heard, E. Recent advances in x-chromosome inactivation. Curr Opin Cell Biol 2004;16:247–255.

388. Turner, C, Dennis NR, Skuse DH, et al. Seven ring (x) chromosomes lacking the xist locus, six with an unexpectedly mild phenotype. Hum Genet 2000;106:93–100.

389. Kuntsi, J, Skuse D, Elgar K, et al. Ring-x chromosomes: Their cognitive and behavioural phenotype. Ann Hum Genet 2000; 64: 295–305.

390. Kubota, T, Wakui K, Nakamura T, et al. The proportion of cells with functional x disomy is associated with the severity of mental retardation in mosaic ring x turner syndrome females. Cytogenet Genome Res 2002;99:276–284.

391. Temple, CM, Carney RA. Intellectual functioning of children with turner syndrome: A comparison of behavioural phenotypes. Dev Med Child Neurol 1993;35:691–698.

392. Lopez Lopez, M, Torres Maldonado LC, Pablo Mendez J, et al. [molecular detection of chromosome y DNA sequences in patients with turner's syndrome]. Rev Invest Clin 1993;45: 233–239.

393. Wegner, RD, Scherer G, Pohlschmidt M, et al. Ring y chromosome: Cytogenetic and molecular characterization. Clin Genet 1992;42:71–75.

394. Rae, C, Joy P, Harasty J, et al. Enlarged temporal lobes in turner syndrome: An x-chromosome effect? Cereb Cortex 2004;14: 156–164.

395. Waber, DP. Neuropsychological aspects of turner's syndrome. Developmental Medicine and Child Neurology 1979;21:58–70.

396. Temple, CM. Oral fluency and narrative production in children with turner's syndrome. Neuropsychologia 2002;40:1419–1427.

397. McCauley, E, Kay T, Ito J, et al. The turner syndrome: Cognitive deficits, affective discrimination, and behavior problems. Child Dev 1987;58:464–473.

398. Romans, SM, Stefanatos G, Roeltgen DP, et al. Transition to young adulthood in ullrich-turner syndrome: Neurodevelopmental changes. Am J Med Genet 1998;79:140–147.

399. Ross, JL, Reiss AL, Freund L, et al. Neurocognitive function and brain imaging in turner syndrome–preliminary results. Horm Res 1993;39 Suppl 2:65–69.

400. Ross, JL, Stefanatos G, Roeltgen D, et al. Ullrich-turner syndrome: Neurodevelopmental changes from childhood through adolescence. Am J Med Genet 1995;58:74–82.

401. Ross, JL, Kushner H, Roeltgen DP. Developmental changes in motor function in girls with turner syndrome. Pediatr Neurol 1996;15:317–322.

402. Rovet, J, Netley C. The mental rotation task performance of turner syndrome subjects. Behav Genet 1980;10:437–443.

403. Rovet, JF. The psychoeducational characteristics of children with turner syndrome. J Learn Disabil 1993;26:333–341.

404. Temple, CM, Carney RA. Patterns of spatial functioning in turner's syndrome. Cortex 1995;31:109–118.

405. Temple, CM, Carney RA, Mullarkey S. Frontal lobe function and executive skills in children with turner's syndrome. Developmental Neuropsychology 1996;12:343–364.

406. Molko, N, Cachia A, Riviere D, et al. Functional and structural alterations of the intraparietal sulcus in a developmental dyscalculia of genetic origin. Neuron 2003;40:847–858.

407. Molko, N, Cachia A, Riviere D, et al. Brain anatomy in turner syndrome: Evidence for impaired social and spatial-numerical networks. Cereb Cortex 2004;14:840–850.

408. Fryer, SL, Kwon H, Eliez S, et al. Corpus callosum and posterior fossa development in monozygotic females: A morphometric mri study of turner syndrome. Dev Med Child Neurol 2003;45: 320–324.

409. Ross, JL, Stefanatos GA, Kushner H, et al. Persistent cognitive deficits in adult women with turner syndrome. Neurology 2002;58:218–225.

410. Ross, JL, Stefanatos GA, Kushner H, et al. The effect of genetic differences and ovarian failure: Intact cognitive function in adult women with premature ovarian failure versus turner syndrome. J Clin Endocrinol Metab 2004;89:1817–1822.

411. Ross, JL, Roeltgen D, Stefanatos GA, et al. Androgen-responsive aspects of cognition in girls with turner syndrome. J Clin Endocrinol Metab 2003;88:292–296.

412. Temple, CM, Carney R. Reading skills in children with turner's syndrome: An analysis of hyperplexia. Cortex 1996;32:335–345.

413. Rovet, J, Szekely C, Hockenberry MN. Specific arithmetic calculation deficits in children with turner syndrome. J Clin Exp Neuropsychol 1994;16:820–839.

414. Mazzocco, MM. Math learning disability and math ld subtypes: Evidence from studies of turner syndrome, fragile x syndrome, and neurofibromatosis type 1. J Learn Disabil 2001;34:520–533.

415. Mazzocco, MM. A process approach to describing mathematics difficulties in girls with turner syndrome. Pediatrics 1998;102: 492–496.

416. Bruandet, M, Molko N, Cohen L, et al. A cognitive characterization of dyscalculia in turner syndrome. Neuropsychologia 2004; 42:288–298.

417. Good, CD, Lawrence K, Thomas NS, et al. Dosage-sensitive x-linked locus influences the development of amygdala and orbitofrontal cortex, and fear recognition in humans. Brain 2003; 126:2431–2446.

418. Lawrence, K, Kuntsi J, Coleman M, et al. Face and emotion recognition deficits in turner syndrome: A possible role for x-linked genes in amygdala development. Neuropsychology 2003;17: 39–49.

419. Lawrence, K, Campbell R, Swettenham J, et al. Interpreting gaze in turner syndrome: Impaired sensitivity to intention and emotion, but preservation of social cueing. Neuropsychologia 2003; 41:894–905.

420. Elgar, K, Campbell R, Skuse D. Are you looking at me? Accuracy in processing line-of-sight in turner syndrome. Proc R Soc Lond B Biol Sci 2002;269:2415–2422.

421. Rourke, BP. The nld syndrome and the white matter model. In: Rourke, BP, ed. *Syndrome of nonverbal learning disabilities: Neurodevelopmental manifestations.* New York: The Guilford Press, 1995:1–26.

422. Murphy, DG, Allen G, Haxby JV, et al. The effects of sex steroids, and the x chromosome, on female brain function: A study of the neuropsychology of adult turner syndrome. Neuropsychologia 1994;32:1309–1323.

423. Skuse, DH, James RS, Bishop DVM, et al. Evidence from turner's syndrome of an imprinted x-linked locus affecting cognitive function. Nature 1997;587:705–708.

424. Donnelly, SL, Wolpert CM, Menold MM, et al. Female with autistic disorder and monosomy x (turner syndrome): Parent-of-origin effect of the x chromosome. Am J Med Genet 2000;96: 312–316.

425. El Abd, S, Patton MA, Turk J, et al. Social, communicational, and behavioral deficits associated with ring x turner syndrome. Am J Med Genet 1999;88:510–516.

426. Rovet, J, Holland J. Psychological aspects of the canadian randomized controlled trial of human growth hormone and low-dose ethinyl oestradiol in children with turner syndrome. The canadian growth hormone advisory group. Horm Res 1993;39 Suppl 2:60–64.

427. McCauley, E, Feuillan P, Kushner H, et al. Psychosocial development in adolescents with turner syndrome. J Dev Behav Pediatr 2001;22:360–365.

428. Lesniak-Karpiak, K, Mazzocco MM, Ross JL. Behavioral assessment of social anxiety in females with turner or fragile x syndrome. J Autism Dev Disord 2003;33:55–67.

429. McCauley, E, Sybert VP, Ehrhardt AA. Psychosocial adjustment of adult women with turner syndrome. Clin Genet 1986;29: 284–290.

430. Money, J, Mittenthal S. Lack of personality pathology in turner's syndrome: Relation to cytogenetics, hormones and physique. Behav Genet 1970;1:43–56.

431. McCauley, E, Ross JL, Kushner H, et al. Self-esteem and behavior in girls with turner syndrome. J Dev Behav Pediatr 1995;16: 82–88.

432. Pavlidis, K, McCauley E, Sybert VP. Psychosocial and sexual functioning in women with turner syndrome. Clin Genet 1995;47: 85–89.

433. Kates, WR, Mostofsky SH, Zimmerman AW, et al. Neuroanatomical and neurocognitive differences in a pair of monozygous twins discordant for strictly defined autism. Ann Neurol 1998;43:782–791.

434. Reiss, AL, Mozzocco MMM, Greenlaw R, et al. Neurodevelopmental effects of x monosomy: A volumetric imaging study. Ann Neurol 1995;38:731–738.

435. Brown, WE, Kesler SR, Eliez S, et al. A volumetric study of parietal lobe subregions in turner syndrome. Dev Med Child Neurol 2004;46:607–609.

436. Brown, WE, Kesler SR, Eliez S, et al. Brain development in turner syndrome: A magnetic resonance imaging study. Psychiatry Res 2002;116:187–196.

437. Kesler, SR, Blasey CM, Brown WE, et al. Effects of x-monosomy and x-linked imprinting on superior temporal gyrus morphology in turner syndrome. Biol Psychiatry 2003;54:636–646.

438. Howard, MA, Cowell PE, Boucher J, et al. Convergent neuroanatomical and behavioural evidence of an amygdala hypothesis of autism. Neuroreport 2000;11:2931–2935.

439. Kesler, SR, Garrett A, Bender B, et al. Amygdala and hippocampal volumes in turner syndrome: A high-resolution mri study of x-monosomy. Neuropsychologia 2004;42:1971–1978.

440. Reiss, AL, Freund L, Plotnick L, et al. The effects of x monosomy on brain development: Monozygotic twins discordant for turner's syndrome. Ann Neurol 1993;34:95–107.

441. Murphy, DG, DeCarli C, Daly E, et al. X-chromosome effects on female brain: A magnetic resonance imaging study of turner's syndrome. Lancet 1993;342:1197–1200.

442. Clark, C, Klonoff H, Hayden M. Regional cerebral glucose metabolism in turner syndrome. Can J Neurol Sci 1990;17:140–144.

443. Murphy, DG, Mentis MJ, Pietrini P, et al. A pet study of turner's syndrome: Effects of sex steroids and the x chromosome on brain. Biol Psychiatry 1997;41:285–298.

444. Dehaene, S, Spelke E, Pinel P, et al. Sources of mathematical thinking: Behavioral and brain-imaging evidence. Science 1999; 284:970–974.

445. Kesler, SR, Haberecht MF, Menon V, et al. Functional neuroanatomy of spatial orientation processing in turner syndrome. Cereb Cortex 2004;14:174–180.

446. Haberecht, MF, Menon V, Warsofsky IS, et al. Functional neuroanatomy of visuo-spatial working memory in turner syndrome. Hum Brain Mapp 2001;14:96–107.

447. Cassidy, SB. Prader-willi syndrome. Characteristics, management, and etiology. Ala J Med Sci 1987;24:169–175.

448. Butler, MG. Prader-willi syndrome: Current understanding of cause and diagnosis. Am J Med Genet 1990;35:319–332.

449. Burd, L. Letter to the editor. Military Medicine 1990;155:A19.

450. Whittington, JE, Holland AJ, Webb T, et al. Population prevalence and estimated birth incidence and mortality rate for people with prader-willi syndrome in one uk health region. J Med Genet 2001;38:792–798.

451. Mitchell, TV, Quittner AL. Multimethod study of attention and behavior problems in hearing-impaired children. J Clin Child Psychol 1996;25:83–96.

452. Butler, MG. Hypopigmentation: A common feature of prader-labhart-willi syndrome. Am J Hum Genet 1989;45:140–146.

453. Cassidy, SB, Forsythe M, Heeger S, et al. Comparison of phenotype between patients with prader-willi syndrome due to deletion 15q and uniparental disomy 15. Am J Med Genet 1997;68: 433–440.

454. Hittner, HM, King RA, Riccardi VM, et al. Oculocutaneous albinoidism as a manifestation of reduced neural crest derivatives in the prader-willi syndrome. Am J Ophthalmol 1982;94:328–337.

455. Wiesner, GL, Bendel CM, Olds DP, et al. Hypopigmentation in the prader-willi syndrome. Am J Hum Genet 1987;40:431–442.

456. Schinzel, A, Kaufmann U. The acrocallosal syndrome in sisters. Clinical Genetics 1986;30:399–405.

457. Donaldson, MD, Chu CE, Cooke A, et al. The prader-willi syndrome. Arch Dis Child 1994;70:58–63.

458. Holm, VA, Cassidy SB, Butler MG, et al. Prader-willi syndrome: Consensus diagnostic criteria. Pediatrics 1993;91:398–402.

459. Gunay-Aygun, M, Schwartz S, Heeger S, et al. The changing purpose of prader-willi syndrome clinical diagnostic criteria and proposed revised criteria. Pediatrics 2001;108 e92.

460. Olander, E, Stamberg J, Steinberg L, et al. Third prader-willi syndrome phenotype due to maternal uniparental disomy 15 with mosaic trisomy 15. Am J Med Genet 2000;93:215–218.

461. Russo, L, Mariotti P, Sangiorgi E, et al. A new susceptibility locus for migraine with aura in the 15q11-q13 genomic region containing three gaba-a receptor genes. Am J Hum Genet 2005; 76:327–333.

462. Papadimitriou, GN, Dikeos DG, Karadima G, et al. Gaba-a receptor beta3 and alpha5 subunit gene cluster on chromosome 15q11-q13 and bipolar disorder: A genetic association study. Am J Med Genet 2001;105:317–320.

463. Sander, T, Kretz R, Williamson MP, et al. Linkage analysis between idiopathic generalized epilepsies and the gaba(a) receptor

alpha5, beta3 and gamma3 subunit gene cluster on chromosome 15. Acta Neurol Scand 1997;96:1–7.

464. Greger, V, Knoll JH, Woolf E, et al. The gamma-aminobutyric acid receptor gamma 3 subunit gene (gabrg3) is tightly linked to the alpha 5 subunit gene (gabra5) on human chromosome 15q11–q13 and is transcribed in the same orientation. Genomics 1995;26:258–264.

465. Sinnett, D, Woolf E, Xie W, et al. Identification of a putative DNA replication origin in the gamma-aminobutyric acid receptor subunit beta3 and alpha5 gene cluster on human chromosome 15q11–q13, a region associated with parental imprinting and allele-specific replication timing. Gene 1996;173:171–177.

466. Gillessen-Kaesbach, G, Demuth S, Thiele H, et al. A previously unrecognised phenotype characterised by obesity, muscular hypotonia, and ability to speak in patients with angelman syndrome caused by an imprinting defect. Eur J Hum Genet 1999;7:638–644.

467. Ozcelik, T, Leff S, Robinson W, et al. Small nuclear ribonucleoprotein polypeptide n (snrpn), an expressed gene in the prader-willi syndrome critical region. Nat Genet 1992;2:265–269.

468. Gallagher, RC, Pils B, Albalwi M, et al. Evidence for the role of pwcr1/hbii-85 c/d box small nucleolar rnas in prader-willi syndrome. Am J Hum Genet 2002;71:669–678.

469. Whittington, J, Holland A, Webb T, et al. Academic underachievement by people with prader-willi syndrome. J Intellect Disabil Res 2004;48:188–200.

470. Curfs, LM, Wiegers AM, Sommers JR, et al. Strengths and weaknesses in the cognitive profile of youngsters with prader-willi syndrome. Clin Genet 1991;40:430–434.

471. Taylor, RL. Cognitive and behavioral characteristics. In Caldwell, ML and Taylor, RL, *Prader-Willi Syndrome: Selected Research and Management Issues*. New York: Springer-Verlag, 1988:29–43.

472. Dykens, EM. Are jigsaw puzzle skills 'spared' in persons with prader-willi syndrome? J Child Psychol Psychiatry 2002;43:343–352.

473. Branson, C. Speech and language characteristics of children with prader-willi syndrome. In Holm, VA, Sulzbacher, S and Pipes, PL, eds. *The Prader-Willi Syndrome*. Baltimore, MD: University Park Press, 1981:174–183.

474. Kleppe, SA, Katayama KM, Shipley KG, et al. The speech and language characteristics of children with prader-willi syndrome. J Speech Hear Disord 1990;55:300–309.

475. Dyson, AT, Lombardino LJ. Phonological abilities of a preschool child with prader-willi syndrome. J Speech Hear Disord 1989;54:44–48.

476. Sundheim, S, Voeller KKS. Psychiatric implications of language disorders and learning disabilities: Risks and management. Journal of Child Neurology 2004;19:814–826.

477. Burd, L, Kerbeshian J. Hyperlexia in prader-willi syndrome. Lancet 1989;2:983–984.

478. Whittington, J, Holland A, Webb T, et al. Cognitive abilities and genotype in a population-based sample of people with prader-willi syndrome. J Intellect Disabil Res 2004;48:172–187.

479. Butler, MG, Bittel DC, Kibiryeva N, et al. Behavioral differences among subjects with prader-willi syndrome and type i or type ii deletion and maternal disomy. Pediatrics 2004;113:565–573.

480. Veltman, MW, Thompson RJ, Roberts SE, et al. Prader-willi syndrome—a study comparing deletion and uniparental disomy cases with reference to autism spectrum disorders. Eur Child Adolesc Psychiatry 2004;13:42–50.

481. Dykens, EM, Cassidy SB. Correlates of maladaptive behavior in children and adults with prader-willi syndrome. Am J Med Genet 1995;60:546–549.

482. Dykens, EM. Maladaptive and compulsive behavior in prader-willi syndrome: New insights from older adults. Am J Ment Retard 2004;109:142–153.

483. Steinhausen, HC, Eiholzer U, Hauffa BP, et al. Behavioural and emotional disturbances in people with prader-willi syndrome. J Intellect Disabil Res 2004;48:47–52.

484. Wigren, M, Hansen S. Rituals and compulsivity in prader-willi syndrome: Profile and stability. J Intellect Disabil Res 2003; 47:428–438.

485. Dykens, EM, Leckman JF, Cassidy SB. Obsessions and compulsions in prader-willi syndrome. J Child Psychol Psychiatry 1996;37:995–1002.

486. Stein, DJ, Keating J, Zar HJ, et al. A survey of the phenomenology and pharmacotherapy of compulsive and impulsive-aggressive symptoms in prader-willi syndrome. J Neuropsychiatry Clin Neurosci 1994;6:23–29.

487. Whitman, BY, Myers S, Carrel A, et al. The behavioral impact of growth hormone treatment for children and adolescents with prader-willi syndrome: A 2-year, controlled study. Pediatrics 2002;109:E35.

488. Vogels, A, Matthijs G, Legius E, et al. Chromosome 15 maternal uniparental disomy and psychosis in prader-willi syndrome. J Med Genet 2003;40:72–73.

489. Boer, H, Holland A, Whittington J, et al. Psychotic illness in people with prader willi syndrome due to chromosome 15 maternal uniparental disomy. Lancet 2002;359:135–136.

490. Clarke, DJ. Prader-willi syndrome and psychoses. Br J Psychiatry 1993;163:680–684.

491. Verhoeven, WM, Tuinier S, Curfs LM. Prader-willi syndrome: The psychopathological phenotype in uniparental disomy. J Med Genet 2003;40:e112.

492. Vogels, A, De Hert M, Descheemaeker MJ, et al. Psychotic disorders in prader-willi syndrome. Am J Med Genet 2004;127A:238–243.

493. Symons, FJ, Butler MG, Sanders MD, et al. Self-injurious behavior and prader-willi syndrome: Behavioral forms and body locations. Am J Ment Retard 1999;104:260–269.

494. Whitman, BY, Accardo P. Emotional symptoms in prader-willi syndrome adolescents. Am J Med Genet 1987;28:897–905.

495. Bhargava, SA, Putnam PE, Kocoshis SA, et al. Rectal bleeding in prader-willi syndrome. Pediatrics 1996;97:265–267.

496. Schepis, C, Failla P, Siragusa M, et al. Skin-picking: The best cutaneous feature in the recognition of prader-willi syndrome. Int J Dermatol 1994;33:866–867.

497. Hellings, JA, Warnock JK. Self-injurious behavior and serotonin in prader-willi syndrome. Psychopharmacol Bull 1994;30:245–250.

498. Warnock, JK, Kestenbaum T. Pharmacologic treatment of severe skin-picking behaviors in prader-willi syndrome. Two case reports. Arch Dermatol 1992;128:1623–1625.

499. Pirker, S, Schwarzer C, Wieselthaler A, et al. Gaba(a) receptors: Immunocytochemical distribution of 13 subunits in the adult rat brain. Neuroscience 2000;101:815–850.

500. Bohme, I, Rabe H, Luddens H. Four amino acids in the alpha subunits determine the gamma-aminobutyric acid sensitivities of gabaa receptor subtypes. J Biol Chem 2004;279:35193–35200.

501. Rudolph, U, Crestani F, Benke D, et al. Benzodiazepine actions mediated by specific gamma-aminobutyric acid(a) receptor subtypes. Nature 1999;401:796–800.

502. Fritschy, JM, Mohler H. Gabaa-receptor heterogeneity in the adult rat brain: Differential regional and cellular distribution of seven major subunits. J Comp Neurol 1995;359:154–194.

503. Lujan, R, Shigemoto R, Lopez-Bendito G. Glutamate and gaba receptor signalling in the developing brain. Neuroscience 2005;130:567–580.

504. Steiger, JL, Russek SJ. Gabaa receptors: Building the bridge between subunit mrnas, their promoters, and cognate transcription factors. Pharmacol Ther 2004;101:259–281.

505. Dawson, GR, Collinson N, Atack JR. Development of subtype selective gabaa modulators. CNS Spectr 2005;10:21–27.

506. Bormann, J. The 'abc' of gaba receptors. Trends Pharmacol Sci 2000;21:16–19.

507. Marowsky, A, Fritschy JM, Vogt KE. Functional mapping of gaba a receptor subtypes in the amygdala. Eur J Neurosci 2004; 20:1281–1289.

508. Skolnick, P, Hu RJ, Cook CM, et al. [3h]ry 80: A high-affinity, selective ligand for gamma-aminobutyric acida receptors containing alpha-5 subunits. J Pharmacol Exp Ther 1997;283:488–493.

509. Wisden, W, Laurie DJ, Monyer H, et al. The distribution of 13 gabaa receptor subunit mrnas in the rat brain. I. Telencephalon, diencephalon, mesencephalon. J Neurosci 1992;12:1040–1062.

510. Sur, C, Fresu L, Howell O, et al. Autoradiographic localization of alpha5 subunit-containing gabaa receptors in rat brain. Brain Res 1999;822:265–270.

511. Ortinski, PI, Lu C, Takagaki K, et al. Expression of distinct alpha subunits of gabaa receptor regulates inhibitory synaptic strength. J Neurophysiol 2004;92:1718–1727.

512. Barberis, A, Lu C, Vicini S, et al. Developmental changes of gaba synaptic transient in cerebellar granule cells. Mol Pharmacol 2005;67:1221–1228.

513. Fritschy, JM, Paysan J, Enna A, et al. Switch in the expression of rat gabaa-receptor subtypes during postnatal development: An immunohistochemical study. J Neurosci 1994;14:5302–5324.

514. Killisch, I, Dotti CG, Laurie DJ, et al. Expression patterns of gabaa receptor subtypes in developing hippocampal neurons. Neuron 1991;7:927–936.

515. LoTurco, JJ, Owens DF, Heath MJ, et al. Gaba and glutamate depolarize cortical progenitor cells and inhibit DNA synthesis. Neuron 1995;15:1287–1298.

516. Haydar, TF, Wang F, Schwartz ML, et al. Differential modulation of proliferation in the neocortical ventricular and subventricular zones. J Neurosci 2000;20:5764–5774.

517. Khazipov, R, Esclapez M, Caillard O, et al. Early development of neuronal activity in the primate hippocampus in utero. J Neurosci 2001;21:9770–9781.

518. Behar, TN, Schaffner AE, Scott CA, et al. Differential response of cortical plate and ventricular zone cells to gaba as a migration stimulus. J Neurosci 1998;18:6378–6387.

519. Fritschy, JM, Brunig I. Formation and plasticity of gabaergic synapses: Physiological mechanisms and pathophysiological implications. Pharmacol Ther 2003;98:299–323.

520. Meier, J, Akyeli J, Kirischuk S, et al. Gaba(a) receptor activity and pkc control inhibitory synaptogenesis in cns tissue slices. Mol Cell Neurosci 2003;23:600–613.

521. Jelitai, M, Anderova M, Marko K, et al. Role of gamma-aminobutyric acid in early neuronal development: Studies with an embryonic neuroectodermal stem cell clone. J Neurosci Res 2004; 76:801–811.

522. Fagiolini, M, Fritschy JM, Low K, et al. Specific gabaa circuits for visual cortical plasticity. Science 2004;303:1681–1683.

523. Wallenstein, GV, Eichenbaum H, Hasselmo M. The hippocampus as an associator of discontigous events. Trends Neurosci 1998;21:317–323.

524. Paulsen, O, Moser EI. A model of hippocampal memory encoding and retrieval: Gabaergic control of synaptic plasticity. Trends Neurosci 1998;21:273–278.

525. Collinson, N, Kuenzi FM, Jarolimek W, et al. Enhanced learning and memory and altered gabaergic synaptic transmission in mice lacking the alpha 5 subunit of the gabaa receptor. J Neurosci 2002;22:5572–5580.

526. Crestani, F, Keist R, Fritschy JM, et al. Trace fear conditioning involves hippocampal alpha5 gaba(a) receptors. Proc Natl Acad Sci U S A 2002;99:8980–8985.

527. Maubach, K. Gaba(a) receptor subtype selective cognition enhancers. Curr Drug Targets CNS Neurol Disord 2003;2:233–239.

528. Caraiscos, VB, Elliott EM, You-Ten KE, et al. Tonic inhibition in mouse hippocampal ca1 pyramidal neurons is mediated by alpha5 subunit-containing gamma-aminobutyric acid type a receptors. Proc Natl Acad Sci U S A 2004;101:3662–3667.

529. Ebert, MH, Schmidt DE, Thompson T, et al. Elevated plasma gamma-aminobutyric acid (gaba) levels in individuals with either prader-willi syndrome or angelman syndrome. J Neuropsychiatry Clin Neurosci 1997;9:75–80.

530. Keverne, EB. Gaba-ergic neurons and the neurobiology of schizophrenia and other psychoses. Brain Res Bull 1999;48: 467–473.

531. Holsen, L, Thompson T. Compulsive behavior and eye blink in prader-willi syndrome: Neurochemical implications. Am J Ment Retard 2004;109:197–207.

532. Lucignani, G, Panzacchi A, Bosio L, et al. Gaba a receptor abnormalities in prader-willi syndrome assessed with positron emission tomography and [11c]flumazenil. Neuroimage 2004;22: 22–28.

533. Holland, AJ, Treasure J, Coskeran P, et al. Characteristics of the eating disorder in prader-willi syndrome: Implications for treatment. J Intellect Disabil Res 1995;39 :373–381.

534. Holland, AJ, Treasure J, Coskeran P, et al. Measurement of excessive appetite and metabolic changes in prader-willi syndrome. Int J Obes Relat Metab Disord 1993;17:527–532.

535. Eiholzer, U, Blum WF, Molinari L. Body fat determined by skinfold measurements is elevated despite underweight in infants with prader-labhart-willi syndrome. J Pediatr 1999;134:222–225.

536. Carrel, AL, Allen DB. Effects of growth hormone on adipose tissue. J Pediatr Endocrinol Metab 2000;13 Suppl 2:1003–1009.

537. Shapira, NA, Lessig MC, He AG, et al. Satiety dysfunction in prader-willi syndrome demonstrated by fmri. J Neurol Neurosurg Psychiatry 2005;76:260–262.

538. Tauber, M, Conte Auriol F, Moulin P, et al. Hyperghrelinemia is a common feature of prader-willi syndrome and pituitary stalk interruption: A pathophysiological hypothesis. Horm Res 2004; 62:49–54.

539. DelParigi, A, Tschop M, Heiman ML, et al. High circulating ghrelin: A potential cause for hyperphagia and obesity in prader-willi syndrome. J Clin Endocrinol Metab 2002;87:5461–5464.

540. Haqq, AM, Stadler DD, Rosenfeld RG, et al. Circulating ghrelin levels are suppressed by meals and octreotide therapy in children with prader-willi syndrome. J Clin Endocrinol Metab 2003;88: 3573–3576.

541. Tan, TM, Vanderpump M, Khoo B, et al. Somatostatin infusion lowers plasma ghrelin without reducing appetite in adults with prader-willi syndrome. J Clin Endocrinol Metab 2004;89: 4162–4165.

542. Angulo, M, Castro-Magana M, Uy J. Pituitary evaluation and growth hormone treatment in prader-willi syndrome. J of Pediatr Endocrinol 1991;4:167–173.

543. Stevenson, DA, Anaya TM, Clayton-Smith J, et al. Unexpected death and critical illness in prader-willi syndrome: Report of ten individuals. Am J Med Genet 2004;124A:158–164.

544. Vestergaard, P, Kristensen K, Bruun JM, et al. Reduced bone mineral density and increased bone turnover in prader-willi syndrome compared with controls matched for sex and body mass index—a cross-sectional study. J Pediatr 2004;144:614–619.

545. Sakai, K, Mansari EL, Lin JS. The posterior hypothalamus in the regulation of wakefulness and paradoxical sleep. In Mancia, M and Marini, G, eds. The Diencephalon and Sleep. New York: Raven, 1990:171–198.

546. Stores, G. Sleep studies in children with a mental handicap. J Child Psychol Psychiatry 1992;33:1303–1317.

547. Vela-Bueno, A, Kales A, Soldatos CR, et al. Sleep in the prader-willi syndrome. Clinical and polygraphic findings. Arch Neurol 1984;41:294–296.

548. Holland, AJ, Wong J. Genetically determined obesity in prader-willi syndrome: The ethics and legality of treatment. J Med Ethics 1999;25:230–236.

549. Hoffman, CJ, Aultman D, Pipes P. A nutrition survey of and recommendations for individuals with prader-willi syndrome who live in group homes. J Am Diet Assoc 1992;92:823–830, 833.

550. Silverthorn, KH, Hornak JE. Beneficial effects of exercise on aerobic capacity and body composition in adults with prader-willi syndrome. Am J Ment Retard 1993;97:654–658.

551. Page, TJ, Finney JW, Parrish JM, et al. Assessment and reduction of food stealing in prader-willi children. Appl Res Ment Retard 1983;4:219–228.

552. Mullins, JB, Vogl-Maier B. Weight management of youth with prader-willi syndrome. Int J Eat Disord 1987;6:419–425.

553. Allen, DB, Carrel AL. Growth hormone therapy for prader-willi syndrome: A critical appraisal. J Pediatr Endocrinol Metab 2004; 17 Suppl 4:1297–1306.

554. Whitman, B, Carrel A, Bekx T, et al. Growth hormone improves body composition and motor development in infants with prader-willi syndrome after six months. J Pediatr Endocrinol Metab 2004;17:591–600.

555. Carrel, AL, Myers SE, Whitman BY, et al. Benefits of long-term gh therapy in prader-willi syndrome: A 4-year study. J Clin Endocrinol Metab 2002;87:1581–1585.

556. Wilson, TA, Rose SR, Cohen P, et al. Update of guidelines for the use of growth hormone in children: The lawson wilkins pediatric endocrinology society drug and therapeutics committee. J Pediatr 2003;143:415–421.

557. Tezenas Du Montcel, S, Mendizabai H, Ayme S, et al. Prevalence of 22q11 microdeletion. J Med Genet 1996;33:719.

558. Oskarsdottir, S, Vujic M, Fasth A. Incidence and prevalence of the 22q11 deletion syndrome: A population-based study in western sweden. Arch Dis Child 2004;89:148–151.

559. Shprintzen, RJ, Goldberg RB, Young D, et al. The velo-cardio-facial syndrome: A clinical and genetic analysis. Pediatrics 1981; 67:167–172.

560. Marino, B, Digilio MC, Toscano A, et al. Anatomic patterns of conotruncal defects associated with deletion 22q11. Genet Med 2001;3:45–48.

561. Vantrappen, G, Devriendt K, Swillen A, et al. Presenting symptoms and clinical features in 130 patients with the velo-cardio-facial syndrome. The leuven experience. Genet Couns 1999; 10:3–9.

562. Havkin, N, Tatum SA, Shprintzen RJ. Velopharyngeal insufficiency and articulation impairment in velo-cardio-facial syndrome: The influence of adenoids on phonemic development. Int J Pediatr Otorhinolaryngol 2000;54:103–110.

563. Shprintzen, RJ. Velo-cardio-facial syndrome: A distinctive behavioral phenotype. Ment Retard Dev Disabil Res Rev 2000;6: 142–147.

564. Digilio, MC, Angioni A, De Santis M, et al. Spectrum of clinical variability in familial deletion 22q11.2: From full manifestation to extremely mild clinical anomalies. Clin Genet 2003;63: 308–313.

565. Bassett, AS, Chow EW, AbdelMalik P, et al. The schizophrenia phenotype in 22q11 deletion syndrome. Am J Psychiatry 2003; 160:1580–1586.

566. Gothelf, D, Frisch A, Munitz H, et al. Velocardiofacial manifestations and microdeletions in schizophrenic inpatients. Am J Med Genet 1997;72:455–461.

567. Gothelf, D, Frisch A, Munitz H, et al. Clinical characteristics of schizophrenia associated with velo-cardio-facial syndrome. Schizophrenia Research 1999;35:105–112.

568. Sergi, C, Serpi M, Muller-Navia J, et al. Catch 22 syndrome: Report of 7 infants with follow-up data and review of the recent advancements in the genetic knowledge of the locus 22q11. Pathologica 1999;91:166–172.

569. Shaikh, TH, Kurahashi H, Saitta SC, et al. Chromosome 22-specific low copy repeats and the 22q11.2 deletion syndrome: Genomic organization and deletion endpoint analysis. Hum Mol Genet 2000;9:489–501.

570. Budarf, ML, Collins J, Gong W, et al. Cloning a balanced translocation associated with digeorge syndrome and identification of a disrupted candidate gene. Nat Genet 1995;10:269–278.

571. Ensenauer, RE, Adeyinka A, Flynn HC, et al. Microduplication 22q11.2, an emerging syndrome: Clinical, cytogenetic, and molecular analysis of thirteen patients. Am J Hum Genet 2003; 73:1027–1040.

572. McDermid, HE, Morrow BE. Genomic disorders on 22q11. Am J Hum Genet 2002;70:1077–1088.

573. Shaikh, TH, Kurahashi H, Emanuel BS. Evolutionarily conserved low copy repeats (lcrs) in 22q11 mediate deletions, duplications, translocations, and genomic instability: An update and literature review. Genet Med 2001;3:6–13.

574. Nimmakayalu, MA, Gotter AL, Shaikh TH, et al. A novel sequence-based approach to localize translocation breakpoints identifies the molecular basis of a t(4;22). Hum Mol Genet 2003; 12:2817–2825.

575. Edelmann, L, Spiteri E, Koren K, et al. At-rich palindromes mediate the constitutional t(11;22) translocation. Am J Hum Genet 2001;68:1–13.

576. Saitta, SC, Harris SE, Gaeth AP, et al. Aberrant interchromosomal exchanges are the predominant cause of the 22q11.2 deletion. Hum Mol Genet 2004;13:417–428.

577. Vincent, MC, Heitz F, Tricoire J, et al. 22q11 deletion in dgs/vcfs monozygotic twins with discordant phenotypes. Genet Couns 1999;10:43–49.

578. Maynard, TM, Haskell GT, Peters AZ, et al. A comprehensive analysis of 22q11 gene expression in the developing and adult brain. Proc Natl Acad Sci U S A 2003;100:14433–14438.

579. Gottlieb, S, Emanuel BS, Driscoll DA, et al. The digeorge syndrome minimal critical region contains a goosecoid-like (gscl) homeobox gene that is expressed early in human development. Am J Hum Genet 1997;60:1194–1201.

580. Gottlieb, S, Hanes SD, Golden JA, et al. Goosecoid-like, a gene deleted in digeorge and velocardiofacial syndromes, recognizes DNA with a bicoid-like specificity and is expressed in the developing mouse brain. Hum Mol Genet 1998;7:1497–1505.

581. De Luca, A, Pasini A, Amati F, et al. Association study of a promoter polymorphism of ufd11 gene with schizophrenia. Am J Med Genet 2001;105:529–533.

582. Saito, T, Stopkova P, Diaz L, et al. Polymorphism screening of pik4ca: Possible candidate gene for chromosome 22q11-linked psychiatric disorders. Am J Med Genet B Neuropsychiatr Genet 2003;116:77–83.

583. Jacquet, H, Demily C, Houy E, et al. Hyperprolinemia is a risk factor for schizoaffective disorder. Mol Psychiatry 2005;10: 479–485.

584. GrandPre, T, Li S, Strittmatter SM. Nogo-66 receptor antagonist peptide promotes axonal regeneration. Nature 2002;417: 547–551.

585. Mingorance, A, Fontana X, Sole M, et al. Regulation of nogo and nogo receptor during the development of the entorhino-hippocampal pathway and after adult hippocampal lesions. Mol Cell Neurosci 2004;26:34–49.

586. Sun, ZY, Wei J, Xie L, et al. The cldn5 locus may be involved in the vulnerability to schizophrenia. Eur Psychiatry 2004;19:354–357.

587. Forrester, S, Kovach MJ, Smith RE, et al. Kousseff syndrome caused by deletion of chromosome 22q11–13. Am J Med Genet 2002;112:338–342.

588. Kao, A, Mariani J, McDonald-McGinn DM, et al. Increased prevalence of unprovoked seizures in patients with a 22q11.2 deletion. Am J Med Genet 2004;129A:29–34.

589. Swillen, A, Devriendt K, Legius E, et al. The behavioural phenotype in velo-cardio-facial syndrome (vcfs): From infancy to adolescence. Genet Couns 1999;10:79–88.

590. Niklasson, L, Rasmussen P, Oskarsdottir S, et al. Chromosome 22q11 deletion syndrome (catch 22): Neuropsychiatric and neuropsychological aspects. Dev Med Child Neurol 2002;44: 44–50.

591. Gerdes, M, Solot C, Wang PP, et al. Taking advantage of early diagnosis: Preschool children with the 22q11.2 deletion. Genet Med 2001;3:40–44.

592. Scherer, NJ, D'Antonio LL, Kalbfleisch JH. Early speech and language development in children with velocardiofacial syndrome. Am J Med Genet 1999;88:714–723.

593. Glaser, B, Mumme DL, Blasey C, et al. Language skills in children with velocardiofacial syndrome (deletion 22q11.2). J Pediatr 2002;140:753–758.

594. Moss, EM, Batshaw ML, Solot CB, et al. Psychoeducational profile of the 22q11.2 microdeletion: A complex pattern. J Pediatr 1999;134:193–198.

595. Gerdes, M, Solot C, Wang PP, et al. Cognitive and behavior profile of preschool children with chromosome 22q11.2 deletion. Am J Med Genet 1999;85:127–133.

596. Eliez, S, Schmitt JE, White CD, et al. Children and adolescents with velocardiofacial syndrome: A volumetric mri study. Am J Psychiatry 2000;157:409–415.

597. Eliez, S, Blasey CM, Schmitt EJ, et al. Velocardiofacial syndrome: Are structural changes in the temporal and mesial temporal regions related to schizophrenia? Am J Psychiatry 2001;158: 447–453.

598. De Smedt, B, Swillen A, Ghesquiere P, et al. Pre-academic and early academic achievement in children with velocardiofacial syndrome (del22q11.2) of borderline or normal intelligence. Genet Couns 2003;14:15–29.

599. Bearden, CE, Woodin MF, Wang PP, et al. The neurocognitive phenotype of the 22q11.2 deletion syndrome: Selective deficit in visual-spatial memory. J Clin Exp Neuropsychol 2001;23: 447–464.

600. Swillen, A, Vandeputte L, Cracco J, et al. Neuropsychological, learning and psychosocial profile of primary school aged children with the velo-cardio-facial syndrome (22q11 deletion): Evidence for a nonverbal learning disability? Neuropsychol Dev Cogn C Child Neuropsychol 1999;5:230–241.

601. Henry, JC, van Amelsvoort T, Morris RG, et al. An investigation of the neuropsychological profile in adults with velo-cardio-facial syndrome (vcfs). Neuropsychologia 2002;40:471–478.

602. Bearden, CE, Jawad AF, Lynch DR, et al. Effects of a functional comt polymorphism on prefrontal cognitive function in patients with 22q11.2 deletion syndrome. Am J Psychiatry 2004;161: 1700–1702.

603. Gothelf, D, Presburger G, Levy D, et al. Genetic, developmental, and physical factors associated with attention deficit hyperactiv-

ity disorder in patients with velocardiofacial syndrome. Am J Med Genet 2004;126B:116–121.

604. Arnold, PD, Siegel-Bartelt J, Cytrynbaum C, et al. Velo-cardio-facial syndrome: Implications of microdeletion 22q11 for schizophrenia and mood disorders. Am J Med Genet 2001;105: 354–362.

605. Sobin, C, Kiley-Brabeck K, Daniels S, et al. Networks of attention in children with the 22q11 deletion syndrome. Dev Neuropsychol 2004;26:611–626.

606. Sobin, C, Kiley-Brabeck K, Karayiorgou M. Associations between prepulse inhibition and executive visual attention in children with the 22q11 deletion syndrome. Mol Psychiatry 2005;10: 553–562.

607. Eliez, S, Palacio-Espasa F, Spira A, et al. Young children with velo-cardio-facial syndrome (catch-22). Psychological and language phenotypes. Eur Child Adolesc Psychiatry 2000;9:109–114.

608. Swillen, A, Devriendt K, Ghesquiere P, et al. Children with a 22q11 deletion versus children with a speech-language impairment and learning disability: Behavior during primary school age. Genet Couns 2001;12:309–317.

609. Heineman-de Boer, JA, Van Haelst MJ, Cordia-de Haan M, et al. Behavior problems and personality aspects of 40 children with velo-cardio-facial syndrome. Genet Couns 1999;10:89–93.

610. Papolos, DF, Faedda GL, Veit S, et al. Bipolar spectrum disorders in patients diagnosed with velo-cardio-facial syndrome: Does a hemizygous deletion of chromosome 22q11 result in bipolar affective disorder? Am J Psychiatry 1996;153:1541–1547.

611. Papolos, DF, Veit S, Faedda GL, et al. Ultra-ultra rapid cycling bipolar disorder is associated with the low activity catecholamine-o-methyltransferase allele. Mol Psychiatry 1998;3:346–349.

612. Lachman, HM, Kelsoe J, Moreno L, et al. Lack of association of catechol-o-methyltransferase (comt) functional polymorphism in bipolar affective disorder. Psychiatr Genet 1997;7:13–17.

613. Gothelf, D, Presburger G, Zohar AH, et al. Obsessive-compulsive disorder in patients with velocardiofacial (22q11 deletion) syndrome. Am J Med Genet 2004;126B:99–105.

614. Murphy, KC, Jones LA, Owen MJ. High rates of schizophrenia in adults with velo-cardio-facial syndrome. Arch Gen Psychiatry 1999;56:940–945.

615. Pulver, AE, Nestadt G, Goldberg R, et al. Psychotic illness in patients diagnosed with velo-cardio-facial syndrome and their relatives. J Nerv Ment Dis 1994;182:476–478.

616. Murphy, KC, Owen MJ. Velo-cardio-facial syndrome: A model for understanding the genetics and pathogenesis of schizophrenia. Br J Psychiatry 2001;179:397–402.

617. Sugama, S, Namihira T, Matsuoka R, et al. Psychiatric inpatients and chromosome deletions within 22q11.2. J Neurol Neurosurg Psychiatry 1999;67:803–806.

618. Arinami, T, Ohtsuki T, Takase K, et al. Screening for 22q11 deletions in a schizophrenia population. Schizophr Res 2001;52: 167–170.

619. Liu, H, Heath SC, Sobin C, et al. Genetic variation at the 22q11 prodh2/dgcr6 locus presents an unusual pattern and increases susceptibility to schizophrenia. Proc Natl Acad Sci U S A 2002; 99:3717–3722.

620. Liu, H, Abecasis GR, Heath SC, et al. Genetic variation in the 22q11 locus and susceptibility to schizophrenia. Proc Natl Acad Sci U S A 2002;99:16864–16864.

621. Eliez, S, Schmitt JE, White CD, et al. A quantitative mri study of posterior fossa development in velocardiofacial syndrome. Biol Psychiatry 2001;49:540–546.

622. van Amelsvoort, T, Daly E, Robertson D, et al. Structural brain abnormalities associated with deletion at chromosome 22q11: Quantitative neuroimaging study of adults with velo-cardio-facial syndrome. Br J Psychiatry 2001;178:412–419.

623. Chow, EW, Mikulis DJ, Zipursky RB, et al. Qualitative mri findings in adults with 22q11 deletion syndrome and schizophrenia. Biological Psychiatry 1999;157:409–415.

624. Mitnick, RJ, Bello JA, Shprintzen RJ. Brain anomalies in velo-cardio-facial syndrome. Am J Med Genet 1994;54:100–106.

625. Lynch, DR, McDonald-McGinn DM, Zackai EH, et al. Cerebellar atrophy in a patient with velocardiofacial syndrome. J Med Genet 1995;32:561–563.

626. van Amelsvoort, T, Daly E, Henry J, et al. Brain anatomy in adults with velocardiofacial syndrome with and without schizophrenia: Preliminary results of a structural magnetic resonance imaging study. Arch Gen Psychiatry 2004;61:1085–1096.

627. Bird, LM, Scambler P. Cortical dysgenesis in 2 patients with chromosome 22q11 deletion. Clin Genet 2000;58:64–68.

628. Bingham, PM, Lynch D, McDonald-McGinn D, et al. Polymicrogyria in chromosome 22 delection syndrome. Neurology 1998; 51:1500–1502.

629. Bingham, PM, Zimmerman RA, McDonald-McGinn D, et al. Enlarged sylvian fissures in infants with interstitial deletion of chromosome 22q11. Am J Med Genet 1997;74:538–543.

630. Vataja, R, Elomaa E. Midline brain anomalies and schizophrenia in people with catch 22 syndrome. Br J Psychiatry 1998;172: 518–520.

631. Nopoulos, PC, Giedd JN, Andreasen NC, et al. Frequency and severity of enlarged cavum septi pellucidi in childhood-onset schizophrenia. Am J Psychiatry 1998;155:1074–1079.

632. Nopoulos, P, Krie A, Andreasen NC. Enlarged cavum septi pellucidi in patients with schizophrenia: Clinical and cognitive correlates. J Neuropsychiatry Clin Neurosci 2000;12:344–349.

633. Galarza, M, Merlo AB, Ingratta A, et al. Cavum septum pellucidum and its increased prevalence in schizophrenia: A neuroembryological classification. J Neuropsychiatry Clin Neurosci 2004;16:41–46.

634. Kasai, K, McCarley RW, Salisbury DF, et al. Cavum septi pellucidi in first-episode schizophrenia and first-episode affective psychosis: An mri study. Schizophr Res 2004;71:65–76.

635. Kwon, JS, Shenton ME, Hirayasu Y, et al. Mri study of cavum septi pellucidi in schizophrenia, affective disorder, and schizotypal personality disorder. Am J Psychiatry 1998;155:509–515.

636. Barnea-Goraly, N, Menon V, Krasnow B, et al. Investigation of white matter structure in velocardiofacial syndrome: A diffusion tensor imaging study. Am J Psychiatry 2003;160: 1863–1869.

637. Kates, WR, Burnette CP, Bessette BA, et al. Frontal and caudate alterations in velocardiofacial syndrome (deletion at chromosome 22q11.2). J Child Neurol 2004;19:337–342.

638. Eliez, S, Barnea-Goraly N, Schmitt JE, et al. Increased basal ganglia volumes in velo-cardio-facial syndrome (deletion 22q11.2). Biol Psychiatry 2002;52:68–70.

639. Shashi, V, Muddasani S, Santos CC, et al. Abnormalities of the corpus callosum in nonpsychotic children with chromosome 22q11 deletion syndrome. Neuroimage 2004;21:1399–1406.

640. Usiskin, SI, Nicolson R, Krasnewich DM, et al. Velocardiofacial syndrome in childhood-onset schizophrenia. J Am Acad Child Adolesc Psychiatry 1999;38:1536–1543.

641. Eliez, S, Blasey CM, Menon V, et al. Functional brain imaging study of mathematical reasoning abilities in velocardiofacial syndrome (del22q11.2). Genet Med 2001;3:49–55.

642. Kok, LL, Solman RT. Velocardiofacial syndrome: Learning difficulties and intervention. J Med Genet 1995;32:612–618.

643. Swillen, A, Devriendt K, Legius E, et al. Intelligence and psychosocial adjustment in velocardiofacial syndrome: A study of 37 children and adolescents with vcfs. J Med Genet 1997;34: 453–458.

644. Graf, WD, Unis AS, Yates CM, et al. Catecholamines in patients with 22q11.2 deletion syndrome and the low-activity comt polymorphism. Neurology 2001;57:410–416.

645. O'Hanlon, JF, Ritchie RC, Smith EA, et al. Replacement of antipsychotic and antiepileptic medication by l-alpha-methyldopa in a woman with velocardiofacial syndrome. Int Clin Psychopharmacol 2003;18:117–119.

646. Gothelf, D, Gruber R, Presburger G, et al. Methylphenidate treatment for attention-deficit/hyperactivity disorder in children and adolescents with velocardiofacial syndrome: An open-label study. J Clin Psychiatry 2003;64:1163–1169.

Genetic Syndromes

9

Chiara Pantaleoni, MD   *Stefano D'Arrigo, MD*
Sara Bulgheroni, DN   *Daria Riva, MD*

Genetic syndromes, also called dysmorphic-genetic syndromes, are complex conditions characterized by the association of genetic abnormalities with severe or mild dysmorphisms, in which staturo-ponderal growth problems, psychomotor delay, mental retardation, and behavioral disorders are frequent (1,2). Patients presenting these characteristics are often referred to a specialist in pediatric neurology or to a child psychiatry unit. Clearly, those operating in such settings need to possess specific diagnostic expertise, not only to ensure targeted therapeutic and rehabilitative interventions (3), but also to be able to inform families as to the risk of recurrence (4).

On a causal level, the various genetic syndromes can be secondary to chromosomal abnormalities, numerical or structural, or to the mutation of a single gene (5). Frequently, the underlying abnormality is not known and, without the opportunity for laboratory confirmation, the diagnosis is based exclusively on clinical data (6). Thus, diagnosing these syndromes means following a rigorous procedure in which the first step is collection of a detailed history of the family (reconstruction of the family tree must go back at least three generations) and of the patient himself: prenatal, neonatal, physiological, and pathological (7). This is followed by the clinical investigation, which involves not only neurological examination (including exploration of intellectual and behavioral aspects), but also assessment of dysmorphological features; that is, measurement of auxological parameters and careful detection of all those minor abnormalities (dysmorphisms) that constitute the gestalt of dysmorphic syndromes (8). It must be pointed out that the presence of a single minor abnormality cannot be deemed to have clinical significance; at least three are needed (9). It is also important to stress that the collection of photographic evidence is useful for reassessing a patient over time (10).

Once collection of the history is complete, a diagnostic hypothesis can be formulated, also with the help of special computerized systems such as the Possum database (11) and London Dysmorphology (12). These systems are undoubtedly important diagnostic aids but they are intended to be used by experts; that is, by those with specific expertise in selecting search criteria and in interpreting results (13).

At this point, instrumental investigations can be carried out, the choice of investigations being guided by the clinical suspicion. Of the various available instrumental tests, brain magnetic resonance imaging (MRI), to verify the presence of structural abnormalities of the central nervous system (14), and an electroencephalogram (EEG) are, in our view, indispensable. Neurophysiological investigations (evoked potentials, electromyography) may also be useful for diagnostic purposes and again must be performed to investigate a definite clinical suspicion. Similarly, the choice of tests for the diagnosis of metabolic diseases must be guided by the patient's clinical picture (15).

With regard to the more strictly genetic analyses, all patients with a suspected dysmorphic-genetic syndrome should undergo standard karyotype analysis at 500-band level (16). Importantly, given the rapid evolution of cytogenetic techniques, it may be deemed opportune to repeat this analysis if the last one performed dates back more than 5 years (17).

Cytogenetic analyses, such as high-resolution karyotype, fluorescence in situ hybridization (FISH), and karyotype analysis of dermal fibroblasts, are indicated only if performed in order to confirm a clinical suspicion (18).

Molecular analysis of DNA or RNA samples, conducted to identify the gene defect responsible for the disease, should be performed only to confirm a clinical hypothesis: the only exception to this is, in our view, molecular analysis for fragile-X syndrome, which is warranted in all cases of unclassified mental retardation, regardless of the sex of the patient (17).

The most recent evolutions in molecular cytogenetics and molecular biology have been directed toward two groups of genetic abnormalities: uniparental disomies and subtelomeric rearrangements. Uniparental disomy is present when a patient has inherited both copies (or parts thereof) of a particular chromosome from only one parent. In addition to patients suspected of having a clinical condition in which uniparental disomy is a known feature (Angelman syndrome, Prader-Willi syndrome), testing for uniparental disomy is also indicated in patients presenting association of mental retardation, dysmorphisms and growth delay (pre- or postnatal) of unknown etiology (17).

According to the most recent data, subtelomeric rearrangements are responsible for around 5% of cases of mental retardation (19). Screening for these rearrangements is indicated in the presence of several factors: family history of mental retardation, intrauterine growth delay, postnatal growth abnormalities (excessive or deficient growth), at least two facial dysmorphisms, one or more nonfacial dysmorphism and/or congenital malformations (19).

Recently a new technique, called microarray-based comparative genomic hybridization (array CGH) has been introduced, enabling analysis of the whole genome in a single experiment. It can be used for the screening of known submicroscopic aberrations in human genetic diseases, but is also suitable for identification of yet unidentified abnormalities (20).

Let us now consider the dysmorphic-genetic syndromes most frequently encountered by the pediatric neurologist.

FRAGILE-X SYNDROME

Fragile-X syndrome is the most frequent inherited cause of mental retardation: its prevalence has been estimated at around 1/2,000–1/3,000. The syndrome is caused by a mutation of the FMR1 (Fragile-X mental retardation 1) gene on chromosome X (X q27.3). The mutation is associated with expansion CGG repeats, which determines a deficit of FMR1-protein (21). FMR1 is, to date, the only gene known to be associated with fragile-X syndrome. Genetic tests for mutation of the gene generally focus on the number of CGG repeats, and the FMR1 alleles are usually categorized according to this number:

(a) Normal alleles: the number of repeats ranges from 5 to 44: normal alleles are transmitted without modification of the number of repeats
(b) Intermediate alleles: the number of repeats ranges from 45 to 58: transmission of intermediate alleles can (occasionally) result in slight modification of the number of repeats
(c) Premutation alleles: the number of repeats ranges from 59 to 200: females in this group are considered to be at risk of having affected offspring, due to a potential expansion of the number of repeats
(d) Full mutation alleles: over 200 repeats (22).

Fragile-X syndrome shows a clear genotype-phenotype correlation. In male full mutation patients (hemizygotes), the prepubertal clinical picture is characterized by psychomotor retardation, prevalently affecting language, and by craniofacial dysmorphisms: long face, prominent forehead, large or prominent ears, prognathism. Mental retardation is moderate (IQ 30–50). It is often associated with behavioral disorders: hypersensitivity to sensory stimuli, hyperactivity, stereotyped movements (hand flapping, hand biting), gaze avoidance, social anxiety. Some patients present some or all the symptoms of autism: Rogers et al (23), investigating a series of 27 fragile-X children, found that 8% fulfilled the diagnostic criteria for autism. On the other hand, the incidence of fragile-X syndrome in autistic patients has been reported, in different studies, to be between 2.5 and 6%. Although some of the symptoms appear very reminiscent of autism, one important behavioral difference does in fact separate these two groups of children: the ability of fragile-X children to recognize human facial expressions of emotion (an ability severely impaired in autistic children) has been shown to be comparable to that of the general population. This explains the tendency of the fragile-X child to maintain an adequate preferential relationship with his main caregivers.

Epileptic seizures are present in around 20% of patients (24): typically these have onset in early infancy, with children presenting generalized tonic-clonic, absence, partial motor, and temporal lobe seizures. The seizures generally respond to common antiepileptic medication and they occur less and less frequently over time, usually disappearing in adolescence (even though they can occasionally persist until adulthood). The main postpubertal phenotypic characteristics are macrocrania, strabismus, prognathism, macroorchidism, joint hyperextensibility, subluxation of the thumb, flat foot. The cognitive deficit persists and, from the behavioural point of view, it is possible to observe an increase of the hyperactivity and social anxiety, and onset of obsessive-compulsive disorder and, in the most severe cases, psychotic symptoms (25). Mitral valve prolapse has been observed in 50% of adult patients.

Female full mutation patients (heterozygotes) show similar (but less severe) physical and behavioral characteristics (26). Premutation patients generally have a normal appearance and normal intelligence. Some may present slight cognitive or behavioral disorders, learning difficulty and social anxiety.

Female premutation carriers can have a premature menopause, while a late-onset ataxic syndrome with tremor has been reported in premutation male carriers (27). Brain MRI can reveal cerebellar vermis hypoplasia and, more rarely, malformations of other areas: enlarged hippocampus, caudate nucleus and thalamus (28).

Finally, another condition, characterized by less severe mental delay and by less marked somatic traits, has been described in males with expansion of CCG repeats in the FRAXE fragile site (clearly distinct from FRAXA, the fragile site associated with the more common fragile-X syndrome) in the FMR2 gene. Given that mutations in FRAXE are far less common, routine testing for them in subjects with mental retardation is not deemed opportune. (29)

ANGELMAN SYNDROME

Angelman syndrome is a disease associated with a chromosome 15 (15q11–13) abnormality. In most cases this abnormality is a deletion of the maternal derived chromosome, while in 3 to 5% it is a paternal uniparental disomy (i.e., both the alleles of that specific location on chromosome 15 have been inherited from the father). In 4 to 6% of cases it is due to an imprinting center defect or to a defect of the E6-P ubiquitin-protein ligase (UBE3A) gene (30). The region 15q11–13 contains the genes for the subunits β3, α5 and γ3 of the receptor of the main inhibitory neurotransmitter system, gamma-aminobutyric acid type-A receptor (GABA(A)R.) (31). A link between the β3 subunit gene and susceptibility to autism has recently been suggested (32). In 20% of cases, no genetic abnormality is demonstrated and the diagnosis remains clinical. The prevalence of the disease is estimated at around 1/12,000. From a clinical point of view (33), patients present severe psychomotor retardation and gait ataxia: gait is stiff, extremely hesitant, and irregular. Impairment of language, mainly expressive language, is again a feature: nonverbal performances can vary widely; some children are able to learn sign language and to use alternative methods of communication. A frank behavioral disorder constitutes another constant feature: these children have been dubbed "happy puppets" on account of their manner; they are typically cheerful, excitable, hyperactive and inattentive, a profile associated with stereotyped "hand fluttering" movements. More than 80% of patients also present acquired microcephaly, epilepsy and a characteristic EEG pattern (high-amplitude slow-wave activities prominent in the frontal region and spike-and-slow-wave multifocal activity prominent in occipitofrontal areas). Epileptic seizures generally have onset after the first year of life, usually after the age of three years. Patients with the deletion may present drug-resistant epilepsy, characterized by atypical absence or myoclonic seizures (34). Brain MRI generally confirms the finding of microcephaly, but fails to reveal other abnormalities, with the exception of mild cortical atrophy, mild ventriculomegaly, and thin corpus callosum. Other findings occasionally described include cerebellar hypoplasia, unilateral temporal lobe hypoplasia, and vermian cysts (33).

Less common signs (20 to 80% of cases) include flat occiput, strabismus, macrostomia, widely spaced teeth, prominent jaw and hypopigmentation of skin and eyes.

From a behavioral point of view, these subjects display hypersensitivity to heat, attraction to water, and a sleep disorder characterized by reduced need for sleep and altered sleep-wake rhythms. Some behavioral aspects of the syndrome fulfill perfectly two of the DSM-IV classification's three essential criteria for autism: stereotyped behaviors and absence of language (35). Social interaction appears to be relatively conserved in these children, and they seek relationships with others. Williams et al. (36), in a report on the differential diagnosis of the syndrome, maintains that children with a clinical diagnosis of Angelman syndrome who give negative results in genetic laboratory tests for the four known types of genetic anomaly must be considered affected by a pervasive developmental disorder not otherwise specified (PDD NOS), in accordance with the criteria of the DSM-IV. Longitudinal evaluation of these children in fact revealed that the phenotypic characteristics of the syndrome became less clearly defined over the years, while the opposite was true of the behavioral disorder.

WILLIAMS SYNDROME

Williams syndrome is due to a submicroscopic deletion of a segment of chromosome 7 (7q11.23): the deleted region spans approximately 1.5 megabases and 14 genes have been mapped to it. Many of the syndrome's clinical manifestations are caused by the deletion of the elastin (ELN) gene, which results in abnormal elastin production and thus connective tissue alterations (37). LIM kinase 1 (LIMK1), a gene contiguous to ELN, is the second gene recognized as implicated in the syndrome. In particular, the cognitive profile of the syndrome seems to be attributable to the deletion of LIMK1: the gene is expressed at brain level and could be involved in the development of the neural pathways responsible for visuospatial integration. The true prevalence of the syndrome is not known, although it is estimated to be between 1/10,000 and 1/20,000. Clinical diagnosis is made on the basis of the presence of a characteristic pattern of facial dysmorphisms, mental retardation, short stature, connective tissue abnormalities, a distinctive cognitive profile and typical behavioral phenotype. The facial characteristics are distinctive: younger children present a broad forehead with bitemporal narrowing bilaterally, periorbital edema, stellate iris, strabismus, low-set nasal root, bulbous nasal tip, flattened cheekbones, prominent earlobes, long philtrum, wide mouth and full lips, patho-occlusion with small widely-spaced teeth, and micrognathia. In older children and adults, there are other distinctive features (prominent supraorbital ridge, narrowing of the nasal root and long neck) and the face has, overall, a less chubby appearance. The main connective tissue abnormality is a cardiovascular alteration, in most cases supravalvular aortic stenosis; other possible findings include vesical or intestinal diverticula, hernias, joint laxity, phonation disorder (i.e., deep voice), and loose skin. The earliest reports consistently described idiopathic hypercalcemia, but this is actually documented in only 15% of cases.

From the neurological viewpoint, hypotonia is a common early sign, which can be followed at a later stage by limb hypertonia and hyperreflexia. Brain MRI can reveal reduced cerebral volume, while the cerebellum is normal size; it is even possible to observe hyperplasia of the cerebellar vermis lobules VI-VII and VIII-X (38); sporadic cases of associated Chiari I malformation (39) and of cerebrovascular accidents attributable to multiple intracranial arterial stenoses (40) have also been reported. We described a personal case of Williams syndrome with olygogyric microcephaly (41).

Most affected subjects present mental retardation ranging from severe to mild (the latter being relatively more frequent). The cognitive phenotype is extremely distinctive (42): in intelligence scales, high scores are recorded on the verbal subtests, exceeding IQ-based expectations, good scores on the sentence repetition memory tests, and lower-than-expected scores on the nonverbal tests; there also emerges a significant impairment of visuospatial organization and integration (43). Writing and drawing skills are found to be significantly impaired, as is the ability to reconstruct models. Since visuomotor skills are processed by the occipital-parietal visual pathway, it is possible, in this syndrome, to hypothesize gene involvement in the development of this neural circuit. Conversely, visuoperceptual abilities, processed by the occipital-temporal pathway, are relatively spared (44).

The behavioral profile is distinctive: a high percentage of cases present an attention disorder which may or may not be associated with hyperactivity (45) and an excessively sociable and friendly attitude to strangers. Compared with other children of similar intelligence, the incidence of behavioral problems (such as anxiety, worry, attention deficit) in these subjects is high; they also show impaired capacity for autonomy.

VELO-CARDIO-FACIAL SYNDROME

This syndrome, which shows marked phenotypic variability, is caused by a microdeletion of Chr 22q 11.2, and characterized by involvement of the face, palate and heart, as well as possible involvement of other organs (46). Its prevalence is difficult to establish, partly because the condition has been called by different names (DiGeorge sequence, CATCH 22, Shprintzen syndrome); nevertheless, its prevalence is estimated to be around 1/4,000. Although more than 150 clinical characteristics have been reported in connection with this syndrome, none has been found to be present in 100% of the cases and thus pathognomic; but several characteristics do give rise to clinical suspicion: in particular, in small children, the association of palatoschisis with conotruncal cardiac defects. The most common cardiac malformations are alterations of the aortic arch, ventricular septal defects, pulmonary atresia or stenosis, and tetralogy of Fallot. The suspicion becomes stronger if these signs are associated with other malformations such as facial asymmetry, hypocalcemia, equinus foot, laryngoma-lacia, inguinal or umbilical hernias, and hypospadia. Later on, the clinical phenotype becomes even more evident, thanks in particular to the appearance of the classic behavioral and personality traits. Mental delay is found in only a minority of patients, and IQ is generally borderline or slightly below normal. Children initially present psychomotor retardation, but good recovery around the age of four years. A language delay is also present, attributable in part to the phonation and articulation problems caused by the malformations. The psychiatric disorders evident in the affected adult are preceded by prodromes in childhood: attention deficit with hyperactivity, obsessive-compulsive disorder, dysthymia and cyclothymia. Bipolar disorder and schizophrenia have also been reported in adults and in general it is estimated that around 20% of affected subjects present psychosis in adulthood. In a recent study (47), brain MR investigations in patients affected by the syndrome have revealed structural abnormalities in the temporal and temporomesial regions also involved in schizophrenia. It is thus suggested that the effects of deletion 22q11.2 and the complex pathogenetic alterations underlying schizophrenia share a common etiology.

From the neurological point of view, epileptic seizures can present even as an early manifestation of the syndrome, generally symptomatic of hypocalcemia, stroke or cortical atrophy; febrile convulsions are also common. Other common neurological signs are chronic lower limb pain and nocturnal leg cramps; tethered cord has been found in some cases, while equinus-varus deformity of the foot is present in around 10%.

SMITH-MAGENIS SYNDROME

Smith-Magenis syndrome is due to an interstitial deletion of the short arm of chromosome 17 (17p11.2); its prevalence is estimated to be around 1/25,000. The symptomatic phenotype varies with age: in infancy (0–3 years), facial dysmorphisms are very mild, the face having a characteristic "cherubic" appearance, with full, prominent cheeks, upslanting palpebral fissures, depressed nasal root, and micrognathia (48). The shape of the mouth is very distinctive, with a "Cupid's bow" upper lip and pronounced philtrum. In childhood (3–10 years), the facial traits become coarser and "Down's-like" owing to hypotonic facial muscles, brachycephaly, flattened face, and short broad nose. After the age of 10 years, the facial traits become even more distinctive: facial hypoplasia and a wide, prognathic jaw (49). The cognitive phenotype is characterized by mental retardation of extremely variable degree: patients with borderline IQ have been reported, but also ones with very low IQ. As regards to language, impairment of expressive language predominates. The behavioral phenotype is very distinctive: maladaptive disorders are reported, such as self-harm, impulsivity, rage attacks, and onychotillomania. These are also associated with stereotyped behaviors: the self-hugging phenomenon is common, but these subjects can also present body rocking and object spinning. Udwin et al. (50), studying 50 patients, and Willekens et al. (51), studying a sample of just 3, both encountered very clinging and dependent behaviors, toward both family members and strangers: this finding allows this syndrome to be distinguished from classic autism.

Epileptic seizures are present in 10 to 30% of cases, while EEG abnormalities in the absence of seizures are reported in around 20%. In 75% of cases, there are clinical signs of peripheral neuropathy: anatomical-pathological studies highlight a picture of segmental demyelination and remyelination similar to that found in hereditary Carchot-Marie-Tooth 1A (CMT1A) neuropathy, although the PMP22 mutation typical of CMT1A is not found in patients with Smith-Magenis syndrome. Brain MRI can reveal cerebral malformations: ventriculomegaly, mega cisterna magna, cerebellar vermis hypoplasia (49).

CHROMOSOME 15 INVERSION-DUPLICATION SYNDROME

Chromosome 15 inversion-duplication (inv-dup 15) syndrome is a genetic condition that can, in most cases, be diagnosed with standard karyotype analysis. The syndrome is characterized by psychomotor retardation, ranging from mild to severe, hypotonia, and ataxia and dyspraxia. Many affected subjects are epileptic, presenting generalized myoclonic or atonic seizures, or focal seizures. These patients show a measure of resistance to antiepileptic drug therapy. Not all patients have epileptic seizures, but even those who do not present them typically have an electroencephalogram showing diffuse rapid activity and focal paroxysms bilaterally (52). These patients are also characterized by mild facial dysmorphisms: flat nasal root with upslanting nostrils, downslanting palpebral fissues, migrognathia, low-set ears, and flat occiput. These patients typically show an autistic-like behavioral phenotype. A recent study (53) examined six patients with inv-dup 15 syndrome: two fulfilled the diagnostic criteria for classic autism, while the other four were diagnosed with PDD NOS in accordance with the DSM-IV criteria. These patients indeed presented severe impairment of social interaction and communication, but no repetitive or stereotyped behaviors were either reported or observed. Brain MRI in these patients generally gave normal findings, even though there exist sporadic reports of mild cerebral atrophy (53).

OTHER SYNDROMES

We will now describe some of the peculiar characteristics of syndromes sometimes brought to the attention of pediatric neurologists due to the presence of neurological, cognitive, and behavioral signs: Rett syndrome, which the DSM-IV classifies under Pervasive Developmental Disorders, and the syndromes of Turner, Sotos, Cohen, and Noonan.

Rett syndrome is a genetic condition associated with various mutations of the MECP2 gene on chromosome X. The syndrome has an estimated prevalence of 1/10,000, and typically (but not exclusively) affects females, who, in the classic form, present a typically autistic phenotype (54). These patients' most striking phenotypic characteristic is their gentle gaze and dreamy expression. Their laughter is distinctive, typically having a circadian pattern of manifestation and occurring prevalently in the evening, which contrasts with the laughter in patients with Angelman syndrome in whom it is practically constant (throughout the day). In classic Rett syndrome, language is absent, but there exists a variant form in which patients do acquire, over time, the ability to produce simple or even more structured sentences; this growing ability being accompanied by a reduction in their stereotyped hand movements (55).

Turner syndrome, which has a prevalence of 1/5,000, is due to the loss of part or all of the second X chromosome (45X0), frequently accompanied by cell-line mosaicism. Features of the syndrome are: low birthweight, neonatal lymphoedema of the extremities, low stature, pterygium colli, broad chest, valgus deformity of the upper limbs, cardiac malformations (bicuspid aortic valve, mitral valve prolapse, coarctation of the aorta), kidney malformations, primary amenorrhoea and sterility. IQ is generally normal, although visuospatial organization difficulties have been reported. Brain MRI gives normal findings (56).

Sotos syndrome (prevalence 1/100,000) is characterized by accelerated somatic growth, which is most marked in the first five years of life. Children affected by Sotos syndrome present dolichocephaly and macrocephaly, frontal bossing, high forehead, downslanting palpebral fissures and prognathism. Bone age is typically, although not necessarily, higher than chronological age. Patients can be cognitively normal or present an intellectual impairment of varying degree (ranging from mild to severe). From the behavioral point of view, they can present phobic traits, sleep disorders, hyperphagia, and aggressiveness. Morrow et al. (57) described an autistic disorder in a child with Sotos syndrome. Around 50% of patients present a genetic abnormality (deletion or intragenic mutation) of the long arm of chromosome 5 (5q35). The neuroradiological findings include ventriculomegaly and midline defects (hypoplasia of the corpus callosum) (58).

Howlin (59) found a diagnosis of autism in 19 out of 33 patients affected by Cohen syndrome, a condition characterized by low birthweight, microcephaly and psychomotor retardation of varying degree (ranging from mild to severe). The prevalence of Cohen syndrome is 1/100,000. Patients present maxillary hypoplasia, large ears, prominent upper incisors, tapered fingers, trunk obesity and scoliosis. They may also present neutropenia and chorioretinal dystrophy or optic atrophy. The syndrome is caused by a mutation in the COH1 gene on chromosome 8 (8q22).

Central nervous system abnormalities are not generally reported, even though a case with focal polymicrogyria was recently described (60).

Another frequent syndrome is Noonan's syndrome. Known to have a prevalence 1/2,000, it is characterized by short stature, pterygium colli, epicanthic folds, low-set and malformed ears, micrognathia, and association, in 50% to 80% of cases, with congenital cardiopathy (frequently pulmonary stensosis). Patients are cognitively normal, or may present a mild-moderate cognitive deficit. Behavioral disorders include sleep disorder and aggressiveness, anxiety, and an association with autism has also been described (61). Fifty percent of cases present a missense mutation of the PTPN11 gene on chromosome 12 (12q24.1). From the neuroradiological point of view, the syndrome may present associations with syringomyelia, Chiari I malformation, Dandy-Walker syndrome, and arteriovenous malformations.

REFERENCES

1. Gorlin RJ, Cohen MM Jr, Hennekam RCM, eds. Syndromes of the head and neck. 4th ed. New York: Oxford University Press, 2001.
2. Jones KL, ed. Smith's recognizable pattern of human malformations. 5th ed. Philadelphia: WB Saunders, 1997.
3. Cassidy SB, Allanson JE, eds. Management of genetic syndromes. New York: John Wiley & Sons, 2001.
4. Hunter AGW. Medical genetics: 2. The diagnostic approach to the child with dysmorphic signs. CMAJ 2002;167:367–372.
5. Hunter AGW. Outcome of the routine assessment of patients with mental retardation in a genetic clinic. Am J Med Genet 2000;90: 60–68.
6. Van Buggenhout GJ, van Ravenswaaij-Arts C, Mieloso H, et al. Dysmorphology and mental retardation: molecular cytogenetic studies in dysmorphic mentally retarded patients. Ann Genet 2001;44:89–92.
7. Sullivan PK, Tattini CD. Early evaluation and management of craniofacial dysmorphology. Med Health RI 2001;84:392–394.
8. Merks JHM, van Karnebeek CDM, Caron HN, et al. Phenotypic abnormalities: terminology and classifications. Am J Med Genet 2003;123A:211–230.
9. Winter RB, Donnai D, eds. Congenital malformation syndromes. London: Chapman & Hall Medical, 1995.
10. Dysmorphology Subcommittee of the Clinical Practice Committee, American College of Medical Genetics. Informed consent for medical photographs. Dysmorphology Subcommittee of the Clinical Practice Committee, American College of Medical Genetics. Genet Med 2000;2:353–355.
11. POSSUM. Version 5.6 Melbourne (Australia): Murdoch Institute, 2002.
12. Winter RM, Baraister M. Dysmorphology photo library on CD-ROM. Version 2.2. Oxford Medical Databases. Oxford: Oxford University Press, 2000.
13. Pelz J, Arendt V, Kunze J. Computer assisted diagnosis of malformation syndromes: an evaluation of three databases (LDDB, POSSUM and SYNDROC). Am J Med Genet 1996;63:257–267.
14. Battaglia A. Neuroimaging studies in the evaluation of developmental delay/mental retardation. Am J Med Genet 2003;117C: 25–30.
15. Ayme S. Bridging the gap between molecular genetics and metabolic medicine: access to genetic information. Eur J Pediatr 2000;159:S183–185.
16. Battaglia A, Carey JC. Diagnostic evaluation of developmental delay/mental retardation. Am J Med Genet 2003;117C:3–14.
17. Curry CJ, Stevenson RE, Aughton D, et al. Evaluation of mental retardation: recommendations of a consensus conference. Am J Med Genet 1997;72:468–477.
18. Stevenson RE, Procopio-Allen AM, Schroer RJ et al. Genetic syndromes among individuals with mental retardation. Am J Med Genet 2003;123A:29–32.
19. de Vries BBA, Winter R, Schinzel A, et al. Telomeres: a diagnosis at the end of the chromosome. J Med Genet 2003;40:385–398.
20. Vissers LE, de Vries BB, Osoegawa K, et al. Array-based comparative genomic hybridization for the genomewide detection of submicroscopic chromosomal abnormalities. Am J Hum Genet 2003; 73:1261–1270.
21. Oostra BA, Willemsen R. The X chromosome and fragile X mental retardation. Cytogenet Genome Res 2002;99:257–264.
22. Song FJ, Barton P, Sleightholme V, et al. Screening for fragile X syndrome: a literature review and modelling study. Health Technol Assess 2003;7:1–106.
23. Rogers SJ, Wehner DE, Hagerman R. The behavioral phenotype in fragile X: symptoms of autism in very young children with fragile X syndrome, idiopathic autism, and other developmental disorders. J Dev Behav Pediatr 2001;22:409–417.
24. Musumeci SA, Hagerman RS, Ferri R, et al. Epilepsy and EEG findings in males with fragile X syndrome. Epilepsia 1999;40: 1092–1099.
25. Hatton HH, Hooper SR, Bailey DB, et al. Problem behavior in boys with fragile X syndrome. Am J Med Genet 2002;108: 105–116.
26. Hessl D, Dyer-Fiedman J, Glaser B, et al. The influence of environmental and genetic factors on behavior problems and autistic symptoms in boys and girls with fragile X syndrome. Pediatrics 2001;108:E88.
27. Brunberg JA, Jacquemont S, Hagerman RJ, et al. Fragile X permutations carriers: characteristic MR imaging findings of adult male patients with progressive cerebellar and cognitive dysfunctions. Am J Neuroradiol 2002;23:1757–1766.
28. Eliez S, Blasey CM, Freund LS, et al. Brain anatomy, gender and IQ in children and adolescents with fragile X syndrome. Brain 2001; 124:1610–1618.
29. Brown TW. The FRAXE syndrome: is it time for routine screening? Am J Hum Genet 1996;58:903–905,
30. Nurmi EL, Bradford Y, Chen Y, et al. Linkage disequilibrium at the Angelman syndrome gene UBE3A in autism families. Genomics 2001;77:105–113.
31. Sinkkonen ST, Homanics GE, Korpi ER. Mouse models of Angelman syndrome, a neurodevelopmental disorder, display different brain regional GABA(A) receptor alterations. Neurosci Lett 2003; 17:205–208.
32. Buxbaum JD, Silverman JM, Smith CJ, et al. Association between a GABRB3 polymorphism and autism. Mol Psychiatry 2002;7: 311–316.
33. Clayton-Smith J, Laan L. Angelman syndrome: a review of the clinical and genetics aspects. J Med Genet 2003;40:87–95.
34. Buoni S, Grosso S, Pucci L. Diagnosis of Angelman syndrome: clinical and EEG criteria. Brain Dev 1999;21:296–302.
35. Steffenburg, S, Gillberg CL, Steffenburg U, et al. Autism in Angelman syndrome: a population-based study. Pediatr Neurol 1996; 14:131–136.
36. Williams CA, Lossie A, Driscoll D. Angelman syndrome: mimicking conditions and phenotypes. Am J Med Genet 2001;101: 59–64.
37. Bayes M, Magano LF, Rivera N, et al. Mutational mechanism of Williams-Beuren syndrome deletions. Am J Hum Genet 2003;73; 131–151.
38. Schmitt JE, Eliez S, Warsofsky IS, et al. Enlarged cerebellar vermis in Williams syndrome. J Psychiatr Res 2001;35:225–229.
39. Wang PP, Hesselink JR, Jernigan TL, et al. Specific neurobehavioral profile of Williams syndrome is associated with neocerebellar hemispheric preservation. Neurology 1992;42:1999–2002
40. Wollack JB, Kaifer M, LaMonte MP, et al. Stroke in Williams syndrome. Stroke 1996;27:143–146.
41. Faravelli F, D'Arrigo S, Bagnasco I, et al. Olygogyric microcephaly in a child with Williams syndrome. Am J Med Genet 2003;117A: 169–171.
42. Levy Y, Bechar T. Cognitive, lexical and morpho-syntactit profiles of Israeli children with Williams syndrome. Cortex 2003;39: 255–271.

43. Farran EK, Jarrold C. Visuospatial cognition in Williams syndrome: reviewing and accounting for the strengths and weaknesses in performance. Dev Neuropsychol 2003;23:173–200.

44. Atkinson J, Braddick O, Anker S, et al. Neurobiological models of visuospatial cognition in children with Williams syndrome: measures of dorsal-stream and frontal function. Dev Neuropsychol 2003;23:139–172.

45. Greer MK, Brown FR, Pai GS, et al. Cognitive, adaptative and behavioral characteristics of Williams syndrome. Am J Med Genet 1997;4:521–525.

46. Perez E, Sullivan KE. Chromosome 22q11.2 deletion sindrome (DiGeorge and velocardiofacial syndromes). Curr Opin Pediatr 2002;14:678–683.

47. Eliez S, Blasey CM, Schmitt Ej, et al. velocardiofacial syndrome: are structural changes in the temporal and mesial temporal regions related to schizophrenia? Am J Psychiatry 2001;158:447–453.

48. Potocki L, Shaw CJ, Stankiewicz P, et al. Variability in clinical phenotype despite common chromosoamal deletion in Smith-Magenis sindrome [del(17)(p11.2p11.2)]. Genet Med 2003;5:430–434.

49. Greenberg F, Lewis RA, Potocki L, et al. Multi-disciplinary clinical study of Smith-Magenis syndrome (deletion 17p11.2). Am J Med Genet 1996;62:247–254.

50. Udwin O, Webber C, Horn I. Abilities and attainment in Smith-Magenis syndrome. Dev Med Child Neurol 2001;43:823–828.

51. Willekens D, De Cock P, Fryns JP. Three young children with Smith-Magenis syndrome: their distinct, recognisable behavioural

52. Buoni S, Sorrentino L, Farnetani MA, et al. The syndrome of Inv Dup (15): clinical, electroencephalographic, and imaging findings. J Child Neurol 2000;15:380–385.

53. Borgatti R, Piccinelli P, Passoni D, et al. Relationship between clinical and genetic features in "inverted-duplicated chromosome 15" patients. Pediatr Neurol 2001;24:111–116.

54. Mount RH, Charman T, Hastings RP, et al. Features of autism in Rett syndrome and severe mental retardation. J Autism Dev Disord 2003;33:435–442.

55. Zappella M, Meloni I, Longo I, et al. Preserved speech variants of the Rett syndrome: molecular and clinical analysis. Am J Med Genet 2001;104:14–22.

56. Ranke MB, Saenger P. Turner's syndrome. Lancet 2001;358:309–314.

57. Morrow JD, Whitman BY, Accardo PJ. Autistic disorder in Sotos syndrome: a case report. Eur J Pediatr 1990;149:567–569.

58. Schaefer GB, Bodesteiner JB, Buehler BA, et al. The neuroimaging findings in Sotos syndrome. Am J Med Genet 1997;68:462–465.

59. Howlin P. Autistic features in Cohen syndrome: a preliminary report. Dev Med Child Neurol 2001;43:692–696.

60. Coppola G, Federico RR, Epifanio G, et al. Focal polymicrogyria, continuous spike-and-wave discharges during slow-wave sleep and Cohen syndrome: a case report. Brain Dev 2003;25:446–449.

61. Ghaziuddin M, Bolyard B, Alessi N. Autistic disorder in Noonan syndrome. J Intellect Disabil Res 1994;38:67–72.

phenotype as the most important clinical symptoms. Genet Couns 2000;11:103–110.

10

Neuropsychiatric Aspects of Autistic Spectrum Disorders and Childhood-Onset Schizophrenia

Natacha Akshoomoff, PhD

The autistic spectrum disorders and childhood-onset schizophrenia are complex disabling neuropsychiatry disorders. Children with schizophrenia share some symptoms with, and may be mistaken for, children who suffer from autistic spectrum disorders, which are more common. The pervasive and disabling symptoms associated with these disorders typically necessitate lifelong specialized educational, family, and adult services which cost billions of dollars each year. Early identification and effective interventions can potentially reduce human suffering and costs with the potential of significantly improved functioning and personal independence for individuals with these disorders. As will be discussed in this chapter, recent studies have identified a number of brain development abnormalities and genetic factors associated with these disorders.

Childhood-onset schizophrenia (COS) has been recognized since before the time of Kraeplin (1). It is a rare but disabling condition. Both Kanner (2) and Asperger (3) independently provided the first accounts of autism, describing children with a "disturbance of contact," unusual communication skills, and movement stereotypes, with an onset of symptoms before age three. Despite the notice paid to Kanner's landmark paper, autistic disorder was not formally distinguished from COS for many years. In the

DSM-II (4), the diagnosis of childhood-onset schizophrenia included all psychiatric disorders in children as well as autistic disorder. Autistic disorder and childhood-onset schizophrenia were separately classified with the publication of the DSM-III (5) after studies made it clear that the symptoms of childhood schizophrenia are much more similar to those of adult-onset schizophrenia than autistic disorder (6, 7). The history of the concept of COS has been reviewed in more detail elsewhere (e.g., 1, 8, 9).

AUTISTIC SPECTRUM DISORDERS

In the past, autism was viewed as a very rare disorder (estimated 4 to 5 per 10,000 births). Autism is now more commonly seen as part of a spectrum of disorders with significant social deficits and the presence of repetitive behaviors and restricted interests (10–12). Variations in severity, particularly with regard to a history of early language delays and degree of communication difficulties, are the primary differences in the criteria for the autistic spectrum disorders, which include Autistic Disorder, Asperger's Disorder, and Pervasive Developmental Disorder-NOS (PDD-NOS) and which are included as pervasive developmental disorders in DSM-IV-TR (13).

Recent epidemiological studies suggest that the prevalence of autistic spectrum disorders is approximately 60 per 10,000, while the prevalence of Autistic Disorder specifically is estimated to be 8 to 30 per 10,000 (14–17). From a clinical and service perspective, there are many more children identified with "autism" today than 10 or 20 years ago. This increased rate of referrals has led parents, clinicians, researchers, and the public to question a possible "epidemic" of autism. Although recent epidemiological studies have generally been in agreement regarding the best estimate for the prevalence of autism and related disorders (15), the precise estimate is difficult to determine due to changing definitions of the disorders and differences in survey methodology (e.g., studies using multiple sources of ascertainment and direct diagnostic procedures yield higher rates). The National Center on Birth Defects and Developmental Disabilities (a division of the Centers for Disease Control and Prevention) is developing a surveillance system which will ultimately provide more reliable epidemiological data (18).

Diagnosis and Appropriate Assessment Strategies

The DSM-IV-TR (13) criteria for autistic disorder require that the individual exhibits six (or more) symptoms, with at least two in the area of social interaction (e.g., impaired use of nonverbal behaviors to regulate social interaction, such as eye-to-eye gaze or gestures; failure to develop peer relationships appropriate to developmental level), one in the area of communication (e.g., delay in the development of language; impaired ability to initiate or sustain conversation), and one in the area of restricted repetitive and stereotyped patterns of behavior (e.g., motor mannerisms; restricted interests; inflexible adherence to routines). Prior to age 3, the child must have exhibited abnormal functioning in social interaction, language as used for social communication, or symbolic/imaginative play. Lower functioning and younger individuals tend to be more aloof in social interactions (such as those described by Kanner), while higher functioning and older individuals are more likely to be described as passive or odd (19). Autistic disorder is more common in males than females (approximately 4:1) and the majority of individuals have Intelligence Quotient (IQ) and adaptive behavior skills that fall in the mentally retarded range (IQ <70).

The diagnosis of PDD-NOS (or "atypical autism") is used with those individuals who do not meet criteria for autistic disorder but exhibit at least two symptoms in the area of social interaction and one in the area of communication or one in the area of restricted repetitive and stereotyped patterns of behavior. This diagnosis is often used to describe very young children who appear to have autism. As children get older, it does appear to be a fitting description for children with the social deficits common to Autistic Disorder and Asperger's Disorder but who have fewer

repetitive behaviors, or high functioning children with early language delay or mild cognitive impairment (20).

The DSM-IV criteria for Asperger's Disorder require that the individual does not meet criteria for Autistic Disorder but exhibits at least two symptoms in the area of social interaction and one in the area of restricted repetitive and stereotyped patterns of behavior. Additional requirements are that the individual did not exhibit significant delays in language (i.e., single words used by age 2 years, communicative phrases used by age 3 years) and does not have delayed cognitive skills. If strict DSM-IV-TR criteria are applied, a diagnosis of Asperger's disorder becomes unlikely (21–24). This issue has led researchers and clinicians to adopt the term *Asperger syndrome* to distinguish those individuals who share many of the features of autism but who had relative preservation of language and cognitive abilities early in life. The direct clinical or educational benefits of this distinction from "high functioning autism" are not yet clear (25–27). Most individuals with Asperger syndrome are not identified with significant difficulties until after age 3, most commonly after having attended school (28). While formal language skills are normal and may develop early, individuals with Asperger syndrome have more difficulty understanding the nuances of language and the use of language in social interactions ("pragmatics"). These children typically appear to want to interact with others but tend to do so in odd, unusual, awkward, and inappropriate ways. Most of these individuals are highly verbal and have a tendency to become very interested in and preoccupied with particular subjects, which can interfere with other activities and social relationships. They are often less anxious when they can adhere to specific routines and may have difficulty with change.

The American Academy of Neurology and the Child Neurology Society have jointly developed a guideline on screening and diagnosis for autism (29). Based upon the empirical evidence, the guideline gives specific recommendations for a dual process:

1. Routine developmental surveillance screening specifically for autism should be performed (using recommended instruments) on all children to identify those at risk for any type of atypical development (especially siblings of children with autism), and to identify those specifically at risk for autism:
   a) screening (with either the CHAT (30) or the Social Communication Questionnaire (31) specifically for autism should be performed on all children failing routine developmental surveillance.
   b) recommended laboratory investigations for any child with developmental delay or autism should include audiologic assessment and lead screening.
2. Specific assessments should be performed to diagnose and evaluate autism, including genetic testing (e.g., karotype and DNA analysis for fragile X) and selective metabolic testing as indicated by clinical findings. Routine clinical brain imaging is not recommended (even in

the presence of megalencephaly) and EEG should be reserved for patients with a regression (see below) or possible seizures. There is inadequate evidence supporting other laboratory studies.

Much progress has been made in the early identification of children with autism so that most children today are identified during the preschool period (29, 32–34). Earlier identification is related to improvements in the recognition of the early features of autism among primary health care providers and other professionals who interact with very young children, as well as the development of appropriate screening tools (16, 35, 36). Research has demonstrated that the use of standardized test instruments by experienced clinicians results in a relatively stable early diagnosis in children as young as two years (37). Another apparent reason behind the decrease in the age of referral and diagnosis for autism is due to a general consensus that appropriately targeted early intervention improves outcome (38).

While the National Research Council's Committee on Educational Interventions for Children with Autism recommended that early diagnosis should be emphasized, children under the age of four who appear to have an ASD should be considered to have a "provisional diagnosis" (38, 39). Although a clinical diagnosis of autism is often sensitive and stable over time in children, stability increases when a spectrum approach is used (37, 40, 41). That is, a proportion of the children identified with possible autism before age three years may not meet criteria for DSM-IV-TR Autistic Disorder at later follow-up but are highly likely to meet criteria for PDD-NOS, a less severe form of autism. Alternatively, a proportion of children under the age of three who do not meet criteria for autism on a standardized parent report measure, such as the Autism Diagnostic Interview-Revised (ADI-R (42)) may nonetheless receive a clinical diagnosis of Autistic Disorder at a later follow-up (37, 40, 41). Studies of young children have demonstrated that the use of a standardized observation of social and communicative behavior and play, such as the Autism Diagnostic Observation Schedule (ADOS: WPS Edition; 43, 44), may be more sensitive and stable over time than a standardized parent report measure alone. It is also important to note that very young children with ASD may not show significant evidence of repetitive and stereotyped behaviors and restricted patterns of interest, as required to meet the cutoff for autism on the ADI-R or to meet DSM-IV-TR criteria. In one study of two-year-olds suspected of having autism, use of instruments that relied on the clinician's ratings of the child, instead of the ADI-R alone, allowed for the inclusion of children who appeared to meet the social and communication criteria for autism but did not yet show significant evidence of restricted or repetitive behaviors (45). A follow-up assessment confirmed the diagnosis of autism in the vast majority of these children. At the earliest ages, experienced clinical judgment using information from a variety of sources is more reliable for deter-

mination of diagnosis than the use of standard assessment instruments alone (14, 33, 37).

Although impairments in social interaction, communication, and a restricted repertoire of interests, behaviors, and activities are core domains in ASD, there are several additional domains that can be affected and influence the manifestation of the disability. It is therefore often recommended that an evaluation for ASD should include a formal multidisciplinary evaluation of social behavior, language and nonverbal communication, adaptive behavior, motor skills, atypical behaviors, and cognitive status by a team of professionals experienced with autistic spectrum disorders (29, 33, 38, 46). This evaluation will typically include an experienced clinical psychologist or school psychologist, a speech/language pathologist, and an occupational therapist. A complete physical examination is critical to rule out any other possible explanations for delayed and abnormal behavior. Many children with ASD experience difficulties with fine motor coordination, low muscle tone, behavior control and aggression, and/or the presence of a seizure disorder, warranting a consultation with an experienced pediatric neurologist or child psychiatrist (29).

Both the ADI-R and the ADOS operationally define current DSM-IV and ICD-10 criteria, and quantify separately the three domains that define autistic spectrum disorders: social reciprocity, communication, and restricted, repetitive behaviors and interests. The ADI-R is a semi-structured interview that is conducted with the parents or primary caregiver and is designed to elicit a full range of information needed to produce a diagnosis of autism or an autistic spectrum diagnosis (42, 47). The assessed individuals can be of any age, as long as their mental abilities are at a developmental level of at least 24 months. Diagnostic decisions are based on algorithm items. The ADOS is a standardized observation of social behavior in naturalistic and communicative contexts, with different modules and tasks for children of different ages and language levels (43, 44, 48, 49). The ADOS yields scores that fall within a range from autism to autism spectrum disorder, and so may be particularly helpful with difficult to diagnose cases. Inter–rater and test–retest reliability as well as internal validity have been demonstrated for both instruments and they, and their previous versions, have been widely used in research and in academic centers for about 15 years. The authors of the ADI-R and ADOS originally intended that experienced clinicians would use them after obtaining training in their use and achieving administration and scoring reliability.

The Gilliam Autism Rating Scale (GARS; 50) is another standardized instrument that can be used to assist in diagnosis. The GARS appears to have limited use for diagnostic purposes and appears to be better used as a screening device. The child's primary caregiver or teacher can complete the GARS. Screening questionnaires were never intended to be a diagnostic gold standard, particularly for low base rate disorders (51). The Social Communication Questionnaire (SCQ; 31) is a brief instrument that helps evaluate communication skills and social functioning in children who may have autism. This instrument, formerly known as the Autism Screening Questionnaire, has good discriminative validity with respect to the separation of ASD from non-ASD diagnoses at all IQ levels (52, 53). It can be used with any individual over 4 (with a mental age exceeding 2 years of age). An experienced professional rates the child's behavior on the GARS (54), which requires direct observation of the child but does not provide guidelines on a standardized method of observation. The GARS has fair agreement with the ADI-R (55). Some argue that the GARS may be best used as a screening measure (46).

Neuropsychological Findings and Theories

Although the majority of children with autistic disorder are mentally retarded, this is less often the case when one looks across children with diagnoses in the autistic spectrum (16). By definition, individuals with Asperger syndrome have intellectual abilities that are within the average range. Some individuals may have IQs that fall in the superior range and yet they have significant social disability. It is thought that while children with ASD are able to perform a variety of tasks, they may do so in ways different from typically developing children.

Neuropsychological studies have demonstrated that individuals with autism are able to perform certain types of tasks better than others. Using standardized intelligence tests, such as the Wechsler Intelligence Test for Children (56, 57), children with autism were reported to perform better on tests of visual pattern matching and rote auditory memory and more poorly on tests of commonsense social reasoning (58, 59). However, more recent studies suggest that a variety of profiles exist, such that some children may have more even nonverbal and verbal skills and some may perform better on verbal tests compared to nonverbal tests (60). Older children with nonverbal skills that are significantly higher than their verbal skills tend to have more social difficulties.

It appears that individuals with autism tend to disregard context and use this to their advantage on certain types of cognitive tests and in certain situations. This is in contrast to individuals with less formal schooling, who tend to perform poorly on tests with relatively little context (61). Even less able children with autism may have remarkable rote memory skills. The difficulty is that they are not able to use these skills to extract meaning as needed for learning important skills and procedures. This difficulty has been termed weak central coherence (61).

It is important to note that while ASD is typically associated with developmental delays and even mental retardation, the social deficits distinguish this disorder from more general cases of learning disability or mental retardation. Reciprocal social skills develop early in life and contribute to the development of a variety of cognitive skills, particularly language. Individuals with ASD appear to have early difficulties in understanding the mental states of other individuals, specifically that others have a mind capable of understanding things the same way they do. This ability has been termed *theory of mind* (62) or *mentalizing* (61). In the time since first described by Simon Baron-Cohen and colleagues as a deficit in autism, many studies have replicated this finding. However, while individuals with ASD are significantly delayed in mentalizing, they are not incapable of acquiring knowledge about mental states. Difficulties with mentalizing may explain why young children with autism typically do not appear interested in sharing things that interest them with others or respond infrequently when others try to attract their attention to things of interest. As they develop, children with ASD may approach others to share things, particularly related to their restricted interests, but have limited interest in learning about the interests of others.

Some children with ASD appear to compensate for this difficulty in mentalizing by employing logic to understand why other people respond in certain ways to certain situations. However, in real-life situations or when under stress, they may continue to have significant difficulties. It is important to note that while many individuals with ASD want companionship and often approach others, they typically have significant difficulty interpreting the actions of others and responding appropriately in different situations. When others do not respond in the expected manner, individuals with ASD often have limited insight regarding how their actions affected the situation. This may lead to social withdrawal, anxiety, or mood disturbance.

Several of the diagnostic features of autism, as well as findings from psychological testing and experiments, have pointed toward deficits in executive function in autism. Executive abilities are not required for routine events or actions but rather when one has to switch between tasks or deal with the unexpected. Difficulties with tests of executive functioning such as the Wisconsin Card Sorting Test, the Tower of Hanoi, and the Trail Making Test have been reported for high functioning individuals with autistic disorder and Asperger syndrome (63–70). Individuals with ASD often exhibit repetitive actions, restricted interests, and have a desire for the "maintenance of sameness." Difficulty with flexible thoughts and actions, reflecting deficits in executive functions, may help to explain why these behavioral features are so prominent and problematic for individuals with ASD.

Etiology

Although autistic characteristics are associated with some neurodevelopmental disorders (e.g., fragile X and other chromosomal abnormalities), the etiology in the vast majority of cases is unknown. There is some evidence of increased prenatal and perinatal risk factors, although how these may relate to the etiology of the disorder is not clear (71).

Neuroanatomy

The neuroanatomical abnormalities associated with autism have been the focus of many investigations that have included the use of structural brain magnetic resonance imaging (MRI), neuropathology, as well as neurophysiological and functional brain MRI techniques. Most studies have included older children, adolescents, and adults, although a few recent studies have focused on children who were studied soon after initial diagnosis.

Although head circumference at birth generally falls within the average range, recent evidence suggests that the trajectory of head growth occurs more rapidly than normal in the first few years of life in children with autism (72, 73). Figure 10.1 shows that head circumference measurements at the time of birth for children later diagnosed with autism were close to or slightly below the population mean. However, head circumference measurements taken between 6 and 14 months of age for those same children were more typically above the population mean, indicating that the relative rate of head growth was abnormally large during the first year of life. It is interesting to note that the abnormally rapid increase in head circumference in the first year of life in children with autism was strongly correlated with abnormal cerebral and cerebellar volumes from brain MRI data by two to five years of age (72). Whole brain volume has been found to be significantly larger than normal in two- to five-year-old children with autism (73, 74). More specifically, cerebellar white matter volume was abnormally large, and within the cerebral cortex, there was an anterior to posterior gradient in degree of abnormality: largest at the frontal lobes and closer to normal in the occipital lobes (75). Head circumference measures are strongly correlated with brain

size in the first few years of life while abnormally large head circumference measures later in life is less likely to be correlated with underlying brain volumes (76).

The degree of overgrowth abnormality during early life may be correlated with later outcome for children with ASD. Two- to five-year-olds with signs of ASD were scanned and sorted into three groups, when diagnoses were confirmed after age five: lower functioning children with autism, higher functioning children with autism, and higher functioning children with PDD-NOS (77). Discriminant function analysis revealed that the groups could be successfully discriminated from typically developing children using a combination of brain MRI measures. Cerebellar white matter volume was significantly larger in all three patient groups compared to the control group, but the posterior cerebellar vermis was smaller than normal in the lower functioning children and the anterior cerebellar vermis was larger than normal in the higher functioning children with autism. Brain MRI studies of high functioning older children and adults with autism have reported no significant differences in the size of the anterior and posterior cerebellar vermis from normal (78, 79) while studies that included both low and high functioning individuals consistently report decreased size of the posterior cerebellar vermis (80–82). Less loss in the posterior cerebellar vermis early in life may therefore be associated with better functional outcome, while early abnormalities in terms of increased white matter in the cerebellum and early overgrowth of the cerebrum may be associated with the persistent autistic symptoms observed across children.

In terms of gross anatomy, there appears to be a changing process with age, with rapid growth early in development preceding the onset of symptoms, and later changes

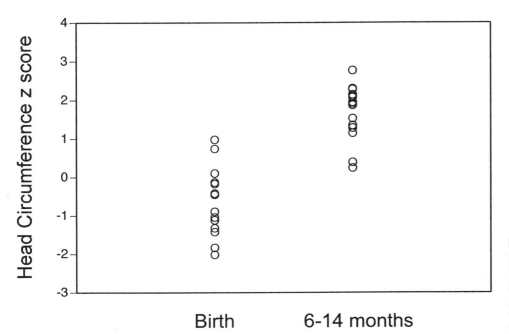

Figure 10.1 Increase in head circumference from birth to 6 to 14 months of age in infants later diagnosed with autistic disorder. Modified from Courchesne, Carper, & Akshoomoff (2003) with permission from the American Medical Association.

that may include abnormally slow brain growth, compensatory overpruning of connections, or abnormal neuron loss (83–86). Rapid growth is only one possible explanation for these findings. Abnormally large brain volume may reflect an excessive number of neurons or glial cells, an excessive number of minicolumns, an excessive and early expansion of dendritic and axonal arbors, an excessive number of axonal connections, premature myelination, or an excessive rate of growth of the neurons or glial cells (72, 87, 88). These abnormal processes could reflect an abnormal acceleration of postnatal growth processes and/or a failure of the late prenatal and early postnatal regressive or "pruning" processes.

Abnormally large brain volume is not a typical finding among school-age children and adolescents with autism (73; for review, see 89). Cerebellar white matter volume also generally falls within the normal range, as well as measures of cerebral gray and white matter volume (73). Cerebellar pathology has been found in 21 of 22 postmortem (primarily adult) cases and appears consistent with prenatal or early postnatal abnormalities in neuronal development (90–93). Specific structures may be affected early in development and appear abnormally small in size compared to normal throughout development. Brain MRI data suggests that the cross-sectional size of the posterior corpus callosum is reduced compared to normal (94–96). Inconsistent findings have been reported with regard to amygdala (97–99) and hippocampal (100, 101) volumes, although there is postmortem evidence of abnormalities at the cellular level in the hippocampus and amygdala (90, 91, 102, 103). A recent study of 7 to 11 year-old high-functioning children with autism found white matter volume was larger than normal while measures of the cortical gray matter and hippocampus/amygdala were smaller than normal (104). Inconsistencies in volumetric abnormalities across studies are likely due to a number of factors. These include the ages of participants, relative sample sizes, the level of functioning of participants (i.e., level of mental retardation), selection criteria for control groups, and other potential confounds (e.g., history of seizures, long-term medication use).

Neurofunctional Findings

Early widespread neuroanatomic defects in autism, including white matter overgrowth and hypoplasia of specific structures, would likely lead to abnormal development of functional systems. Neurophysiological and functional brain MRI studies have revealed abnormal patterns of brain activity during attention and other cognitive tasks, even when relatively high-functioning adolescents and adults with autism are normal in their behavioral performance in these tasks (for review, see 89). For example, individuals with autism have reduced activation in the brain regions typically associated with performing attention, motor, and face processing tasks while showing increased activation in other regions not primarily utilized by normal subjects

(105–109). In a $H_2(15)O$ PET study of five high-functioning adults with autism, brain activation patterns were evaluated while the participants were listening to tones and sentences, and generating sentences (110). Reduced or reversed dominance activation was found over temporal regions associated with language perception and reduced activation of auditory cortex and cerebellum were found during acoustic stimulation. Further analysis showed that during sentence generation, the left dorsolateral prefrontal cortex (Brodmann area 46) and left thalamus and the right dentate nucleus of the cerebellum showed less activation in the males with autism (111). During sentence repetition, greater increases in blood flow in the left frontal cortex and right dentate nucleus were found in the males with autism compared to controls.

Many of the structures that are affected in autism mediate the development of more than one function. Since typical brain development involves competition between functions (or functional inputs) as the natural process of functional specialization, the early neural defects in autism may differentially affect the cerebral and cerebellar organization of different functional domains, with greater abnormalities for some functions than for others, and to a greater degree in some individuals than others (89). It has been hypothesized that the early development of basic skills, such as rapid shifting of attention, are affected to some degree in autism, leading to delays in the development of other skills reliant on these skills, such as joint social attention. As the child develops, these basic skills improve but behavioral and functional neuroimaging data suggest that the development of these skills occurs in an atypical fashion (105, 112, 113).

Functional neuroimaging studies have provided information about abnormal brain metabolism in autism. These studies are useful not only in improving our understanding of structure-function relationships but also to understand developmental changes in biochemistry and therefore lead to more rational design of drug treatments of children of different ages (114). In a positron emission tomography (PET) study using $\alpha[^{11}C]$methyl-L-tryptophan, whole brain serotonin synthesis capacity in children was over 200% of adult values until 5 years of age when it declined to adult values (115). In contrast, serotonin synthesis capacity in children with autism increased gradually from 2 to 15 years of age, reaching 1 to 1.5 times adult normal values. It thus appears that in normal brain development, there is a period of high brain serotonin synthesis capacity during childhood. There is also evidence that serotonin regulates neuronal differentiation, neurite outgrowth and synaptogenesis (116). These data, in conjunction with the brain MRI volumetric data from young children with autism, suggest that the normal developmental process, specifically the regulation of trophic effects, is disrupted in autism. In another study that included a subset of these participants, regional brain alterations in brain serotonin synthesis were observed, namely gross asymmetries in frontal cortex, thalamus, and cerebellum (117). Decreased serotonin synthesis was observed in the left frontal cortex and thalamus accompanied by increased serotonin synthesis in the right cerebellum.

In a study of 14 medication-free children with autism, dopamine metabolism was studied with PET using 18F fluorodopa (118). There was a 39% reduction of dopamine activity in the anterior medial prefrontal cortex compared with activity in the occipital cortex in the children with autism compared with healthy children.

A 31P magnetic resonance spectroscopy (MRS) study of phosphorus metabolites in dorsal prefrontal cortex was conducted with 11 high-functioning adolescent and young adult men with autism (119). Decreased levels of phosphomonoesters, increased levels of phosphodiesters, and decreased levels of ATP were noted. In the autism group, alterations in brain energy and phospholipid metabolism were correlated with neuropsychological and language test scores. The authors suggested that the findings indicate a hypermetabolic energy state and undersynthesis of brain membranes in autism. N-acetylaspartate (NAA) was significantly lower in the cerebellum of 9 children with autism compared to sibling control subjects using MRS (120). NAA levels in the frontal and temporal lobes did not differ between the two groups. An MRS study of 3- and 4-year-olds with ASD revealed widespread alterations in brain chemistry (121). Compared to age-matched developmentally delayed and typically developing control children, decreased metabolism of NAA, creatine plus phosphocreatine, and myo-inositol were found in a variety of brain regions, including the frontal and temporal lobes, cingulate gyrus, and a number of subcortical structures. Another recent MRS study of 5- to 16-year-old children with autism revealed altered metabolism in the left anterior cingulated gyrus, caudate nucleus, and right occipital cortex of NAA, choline compounds, and creatine plus phosphocreatine (122).

Additional studies are needed to determine how metabolic rates are related to cerebral volume increases in young children with ASD and how regional abnormalities may vary as a function of techniques, age, and level of functioning. While direct correlations between measures of brain structures and rates of metabolic activity have not been conducted, many of these findings are consistent with the results from neuroanatomical studies of autism. Measures of levels of activation in specific brain structures using functional MR imaging, PET, and SPECT, may eventually be used in drug treatment trials to assess changes in neural activation patterns in conjunction with behavioral changes (114).

Genetics

Identification of the biological defects has significant implications for quantitative trait genetic linkage analyses and animal models of the neurodevelopmental abnormalities in ASD. These findings may also serve as a component of subject characterization in clinical treatment trials with young children to assist in determining how a child's level

of functioning and biological characteristics may be predictive of treatment response (114).

Data from twin and family studies indicate that genetic factors play an important role in the development of autistic spectrum disorders (123, 124). Concordance among dizygotic twins range from 0 to 25% while the rate of concordance for a diagnosis of autism or an ASD diagnosis among monozygotic twins is higher (40–90%). The concordance rate among siblings (2–6%) is significantly higher than the estimated population prevalence. It is clear that the autistic spectrum disorders are complex and the result of a number of genetic and environmental factors.

A number of recent studies have focused on identifying the specific genes that appear to be important in the development of autism and related disorders. For example, a genomewide scan with DNA markers was conducted in 345 multiplex families, each with at least two siblings affected with autism or an ASD phenotype (125). Evidence for linkage was found on chromosomes 17, 5, 11, 4, and 8. It is important to note that the linkage region implicated on chromosome 17q included the serotonin transporter (5-HTT) gene locus (SLC6A4), which has previously been implicated as a candidate gene for autism on the basis of some association studies (126–129). There is also some evidence of elevated blood serotonin levels both in patients with autism and in their unaffected first-degree relatives (130). A recent study sought to identify a susceptibility gene for autism in the chromosome region 2q24–q33 (131). Linkage and association was identified between two single nucleotide polymorphisms and autism. This region is known to be important for mitochondrial function and ATP synthesis in neurons. Future studies to identify the genes that act together to cause the autism phenotype would be improved by a focus on larger samples, more homogeneous samples, detailed phenotype information that is collected in a consistent manner, selection of candidate genes on the basis on recent neurobiological findings, and the use of knockout models (132, 133).

Other Theories

The first report of an unexpected intestinal lesion associated with gastrointestinal problems in a group of 12 children with pervasive developmental disorders has been associated with a great deal of controversy (134). Specifically, the authors of the report raised the possibility of a link, on the basis of parental and medical histories, between the newly described syndrome of bowel disease and autism and the measles, mumps, and rubella (MMR) vaccine. This suggestion led to a great deal of concern in the United Kingdom and the United States, among other countries, regarding the safety of the MMR vaccine (135). Of particular concern was the suggestion that the MMR vaccine was a contributing factor to early loss or regression (134).

Regression is typically used to refer to the losses of already established skills (136). This is a phenomenon that has been documented for several decades and occurs in approximately 20 to 33% of all cases of autism (136–138). Regression is most commonly identified as occurring between 18 and 24 months of age (137–143). One of the most striking features of regression is word loss. That is, the child may have produced several words and then stopped saying those words altogether for months or even years (142, 144). Children with word loss are also more likely to be described by their caregivers as showing more gestures, greater participation in social games and better receptive language before the time of the word loss (145).

A possible causal relationship between vaccines and autism has been of concern to some clinicians and parents, particularly with reports of increasing prevalence of autism and the increasing number of vaccines given to infants. However, epidemiological studies have not supported the relationship between prevalence of autism and the MMR vaccine (140, 146–149). Ten of the authors of the original study that suggested the possibility between the MMR vaccine and autism (134) have recently published a retraction of that interpretation of their data (150).

Treatment

Behavioral and Educational Treatment

The majority of evidence-based interventions for children with ASD are behavioral and educational in nature (38). Early intervention programs (between 2 and 4 years of age) are the most effective for helping improve the outcome in children with autism (151). Several intensive behavioral treatments are supported by empirical investigations, such as behavior modification or the "Lovaas method," discrete trial training, incidental teaching, and pivotal response training, as well as structured programs such as TEACCH and the Denver Model (152–154). A large number of other treatment programs exist, such as "floor time" developed by Greenspan and colleagues (155). It is important to note that outcome data are limited making it difficult to adequately evaluate the effectiveness of the treatment programs available and in use (156). It is also important to note outcome among children with ASD is variable, in part due to the fact that the needs and strengths of these children are very heterogeneous (38). Speech and language therapy is essential for assisting young children who are delayed in their use of language, as well as older, higher-functioning children in assisting them with pragmatics and the social use of language. Occupational therapy is often helpful for assisting with sensory integration issues as well as the development of fine motor coordination and self-help skills. Physical therapy is often needed, as well as adapted physical education programs.

The Individualized Education Plan (IEP) and the Individual Family Service Plan (IFSP) should be utilized for planning and implementing the educational objectives of children with ASD (38). Learning objectives should be observable, measurable behaviors and skills that are accomplished within one year, including the development of social skills, language and communication skills, developmentally appropriate tasks and play, cognitive skills, and fine and gross motor skill development. The National Research Council's Committee on Educational Interventions for Children with Autism recommended that educational services should include a minimum of 25 hours a week, 12 months a year, and be based on an individualized plan. Until more data are available, particularly with regard to the relative merit of one program model over another, a wider range of outcome variables, and specific approaches for specific needs, the Council suggested that it may be more important to consider how the environment and educational strategies associated with a particular program allow implementation of the goals for a child and family.

Medications

The medications most commonly used in the treatment of individuals with ASD are directed toward amelerioriating the associated rather than core symptoms of the disorder (157). Medications may be prescribed when children are having significant difficulty with hyperactivity, aggression, irritability and agitation, repetitive behaviors, and so on to increase the likelihood that the individual will benefit from behavioral and educational programs. Some aspects of social behavior may also improve as a result of the reduction in these problematic symptoms (158).

Early drug treatment studies included the use of fenfluramine, haloperidol, and naltrexone (158). Haloperidol, in doses of 1 to 2 mg/day, was more effective than placebo for relieving temper outbursts, hyperactivity, withdrawal, stereotypy, anger, and affective lability but acute dystonic reactions and withdrawal and tardive dyskinesias occurred relatively frequently (159, 160). Large controlled studies of naltrexone failed to find improvement of maladaptive behaviors except for motor hyperactivity (161). More recent, well-controlled studies have focused on the atypical antipsychotics, including clozapine, risperidone, olanzapine, and quietiapine (162). Risperidone has received the most attention. In the largest controlled drug treatment study in autistic disorder to date, the National Institute of Mental Health (NIMH)-sponsored Research Units on Pediatric Pychopharmacology (RUPP) Autism Network completed a randomized controlled trial of risperidone in 101 children with autistic disorder (163). Treatment for eight weeks was effective in reducing tantrums, aggression, or self-injurious behavior in children with autistic disorder. An average weight gain of 2.7+/−2.9 kg (as compared with 0.8+/−2.2 kg with placebo) was observed; increased appetite, fatigue, drowsiness, dizziness, and drooling were also associated with risperidone. In an open-label, naturalistic study of preschoolers with autistic disorder or PDD-NOS, low-dose risperidone was associated with reducing behavior problems and affect dysregulation in the short-term, but also in the long-term period (164). Increased prolactin levels without clinical signs and increased appetite were the most frequent side effects. Response was associated with higher doses and weight gain. In general, risperidone appears favorable in reducing symptoms of most concern to parents (165).

Serotonin reuptake inhibitors have also been the focus of investigations on clinical response and side effects in children, adolescents, and adults with ASD. Although a number of studies of clomipramine have been published (166) the selective serotonin reuptake inhibitors (SSRIs) have received more recent attention due to the less severe side effects associated with the SSRIs (158). Few controlled studies have been completed. Studies of fluvoxamine suggest that it may be less efficacious and less tolerated in children and adolescents with ASD than adults (167). Studies of fluoxetine indicate favorable results, although drug-induced side effects, such as hyperactivity, agitation, decreased appetite, and aggression, led to discontinuation in some cases (168). Fewer studies have been conducted to date with sertraline and paroxetine.

Some individuals with a diagnosis of autistic disorder or other ASD may also meet the DSM-IV-TR criteria for attention-deficit/hyperactivity disorder (ADHD). However, the DSM-IV-TR specifies that in order to meet criteria for ADHD, the symptoms do not occur exclusively during the course of a pervasive developmental disorder or schizophrenia. Hyperactivity and impaired attention are more prominent in younger children and can interfere with the implementation of critical early intervention programs. The use of psychostimulants for the treatment of motor hyperactivity and poor attention in ASD has generally resulted in mixed results (169). While these symptoms may improve in some children, adverse effects, notably aggression, irritability, have been noted in children with autism as a result of methylphenidate. There is some interest in the use of clonidine and other α-adrenergic agonists such as guanfacine, particularly for those children and adolescents with ASD who are nonresponders to methylphenidate and other psychostimulants (169).

There has been a great deal of interest in more novel types of treatment strategies for children with ASD, particularly those directed toward gastrointestinal and immune functions. Secretin is a hormone that is secreted in response to food passage by the gut and stimulates the pancreas, resulting in decreased gastrointestinal motility. It is commonly used in gastrointestinal endoscopies. It became a focus of much interest after a report indicated that three boys with ASD demonstrated improvement in autistic symptoms following secretin injection associated with an endoscopy procedure (170). Many children with ASD received treatment with secretin before formal research studies were conducted. A series of double-blind placebo-controlled studies with single dose secretin in children with ASD (with more than 300 children total) have indicated no consistent significant differences in primary outcome measures (171–177). While there is some speculation that

multiple doses are perhaps needed, or secretin may prove helpful with a certain subset of children with ASD (178), others believe that the results indicate that there is a strong placebo effect associated with secretin and no scientific evidence to support its use as a treatment for autism (179).

A limited number of studies have been conducted with drugs that have direct effects on immune function that may warrant further investigation. The use of alternative treatments is increasing among families who have a child with an ASD and therefore physicians should discuss the efficacy and potential side effects of such treatments with parents (180). Although no comprehensive scale has been developed to date to assess change in maladaptive behaviors during treatment, a number of scales have been utilized by the (RUPP) Autism Network (158, 181). These include the Aberrant Behavior Checklist, the Clinical Global Impressions scale, and the Children's Yale–Brown Obsessive Compulsive Scale. There are currently no measures available to adequately assess changes in core symptoms, such as social behavior or restricted/repetitive behaviors, appropriate for drug treatment trials (182). Current information about the individual's cognitive and adaptive skills is also helpful.

Course and Mortality

It is important to consider issues related to outcome and long-term care when working with individuals with ASD. The symptoms of ASD differ over the course of life. These differences reflect developmental interactions with the core symptoms of autism, environmental influences, and individual differences in background variables. The patterns of autism were assessed using the ADI-R in 405 individuals with ASD, ages 10 to 53 years (183). Although the patients met criteria for autistic disorder based on childhood criteria, only 54.8% would have met criteria based on their current behavior. The greatest amount of improvement was observed in development of phrase speech while there was limited change in having friendships.

Individuals with autism are subject to increased mortality risk (184). A database study revealed the causes of mortality and relative risk for individuals who were diagnosed with autism and received any services from the California Department of Developmental Services between 1983 and 1997 (185). Among those with no or mild mental retardation, deaths by seizures, nervous system dysfunction, drowning, and suffocation were all more than three times higher than expected in the general population. Excess mortality was marked for individuals with severe mental retardation but life expectancy was also reduced for individuals who were fully ambulatory with only mild mental retardation.

CHILDHOOD-ONSET SCHIZOPHRENIA

The onset of symptoms in schizophrenia most commonly occurs during late adolescence and early adulthood (13).

Onset of symptoms between the ages of 5 and 14 is commonly referred to as "childhood-onset schizophrenia" (186, 187). Kraeplin reported that only about 6% of his sample of more than 1,000 cases with schizophrenia had an onset of psychotic symptoms before 15 years of age (61). Although epidemiological data are limited, it is estimated that less than 1 child in 10,000 suffers from COS, making it a rare disorder compared to adult schizophrenia, which affects approximately 1 in 100 (188). COS is more common among males than females until adolescence, when the ratio of males to females is more similar. Although this is a rare developmental disorder, COS has increasingly become the focus of research investigations because it is thought that enhanced understanding of developmental changes in the brain could lead to an improved understanding of the neurobiology of schizophrenia.

Diagnosis and Appropriate Assessment Strategies

The DSM-IV-TR (13) criteria for schizophrenia are as follows. The characteristic psychotic symptoms must be present for a significant portion of the time during a one-month period (or less, if successfully treated). Two or more of the core symptoms of schizophrenia must be present, namely delusions, hallucinations, formal thought disorder, grossly disorganized behavior, and negative symptoms (flat affect and anhedonia). However, only one symptom is required if delusions are bizarre or hallucinations consist of a running commentary on the person's behavior or thoughts or two or more conversing voices. There must be deterioration in functioning or failure to achieve the expected level of interpersonal, academic, or occupational achievement. The boundaries between schizophrenia and mood disorders, schizoaffective disorder, organic disorders, and pervasive developmental disorder are specified and should be carefully considered in making a diagnosis. The duration of disturbance, prodromal features, and residual features are also defined in DSM-IV-TR.

Several independent studies have concluded that schizophrenia in childhood can be reliably diagnosed using the same criteria for adults (for review, see 189). However, developmental differences do exist in symptom presentation. Hallucinations, delusions, and formal thought disorders are rare or difficult to diagnose in children younger than age 7 (190). The distinction between schizophrenic symptoms and features of typical children can be difficult in some cases, such as distinguishing between delusions and the imaginative fantasies typical of young children. Of concern is a more persistent pattern of such behaviors, such as a child who often hears voices saying derogatory things about him or her, or hears voices conversing with one another, talks to himself or herself, imagines seeing scary things (such as snakes, spiders, or shadows), and shows no interest in friendships (191). It is important to note that a child with more limited language and cognitive skills may have difficulty accurately describing their experiences and distinguishing them from pretend or fantasy (1).

After age 7, hallucinations are the most common symptom of COS, with auditory hallucinations more common than visual hallucinations (192). It may be difficult to accurately assess disorganized speech or formal thought disorder in children and adolescents with schizophrenia. Blunted affect is fairly common.

Childhood-onset schizophrenia typically presents with an insidious rather than acute onset, with a number of associated symptoms and problems (1, 192). The prodromal symptoms are similar to those observed in adult-onset schizophrenia but language impairments and transient autistic-like and nonspecific symptoms are more common (187). The onset of psychotic symptoms is often preceded by social abnormalities; many children are described as odd prior to the onset of psychotic symptoms. Developmental disturbances are common, such as lags in motor and speech/language development (193). Children with more pronounced early developmental abnormalities tend to have a poorer outcome. The most common type of communication difficulty is poor pragmatic skills. During the early school-age period, difficulties with attention and behavior often affect school functioning (194). Other symptoms include depression, oppositional behavior, and conduct problems.

Researchers have identified other disorders that fall within or similar to the schizophrenia spectrum. Children with "multidimensionally impaired syndrome" exhibit psychosis, poor affect regulation, and difficulty with attention and impulse control (187). These children can be distinguished from children with schizophrenia. Although they are likely to develop more specifically defined psychiatric disorders, such as bipolar disorder, schizoaffective disorder, or a disruptive behavior disorder, longitudinal follow-up studies do not suggest they are likely to be diagnosed later with schizophrenia. Follow-up of children with schizoaffective disorder or schizotypal personality disorder reveals that although the development of full-blown schizophrenia is rare, the majority of children will continue to exhibit a schizophrenia spectrum disorder (195).

The outcome of children with schizophrenia is generally poor and possibly worse than those with adult-onset (196). Eggers and Bunk (197) conducted a 42-year follow-up of a group of 44 patients with COS. They found that 50% of the sample had continuous symptoms and 25% had partial remission. Studies with shorter follow-up periods have reported similar results.

Uncertainty about diagnosis is common among children with schizophrenia and therefore it is important to consider a variety of factors to reduce the misclassification of cases. Although it may appear that the distinction between childhood-onset schizophrenia and an autistic spectrum disorder is fairly apparent, the differential symptoms and similarities should be considered. Childhood-onset schizophrenia is distinguished from autism by the persistence of hallucinations and delusions for at least 6 months, and a later age of onset. Autistic Disorder is most typically identified before age 5 and results in more major intellectual deficits than COS (6, 7). It is interesting to note that in adulthood some individuals with autism exhibit, in their surface behavior, some symptoms characteristic of schizophrenia (61). They may show negative signs, such as little or no speech or facial expressions, little or no interest in social contact or communication, and they may exhibit simple movement stereotypies. However, articulate individuals with autism who have reported their experiences give accounts quite different from those of individuals with schizophrenia; most notably the absence of hallucinations and delusions. Furthermore, in schizophrenia, phases of acute illness often alternate with long periods of symptom remission, which is different from autistic spectrum disorders. It is interesting to note that the term autistic was first coined by Ernst Bleuler to apply to thought processes in schizophrenia. Both autism and schizophrenia result in some sort of social impairment. If children show any interest in friendships, even if they fail at maintaining them, it is unlikely that they have schizophrenia (191).

As part of the ongoing study of childhood-onset schizophrenia at the NIMH, more than 1,300 children and adolescents have been referred to the study since 1990. After the initial screening process, 215 cases were interviewed to identify those that met criteria for COS (198). Many of the cases referred to the study were judged to have psychotic mood disorders rather than schizophrenia. The clinical presentations included mood-congruent hallucinations, the absence of grossly disorganized behavior or speech, and comorbid disorders commonly seen in patients with mood disorders (e.g., anxiety disorders, attention-deficit/hyperactivity disorder). As the authors discuss, it is important to note that the rarity of COS makes it difficult for clinicians to have the experience of the NIMH team in diagnosing COS, as well as the time needed for a comprehensive, structured diagnostic assessment. These results also suggest that it is not uncommon for children with bipolar disorder or major depressive disorder with psychotic features to be diagnosed with schizophrenia initially. The distinction between schizoaffective disorder and schizophrenia was more difficult to achieve reliably, as has been noted in previous studies (199, 200). The acute onset of manic episodes in bipolar disorder may be mistaken for schizophrenia. Children who have experienced abuse or who suffer from posttraumatic stress disorder may sometimes claim to hear voices or see visions associated with abuse or a traumatic event. Due to these issues in misdiagnosis, clinicians should not rely on cross-sectional assessments of children and adolescents with psychotic symptoms (187). It may also be important to consider whether a child develops additional symptoms that may signify an additional diagnosis or perhaps different subtypes. These distinctions are important considerations for neurobiological studies.

A number of standardized assessment tools exist for use with children and adolescents with suspected psychotic dis-

orders (for reviews, see 201, 202). The diagnostic interviews have been developed in order to obtain a categorical diagnosis according to the DSM or ICD systems. These tools include the Schedule for Affective Disorders and Schizophrenia for School-age Children (K-SADS) (203), the Interview for Childhood Disorders and Schizophrenia (ICDS) (204), and the NIMH Diagnostic Interview Schedule for Children (NIMH DISC) (205). Symptom rating scales are broader in focus and assess severity of psychopathological symptoms on a continuous scale. These scales include the Positive and Negative Syndrome Scale for Children and Adolescents (K-PANSS) (206), the Children's Psychiatric Rating Scale (CPRS), the Brief Psychiatric Rating Scale, and the Children's Global Assessment Scale (C-GAS) (207). Caplan and colleagues developed the Kiddie Formal Thought Disorder Rating Scale and Story Game (K-FTDS), which provides a structured evaluation of thinking disturbance (208).

It is essential to obtain information from parents and teachers as well as careful observation of the child (209). The most valid diagnosis is likely to be obtained using a "best estimate" approach, taking into consideration all sources of information and using a prospective approach (202).

The American Academy of Child and Adolescent Psychiatry published a practice parameter for the assessment and treatment of children and adolescents with schizophrenia (210). Based upon the empirical evidence, the practice parameter gives specific recommendations:

1. Assessment
   (a) A comprehensive diagnostic assessment, which includes, when possible, interviews with the child/adolescent and the family, plus a review of past records and other available ancillary information.
   (b) Physical assessment to rule out general medical causes of psychotic symptoms.
   (c) An intellectual assessment or cognitive testing to evaluate possible developmental delays and degree of impairment associated with the illness.
   (d) Recognition of the various phases of the disorder (prodome, acute phase, recovery phase, residual phase, and chronic impairment).
   (e) Psychiatric formulation to establish diagnosis and rule out other disorders. Reassessment longitudinally is recommended.
2. Treatment
   (a) Antipsychotic agents are recommended for the treatment of the psychotic symptoms associated with schizophrenia. Guidelines are provided for the procedures for medication administration and management.
   (b) Psychoeducational therapy for the patient (e.g., education about the illness, social skills training) and for the family.
   (c) Specialized educational program and/or vocational training programs may be indicated.

Etiology

Schizophrenia in childhood appears to have a particularly strong biological predisposition and may possibly represent a more homogeneous genetic form of the disorder. Data from various medical disorders indicate that unusually early onset is associated with greater heritability and disease severity (211). Also the excess of males in younger age groups may indicate a particular biological vulnerability. Childhood-onset schizophrenia may be a more severe and familial variant of schizophrenia, giving hope that the etiology may be more easily discerned in cases with childhood rather than adult-onset. Studies of children with schizophrenia may also provide more information about etiology due to limited history of neuroleptic treatment and years of dysfunction. It is important to note, however, that the children who participated in the NIMH study were selected because they did not respond to traditional neuroleptic medications and therefore have a history of multiple medication use.

The causes of schizophrenia are still unknown. Weinberger (212) proposed a "neurodevelopmental model" of schizophrenia. While COS is rare compared to the typical profile of onset during late adolescence and early adulthood, Weinberger's neurodevelopmental model may be particularly applicable to the early onset cases. Children with schizophrenia are more likely to manifest impairments in language and motor development before the onset of psychotic symptoms, which may reflect early manifestations of the underlying brain abnormalities. Children with schizophrenia often exhibit difficulties with social behavior early in development, more so than children with major depression and other psychiatric conditions (195, 196). It is important to note that these early developmental difficulties in language and social development appear to be distinguishable from the early symptoms of autism.

Genetic Risks

Two classic studies suggested significantly higher rates of schizophrenic disorders (schizophrenia, schizoaffective disorder, schizotypal disorder, schizotypal personality disorder, and paranoid personality disorder) among the first-degree relatives of children with schizophrenia compared to those of adults with schizophrenia (7, 213). Using a larger sample and more rigorous methods, the UCLA Family Study (214) compared the diagnoses of first-degree relatives of probands with COS (N=148) with those of first-degree relatives of probands with attention-deficit hyperactivity disorder (ADHD; N=368) and community control probands (N=206). The families of probands with COS were significantly more likely to have at least one first-degree relative with a diagnosis of schizophrenia, or schizotypal or paranoid personality disorder than the other two groups. An unexpected finding was that the parents with a diagnosis of schizophrenia had an early age of first onset

(mean = 20.8 years) compared to the typical age of first onset for schizophrenia.

The results from the UCLA Family Study (214) suggested that the relative risk for schizophrenia in the parents of probands with COS was higher than that observed in adult-onset schizophrenia. This finding was directly compared as part of the study of COS at the NIMH (215). Indeed, the parents of patients with COS had a significantly higher risk of schizophrenia spectrum disorders (24.74%) than parents of patients with adult-onset schizophrenia (11.35%). The rates of mood disorders, substance use disorders, and schizoid personality disorder did not differ among the two groups and the control group. These results suggest that there is a more specific risk, rather than risk of psychopathology in general. It is also interesting to note that the patients with COS in the NIMH study who had relatives with schizophrenia or spectrum disorder were more likely to have a premorbid language disorder (187). The authors from both the UCLA and NIMH studies conclude that COS may be a more familial, possibly more genetic, form of schizophrenia than adult-onset schizophrenia.

In addition to a family history of a schizophrenia spectrum diagnosis, other factors are useful for developing a clinical phenotype of schizophrenia for genetic linkage studies. In one study, performance on neurocognitive tests was compared in three groups: parents of probands with COS, parents of probands with ADHD and parents of community controls (216). Only parents without a diagnosis of psychosis were included. Parents of probands with COS performed worse than parents of probands with ADHD and community controls on the Degraded Stimulus Continuous Performance Test and the Trail Making Test. The results suggest that neurocognitive impairments index the liability to schizophrenia in nonpsychotic relatives but neurocognitive impairments are not a significant factor among relatives of children with ADHD.

Neuropsychological Findings

Neuropsychological studies indicate that children with schizophrenia have difficulty allocating attention, have limited processing resources, show deficits on tests of executive functions, and have deficits in both verbal and nonverbal memory (187, 217). They also show difficulty with visual-motor coordination and fine motor speed. Other anomalies associated with adult schizophrenia, such as smooth pursuit eye movement abnormalities, are also found in children with schizophrenia and their first-degree relatives (187, 218, 219). The abnormal leading saccade phenotype may prove useful as a marker that is present by age 6 for individuals at risk for developing schizophrenia. A number of studies have been conducted with adolescents and adults at risk for schizophrenia in order to identify neurobehavioral markers associated with risk. Studies have implicated a specific type of eye-tracking dysfunction that is associated with prefrontal cortex function and appears to be specific to schizophrenia (220). Prospective neurobehavioral studies of the children of schizophrenic parents have identified variables that may be associated with the genetic liability of schizophrenia and related disorders, including anticipatory saccades (221). It is also important to note that the early course of neuropsychological dysfunction in patients who have not yet received antipsychotic medication treatment suggests that the neuropsychological dysfunction associated with schizophrenia is neurodevelopmental, rather than neurodegenerative, in nature (222).

Neuroanatomy

MRI abnormalities have been found in many of the same brain regions in childhood-onset schizophrenia as in adult schizophrenia. The ongoing NIMH study of childhood-onset schizophrenia includes children who experienced an onset of psychotic symptoms before the age of 12 and were selected because they did not respond to traditional neuroleptic medications.

In a series of publications, brain MRI data from these children has revealed significant differences in brain anatomy compared with age-matched typically developing children (223–225) (for reviews, see (187, 226). Most notably, the volume of the lateral ventricles is enlarged, and the area of the midsagittal vermis of the cerebellum and the area of the midsagittal thalamus is significantly smaller than normal in the children with schizophrenia. It is important to note that reduction of the thalamus is a consistent finding in adult patients with schizophrenia, including those who have not received neuroleptic medications, as well as the healthy relatives of patients with schizophrenia.

The UCLA group has also reported significant ventricular volume enlargement in their sample, particularly in the poster region of the ventricles (227, 228). Results from the UCLA group, using statistical parametric mapping, are shown in Figure 10.2. Both research groups have also reported reductions of total gray matter volume. These differences appear to be more striking for the cases with COS than has been reported in adults with schizophrenia (226). Both the UCLA and NIMH groups have reported volume increases in basal ganglia structures. This finding may be related to exposure to typical neuroleptic medications. One study reported that after two years of clozapine treatment, the volume of the caudate decreased to normal (229). Differences in caudate volume as a function of age are not clear. Decreased caudate volumes have been reported in adult patients with schizophrenia who did not have a history of neuroleptic medication treatment (230).

Longitudinal data from the NIMH sample of patients with COS have revealed progressive changes in volumetric measures during childhood and adolescence. The volume

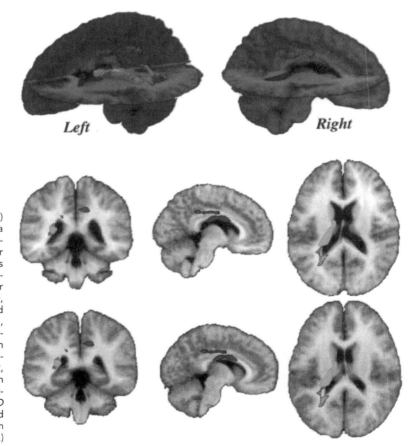

Left   *Right*

Figure 10.2 Statistical parametric mapping (SPM) results from the UCLA childhood-onset schizophrenia study. The <u>top panel</u> shows the three-dimensional renderings of the significant clusters from the gray matter (blue), white matter (red), and CSF (green). SPMs mapped into the average brain space of the nine subjects with COS. Significant voxels from the gray matter (in blue; voxel threshold $p < .01$, corrected at $p = .05$), white matter (in red; voxel threshold $p < .01$, corrected at $p = .05$), and CSF (in green; voxel threshold $p < .01$, corrected at $p = .10$) SPMs are mapped onto three orthogonal slices from the average schizophrenic brain (<u>middle panel</u>) and over the same three slices of the average control brain (<u>bottom panel</u>). From: Sowell ER, Toga AW, Asarnow R. Brain abnormalities observed in childhood-onset schizophrenia: A review of the structural magnetic resonance imaging literature. *MRDD Res. Rev.* 2000;6:180–185. Copyright @ 2000. Reprinted by permission of Wiley-Liss, Inc., a subsidiary of John Wiley & Sons, Inc. (For color detail, see full color insert.)

of temporal lobe structures may not differ from normal when children COS are scanned in late childhood or early adolescence (224, 231). However, a two-year follow-up of brain MRI data from the NIMH study revealed significantly greater decreases in temporal lobe volume, even after taking the 4.6% decrease in total cerebral volume into consideration (232). Reduction of right posterior superior temporal gyrus volume was also associated with increased symptom severity. Longitudinal data obtained from 55 patients with COS also revealed abnormal changes in the corpus callosum (233). At the time of the initial scans, no differences from normal were seen. However, among the patients with schizophrenia the developmental trajectory of the area of the splenium was significantly different from normal. The splenium was significantly smaller than normal in patients with COS.

In a study of a small sample of the children with COS from the NIMH study, healthy controls, and a comparison group of nonschizophrenic patients matched for IQ and drug treatment status, three-dimensional maps of brain change were derived from high-resolution longitudinal brain MRI scans (186). By early adolescence, a "dynamic wave" of gray matter loss occurred. The loss started in the parietal association cortices and continued to the dorsolateral prefrontal cortex and temporal cortex. Significant progressive loss of cerebellar volume has also been reported from the longitudinal NIMH study (234). The loss appears to occur at the same time as cerebral volume loss, despite the fact that the cerebellum appears to reach its peak in total volume later than total cerebral volume. These data suggest that structural changes continue after the early onset of psychotic symptoms and continue well into adolescence. The changes observed in cortical volume are consistent with changes in ventricular enlargement.

These results, as well as a recent report of progressive gray matter volume loss in a larger sample of longitudinal subjects from the NIMH COS study (235), support the concept of schizophrenia as a progressive neurodevelopmental disorder with both early and late developmental abnormalities. While these brain MRI results do not have any immediate clinical implications, they may provide useful information for understanding the underlying pathophysiology.

The progressive loss of neural tissue seen in COS does not appear to be common to other developmental disorders. For example, although there is evidence for early developmental abnormality of cerebellar-striatal-prefrontal circuitry in ADHD, longitudinal data indicate that the developmental trajectory of brain volume is normal in children with ADHD (236, 237). Rapoport and colleagues speculate that in COS, the earlier tissue loss may trigger the onset of psychosis in childhood.

The underlying causes of the brain MRI abnormalities are not clear. There may be abnormalities in neuronal migration, or a disturbance in the process of normal synaptic pruning that follows the peak of synaptic production during the preschool period (212, 238, 239), particularly the prefrontal corticocortical, and corticosubcortical synapses (240). The progressive loss may indicate a late neurodevelopmental disorder that may be correlated with clinical symptoms and pathophysiology of the illness. It is interesting to note that healthy siblings of patients with COS share some of the brain MRI abnormalities as their affected siblings (241). The healthy siblings had smaller than normal total and parietal gray matter volumes than normal comparison subjects. Unlike the patients, however, there was no evidence of ventricular enlargement. These results may suggest that some of the brain abnormalities associated with COS are genetic trait markers, just as has been suggested from similar results from siblings of patients with adult-onset schizophrenia.

Two MRS studies (Bertolino et al., 1998 and Brooks et al., 1998) suggest anterior cingulate and frontal metabolite abnormalities in childhood-onset schizophrenia, including below-normal NAA/Cr (242, 243). In a MRS study of 11 patients with childhood-onset schizophrenia, above-normal levels of creatine plus phosphocreatine were found in the superior anterior cingulate, and above-normal levels of choline compounds were found in the superior anterior cingulate, frontal cortex, and head of the caudate nucleus (244). In the thalamus, NAA was lower in male but not female subjects with COS. Elevated creatine suggests abnormal local cell-energy demand and elevated choline may indicate that patients with COS exhibit phospholipid membrane disturbances (244). Low NAA may reflect diminished neuronal integrity.

Treatment

Patients with childhood-onset schizophrenia appear to be less responsive to medication treatment than adults with schizophrenia and may experience more adverse drug side effects. It is possible that these effects reflect the earlier, more severe nature of their neurodevelopmental abnormalities (188).

As with adults, antipsychotic medications may be beneficial in reducing hallucinations and delusions. The newer generation "atypical" antipsychotics, such as olanzapine and clozapine, may also reduce negative symptoms, such as improving motivation and emotional expressiveness (187). Due to the increased risk of side effects associated with the typical antipsychotics, atypical antipsychotics are preferred in the initial treatment of COS (202, 245). However, side effects are also associated with these newer medications, including excess weight gain, neutropenias, and seizures, and therefore all children should be carefully monitored and administered the lowest effective dose possible. The majority of studies conducted with children and adolescents have been open label studies. The largest number of studies included clozapine or olanzapine. Less data are available on the effectiveness of risperidone (two open label studies), amisulpride (one controlled study), and quietiapine (one open label study) (202).

The NIMH group has conducted studies with patients with COS who were neuroleptic nonresponders. In a double-blind comparison of haloperidol and clozapine, clozapine was found to be superior in reducing both positive and negative symptoms (246). Other studies have also reported positive effects with clozapine (187, 202). Studies comparing clozapine with olanzapine have revealed that olanzapine has a more benign side effect profile but clozapine has superior efficacy for positive and negative symptoms (187). Due to the increased risk of serious side effects, clozapine is not recommended as a first-line antipsychotic medication (1). Clozapine requires daily monitoring. In this era where several atypical neuroleptic medications are available to target negative and positive symptoms, traditional neuroleptic medications, such as haloperidol, are not typically thought of as first line medications.

Schizophrenia impacts a wide range of domains therefore treatment must be multimodal. In addition to medication treatment, it is important to consider the benefits of psychosocial intervention for children and adolescents suffering from schizophrenia (1, 202). An integrated intervention package that combines psychotropic medication to reduce acute symptoms and vulnerability, and psychosocial interventions to reduce stress and build coping strategies is ideal but has not been systematically investigated (209). It is important to consider the impact of developmental level on the treatment process, the necessary case management skills in working with family members and school systems, potential comorbid symptoms, and the chronic nature of this disorder. Given the deficits in attention, verbal learning, and executive functions among children with schizophrenia, neuropsychological assessment can be helpful for treatment and academic planning. Special school programs are often needed. Social skills training and improvement of problem-solving skills may also be warranted (1). Currently, more children are treated within their families and communities rather than long-term hospitalization. The attributes of the family may have an impact on the child's illness, and the needs of the child can also have a significant impact on the rest of the family. Behavioral family treatment is therefore an important consideration.

Acknowledgment: The author was supported by a grant from the National Institutes of Health (NINDS R01 NS042639, P.I.: Jeanne Townsend, Ph.D.).

REFERENCES

1. Asarnow JR, Asarnow RF. Childhood-onset schizophrenia. In: Mash EJ, Barkley RA, eds. *Child psychopathology*, 2nd ed. New York: Guilford; 2003;455–485.
2. Kanner L. Autistic disturbances of affective contact. *Nervous Child*. 1943;2:217–250.
3. Asperger H. Die autistischen Psychopathen im Kindesalter. *Archiv für Psychiatrie und Nervenkrankheiten*. 1944;117:76–136.
4. American Psychiatric Association. *Diagnostic and Statistical Manual of Mental Disorders*. 2nd ed. Washington, DC: American Psychiatric Association; 1968.
5. American Psychiatric Association. *Diagnostic and Statistical Manual of Mental Disorders*. 3rd ed. Washington, DC: American Psychiatric Association; 1980.
6. Green WH, Campbell M, Hardesty AS, et al. A comparison of schizophrenic and autistic children. *Journal of the American Academy of Child and Adolescent Psychiatry*. 1984;23:399–409.
7. Kolvin I. Studies in the childhood psychoses: I. Diagnostic criteria and classification. *British Journal of Psychiatry*. 1971;118:381–384.
8. Eisenberg L. The course of childhood schizophrenia. *Archives of Neurological Psychiatry*. 1957;78:69–83.
9. Werry JS. Childhood schizophrenia. In: Volkmar FR, ed. *Psychoses and pervasive developmental disorders in childhood and adolescence*. Washington, D.C.: American Psychiatric Press; 1996.
10. Lord C, Bailey A. Autism Spectrum Disorders. In: Rutter M, Taylor E, eds. *Child and Adolescent Psychiatry: Modern Approaches, Fourth Edition*. Oxford: Blackwell Publications; 2002:636–663.
11. Wing L. Autistic spectrum disorders. *BMJ*. 1996;312:327–328.
12. Tanguay PE. Commentary: categorical versus spectrum approaches to classification in pervasive developmental disorders. *Journal of the American Academy of Child and Adolescent Psychiatry*. 2004;43:181–182.
13. American Psychiatric Association. *Diagnostic and Statistical Manual of Mental Disorders, 4th ed, Text Revision*. Washington, DC: American Psychiatric Association; 2000.
14. Chakrabarti S, Fombonne E. Pervasive developmental disorders in preschool children. [Comment In: JAMA. 2001 Jun 27;285 (24):3141–2]. *JAMA*. 2001;285(24):3093–3099.
15. Fombonne E. The prevalence of autism. *Journal of the American Medical Association*. 2003;289(1):87–89.
16. Baird G, Charman T, Baron-Cohen S, et al. A screening instrument for autism at 18 months of age: A six-year follow-up study. *Journal of the American Academy of Child and Adolescent Psychiatry*. 2000;39:694–702.
17. Yeargin-Allsopp M, Rice C, Karapurkar T, Doernberg N, Boyle C, Murphy C. Prevalence of autism in a US metropolitan area. *Journal of the American Medical Association*. 2003;289:49–55.
18. Vastag B. National autism summit charts a path through a scientific, clinical wilderness. *JAMA*. 2004;291:29–31.
19. Wing L, Gould J. Severe impairments of social interaction and associated abnormalities in children: Epidemiology and classification. *Journal of Autism and Developmental Disorders*. 1979;9:11–29.
20. Walker DR, Thompson A, Zwaigenbaum L, et al. Specifying PDD-NOS: a comparison of PDD-NOS, Asperger syndrome, and autism. *Journal of the American Academy of Child and Adolescent Psychiatry*. 2004;43:172–180.
21. Eisenmajer R, Prior M, Leekam S, et al. Comparison of clinical symptoms in autism and Asperger's disorder. *Journal of the American Academy of Child and Adolescent Psychiatry*. 1996; 35:1523–1531.
22. Howlin P. Outcome in high-functioning adults with autism with and without early language delays: implications for the differentiation between autism and Asperger syndrome. *Journal of Autism and Developmental Disorders*. 2003;33:3–13.
23. Mayes SD, Calhoun SL, Crites DL. Does DSM-IV Asperger's disorder exist? *Journal of Abnormal Child Psychology*. 2001;29:263–271.
24. Szatmari P. The classification of autism, Asperger's syndrome, and pervasive developmental disorder. *Canadian Journal of Psychiatry*. 2000;45:731–738.
25. Klin A, Volkmar FR. Asperger syndrome: diagnosis and external validity. *Child and Adolescent Psychiatric Clinics of North America*. 2003;12:1–13.
26. Schopler E, Mesibov GB, Kunce LJ. *Asperger syndrome or high functioning autism?* New York: Plenum Press; 1998.
27. Willemsen-Swinkels SHN, Buitelaar JK. The autistic spectrum: subgroups, boundaries, and treatment. *Psychiatric Clinics of North America*. 2002;25(4):811–836.
28. Volkmar FR, Klin A. Diagnostic issues in Asperger syndrome. In: Klin A, Volkmar FR, Sparrow SS, eds. *Asperger Syndrome*. New York: Guilford Press; 2000:25–71.
29. Filipek PA, Accardo PJ, Ashwal S, et al. Practice parameter: screening and diagnosis of autism: report of the Quality Standards Subcommittee of the American Academy of Neurology and the Child Neurology Society. *Neurology*. 2000;55(4):468–479.

30. Baron-Cohen S, Cox A, Baird G, et al. Psychological markers in the detection of autism in infancy in a large population. *British Journal of Psychiatry.* 1996;168(2):158–163.

31. Rutter M, Bailey A, Lord C. *Social Communication Questionnaire.* Los Angeles: Western Psychological Services; 2003.

32. Baird G, Charman T, Cox A, et al. Screening and surveillance for autism and pervasive developmental disorders. *Archives of Diseases in Childhood.* 2001;84:468–475.

33. Charman T, Baird G. Practitioner review: Diagnosis of autism spectrum disorder in 2- and 3-year-old children. *Journal of Child Psychology & Psychiatry.* 2002;43(3):289–305.

34. Rogers S. Diagnosis of autism before the age of 3. *International Review of Mental Retardation.* 2001;23:1–31.

35. Robins DL, Fein D, Barton ML, Green JA. The Modified-Checklist for Autism in Toddlers: An initial study investigating the early detection of autism and pervasive developmental disorders. *Journal of Autism and Developmental Disorders.* 2001;31:131–144.

36. Siegel B. Detection of autism in the 2nd and 3rd years: The Pervasive Developmental Disorders Screening Test (PDDST). Paper presented at: the biennial meeting of the Society for Research in Child Development, 1999; Albuquerque, NM.

37. Lord C. Follow-up of two-year-olds referred for possible autism. *Journal of Child Psychology and Psychiatry.* 1995;36(8):1365–1382.

38. National Research Council. *Educating Children with Autism. Committee on Educational Interventions for Children with Autism. Division of Behavioral and Social Sciences and Education.* Washington, DC: National Academy Press; 2001.

39. Lord C, Risi S. Frameworks and methods in diagnosing autism spectrum disorders. *MRDD Res. Rev.* 1998;4:90–96.

40. Cox A, Klein K, Charman T, et al. Autism spectrum disorders at 20 and 42 months of age: stability of clinical and ADI-R diagnosis. *Journal of Child Psychology and Psychiatry and Allied Disciplines.* 1999;40(5):719–732.

41. Stone WL, Lee EB, Ashford L, et al. Can autism be diagnosed accurately in children under 3 years? *Journal of Child Psychology and Psychiatry and Allied Disciplines.* 1999;40(2):219–226.

42. Lord C, Rutter M, Le Couteur A. Autism Diagnostic Interview-Revised: a revised version of a diagnostic interview for caregivers of individuals with possible pervasive developmental disorders. *Journal of Autism and Developmental Disorders.* 1994;24(5):659–685.

43. Lord C, Risi S, Lambrecht L, et al. The Autism Diagnostic Observation Schedule–Generic: A Standard Measure of Social and Communication Deficits Associated with the Spectrum of Autism. *Journal of Autism and Developmental Disorders.* 2000;30(3):205–223.

44. Lord C, Rutter M, DiLavore PC, Risi S. *Autism Diagnostic Observation Schedule.* Los Angeles: Western Psychological Services; 2001.

45. Lord C, Risi S. Diagnosis of autism spectrum disorders in young children. In: Wetherby A, Prizant B, eds. *Autism spectrum disorders: A transactional developmental perspective.* Baltimore: Paul H. Brookes Publishing Co.; 2000:167–190.

46. Shriver MD, Allen KD, Matthews JR. Effective assessment of the shared and unique characteristics of children with autism. *School Psychology Review.* 1999;28(4):538–558.

47. Rutter M, Le Couteur A, Lord C. *ADI-R. Autism Diagnostic Interview-Revised. WPS Edition.* Los Angeles: Western Psychological Services; 2003.

48. Lord C, Rutter M, Goode S, et al. Autism diagnostic observation schedule: a standardized observation of communicative and social behavior. *Journal of Autism and Developmental Disorders.* 1989;19:185–212.

49. DiLavore PC, Lord C, Rutter M. The pre-linguistic autism diagnostic observation schedule. *Journal of Autism and Developmental Disorders.* 1995;25(4):355–379.

50. Gilliam JE. *Gilliam Autism Rating Scales.* Austin (Texas): Pro-Ed; 1995.

51. Clark A, Harrington R. On diagnosing rare disorders rarely: Appropriate use of screening instruments. *Journal of Child Psychology & Psychiatry.* 1999;40(2):287–290.

52. Berument SK, Rutter M, Lord C, Pickles A, Bailey A. Autism screening questionnaire: diagnostic validity. *British Journal of Psychiatry.* 1999;175:444–451.

53. Bishop DVM, Norbury CF. Exploring the borderlands of autistic disorder and specific language impairment: a study using standardized instruments. *Journal of Child Psychology & Psychiatry.* 2002;43(7):917–929.

54. Schopler E, Reichler RJ, Rochen Renner B. *The Childhood Autism Rating Scale*: Western Psychological Services; 1988.

55. Saemundsen E, Magnusson P, Smari J, Sigurdardottir S. Autism Diagnostic Interview-Revised and the Childhood Autism Rating Scale: convergence and discrepancy in diagnosing autism. *Journal of Autism and Developmental Disorders.* 2003;33:319–328.

56. Wechsler D. *Wechsler Intelligence Scale for Children—Revised.* San Antonio: Psychological Corporation; 1974.

57. Wechsler D. *Wechsler Intelligence Scale for Children, Third Edition.* San Antonio: The Psychological Corporation; 1991.

58. Lincoln AJ, Courchesne E, Kilman BA, Elmasian R, Allen M. A study of intellectual abilities in high-functioning people with autism. *Journal of Autism and Developmental Disorders.* 1988;18(4).

59. Siegel DJ, Minshew NJ, Goldstein G. Wechsler IQ profiles in diagnosis of high-functioning autism [see comments]. *Journal of Autism and Developmental Disorders.* 1996;26(4):389–406.

60. Joseph RM, Tager-Flusberg H, Lord C. Cognitive profiles and social-communicative functioning in children with autism spectrum disorder. *Journal of Child Psychology and Psychiatry.* 2002;43(6):807–821.

61. Frith U. *Autism: explaining the enigma.* 2nd ed. Malden, MA: Blackwell Publishing; 2003.

62. Baron-Cohen S, Leslie AM, Frith U. Does the autistic child have a "theory of mind"? *Cognition.* 1985;21(1):37–46.

63. Minshew NJ, Meyer J, Goldstein G. Abstract reasoning in autism: a dissociation between concept formation and concept identification. *Neuropsychology.* 2002;16:327–334.

64. Ozonoff S, Pennington BF, Rogers SJ. Executive function deficits in high-functioning autistic individuals: relationship to theory of mind. *Journal of Child Psychology and Psychiatry.* 1991;32:1081–1105.

65. Pennington BF, Rogers SJ, Bennetto L, Griffith EM, Reed DT, Shyu V. Validity tests of the executive dysfunction hypothesis of autism. In: Russell J, ed. *Autism as an executive disorder.* Oxford: Oxford University Press; 1997:143–178.

66. Bennetto L, Pennington BF, Rogers SJ. Intact and impaired memory functions in autism. *Child Development.* 1996;67(4):1816–1835.

67. Liss M, Harel B, Fein D, et al. Predictors and correlates of adaptive functioning in children with developmental disorders. *Journal of Autism & Developmental Disorders.* 2001;31:219–230.

68. Prior M, Hoffman W. Neuropsychological testing of autistic children through an exploration with frontal lobe tests. *Journal of Autism and Developmental Disorders.* 1990;20:581–590.

69. Rumsey JM. Neuropsychological studies of high-level autism. In: Schopler E, Mesibov G, eds. *High-functioning Individuals with Autism.* New York: Plenum Press; 1992:41–64.

70. Pennington BF, Ozonoff S. Executive functions and developmental psychopathology. *Journal of Child Psychology and Psychiatry and Allied Disciplines.* 1996;37(1):51–87.

71. Juul-Dam N, Townsend J, Courchesne E. Prenatal, perinatal, and neonatal factors in autism, pervasive developmental disorder-not otherwise specified, and the general population. *Pediatrics.* 2001;107:E63.

72. Courchesne E, Carper R, Akshoomoff N. Evidence of brain overgrowth in the first year of life in autism. *Journal of the American Medical Association.* 2003;290:337–344.

73. Courchesne E, Karns C, Davis HR, et al. Unusual Brain Growth Patterns in Early Life in Patients with Autistic Disorder: An MRI Study. *Neurology.* 2001;57:245–254.

74. Sparks BF, Friedman SD, Shaw DW, et al. Brain structural abnormalities in young children with autism spectrum disorder. *Neurology.* 2002;59:184–192.

75. Carper RA, Moses P, Tigue ZD, Courchesne E. Cerebral lobes in autism: Early hyperplasia and abnormal age effects. *Neuroimage.* 2002;16:1038–1051.

76. Bartholomeusz HH, Courchesne E, Karns C. Relationship between head circumference and brain volume in healthy normal toddlers, children, and adults. *Neuropediatrics.* 2002;33:239–241.

77. Akshoomoff N, Lord C, Lincoln AJ, et al. Outcome classification of preschoolers with autism spectrum disorders using MRI brain measures. *Journal of the American Academy of Child and Adolescent Psychiatry.* 2004;43:349–357.

78. Hardan AY, Minshew NJ, Harenski K, Keshavan MS. Posterior fossa magnetic resonance imaging in autism. *Journal of the American Academy of Child and Adolescent Psychiatry.* 2001;40(6):666–672.

79. Piven J, Saliba K, Bailey J, Arndt S. An MRI study of autism: the cerebellum revisited. *Neurology.* 1997;49(2):546–551.

80. Courchesne E, Yeung-Courchesne R, Press GA, Hesselink JR, Jernigan TL. Hypoplasia of cerebellar vermal lobules VI and VII in autism. *New England Journal of Medicine.* 1988;318(21):1349–1354.

81. Courchesne E, Townsend J, Saitoh O. The brain in infantile autism: posterior fossa structures are abnormal [see comments]. *Neurology.* 1994;44(2):214–223.

82. Hashimoto T, Tayama M, Murakawa K, et al. Development of the brainstem and cerebellum in autistic patients. *Journal of Autism and Developmental Disorders.* 1995;25(1):1–18.

83. Aylward EH, Minshew NJ, Field K, Sparks BF, Singh N. Effect of age on brain volume and head circurmference in autism. *Neurology.* 2002;59(2):175–183.

84. Courchesne E, Press GA, Yeung-Courchesne R. Parietal lobe abnormalities detected with MR in patients with infantile autism. *American Journal of Roentgenology.* 1993;160(2):387–393.

85. Bauman ML, Kemper TL. The neuropathology of the autism spectrum disorders: what have we learned? *Novartis Found Symp.* 2003;251:112–122.

86. Townsend J, Courchesne E. Parietal damage and narrow "spotlight" spatial attention. *Journal of Cognitive Neuroscience.* 1994; 6(3):220–232.

87. Nelson KB, Grether JK, Croen LA, et al. Neuropeptides and neurotrophins in neonatal blood of children with autism or mental retardation. *Annals of Neurology.* 2001;49(5):597–606.

88. Casanova MF, Buxhoeveden DP, Switala AE, Roy E. Minicolumnar pathology in autism. *Neurology.* 2002;58:428–432.

89. Akshoomoff N, Pierce K, Courchesne E. The neurobiological basis of autism from a developmental perspective. *Development and Psychopathology.* 2002;14:613–634.

90. Bailey A, Luthert P, Dean A, et al. A clinicopathological study of autism. *Brain.* 1998;121:889–905.

91. Bauman ML, Kemper TL. Neuroanatomic observations of the brain in autism. In: Bauman ML, Kemper TL, eds. *The Neurobiology of Autism.* Baltimore: Johns Hopkins UP; 1994:119–145.

92. Ritvo ER, Freeman BJ, Scheibel AB, et al. Lower Purkinje cell counts in the cerebella of four autistic subjects: initial findings of the UCLA-NSAC Autopsy Research Report. *American Journal of Psychiatry.* 1986;143(7):862–866.

93. Williams RS, Hauser SL, Purpura DP, DeLong GR, Swisher CN. Autism and mental retardation: neuropathologic studies performed in four retarded persons with autistic behavior. *Archives of Neurology.* 1980;37(12):749–753.

94. Egaas B, Courchesne E, Saitoh O. Reduced size of corpus callosum in autism. *Archives of Neurology.* 1995;52(8):794–801.

95. Manes F, Piven J, Vrancic D, Nanclares V, Plebst C, Starkstein SE. An MRI study of the corpus callosum and cerebellum in mentally retarded autistic individuals. *Journal of Neuropsychiatry and Clinical Neurosciences.* 1999;11(4):470–474.

96. Piven J, Bailey J, Ranson BJ, Arndt S. An MRI study of the corpus callosum in autism. *American Journal of Psychiatry.* 1997; 154(8):1051–1055.

97. Aylward E, Minshew N, Goldstein G, et al. MRI volumes of amygdala and hippocampus in non-mentally retarded autistic adolescents and adults. *Neurology.* 1999;53(9):2145–2150.

98. Haznedar MM, Buchsbaum MS, Wei T-C, et al. Limbic circuitry in patients with autism spectrum disorders studied with positron emission tomography and magnetic resonace imaging. *American Journal of Psychiatry.* 2000;157:1994–2001.

99. Howard M. Convergent neuroanatomical and behavioural evidence of an amygdala hypothesis of autism. *Neuroreport.* 2000; 11(13):2931–2935.

100. Piven J, Bailey J, Ranson BJ, Arndt S. No difference in hippocampus volume detected on magnetic resonance imaging in autistic individuals. *Journal of Autism and Developmental Disorders.* 1998;28:105–110.

101. Saitoh O, Karns C, Courchesne E. Development of the hippocampal formation from 2 to 42 years: MRI evidence of smaller area dentata in autism. *Brain.* 2001;124:1317–1324.

102. Kemper T, Bauman M. Neuropathology of infantile autism. *Journal of Neuropathology and Experimental Neurology.* 1998; 57(7):645–652.

103. Raymond GV, Bauman ML, Kemper TL. Hippocampus in autism: a Golgi analysis. *Acta Neuropathologica.* 1996;91(1): 117–119.

104. Herbert MR, Ziegler DA, Deutsch CK, et al. Dissociations of cerebral cortex, subcortical and cerebral white matter volumes in autistic boys. *Brain.* 2003;126:1182–1192.

105. Allen G, Courchesne E. Differential effects of developmental cerebellar abnormality on cognitive and motor functions in the cerebellum: an fMRI study of autism. *American Journal of Psychiatry.* 2003;160:262–273.

106. Belmonte MK, Yurgelun-Todd DA. Functional anatomy of impaired selective attention and compensatory processing in autism. *Cognitive Brain Research.* 2003;17:651–664.

107. Pierce K, Müller R-A, Ambrose J, Allen G, Courchesne E. Face processing occurs outside the fusiform 'face area' in autism: evidence from functional MRI. *Brain.* 2001;124:2059–2073.

108. Müller R-A, Pierce K, Ambrose JB, Allen G, Courchesne E. Atypical cerebral motor activations in autism: an fMRI study. *Journal of Cognitive Neuroscience.* 2000(Suppl.):85.

109. Muller RA, Kleinhans N, Kemmotsu N, Pierce K, Courchesne E. Abnormal variability and distribution of functional maps in autism: an FMRI study of visuomotor learning. *American Journal of Psychiatry.* 2003;160:1847–1862.

110. Müller RA, Behen ME, Rothermel RD, et al. Brain mapping of language and auditory perception in high-functioning autistic adults: a PET study. *Journal of Autism and Developmental Disorders.* 1999;29:19–31.

111. Müller RA, Chugani DC, Behen ME, et al. Impairment of dentato-thalamo-cortical pathway in autistic men: language activation data from positron emission tomography. *Neuroscience Letters.* 1998;27:1–4.

112. Akshoomoff N. Neurological underpinnings of autism. In: Wetherby AM, Prizant BM, eds. *Autism spectrum disorders: A transactional developmental perspective.* Baltimore: Paul H. Brookes Publishing Co.; 2000:167–190.

113. Townsend J, Westerfield M, Leaver E, et al. Event-related brain response abnormalities in autism: evidence for impaired cerebello-frontal spatial attention networks. *Cognitive Brain Research.* 2001;11:127–145.

114. Anderson GM, Zimmerman AW, Akshoomoff N, Chugani DC. Autism clinical trials: Biological and medical issues in patient selection and treatment response. *CNS Spectrums.* 2004;9:57–64.

115. Chugani DC, Muzik O, Behen M, et al. Developmental changes in brain serotonin synthesis capacity in autistic and nonautistic children. *Annals of Neurology.* 1999;45(3):287–295.

116. Chugani DC. Role of altered brain serotonin mechanisms in autism. *Molecular Psychiatry.* 2002;7:S16–S17.

117. Chugani DC, Muzik O, Rothermel RD, et al. Altered serotonin synthesis in the dentato-thalamo-cortical pathway in autistic boys. *Annals of Neurology.* 1997;14:666–669.

118. Ernst M, Zametkin AJ, Matochik JA, Pascualvaca D, Cohen RM. Low medial prefrontal dopaminergic activity in autistic children. *Lancet.* 1997;350:638.

119. Minshew NJ, Goldstein G, Dombrowski SM, Panchalingam K, Pettegrew JW. A preliminary 31P MRS study of autism: evidence for undersynthesis and increased degradation of brain membranes. *Biological Psychiatry.* 1993;33(11–12):762–773.

120. Chugani DC, Sundram BS, Behen M, Lee M-L, Moore GJ. Evidence of altered energy metabolism in autistic children. *Prog. Neuro-Psychopharmacol. & Biol. Psychiat.* 1999;23:635–641.

121. Friedman SD, Shaw DW, Artru AA, et al. Regional brain chemical alterations in young children with autism spectrum disorder. *Neurology.* 2003;60:100–107.

122. Levitt JG, O'Neill J, Blanton RE, et al. Proton magnetic resonance spectroscopic imaging of the brain in childhood autism. *Biological Psychiatry.* 2003;54:1355–1366.

123. Folstein S, Rutter M. Infantile autism: a genetic study of 21 twin pairs. *Journal of Child Psychology and Psychiatry and Allied Disciplines.* 1977;18(4).

124. Bailey A, Le Couteur A, Gottesman I, et al. Autism as a strongly genetic disorder: evidence from a British twin study. *Psychological Medicine.* 1995;25(1):63–77.

125. Yonan AL, Alarcon M, Cheng R, et al. A genomewide screen of 345 families for autism-susceptibility loci. *Am J Hum Gen.* 2003; 73(886–897).

126. Cook EH, Jr., Courchesne R, Lord C, et al. Evidence of linkage between the serotonin transporter and autistic disorder. *Molecular Psychiatry.* 1997;2(3):247–250.

127. Klauck SM, Poustka F, Benner A, Lesch KP, Poustka A. Serotonin transporter (5-HTT) gene variants associated with autism? *Human Molecular Genetics.* 1997;6(13):2233–2238.

128. Yirmiya N, Pilowsky T, Nemanov L, et al. Evidence for an association with the serotonin transporter promoter region polymorphism and autism. *American Journal of Medical Genetics.* 2001; 105:381–386.

129. Kim SJ, Cox N, Courchesne R, et al. Transmission disequilibrium mapping at the serotonin transporter gene (SLC6A4) region in autistic disorder. *Molecular Psychiatry.* 2002;7:278–288.

130. Cook EH, Leventhal BL. The serotonin system in autism. *Current Opinion in Pediatrics.* 1996;8:348–354.

131. Ramoz N, Reichert JG, Smith CJ, et al. Linkage and association of the mitochondrial aspartate/glutamate carrier SLC25A12 gene with autism. *American Journal of Psychiatry.* 2004;161: 662–669.

132. Folstein SE, Dowd M, Mankoski R, Tadevosyan O. How might genetic mechanisms operate in autism? *Novartis Found Symp.* 2003;251:70–80.

133. Klin A, Jones W, Schultz R, Volkmar F, Cohen D. Defining and quantifying the social phenotype in autism. *American Journal of Psychiatry.* 2002;159:895–908.

134. Wakefield AJ, Murch SH, Anthony A, et al. Ileal-lymphoid-nodular hyperplasia, non-specific colitis, and pervasive developmental disorder in children. *Lancet.* 1998;351:637–641.

135. Horton R. The lessons of MMR. *Lancet.* 2004;363:747–749.

136. Goldberg W, Osann K, Filipek P, et al. Language and other regression: Assessment and timing. *Journal of Autism and Developmental Disorders.* 2003;33:607–616.

137. Rapin I, Katzman R. Neurobiology of autism. *Annals of Neurology.* 1998;43:7–14.

138. Rutter M, Lord C. Language disorders associated with psychiatric disturbance. In: Yule W, Rutter M, eds. *Language Development and Disorders.* Philadelphia, PA: J.B. Lippincott Co.; 1987: 206–233.

139. Davidovitch M, Glick L, Holtzman G, Tirosh E, Safir MP. Developmental regression in autism: Maternal perception. *Journal of Autism and Developmental Disorders.* 2000;30:113–119.

140. Fombonne E, Chakrabarti S. No evidence for a new variant of measles-mumps-rubella-induced autism. *Pediatrics.* 2001; 108:e58.

141. Kurita H. Infantile-Autism with Speech Loss before the Age of 30 Months. *Journal of the American Academy of Child and Adolescent Psychiatry.* 1985;24:191–196.

142. Shinnar S, Rapin I, Arnold S, et al. Language regression in childhood. *Pediatric Neurology.* 2001;24:183–189.

143. Wilson S, Djukic A, Shinnar S, Dharmani C, Rapin I. Clinical characteristics of language regression in children. *Developmental Medicine and Child Neurology.* 2003;45:508–514.

144. Lord C, Shulman C, DiLavore P. Regression and Word Loss in Autism Spectrum Disorder. *Journal of the American Academy of Child and Adolescent Psychiatry.* 2004;45:1–21.

145. Luyster R, Richler J, Risi S, et al. Early Regression in Social Communication in Autistic Spectrum Disorders: A CPEA study. *Developmental Neuropsychology.* 2005;27:311–336.

146. Institute of Medicine. *Immunization Safety Review: Measles-Mumps-Rubella Vaccine and Autism.* Washington, D.C.: National Academy Press; 2001.

147. Madsen K, Hviid A, Vestergaard M, et al. A population-based study of measles, mumps, and rubella vaccination and autism. *New England Journal of Medicine.* 2002;347:1477–1482.

148. Taylor B, Miller E, Farrington CP, et al. Autism and measles, mumps, and rubella vaccine: no epidemiological evidence for a causal association. *Lancet.* 1999;353:2026–2029.

149. Taylor B, Miller E, Lingam R, Andrews N, Simmons A, Stowe J. Measles, mumps, and rubella vaccination and bowel problems or developmental regression in children with autism: Population study. *British Medical Journal.* 2002;324:393–396.

150. Murch SH, Anthony A, Casson DH, et al. Retraction of an interpretation. *Lancet.* 2004;363:750.

151. Rogers SJ. Brief report: early intervention in autism. *Journal of Autism and Developmental Disorders.* 1996;26(2):243–246.

152. Schreibman L. Intensive behavioral/psychoeducational treatments for autism: Research needs and future directions. *Journal of Autism and Developmental Disorders.* 2000;30(373–378).

153. Rogers S. Neuropsychology of autism in young children and its implications for early intervention. *MRDD Res. Rev.* 1998;4: 104–112.

154. Siegel B. *Helping children with autism learn.* New York: Oxford University Press; 2003.

155. Wieder S, Greenspan SI. Climbing the symbolic ladder in the DIR model through floor time/interactive play. *Autism.* 2003;7:425–435.

156. Howlin P. Practitioner review: Psychological and educational treatments for autism. *Journal of Child Psychology & Psychiatry.* 1998;39(3):307–322.

157. Siegel B. *The world of the autistic child.* New York: Oxford University Press; 1996.

158. McDougle CJ, Posey DJ. Autistic and other pervasive developmental disorders. In: Martin A, Scahill L, Charney DS, Leckman JF, eds. *Pediatric psychopharmacology.* New York: Oxford University Press; 2003:563–579.

159. Anderson LT, Campbell M, Grega DM, Perry R, Small AM, Green WH. Haloperidol in the treatment of infantile autism: effects on learning and behavioral symptoms. *American Journal of Psychiatry.* 1984;141(10):1195–1202.

160. Campbell M, Perry R, Small AM, Green WH. Overview of drug treatment in autism. In: Schopler E, Mesibov GB, eds. *Neurobiological issues in autism.* New York: Plenum Press,; 1987:341–356.

161. Willemsen-Swinkels SHN, Buitelaar JK, van Engeland H. The effects of chronic naltrexone treatment in young autistic children: a double-blind placebo-controlled crossover study. *Biological Psychiatry.* 1996;39:1023–1031.

162. McDougle CJ, Scahill L, McCracken JT, et al. Research Units on Pediatric Psychopharmacology (RUPP) Autism Network: background and rationale for an initial controlled study of respiridone. *Child and Adolescent Psychiatric Clinics of North America.* 2000;9:201–224.

163. McCracken JT, McGough J, Shah B, et al. Risperidone in children with autism and serious behavioral problems. *New England Journal of Medicine.* 2002;347:314–321.

164. Masi G, Cosenza A, Mucci M, Brovedani P. A 3-year naturalistic study of 53 preschool children with pervasive developmental disorders treated with risperidone. *Journal of Clinical Psychiatry.* 2003;64:1039–1047.

165. Arnold LE, Vitiello B, McDougle C, et al. Parent-defined target symptoms respond to risperidone in RUPP autism study: customer approach to clinical trials. *Journal of the American Academy of Child and Adolescent Psychiatry.* 2003;42:1443–1450.

166. Gordon CT, State RC, Nelson JE, Hamburger SD, Rapoport JL. A double-blind comparison of clomipramine, desipramine, and placebo in the treatment of autistic disorder. *Archives of General Psychiatry.* 1993;50(6).

167. McDougle CJ, Naylor ST, Cohen DJ, Volkmar FR, Heninger GR, Price LH. A double-blind, placebo-controlled study of fluvoxamine in adults with autistic disorder [see comments]. *Archives of General Psychiatry.* 1996;53(11):1001–1008.

168. Cook E, Rowlett R, Jaselskis C, Leventhal B. Fluoxetine treatment of patients with autism and mental retardation. *Journal of the American Academy of Child and Adolescent Psychiatry.* 1992; 31:739–745.

169. McDougle CJ, Posey D. Genetics of childhood disorders: XLIV. autism, part 3: psychopharmacology of autism. *Journal of the American Academy of Child and Adolescent Psychiatry.* 2002;41: 1380–1383.

170. Horvath K, Stefanos G, Sokolski K, Wachtel R, Nabors L, Tildon J. Improved social and language skills after secretin administration in patients with autistic spectrum disorders. *Journal of the Association for Academic Minority Physicians.* 1998;9:9–15.

171. Sandler AD, Sutton KA, DeWeese J, Girardi MA, Sheppard V, Bodfish JW. Lack of benefit of a single dose of synthetic human secretin in the treatment of autism and pervasive developmental

disorder [see comments]. *New England Journal of Medicine.* 1999;341:1801–1806.

172. Owley T, McMahon W, Cook EH, et al. Multisite, double-blind, placebo-controlled trial of porcine secretin in autism. *Journal of the American Academy of Child and Adolescent Psychiatry.* 2001;40:1293–1299.

173. Chez MG, Buchanan CP, Bagan BT, et al. Secretin and autism: A two-part clinical investigation. *Journal of Autism and Developmental Disorders.* 2000;30:87–94.

174. Coniglio SJ, Lewis JD, Lang C, et al. A randomized, double-blind, placebo-controlled trial of single-dose intravenous secretin as treatment for children with autism. *Journal of Pediatrics.* 2001;138:649–655.

175. Dunn-Geier J, Ho HH, Auersperg E, et al. Effect of secretin on children with autism: A randomized controlled trial. *Developmental Medicine and Child Neurology.* 2000;42:796–802.

176. Molloy CA, Manning-Courtney P, Swayne S, et al. Lack of benefit of intravenous synthetic human secretin in the treatment of autism. *Journal of Autism and Developmental Disorders.* 2002;32:545–551.

177. Unis AS, Munson JA, Rogers SJ, et al. A randomized, double-blind, placebo-controlled trial of porcine versus synthetic secretin for reducing symptoms of autism. *Journal of the American Academy of Child and Adolescent Psychiatry.* 2002;41:1315–1321.

178. Kern JK, Espinoza E, Trivedi MH. The effectiveness of secretin in the management of autism. *Expert Opinion in Pharmacotherapy.* 2004;5:379–387.

179. Tanguay PE. Commentary: the primacy of the scientific method. *Journal of the American Academy of Child and Adolescent Psychiatry.* 2002;41:1322–1323.

180. Levy SE, Hyman SL. Use of complementary and alternative treatments for children with autistic spectrum disorders is increasing. *Pediatric Annals.* 2003;32:685–691.

181. Arnold LE, Aman MG, Martin A, et al. Assessment in multisite randomized clinical trials of patients with autistic disorder: the Autism RUPP Network. Research Units on Pediatric Psychopharmacology. *Journal of Autism and Developmental Disorders.* 2000;30:99–111.

182. Aman MG, Novotny S, Samango-Sprouse C, et al. Outcomes measures for clinical drug trials in autism. *CNS Spectrums.* 2004;9:36–47.

183. Seltzer MM, Krauss MW, Shattuck PT, Orsmond G, Swe A, Lord C. The symptoms of autism spectrum disorders in adolescence and adulthood. *Journal of Autism and Developmental Disorders.* 2003;33(6):565–581.

184. Shavelle RM, Strauss D. Comparative mortality of persons with autism in California, 1980–1996. *Journal of Insurance Medicine.* 1998;30(4):220–225.

185. Shavelle RM, Strauss DJ, Pickett J. Causes of death in autism. *Journal of Autism and Developmental Disorders.* 2001;31:569–576.

186. Thompson PM, Vidal C, Giedd JN, et al. Mapping adolescent brain change reveals dynamic wave of accelerated gray matter loss in very early-onset schizophrenia. *Proceedings of the National Academy of Sciences of the United States of America.* 2001;98:11650–11655.

187. Kumra S, Nicolson R, Rapoport JL. Childhood-onset schizophrenia. In: Zipursky RB, Schulz SC, eds. *The early stages of schizophrenia.* Washington, D.C.: American Psychiatric Publishing, Inc.; 2002:161–190.

188. Nicolson R, Rapoport JL. Neurobiology of childhood schizophrenia and related disorders. In: Martin A, Scahill L, Charney DS, Leckman JF, eds. *Pediatric psychopharmacology.* New York: Oxford University Press; 2003:184–194.

189. Werry JS. Child and adolescent (early onset) schizophrenia: New directions. *Journal of Autism and Developmental Disorders.* 1992;22:601–624.

190. Caplan R. Communication deficits in childhood schizophrenia spectrum disorders. *Schizophrenia Bulletin.* 1994;20:671–684.

191. National Institute of Mental Health. Childhood-Onset Schizophrenia: An Update from the National Institute of Mental Health. Available at: http://www.nimh.nih.gov/publicat/schizkids.cfm.

192. Dunn DW, McDougle CJ. Childhood-onset schizophrenia. In: Brier A, Tran PV, Herrera JM, Tollefson GD, Bymaaster FP, eds.

Current issues in the psychopharmacology of schizophrenia. Philadelphia: Lippincott Williams & Wilkins; 2001:375–388.

193. Nicolson R, Lenane M, Singaracharlu S, et al. Premorbid speech and language impairments in childhood-onset schizophrenia: association with risk factors. *American Journal of Psychiatry.* 2000;157:794–800.

194. Schaeffer JL, Ross RG. Childhood-onset schizophrenia: Premorbid and prodromal diagnostic and treatment histories. *Journal of the American Academy of Child and Adolescent Psychiatry.* 2002;41:538–545.

195. Asarnow JR, Tompson M, Goldstein MJ. Childhood-onset schizophrenia: A follow-up study. *Schizophrenia Bulletin.* 1994;20:599–618.

196. Hollis C. Adult outcomes of child- and adolescent-onset schizophrenia: diagnostic stability and predictive validity. *American Journal of Psychiatry.* 2000;157:1652–1659.

197. Eggers C, Bunk D. The long-term course of childhood-onset schizophrenia: A 42-year followup. *Schizophrenia Bulletin.* 1997;23:105–117.

198. Calderoni D, Wudarsky M, Bhangoo R, et al. Differentiating childhood-onset schizophrenia from psychotic mood disorders. *Journal of the American Academy of Child and Adolescent Psychiatry.* 2001;40(10):1190–1196.

199. Levitt JJ, Tsuang MT. The heterogeneity of schizoaffective disorder: implications for treatment. *American Journal of Psychiatry.* 1988;145:926–936.

200. Werry JS, McClellan JM, Chard L. Childhood and adolescent schizophrenic, bipolar, and schizoaffective disorders: a clinical and outcome study. *Journal of the American Academy of Child and Adolescent Psychiatry.* 1991;30:457–465.

201. Hollis C. Diagnosis and differential diagnosis. In: Remschmidt H, ed. *Schizophrenia in children and adolecents.* Cambridge, U.K.: Cambridge University Press; 2001:82–118.

202. Remschmidt H, Hebebrand J. Early-onset schizophrenia. In: Martin A, Scahill L, Charney DS, Leckman JF, eds. *Pediatric psychopharmacology.* New York: Oxford University Press; 2003:543–562.

203. Ambrosini PJ. Historical development and present status of the schedule for affective disorders and schizophrenia for school-age children (K-SADS). *Journal of the American Academy of Child and Adolescent Psychiatry.* 2000;39:49–58.

204. Russell AT, Bott L, Sammons C. The phenomenology of schizophrenia occurring in childhood. *Journal of the American Academy of Child and Adolescent Psychiatry.* 1989;28:399–407.

205. Shaffer D, Fisher P, Lucas CP, Dulcan MK, Schwab-Stone ME. NIMH Diagnostic Interview Schedule for Children Version IV (NIMH DISC-IV): description, differences from previous versions, and reliability of some common diagnoses. *Journal of the American Academy of Child and Adolescent Psychiatry.* 2000;39:28–38.

206. Fields JH, Grochowski S, Lindenmayer JP, et al. Assessing positive and negative symptoms in children and adolescents. *American Journal of Psychiatry.* 1994;151:249–253.

207. Shaffer D, Gould MS, Brasic J, et al. A children's global assessment scale (CGAS). *Archives of General Psychiatry.* 1983;40:1228–1231.

208. Caplan R, Guthrie D, Fish B, Tanguay PE, David-Lando G. The Kiddie Formal Thought Disorder Rating Scale: Clinical assessment, reliability, and validity. *Journal of the American Academy of Child and Adolescent Psychiatry.* 1989;28:408–416.

209. Tompson MC, Asarnow JR. Conceptualization and treatment of childhood-onset schizophrenia. In: Orvaschel H, Faust J, Hersen M, eds. *Handbook of conceptualization and treatment of child psychopathology.* Amsterdam, Netherlands: Pergamon/Elsevier Science Inc.; 2001:417–435.

210. American Academy of Child and Adolescent Psychiatry. Practice parameter for the assessment and treatment of children and adolescents with schizophrenia. American Academy of Child and Adolescent Psychiatry. *Journal of the American Academy of Child and Adolescent Psychiatry.* 2001;40((7 Suppl)):4S–23S.

211. Tsuang MT, Stone WS, Faraone SV. Genes, environment and schizophrenia. *British Journal of Psychiatry Suppl.* 2001;40:s18–24.

212. Weinberger DR. Implications of normal brain development for the pathogenesis of schizophrenia. *Archives of General Psychiatry.* 1987;44:660–669.

213. Kallman FJ, Roth B. Genetic aspects of pre-adolescent schizophrenia. *American Journal of Psychiatry.* 1956;112:599–606.

214. Asarnow RF, Nuechterlein KH, Fogelson DL, et al. Schizophrenia and schizophrenia-spectrum personality disorders in the first-degree relatives of children with schizophrenia: The UCLA Family Study. *Archives of General Psychiatry.* 2001;58:581–588.

215. Nicolson R, Brookner FB, Lenane M, et al. Parental schizophrenia spectrum disorders in childhood-onset and adult-onset schizophrenia. *American Journal of Psychiatry.* 2003;160: 490–495.

216. Asarnow RF, Nuechterlein KH, Subotnik KL, et al. Neurocognitive impairments in nonpsychotic parents of children with schizophrenia and attention-deficit/hyperactivity disorder. *Archives of General Psychiatry.* 2002;59:1053–1060.

217. Asarnow RF, Asamen J, Granholm E, Sherman T, Watkins J, Williams M. Cognitive/neuropsychological studies of children with a schizophrenic disorder. *Schizophrenia Bulletin.* 1994;20: 647–670.

218. Ross RG. Early expression of a pathophysiological feature of schizophrenia: saccadic intrusions into smooth-pursuit eye movements in school-age children vulnerable to schizophrenia. *Journal of the American Academy of Child and Adolescent Psychiatry.* 2003;42:468–476.

219. Ross RG, Olincy A, Harris JG, et al. Evidence for bilineal inheritance of physiological indicators of risk in childhood-onset schizophrenia. *American Journal of Medical Genetics.* 1999;88: 88–99.

220. Park S, Holzman PS. Association of working memory deficit and eye tracking dysfunction in schizophrenia. *Schizophrenia Research.* 1993;11:55–61.

221. Erlenmeyer-Kimling L. Neurobehavioral deficits in offspring of schizophrenic parents: liability indicators and predictors of illness. *American Journal of Medical Genetics.* 2000;97:65–71.

222. Hill SK, Schuepbachb D, Herbener ES, Keshavan MS, Sweeney JA. Pretreatment and longitudinal studies of neuropsychological deficits in antipsychotic-naive patients with schizophrenia. *Schizophrenia Research.* 2004;68:49–63.

223. Frazier JA, Giedd JN, Hamburger SD, et al. Brain anatomic magnetic resonance imaging in childhood-onset schizophrenia. *Archives of General Psychiatry.* 1996;53:617–624.

224. Jacobsen LK, Giedd JN, Vaituzis AC, et al. Temporal lobe morphology in childhood-onset schizophrenia. *American Journal of Psychiatry.* 1996;155:678–685.

225. Jacobsen LK, Giedd JN, Berquin PC, et al. Quantitative morphology of the cerebellum and fourth ventricle in childhood-onset schizophrenia. *American Journal of Psychiatry.* 1997;154 (12):1663–1669.

226. Nicolson R, Lenane M, Hamburger SD, Fernandez T, Bedwell J, Rapoport JL. Lessons from childhood-onset schizophrenia. *Brain Research Reviews.* 2000;31:147–156.

227. Sowell ER, Toga AW, Asarnow R. Brain abnormalities observed in childhood-onset schizophrenia: A review of the structural magnetic resonance imaging literature. *MRDD Res. Rev.* 2000; 6:180–185.

228. Sowell ER, Levitt J, Thompson PM, et al. Brain abnormalities observed in childhood-onset schizophrenia spectrum disorder observed with statistical parametric mapping of structural magnetic resonance images. *American Journal of Psychiatry.* 2000;157: 1475–1484.

229. Frazier JA, Giedd JN, Kaysen D, et al. Childhood-onset schizophrenia: brain MRI rescan after 2 years of clozapine maintenance treatment. *American Journal of Psychiatry.* 1996; 153:564–566.

230. Keshavan MS, Rosenberg D, Sweeney JA, Pettegrew JW. Decreased caudate volume in neuroleptic-naive psychotic patients. *American Journal of Psychiatry.* 1998;155:774–778.

231. Levitt JG, Blanton RE, Caplan R, et al. Medial temporal lobe in childhood-onset schizophrenia. *Psychiatry Research: Neuroimaging Section.* 2001;108:17–27.

232. Jacobsen LK, Giedd JN, Castellanos X, et al. Progressive reduction of temporal lobe structures in childhood-onset schizophrenia. *American Journal of Psychiatry.* 1998;155:678–685.

233. Keller A, Jeffries NO, Blumenthal J, et al. Corpus callosum development in childhood-onset schizophrenia. *Schizophrenia Research.* 2003;62:105–114.

234. Keller A, Castellanos FX, Vaituzis AC, Jeffries NO, Giedd JN, Rapoport JL. Progressive loss of cerebellar volume in childhood-onset schizophrenia. *American Journal of Psychiatry.* 2003; 160:128–133.

235. Sporn AL, Greenstein DK, Gogtay N, et al. Progressive brain volume loss during adolescence in childhood-onset schizophrenia. *American Journal of Psychiatry.* 2003;160:2181–2189.

236. Gogtay N, Giedd JN, Rapoport JL. Brain development in healthy, hyperactive, and psychotic children. *Archives of Neurology.* 2002; 59:1244–1248.

237. Castellanos FX, Lee PP, Sharp W, et al. Developmental trajectories of brain volume abnormalities in children and adolescents with attention-deficit/hyperactivity disorder. *Journal of the American Medical Association.* 2002;288:1740–1748.

238. Feinberg I. Cortical pruning and the development of schizophrenia. *Schizophrenia Bulletin.* 1990;16:567–570.

239. Huttenlocher PR, Dabholkar AS. Regional differences in synaptogenesis in human cerebral cortex. *Journal of Comparative Neurology.* 1997;387(2):167–178.

240. Keshavan MS, Anderson S, Pettegrew JW. Is schizophrenia due to excessive synaptic pruning in the prefrontal cortex? The Feinberg hypothesis revisited. *Journal of Psychiatry Research.* 1994; 28: 239–265.

241. Gogtay N, Sporn AL, Clasen LS, et al. Structural brain MRI abnormalities in healthy siblings of patients with childhood-onset schizophrenia. *American Journal of Psychiatry.* 2003;160: 569–571.

242. Bertolino A, Kumra S, Callicott JH, et al. Common pattern of cortical pathology in childhood-onset and adult-onset schizophrenia as identified by proton magnetic resonance spectroscopic imaging. *American Journal of Psychiatry.* 1998; 155:1376–1383.

243. Brooks WM, Hodde-Vargas J, Vargas LA, Yeo RA, Ford CC, Hendren RL. Frontal lobe of children with schizophrenia spectrum disorders: a proton magnetic resonance spectroscopic study. *Biological Psychiatry.* 1998;43:263–269.

244. O'Neill J, Levitt J, Caplan R, et al. 1H MRSI evidence of metabolic abnormalities in childhood-onset schizophrenia. *Neuroimage.* 2004;21:1781–1789.

245. Clark AF, Lewis SW. Treatment of schizophrenia in childhood and adolescence. *Journal of Child Psychology & Psychiatry.* 1998; 39:1071–1081.

246. Kumra S, Frazier JA, Jacobsen LK, et al. Childhood-onset schizophrenia. A double-blind clozapine-haloperidol comparison. *Archives of General Psychiatry.* 1996;53:1090–1097.

Attention Deficit–Hyperactivity Disorder

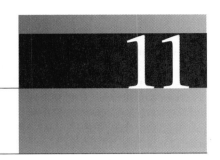

Kytja K. S. Voeller, MD

EPIDEMIOLOGY OF ATTENTION DEFICIT–HYPERACTIVITY DISORDER

Attention deficit–hyperactivity disorder (ADHD) is the most common neuropsychiatric disorder in the pediatric age group, with a worldwide prevalence in the range of 7 to 17% of school-aged children (1,2). This disorder has a long history. The first description of ADHD is attributed to Sir George Still, who in 1902, described children with "morbid deficits in moral control" (3). The disorder was also described in association with the residual effects of encephalitis and traumatic brain injury. In 1937, the efficacy of psychostimulants in the treatment of hyperactivity was described (4). Terms such as "minimal brain damage/dysfunction, minimal/minor cerebral dysfunction and hyperkinetic syndrome or hyperactive child syndrome" were also common descriptors at the time. The diagnosis of ADHD has undergone considerable evolution since the first clinically-based behavioral descriptions were put forth. It has now been recognized as a neuropsychiatric disorder with a strong genetic basis.

Two large-scale studies have provided considerable information about the clinical presentation of ADHD. The first, sponsored by the National Institute of Mental Health, was undertaken as part of the DSM-IV field trials. The study was based on 380 clinic-referred children and adolescents, ranging in age from 4 to 17 years. Structured diagnostic interviews were conducted with multiple informants and standardized clinician's diagnoses of ADHD were obtained to assess agreement. The study was also directed at definitional criteria for "impairment" (8). A second study, the NIMH Collaborative Multisite Multimodal Treatment Study of Children with ADHD, was conducted at six different sites across the country and enrolled 579 children with ADHD combined type, aged 7 years to 9 years 9 months. The subjects were randomly assigned to one of four different treatment conditions and followed for a period of 14 months. Both of these studies, although not without some limitations, provide a rich source of data regarding the clinical presentation of ADHD.

DIAGNOSIS AND CLINICAL PRESENTATION OF ATTENTION DEFICIT–HYPERACTIVITY DISORDER: INATTENTIVE, HYPERACTIVE/IMPULSIVE, AND COMBINED SUBTYPES

Currently, DSM-IV defines three subtypes of ADHD: the predominantly inattentive type, the predominantly hyperactive/inattentive type, and the combined type. To be given a specific diagnosis, a child must meet six of nine criteria for each of the subtypes. However, this is of questionable clinical utility, particularly if ADHD is a biological phenomenon with gradations of severity. A child would technically not be considered to have met diagnostic criteria of ADHD if only five of the nine behaviors were identified, even in the presence of serious impairment in daily life. Moreover, even though there is often relatively good agreement between observers, the diagnosis is based on behavioral manifestations and these observations are, of course, subject to observer bias and definitional criteria. (Some raters have a much lower threshold for "hyperactivity" or "impulsivity" than others.) The inattentive and hyperactive/impulsive subtypes differ in terms of age of onset, gender, and associated comorbid psychiatric conditions and learning disabilities. In general, the agreement between DSM-III-R and DSM-IV criteria is high (positive predictive power 93%) (9).

In 1987, Lahey and colleagues described a group of children, with a "sluggish cognitive tempo." These behaviors are typically seen in children who fall into the inattentive group and are not hyperactive or impulsive. They had difficulty initiating behaviors and were often disorganized and, if anything, apathetic (10). Although these symptoms demonstrated high positive predictive power in the DSM-IV field trials, they did not have high negative predictive power; that is, they were strongly associated with inattention but their absence did not predict absence of inattention. In addition, because the sluggish cognitive tempo subtype had a low base rate (that is, it was observed relatively infrequently in the study population), it was not included in the final symptom list (8).

Since the publication of DSM-IV in 1994, this issue has been reconsidered by several research groups. Several studies supported the validity of the sluggish cognitive tempo subtype. In a study of 692 clinic-referred children, a factor analysis indicated that the sluggish cognitive tempo items were most strongly associated with the severe end of the inattention spectrum. When the hyperactive/impulsive items and the inattention items were analyzed separately, the inattention symptoms could be broken down into two components: the sluggish cognitive tempo items plus forgetfulness and the DSM inattention items. These authors noted that their results challenged the two factor structure of DSM-IV (hyperactivity/impulsivity and inattention) and also observed that DSM-III inattention and DSM-IV inattention were not necessarily the same disorder. They concluded that DSM-IV inattention was a "perhaps overly heterogeneous group of children" and the inclusion of the sluggish cognitive tempo criteria might be helpful (11).

Carlson and Mann constructed a sluggish cognitive tempo scale based on the Achenbach Teacher Rating Scale (Achenbach 1991) and compared children with the combined ADHD subtype and the inattentive type. The sluggish cognitive tempo group was more prominently apathetic, underactive and day-dreaming, and prone to more social-emotional difficulties and withdrawal. Not surprisingly, they received lower teacher ratings for externalizing behaviors (12).

In contrast to the two previous studies, a large population-based study of 2,944 Australian twins, based on parent report found little selectivity for sluggish cognitive tempo symptoms based on latent class analysis. However, using a principal components factor analysis, there were striking gender differences. In boys, the sluggish cognitive tempo symptoms formed a separate factor, whereas in girls the sluggish cognitive tempo items loaded strongly on an inattentive factor. They concluded that the overall pattern of ADHD behaviors was not altered by this factor, but there were distinct gender differences (13).

In a study on a school population based on teacher ratings, Gaub and Carlson observed that children with DSM-IV combined type were severely impaired in academic and behavioral spheres, whereas those with the inattentive type had fewer externalizing behavior problems than those with the hyperactive/impulsive or combined types. The hyperactive/impulsive type had externalizing and social problems but did not have learning problems or internalizing problems (14). This study was based on teacher ratings. In some cases teachers attribute poor school performance to behavior problems but, there may also be a subtle comorbid learning disability. In a chart review comparing 143 cases of ADHD-inattentive type and 133 cases of combined type, the inattentive group tended to be older, have a higher proportion of girls, had more comorbid internalizing disorders, more academic difficulty and learning disabilities, particularly in the realm of speech and language problems. Although some of these children also had clinically significant hyperactivity and impulsivity, they did not meet formal diagnostic criteria (15).

A different approach to categorization of ADHD subtypes has been suggested by researchers in the Colorado group. Chhabildas examined the neuropsychological profiles associated with the three ADHD subtypes (inattentive, hyperactive/impulsive, and combined) as well as nonADHD controls. Subjects were drawn from a community sample of twins evaluated for reading disability, ADHD, and comorbid disorders. Somewhat counterintuitively, every dependent measure was best predicted by symptoms of inattention. The hyperactive/impulsive type resembled the controls in many respects, whereas the inattentive type performed more poorly than the other groups on almost all of the neuropsychological tasks (16). In another study by this group, extreme scores on the hyperactivity/inattention dimension were highly heritable only when the proband also exhibited a concurrent elevation of inattention. If the child did not meet criteria for inattention the hyperactive/inattentive scores were not heritable (17).

Electrophysiological studies also provide some support for these different subtypes. In boys with ADHD, two distinct electroencephalography (EEG) clusters were identified in the boys with ADHD of the inattentive type. One was characterized by high-amplitude theta with decreased delta/beta activity, and the other by increased slow-wave and decreased fast-wave activity. These different patterns of EEG activity were felt to reflect two physiologically different subgroups: those who were hypoaroused and those who had a more immature pattern ("developmental lag") (18). In an event-related potential study in which children and adolescents with ADHD were compared to controls, a stepwise discriminant function analysis demonstrated different response patterns between the combined type, inattentive type, and controls. The discrimination of the adolescent groups was not at all as robust, but it would appear that event-related potentials might be combined with other clinical information to enhance differentiation (19). A time-frequency analysis revealed event-related slow-wave activity that was reduced in the combined type group but not the inattentive group. Activity in the 1- to 12-Hz range was different in the control group and the ADHD group but not between the ADHD subtypes (20).

Age of Onset

There are significant differences between the hyperactive/impulsive type and the inattentive type in terms of the age at which symptoms emerge. Based on a retrospective parent report, children with ADHD become noticeably impaired around the age of 3½ years, with the median age of onset of the first ADHD symptom appearing around 1 year of age. The age of onset of the hyperactive type (mean = 4.21 years) is earlier than that of the combined type (mean = 4.88 years), and both are considerably earlier than the inattentive type. Virtually all (193 of 199 children in the DSM-IV field trials—98%) of the children with the hyperactive-impulsive type of ADHD, and 82% of those with the combined type are considered impaired before they reach the age of 7 years. By age 9 years, all would have met formal ADHD diagnostic criteria.

In contrast, the developmental pathway characterizing the inattentive type is quite different: ADHD of the inattentive type is often not apparent until around the first grade (mean age = 6.13 years) and in the DSM-IV field trials, some subjects did not become symptomatic until age 14 years. In the preschool years, symptoms of inattention without hyperactivity and impulsivity are less obvious and become impairing in half of the children with inattentive type at some point in the first grade. Based on the Great Smoky Mountains Study, Willoughby and colleagues noted a similar pattern of age of onset (21). Although most (85%) of children with the inattentive type manifest at least one symptom before the age of 7 years, only about half (43%) are considered impaired after age 7 years. (Moreover, astute clinicians not infrequently identify an adult with the inattentive type who may have been able to function adequately enough to miss detection until they embark on a demanding academic program in graduate school or in a profession or they change professions.)

Using appropriate assessments, the characteristic motivational and cognitive profile seen in the older individual with ADHD can also be observed in the preschool child (22). Moreover, children who meet full DSM-IV criteria for ADHD in the preschool years continue to manifest these symptoms into the school years (23). In one study involving 156 preschool children (aged 3 to 5½ years) executive dysfunction (working memory, planning, and set shifting)

as well as aversion to delay of gratification were predictive of ADHD symptoms (24).

These findings are of considerable importance to the clinician. One should be able to make the diagnosis of ADHD with hyperactivity/impulsivity in the preschool child. On the other hand, the age-of-onset criteria specified in DSM-IV for ADHD of the inattentive type, which indicates that some symptoms are "present before age 7 years," should not be taken too seriously, as evidence of impairment may not be apparent until much later, when the child is required to perform in an autonomous fashion (25). Thus, the way the symptoms are expressed may differ with age. Children with ADHD present in preschool with hyperactivity and impulsivity. As the demands for autonomous self-regulation increase, the inattentive profile becomes more prominent and more impairing.

Gender

It is only in the last decade that it has been recognized that boys and girls are at much the same risk for ADHD and that the clinical manifestations of the disorder are not gender-related. If anything, they may be an artifact of referral source. In earlier studies, substantial differences with ratios of boys to girls ranging from 6 to 12 to 1 were reported. In epidemiologic samples, the ratio is closer to 3 to 1. With more finely tuned diagnostic strategies, the ratio may become even lower. The clinical presentation of boys and girls with ADHD has also appeared to be different. In clinic-referred populations, girls with ADHD are more likely to have inattention and internalizing behaviors, and less peer aggression than boys with ADHD. Gaub and Carlson conducted a meta-analysis comparing ADHD symptoms, intellectual and academic functioning, comorbid behavior problems, social behavior, and family variables in boys and girls. They found no differences in impulsivity, academic performance, social functioning, fine motor skills, parental education, or parental depression. Girls with ADHD were not as hyperactive, and had fewer externalizing behaviors, but were more intellectually impaired. In some cases these differences were attributable to referral source (26). Boys manifest much higher rates of conduct disorder and oppositional defiant disorder than girls, which may explain the higher rate of referral to mental health clinics. In contrast, girls are more likely to have higher rates of depression and anxiety, poor self-esteem, a sense of limited control, and significant difficulties in the social sphere (27). Based on a large non-referred sample (577 subjects), Biederman and colleagues were unable to identify gender-based differences in full scale IQ, rates of learning disabilities, school performance, or social adjustment (28).

There are no gender differences in prefrontal executive function in boys and girls with ADHD (29, 30). When girls with ADHD are compared to controls, their ratings on the Global Assessment of Functioning Scale, cognitive functioning, and academic performance are all impaired. They have higher rates of disruptive behavior disorders, are vulnerable to alcohol and drug dependence, and are at risk for academic failure (31, 32). In a study of girls aged 6 to 12 years, 93 with ADHD-combined type, 47 with inattentive type, and 88 controls, the ADHD group had more speech and language problems and academic problems (repeating grades), externalizing/internalizing behaviors, and psychiatric comorbidities than the controls, and were more likely to be adopted. Girls with the combined type were more likely to be abused. Although girls with the inattentive type were more likely to be socially isolated, those with the combined type suffered more social rejection (33). In terms of performance on a neuropsychological test battery, there were robust differences between the girls with ADHD-combined and the control group, but differences between girls with the inattentive type and controls were much less prominent, and few differences were noted between the combined and inattentive types (34).

In a review of the effects of gender on ADHD, Biederman and Faraone concluded that ADHD is expressed similarly in both boys and girls. The differences in comorbid psychiatric disorders, learning disability, and inattention in boys and girls was not the result of effect modification of ADHD but rather were features of gender differences per se. Gender and ADHD were felt to be independent risk factors for comorbid psychopathology. The only significant gender-by-ADHD interaction that was identified in this study was the higher risk of alcohol or drug-dependence in females with ADHD compared to males with ADHD (35). However, in the study described previously, consisting of somewhat younger subjects, the propensity for drug dependence in girls with ADHD was not replicated (28).

Comorbid Disorders and Attention Deficit–Hyperactivity Disorder

There is a very high rate of comorbid psychiatric disorders in children and adults with ADHD. Conduct disorder, oppositional defiant disorder, depression and bipolar disorder, anxiety disorder, obsessive-compulsive disorder (OCD), Tourette's disorder, and learning disabilities are present in many children with ADHD. This risk is not limited to affected children, but also extends to the first-degree relatives of children with ADHD who are also at higher risk for neuropsychiatric disorders than control families (36, 37). Moreover, when followed over a number of years, comorbid conditions can emerge in children who previously did not meet diagnostic criteria.

The specific comorbidity is related to the subtype profile. Children with comorbid oppositional defiant or conduct disorder are rated as more impulsive than inattentive. Children with comorbid anxiety disorder have higher inattention than impulsivity ratings (38). Children with ADHD of both sexes are at risk for oppositional and conduct disorder.

In a follow-up study in which 207 caucasian boys (ages 6 to 12 years) who did not have a conduct disorder diagnosis in childhood were then re-evaluated at age 18 years by clinicians who were blind to childhood status. A control group of nonADHD adolescents was also evaluated. There was no specific single conduct disorder or oppositional disorder behavior which predicted later outcome. However, even the boys who had minimal evidence of conduct disorder in childhood were at significantly increased risk in adolescence. In addition, the presence of conduct disorder and oppositional defiant disorder also was associated with antisocial personality in adulthood (39).

Mood disorders are also associated with ADHD and tend to cluster in families. Depression and anxiety do not appear to be related to the particular subtype of ADHD and are present in both the combined and inattentive types to the same degree (40). However, Vance and colleagues reported that dysthymic disorder and ADHD combined type contributed in the multiple regression analysis to the prediction of oppositional defiant disorder (41). They made the point that dysthymic disorder often emerges in early childhood and might be regarded as a risk factor. Bipolar disorder is also not only a comorbidity of ADHD but can be part of the differential diagnosis. However, the association of bipolar disorder and ADHD is still somewhat controversial. In a study comparing well-functioning youths with bipolar disorder, unipolar depression, and normal controls, only 6.8% of those with bipolar disorder, 10% of those with depression and none of the controls reported a previous diagnosis of ADHD. Results of a test battery involving neuropsychological assessments of attention, did not reveal any objective differences in performance between the groups. However, the patients with bipolar disorder reported subjective attentional disturbance (42). In contrast to these observations, in a study of young adults with bipolar disorder, 67% had impaired performance on the Wisconsin Card Sorting Test when previously assessed as adolescents, in comparison to those with unipolar depression (19%) or those without major mood disorder (17%). Attention problems in adolescence were not associated with later bipolar disorder (43).

Anxiety disorder is also associated with ADHD and often makes treatment challenging as some children become more anxious on psychostimulants. In the MTA study, 33% of the children with ADHD met DSM-III-R criteria for an anxiety disorder (excluding simple phobias). More than half of these children also met DSM-III-R criteria for comorbid oppositional-defiant or conduct disorder (44). In one study, 146 medication-naïve elementary school children with ADHD combined type were grouped into those with and without dysthymic disorder. The group with dysthymic disorder had a higher incidence of anxiety disorder (41, 45).

Epidemiological studies have revealed a consistent and rather complex association between ADHD, OCD, and Tourette's disorder. When viewed in longitudinal studies, tics in early childhood and adolescence were associated with increasing OCD symptoms with maturation. ADHD in adolescence predicted an increase in OCD symptoms in early adulthood, and OCD in adolescence predicted more ADHD symptoms in adulthood (46). This close association is not surprising, given that all three disorders involve frontal-subcortical pathways and disruption of catecholamine neurotransmission (47).

Many individuals with mental retardation and autistic-spectrum disorders (that is pervasive developmental disorder, autistic disorder, Asperger's disorder, and nonverbal learning disability) are found to have associated attention deficit and impulsivity although these are considered exclusionary criteria.

NEUROLOGY OF ATTENTION DEFICIT–HYPERACTIVITY DISORDER

ADHD is a disorder of self-regulation reflecting dysfunction in frontal-subcortical systems that control attention, intention, and emotional arousal. Children and adults with ADHD have great difficulty following through on their intention to perform certain tasks. Although they typically know what needs to be done, they have difficulty initiating work on a task (in fact, they are often skilled procrastinators) and do not complete the task in a satisfactory manner. They may perform the task so slowly or ineffectively that they are quite frustrating to those around them. They may rush through the task in a sloppy manner. Parents complain that a child with ADHD requires constant monitoring when performing routine tasks, and disrupts family functioning by being unable to get dressed or complete homework without constant supervision. This is often accompanied by a striking lack of awareness of the difficulty.

In this section, some of the brain mechanisms that underlie the regulation of attention, motor intention (activity, response time, inhibition and intention), and arousal and motivation will be discussed.

Attention

We are bombarded by stimuli all the time, but not everything in the world around us is of equal importance at a given moment. Attention is an active process which enables organisms to screen out irrelevant stimuli and to focus on (or pay attention to) stimuli that are relevant. The metaphor that attention is like a spotlight has been used—one may scan the environment with a broad beam but then focus the beam very narrowly on a few important details, or shift from one aspect of the scene to another. Shifts in attention can be *overt*—that is a shift in direction of gaze, or *covert*—changing the focus of attention without shifting gaze. Attentional behaviors also need to be relatively constant during wakefulness (vigilance). Thus, adequate function, if not survival, depends on being able to detect important stimuli, identify

new stimuli, shift attention as necessary, and ignore irrelevant stimuli. In the classroom, a child is expected to attend to the teacher and the task at hand and *not* pay attention (or at least pay less attention) to what Jimmy is doing in the next seat, or what is happening in the hall. This also involves regulating one's own cognitive processes. One child that we worked with talked about his "green ideas"; namely, a flood of rich associations about the topic at hand, or possibly other matters, which, although undeniably brilliant and creative, definitely impaired his ability to concentrate on the immediate task. In addition, the child is expected to be aware of important internal and external stimuli—a precipitous dash to the bathroom is appropriate in a three-year-old, but would suggest inadequate monitoring in an eight-year-old.

The best model for understanding the neurophysiological processes underlying attention involves the visual system, which has been extensively studied. The essential feature of the processing of sensory information is that there are top-down attentional control functions at all levels of the system.

Visual information flows from the retina, through the optic nerve, to the lateral geniculate nucleus. In the lateral geniculate, a six-layered structure, visual information is sorted into two systems. One system is specialized for motion detection (analysis of speed and direction or movement, and depth perception and is closely linked to the extraocular system that controls eye movements). This system, the magnocellular system, feeds into layers one and two which have large cell sizes. The other system, which feeds into the other four layers consisting of smaller size neurons ("parvocellular"), is specialized for the analysis of shape, color, fine details, and fine depth perception. Both of these streams then project into different layers in primary visual cortex (V1 or Brodmann's area 17). The magnocellular system projects into area 4B and the parvocellular system to area 4A. Neurons in V1 do not identify objects or movements, but rather bars of light. The information then flows into visual association cortex—initially areas 18 and 19. The motion detection pathway (also called the dorsal pathway) is divided into two separate streams. The dorsodorsal stream arises in area V6 and projects to the superior parietal lobule. This is part of a broader system involved in the integration of sensory motor information; there are a multitude of connections to motor cortex and subcortical structures, involved in the guidance of arm movements, and the integration of arm, eye, and head movements. Damage results in optic ataxia. The ventral dorsal stream flows from the middle temporal visual area (area MT) and projects to the inferior parietal lobule, and processes visual motion (48). The ventral pathway (or "what?" pathway) travels into the temporal lobe where information relating to objects and faces is processed. By the time a stimulus reaches the level of awareness, it has been cataloged as to identity (*what* it is), location/orientation (*where* it is), the features relevant to its movement, familiarity (memory), and significance (its motivational/emotional valence). The stimulus itself may be subjected to closer inspection (selective attention). In real-world situations, the attentional focus must be constantly readjusted to either scan a broad area or focus in on a small detail. This has been referred to as "the zoom lens model" (49).

During this sequential process of visual stimuli, attention plays a critical role (50–52). *Enhancement* is a term used by neurophysiologists to label this effect of attention on the firing pattern of neurons. Attention increases the firing rate of certain neurons and decreases the firing of others. In a classical experiment, monkeys were trained to release a lever when the light dimmed to receive a juice reward. The firing of a single neuron in the visual system was increased if the stimulus (a central spot of light) was important to the monkey, because upon release of the lever, the monkey would get the juice. A second neuron responded with only a brief burst of firing when another light stimulus, not linked to the juice reward, was presented to the monkey. However, when the second spot of light was then linked to the juice reward, the firing rate of the second neuron increased significantly. Thus, the rate of neuronal firing was modulated by the motivational significance of the stimulus specific to a given context (53). In humans, a combination of functional magnetic resonance imaging (fMRI) and evoked potential techniques have demonstrated that the initial arrival of visual information to primary visual cortex is not attended, but within 70 to 75 milliseconds, attentional modulation becomes engaged (54). In a fMRI study, subjects were asked to fixate on one target and pay covert attention (that is, without shifting gaze) to another location. Activation (or enhanced neural activity) was observed in the brain area corresponding to the attended location and was greater in parietal and frontal areas than in visual areas (55). Moreover, in a difficult task in which subjects were required to detect specific patterns, there was a clear relationship between the extent of activation in visual cortex and adequacy of task performance (56). However, attention is not an infinite resource and there are distinct limits to attentional capacity. As attentional resources are deployed over a broader area, the capacity of the attentional system is taxed and task performance became more difficult. This was demonstrated in an fMRI study. As the size of the attended field increased, the activation in the visual cortex decreased, and subjects made more errors and reaction time was increased. The investigators felt this provided substantiation of the "zoom lens model" as well as the limited capacity notion (57).

Attention involves different processes that are instantiated in different brain areas. A large, widely distributed neural network, which involves posterior and frontal association cortex, is involved in guiding visual spatial attention as well as linking working memory into the attentional system. Voluntary attention is controlled by superior frontal, inferior parietal, and superior temporal cortices (58). The interparietal sulcus contains four different areas, each integrating a specific aspect of attention, sensory input, and representations of movement through space as well as motor exploration of space. Frontal eye fields are more involved in the motor exploration aspect. This region appears to play a crucial role in processing the sensory aspects of covert spatial attention. In a study in which some of the confounding variables were controlled, it was apparent that the parietal lobe was involved in the representation of sensory information (the banks of the interparietal sulcus and the temporo-occipital region were activated to a much greater extent than frontal areas), whereas the frontal areas were involved in the motor aspects of visual exploration. There was also evidence that the parietal cortex may engage visual and frontal cortex in the attentional processes (58).

Selective attention involves anticipatory attending to a specific location before presentation of a visual target. It is associated with activation of the intraparietal sulcus. When an unexpected target is detected, there is activation in the right temporoparietal junction (59). In another study, a group of neurons in area 7a of the parietal lobe responded preferentially to stimuli that require reorienting attention (60). In addition to the posterior parietal areas, attending to representations of external space involves lateral premotor, dorsal prefrontal, and cingulate cortices. Working memory is intimately linked to the efficient deployment of selective attention and is subserved by a distributed system involving intraparietal sulcus and frontal eye fields that mediates the on-line storage of location information (61).

However, attention is also directed to internal mental representation in the absence of any "real" extrapersonal object. In one fMRI study, subjects were asked to orient attention to a location that existed only as a mental representation held in working memory. (The task was complex in that a spatial array was presented which then disappeared and the subjects had to hold both color and location characteristics in working memory.) The neuroanatomical areas that were activated in this study overlapped to a great extent with those related to attending to spatial locations, but the mental representation also resulted in activation of frontal regions (62).

Lesions of the parietal lobe and transcranial magnetic stimulation of the parietal lobe both produce *neglect*—unawareness of stimuli in contralateral space—or deficits in disengaging visual attention from one location and shifting it to another (63–65). Similarly, transcranial magnetic stimulation of the parietal lobe results in neglect in contralateral hemispace (Fierro 2000; Bjoetomt 2002). When ADHD children were tested using paradigms that had been sensitive to neglect in adults, the children's profile was similar to that to adults who had sustained right hemisphere lesions (66).

To summarize, attention is an active process that includes detecting important stimuli in the environment, being able to focus on it, controlling distractibility, and shifting attention rapidly when it is necessary to do so. Thus, long before one becomes conscious of a specific item in one's environment, the nervous system has surveyed the environment, selected relevant stimuli, and decreased attention paid to unimportant stimuli. One can see that if the attention system is not working well, an important stimulus might not be recognized (neglect), or attending to an important stimulus may be disrupted by distraction, or the inability to sustain attention as long as is necessary.

Hyperactivity

Hyperactivity is a common manifestation of ADHD; children can show high levels of motor activity, fiddle with objects, and move and shift their bodies. Older children can appear very restless and adults with ADHD can have an uncomfortable sense that they have to move. Hyperactivity in children with ADHD has been documented in numerous studies using a variety of motion detection devices (67–69). From a neurological perspective, patients with lesions in orbitofrontal cortex are restless and engage in random and purposeless movements. Some children with ADHD manifest "utilization behavior." This is behavior that is initiated by a common object (such as a pencil or a knife) and the patient performs the activity even when it is grossly inappropriate (70). It is important to emphasize that not all frontal lobe lesions result in hyperactivity. Patients with lesions in the anterior cingulate area are often hypoactive and abulic. Lesions involving the caudate nucleus and the mesolimbic system also result in hyperactivity (Davis, 1958; Koob et al. 1981). In rodents, the hippocampal-accumbens-subpallidal circuit appears to be associated with increased locomotor activity (Mogenson, 1984). In a study involving the selective breeding of mice with a propensity to "voluntary" wheel-running, a total of 11,904 genes were screened using high-density oligonucleotide arrays. Increased wheel-running was associated with a significant increase in expression of 30 genes (primarily involved in transcription and translation) and, more specifically, a 20% increase in the expression of dopamine D2 and D4 receptor mRNA in the hippocampus (71). The major neurotransmitter implicated in hyperactive behaviors is dopamine; for example, akathisia is noted in patients with Parkinson's disease (Lang and Johnson 1987). Tassin and colleagues (1978) reported that motor restlessness in rats was inversely correlated with prefrontal cortical dopamine. The "knockout" mouse that lacks the dopamine transporter gene, which then results in increased extracellular dopamine, manifests a remarkably high level of motor activity (Giros et al. 1996). Jucaite and colleagues conducted a PET-scan study that involved adolescents with ADHD and young adults, who served as controls. The study used selective radioligands to assess the relationships between the binding potential of dopamine transporter and dopamine receptor D2 density in various brain regions to levels of attention and hyperactivity. There were no group differences noted in radioligand binding in the striatum, but the binding potential of the dopamine transporter in the midbrain was significantly lower in the ADHD group. Dopamine receptor D2 binding in the right caudate showed a significant positive correlation with hyperactivity (72). Thus, although the neural circuitry underlying hyperactivity has not been as clearly defined in humans, it appears to be related to several different areas all of which involve dopaminergic neurotransmission.

Impulsivity

In DSM-IV, impulsivity is defined by three criteria—blurting out answers before questions have been completed, having difficulty awaiting turn, and interrupting or intruding on others. More broadly, impulsivity involves not waiting for complete information before plunging into a task, not considering undesirable consequences, proceeding with an action based on limited information, and difficulty inhibiting an inappropriate response. Psychiatrists include an even broader array of complex behaviors such as suicide, pathological gambling, kleptomania, intermittent explosive disorder, and addiction under the rubric of impulsivity. Impulsivity also includes a broad range of behaviors such as inability to tolerate delays, and a tendency to perseverate. From a neurological viewpoint, impulsivity is a deficit in controlling responses to stimuli. In this context, impulsivity is defined as a deficit in response inhibition. However, on analysis, in addition to inhibitory control, impulsivity can also be viewed as an aversion to delay.

There are a number of experimental paradigms that are used to measure impulsivity in individuals with ADHD. The Stop Signal Paradigm assesses inhibitory control. The Choice-Delay Task monitors delay aversion. The Go–No Go task assesses the ability to withhold a response, particularly in a situation in which a prepotent response pattern has been established. The Gambling task monitors delay aversion in a context which requires weighing highly motivating factors. Solanto and colleagues studied a group of 7.0- to 9.9-year-old children with ADHD using the Choice-Delay and Stop Signal tasks. ADHD subjects performed significantly more poorly on both tasks, and both were associated with ADHD, suggesting that aversion to delay and inability to inhibit responses were features of ADHD. The Choice-Delay task correlated with teacher ratings of impulsivity, hyperactivity, conduct problems, and aggression as well as the ADHD composite score. This suggests that delay aversion is associated with a broad range of ADHD behaviors. In contrast, the Stop Signal task correlated with the behavioral observations, and appears to tap executive control. One neurological experimental model involves the inability to inhibit gaze to a visual target. In this context, distractibility would be considered an intentional motor deficit rather than an attentional deficit. Deficits on contrasaccade tasks are associated with medial frontal lesions (Butter et al. 1988, Guitton et al. 1985). Difficulties inhibiting gaze have been described in children with ADHD. In a study which required subjects to delay before shifting gaze to a target held in working memory, children with ADHD performed more poorly than controls in the inhibition component of the task, but had no difficulty in response preparation or in the memory component (Ross et al. 1994). Similarly, children with ADHD had much greater difficulty in contrast to controls in inhibiting gaze to a visual stimulus (Voeller et al. 1990).

There is a strong link between impulsivity and dysfunction of the frontal-subcortical circuits, particularly the right orbitofrontal area (73). The amygdala, which is highly interconnected with prefrontal cortex, is also involved with impulsivity (74). Lesions of the subcortical nuclei, which receive orbitofrontal projections, are also associated with impulsive behaviors. For example, individuals with Sydenham's chorea manifest significant impulsivity (75). In a study of the Go–No Go task performed by normal subjects who had undergone extensive assessments of impulsive traits, neural response inhibition activated right lateral orbitofrontal cortex and was strongly correlated with Eysenck's impulsivity score. Other cortical areas—the superior temporal gyrus, medial orbitofrontal cortex, cingulate gyrus, and inferior parietal lobule, more on the right than left—were also activated. Subjects who had higher impulsivity ratings and made more errors had greater activation of paralimbic areas during response inhibition, while less impulsive individuals and those with least errors activated higher order association areas.

In terms of neurotransmitters and pharmacology, numerous reports have linked decreased central nervous system serotonin to impulsive behaviors. However, Winstanley, in a study on rats that had depleted forebrain serotonin levels, noted only a subset of behaviors that could be construed as impulsive, suggesting that impulsivity is not a unitary construct (76). However, there also appears to be a role for dopamine as one of the neurotransmitters involved in impulsive responding (77). Hershey and colleagues studied eight neuroleptic-naive adults with tic disorders and controls on a Go–No Go task before and during IV levodopa infusion. In the baseline condition, higher cerebellar activations were associated with faster reaction times and higher parietal activation with higher error rates. There was no difference in actual task performance, but the study indicated that lower levels of activation were required in the presence of this dopamine agonist (78).

In summary, impulsivity is a less well-defined entity, both behaviorally and neurologically than other aspects of ADHD. There is a body of research indicating that it is instantiated in orbitofrontal cortex and related subcortical circuits. There is evidence that impulsive behaviors are at least in part related to genetic makeup. Serotonin likely plays an important role in regulating impulsivity. However, both dopamine as well as other neurotransmitters interact in a complex way with serotonin.

Regulation of Arousal

Arousal refers to a state of physiological readiness that enables the organism to respond to incoming stimuli and develop appropriate responses. Although arousal is often triggered by novel or exciting environmental stimuli, the ability to regulate one's level of arousal with relative autonomy so that it is appropriate to the situation is an important adaptive strategy. If a child is working on a long and boring task, maintaining alertness and persevering is very helpful. On the other hand, the ability to remain calm and decrease the impact of unpleasant and distracting stimuli in certain situations is also an advantage. Arousal is closely linked to motivation and the ability to sustain attention and persist in performance when confronted with a difficult or boring task. The regulation of one's internal arousal is not one of the DSM criteria for ADHD, but it has considerable clinical relevance, particularly when dealing with children in an educational setting. Children with ADHD appear to have difficulty regulating their internal emotional states.

The concept of "sensory integration," a term used by occupational therapists, is another aspect of arousal. Occupational therapists note that some children are hypersensitive whereas others are quite unaware of stimuli in some or all sensory modalities. Some children may find tactile stimuli such as rough carpet, sand or grass on bare feet, or scratchy clothing tags or sweaters particularly unpleasant. Noises and visual stimuli can be particularly distracting. Other children appear to have very high sensory thresholds and are often unaware of stimuli. Some of these children may use motor activity to enhance stimulation. A preferred term for "sensory integration disorder" might be "sensory modulation disorder," which would include sensory overresponsiveness, sensory under-responsiveness, and sensation seeking/craving (personal communication, L. Miller). From the point of view of a clinician who deals with children with ADHD as well as those sensory modulation disorders, they appear to be close cousins, if not reflections of the same dysfunctional attention/sensory processing system that is seen in ADHD. Sensory overresponsiveness could be viewed from a neurological perspective as an impairment in the ability to downregulate incoming sensory stimuli and would be related to a failure to not only modulate and habituate to sensory stimuli, but to inhibit response, which would map on to distractibility. Sensory underresponsiveness, like inattention, is a failure to detect stimuli. This lack of awareness of external stimuli is often coupled with underarousal. These children clinically resemble Lahey's "sluggish cognitive tempo" type. One might speculate that sensation seeking/craving is another manifestation of inattention and underarousal, and these children are attempting to enhance sensory input and maintain arousal by movement. Some children with ADHD manifest extreme restlessness and are in constant motion at the same time they appear quite drowsy and underaroused (they yawn profusely).

Representation and Awareness of Time

Although the representation of time is not a DSM-IV diagnostic criterion for ADHD a number of studies have presented evidence that individuals with ADHD have difficulty with time estimation. This idea was introduced by Barkley (79), and although there has been some controversy, a number of subsequent studies have supported this notion (80). A widely distributed neural network is involved in time estimation, which includes the frontal, parietal, cortices basal ganglia, and the cerebellum (81, 82).

Subtle Deficits in Motor Performance in Attention Deficit–Hyperactivity Disorder

There is a considerable body of information relating to motor performance in children with ADHD. In the absence of any classical neurological deficits, children with ADHD as a group manifest deficits in the regulation of motor performance. In one study, a discriminant function analysis classified 89% of boys who were hyperactive versus controls based on speed, rhythm, and overflow (83). Differences in velocity, coordination, and accuracy were observed in children with ADHD and controls during the performance of bimanual movements (84) as well as when programming goal-directed arm movement, particularly in the absence of visual feedback (85). In a prospective study of 5- and 6-year-old children, those who, when assessed several years later met criteria for ADHD, manifested much greater difficulty in regulating motor performance (86). They were more inaccurate and much more variable in performance. It may be that this type of variability in motor performance is more prominent in the preschool child with ADHD and becomes less apparent with age. Adults with prefrontal lesions typically manifest variability in motor performance (87).

NEUROIMAGING STUDIES

There are numerous morphometric MRI studies that have identified relatively consistent differences in the brains of children with ADHD compared to normal controls. A particularly informative study is a large, longitudinal NIMH study involving children with ADHD and age- and gender-matched controls (Castellanos, 2002). The mean total cerebral volume in children with ADHD is slightly (approximately 5%) but significantly smaller than controls (88–93) (Fillipek 1997). In one study in which unaffected sibling of boys with ADHD were examined, the unaffected siblings also showed a slight (but statistically significant trend) amounting to 3.4% reduction in total cerebral volume (89).

Various components of the cortical-striatal-thalamo-cortical circuits and cerebellum have been reported, with fair consistency, to be affected in most studies. These include frontal lobe (88, 91, 93–95) (Castellanos 2002), caudate nucleus (88, 96) (Castellanos 2002, Filipek 1997) as well as other basal ganglia structures (97, 98) and cerebellum (88, 90, 99, 100) (Castellanos 2002, Filipek 1997). In normally developing children, the caudate appears to decrease in size as the child matures (consistent with neuronal pruning, which is seen in many different areas in the course

of normal development) (88, 101) (Castellanos 2002). The decrease in size of the caudate is present early in development, suggesting that there is specific disruption of normal neuronal growth. Moreover, there is evidence that right hemisphere structures are affected to a greater extent than left hemisphere structures (88–90, 98, 102, 103) (Castellanos 2002, Filipek 1997). This is interesting, given the role of the right hemisphere in regulating sensory attention and motor intention in the majority of humans (66, 104).

Functional neuroimaging is consistent with the morphometric findings in that these studies reveal anomalous patterns of function in the prefrontal-subcortical circuits, often more prominent in the right hemisphere (105, 106). Early studies, which were not consistently replicated, suggested a complex interaction between gender, age, and hormonal effects (107–109).

When children are asked to perform a task that places demands on the frontal executive system, those with ADHD have atypical patterns of activation. In one study, children with ADHD and controls were studied using fMRI during a Go–No Go task. In general, fMRI scans on children performing tasks that demand executive function control have somewhat different patterns of activation than those seen in adults (110). However, when compared to age-matched controls, children with ADHD do not activate frontostriatal networks to the same extent as those without ADHD, but rather manifest a more diffuse activation pattern, suggesting a delay in the development of frontostriatal circuits (111). In another fMRI study involving children with ADHD and controls performing two somewhat different types of Go–No Go tasks, children with ADHD made more errors than controls. In one task, children with ADHD activated frontal areas to a greater extent than controls. Although this is not consistent with the findings in other studies, it is possible that in that specific paradigm, subjects with ADHD had to exert more effort than controls. (In this study, other brain regions were not examined so that there was no opportunity to see the diffuse activation pattern described in the Durston study.) After receiving methylphenidate, there was a decrease in the number of errors, particularly in the ADHD group. Both the controls and the children showed increased frontal activation. Striatal activation was increased in the children with ADHD, but decreased in the controls (112).

Schulz and colleagues examined male adolescents who had been diagnosed with ADHD at an earlier age, and divided them into "persisters" (those who continued to meet DSM-IV diagnostic criteria), "remitters" (those who no longer met DSM-IV criteria), and a group of matched controls who had never had ADHD. The subjects performed a Go–No Go task with fMRI monitoring. All groups activated ventrolateral prefrontal cortex to some extent, but there was a difference between the groups in both the number of commission errors and extent of activation. Commission errors ranged from 33% in the subjects who continued to meet full DSM-IV diagnostic criteria, to 13% in the control group. The remitters made 24% errors. There was much greater activation in the persister group than in the controls (113–115).

In a study comparing adolescents with ADHD, those with dyslexia, those with ADHD and dyslexia, and controls, subjects with ADHD and dyslexia activated left ventral basal ganglia significantly less than did the controls. Methylphenidate decreased the level of activation but did not significantly change performance (116).

A technical issue of relevance to the interpretation of these studies is the concept of *deactivation*: the suspension or inhibition of ongoing background neuronal activity during the performance of tasks requiring increased cognitive activity (117). The computation involves subtracting the cognitive task condition from the control or baseline condition. This is the opposite of activation (cognitive task condition minus baseline) and is observed in normal individuals.

In a Go–No Go study, a number of methodological issues in the paradigm were carefully controlled so that it was possible to discriminate activation during the segments of the task in which inhibition was required. There were significantly more omission and commission errors made by the ADHD subjects than by the controls. This was accompanied by marked hypoactivation of the anterior/midcingulate cortex extending to the supplementary motor area. It was also noted that the left temporal gyrus was hyperactivated (118).

Dysfunction in the frontal-subcortical system has been supported by magnetic resonance spectroscopy (MRS) studies. Two of these studies have revealed an increase in the glutamate/glutamine/ GABA ratio in frontal-striatal circuits of children with ADHD (Macmaster et al. 2001; Courvoisie et al. 2004). This can be interpreted as reflecting an imbalance between excitatory (glutamate) and inhibitory (GABA) neurotransmission, particularly at various nodes in the frontal-striatal system, which has been implicated in ADHD. This imbalance can be interpreted as either due to increased excitation or reduced inhibition. There has been less consistency related to N-acetylaspartate with some investigators reporting no difference (McMaster et al. 2003), a unilateral (right frontal) increase (Courvoisie et al. 2004) or a bilateral decrease in the basal ganglia (Jin et al. 2001; Sun et al. 2005). Jin et al. (2001) suggested that there might be a neuronal loss in the striatum as well as an increase in cholinergic activity. N-acetyl aspartate is generally considered a marker for neuronal viability, although, arguably, it may reflect formation and maintenance of myelin. In the study by Sparkes et al. (2004) there was a positive correlation between N-acetyl aspartate /creatine and mean reaction time in the controls which was significantly different from the negative correlation of the same magnitude in the ADHD group (Sparkes 2004). Interestingly, the subgroup of children with ADHD whose N-acetyl aspartate /creatine ratios were close to that of controls still had longer reaction times than controls. In one study, a decreased N-acetyl aspartate/creatine ratio in girls with ADHD was noted relative to both controls and boys (Yeo et al. 2003). These studies

are intriguing but should be interpreted with caution because of the relatively small sample sizes and resulting limited statistical power.

NEUROTRANSMITTERS, TRANSPORTERS, AND RECEPTORS RELATED TO ATTENTION DEFICIT–HYPERACTIVITY DISORDER

Synapses are the basic structures underlying neurotransmission and brain function. A synapse is composed of a presynaptic neuron and a postsynaptic neuron which are separated by a synaptic cleft. Neurotransmitters are synthesized and packaged into synaptic vesicles in the presynaptic neuronal terminal. In response to a nerve impulse, the vesicles are extruded into the synaptic cleft; approximately 1,000 molecules of neurotransmitter per terminal. The neurotransmitter then binds to the cell membrane of the postsynaptic neuron, triggering a nerve impulse. Neurotransmitter in the synaptic cleft is then either recaptured by specialized monoamine transporter proteins, located in the plasma membrane of the presynaptic neuron and repackaged into synaptic vesicles; or the neurotransmitter is degraded by enzymes, such as the monoamine oxidases, or catechol-o-methyltransferase. These transporters and enzymes are the targets for many psychiatric drugs, which modify the amount of neurotransmitter available and modify brain function. Dopamine, norepinephrine, and serotonin belong to a family of monoamine transporters, part of a larger group of Na^+- and Cl^--dependent transporters. This section will focus on dopamine and norepinephrine, which have been extensively studied in relation to ADHD. However, it is apparent that a number of other neurotransmitters (glutamate, gamma-aminobutyric acid (119), and acetylcholine) figure prominently in modulating dopaminergic and adrenergic neurotransmission. In addition, growth factors, such as brain-derived neurotrophic factor, and other regulators of synaptic function play an important role in regulating the neural networks that are involved in ADHD.

The Dopaminergic System

Dopamine has long been thought to be a neurotransmitter that plays an essential role in the pathophysiology of ADHD. Dopamine is evolutionarily a highly conserved neurotransmitter, being found in very primitive organisms. Dopaminergic neurons are involved in learning, as well as maintaining trained/conditioned responses, and motivated, goal-directed behavior (120–122). (Schultz 1986, 1993). Dopamine appears to serve a special function in the extraction of reward-related information from an array of environmental stimuli and in using this information in programming goal-directed behaviors (123, 124). Dopamine also plays an important role in the prefrontal circuits that subserve working memory; the ability to "keep something in mind" for a brief time (125, 126). Prefrontal cortex is highly dependent on a relatively narrow range of dopamine for adequate functioning: too little dopamine impairs working memory (127), too much dopamine disrupts cognitive function (128). However, in contrast to the abundant dopaminergic innervation of the striatum, dopaminergic neurons are not as dense and have a high firing rate and a much higher rate of dopamine turnover than dopaminergic neurons in the striatum (129, 130). Moreover, the dopamine transporter is not at all as prevalent as it is in other areas.

There are two dopaminergic systems: the nigrostriatal system, which arises from the substantia nigra and projects to the caudate and putamen (relay stations in the cortical-striatal-thalamo-cortical circuits); and the mesolimbic system, which arises from cell bodies in the mesencephalic ventral tegmental area of Tsai (A10), the substantia nigra pars compacta (A9), and the caudolateral cell group (A8), and projects to the nucleus accumbens and the ventro-medial sector of the striatum, which in turn receives projections from the limbic system (131). Dopaminergic projections to the cortex involve primary motor cortex, and association neocortex (dorsomedial prefrontal cortex and inferior parietal cortex) (132), with relatively sparse innervation of primary visual, auditory, and somatosensory cortices (133, 134).

The human dopamine transporter is a protein consisting of 620 amino acids forming 12 putative transmembrane domains. It maps to chromosome 5p15.3 (135, 136). The coding region of the DAT-1 gene (also referred to SLC6A3) is of fixed length–a 2-kb coding region, consisting of 15 exons distributed across an over a 64-kb gene, that has little genetic variability (137). However, there is considerable variation in the length of the 3'-untranslated region (3'UTR) due to a variable number of tandem repeats (VNTRs) (135, 136, 138).

The dopamine receptors are part of a family of "G-proteins" (guanosine triphosphate binding proteins). These proteins traverse the cell wall membrane of the neuron and contain seven transmembrane domains. Once dopamine is bound to the receptor, it activates a cascade of biochemical events inside the cell, which either enhance or inhibit cyclic adenosine monophosphate (cAMP) production. In this complex sequence transcription factors are activated and early immediate genes are expressed, which in turn activate the expression of other genes. It is likely that the dopamine in humans originally arose from two gene subfamilies, the D1-like (consisting of D1 and D5) and the D2-like (D2, D3, D4) receptor genes. D1-like receptor genes do not contain introns in their protein coding regions, whereas the D2-like genes do. D1 and D5 receptors are excitatory, whereas D2, D3, D4 receptors are inhibitory. Based on positron emission tomography (PET) scan studies using radioligands as well as the distribution of mRNAs, it has been observed that dopamine receptor subtypes types are concentrated in different brain areas: D1 and D2 receptor mRNAs are found in the caudate and putamen, whereas the D3 and D4 receptors are clustered in limbic areas, and D5 receptor distribution is restricted to hippocampus, the hypothalamus, and the parafascicular nucleus of the thalamus (139–141).

However, there is yet an additional level of variability. Each receptor subtype also has different genetic variants, which behave in physiologically different ways, with different binding affinities. For example, there are three dopamine D5 receptor subtypes. The "standard" dopamine D5 receptor, which consists of 477 amino acids, and two other dopamine D5 receptor subtypes coded by "pseudogenes." These shorter D5 receptor variants are composed of only 154 amino acids and likely function very differently. There are "short" (414 amino acids) and "long" (443 amino acids) versions of the D2 receptor, as well as several other D2 receptors which vary because of different amino acids inserted at different points in the protein. Similarly, there are several different variants of the dopamine D3 receptor. Ten different D4 receptor subtypes have been identified; they differ in the number of 48 base-pair repeats in the putative third cytoplasmic loop, ranging from one to ten repeats. These various receptor subtypes also show differences of variable clinical significance. Two examples of this phenomenon should provide some insight into the complexity of the process. One patient, with the D4Valine194Glycine variant was reported as being strikingly less sensitive to dopamine, clozapine and olanzapine (142). Similarly, the long and short dopamine D2 receptor variants show different patterns of response to prior activation of protein kinase C without changing dopamine-induced inhibition (143). In rats, Martres and colleagues demonstrated a 70% increase in striatal D2 mRNA levels following a 15-day treatment with haloperidol, but no change in mRNA levels in cerebral cortex or brainstem. In contrast, the amount of long D2 receptor mRNA was decreased to a greater extent than the short D2 receptor following 6-hydroxydopamine treatment in the substantia nigra (144).

Several polymorphisms of the dopamine D4 gene have been identified. There have been numerous studies (145–153) and several meta-analyses (154, 155) supporting the association between the dopamine D4 48 base-pair seven-repeat allele in exon 3 and ADHD. However, some studies did not support the association (156–160). Another 120 base pair repeat promoter polymorphism, upstream of the 5' transcription initiation site, may be associated with ADHD, particularly the inattentive type (161). Leung and colleagues conducted a study in the Chinese Han population. Rather than the expected increase in the seven-repeat allele, they found an unexpected 1.65 times increase in the two-repeat allele, which can be interpreted as supporting the association between the dopamine receptor D2 and ADHD, but with differences in the number of repeats that are specific to a given ethnic group (162).

Recently a series of studies examined the relationship between performance on cognitive tasks assessing attention and impulsivity, independent of a specific diagnosis of ADHD. This approach has yielded some interesting results and provided evidence that specific genotypes are related to specific cognitive profiles. Langley and colleagues examined the effect of the dopamine D4 receptor seven-repeat allele in 133 drug-naive children ranging in age from 6 to 13 years on a series of neurological tasks sensitive to inattention, impulsivity, response inhibition, and monitored activity level. The patients were divided into two groups: those with one or more dopamine D4 receptor seven-repeat alleles (38.3%) and those without (61.7%). The groups did not differ significantly in age or IQ. Although the children with the seven-repeat allele had a significantly higher total number of ADHD symptom than those without, the groups did not differ when the symptoms were subdivided into inattention or hyperactivity/impulsivity. The children with the seven-repeat allele showed significantly higher rates of oppositional defiant disorder and conduct disorder than those without. The children with the seven-repeat allele also tended to trade speed for accuracy (they were faster but more impulsive and more error-prone) and were more hyperactive. Interestingly, there was little difference between children with ADHD and the seven-repeat allele and those with ADHD without the seven-repeat allele, but these subjects differed significantly from the nonADHD control subjects (163).

Norepinephrine

Norepinephrine (noradrenaline) is involved in regulating alertness and attention. Norepinephrine neurons arise from the locus coeruleus and innervate the dorsomedial and anterior cingulate regions (cortical regions heavily involved in attention) (164–166). Norepinephrines are also preferentially found in layers V and VI, which receive thalamocortical afferent fibers (167). Prefrontal cortex is reciprocally connected with the locus coeruleus, which enables prefrontal cortex to exert top-down control on attention (168). There is also a peripheral noradrenergic system, which regulates the cardiovascular system controlling blood pressure and heart rate (the "fight or flight" response).

The norepinephrine system plays a key role in stimulus detection and alertness. Neurons in the locus coeruleus respond to environmental stimuli (particularly novel stimuli), are quiet during sleep, and do not respond to automatic grooming and feeding behaviors (169, 170). There are four main types of central noradrenergic receptors: alpha-1, alpha-2, beta-1, and beta-2. Alpha-1 and the beta-1 and -2 receptors are primarily postsynaptic, whereas alpha-2 receptors are found at both presynaptic and postsynaptic sites. The presynaptic receptors are *autoreceptors*; that is, in response to an agonist, they downregulate noradrenergic activity by a negative feedback mechanism.

Although it was previously believed that a nerve terminal could store only one neurotransmitter, it is now recognized

that two neurotransmitters may be colocalized in one neuron (e.g., dopamine 1 and dopamine 2 may colocalize in neostriatal neurons) (171). In prefrontal cortex, Sawaguchi observed that about one-third of the neurons in prefrontal cortex responded to both dopamine and norepinephrine. However, the two neurotransmitters elicited quite different responses: dopamine was involved in the modulation of goal-directed motor performance guided by external cues, whereas norepinephrine appeared to modulate visual perception and behavioral arousal (124).

The norepinephrine transporter (NET1) functions to block the reuptake of norepinephrine into the presynaptic neuron, thus increasing available norepinephrine at the synapse. Atomoxetine is a selective NET1 inhibitor. Thus, the norepinephrine transporter is an attractive susceptibility factor in ADHD. A transmission disequilibrium test revealed a significant association between two *NET1* single nucleotide polymorphisms (SNPs) and ADHD (172). However, another study yielded what might be a small effect, but no evidence of a significant association (173).

Serotonin

Serotonin has been implicated in a broad range of neuropsychiatric disorders, mood disorders, OCD, drug abuse, and impulsive/aggressive behaviors, all of which are also frequently observed in children and adults with ADHD. The serotonin transporter is the target for the selective serotonin reuptake inhibitors, which have become central to the treatment of many psychiatric disorders. Serotonin modulates the function of dopaminergic neurons (174), as well as that of other neurotransmitters (175). Dysregulation of the serotonergic system results in hyperactivity (176). Moreover, in DAT-1 knockout mice who are markedly hyperactive, reduction in hyperactivity following psychostimulant treatment requires a functioning serotonergic system (177). For all these reasons, a number of studies assessing the relationship of the serotonin transporter and specific serotonin receptors to ADHD have been conducted.

Susceptibility to ADHD has been linked to various polymorphisms of the serotonin transporter. A common 44 base pair deletion in the promoter region of the serotonin transporter gene (*5-HTTLPR*) results in reduced transcription and lower transporter protein levels. The homozygous L/L polymorphism results in higher levels of serotonin, which is associated with severe hyperactivity in animal studies. Several studies have reported a significant association between the long allele of the *5-HTTLPR* gene and ADHD (178–183). In some studies, there was also an association of the L/L polymorphism with conduct disorder as well (180).

A possible association between polymorphisms of the serotonin *HTR2A* receptor and the *5-HT1B* receptor genes and ADHD has also been reported (184–186). In a study of the T102C polymorphism of the *HTR2A* gene in a group of older women with seasonal affective disorder, those women who were homozygous for the C polymorphism had a significantly higher score for retrospectively assessed ADHD behaviors than those with the T/T or T/C genotype (187). However, these associations vary with the particular ethnic group studied, and, not surprisingly, some studies have failed to show associations between these genes and ADHD (188–190).

Glutamate

L-Glutamate, the most abundant excitatory neurotransmitter is involved in prefrontal-striatal and as thalamocortical projections. There are two types of glutamate receptors: metabotropic and ionotropic. Metabotropic receptors are members of the G-protein family (guanine nucleotide binding proteins) and trigger neural impulses through a biochemical cascade that is slower and longer-lasting than ionotropic receptors. Ionotropic receptors are ligand-gated ion channels and mediate rapid transmission. They consist of N-methyl D-aspartate (NMDA) receptors and closely related alpha-amino-3-hydroxy-5-methyl-4-isoxazolepropionic acid receptors (AMPA) and kainate receptors. These receptors play a crucial role in enhancing cognition by promoting synaptic plasticity and increasing the production of trophic factors. Glutamate has been implicated in ADHD in a number of clinical and preclinical studies. The glutamatergic and dopaminergic systems have a complex pattern of interaction. Glutamate may also be involved in the treatment response to psychostimulants, as magnetic resonance spectroscopy studies have revealed a significant decrease in the striatal glutamate/glutamine/GABA-to-creatine ratio following treatment with psychostimulants (191) (Carrey 2003).

The ionotropic glutamate receptor N-methyl D-aspartate *2A GRIN2A* (*NMDA-2A*) gene that encodes the N-methyl D-aspartate receptor subunit 2A (NMDA2A) maps to chromosome 16p13. One study reported linkage between 16p13 and ADHD (192) Other studies have reported a positive association of the *GRIN2A* exon 5 polymorphism with ADHD (160), whereas others have not (193). Another study demonstrated linkage between the SLC1A3 (Solute Carrier Family 1, member 3) gene (encoding a glial glutamate transporter), which maps to chromosome 5p12 (194). Genome-wide scans have also implicated this region as one possibly related to ADHD. (However, this is also close to the locus of the dopamine transporter gene.) This locus is thus both a functional and positional candidate for ADHD.

Gamma-Amino Butyric Acid

GABA is an inhibitory neurotransmitter in the mature brain. There are numerous types of GABA receptors. GABA (A) receptors in prefrontal cortex regulate prefrontal cortical neurons by continuous "silent" task-related inhibition, which appears to contribute to behavioral organization

(195). There are also an array of GABA polymorphisms that have a variable effect on behaviors mediated by prefrontal cortex, particularly dopamine. Although GABA plays an important role in the regulation of these networks, it has not been examined in relation to ADHD. The noteworthy aspect of this neurotransmitter is its double life: in the developing brain, it is the first neurotransmitter to become functional and at that time, it behaves as an *excitatory* neurotransmitter through a diffuse, paracrine nonsynaptic mode of action. At this early stage, it plays an important role in neuronal proliferation, migration, dendritic arborization, and synaptic modeling. GABAergic synapses also interact with developing glutamatergic synapses (196).

Other Aspects of Synaptic Function Possibly Related to Attention Deficit–Hyperactivity Disorder

An important aspect of synaptic function involves the formation of synaptic vesicles and the extrusion of neurotransmitter into the synaptic cleft. Numerous factors regulate synaptic function in addition to the transporters and receptor–vesicle docking proteins, agrins, which control clustering of receptors, and synapsins, which regulate neurotransmitter release.

One of the important components of this process is synaptosomal protein synaptic vesicle docking fusion protein 25 kDa (SNAP-25), which belongs to a family of soluble N-ethylmaleimide-sensitive factor attachment (SNARE) proteins that form complexes bridging the two cellular membranes and play an important role in presynaptic neurotransmitter release in association with the other vesicle-associated membrane proteins (VAMP)—syntaxin and synaptobrevin. Any disturbance of SNAP-25 would thus be expected to impair neurotransmitter release. The hyperactive coloboma mouse is hemizygous for a deletion of the *SNAP-25* gene. These mice have a selective deficit of dopamine release in the dorsal striatum coupled with a significant increase in norepinephrine concentration in the striatum and nucleus accumbens (Jones 2001; Wilson 2000). A number of studies in humans have supported the association between *SNAP-25* (on 20p11.2) and ADHD. There is some evidence that the gene is imprinted and preferentially inherited from the father (198, 199; Barr 2000, Mill 2002, 2004). However, not all studies have supported this association.

Dopamine- and cAMP-regulated phosphoprotein of 32 kDa (DARPP-32)

DARPP-32 integrates various neurotransmitter, neuromodulator, and neuropeptide signaling pathways in the striatum and, depending on the state of phosphorylation, serves as a molecular switch. There is a very complex response to glutamate (201). DARPP-32 is thought to play a central role in dopaminergic reward pathways and to be involved in response to a number of drugs of abuse (202).

Although DARPP-32 has been postulated as possibly being associated with ADHD, studies in humans have not been conducted (203).

Brain-Derived Neurotrophic Factor

Brain-derived neurotrophic factor (BDNF), which is involved in neuronal plasticity and survival, increases spine density on pyramidal neurons and enhances the synaptic efficacy of glutamate, has been mapped to 11p14 (204). BDNF is found in high concentration in the hippocampus and prefrontal cortex, and appears to play an important role in memory and prefrontal function. A number of studies have implicated *BDNF* polymorphisms in mood disorders (particularly bipolar disorder), schizophrenia, and OCD (205). An MRI morphometry study on a group of normal individuals indicated that the val66met polymorphism results in anomalies in prefrontal cortex and hippocampus (206). Kent and colleagues reported preferential transmission of the *BDNF* valine (G) allele to offspring with ADHD. There were significantly more paternal than maternal transmissions (207).

Catecholamine-O-methyl Transferase

Catecholamine-O-methyl transferase (COMT) degrades catecholamines by converting dopamine to 3-methyoxytyramine, thus playing a major role in prefrontal function. This gene is located on chromosome 22q11. The polymorphism in which there is a valine to methionine substitution results in a three- to fourfold difference in enzyme activity. Individuals who are homozygous for the methionine allele degrade dopamine more slowly and therefore have higher levels of dopamine in prefrontal cortex. In one study they made significantly fewer perseverative errors on the Wisconsin Card Sorting Test than subjects with one or two valine alleles (208). In a study examining the effect of these two polymorphisms on attentional control and anterior cingulate activity, monitored with fMRI, there was a distinct gradient noted, with those homozygous for the valine allele performing more poorly and showing more activation of cingulate cortex than the heterozygotes, who performed more poorly and manifested greater fMRI activation than subjects homozygous for the methionine allele (209).

In another study performance of subjects with these different genotypes was monitored following administration of dextroamphetamine. Subjects were initially tested on the Wisconsin Card Sorting Test and then performed a working memory task while undergoing fMRI scanning. On the Wisconsin Card Sorting Test, subjects who were homozygous for the methionine alleles made fewer perseverative errors in the baseline condition than those who had two copies of the valine alleles, but their performance deteriorated following administration of dextroamphetamine, whereas those with two valine alleles showed a slight improvement. On the less demanding working memory task, subjects who were homozygous for the methionine allele did not show any change following

dextroamphetamine, but their performance deteriorated on the most demanding working memory task and there was an increase in prefrontal cortical activation indicating a less efficient performance. In contrast, subjects with two copies of the valine allele showed improved performance and enhanced prefrontal efficiency relative to baseline in response to dextroamphetamine (210).

Diamond and colleagues examined children who were 8.2 to 14.6 years old on tasks demanding working memory and inhibition. Children who had two copies of the methionine polymorphism performed far better on a task requiring both working memory and inhibition, whereas there was no difference on the self-ordered pointing or recall memory tasks. On the mental rotation task, children with two copies of valine polymorphism performed better (211). However, in another study that assessed working memory, attention and speed, impulsiveness and response inhibition in children with ADHD, no association with COMT was identified (212).

Monoamine Oxidase

Monoamine oxidase (MAO-A, MAO-B) genes are mapped to Xp11.23 and code for enzymes that deaminate catecholamines. Brunner and colleagues described a large Dutch kindred in which affected males presented with mild mental retardation and impulsive, aggressive, antisocial behavior (arson, attempted rape, and exhibitionism) (213). This was related to a point mutation in the eighth exon of the *MAO-A* gene, which changed a glutamine to a termination codon (214). In a Chinese population, there is evidence of an association and linkage between ADHD and the monoamine oxidase genes (215, 216). In an Irish population, no association was noted with *MAO-B*, but certain *MAO-A* markers were significantly associated with ADHD (217). Children with certain *MAO-A* alleles who have been abused in early childhood are at greater risk for subsequent aggressive behaviors (218).

Enzymes Involved in the Biosynthesis of Catecholamines

This section would not be complete without a brief mention of the enzymes that are involved in the production of catecholamines. The rationale for including these enzymes is that if the pathways leading to dopamine and norepinephrine are not totally functional, this might result in decreased levels of neurotransmitter. Enzymes in this pathway include tyrosine hydroxylase (mapped to 11p15.5), which is involved in the synthesis of dihydroxyphenylalanine (DOPA) from tyrosine. Deficiency of tyrosine hydroxylase in its autosomal dominant form results in L-dopa responsive dystonia, and involves the basal ganglia. DOPA decarboxylase (gene locus 7p11) converts DOPA to dopamine. A possible relationship to ADHD and a paternal pattern of transmission suggesting imprinting has been described (219). DOPA concentration is elevated in the right brainstem areas of children with ADHD compared to controls, which may be the result of dysfunction in this system (109, 220). Dopamine β-hydroxylase (on 9q34) catalyzes the production of norepinephrine from DOPA and is associated with a disorder of cardiovascular regulation that is particularly severe in the young infant. Some studies have supported an association with ADHD (221–224) (Roman 2002), whereas others have not (225, 226).

ETIOLOGY OF ATTENTION DEFICIT–HYPERACTIVITY DISORDER

Genetic Factors

There is little question that genetic factors are extremely important in the etiology of ADHD. There are now well over 200 studies, consisting of relatively small samples, using different genetic tests of association, and carried out in different ethnic populations. As is clear from the previous review, there is far from total agreement across all these studies. However, there is evidence across many of these studies that some genetic perturbation of catecholaminergic systems is involved in the pathogenesis of ADHD. In addition to the issues of varying strategies in approaching the association, there is also the problem that one would not necessarily expect different ethnic populations to have the same gene pool. It is also unlikely that a single gene will be identified as the cause of ADHD. Like most neuropsychiatric disorders, it is likely that the disorder is polygenic. Thus, there is now an emerging trend to sample multiple candidate genes simultaneously and to increase the size of the population and use a variety of tests to determine if an association exists. Moreover, the inclusion of genes other than the classical neurotransmitters may strengthen these studies as patients may manifest symptoms of ADHD only when function of the transporters or the receptors is compromised by other factors. Moreover, it is possible that some of these genetic factors may interact with psychosocial or biological environmental factors.

Nongenetic and Acquired Forms of Attention Deficit–Hyperactivity Disorder

ADHD has an undisputed genetic basis, but can also be the result of acquired brain injury or dysfunction of the frontal-subcortical system. In some individuals, both factors can be operative. DSM-IV diagnostic criteria do not distinguish between these various etiologies for ADHD. For the clinician, this distinction may not appear to be totally relevant because there appears to be no consistently different response to psychostimulant medications. However, as information relating to pharmacogenetics expands, different etiologies of ADHD are likely to become increasing important to the treating physician.

Prenatal Factors

A number of prenatal factors appear to place a child at risk for ADHD-like behaviors. Maternal cigarette smoking during pregnancy is one such factor. Twenty-two percent of the children with ADHD had a history of maternal smoking during pregnancy, compared with only 8% in the control group (227). This is an interesting association, given the effect of nicotine on the dopaminergic system and its effect on improving inhibition (228). Moreover, one cannot eliminate the possibility of a potential genetic confound, given the association of cigarette smoking and the DRD2 TaqI A1 allele (229). However, in a study in which the contribution of genetic factors (that is, maternal ADHD) was assessed in comparison to exposure to cigarette smoke inutero, Milberger demonstrated that maternal smoking was associated with a fourfold higher risk of ADHD in the offspring than in controls, even after controlling for maternal ADHD (230). A subsequent study by Mick and colleagues, using Milberger's data and adding information from girls, reported a 2 to 1 risk. In 2003, Thapar and colleagues also noted that maternal smoking increased the risk of ADHD in the offspring in addition to any specific genetic effect (231).

Fetal alcohol syndrome is also associated with ADHD but typically occurs in the context of neurocognitive deficits and microcephaly. In a meta-analysis of studies on maternal smoking, alcohol ingestion, caffeine and psychosocial stress published between 1973 and 2002, the authors reported that the findings on alcohol were contradictory, and studies on caffeine inconclusive. There was a possible modest contribution of stress to ADHD symptoms in offspring. However, maternal smoking during pregnancy appeared to place offspring at a greater risk for ADHD. Sowell and colleagues reported MRI morphometric studies in children exposed to heavy maternal alcohol ingestion that reveal widespread effects, including decrease in size of prefrontal cortex (232).

Prematurity

Prematurity is often associated with ADHD. This can be relatively subtle in older children. In one study, very-low birthweight prematures who were free of major cognitive or neurological impairment and did not manifest a classical ADHD-profile when tested on a CPT task at the age of 17 years nonetheless continued to show lingering emotional and neuropsychological deficits (233). A number of factors might explain the high incidence of ADHD-spectrum symptoms in this population.

First, the dopaminergic system, particularly in the developing brain, is easily damaged by hypoxia. Small premature infants are at high risk for recurrent apneic attacks. In a study on hypoxia in neonatal rats, Dell'Anna and colleagues reported that exposure to a hypoxic environment resulted in alterations in dopamine, norepinephrine, and serotonin in various areas of the brain (234, 235) and also observed that hypoxia affected the mesotelencephalic pathways involved in sleep, wakefulness, locomotion, and executive function. A small group of ex-premature infants who had been examined with cerebral blood flow measures at birth and in whom ADHD later developed were re-examined at the age of 12 to 14 years. Dopamine receptor binding was examined, using PET with [11C] raclopride, which preferentially binds to dopamine receptors. They found that low neonatal cerebral blood flow was associated with increased dopamine receptor availability in adolescence ("empty receptors") (236). In other words, damage to the dopaminergic system early in development resulted in the availability of an increased number of "empty receptors."

Damage to white matter pathways also occurs in the small premature infant. Periventricular leukomalacia involves focal cystic necrosis of axons and white matter tracts lying deep in the brain around the lateral ventricles. There is also a more diffuse injury to white matter resulting from damage to oligodendrocytes, which ultimately are the source of the myelinated pathways (237). This diffuse white matter damage also disrupts normal gray matter growth. Inder and colleagues conducted an MRI study on premature infants and observed that gray matter abnormalities were correlated with the extent of white matter abnormality, so that cortical atrophy and immature gyral development were found in the vast majority of infants born at less than 26 weeks' gestational age. Factors that contributed to this picture included infection in the perinatal period and hypotension requiring inotrope use (238).

Hyperbilirubinemia (jaundice) occurs in children who are premature as well as those who have blood group incompatibility. Bilirubin appears to function as a specific neuronal poison for neurons in the basal ganglia. Although the mechanism by which bilirubin damages neurons is not entirely clear, one possible mechanism is the excitotoxic effects of NMDA. The basal ganglia, certain brainstem nuclei, and the Purkinje cells are highly sensitive to damage. Before the use of exchange transfusions and RhoGAM, hyperbilirubinemia could result in devastating choreoathetoid cerebral palsy and deafness. Hyperbilirubinemia is a particular problem in the small premature infant, who lacks the ability to conjugate bilirubin and is at risk for hypoxia, which increases the potential for neuronal damage. Even full-term infants who are jaundiced at birth may have subtle attentional dysfunction, suggesting that in susceptible children, hyperbilirubinemia may not be all that benign (239).

Finally, focal lesions early in development may affect more distant cerebral regions and result in an ADHD-like picture. Saunders and Merjanian found that temporal lobe lesions in monkeys in the neonatal period disrupted dopamine regulation in the dorsolateral prefrontal cortex (240). Interestingly, Milichap described ADHD-like symptoms in children who had temporal lobe cysts (241).

Epilepsy

ADHD is also more prevalent in children with epilepsy. Although there has been some controversy surrounding this point, whether or not it is a side effect of treatment, there is

evidence of an association between epilepsy and ADHD. One study from Iceland reported by Hesdorffer found that ADHD was 2.5 times more common in children with newly diagnosed seizures than in controls. This was most prominent in ADHD, predominantly inattentive type whereas the hyperactive impulsive or combined types were not as closely associated. There was no particular relationship to seizure type, ideology, gender, or seizure frequency at the time of diagnosis. In a study of 175 children ranging in age from 9 to 14 years with at least a 6-month history of epilepsy, Dunn and colleagues noted that 24% met DSM-IV criteria for ADHD, predominantly inattentive type. This was unrelated to gender, seizure type, or seizure focus (242). Holtmann and colleagues described a group of children who had ADHD-like symptoms and had an unusually high incidence of Rolandic spikes. The subjects included 483 patients between the ages of 2 and 16 years who met DSM-IV criteria for ADHD. Rolandic spikes were observed in the electroencephalographs of 5.6% of the children (243).

Medical Illness

Another disorder that has been associated with ADHD is celiac disease, a multisystem autoimmune disorder, which has been associated with a broad spectrum of central nervous system symptoms. In adults, celiac disease is a important cause of cerebellar ataxia, and white matter lesions and cerebellar atrophy are often noted (244). In children, epilepsy, occipital calcifications surrounded by hypodense areas on CT scan, and diffuse white matter lesions have been reported (245, 246). This may be related either to an autoimmune demyelinating process or a vasculopathy. Celiac disease has been implicated in stroke in children (247). Developmental delay, ataxia, and hypotonia are prominent, but more subtle presentations, such as inattention and other ADHD-like symptoms, may be noted in approximately 20% of children (248). Although many of these children typically have gastrointestinal symptoms and failure to thrive, cases with few of these GI symptoms have also been observed. There are several possible explanations for the association between celiac disease and ADHD-like symptoms; the vasculopathy, white matter lesions, and cerebellar involvement (with secondary effectives on frontal-executive function) come to mind.

ADHD has also been associated with other autoimmune disorders involving a vasculitis. Following a Group A beta-hemolytic streptococcal infection that appears to specifically involve the basal ganglia, ADHD, often in association with Tourette disorder and OCD, have been reported. This syndrome is called Pediatric Autoimmune Neuropsychiatric Disorders Associated with Streptococcus (PANDAS). There is controversy whether PANDAS and Sydenham chorea are different entities.

Phenylketonuria (PKU) is an inborn error of metabolism that results in significant ADHD symptoms. Although there are numerous gene mutations that disrupt the metabolism of phenylalanine, classically the absence of phenylalanine hydroxylase, the enzyme involved in the conversion of phenylalanine to tyrosine which is an important step in the production of dopamine, results in varying degrees of hypodopaminergia. Any factor that reduces dopamine in prefrontal cortical neurons is likely to result in an ADHD-like picture. A gradient effect was noted in that exposure during fetal development (occurring in phenylketonuric mothers) resulted in hyperactivity/impulsivity and inattention while postnatal exposure was associated with inattention (249). Despite very tight control of phenylalanine during pregnancy, children with PKU who are then treated early and vigorously perform poorly on tasks demanding frontal executive resources and manifest hyperactivity, impulsivity, and inattention. Diamond observed that preschool children with elevated phenylalanine levels showed deficits in working memory and inhibitory control functions dependent upon dorsolateral prefrontal cortex, suggesting that dopamine played an important role in the maturation of that area (250).

Environmental Toxins

Environmental toxins have received relatively little attention as contributing to the ADHD phenotype. The issue is complex because of the need to untangle various other factors, for example, socioeconomic and genetic. Probably the most extensively studied environmental toxin is lead. The severe encephalopathy that occurs in children with blood levels in the range of 60 mcg/dL has been well documented, but the more subtle effects of exposure to lower lead levels have been less obvious. Moreover, lead poisoning usually is found in specific populations and in restricted geographic areas. There is evidence that relatively minimal blood lead levels (above 10 mcg/dL) puts a child at risk for hyperactivity and subtle impairment of executive function (251, 252). In lead-exposed rats, striatal dopamine uptake as well as behavioral changes have been noted (253). Increased mercury ingestion also appears to target dopaminergic systems (254). Other environmental toxins such as polychlorinated biphenyls (PCBs) may also contribute to ADHD-like behaviors, particularly since exposure occurs not only during fetal development, but also during breastfeeding. Nigg has provided a thoughtful review of the issue of the role of environmental contaminants in ADHD (255).

Acquired Brain Injury

Traumatic brain injury, particularly when there is damage to frontal subcortical circuits also produces ADHD-like behaviors (256–259). Because many types of traumatic injury involve damage to the frontal poles or shearing of white matter tracts, this is not an uncommon outcome.

Similarly, children who have suffered strokes not infrequently manifest ADHD-like behaviors, which had not existed before the stroke, and typically involve inattention and apathy. Max and colleagues noted that in their sample

of children with stroke, compared to matched controls with clubfoot or scoliosis, nearly half (46%) had ADHD-like traits following stroke. They performed poorly on a task that required alert, sensory orientation. Two factors were also important in determining severity of attentional disturbance: size of lesion in the attention/arousal network (but not executive attention) (260–264).

Castellanos and colleagues recruited nine carefully studied monozygotic twin pairs discordant for DSM-IV ADHD. Total caudate volume of the affected twin was significantly smaller than that of the unaffected co-twin. No significant differences within the twin pairs were found with regard to volume differences in other brain regions. The caudate volume differences did not correlate significantly with parent/teacher Conner's rating of hyperactivity severity, differences in birth weight, or duration of stimulant exposure (265).

Meningitis and encephalitis can result in ADHD-like behaviors, particularly when the basal ganglia are affected. Autoimmune disorders have also been implicated in triggering ADHD-like symptoms in susceptible patients. PANDAS are linked to Tourette disorder, OCD, and ADHD (266, 267). Lyme disease has also been associated with a number of neuropsychiatric symptoms, including those of ADHD (268).

Psychosocial Factors

Although environmental factors may not directly cause ADHD, there is little question than the more adverse the environment, the more severe the symptoms are likely to be. Children who grow up in "adverse" environments (i.e., poverty, maternal psychopathology, paternal criminality) are at much greater risk for ADHD, and the risk is in proportion to the number of adverse factors that are present (269). Children with reactive attachment are often hyperactive and inattentive, and ADHD is one of the differential diagnostic considerations in these children. Children who are genetically at risk for ADHD would seem to be much more likely to be severely impaired if they grow up in chaotic, unstructured households. However, there is clearly a need for further research in this area (270).

TREATMENT OF ATTENTION DEFICIT–HYPERACTIVITY DISORDER

The impressive effect of psychostimulants on ADHD symptoms has been known since 1937 when Bradley observed its remarkable effect on a classroom of children with ADHD (4). At present there are now a variety of drugs and delivery systems available for the treatment of ADHD. The most thoroughly studied and those that have been used for the treatment of ADHD for half a century or more are dextroamphetamine and methylphenidate. Both of these drugs increase available dopamine and norepinephrine at central synapses through somewhat different mechanisms.

Volkow and colleagues have provided a convincing demonstration that dopamine release at central synapses is enhanced when presented in the context of a salient stimulus. Methylphenidate, in the absence of such a stimulus, does not reliably enhance dopaminergic release (271, 272).

Not all patients respond equally well to these medications. Some show dramatic positive responses, whereas others are helped to some extent but often continue to experience unacceptable side effects. The most common side effects are decreased appetite and disrupted sleep, although some patients report improved sleep. Other side effects include dyspepsia, autonomic arousal and increased anxiety, and headache. Rare side effects include vermification or hallucinations.

Although a carefully executed double-blind crossover study reported a response rate of 98% to methylphenidate and/or dextroamphetamine (25% responded to only one agent) (273), this does not seem to concur with clinical experience, nor does it explain the substantial number of patients who drop out of treatment. A more reasonable estimate, based on 155 controlled studies involving 5,768 subjects, indicated a response in the 70% range (274). However, longterm adherence to psychostimulant medication can range from 52% to close to 90%. Adherence does not appear to be related to the effectiveness of the treatment. In a multicenter study involving 407 children treated with OROS MPH, 71% of the subjects remained on medication after 12 months. This is surprising as the children were responders and had been titrated to an appropriate dose and were followed closely (275). In the NIMH Collaborative Multisite Multimodal Treatment Study of Children With ADHD (MTA), 88% of the 198 children for whom MPH was the optimal treatment remained on medication. These children were followed monthly and received dose adjustments as needed (276). In a longterm follow-up study of children treated with methylphenidate, 52% continued to take medication at least 5 days a week at the 3-year mark. Adherence was predicted by absence of oppositional defiant disorder and more ADHD symptoms (based on teacher ratings), as well as a younger age at the start of program (277). Although continued treatment is associated with good response, side effects do not change. In a somewhat longer (5-year follow-up study) involving 79 children treated with methylphenidate with annual evaluations for 5 years, subjects who remained on medication had consistently greater improvement in teacher-reported symptoms than those who took medication inconsistently or took none at all. However, side effects in these treated children continued to persist (278).

In the past few years, a number of new drugs and new delivery devices have become available so that the physician now has an array of options. A number of extended release forms with a duration of action ranging from 8 to 12 hours are now available in an array of doses. The purified D-isomer of methylphenidate (dexmethylphenidate hydrochloride, D-MPH is available in a variety of doses

(279, 280). Transdermal methylphenidate has also been used in experimental settings with good results (281).

Atomoxetine, a specific norepinephrine transport inhibitor, was originally developed as an antidepressant but was never marketed as such. It was then later reevaluated as a potential treatment for ADHD. A desirable feature is that once a day dosing provides 24 hour coverage. Atomoxotine has a low abuse potential and is considered a nonstimulant approved by the US Food and Drug Administration for treatment of ADHD. An important metabolic pathway for atomoxetine involves cytochrome P450 (CYP) 2D6. In extensive metabolizers, atomoxetine has a plasma half-life of 5.2 hours, while in poor metabolizers, atomoxetine has a plasma half-life of 21.6 hours. Once a steady state has been reached, the average steady-state plasma concentrations are approximately ten times higher in poor metabolizers than in extensive metabolizers. However, on the same dose, the incidence of side effects does not seem to differ in the two groups. Atomoxetine does not inhibit or induce the clearance of other drugs metabolized by P450 (CYP) 2D6 enzymes (282). In one study, the discontinuation rate was 3.5% and appeared to be dose-dependent, with higher discontinuation rates at dosages over 1.5 mg/kg day. In children and adolescents, nausea, vomiting, decreased appetite, and weight loss are common side effects. Several interesting preclinical studies have supported the use of atomoxetine as a treatment for ADHD. In the model of neonatal 6-hydroxydopamine lesions in neonatal rats, atomoxetine resulted in marked reduction of motor activity in these animals. In contrast, there was only a transient sedative effect in sham controls. The important aspect of atomoxetine is its effect on CYP 2D6 (283).

Another drug that has shown some promise in the treatment of some individuals with ADHD is modafinil, originally developed as a treatment for narcolepsy. This is also a nonstimulant and its mechanism of action is largely unknown. It has a different mechanism of action than psychostimulants, and does not increase dopamine or norepinephrine either by inhibiting reuptake or enhancing release. The mechanism of action that promotes alertness is not related to the locus coeruleus projections to the forebrain, but rather involves the hypothalamus, probably the tuberomammillary nucleus and hypocretin/orexin neurons in the perifornical area (284). These hypocretin/orexin neurons play an important role in hypothalamic arousal. Interestingly, low-dose modafinil also appeared to affect neurons in the amygdala as well. The input to the hypothalamic neurons appears to involve dopamine-dependent norepinephrine signaling (285), although the hypocretin/orexin neurons are also modulated by glutamatergic input (286).

Behavioral Treatment

Behavioral treatments are also of value. Many children with ADHD need to have "accessory frontal lobes" and benefit immensely from being provided with routines and scripts and being given tools that enable them to organize themselves. Pelham and colleagues reported that the combination of behavioral treatment and low doses of medication has been successful (281). The MTA study provided strong support for the efficacy of psychostimulants in the treatment of ADHD. In the short range, medication alone appeared to be more efficacious than the combination of medical and behavioral treatment, but the combination of medicine and behavioral management was associated with a better 2-year outcome than the medication group alone. In the long run, the difference (68% versus 56%) was relatively small but was significantly better compared to behavioral treatment alone and community care. The behavioral treatment was extremely intense and involved (1) parent training, (2) individual work with the child, (3) integration of the school into the behavior program, and (4) a daily report card completed by the teacher that was then used by the parents to deliver consequences. This large, well-designed study strongly supports the use of medication integrated with a behavioral program.

Pharmacogenomics

Given the variability in the clinical responses of patients and the burgeoning information in the genetics of ADHD, the notion of developing systematic pharmacogenomic approaches to the treatment of ADHD is especially attractive. Unfortunately, this undertaking is still in its infancy. Current research studies involve small sample sizes, varying ethnic gene pools, and thus may not be applicable to all populations. Nonetheless the information available is tantalizing.

Most studies in this area have been limited to methylphenidate and most have involved the *DAT-1* gene. There are two common alleles, the 9-9-repeat and the more common 10-repeat. The *DAT-1* 10-repeat (480-base pair) polymorphism and the D4 dopamine receptor-7-repeat allele have been the subject of many genetic studies. Both of these genes have been demonstrated (albeit not consistently) to be associated with ADHD. The efficacy of methylphenidate is related to its ability to inhibit the function of DAT-1 to recycle dopamine from the synaptic cleft back into the presynaptic neuron. In a single photon emission spectroscopy study, using a ligand for the dopamine transporter, subjects with the 9-9 repeat or 9-10 repeat genotype had significantly higher DAT availability in the caudate and putamen than those homozygous for the 10-repeat (287).

With regard to D4, a preclinical study has suggested that the D4 dopamine receptor -7-repeat allele is less responsive to dopamine. (The assumption that the *DRD4-7* repeat polymorphism responds differently is based on a study by Asghari and colleagues that indicated that there was a twofold reduction in the D4-7 repeat polymorphism in the inhibition of cAMP formation compared to the dopamine 4 receptor with 2- and 4- repeats. [288]). The question

addressed in these pharmacogenomic studies is whether patients with these different genotypes manifest a differential response to methylphenidate.

In 1999, Winsberg and Cummings evaluated the interaction between genotype (*DAT-1*, and dopamine receptors D2 and D4) and response to methylphenidate in a group of 30 African American children. Methylphenidate was titrated to the point that a behavioral change was achieved, or a maximum tolerated dose was reached (the dose did not exceed 60 mg [approximately 0.7 mg/kg]). Eighty-six percent of nonresponders were homozygous for the 10-copy allele of the *DAT-1* gene in contrast to 31% of responders. The response rate in this group of children was only 53%, much less than that reported in most studies. No difference in response pattern was detected for the Taq 1A dopamine D2 receptor or the dopamine D4 receptor (289).

The lack of response to methylphenidate in children with two copies of the 10-copy allele of the *DAT-1* gene was replicated in a study on 50 male Brazilian youths. More (75%) of the boys who were not homozygous for the 10-repeat allele showed improvement compared to 47% of those who had two copies (290). In a single photon emission computerized tomography (SPECT) study involving children who demonstrated at least a moderate response to methylphenidate, those with the 10-repeat *DAT-1* allele showed significantly higher regional blood flow in the medial frontal and left basal ganglia (291). In a study on a small group of Korean children with ADHD, only about one third (28.6%) of the children homozygous for the 10-repeat *DAT-1* manifested a good response to methylphenidate. In contrast, all children without the 10/10 genotype manifested a good response to treatment. Moreover, the children homozygous for the 10/10 genotype also showed a significantly greater increase in DAT density in the basal ganglia compared to those without the 10/10 genotype (292).

However, the exact opposite finding was reported in a study involving 119 Irish children; namely that individuals with two copies of the 10-repeat allele showed a good response to methylphenidate in comparison to those who did not. The hypothesis on which this study was based was that the 10-repeat *DAT-1* allele resulted in an overactive transporter, and the investigators suggested that this might heighten the response to methylphenidate (293).

In a study of 47 children with ADHD treated with a placebo-controlled, double-blind crossover dosing schedule that involved three dose levels of OROS methylphenidate (18 mg, 36 mg, and 54 mg), it was noted that children who were homozygous for the *DAT-1* 9-repeat 1 3′ UTR genotype (this is relatively rare) did not show a linear improvement as the dose was increased (294).

In a study comparing the magnitude of methylphenidate dose required to achieve behavioral responses (measured by rating scales), subjects with the *DRD4* receptor 7-repeat polymorphism required 1.5 times as much methylphenidate (with doses up to 1.70 mg/kg) compared to those without that polymorphism (295). This study supports the hypothesis that the 7-repeat *DRD 4* allele results in a less efficient dopamine receptor.

Tahir and colleagues reported that the *DRD4* 7-repeat allele was associated with a better response to methylphenidate. This Turkish study population included 104 trios and 7 dyads, and the analysis involved the transmission disequilibrium test (296).

Given the importance of serotonin and dopamine in psychopathology, and the possibility that serotonin is associated with ADHD (178), as well as the complex interaction of these two neurotransmitters at a neuronal level, examination of the methylphenidate response in individuals with differing dopamine and serotonin receptors is an important undertaking. Individuals who are homozygous for the long allele (L/L) manifest increased serotonin levels compared to the heterozygous (L/S) or those with two short alleles (SS). Prolactin release is inhibited by dopamine and enhanced by serotonin. Seeger and colleagues examined the methylphenidate response in 47 children with ADHD whose *DRD4* and *5-HTT* genotypes were known. Those who were homozygous for both the 7-repeat dopamine *DRD4* polymorphism and the long serotonin receptor had the smallest response to methylphenidate and the highest level of prolactin release. Moreover, children with the two long alleles had a higher incidence of conduct disorder (180).

Several other genes have been evaluated with regard to response to methylphenidate. One study reported a significant association between the norepinephrine transporter gene *G1287A* genotypes and response to methylphenidate. Chinese Han children with ADHD with the G/G or G/A genotype showed highly significant reductions in hyperactive/impulsive scores but not inattention scores. Those with the A/A genotype showed minimal response (297). There is also some support from preclinical studies for the specific reduction of hyperactivity/impulsivity in these children. In rats with 6-OHDA-induced lesions in the neonatal period, there is a marked reduction in hyperactivity following administration of atomoxetine, a specific norepinephrine inhibitor (283).

REFERENCES

1. Szatmari, P, Boyle M, Offord DR. ADDH and conduct disorder: degree of diagnostic overlap and differences among correlates. J Am Acad Child Adolesc Psychiatry 1989;28:865–872.
2. Szatmari, P. The epidemiology of attention-deficit hyperactivity disorders. In: *Child and Adolescent Psychiatry Clinics of North America: Attention Deficit Disorder.* Philadelphia: WB Saunders, 1992:361–372.
3. Still, GF. The Coulstonian Lectures on some abnormal physical conditions in children. Lancet 1902;1:1008–1012, 1077–1082, 1163–1168.
4. Bradley, C. The behavior of children receiving benzedrine. Am J Psychiatry 1937;94:577–585.
5. American Psychiatric Association. *Diagnostic and Statistical Manual of Mental Disorders,* 3rd Ed. (DSM-III). Washington, D.C.: American Psychiatric Association, 1980.
6. American Psychiatric Association. *Diagnostic and Statistical Manual of Mental Disorders,* 4th Ed. (DSM-IV). Washington, D.C.: American Psychiatric Association, 1994.
7. Lahey, BB, Applegate B, McBurnett K, et al. DSM-IV field trials for attention deficit/hyperactivity disorder in children and adolescents. Am J Psychiatry 1994;151:1673–1685.
8. Frick, PJ, Lahey BB, Applegate B, et al. DSM-IV field trials for the disruptive behavior disorders: Symptom utility estimates. J Am Acad Child Adolesc Psychiatry 1994;33:529–539.
9. Biederman, J, Faraone SV, Weber W, et al. Correspondence between DSM-III-R and DSM-IV attention-deficit/hyperactivity disorder. J Am Acad Child Adolesc Psychiatry 1997;36:1682–1687.
10. Lahey, BB, Schaughency EA, Hynd GW, et al. Attention deficit disorder with and without hyperactivity: comparison of behavioral characteristics of clinic-referred children. J Am Acad Child Adolesc Psychiatry 1987;26:718–723.
11. McBurnett, K, Pfiffner LJ, Frick PJ. Symptom properties as a function of ADHD type: an argument for continued study of sluggish cognitive tempo. J Abnorm Child Psychol 2001;29:207–213.
12. Carlson, CL, Mann M. Sluggish cognitive tempo predicts a different pattern of impairment in the attention deficit hyperactivity disorder, predominantly inattentive type. J Clin Child Adolesc Psychol 2002;31:123–129.
13. Todd, RD, Rasmussen ER, Wood C, et al. Should sluggish cognitive tempo symptoms be included in the diagnosis of attention-deficit/hyperactivity disorder? J Am Acad Child Adolesc Psychiatry 2004;43:588–597.
14. Gaub, M, Carlson CL. Behavioral characteristics of DSM-IV ADHD subtypes in a school-based population. J Abnorm Child Psychol 1997;25:103–111.
15. Weiss, M, Worling D, Wasdell M. A chart review study of the inattentive and combined types of ADHD. J Atten Disord 2003;7:1–9.
16. Chhabildas, N, Pennington BF, Willcutt EG. A comparison of the neuropsychological profiles of the DSM-IV subtypes of ADHD. J Abnorm Child Psychol 2001;29:529–540.
17. Willcutt, EG, Pennington BF, DeFries JC. Etiology of inattention and hyperactivity/impulsivity in a community sample of twins with learning difficulties. J Abnorm Child Psychol 2000;28: 149–159.
18. Clarke, AR, Barry RJ, McCarthy R, et al. EEG evidence for a new conceptualisation of attention deficit hyperactivity disorder. Clin Neurophysiol 2002;113:1036–1044.
19. Smith, JL, Johnstone SJ, Barry RJ. Aiding diagnosis of attention-deficit/hyperactivity disorder and its subtypes: discriminant function analysis of event-related potential data. J Child Psychol Psychiatry 2003;44:1067–1075.
20. Johnstone, SJ, Barry RJ, Dimoska A. Event-related slow-wave activity in two subtypes of attention-deficit/hyperactivity disorder. Clin Neurophysiol 2003;114:504–514.
21. Willoughby, MT, Curran PJ, Costello EJ, et al. Implications of early versus late onset of attention-deficit/hyperactivity disorder symptoms. J Am Acad Child Adolesc Psychiatry 2000;39:1512– 1519.
22. Lahey, BB, Pelham WE, Stein, MA., et al. Validity of DSM-IV attention-deficit/hyperactivity disorder for younger children. J Am Acad Child Adolesc Psychiatry 1998;37:695–702.
23. Lahey, BB, Pelham WE, Loney J, et al. Three-year predictive validity of DSM-IV attention deficit hyperactivity disorder in children diagnosed at 4–6 years of age. Am J Psychiatry 2004; 161: 2014–2020.
24. Sonuga-Barke, EJ, Dalen L, Remington B. Do executive deficits and delay aversion make independent contributions to preschool attention-deficit/hyperactivity disorder symptoms? J Am Acad Child Adolesc Psychiatry 2003;42:1335–1342.
25. Applegate, B, Lahey BB, Hart EL, et al. Validity of age-of-onset criterion for ADHD: A report from the DSM-IV field trials. J Am Acad Child Adolesc Psychiatry 1997;36:1211–1221.
26. Gaub, M, Carlson CL. Gender differences in ADHD: a meta-analysis and critical review. J Am Acad Child Adolesc Psychiatry 1997;36:1036–1045.
27. Greene, RW, Biederman J, Faraone SV, et al. Social impairment in girls with ADHD: patterns, gender comparisons, and correlates. J Am Acad Child Adolesc Psychiatry 2001;40:704–710.
28. Biederman, J, Kwon A, Aleardi M, et al. Absence of gender effects on attention deficit hyperactivity disorder: findings in nonreferred subjects. Am J Psychiatry 2005;162:1083–1089.

29. Castellanos, FX, Marvasti FF, Ducharme JL, et al. Executive function oculomotor tasks in girls with ADHD. J Am Acad Child Adolesc Psychiatry 2000;39:644–650.
30. Seidman, LJ, Biederman J, Monuteaux MC, et al. Impact of gender and age on executive functioning: do girls and boys with and without attention deficit hyperactivity disorder differ neuropsychologically in preteen and teenage years? Dev Neuropsychol 2005;27:79–105.
31. Faraone, SV, Biederman J, Mick E, et al. Family study of girls with attention deficit hyperactivity disorder. Am J Psychiatry 2000; 157:1077–1083.
32. Rucklidge, JJ, Tannock R. Psychiatric, psychosocial, and cognitive functioning of female adolescents with ADHD. J Am Acad Child Adolesc Psychiatry 2001;40:530–540.
33. Hinshaw, SP. Preadolescent girls with attention-deficit/hyperactivity disorder: I. Background characteristics, comorbidity, cognitive and social functioning, and parenting practices. J Consult Clin Psychol 2002;70:1086–1098.
34. Hinshaw, SP, Carte ET, Sami N, et al. Preadolescent girls with attention-deficit/hyperactivity disorder: II. Neuropsychological performance in relation to subtypes and individual classification. J Consult Clin Psychol 2002;70:1099–1111.
35. Biederman, J, Faraone SV. The Massachusetts General Hospital studies of gender influences on attention-deficit/hyperactivity disorder in youth and relatives. Psychiatr Clin North Am 2004; 27:225–232.
36. Biederman, J, Munir K, Knee D, et al. High rate of affective disorders in probands with attention deficit disorder and in their relatives: a controlled family study. Am J Psychiatry 1987;144: 330–333.
37. Biederman, J, Faraone SV, Keenan K, et al. Further evidence for family-genetic risk factors in attention deficit hyperactivity disorder: patterns of comorbidity in probands and relatives in psychiatrically and pediatrically referred samples. Arch Gen Psychiatry 1992;49:728–738.
38. Newcorn, JH, Halperin JM, Jensen PS, et al. Symptom profiles in children with ADHD: effects of comorbidity and gender. J Am Acad Child Adolesc Psychiatry 2001;40:137–146.
39. Mannuzza, S, Klein RG, Abikoff H, et al. Significance of childhood conduct problems to later development of conduct disorder among children with ADHD: a prospective follow-up study. J Abnorm Child Psychol 2004;32:565–573.
40. Power, TJ, Costigan TE, Eiraldi RB, et al. Variations in anxiety and depression as a function of ADHD subtypes defined by DSM-IV: do subtype differences exist or not? J Abnorm Child Psychol 2004;32:27–37.
41. Vance, A, Sanders M, Arduca Y. Dysthymic disorder contributes to oppositional defiant behaviour in children with attention deficit hyperactivity disorder, combined type (ADHD-CT). J Affect Disord 2005;86:329–333.
42. Robertson, HA, Kutcher SP, Lagace DC. No evidence of attentional deficits in stabilized bipolar youth relative to unipolar and control comparators. Bipolar Disord 2003;5:330–339.
43. Meyer, SE, Carlson GA, Wiggs EA, et al. A prospective study of the association among impaired executive functioning, childhood attentional problems, and the development of bipolar disorder. Dev Psychopathol 2004;16:461–476.
44. March, JS, Swanson JM, Arnold LE, et al. Anxiety as a predictor and outcome variable in the multimodal treatment study of children with ADHD (MTA). J Abnorm Child Psychol 2000;28:527–541.
45. Vance, A, Harris K, Boots M, et al. Which anxiety disorders may differentiate attention deficit hyperactivity disorder, combined type with dysthymic disorder from attention deficit hyperactivity disorder, combined type alone? Aust N Z J Psychiatry 2003;37: 563–569.
46. Peterson, BS, Pine DS, Cohen P, et al. Prospective, longitudinal study of tic, obsessive-compulsive, and attention-deficit/hyperactivity disorders in an epidemiological sample. J Am Acad Child Adoles Psychiatry 2001;40:685–695.
47. Sheppard, DM, Bradshaw JL, Purcell R, et al. Tourette's and comorbid syndromes: obsessive compulsive and attention deficit hyperactivity disorder. A common etiology? Clin Psychol Rev 1999;19:531–552.
48. Rizzolatti, G, Matelli M. Two different streams form the dorsal visual system: anatomy and functions. Exp Brain Res 2003;153: 146–157.
49. Eriksen, CW, St James JD. Visual attention within and around the field of focal attention: a zoom lens model. Percept Psychophys 1986;40:225–240.
50. Van Essen, DC, Anderson CH, Felleman DJ. Information processing in the primate visual system: an integrated systems perspective. Science 1992;255:419–423.
51. Maunsell, JHR. The brain's visual world: representation of visual targets in cerebral cortex. Science 1995;270:764–769.
52. Ungerleider, LG. Functional brain imaging studies of cortical mechanisms for memory. Science 1995;270:769–773.
53. Goldberg, ME, Wurtz RH. Activity of superior colliculus in behaving monkey: I. The effect of attention on neuronal responses. J Neurophysiol 1972;35:575–586.
54. Martinez, A, Anllo-Vento L, Sereno MI, et al. Involvement of striate and extrastriate visual cortical areas in spatial attention. Nat Neurosci 1999;2:364–369.
55. Kastner, S, Pinsk MA, De Weerd P, et al. Increased activity in human visual cortex during directed attention in the absence of visual stimulation. Neuron 1999;22:751–761.
56. Ress, D, Backus BT, Heeger DJ. Activity in primary visual cortex predicts performance in a visual detection task. Nat Neurosci 2000;3:940–945.
57. Muller, NG, Bartelt OA, Donner TH, et al. A physiological correlate of the "Zoom Lens" of visual attention. J Neurosci 2003;23: 3561–3565.
58. Hopfinger, JB, Buonocore MH, Mangun GR. The neural mechanisms of top-down attentional control. Nat Neurosci 2000;3: 284–291.
59. Corbetta, M, Kincade JM, Ollinger JM, et al. Voluntary orienting is dissociated from target detection in human posterior parietal cortex. Nat Neurosci 2000;3:292–297.
60. Steinmetz, MA, Constantinidis C. Neurophysiological evidence for a role of posterior parietal cortex in redirecting visual attention. Cereb Cortex 1995;5:448–456.
61. Awh, E, Anllo-Vento L, Hillyard SA. The role of spatial selective attention in working memory for locations: evidence from event-related potentials. J Cogn Neurosci 2000;12:840–847.
62. Nobre, AC, Coull JT, Maquet P, et al. Orienting attention to locations in perceptual versus mental representations. J Cogn Neurosci 2004;16:363–373.
63. Posner, MI, Walker JA, Friedrich FA, et al. Effects of parietal lobe injury on covert orienting of attention. J Neurosci 1984;4:1863–1874.
64. Posner, MI, Walker JA, Friedrich FA, et al. How do the parietal lobes direct covert attention? Neuropsychologia 1987;25: 135–145.
65. Rapcsak, SZ, Verfaellie M, Fleet WS, et al. Selective attention in hemispatial neglect. Archives of Neurology 1989;46:178–182.
66. Voeller, KKS, Heilman KM. Attention deficit disorder in children: A neglect syndrome? Neurology 1988;38:806–808.
67. Heiser, P, Frey J, Smidt J, et al. Objective measurement of hyperactivity, impulsivity, and inattention in children with hyperkinetic disorders before and after treatment with methylphenidate. Eur Child Adolesc Psychiatry 2004;13:100–104.
68. Porrino, LJ, Rapoport JL, Behar D, et al. A naturalistic assessment of the motor activity of hyperactive boys. Arch Gen Psychiatry 1983;40:688–693.
69. Teicher, MH, Ito Y, Glod CA, et al. Objective measurement of hyperactivity and attentional problems in ADHD. J Am Acad Child Adolesc Psychiatry 1996;35:334–342.
70. Lhermitte, F. 'Utilization behaviour' and its relation to lesions of the frontal lobes. Brain 1983;106:237–255.
71. Bronikowski, AM, Rhodes JS, Garland T, Jr., et al. The evolution of gene expression in mouse hippocampus in response to selective breeding for increased locomotor activity. Evolution Int J Org Evolution 2004;58:2079–2086.
72. Jucaite, A, Fernell E, Halldin C, et al. Reduced midbrain dopamine transporter binding in male adolescents with attention-deficit/hyperactivity disorder: association between striatal dopamine markers and motor hyperactivity. Biol Psychiatry 2005;57:229–238.

73. Berlin, HA, Rolls ET, Kischka U. Impulsivity, time perception, emotion and reinforcement sensitivity in patients with orbitofrontal cortex lesions. Brain 2004;127:1108–1126.

74. Winstanley, CA, Theobald DE, Cardinal RN, et al. Contrasting roles of basolateral amygdala and orbitofrontal cortex in impulsive choice. J Neurosci 2004;24:4718–4722.

75. Casey, BJ, Vauss YC, Chused A, et al. Cognitive functioning Sydenham's chorea: Part 2. Executive functioning. Dev Neuropsychol 1994;10:89–96.

76. Winstanley, CA, Dalley JW, Theobald DE, et al. Fractionating impulsivity: contrasting effects of central 5-ht depletion on different measures of impulsive behavior. Neuropsychopharmacology 2004;29:1331–1343.

77. Winstanley, CA, Theobald DE, Dalley JW, et al. Interactions between serotonin and dopamine in the control of impulsive choice in rats: therapeutic implications for impulse control disorders. Neuropsychopharmacology 2005;30:669–682.

78. Hershey, T, Black KJ, Hartlein J, et al. Dopaminergic modulation of response inhibition: an fMRI study. Brain Res Cogn Brain Res 2004;20:438–448.

79. Barkley, RA, Koplowitz S, Anderson T, et al. Sense of time in children with ADHD: three preliminary studies. J Int Neuropsychol Soc 1997;3:359–369.

80. West, J, Douglas G, Houghton S, et al. Time perception in boys with attention-deficit/hyperactivity disorder according to time duration, distraction and mode of presentation. Neuropsychol Dev Cogn Child Neuropsychol 2000;6:241–250.

81. Pouthas, V, George N, Poline JB, et al. Neural network involved in time perception: An fMRI study comparing long and short interval estimation. Hum Brain Mapping 2005;25:433–441.

82. Meck, WH. Neuropsychology of timing and time perception. Brain Cogn 2005;58:1–8.

83. Denckla, MB, Rudel RG. Anomalies of motor development in hyperactive boys. Ann Neurol 1978;3:231–233.

84. Klimkeit, EI, Sheppard DM, Lee P, et al. Bimanual coordination deficits in attention deficit/hyperactivity disorder (ADHD). J Clin Exp Neuropsychol 2004;26:999–1010.

85. Eliasson, AC, Rosblad B, Forssberg H. Disturbances in programming goal-directed arm movements in children with ADHD. Dev Med Child Neurol 2004;46:19–27.

86. Kalff, AC, de Sonneville LM, Hurks PP, et al. Low- and high-level controlled processing in executive motor control tasks in 5–6-year-old children at risk of ADHD. J Child Psychol Psychiatry 2003;44:1049–1057.

87. Stuss, DT, Murphy KJ, Binns MA, et al. Staying on the job: the frontal lobes control individual performance variability. Brain 2003;126:2363–2380.

88. Castellanos, FX, Giedd JN, Marsh WL, et al. Quantitative brain magnetic resonance imaging in attention-deficit hyperactivity disorder. Arch Gen Psychiatry 1996;53:607–616.

89. Durston, S, Hulshoff Pol HE, Schnack HG, et al. Magnetic resonance imaging of boys with attention-deficit/hyperactivity disorder and their unaffected siblings. J Am Acad Child Adolesc Psychiatry 2004;43:332–340.

90. Hill, DE, Yeo RA, Campbell RA, et al. Magnetic resonance imaging correlates of attention-deficit/hyperactivity disorder in children. Neuropsychology 2003;17:496–506.

91. Kates, WR, Frederikse M, Mostofsky SH, et al. MRI parcellation of the frontal lobe in boys with attention deficit hyperactivity disorder or Tourette syndrome. Psychiatry Res 2002;116: 63–81.

92. Mataro, M, Garcia-Sanchez C, Junquç C, et al. Magnetic resonance imaging measurement of the caudate nucleus in adolescents with attention-deficit hyperactivity disorder and its relationship with neuropsychological and behavioral measures. Arch Neurol 1997;54:963–969.

93. Mostofsky, SH, Cooper KL, Kates WR, et al. Smaller prefrontal and premotor volumes in boys with attention-deficit/hyperactivity disorder. Biol Psychiatry 2002;52:785–794.

94. Hesslinger, B, Tebartz van Elst L, Thiel T, et al. Frontoorbital volume reductions in adult patients with attention deficit hyperactivity disorder. Neurosci Lett 2002;328:319–321.

95. Sowell, ER, Thompson PM, Welcome SE, et al. Cortical abnormalities in children and adolescents with attention-deficit hyperactivity disorder. Lancet 2003;362:1699–1707.

96. Hynd, GW, Hern KL, Novey ES, et al. Attention deficit-hyperactivity disorder and asymmetry of the caudate nucleus. J Child Neurol 1993;8:339–347.

97. Aylward, EH, Reiss AL, Reader MJ. Basal ganglia volumes in children with attention-deficit hyperactivity disorder. J Child Neurol 1996;11:112–115.

98. Overmeyer, S, Bullmore ET, Suckling J, et al. Distributed grey and white matter deficits in hyperkinetic disorder: MRI evidence for anatomical abnormality in an attentional network. Psychol Med 2001;31:1425–1435.

99. Berquin, PC, Giedd JN, Jacobsen LK, et al. Cerebellum in attention-deficit hyperactivity disorder: a morphometric MRI study. Neurology 1998;50:1087–1093.

100. Mostofsky, SH, Reiss AL, Lockhart P, et al. Evaluation of cerebellar size in attention-deficit hyperactivity disorder. J Child Neurol 1998;13:434–439.

101. Jernigan, TL, Trauner DA, Hesselink JR, et al. Maturation of human cerebrum observed in vivo during adolescence. Brain 1991;114:2037–2049.

102. Hynd, GW, Semrud-Clikeman M, Lorys AR, et al. Brain morphology in developmental dyslexia and attention deficit disorder/hyperactivity. Arch Neurol 1990;47:919–926.

103. Castellanos, FX, Giedd JN, Eckburg P, et al. Quantitative morphology of the caudate nucleus in attention deficit hyperactivity disorder. Am J Psychiatry 1994;151:1791–1796.

104. Stefanatos, GA, Wasserstein J. Attention deficit/hyperactivity disorder as a right hemisphere syndrome. Selective literature review and detailed neuropsychological case studies. Ann NY Acad Sci 2001;931:172–195.

105. Lou, HC, Henriksen L, Bruhn P, et al. Striatal dysfunction in attention deficit and hyperkinetic disorder. Arch Neurol 1989;46:48–52.

106. Ernst, M, Zametkin AJ, Phillips RL, et al. Age-related changes in brain glucose metabolism in adults with attention-deficit/hyperactivity disorder and control subjects. J Neuropsychiatry Clin Neurosci 1998;10:168–177.

107. Ernst, M, Liebenauer LL, King AC, et al. Reduced brain metabolism in hyperactive girls. J Am Acad Child Adolesc Psychiatry 1994;33:858–868.

108. Ernst, M, Cohen RM, Liebenauer LL, et al. Cerebral glucose metabolism in adolescent girls with attention-deficit/hyperactivity disorder. J Am Acad Child Adolesc Psychiatry 1997;36:1399–1406.

109. Ernst, M, Zametkin AJ, Matochik JA, et al. DOPA decarboxylase activity in attention deficit hyperactivity disorder adults. A [Fluorine-18] Fluorodopa positron emission tomographic study. J Neurosci 1998;18:5901–5907.

110. Bunge, SA, Dudukovic NM, Thomason ME, et al. Immature frontal lobe contributions to cognitive control in children: evidence from fMRI. Neuron 2002;33:301–311.

111. Durston, S, Tottenham NT, Thomas KM, et al. Differential patterns of striatal activation in young children with and without ADHD. Biol Psychiatry 2003;53:871–878.

112. Vaidya, CJ, Austin G, Kirkorian G, et al. Selective effects of methylphenidate in attention deficit hyperactivity disorder: a functional magnetic resonance study. Proc Natl Acad Sci USA 1998;95:14494–14499.

113. Schulz, KP, Fan J, Tang CY, et al. Response inhibition in adolescents diagnosed with attention deficit hyperactivity disorder during childhood: an event-related FMRI study. Am J Psychiatry 2004;161:1650–1657.

114. Schulz, KP, Newcorn JH, Fan J, et al. Brain activation gradients in ventrolateral prefrontal cortex related to persistence of ADHD in adolescent boys. J Am Acad Child Adolesc Psychiatry 2005;44: 47–54.

115. Schulz, KP, Tang CY, Fan J, et al. Differential prefrontal cortex activation during inhibitory control in adolescents with and without childhood attention-deficit/hyperactivity disorder. Neuropsychology 2005;19:390–402.

116. Shafritz, KM, Marchione KE, Gore JC, et al. The effects of methylphenidate on neural systems of attention in attention deficit hyperactivity disorder. Am J Psychiatry 2004;161:1990–1997.

117. Raichle, ME, MacLeod AM, Snyder AZ, et al. A default mode of brain function. Proc Natl Acad Sci U S A 2001;98:676–682.

118. Tamm, L, Menon V, Ringel J, et al. Event-related FMRI evidence of frontotemporal involvement in aberrant response inhibition and task switching in attention-deficit/hyperactivity disorder. J Am Acad Child Adolesc Psychiatry 2004;43:1430–1440.
119. Seamans, JK, Gorelova N, Durstewitz D, et al. Bidirectional dopamine modulation of GABAergic inhibition in prefrontal cortical pyramidal neurons. J Neurosci 2001;21:3628–3638.
120. Aosaki, T, Graybiel AM, Kimura M. Effect of the nigrostriatal dopamine system on acquired neural responses in the striatum of behaving monkeys. Science 1994;265:412–415.
121. Moore, RY, Bloom FE. Central catecholamine neuron systems: Anatomy and physiology of the dopamine systems. Ann Rev Neurosci 1978;1:129–169.
122. Papp, M, Bal A. Separation of the motivational and motor consequences of 6-hydroxydopamine lesions of the mesolimbic or nigrostriatal system in rats. Behav Brain Res 1987;23:221–229.
123. Hollerman, JR, Tremblay L, Schultz W. Involvement of basal ganglia and orbitofrontal cortex in goal-directed behavior. Prog Brain Res 2000;126:193–215.
124. Sawaguchi, T, Matsumura M, Kubota K. Catecholaminergic effects on neuronal activity related to a delayed response task in monkey prefrontal cortex. J Neurophysiol 1990;63:1385–1400.
125. Funahashi, S, Bruce CJ, Goldman-Rakic PS. Mnemonic coding of visual space in the monkey's dorsolateral prefrontal cortex. J Neurophysiol 1989;61:331–349.
126. Goldman-Rakic, PS. Working memory dysfunction in schizophrenia. J Neuropsychiatry Clin Neurosci 1994;6:348– 357.
127. Brozoski, TJ, Brown RM, Rosvold HE, et al. Cognitive deficit caused by regional depletion of dopamine in prefrontal cortex of rhesus monkey. Science 1979;205:929–932.
128. Seamans, JK, Yang CR. The principal features and mechanisms of dopamine modulation in the prefrontal cortex. Prog Neurobiol 2004;74:1–58.
129. Tam, SY, Elsworth JD, Bradberry CW, et al. Mesocortical dopamine neurons: high basal firing frequency predicts tyrosine dependence of dopamine synthesis. J Neural Transm Gen Sect 1990;81:97–110.
130. Tassin, JP, Stinus L, Simon H, et al. Distribution of dopaminergic terminals in rat cerebral cortex: role of dopaminergic mesocortical system in ventral tegmental area syndrome. Adv Biochem Psychopharmacol 1977;16:21–28.
131. Domesick, VB. Neuroanatomical organization of dopamine neurons in the ventral tegmental area. In: Kalivas, PW and Nemeroff, CB, ed. *The Mesocorticolimbic Dopamine System.* Annals of the NY Acad of Sciences. New York: New York Academy of Sciences, 1988:10–26.
132. Lewis, DA, Morrison JH, Goldstein M. Brainstem dopaminergic neurons project to monkey parietal cortex. Neurosci Lett 1988;86:11–16.
133. Foote, SL, Morrison JH. Development of the noradrenergic, serotonergic, and dopaminergic innervation of neocortex. Curr Top Dev Biol 1987;21:391–423.
134. Bjorklund, A, Lindvall O. Dopamine-containing systems in the CNS. In: Bjorklund, A and Hokfelt, T, ed. *Handbook of Chemical Neuroanatomy.* Vol 2: *Classical neurotransmitters in the CNS, Part I.* Amsterdam: Elsevier, 1984:55–122.
135. Vandenbergh, DJ, Persico AM, Hawkins AL, et al. Human dopamine transporter gene (DAT1) maps to chromosome 5p15.3 and displays a VNTR. Genomics 1992;14:1104–1106.
136. Kawarai, T, Kawakami H, Yamamura Y, et al. Structure and organization of the gene encoding human dopamine transporter. Gene 1997;195:11–18.
137. Grunhage, F, Schulze TG, Muller DJ, et al. Systematic screening for DNA sequence variation in the coding region of the human dopamine transporter gene (DAT1). Mol Psychiatry 2000;5:275–282.
138. Sano, A, Kondoh K, Kakimoto Y, et al. A 40-nucleotide repeat polymorphism in the human dopamine transporter gene. Hum Genet 1993;91:405–406.
139. Hoover, BR, Marshall JF. Molecular, chemical, and anatomical characterization of globus pallidus dopamine D2 receptor mRNA-containing neurons. Synapse 2004;52:100–113.
140. Matsumoto, M, Hidaka K, Tada S, et al. Low levels of mRNA for dopamine D4 receptor in human cerebral cortex and striatum. J Neurochem 1996;66:915–919.
141. Olsson, H, Halldin C, Farde L. Differentiation of extrastriatal dopamine D2 receptor density and affinity in the human brain using PET. Neuroimage 2004;22:794–803.
142. Liu, IS, Seeman P, Sanyal S, et al. Dopamine D4 receptor variant in Africans, D4valine194glycine, is insensitive to dopamine and clozapine: report of a homozygous individual. Am J Med Genet 1996;61:277–282.
143. Liu, YF, Civelli O, Grandy DK, et al. Differential sensitivity of the short and long human dopamine D2 receptor subtypes to protein kinase C. J Neurochem 1992;59:2311–2317.
144. Martres, MP, Sokoloff P, Giros B, et al. Effects of dopaminergic transmission interruption on the D2 receptor isoforms in various cerebral tissues. J Neurochem 1992;58:673–679.
145. Arcos-Burgos, M, Castellanos FX, Konecki D, et al. Pedigree disequilibrium test (PDT) replicates association and linkage between DRD4 and ADHD in multigenerational and extended pedigrees from a genetic isolate. Mol Psychiatry 2004;9:252–259.
146. Curran, S, Mill J, Tahir E, et al. Association study of a dopamine transporter polymorphism and attention deficit hyperactivity disorder in UK and Turkish samples. Mol Psychiatry 2001;6:425–428.
147. Holmes, J, Payton A, Barrett JH, et al. A family-based and case-control association study of the dopamine D4 receptor gene and dopamine transporter gene in attention deficit hyperactivity disorder. Mol Psychiatry 2000;5:523–530.
148. Qian, Q, Wang Y, Zhou R, et al. Family-based and case-control association studies of DRD4 and DAT1 polymorphisms in Chinese attention deficit hyperactivity disorder patients suggest long repeats contribute to genetic risk for the disorder. Am J Med Genet 2004;128B:84–89.
149. Roman, T, Schmitz M, Polanczyk G, et al. Attention-deficit hyperactivity disorder: a study of association with both the dopamine transporter gene and the dopamine D4 receptor gene. Am J Med Genet 2001;105:471–478.
150. Sunohara, GA, Roberts W, Malone M, et al. Linkage of the dopamine D4 receptor gene and attention-deficit/hyperactivity disorder. J Am Acad Child Adolesc Psychiatry 2000;39:1537–1542.
151. Swanson, JM, Sunohara GA, Kennedy JL, et al. Association of the dopamine receptor D4 (DRD4) gene with a refined phenotype of attention deficit hyperactivity disorder (ADHD): a family-based approach. Mol Psychiatry 1998;3:38–41.
152. Smalley, SL, Bailey JN, Palmer CG, et al. Evidence that the dopamine D4 receptor is a susceptibility gene in attention deficit hyperactivity disorder. Mol Psychiatry 1998;3:427–430.
153. El-Faddagh, M, Laucht M, Maras A, et al. Association of dopamine D4 receptor (DRD4) gene with attention-deficit/hyperactivity disorder (ADHD) in a high-risk community sample: a longitudinal study from birth to 11 years of age. J Neural Transm 2004;111:883–889.
154. Faraone, SV, Biederman J, Weiffenbach B, et al. Dopamine D4 gene 7-repeat allele and attention deficit hyperactivity disorder. Am J Psychiatry 1999;156:768–770.
155. Faraone, SV, Doyle AE, Mick E, et al. Meta-analysis of the association between the 7-repeat allele of the dopamine D(4) receptor gene and attention deficit hyperactivity disorder. Am J Psychiatry 2001;158:1052–1057.
156. Hawi, Z, McCarron M, Kirley A, et al. No association of the dopamine DRD4 receptor (DRD4) gene polymorphism with attention deficit hyperactivity disorder (ADHD) in the Irish population. Am J Med Genet 2000;96:268–272.
157. Kotler, M, Manor I, Sever Y, et al. Failure to replicate an excess of the long dopamine D4 exon III repeat polymorphism in ADHD in a family-based study. Am J Med Genet 2000;96:278–281.
158. Mill, JS, Caspi A, McClay J, et al. The dopamine D4 receptor and the hyperactivity phenotype: a developmental-epidemiological study. Mol Psychiatry 2002;7:383–391.
159. Todd, RD, Jong YJ, Lobos EA, et al. No association of the dopamine transporter gene 3' VNTR polymorphism with ADHD subtypes in a population sample of twins. Am J Med Genet 2001;105:745–748.

160. Turic, D, Langley K, Mills S, et al. Follow-up of genetic linkage findings on chromosome 16p13: evidence of association of N-methyl-D aspartate glutamate receptor 2A gene polymorphism with ADHD. Mol Psychiatry 2004;9:169–173.

161. McCracken, JT, Smalley SL, McGough JJ, et al. Evidence for linkage of a tandem duplication polymorphism upstream of the dopamine D4 receptor gene (DRD4) with attention deficit hyperactivity disorder (ADHD). Mol Psychiatry 2000;5: 531–536.

162. Leung, PW, Lee CC, Hung SF, et al. Dopamine receptor D4 (DRD4) gene in Han Chinese children with attention-deficit/ hyperactivity disorder (ADHD): increased prevalence of the 2-repeat allele. Am J Med Genet B Neuropsychiatr Genet 2005;133: 54–56.

163. Langley, K, Marshall L, van den Bree M, et al. Association of the dopamine D4 receptor gene 7-repeat allele with neuropsychological test performance of children with ADHD. Am J Psychiatry 2004;161:133–138.

164. Lewis, DA, Morrison JH. Noradrenergic innervation of monkey prefrontal cortex: a dopamine-beta-hydroxylase immunohistochemical study. J Comp Neurol 1989;282:317–330.

165. Posner, MI, Petersen SE, Fox PT, et al. Localization of cognitive operations in the human brain. Science 1988;240:1627–1631.

166. Corbetta, M, Miezin FM, Dobmeyer S, et al. Attentional modulation of neural processing of shape, color, and velocity in humans. Science 1990;248:1556–1559.

167. Berridge, CW, Arnsten AFT, Foote SL. Noradrenergic modulation of cognitive function: clinical implications of anatomical, electrophysiological and behavioral studies in animal models. Psychol Med 1993;23:557–564.

168. Arnsten, AFT, Goldman-Rakic PS. Selective prefrontal cortical projections to the region of the locus coeruleus and raphe nuclei in the rhesus monkey. Brain Res 1984;306:9–18.

169. Aston-Jones, G, Bloom FE. Norepinephrine containing locus coeruleus neurons in behaving rats exhibit pronounced responses to non-noxious environmental stimuli. J Neurosci 1981;1:887–900.

170. Aston-Jones, G, Rajkowski J, Kubiak P, et al. Locus coeruleus neurons in monkey are selectively activated attended cues in a vigilance task. J Neurosci 1994;14:4467–4480.

171. Aizman, O, Brismar H, Uhlen P, et al. Anatomical and physiological evidence for D1 and D2 dopamine receptor colocalization in neostriatal neurons. Nat Neurosci 2000;3:226–230.

172. Bobb, AJ, Addington AM, Sidransky E, et al. Support for association between ADHD and two candidate genes: NET1 and DRD1. Am J Med Genet B Neuropsychiatr Genet 2005;134: 67–72.

173. Xu, X, Knight J, Brookes K, et al. DNA pooling analysis of 21 norepinephrine transporter gene SNPs with attention deficit hyperactivity disorder: no evidence for association. Am J Med Genet B Neuropsychiatr Genet 2005;134:115–118.

174. Smith, GS, Dewey SL, Brodie JD, et al. Serotonergic modulation of dopamine measured with [11C] raclopride and PET in normal human subjects. Am J Psychiatry 1997;157:1708–1710.

175. Sari, Y. Serotonin1B receptors: from protein to physiological function and behavior. Neurosci Biobehav Rev 2004;28:565– 582.

176. Zhang, K, Davids E, Tarazi FI, et al. Serotonin transporter binding increases in caudate-putamen and nucleus accumbens after neonatal 6-hydroxydopamine lesions in rats: implications for motor hyperactivity. Brain Res Dev Brain Res 2002;137:135–138.

177. Gainetdinov, RR, Wetsel WC, Jones SR, et al. Role of serotonin in the paradoxical calming effect of psychostimulants on hyperactivity. Science 1999;283:397–401.

178. Curran, S, Purcell S, Craig I, et al. The serotonin transporter gene as a QTL for ADHD. Am J Med Genet B Neuropsychiatr Genet 2005;134:42–47.

179. Manor, I, Eisenberg J, Tyano S, et al. Family-based association study of the serotonin transporter promoter region polymorphism (5-HTTLPR) in attention deficit hyperactivity disorder. Am J Med Genet 2001;105:91–95.

180. Seeger, G, Schloss P, Schmidt MH. Functional polymorphism within the promotor of the serotonin transporter gene is associated with severe hyperkinetic disorders. Mol Psychiatry 2001;6: 235–238.

181. Zoroglu, SS, Erdal ME, Alasehirli B, et al. Significance of serotonin transporter gene 5-HTTLPR and variable number of tandem repeat polymorphism in attention deficit hyperactivity disorder. Neuropsychobiology 2002;45:176–181.

182. Kent, L, Doerry U, Hardy E, et al. Evidence that variation at the serotonin transporter gene influences susceptibility to attention deficit hyperactivity disorder (ADHD): analysis and pooled analysis. Mol Psychiatry 2002;7:908–912.

183. Retz, W, Thome J, Blocher D, et al. Association of attention deficit hyperactivity disorder-related psychopathology and personality traits with the serotonin transporter promoter region polymorphism. Neurosci Lett 2002;319:133–136.

184. Hawi, Z, Dring M, Kirley A, et al. Serotonergic system and attention deficit hyperactivity disorder (ADHD): a potential susceptibility locus at the 5-HT(1B) receptor gene in 273 nuclear families from a multi-centre sample. Mol Psychiatry 2002;7:718–725.

185. Quist, JF, Barr CL, Schachar R, et al. Evidence for the serotonin HTR2A receptor gene as a susceptibility factor in attention deficit hyperactivity disorder (ADHD). Mol Psychiatry 2000;5:537–541.

186. Quist, JF, Barr CL, Schachar R, et al. The serotonin 5-HT1B receptor gene and attention deficit hyperactivity disorder. Mol Psychiatry 2003;8:98–102.

187. Levitan, RD, Masellis M, Basile VS, et al. Polymorphism of the serotonin-2A receptor gene (HTR2A) associated with childhood attention deficit hyperactivity disorder (ADHD) in adult women with seasonal affective disorder. J Affect Disord 2002;71:229–233.

188. Langley, K, Payton A, Hamshere ML, et al. No evidence of association of two 5HT transporter gene polymorphisms and attention deficit hyperactivity disorder. Psychiatr Genet 2003;13: 107–110.

189. Li, J, Wang Y, Zhou R, et al. Serotonin 5-HT1B receptor gene and attention deficit hyperactivity disorder in Chinese Han subjects. Am J Med Genet B Neuropsychiatr Genet 2005;132:59–63.

190. Zoroglu, SS, Erdal ME, Erdal N, et al. No evidence for an association between the T102C and 1438 G/A polymorphisms of the serotonin 2A receptor gene in attention deficit/hyperactivity disorder in a Turkish population. Neuropsychobiology 2003;47: 17–20.

191. Carrey, N, MacMaster FP, Sparkes SJ, et al. Glutamatergic changes with treatment in attention deficit hyperactivity disorder: a preliminary case series. J Child Adolesc Psychopharmacol 2002;12:331–336.

192. Smalley, SL, Kustanovich V, Minassian SL, et al. Genetic linkage of attention-deficit/hyperactivity disorder on chromosome 16p13, in a region implicated in autism. Am J Hum Genet 2002; 71:959–963.

193. Adams, J, Crosbie J, Wigg K, et al. Glutamate receptor, ionotropic, N-methyl D-aspartate 2A (GRIN2A) gene as a positional candidate for attention-deficit/hyperactivity disorder in the 16p13 region. Mol Psychiatry 2004;9:494–499.

194. Turic, D, Langley K, Williams H, et al. A family based study implicates solute carrier family 1-member 3 (SLC1A3) gene in attention-deficit/hyperactivity disorder. Biol Psychiatry 2005;57: 1461–1466.

195. Sawaguchi, T. Unmasking of silent "task-related" neuronal activity in the monkey prefrontal cortex by a GABA(A) antagonist. Neurosci Res 2001;39:123–131.

196. Represa, A, Ben-Ari Y. Trophic actions of GABA on neuronal development. Trends Neurosci 2005;28:278–283.

197. Bowen, ME, Engelman DM, Brunger AT. Mutational analysis of synaptobrevin transmembrane domain oligomerization. Biochemistry 2002;41:15861–15866.

198. Brophy, K, Hawi Z, Kirley A, et al. Synaptosomal-associated protein 25 (SNAP-25) and attention deficit hyperactivity disorder (ADHD): evidence of linkage and association in the Irish population. Mol Psychiatry 2002;7:913–917.

199. Kustanovich, V, Merriman B, McGough J, et al. Biased paternal transmission of SNAP-25 risk alleles in attention-deficit hyperactivity disorder. Mol Psychiatry 2003;8:309–315.

200. Hess, EJ, Rogan PK, Domoto M, et al. Absence of linkage of apparently single gene mediated ADHD with the human syntenic region of the mouse mutant Coloboma. Am J Med Genet 1995;60:573–579.

201. Nishi, A, Watanabe Y, Higashi H, et al. Glutamate regulation of DARPP-32 phosphorylation in neostriatal neurons involves activation of multiple signaling cascades. Proc Natl Acad Sci USA 2005;102:1199–1204.

202. Nairn, AC, Svenningsson P, Nishi A, et al. The role of DARPP-32 in the actions of drugs of abuse. Neuropharmacology 2004;47 Suppl 1:14–23.

203. Viggiano, D, Vallone D, Ruocco LA, et al. Behavioural, pharmacological, morpho-functional molecular studies reveal a hyper-functioning mesocortical dopamine system in an animal model of attention deficit and hyperactivity disorder. Neurosci Biobehav Rev 2003;27:683–689.

204. Guillemot, F, Auffray C, Devignes MD. Detailed transcript map of a 810-kb region at 11p14 involving identification of 10 novel human 3' exons. Eur J Hum Genet 1999;7:487–495.

205. Weickert, CS, Hyde TM, Lipska BK, et al. Reduced brain-derived neurotrophic factor in prefrontal cortex of patients with schizophrenia. Mol Psychiatry 2003;8:592–610.

206. Pezawas, L, Verchinski BA, Mattay VS, et al. The brain-derived neurotrophic factor val66met polymorphism and variation in human cortical morphology. J Neurosci 2004;24:10099–10102.

207. Kent, L, Green E, Hawi Z, et al. Association of the paternally transmitted copy of common Valine allele of the Val66Met polymorphism of the brain-derived neurotrophic factor (BDNF) gene with susceptibility to ADHD. Mol Psychiatry 2005.

208. Malhotra, AK, Kestler LJ, Mazzanti C, et al. A functional polymorphism in the COMT gene and performance on a test of prefrontal cognition. Am J Psychiatry 2002;159:652–654.

209. Blasi, G, Mattay VS, Bertolino A, et al. Effect of catechol-O-methyltransferase val158met genotype on attentional control. J Neurosci 2005;25:5038–5045.

210. Mattay, VS, Berman KF, Ostrem JL, et al. Dextroamphetamine enhances 'neural network-specific' physiological signals: a positron-emission tomography rCBF study. J Neurosci 1996;16:4816–4822.

211. Diamond, A, Briand L, Fossella J, et al. Genetic and neurochemical modulation of prefrontal cognitive functions in children. Am J Psychiatry 2004;161:125–132.

212. Mills, S, Langley K, Van den Bree M, et al. No evidence of association between Catechol-O-Methyltransferase (COMT) Val158Met genotype and performance on neuropsychological tasks in children with ADHD: a case-control study. BMC Psychiatry 2004;4:15.

213. Brunner, HG, Nelen M, Breakefield XO, et al. Abnormal behavior associated with a point mutation in the structural gene for monoamine oxidase A. Science 1993;262:578–580.

214. Brunner, HG, Nelen MR, van Zandvoort P, et al. X-linked borderline mental retardation with prominent behavioral disturbance: phenotype, genetic localization, and evidence for disturbed monoamine metabolism. Am J Hum Gen 1993;52:1032–1039.

215. Jiang, S, Xin R, Wu X, et al. Association between attention deficit hyperactivity disorder and the DXS7 locus. Am J Med Genet 2000;96:289–292.

216. Jiang, S, Xin R, Lin S, et al. Linkage studies between attention-deficit hyperactivity disorder and the monoamine oxidase genes. Am J Med Genet 2001;105:783–788.

217. Domschke, K, Sheehan K, Lowe N, et al. Association analysis of the monoamine oxidase A and B genes with attention deficit hyperactivity disorder (ADHD) in an Irish sample: preferential transmission of the MAO-A 941G allele to affected children. Am J Med Genet B Neuropsychiatr Genet 2005;134:110–114.

218. Haberstick, BC, Lessem JM, Hopfer CJ, et al. Monoamine oxidase A (MAOA) and antisocial behaviors in the presence of childhood and adolescent maltreatment. Am J Med Genet B Neuropsychiatr Genet 2005;135:59–64.

219. Hawi, Z, Foley D, Kirley A, et al. Dopa decarboxylase gene polymorphisms and attention deficit hyperactivity disorder (ADHD): no evidence for association in the Irish population. Mol Psychiatry 2001;6:420–424.

220. Ernst, M, Zametkin AJ, Matochik JA, et al. High midbrain [18F]DOPA accumulation in children with attention deficit hyperactivity disorder. Am J Psychiatry 1999;156:1209–1215.

221. Daly, G, Hawi Z, Fitzgerald M, et al. Mapping susceptibility loci in attention deficit hyperactivity disorder: preferential transmission of parental alleles at DAT1, DBH and DRD5 to affected children. Mol Psychiatry 1999;4:192–196.

222. Hawi, Z, Lowe N, Kirley A, et al. Linkage disequilibrium mapping at DAT1, DRD5 and DBH narrows the search for ADHD susceptibility alleles at these loci. Mol Psychiatry 2003;8:299–308.

223. Smith, KM, Daly M, Fischer M, et al. Association of the dopamine beta hydroxylase gene with attention deficit hyperactivity disorder: genetic analysis of the Milwaukee longitudinal study. Am J Med Genet 2003;119B:77–85.

224. Wigg, K, Zai G, Schachar R, et al. Attention deficit hyperactivity disorder and the gene for dopamine Beta-hydroxylase. Am J Psychiatry 2002;159:1046–1048.

225. Inkster, B, Muglia P, Jain U, et al. Linkage disequilibrium analysis of the dopamine beta-hydroxylase gene in persistent attention deficit hyperactivity disorder. Psychiatr Genet 2004;14:117–120.

226. Payton, A, Holmes J, Barrett JH, et al. Examining for association between candidate gene polymorphisms in the dopamine pathway and attention-deficit hyperactivity disorder: a family-based study. Am J Med Genet 2001;105:464–470.

227. Milberger, S, Biederman J, Faraone SV, et al. Is maternal smoking during pregnancy a risk factor for attention deficit hyperactivity disorder in children? Am J Psychiatry 1996;153:1138–1142.

228. Potter, AS, Newhouse PA. Effects of acute nicotine administration on behavioral inhibition in adolescents with attention-deficit/hyperactivity disorder. Psychopharmacology (Berl) 2004;176:182–194.

229. Li, MD, Ma JZ, Beuten J. Progress in searching for susceptibility loci and genes for smoking-related behaviour. Clin Genet 2004;66:382–392.

230. Milberger, S, Biederman J, Faraone SV, et al. Further evidence of an association between maternal smoking during pregnancy and attention deficit hyperactivity disorder: findings from a high-risk sample of siblings. J Clin Child Psychol 1998;27:352–358.

231. Thapar, A, Fowler T, Rice F, et al. Maternal smoking during pregnancy and attention deficit hyperactivity disorder symptoms in offspring. Am J Psychiatry 2003;160:1985–1989

232. Riley, EP, McGee CL, Sowell ER. Teratogenic effects of alcohol: a decade of brain imaging. Am J Med Genet 2004;127C:35–41.

233. Grunau, RE, Whitfield MF, Fay TB. Psychosocial and academic characteristics of extremely low birth weight (< or =800 g) adolescents who are free of major impairment compared with term-born control subjects. Pediatrics 2004;114:e725–732.

234. Dell'Anna, ME, Luthman J, Lindqvist E, et al. Development of monoamine systems after neonatal anoxia in rats. Brain Res Bull 1993;32:159–170.

235. Decker, MJ, Rye DB. Neonatal intermittent hypoxia impairs dopamine signaling and executive functioning. Sleep Breath 2002;6:205–210.

236. Lou, HC, Rosa P, Pryds O, et al. ADHD: increased dopamine receptor availability linked to attention deficit and low neonatal cerebral blood flow. Dev Med Child Neurol 2004;46:179–183.

237. Volpe, JJ. Neurobiology of periventricular leukomalacia in the premature infant. Pediatr Res 2001;50:553–562.

238. Inder, TE, Wells SJ, Mogridge NB, et al. Defining the nature of the cerebral abnormalities in the premature infant: a qualitative magnetic resonance imaging study. J Pediatr 2003;143:171–179.

239. Soorani-Lunsing, I, Woltil HA, Hadders-Algra M. Are moderate degrees of hyperbilirubinemia in healthy term neonates really safe for the brain? Pediatr Res 2001;50:701–705.

240. Saunders, RC, Kolachana BS, Bachevalier J, et al. Neonatal lesions of the medial temporal lobe disrupt prefrontal cortical regulation of striatal dopamine. Nature 1998;393:169–171.

241. Millichap, JG. Temporal lobe arachnoid cyst-attention deficit disorder syndrome: Role of the electroencephalograph in diagnosis. Neurology 1997;48:1435–1439.

242. Dunn, DW, Austin JK, Harezlak J, et al. ADHD and epilepsy in childhood. Dev Med Child Neurol 2003;45:50–54.

243. Holtmann, M, Becker K, Kentner-Figura B, et al. Increased frequency of rolandic spikes in ADHD children. Epilepsia 2003;44:1241–1244.

244. Hadjivassiliou, M, Grunewald R, Sharrack B, et al. Gluten ataxia in perspective: epidemiology, genetic susceptibility and clinical characteristics. Brain 2003;126:685–691.

245. Arroyo, HA, De Rosa S, Ruggieri V, et al. Epilepsy, occipital calcifications, and oligosymptomatic celiac disease in childhood. J Child Neurol 2002;17:800–806.

246. Kieslich, M, Errazuriz G, Posselt HG, et al. Brain white-matter lesions in celiac disease: a prospective study of 75 diet-treated patients. Pediatrics 2001;108:E21.

247. Goodwin, FC, Beattie RM, Millar J, et al. Celiac disease and childhood stroke. Pediatr Neurol 2004;31:139–142.

248. Zelnik, N, Pacht A, Obeid R, et al. Range of neurologic disorders in patients with celiac disease. Pediatrics 2004;113: 1672–1676.

249. Antshel, KM, Waisbren SE. Timing is everything: executive functions in children exposed to elevated levels of phenylalanine. Neuropsychology 2003;17:458–468.

250. Diamond, A. Evidence for the importance of dopamine for prefrontal cortex functions early in life. Philos Trans R Soc Lond B Biol Sci 1996;351:1483–1493; discussion 1494.

251. Brockel, BJ, Cory-Slechta DA. Lead, attention, and impulsive behavior: Changes in a fixed ratio waiting-for-reward paradigm. Pharmacol Biochem Behav 1998;60:545–552.

252. Canfield, RL, Gendle MH, Cory-Slechta DA. Impaired neuropsychological functioning in lead-exposed children. Dev Neuropsychol 2004;26:513–540.

253. NourEddine, D, Miloud S, Abdelkader A. Effect of lead exposure on dopaminergic transmission in the rat brain. Toxicology 2005;207:363–368.

254. Basu, N, Scheuhammer A, Grochowina N, et al. Effects of mercury on neurochemical receptors in wild river otters (*Lontra canadensis*). Environ Sci Technol 2005;39:3585–3591.

255. Nigg, J. What role might environmental contaminants play in ADHD? ADHD Report 2005;13:6–14.

256. Bloom, DR, Levin HS, Ewing-Cobbs L, et al. Lifetime and novel psychiatric disorders after pediatric traumatic brain injury. J Am Acad Child Adolesc Psychiatry 2001;40:572–579.

257. Gerring, JP, Brady KD, Chen A, et al. Premorbid prevalence of ADHD and development of secondary ADHD after closed head injury. J Am Acad Child Adolesc Psychiatry 1998;37:647–656.

258. Herskovits, EH, Megalooikonomou V, Davatzikos C, et al. Is the spatial distribution of brain lesions associated with closed-head injury predictive of subsequent development of attention-deficit/hyperactivity disorder? Analysis with brain-image database. Radiology 1999;213:389–394.

259. Herskovits, EH, Gerring JP. Application of a data-mining method based on Bayesian networks to lesion-deficit analysis. Neuroimage 2003;19:1664–1673.

260. Max, JE, Fox PT, Lancaster JL, et al. Putamen lesions and the development of attention-deficit/hyperactivity symptomatology. J Am Acad Child Adolesc Psychiatry 2002;41:563–571.

261. Max, JE, Mathews K, Lansing AE, et al. Psychiatric disorders after childhood stroke. J Am Acad Child Adolesc Psychiatry 2002;41: 555–562.

262. Max, JE, Mathews K, Manes FF, et al. Attention deficit hyperactivity disorder and neurocognitive correlates after childhood stroke. J Int Neuropsychol Soc 2003;9:815–829.

263. Max, JE, Robin DA, Taylor HG, et al. Attention function after childhood stroke. J Int Neuropsychol Soc 2004;10:976–986.

264. Max, JE, Manes FF, Robertson BA, et al. Prefrontal and executive attention network lesions and the development of attention-deficit/hyperactivity symptomatology. J Am Acad Child Adolesc Psychiatry 2005;44:443–450.

265. Castellanos, FX, Sharp WS, Gottesman RF, et al. Anatomic brain abnormalities in monozygotic twins discordant for attention deficit hyperactivity disorder. Am J Psychiatry 2003;160:1693–1696.

266. Peterson, BS, Leckman JF, Tucker D, et al. Preliminary findings of antistreptococcal antibody titers and basal ganglia volumes in tic, obsessive-compulsive, and attention deficit/hyperactivity disorders. Arch Gen Psychiatry 2000;57:364–372.

267. Swedo, SE, Leonard HL, Mittleman BB, et al. Identification of children with pediatric autoimmune neuropsychiatric disorders associated with streptococcal infections by a marker associated with rheumatic fever. Am J Psychiatry 1997;154:110–112.

268. Fallon, BA. The underdiagnosis of neuropsychiatric Lyme disease in children and adults. Psychiatr Clin North Am 1998;21:693–703.

269. Biederman, J, Milberger S, Faraone SV, et al. Family-environment risk factors for attention-deficit hyperactivity disorder: a test of Rutter's indicators of adversity. Arch Gen Psychiatry 1995;52: 464–470.

270. Moffitt, TE, Caspi A, Rutter M. Strategy for investigating interactions between measured genes and measured environments. Arch Gen Psychiatry 2005;62:473–481.

271. Volkow, ND, Wang GJ, Fowler JS, et al. Evidence that methylphenidate enhances the saliency of a mathematical task by increasing dopamine in the human brain. Am J Psychiatry 2004;161:1173–1180.

272. Volkow, ND, Wang GJ, Fowler JS, et al. Imaging the effects of methylphenidate on brain dopamine: new model on its therapeutic actions for attention-deficit/hyperactivity disorder. Biol Psychiatry 2005;57:1410–1415.

273. Elia, J, Borcherding BG, Rapoport JL, et al. Methylphenidate and dextroamphetamine treatments of hyperactivity: are there true nonresponders? Psychiatry Res 1991;36:141–155.

274. Spencer, T, Biederman J, Wilens T, et al. Pharmacotherapy of attention-deficit hyperactivity disorder across the life cycle. J Am Acad Child Adolesc Psychiatry 1996;35:409–432.

275. Wilens, T, Pelham W, Stein M, et al. ADHD treatment with once-daily OROS methylphenidate: interim 12-month results from a long-term open-label study. J Am Acad Child Adolesc Psychiatry 2003;42:424–433.

276. Vitiello, B, Severe JB, Greenhill LL, et al. Methylphenidate dosage for children with ADHD over time under controlled conditions: lessons from the MTA. J Am Acad Child Adolesc Psychiatry 2001; 40:188–196.

277. Thiruchelvam, D, Charach A, Schachar RJ. Moderators and mediators of long-term adherence to stimulant treatment in children with ADHD. J Am Acad Child Adolesc Psychiatry 2001;40:922–928.

278. Charach, A, Ickowicz A, Schachar R. Stimulant treatment over five years: adherence, effectiveness, and adverse effects. J Am Acad Child Adolesc Psychiatry 2004;43:559–567.

279. Arnold, LE, Lindsay RL, Conners CK, et al. A double-blind, placebo-controlled withdrawal trial of dexmethylphenidate hydrochloride in children with attention deficit hyperactivity disorder. J Child Adolesc Psychopharmacol 2004;14:542–554.

280. Wigal, S, Swanson JM, Feifel D, et al. A double-blind, placebo-controlled trial of dexmethylphenidate hydrochloride and d,l-threo-methylphenidate hydrochloride in children with attention-deficit/hyperactivity disorder. J Am Acad Child Adolesc Psychiatry 2004;43:1406–1414.

281. Pelham, WE, Burrows-Maclean L, Gnagy EM, et al. Transdermal methylphenidate, behavioral, and combined treatment for children with ADHD. Exp Clin Psychopharmacol 2005;13:111–126.

282. Sauer, JM, Ring BJ, Witcher JW. Clinical pharmacokinetics of atomoxetine. Clin Pharmacokinet 2005;44:571–590.

283. Moran-Gates, T, Zhang K, Baldessarini RJ, et al. Atomoxetine blocks motor hyperactivity in neonatal 6-hydroxydopamine-lesioned rats: implications for treatment of attention-deficit hyperactivity disorder. Int J Neuropsychopharmacol 2005;8: 434–444.

284. Scammell, TE, Estabrooke IV, McCarthy MT, et al. Hypothalamic arousal regions are activated during modafinil-induced wakefulness. J Neurosci 2000;20:8620–8628.

285. Wisor, JP, Eriksson KS. Dopaminergic-adrenergic interactions in the wake promoting mechanism of modafinil. Neuroscience 2005;132:1027–1034.

286. Acuna-Goycolea, C, Li Y, Van Den Pol AN. Group III metabotropic glutamate receptors maintain tonic inhibition of excitatory synaptic input to hypocretin/orexin neurons. J Neurosci 2004;24:3013–3022.

287. van Dyck, CH, Malison RT, Jacobsen LK, et al. Increased dopamine transporter availability associated with the 9-repeat allele of the SLC6A3 gene. J Nucl Med 2005;46:745–751.

288. Asghari, V, Sanyal S, Buchwaldt S, et al. Modulation of intracellular cyclic AMP levels by different human dopamine D4 receptor variants. J Neurochem 1995;65:1157–1165.

289. Winsberg, BG, Comings DE. Association of the dopamine transporter gene (DAT1) with poor methylphenidate response. J Am Acad Child Adolesc Psychiatry 1999;38:1471–1477.
290. Roman, T, Szobot C, Martins S, et al. Dopamine transporter gene and response to methylphenidate in attention-deficit/hyperactivity disorder. Pharmacogenetics 2002;12:497–499.
291. Rohde, LA, Roman T, Szobot C, et al. Dopamine transporter gene, response to methylphenidate and cerebral blood flow in attention-deficit/hyperactivity disorder: a pilot study. Synapse 2003;48:87–89.
292. Cheon, KA, Ryu YH, Kim JW, et al. The homozygosity for 10-repeat allele at dopamine transporter gene and dopamine transporter density in Korean children with attention deficit hyperactivity disorder: relating to treatment response to methylphenidate. Eur Neuropsychopharmacol 2005;15:95– 101.
293. Kirley, A, Lowe N, Hawi Z, et al. Association of the 480 bp DAT1 allele with methylphenidate response in a sample of Irish children with ADHD. Am J Med Genet B Neuropsychiatr Genet 2003;121:50–54.
294. Stein, MA, Waldman ID, Sarampote CS, et al. Dopamine transporter genotype and methylphenidate dose response in children with ADHD. Neuropsychopharmacology 2005; 30:1374–1382.
295. Hamarman, S, Fossella J, Ulger C, et al. Dopamine receptor 4 (DRD4) 7-repeat allele predicts methylphenidate dose response in children with attention deficit hyperactivity disorder: a pharmacogenetic study. J Child Adolesc Psychopharmacol 2004;14:564–574.
296. Tahir, E, Yazgan Y, Cirakoglu B, et al. Association and linkage of DRD4 and DRD5 with attention deficit hyperactivity disorder (ADHD) in a sample of Turkish children. Mol Psychiatry 2000;5: 396–404.
297. Yang, L, Wang YF, Li J, et al. Association of norepinephrine transporter gene with methylphenidate response. J Am Acad Child Adolesc Psychiatry 2004;43:1154–1158.

ADDITIONAL REFERENCES

Achenbach, TM. Manual for the teacher's report form and 1991 profile. Burlington VT: University of Vermont, Department of Psychiatry, 1991.
Barr, CL, Feng Y, Wigg K, et al. Identification of DNA variants in the SNAP-25 gene and linkage study of these polymorphisms and attention-deficit hyperactivity disorder. Mol Psychiatry 2000; 5:405–409.
Bjoertomt, O, Cowey A , Walsh V. Spatial neglect in near and far space investigated by repetitive transcranial magnetic stimulation. Brain 2002;125:2012–2022.
Butter, CM, Rapcsak S, Watson RT, et al. Changes in sensory inattention, directional motor neglect and "release" of the fixation reflex following a unilateral frontal lesion: a case report. Neuropsychologia 1988;26:533–545.
Carrey, N, MacMaster FP, Fogel J, et al. Metabolite changes resulting from treatment in children with ADHD: a 1H-MRS study. Clin Neuropharmacol 2003;26:218–221.
Castellanos, FX, Lee PP, Sharp W, et al. Developmental trajectories of brain volume abnormalities in children and adolescents with attention-deficit/hyperactivity disorder. JAMA 2002;288: 1740– 1748.
Courvoisie, H, Hooper SR, Fine C, et al. Neurometabolic functioning and neuropsychological correlates in children with ADHD-H: preliminary findings. J Neuropsychiatry Clin Neurosci 2004; 16:63–69.
Davis, GD. Caudate lesions and spontaneous locomotion in the monkey. Neurology 1958;8:135–139.
Fierro, B, Brighina F, Oliveri M, et al. Contralateral neglect induced by right posterior parietal rTMS in healthy subjects. Neuroreport 2000;11:1519–1521.

Filipek, PA, Semrud-Clikeman M, Steingard RJ, et al. Volumetric MRI analysis comparing subjects having attention-deficit hyperactivity disorder with normal controls. Neurology 1997;48: 589–601.
Giros, B, Jaber M, Jones SR, et al. Hyperlocomotion and indifference to cocaine and amphetamine in mice lacking the dopamine transporter. Nature 1996;379:606–612.
Guitton, D, Buchtel HA , Douglas RM. Frontal lobe lesions in man cause difficulties in suppressing reflexive glances and in generating goal-directed saccades. Exp Brain Res 1985;58:455–472.
Jin, Z, Zang YF, Zeng YW, Zhang L. Wang YF. Striatal neuronal loss or dysfunction and choline rise in children with attention-deficit hyperactivity disorder: a 1H-magnetic resonance spectroscopy study. Neurosci Lett 2001;315:45–48.
Jones, MD, Williams ME , Hess EJ. Expression of catecholaminergic mRNAs in the hyperactive mouse mutant coloboma. Brain Res Mol Brain Res 2001;96:114–121.
Koob, GF, Stinus L, Le Moal M. Hyperactivity and hypoactivity produced by lesions to the mesolimbic dopamine system. Behav Brain Res 1981;3:341–359.
Lang, AE , Johnson K. Akathisia in idiopathic Parkinson's disease. Neurology 1987;37:477–480.
MacMaster, FP, Carrey N, Sparkes S, et al. Proton spectroscopy in medication-free pediatric attention-deficit/hyperactivity disorder. Biol Psychiatry 2003;53:184–187.
Mill, J, Curran S, Kent L, et al. Association study of a SNAP-25 microsatellite and attention deficit hyperactivity disorder. Am J Med Genet 2002;114:269–271.
Mill, J, Richards S, Knight J, et al. Haplotype analysis of SNAP-25 suggests a role in the aetiology of ADHD. Mol Psychiatry 2004; 9:801–810.
Mogenson, GJ, Nielsen M. Neuropharmacological evidence to suggest that the nucleus accumbens and subpallidal region contribute to exploratory locomotion. Behavioral Neural Biology 1984;42: 52–60.
Ross, RG, Hommer D, Breiger D, Varley C, Radant, A. Eye movement task related to frontal lobe functioning in children with attention deficit disorder. J Am Acad Child Adolesc Psychiatry 1994; 33:869–874.
Schultz, W. Responses of midbrain dopamine neurons to behavioral trigger stimuli in the monkey. J Neurophysiol 1986;63: 1401–1412.
Schultz, W, Apicella P, Ljungberg T. Responses of monkey dopamine neurons to reward and conditioned stimuli during successive steps of learning a delayed response task. J Neurosci 1993; 13:900–913.
Sparkes, SJ, MacMaster FP, Carrey NC. Proton magnetic resonance spectroscopy and cognitive function in pediatric attention-deficit/hyperactive disorder. Brain Cogn 2004;54:173–175.
Sun, L, Jin Z, Zang YF, et al. Differences between attention-deficit disorder with and without hyperactivity: a 1H-magnetic resonance spectroscopy study. Brain Dev 2005;27:340–344.
Tassin, JP, Stinus L, Simon H, et al. Relationship between the locomotor hyperactivity induced by A10 lesions and the destruction of the fronto-cortical dopaminergic innervation in the rat. Brain Research 1978;141:267–281.
Voeller, KKS, Alexander, A, Heilman KM. Defective response inhibition in attention deficit hyperactivity disorder. Neurology 1990; 40; S1;410.
Wilson, MC. Coloboma mouse mutant as an animal model of hyperkinesis and attention deficit hyperactivity disorder. Neurosci Biobehav Rev 2000;24:51–57.
Yeo, RA, Hill DE, Campbell RA, et al. Proton magnetic resonance spectroscopy investigation of the right frontal lobe in children with attention-deficit/hyperactivity disorder. J Am Acad Child Adolesc Psychiatry 2003;42:303–310.

Conduct Disorder and Sociopathy

12

Markus J. P. Kruesi, MD   *Kevin Gray, MD*

This chapter reviews the neuropsychiatry of conduct disorder/sociopathy (CD). The term *conduct disorder/sociopathy* emphasizes the life course persistent nature of some conduct disorders and their continuity with antisocial personality disorder (ASP) (Robins 1966; Moffitt 1993).

HISTORICAL OVERVIEW

The emergence of near universal schooling in the early 20th century brought children under the eye of institutions and professionals and the subsequent detection of more subtle forms of disturbance than epilepsy, mental retardation, and gross psychosis (Neve & Turner 2002). This led to a need to deal with troubled or delinquent children as seen in the work of William Healy (1917), an obstetrician, who founded juvenile court clinics in Chicago and Boston. Healy viewed delinquents as suffering from a "psychic constitutional deficiency." In contrast to this internal deficit perspective, conduct disorder has also been viewed as an ecological adaptation to a harsh family or community environment (Steiner et al. 1997). As psychodynamic perspective grew influential, August Aichorn, the principal of Austrian reform schools, described delinquents whose actions were attempts to assuage neurotic guilt via seeking punishment (Aichorn 1935). Although Cleckley in *The Mask of Sanity* (1941) described psychopathy as driven by both environmental and hereditary factors, nature and nurture generally remained oppositional conceptualizations of CD (Steiner et al. 1997).

The groundbreaking evidence for the continuity of conduct disorder and antisocial personality disorder came from the serendipity of juvenile clinic records being stored in space that Lee Robins was to move into. Rather than dispose of the records, she had the perspicacity to investigate those children's outcome. Her longitudinal follow up of those youths, *Deviant Children Grown Up* (1966), provided valuable missing descriptive data analagous to the observations of Kraeplin about psychiatric disorders in adults. Subsequent longitudinal studies of Loeber et al., Trembley et al., Raine et al., and McCord et al. supported the concept that CD is not purely a transient reaction to circumstance. Gradually an appreciation of the costs of the disorder is beginning to emerge along with an interactive perspective on nature nurture relationships.

DEFINITIONS AND NOSOLOGY

Conduct disorder is a psychiatric disorder in the category of disruptive behavior disorders, with criteria listed below. However, a number of other potentially overlapping constructs are pertinent. Many studies use related but non-interchangeable criteria. CD, crime/delinquency, psychopathy, and/or aggression are related but not entirely the same concepts. Delinquency is a legal term. Juvenile delinquents may present with no psychiatric diagnosis at all or with many different diagnoses (Quay 1979). Similarly, aggression has considerable overlap with conduct disorder, but there are conduct disordered individuals who do not display other directed physical aggression. Psychopathy refers to a disorder characterized by two features—an antisocial behavioral dimension which includes instrumental aggression and a wide variety of offenses plus a dimension of emotional impairment such as a lack of guilt and emotional shallowness (Cleckley 1941; Hare 1993). Most psychopaths qualify for an antisocial personality disorder diagnosis, but only 1 in 3 persons who meet criteria for antisocial personality disorder diagnosis meet criteria for psychopathy (Hart & Hare 1996). It is not surprising that inconsistency in findings exist given these discrepant inclusionary criteria. A further potential confound is that some studies examine the broad band of externalizing or disruptive behavior. Although, evidence for the existence of this broad band is substantial, discriminating among the different typologies subsumed under the broad externalizing banner may have considerable prognostic import. For example, ADHD was thought to be a risk for later substance abuse. However, subsequent studies clarified it is comorbid conduct problems that drive the relationship, not ADHD per se (Disney et al. 1999; Chilcoat & Breslau 1999). Review of conduct disorder is complicated by the many studies which concentrate on aggregated measures of antisocial behavior and often include symptoms of ADHD, or more general behavior problems (Burke et al. 2002).

EPIDEMIOLOGY

Prevalence rates for CD are generally reported to be between 1.5 to 3.4% in the general population (AACAP 1997, Manfred et al. 2002) and vary according to age, sex, geographic location, socioeconomic status, and familial structure and attributes. It is generally agreed that the prevalence of CD is greater among males (2.6–8.2%) than among females (0.8–2.8%) (Feehan et al. 1994; Offord et al. 1987; Rutter et al 1970). The association between CD and age remains unclear. Previous findings (Cohen 1987) suggested higher prevalence rates among adolescents than among prepubertal children, but this has more recently come into question (Breton et al. 1999; Cohen et al. 1993; Lewinsohn et al. 1993; Nolan et al. 2001). Symptoms of both conduct disorder and various comorbid disorders fluctuate over time (Lahey et al. 2002). A greater prevalence of CD has been reported among youths from families of low socioeconomic status (Lahey et al. 1999; Rutter et al. 1975; Stanger et al. 1992) and from families with disrupted structure (Esser et al. 1990; Velez et al. 1989). Urban environment has been found to be a risk by some (Tolan and Henry 1996) but not by others (Rutter et al. 1970; Breton et al. 1999). Many youth with conduct disorder have reading problems (Hinshaw 1992), but it is unclear whether a causal relationship exists (Fergusson and Lynskey 1997; Maughan et al. 1996; Bennett et al. 2003).

Epidemiologic studies support a possible distinction between delinquency and conduct disorder. Of 478 individuals in the juvenile justice setting, less than 30% met criteria for conduct disorder in a study that took social, academic, and occupational impairment into account (Garland et al. 2001). In a randomly selected, stratified sample of 1,829 juvenile detainees, only about 40% had conduct disorder (Teplin et al. 2002).

ETIOLOGY

Genetic and Environmental Factors

The field of behavior genetics largely finds origin in the study of animals, as domesticated animals have been selectively bred for a variety of attributes, including temperament (Takeuchi and Houpt 2003). Despite selective breeding, it is well known that individual differences in temperament occur. Correlation with humans leads us to the concept of genetic and environmental interaction. Many individual characteristics may have origins in synergistic genetic and environmental effects, while others may be related solely to genetics or environment.

Twin (Simonoff et al. 1998; Slutske et al. 1997) and adoption (Cadoret et al. 1995) studies support a genetic liability for conduct disorder. In addition, variance in adolescent antisocial behavior may be accounted for in part by conflictual and negative parental behavior directed specifically toward the adolescent (Reiss et al. 1995).

Attempts have been made to correlate behavioral traits with genetic abnormalities of various neurotransmitters, including dopamine, serotonin, and noradrenaline. Behavioral traits often linked to conduct disorder include aggression and novelty seeking. Dopamine DRD2 and DRD4 polymorphisms have been found to associate with novelty seeking behavior (Noble et al. 1998; Ono et al. 1997). Polymorphisms of the gene coding for tryptophan hydroxylase, the rate-limiting enzyme in serotonin biosynthesis, were associated with individual differences in aggressive disposition among 251 adult subjects (Manuck et al. 1999). Comings and colleagues have examined 42 genes using multivariate regression analysis to determine associations with attention deficit hyperactivity disorder (ADHD), oppositional defiant disorder (ODD), and conduct disorder among 326 subjects, 271 of which had a diagnosis of Tourette's syndrome (Comings et al. 2000a, 2000b). They report that some noradrenaline genes may share a role in all of these disorders, while hormone and neuropeptide genes may be linked to CD.

Recent twin studies of adults (Bloningen et al. 2003) and adolescents (Taylor et al. 2003) examined genetic and environmental influences on psychopathy. Both studies revealed a substantial genetic contribution to psychopathy and neither revealed a shared environment effect.

The measure most frequently utilized for evaluating the level of childhood and adolescent aggression in genetic studies is the Child Behavior Checklist (CBCL) (Achenbach 1983). Twin (Ghodesian-Carpy and Baker 1987) and adoption (van den Oord 1994) studies suggest that genetics account for 42 to 90% of variance in CBCL-rated aggression. It should be noted, however, that only two items on the CBCL aggressive subscale refer to physical aggressiveness and that, in a study of disruptive and aggressive children, CBCL aggressive scale scores did not correlate significantly with severity of physical aggressiveness (Kruesi et al. 1994).

Birth Complications: Pre- and Perinatal Toxic Influences

Birth complications and pre- and perinatal toxic exposures can play a substantial role in the development of CD/ASP. Child and adolescent behavioral disturbances have been associated with low birth weight, prematurity, obstetric complications, physical anomalies, maternal illness, nutritional status, and substance and medication use (Rutter et al. 1998). Dutch military psychiatric examinations among those exposed prenatally to German army food supply blockade in 1944 and 1945 revealed that in utero malnutrition during the first and second trimesters is associated with an excess of Antisocial Personality Disorder in the offspring of those pregnancies (Neugebauer et al. 1999).

Toxin exposure is more controversial. Associations between maternal smoking and risk of conduct disorder, behavior problems, and crime have been reported in several studies (Brennan et al. 1999; Fergusson et al. 1993; Fergusson et al. 1998; Orlebeke et al. 1997; Rantakallio et al. 1992; Wakschlag et al. 1997; Weissman et al. 1999; Williams et al. 1998). Some question the role of direct causation and offer the alternative and increasingly accepted explanation that the associations may be attributed to the transmission of a latent conduct disturbance factor from mother to child (Maughan et al. 2001; Silberg et al. 2003). In a 1995 study, prenatal alcohol exposure contributed significantly to CD as an offspring outcome, but having an alcoholic biological parent did not (Cadoret et al. 1995). This finding implies that it was the actual alcohol exposure of the fetus in utero (not the genetic contribution from the parents' alcoholism) that resulted in the development of CD.

In a cohort of 4,269 consecutive live male births, infants who experienced both birth complications and early maternal rejection were more likely than those with only one of these risk factors to become violent offenders in adulthood (Raine et al. 1994). Although only 4.5% of the subjects had both risk factors, this small group accounted for 18% of all violent crimes committed by members of the original cohort. The interactive effect of maternal rejection and birth complications was specific to violence and was not observed for nonviolent criminal offending.

Physical Characteristics

Historical attempts to correlate physical appearance with psychopathology have often come into question. The classic example was phrenology, wherein personality and mental characteristics were thought to be represented by the contours of the skull, and diagnostic interpretations were based on its palpation. With advances in genetic research, however, there has been a renewed interest in physical markers that may correlate with mental disorders. For example, hair whorl patterns and dermatoglyphic abnormalities have been studied in patients with schizophrenia (Alexander et al. 1993; Puri et al. 1995; Rosa et al. 2000) (Table 12.1).

TABLE 12.1

PHYSICAL CHARACTERISTICS POTENTIALLY ASSOCIATED WITH CONDUCT DISORDER, DELINQUENCY, AND CHILDHOOD AGGRESSION

Mesomorphic body type (heavy-boned, muscular)
Large body size
Increased height
Decreased fluctuating asymmetry

Investigation of physical characteristics of delinquents was undertaken in the mid-twentieth century. Sheldon described three major body types, including endomorphic, mesomorphic, and ectomorphic (1949). In both male and female populations, mesomorphs (i.e., heavier boned and muscular subjects) were more commonly found among delinquents than among controls (Epps and Parnell 1952; Glueck and Glueck 1956). A study of somatostatin in cerebrospinal fluid revealed lower levels among subjects with disruptive behavior disorders compared with age-matched subjects with obsessive-compulsive disorder (Kruesi et al. 1990). If the reduced somatostatin concentration correlated with hypothalamic levels, the resultant decreased inhibition of growth hormone might result in increased bone and muscle mass, and thus a more mesomorphic appearance. Large body size and increased height have been linked to child and adolescent aggression, violence, and conduct disorder (Farrington 1989; Ishikawa et al. 2001; Pine et al. 1997; Raine et al. 1998; Tremblay 1998).

Fluctuating asymmetry, which refers to a deviation from bilateral symmetry of physical characteristics, such as ear widths, ear lengths, elbows, wrists, finger lengths, ankles, and foot widths, is described as a reliable measure of developmental instability, defined as "the imprecise expression of a given developmental design because of untoward environmental or genetic perturbations that disrupt developmental processes" (Gangestad and Yeo 1994). Measures of developmental instability, including fluctuating asymmetry, "tell a historical tale of poor or disrupted design, random errors and accidents, or deleterious environments" (Lalumiere et al. 2001). Fluctuating asymmetry is recognized to correlate negatively with fitness across a wide range of taxa other than our own species (Moller 1997). Two recent studies revealed a negative correlation between fluctuating asymmetry of morphological traits and aggression and fighting history among male children and college students (Furlow et al. 1998; Manning and Wood 1998). Given that fluctuating asymmetry reliably measures developmental instability, those male subjects with higher aggression ratings might be seen as more developmentally stable. The implications of these studies may include viewing aggression as a developmentally adaptive behavior in some contexts. Lower rates of fluctuating asymmetry and obstetrical problems were found among male offenders with psychopathy when compared with nonpsychopathic offenders (Lalumiere et al. 2001). These results may support the theory of psychopathy as an evolutionarily stable strategy (Harpending & Sobus 1987; Mealey 1995). Another symmetry analogy, a study comparing successful (e.g., not caught) psychopaths versus unsuccessful psychopaths, found that the successful psychopaths had greater hippocampal symmetry (Raine et al. 2004).

REPRODUCTIVE ADAPTATION

An early attempt to address the evolutionary biologic fit of ASP (MacMillan & Kofoed 1984) proposed that ASP, in sociobiological terms, represented an alternate reproductive strategy—a minimal investment reproductive strategy. A continuum of reproductive strategies ranges from maximal investment characterized by protracted care of the young and minimal numbers of offspring to minimal investment characterized by lack of care for the young and greater numbers of offspring. Larger numbers of offspring, more promiscuous matings (Robins 1966), more abuse/neglect/abandonment of partners and offspring (Robins 1966), and a "cheating" reproductive strategy wherein males misrepresent their position in the dominance heirarchy to mate were cited (MacMillan & Kofoed 1984) as evidence of that alternate strategy. In contrast, nonantisocial individuals were said to be more likely to have a greater investment/fewer offspring strategy.

There is a growing consistency of evidence to support the idea that CD/ASP represents an alternate reproductive adaptation among humans (Kruesi & Showalter, in press). Individuals with ASP differ in their number of sexual partners and for their comparative lack of investment in their young. A study of 55 methadone patients found those with ASP were significantly more likely to be promiscuous—defined as having 10 or more sexual partners in the past year (Gill et al, 1992). A separate study of 351 cocaine abusers also found that those with ASP are more promiscuous (Compton et al., 1995). Another consistent finding is assortative mating among sociopaths: sociopaths tend to mate with other sociopaths (Krueger et al, 1998). Studies of the sexual behavior of juveniles are limited, but also support the theory. A study of 126 boys aged 5 to 11 years at increased risk for the development of conduct-disorder-related behavior re-evaluated 112 of them 15 months later (Meyer-Bahlburg et al, 1999). At both time points, the boys scored higher on the Sex Problems scale as well as on the nonsexual CBCL scales than Achenbach's nonclinical norm sample. Data analyzed from 5,877 respondents aged 15–54 years in the National Comorbidity Survey, a nationally representative household survey, indicated that early-onset psychiatric disorders were associated with subsequent teenage parenthood among both females and males, with odds ratios of 2.0–12.0 and population attributable risk proportions of

6.2–33.7% (Kessler et al, 1997). Because of this risk due to the general category of early onset psychiatric disorder, it is important that studies address psychiatric comorbidity in order to parse out relationships to CD.

Recent studies have shed light on the association between CD and sexual/reproductive behavior by controlling for confounds. Girls with conduct disorder, girls with depression, girls with anxiety, and healthy girls (N = 459) who had been evaluated at age 15 years were followed up at age 21, when reproductive health was assessed (Bardone et al, 1998). After control for potentially confounding variables including prior health, adolescent conduct disorder predicted more medical problems, poorer self-reported overall health, lower body mass index, alcohol and/or marijuana dependence, tobacco dependence, daily smoking, more lifetime sexual partners, sexually transmitted disease, and early pregnancy. In a separate study, 83 girls, 8 to 13 years old at study entry with childhood-onset psychiatric disorders were repeatedly evaluated during an interval of up to 12 years (Kovacs et al, 1994). In the final model, childhood or adolescent onset conduct disorders (but not depressive disorders) were significantly associated with teenage pregnancy. Among the girls with conduct disorders, 54.8% became pregnant teenagers versus 12% of the rest. In addition to earlier sexual initiation, pregnancy and greater numbers of partners, there are indications that other aspects of sexuality differ as well. A birth cohort study of 930 New Zealand residents found that individuals with ASP have a risk ratio of 2.8 for early onset intercourse (prior to age 16), whereas those with depressive disorders have a risk ratio of 1.3 (Ramrakha et al, 2002). This is consistent with the idea that it is CD that is driving the early age of sexual initiation rather than other psychiatric disorders.

Sexual victimization, as victim or as perpetrator, is associated with conduct disorder in community as well as clinical samples. A study of 1,025 females and 1,087 males in grades 7 to 12 in Alberta (Canada) high schools found associations between experiencing a high number of sexual assaults and clinical profiles on measures of conduct disorder for both males and females (Bagley et al, 1995). CD was present in 94% of a clinical sample of 17 adolescents who sexually molested children (Galli et al, 1999). In a study of 499 mentally ill children and adolescents which grouped subjects in four mutually exclusive categories (no inappropriate sexual behavior (n=296), hypersexual (n=82), exposing (n=39), and victimizing (n=82)), an antisocial family history was associated with an increased rate of sexually inappropriate behaviors (Adams et al, 1995). One criterion symptom for conduct disorder is "has forced someone into sexual activity" (DSM-IV), therefore the "victimizing" group might be expected to be associated with antisocial family histories. However, hypersexuality and exposing behaviors were also associated with antisocial family histories suggesting that antisocial family history is associated with a broad range of sexual behavior that differs in qualitative and quantitative ways from that of other youth.

Another facet of reproductive adaptation, parenting, also differs between antisocial and other families: individuals with ASP tend to do less parental monitoring and have greater family conflict and lower family involvement (Patterson et al, 1989; Ary et al 1999). The predictive association between parenting and adolescent adjustment has been assumed to be environmental. However, one recent examination of genetic and environmental contributions suggests a need for greater consideration of genetic contributions. A study of 395 families with adolescent siblings who participated in the Nonshared Environment in Adolescent Development (Reiss et al., 1994) project indicates that the cross-lagged associations between parental conflict-negativity and adolescent antisocial behavior can be explained primarily by genetic factors (Neiderhiser et al, 1999).

NEUROBIOLOGY

Neurochemistry

The most studied neurotransmitter related to CD is serotonin and its major metabolite 5-hydroxyindoleacetic acid (5-HIAA). Recent meta-analysis (Moore et al, 2002) of 20 adult studies of cerebrospinal fluid 5-HIAA concentration where the experimental subjects included adults exhibiting outwardly directed antisocial behavior found a significant overall effect size (d = $-.45$). Lower concentrations are associated with antisocial behavior. A significant moderating effect for age was found, with larger effect sizes for groups under age 30 (weighted d = -1.37). The relative dearth of child CSF 5-HIAA studies necessitated a broader behavioral inclusion definition—the experimental group included children with disruptive behavior or whose parents evidenced antisociality. Again, a significant effect size was found (d = $-.32$). Sixteen of 29 in the initial pediatric CSF 5-HIAA aggression study and follow-up (Kruesi et al 1990, 1992) had conduct disorder. A study of 29 boys with ADHD (11 with CD) did not find the expected low 5-HIAA concentration f aggression relationship (Castellanos et al., 1994). However, those subjects were significantly less aggressive (Kruesi & Jacobsen 1997). More recently, two studies investigated 5-HIAA concentrations in infants and behavioral variables. In one study, the investigators assayed monoamine metabolites in "leftover" spinal fluid from 167 neurologically normal infants (0–3 months of age), and later (at age 18–21 months of age) obtained their family psychiatric histories (Constantino et al, 1999). As calculated by Moore et al (2002), there was a significant but small effect size (d = $-.261$) for the relationship between newborns CSF 5-HIAA and antisociality in the family in the expected direction (lower concentration—more antisocial). In a behavioral follow-up study, leftover CSF from 73 febrile infants (age $\leq$ 3 months) was assayed for 5-HIAA (Clarke et al, 1999). Subjects with 5-HIAA below the median had higher externalizing behavior scores at 30 months than did subjects whose 5-HIAA levels fell above the median ($P = 0.02$).

Relationships between serotonergic measures and psychopathy have been investigated in adults. In the first study, psychopathy as assessed by the Psychopathy Checklist-Revised (PCL-R) (Hare et al 1990) was associated with the ratio of CSF HVA/5-HIAA concentrations in 22 violent offenders undergoing pretrial forensic psychiatric assessment (Soderstrom et al, 2001). 5-HIAA alone was not significantly correlated with PCL-R scores. That finding was replicated in a new group of 28 violent and sexual offenders, where the HVA:5-HIAA ratio was strongly associated with psychopathic traits (r = 0.50, p = 0.010), (Soderstrom et al, 2003). Recently, fifty-one DSM-III-R personality disordered offenders who had a dynamic assessment of 5-HT function (prolactin response to 30 mg d-fenfluramine challenge) were rated on the Psychopathy Checklist: Screening Version (Dolan & Anderson 2003). 5-HT function did not correlate with psychopathy as a unidimensional phenomenon. The impulsive-antisocial component correlates negatively with 5-HT function while the arrogant/deceitful component correlates positively with 5-HT. In line with previous research findings, impulsive-antisocial conduct shows an inverse relationship with 5-HT function. The findings are consistent with genetic studies in supporting some degree of independence for the impulsive antisocial and callous unemotional factors.

Aggression and its associations with CSF 5-HIAA concentrations have been examined in adults, but pediatric age groups have not addressed aggression subtypes. An important early and replicated finding in adult samples is that it is impulsive, affect laden aggression in contrast to the "cold blooded" premeditated aggression that is associated with low concentrations of CSF 5-HIAA. It is *not* crime in general that is linked with low 5-HIAA concentrations, but rather only impulsive, affect laden violent crime that has an association. Pediatric CSF studies have not thus far systematically assessed predatory versus affective/impulsive aggression (Kruesi et al, 2003). However, studies of both youth and of adults indicate that impulsive and premeditated aggression are independent constructs (Dodge and Coie 1987; Vitiello et al, 1990; Barrat 1999).

Pediatric fenfluramine challenge studies present an inconsistent picture of serotonin aggression links. One study of boys with ADHD who were divided into aggressive and nonaggressive subgroups found the aggressive subgroup had a significantly greater prolactin response to the fenfluramine challenge (Halperin et al, 1994). However, another study found fenfluramine-induced prolactin release was not correlated with aggression rating scores in disruptive behavior disorder (DBD) patients and did not differ significantly between adolescent DBD patients and normal controls subjects (Stoff et al 1992). A study of 18 late adolescent/early adult individuals with early onset alcoholism use disorders who were impulsive and aggressive found no significant difference in prolactin response to fenfluramine compared to 19 matched controls (Soloff et al, 2000). A study of 34 younger brothers of convicted delinquents found increasing degrees of aggressive behavior were positively correlated with the prolactin response to fenfluramine challenge (Pine et al, 1997). Furthermore, adverse-rearing circumstances conducive to development of aggressive behavior also exhibited positive correlations with the prolactin response. This association between adverse rearing and the prolactin response was statistically independent of that between aggression and the prolactin response. The inconsistent results may be a product of failing to address predatory versus affective aggression or presence/absence of psychopathy.

A significant caveat in examining relationships between monoamine metabolite concentrations and behavior is that age may alter the relationships. Studies of relationships of certain types of aggression (e.g., suicide and monoamine metabolites) suggest caution in generalizing across age. Although studies of adults are very consistent in finding relationships between low CSF 5-HIAA and suicide (Lester 1995), the two studies of adolescents to date (Kruesi et al, 1992; LL Greenhill personal communication) both found the dopamine metabolite, HVA, a better predictor.

Hormonal Studies

Hormones of adrenal as well as gonadal origin have been implicated in the neurobiology of conduct disorder. In most species, androgens appear to exert a significant influence on the form and degree of aggressive behavior (Rubinow & Schmidt 1996). Steroid hormones are thought to play two distinct roles in modulating behavior: an organizational as well as an activational role. Gonadal steroids act around the time of birth in organizing which brain and other tissues will be steroid responsive. Later in life, the hormone will activate behavioral patterns such as mating behavior.

Body fluid findings have linked testosterone concentrations with aggression in humans. For example, higher CSF testosterone was associated with increased aggression among alcoholic offenders (Virkkunnen et al, 1994). Yet, aggression testosterone relationships are not simple one to one linear relationships. Androgens interact with neurotransmitters in modifying or modulating aggression. For example, the increased aggression evident in genetically altered neuronal nitrous oxide negative male mice appears modulated by testosterone (Dawson 1997). Castration reduced aggression in neuronal nitrous oxide negative mice and wild type mice to equal low levels. Testosterone replacement restored aggression to precastration levels suggesting testosterone dependence. A study of plasma androgens in 15 boys with conduct disorder and 25 normal controls found significantly higher levels of dehydroepiandrosterone sulfate (DHEAS) but not testosterone in CD (van Goozen et al, 1998). Both aggression and delinquency correlated with DHEAS levels.

Another neuroendocrine abnormality associated with antisocial behavior is decreased cortisol secretion. The first study describing low cortisol response to a stressor compared adult male criminals in a maximum security hospital to a criminal control group (Woodman et al, 1978). More recently pediatric studies have documented associations. A study of 38 clinic referred boys with disruptive behavior found low salivary cortisol levels associated with early onset of and persistence of aggression (McBurnett et al, 2000). A study of 47 adolescent girls with conduct disorder and 37 control girls found the girls with CD had lower plasma cortisol levels (Pajer et al, 2001). Girls with CD, who did not have other psychiatric comorbidity, had lower cortisol than those with comorbidity or controls. Salivary cortisol had a significant negative correlation with CD symptom counts in boys and their parents (Vanyukov et al, 1993). However, not all studies have found decreases. Urinary free cortisol (Kruesi et al 1990) and plasma cortisol (Schulz et al 1997) did not differ in boys with ADHD (most of whom had comorbid CD or ODD) compared to normal controls.

Electrophysiology

The most common psychophysiologic measures recorded from antisocial populations have been electroencephalography (EEG), evoked potentials, event related potentials (ERPs), heart rate (HR), and skin conductance (SC) (Scarpa and Raine 1997). Adult psychopathy studies find three relatively consistent abnormalities: (1) Generalized excess theta activity; (2) foci of 6–8/second, 14–16/second bilateral or right temporal activity; (3) localized slow-wave activity in the temporal lobe (Dolan 1994). The comparatively slower EEGs are consistent with underarousal theories of psychopathy. However, often the EEG studies include psychopaths or criminals, but may not represent aggression or the diagnosis of conduct disorder. For example, two prospective studies by Volavka (1987) tracked Scandinavian boys who had had EEG recordings before age 16 and followed up their criminal records. These studies revealed relatively slower EEG frequencies in those with repetitive theft but do not mention a link to violence. However, study of 372 male maximum security mental hospital patients found more EEG abnormalities (slowing and/or sharp waves) in the temporal lobes of the most violent compared to the least violent: 20% versus 2.4% (Wong et al. 1994). Overall rates of EEG abnormalities (meaning without regard to location) were higher (43%) in the most violent compared to less violent patients (24–26%). Clinically, routine EEG screening is of limited value in childhood antisocial behavior problems without clinical evidence of neurologic disorder (Phillips et al. 1993).

Evoked Potentials

Event related potentials (ERP) are averaged changes of the brains electrical activity in response to specific stimuli. The event related potential alternatively referred to as P 300 or P3 describes the third positive peak component of the ERP waveform that occurs at a modal time of 300 msec after presentation of a novel/deviant/unexpected stimulus (Fabiani, Gratton, & Coles 2000). Late, middle, and early components are believed associated with attention, cortical augmenting, and environmental filtering. Earlier studies reviewed by Raine (1993), largely in psychopathic subjects, support three findings: (1) enhanced late latency ERP P300 amplitudes to stimuli of interest suggesting enhanced attention for stimulating events; (2) heightened middle latency ERP amplitudes to stimuli of increasing intensity, consistent with sensation seeking; and (3) long early latency brain stem average evoked responses, consistent with decreased arousal and excessive environmental filtering.

A recent study (Iacono et al, 2002) using a statewide sample of 502 male youth about age 17, identified from Minnesota birth records as members of twin pairs, had their P300 amplitude measured, using a visual oddball paradigm. Structured clinical interviews covering attention deficit hyperactivity disorder, conduct disorder, oppositional defiant disorder, antisocial personality disorder, and substance use disorders were administered to the youth and his parents at the time of the P300 assessment and again to the youth 3 years later. Reduced P300 was associated with disorders and paternal risk for disorders, reflecting a behavioral disinhibition spectrum that included attention deficit hyperactivity disorder, oppositional defiant disorder, conduct disorder, antisocial personality disorder, alcoholism, nicotine dependence, and illicit drug abuse and dependence. Reduced P300 at age 17 predicted the development of substance use disorders at age 20. Most effect sizes associated with these group differences exceeded 0.70, indicating medium to moderately large group differences.

In another ERP study, the subjects were 94 community males, aged 14–19 years, who varied in the type and number of conduct problem behaviors exhibited prior to age 15. Groups were operationally defined by the number (0 versus > or =1) of DSM-IV conduct disorder diagnostic criteria within each of four categories: rules violations, aggression, deceitfulness/theft, and destructiveness. P300 electroencephalographic potentials were recorded while subjects performed a task in which rare auditory stimuli were used to signal a change in stimulus-response mapping during a succeeding set of trials. Analyses revealed that boys with a history of rules violations failed to exhibit the normal maturational increase in P300 amplitude. Topographic analyses suggest that the source of the maturational deficit involved P300 generators within the frontal brain. Parietal generators of P300 matured normally (Bauer & Hesselbrock 2003). See Figure 12.1 from Bauer & Hesselbrock 2003.

Heart rate (HR) reflects sympathetic and parasympathetic activity. The common view is that high HR is associated with anxiety, whereas low HR reflects underarousal. A recent meta-analysis of studies of heart rate and antisocial

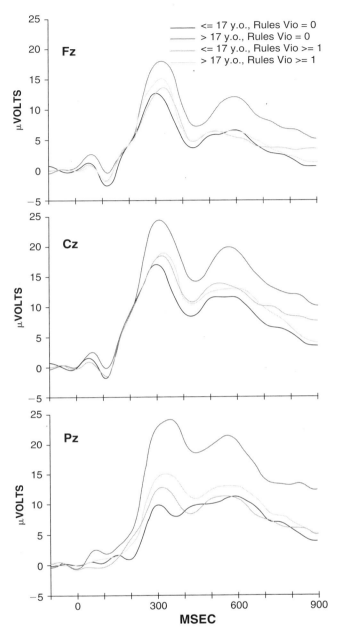

Figure 12.1 Group-averaged event-related potential (ERP) waveforms recorded at three representative electrode sites. The waveforms are sorted by severity of the Rules Violations subtype and age group. Note: Upon first examination, it appears that two late positive (P300) components are present in the group-averaged waveform. However, an examination of ERP waveforms obtained from individual subjects reveals only one prominent positive peak. The erroneous impression of two peaks is the result of averaging data across subjects whose P300 ERPs vary markedly in their peak latencies. (Reprinted from Bauer & Hesselbrock, 2003.)

behavior in children and adolescents found considerable support for relationships between low heart rate and antisocial behavior (Raine et al. 2004). Forty-five independent effect sizes of the resting heart rate–antisocial behavior relationship were obtained from 40 studies conducted between 1971 to 2002 using a total of 5,868 children.

Significant overall effect sizes were found for both resting heart rate ($d = -0.44$, $P < .0001$) and heart during a stressor ($d = -0.76$, $P < .0001$).

There appears to be some specificity to the low heart rate antisocial behavior relationship. Other psychiatric conditions such as hyperactivity, anxiety, depression, schizophrenia or PTSD either do not differ from normal controls or have higher rates (Raine 2002). The specificity of the low heart rate relationship may be greatest for crime/delinquency. The Ortiz & Raine meta-analysis examined broad band "antisocial" behavior. All the studies that used crime as their inclusion criteria reported significant effect sizes and had a 95% confidence interval for their effect size in the direction of lower HR associated with antisocial behavior. In contrast, studies which reported higher heart rate associated with antisocial outcome used samples where crime was not a clear inclusion criteria. For example, two studies which found effects (nonsignificant) in the opposite direction, higher rate associated with greater externalizing behavior used samples which may not have been crime predominant. Zahn & Kruesi (1993) studied a mixed group of ADHD, conduct disorder and oppositional defiant disorder. Pine et al. (1998) studied children at risk for delinquency. A third study (Van Hulle et al. 2000) which did not find a low heart rate association, used a young (age 7) twin sample that lacked significant criminal representation as evidenced by mean scores on the CBCL delinquent subscale that were significantly lower than published norms.

Skin conductance (SC), represents changes in the electrical activity of skin. Sweating increases SC. Resting skin conductance is thought to reflect arousal. There is some evidence for underarousal in antisocial spectrum individuals, but it is linked more to crimes of evasion than violence (Scarpa & Raine 1997).

NEUROANATOMY AND NEUROIMAGING

Where is the neuropathology for conduct disorder localized? Despite the enormous public health impact of this condition (Vostanis et al. 2003; Mandel et al. 2003; Jones et al. 2002; Knapp et al. 2002; Kittelsen et al. 2001), there is relatively little direct anatomic data to answer the question. Most pediatric neuroimaging studies have focused upon diagnoses other than CD (Peterson 1995, Kruesi et al. 2004). Consequently, much of the information this section draws upon is from adult studies that address a variety of related conditions.

Anatomic Evidence

Historically, lesions (often due to accident or tumor), trauma history, and findings on neurological exam or neuropsychological testing have furnished evidence regarding localization. Two regions have most consistently been implicated: prefrontal cortex and temporal lobe.

The *Phineas Gage* case is well known as evidence of traumatic frontal lesion in adulthood leading to impulsivity and rage (Damasio et al. 1994). Subsequent cases, such as those from the Vietnam Head Injury Study offer some confirmation that frontal lesions are associated with hostile, impulsive, aggressive behavior (Grafman et al. 1996). However, that study of Vietnam veterans did not address or control for prehead injury aggression/conduct disorder rendering it unclear how much aggression should be attributed to the head injury (Brower & Price 2001). Violent adult psychopaths display orbitofrontal dysfunction on neuropsychological tests (LaPierre et al. 1995). However, clinical observation suggests that the social inappropriateness of patients with adult-onset prefrontal damage tends not to include violent and criminal behavior (Damasio 2000). Traumatic frontal lobe injury cases have been referred to as acquired sociopathy because of the pattern of irresponsible socially inept behavior seen in the face of normal intellectual abilities. In contrast, early childhood onset of prefrontal cortex lesions (before 16 months) is associated with defective social and moral reasoning in addition to the insensitivity to future consequences of decisions, defective autonomic responses to punishment contingencies and failure to respond to behavioral interventions despite normal basic cognitive abilities picture seen in adult-onset patients (Anderson et al. 1999).

It has long been recognized that temporal lobe epilepsy (TLE) can result in increased aggression (Bear & Fedio 1977). A study of 372 adult male maximum security patients found high violence scores correlated with CT scan and EEG abnormalities in the temporal lobes (Wong et al. 1994).

Frontal and/or temporal locations need to be thought of as interconnected rather than isolated independent structures. This is illustrated by a study of temporal lobe epilepsy patients. Analysis of MRI from 35 control subjects, 24 TLE patients with a history of repeated, interictal episodes of aggression, and 24 patients with TLE without episodes of aggression showed that patients with TLE with aggressive episodes had a decrease of gray matter, most markedly in the left frontal lobe, compared with each of the other groups (Woermann et al. 2000). Although the temporal lobe is a site of obvious pathology, the epileptic focus, findings suggest that structures elsewhere (frontal lobe) underlie the pathophysiology of aggression in TLE.

Pediatric Neuroimaging Studies

There are only three MRI studies of groups of subjects with conduct disorders to date and all address anatomic features (Lyoo et al. 2002; Bussing et al. 2002; Kruesi et al. 2004). The first examined white matter hyperintensities (WMH) on MRI scans in 408 child and adolescent psychiatric inpatients. WMH are believed to represent regions of increased water density (Awad et al. 1986) and are reported to be involved in the pathogenesis of cognitive impairment (Breteler et al. 1994). Study subjects were grouped according to a hierarchical diagnostic system as follows: schizophrenia (n = 42), bipolar disorder (n = 56), unipolar depression (n = 94), conduct disorder/attention deficit disorder (n = 103 of whom 80 met criteria for CD), and other neurotic disorders (n = 30). Subjects without any level 2 diagnoses on structured interview (n = 83) constituted the comparison group. Bipolar disorder, unipolar depression, and conduct disorder/attention deficit disorder groups were significantly more likely to have severe levels of WMH than the controls (prevalence rates: 17.9%, 13.8%, 13.6%, 1.2%). The frontal lobes were the most frequent location for WMH in the conduct disorder/attention deficit disorder group (35.7%). The Bussing et al. study examined a community sample of 12 children with combined subtype ADHD (aged 8–12, 7 of whom had comorbid conduct disorder) and 19 healthy controls matched for age, gender, and handedness. Volume measurements, including left/right asymmetries, were quantified from MRI of the total brain, caudate and cerebellar vermis. No significant differences in total brain volume, caudate volume, asymmetry of the hemispheres or asymmetry of the caudate were found between the groups. Another study used MRI imaging to compare brain anatomy in 10 early onset conduct disorders and 10 age, sex, and handedness matched controls free of psychiatric disorders (Kruesi et al. 2004). Right temporal lobe total and gray matter volumes were smaller in conduct disorder subjects before and after covarying whole brain volume. See Figure 12.2 for an illustration of MRI techniques used.

Smaller frontal lobe volumes were found, but did not reach statistical significance.

Two SPECT studies have examined mixed adolescent and adult subjects with aggression. One study examined a mixed group of 40 aggressive adolescents and adults with various psychiatric disorders (Amen et al. 1996). Findings include significant decreased activity in the prefrontal cortex and increased activity in the anteriomedial portion of the frontal lobe and left side basal/ganglia in the aggressive patients. Focal abnormalities were also seen in the left temporal lobe. The prefrontal cortex is involved in impulse control, critical thinking and concentration. Another SPECT study (Soderstrom et al. 2000) also includes a mixed adolescent and adult sample of 21 nonpsychotic violent offenders. In 16/21 of those subjects some hypoperfusion was noted in the frontal or temporal lobes. Importantly, the abnormalities were as severe in the subgroup (n =7) without major mental disorders or substance abuse as they were in those with those diagnoses.

Adult Neuroimaging

Using MRI, Raine et al. (2000) found an 11% reduction in the prefrontal gray matter volume compared to controls in 21 subjects with ASP to 34 healthy controls, 26 substance abusers, and 21 psychiatric controls. The mean psychopathy scores for subjects suggest many, if not most, of the ASP subjects in that study also meet criteria for psychopathy. A study of 15 antisocial men with high psychopathy scores and 25 matched controls found a large effect size (d = 1.8) for an increase in volume of the corpus callosum in the psychopaths compared to controls (Raine et al. 2003).

A growing body of literature is identifying activity differences in adult psychopaths. A study of 32 violent offenders found correlations between regional cerebral blood

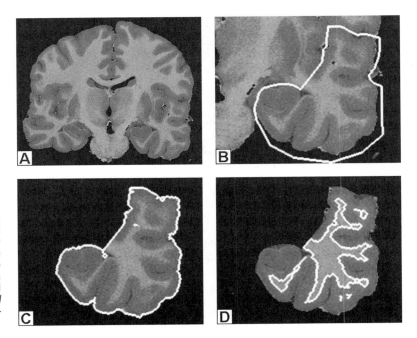

Figure 12.2 The figure (A) illustrates an unenhanced MRI coronal section through a midlevel of the temporal lobe (anterior thalamic nucleus visible). In (B) the temporal lobe has been defined by a boundary function. In the figure (C) a line perpendicular to the axis of the temporal stem connects the Sylvian fissure and the lateral ventricle. An automated edge detection technique defines the outer border of the temporal lobe and corresponding white matter (C and D). *Used with permission from MJP Kruesi, et al. Psychiatry Research: Neuroimaging 132 (2004) 1–11.*

flow and scores on the Psychopathy Checklist–Revised (Soderstrom et al. 2002). Significant negative correlations between frontotemporal perfusion and the interpersonal (callous, unemotional), but not the behavioral (antisocial, impulsive) aspects of psychopathy were seen. The most clearly associated regions of interest were the head of the caudate and the hippocampi. Decreased hippocampal perfusion may also reflect the anatomic finding of another Scandinavian group who reported decreased hippocampal volumes in psychopaths (Laasko et al. 2001). A study of 8 psychopathic criminals, 8 nonpsychopathic criminals and 8 controls used fMRI to examine localized brain activation during performance of an affective memory task (Kiehl et al. 2001). The psychopaths showed significantly less affect-related activity in the amygdala/hippocampus but overactivation in the frontotemporal cortex for processing affective stimuli. An fMRI study of 6 psychopaths and 6 controls found increased right prefrontal and amygdala activation in response to negative emotional pictures among the psychopaths (Muller et al. 2003). Another small sample study with 4 psychopaths, 4 social phobics, and 7 controls used fMRI to examine brain activity during an emotional learning activity (Veit et al. 2002). Results were indicative of hypoactive frontolimbic circuits among the psychopaths during the aversive conditioning.

One important caveat in examining neurobiologic studies of ASP is that substance abuse is a recognized confound. Uncertainty about primary versus acquired deficits is a problem in cross-sectional MRI studies (Franklin et al. 2002). For example in the Raine et al. (2000) MRI study of ASP, cocaine dependence was present in 67% of the ASP group but only 31% of the substance abuse group which raised questions as to whether the prefrontal volume reduction is related to ASP or a product of cocaine dependence (Franklin et al. 2002). Evidence mounts that state dependent brain changes due to substance abuse/dependence or abstinence occur. Brain shrinkage with chronic alcoholism is well acknowledged, but only recently have increases in brain size been shown with abstinence (Liu et al. 2000).

PET scan studies have also identified functional abnormalities associated with violence. Murderers (n = 41) were characterized by reduced glucose metabolism compared to controls in the prefrontal cortex, superior parietal gyrus, left angular gyrus, and the corpus callosum, while abnormal asymmetries of activity (left hemisphere lower than right) were also found in the amygdala, thalamus, and medial temporal lobe (Raine et al. 1997). Some subjects were classified as predatory murderers (N=15) and others as affective murderers (n=9) (Raine et al. 1998). Paralleling studies of predatory versus affective aggression in cats, functional differences were seen between groups: Affective murderers relative to comparisons had lower left and right prefrontal functioning, higher right hemisphere subcortical functioning, and lower right hemisphere prefrontal/subcortical ratios. In contrast, predatory murderers had prefrontal functioning that was more equivalent to comparisons, while also having excessively high right subcortical activity. Results support the hypothesis that emotional, unplanned impulsive murderers are less able to regulate and control aggressive impulses generated from subcortical structures due to deficient prefrontal regulation. The excessive subcortical activity associated with violence is consistent with other suggestions that neural overactivity, such as seen in temporal lobe epilepsy, can increase violence risk.

An imaginal study found rCBF reductions in the ventromedial prefrontal cortex of 15 volunteers during imagined aggressive behavior (Pietrini et al. 2000). This suggests a possible role for functional deactivation of the area during aggression.

A magnetic resonance spectroscopy study examined correlates of repetitive violence to self and others in 13 mildly mentally retarded individuals and 14 controls (Critchley et al. 2000). Concentrations and ratios of N-acetyl aspartate (NAA) and creatine phosphocreatine (Cr+PCr) were assayed. NAA concentration and Cr+PCr concentration reflect neuronal density and high-energy phosphate metabolism respectively. Violent patients had lower prefrontal concentrations of NAA and Cr+PCr and a lower NAA/Cr+PCr ratio in the amygdalo-hippocampal complex than controls. Within the violent group, prefrontal NAA concentration correlated with the frequency of observed aggression.

DIAGNOSIS & CLINICAL FEATURES

Assessment

Assessment of the child with CD needs to include a thorough psychiatric evaluation which should be multidimensional and employ multiple informants (AACAP 1997). Multiple lines of inquiry—diagnosis, symptom severity/diversity, associated features, comorbid conditions and the context within which the disorder is appearing—will influence the methods, intensity, and foci of intervention. The DSM-IV-TR criteria for CD require that the individual repetitively and persistently violates either the basic rights of others or age-appropriate societal norms or rules, as evidenced by at least three of the following criteria in the past year (and at least one criterion present in the past 6 months):

Aggression to people or animals—criteria include bullying or intimidation, physical fights, use of a weapon, physical cruelty to people, physical cruelty to animals, theft while confronting a victim, forcing someone into sexual activity

Destruction of property—criteria include deliberate firesetting or by other means

Deceitfulness or theft—criteria include theft with or without breaking and entering, lying in order to obtain goods or avoid obligation

Serious violation of rules—criteria include staying out at night despite parental objection (beginning before age 13), running away from home, truancy from school (beginning before age 13).

These behaviors must have caused clinically significant impairment in social, academic, or occupational functioning. In addition, if the individual is at least 18 years old, criteria are not met for antisocial personality disorder.

Antisocial personality disorder (ASP) in adulthood requires conduct disorder in childhood. Because ASP is one of the adverse possible outcomes of CD, it is important to recognize when a patient has already met ASP criteria prior to age 18. The DSM-IV-TR criteria for ASP require that the individual be at least 18 years of age, have a history of conduct disorder, and display a pervasive pattern of disregard for and violation of the rights of others occurring since age 15, as evidenced by at least three of the following: (i) repeatedly engaging in unlawful behaviors that are grounds for arrest; (ii) deceitfulness; (iii) impulsivity or failure to plan ahead; (iv) irritability and aggressiveness; (v) reckless disregard for safety of self or others; (vi) consistent irresponsibility (failure to honor obligations); and (vii) lack of remorse. These behaviors must not occur exclusively during the course of a schizophrenic or manic episode.

A careful history, review of systems, psychiatric and medical exam will often determine the need for further investigations. Laboratory examinations are a function of individual history as well as age: for example, adolescents with CD should have a urine drug screen and have screens for sexually transmitted disease but not all prepubertal individuals with CD will need those measures. EEG, MRI, CT and other brain imaging are not routine evaluations for individuals with conduct disorder, but are prompted by neurologic symptoms or history.

The usual clinical use of neuropsychological testing in CD, in the absence of brain damage/focal neurologic findings, is to assess learning disabilities and intellectual ability. Individuals who have committed severe violence (e.g. homicide) may require greater scrutiny because of high rates of head injuries and other CNS insults (Lewis et al. 1988).

Assessment needs to consider features that are not part of the CD diagnosis. For example, strengths and protective factors are important to assess, so they can be mobilized in treatment (U.S. Department of Health and Human Services 1999). Some domains to be assessed are listed in Table 12.2.

Neuropsychological Testing

Intelligence quotient (IQ) has long been related to risk for juvenile delinquency with IQ scores showing associations with juvenile delinquency of the same magnitude as those of class or race (Moffitt 1993). The generally accepted 8 point discrepancy between delinquents and their law abiding peers, is not propelled by those with transient law breaking but a large (e.g. 17 point) difference between habitual offenders and controls (Moffitt 1990).

TABLE 12.2
DOMAINS FOR ASSESSMENT IN CONDUCT DISORDER INDIVIDUALS

- supervision and behavioral management needs;
- history of sexual and physical abuse;
- separation, divorce or death of key attachment figures;
- evidence of attachment capacity;
- intellectual ability, educational potential, disabilities, achievements, and learning style;
- peer relationships, especially the extent peers are reinforcing negative behaviors;
- family problems and strengths;
- environmental factors including disorganized home and lack of supervision;
- presence of neurotoxins such as lead; and
- ability to form and maintain relationships.

Adapted from Steiner et al, 1997 and McMains et al

Although there is substantial agreement about the association between IQ and delinquency, associations between CD and more circumscribed neuropsychological functions are controversial. In the preceding decade, two domains were thought impaired in individuals with CD: "executive" self-control functions and language based verbal skills (Moffitt 1993). Executive cognitive function is defined as a higher order cognitive construct involved in the planning, initiation, and regulation of goal directed behavior (Milner 1995). Executive function is thought to localize in prefrontal cortex and its limbostriatal connections.

Recent evidence suggests executive function problems are not as central to CD as previously thought. Executive function deficits are well documented in ADHD but not in CD without ADHD (Pennington & Ozonoff 1996). Meta-analysis of 39 studies of antisocial behavior which utilized well-defined criteria for executive function: (a) tests had to incorporate at least one of the theoretical domains of executive function (e.g. volition, planning, purposive action, and/or effective performance); and one or more of (b) and (c): (b) the test has been found in brain imaging research to preferentially activate the frontal cortex and/or (c) the test had differentiated patients with frontal lesions from patients with focal lesions in other brain areas or patients with diffuse brain damage delineated the impact of differing antisocial inclusion criteria (Morgan & Lilienfeld 2000). Overall, antisocial groups performed 0.62 standard deviations worse on executive function tests than controls. Significantly, larger effect sizes were seen when crime/ delinquency was the inclusion criteria rather than ASP/CD or psychopathy.

The primacy of verbal cognitive deficits has also been brought into question. Cross-sectional studies support the view that there are verbal, but not spatial, cognitive deficits in antisocial groups (Rutter et al. 1998; Raine 1993; Moffit 1993). In the Morgan & Lilenfeld (2000) meta-analysis of executive function tests and antisocial behavior the largest effect size (d = .8) was seen for a visuospatial measure

(Porteus Mazes) whereas a verbal measure (word fluency) showed a small effect size (d = .26). Until recently studies had not examined which came first. A recent population-based study assessed verbal and spatial abilities at ages 3 and 11 in 330 children whose antisocial behavior was assessed at ages 8 and 17 (Raine et al. 2002). Persistently antisocial individuals had spatial deficits, in the absence of verbal deficits at age 3, independent of social adversity, early hyperactivity, test motivation, or comprehension. This suggests early spatial deficits, as assessed by block assembly and copying shapes, are a precursor to delinquent behavior whereas the verbal deficits may be developmentally acquired or represent a later unfolding of latent neuropathology. Verbal deficits were seen at age 11 but not age 3. Persistent spatial cognitive deficits were specific to persistently antisocial individuals; the childhood limited and adolescent-onset antisocial groups did not show this finding.

COURSE AND PROGNOSIS

Although childhood conduct disturbance is common, it persists into adulthood in only about one third of cases (Rutter 1989). In contrast, ASP is almost always preceded by CD in childhood (Robins 1966, 1978). Thus, the presence of conduct disturbance in childhood is not in itself predictive of chronicity. Moran reports a prevalence rate of antisocial personality disorder between 2 and 3% in the general adult population (1999). Study data on longitudinal course are influenced by the defining characteristics of the sample studied. Clinic-based samples usually differ in important ways from those collected epidemiologically. Thus, care must be taken when generalizing across studies. As previously noted, aggression and delinquency are concepts that overlap with CD but are not synonymous with it. Nonetheless, longitudinal studies of these behavioral dimensions yield information important to our understanding of CD.

Rates of psychiatric comorbidity with CD are known to be high, and may in part explain the significant functional impairment in children with CD. As such, understanding the nature and longitudinal course of comorbidity may be helpful in recognizing and treating children with CD. Six waves of structured diagnostic assessments over a period of seven years in a group of 168 clinic-referred boys, revealed a parallel longitudinal relationship between conduct disorder behaviors and symptoms of ODD, ADHD, depression, and anxiety (Lahey et al. 2002). CD and ODD behaviors were found to be symmetrically associated, in that early CD symptoms presaged ODD symptoms in later waves and vice-versa. In contrast, the CD behavior association with ADHD, depression, and anxiety symptoms was asymmetric. Early high symptom levels of ADHD, depression, and anxiety did not presage high levels of CD behaviors in later waves, though high early levels of CD did presage later high symptom levels of ADHD, depression, and anxiety. The results support the notion that ODD symptoms are often seen as a precursor to later CD symptoms. In a group of 4,500 children, the Great Smoky Mountains Study examined models of the relationship between ODD and CD (Rowe et al. 2002). Over four waves of data collection, ODD was a strong risk factor for CD among boys but not girls.

The landmark study of CD outcome was Lee Robins's longterm follow-up of children who attended a St. Louis, Missouri, child guidance clinic in the 1920s and 1930s (Robins 1966). This study made the important observation that persistence of CD was predicted not by any one specific CD symptom but rather by the quantity of symptoms.

DSM-IV includes subtypes of CD based on age of onset (age 10 or younger versus age 11 or older). These subgroups differ markedly in level of physical aggression: those with early-onset CD are more likely to exhibit aggression than those with late-onset CD (Lahey et al. 1998). Evidence suggests a relatively early onset of CD among boys with ADHD (Biederman et al. 1996; Hinshaw et al. 1993).

Community-based studies in New Zealand (McGee et al. 1992) and Canada (Offord et al. 1992) have provided data on the shorter-term course of CD. In the Canadian study, close to half (45%) of the children with CD at age 4 to 12 years still had CD when followed up 4 years later (Offord et al. 1992). Moreover, the presence of CD also predicted emotional disorder at follow-up in 29% of subjects. Four-year follow-up of the New Zealand birth cohort revealed that the presence of a disruptive behavior disorder (CD, oppositional defiant disorder, or hyperactivity) at age 11 years predicted a disruptive behavior disorder at age 15 years for boys *but not for girls* (McGee et al. 1992).

Childhood-onset aggression is a significantly stable characteristic (Farrington 1991; Loeber 1991; Olweus 1979) that has considerable prognostic import both within CD and for a broad range of (overlapping) poor outcomes: subsequent aggression (Huessmann and Eron 1984; Loney et al. 1981; Pfeffer et al. 1983), illegal drug involvement (Farrington 1991; Loney et al. 1981), criminal activity (Douglas 1966; Ensminger et al. 1983; Farrington 1991; Feldhusen et al. 1976; Huessmann and Eron 1984; Morris et al. 1956; Stattin and Magnusson 1989; Farrington 1991). A significant limitation is the paucity of data on the outcome of aggressive behavior in girls; almost all of the available information derives from studies of males (Offord & Bennett 1994). Early pregnancy and adult diagnosis of antisocial personality disorder are known potential outcomes of girls with CD (Bardone et al. 1996; Kovacs et al. 1994; Robins et al. 1991; Zoccolillo and Rogers 1991).

INTERVENTION

Prevention

Prevention of CD appears to require very early intervention (Webster-Stratton & Taylor 2001). Because pediatric behavioral disturbances have been associated with low birth weight, prematurity, obstetric complications, physical

TABLE 12.3
INTERVENTION FOR CONDUCT DISORDER

1. Thorough assessment using multiple information sources with special attention to risk and resiliency factors. Identify all significant problems. Address severity and course both in terms of past history and of future risk.
2. Identify strength and resilience factors in the environment as well as within the individual to mobilize and build upon for treatment. Consider the fit of the behavior within its environmental context.
3. Identify all significant problem domains and plan for each of them. Prioritize impact.
4. Mobilize, strengthen and support parenting of the youth.
5. Address supervision and behavioral management needs.
6. Treat comorbidity.
7. Consider pharmacotherapy as an adjunct for certain targeted behaviors (e.g. affective aggression).

Source: Adapted from AACAP practice parameters for Conduct Disorder (Steiner et al, 1997)

anomalies, maternal illness, child maltreatment, poor nutritional status, parental substance use, weak or harsh parenting, and maternal rejection it is logical that efforts to minimize such risks may help prevent CD. Home visitation is an instructive example. Early childhood home visitation programs have parents and their children visited in home by trained personnel during the first 2 years of the child's life. Support, information or training about child development, health and care are the usual elements. Review of 21 studies found home visitation of young mothers reduced child maltreatment by about 40% compared to controls, but insufficient evidence was available to determine the effectiveness in preventing violence by the children who had been visited (Hahn et al. 2003).

Intervention

Broad guidelines for the treatment of conduct disorder are presented in Table 12.3 as adapted from the American Academy of Child and Adolescent Psychiatry's Practice Parameters (AACAP 1997), the Surgeon Generals Report on Mental Health (US Dept of Health and Human Services 1999), and Vermont State Interagency Team recommendations for treatment of Conduct Disorder (McMains et al. 2003).

Psychosocial Intervention

Psychosocial interventions are first line treatments that must address a wide array of features, including CD symptoms, comorbid diagnoses, other concurrent problems, and the context in which the child lives. A spectrum of interventions may be needed, depending on the severity of the disorder, the individual's response to less intense treatment, and the risk he or she presents to self, others, and the community. Wide-ranging intervention strategies have

been termed *multimodal* or *multisystemic*, indicating that a variety of therapeutic modalities are to be applied to a range of systems that relate to or interface with the child (Henggeler et al. 1998).

Interventions for CD in pediatric age groups take advantage of the fact that CD is more environmentally responsive than adult ASP (Cadoret et al. 1995; Lyons et al. 1995; Reiss et al. 1995). Among the components of CD interventions, efforts that support parenting and behavioral monitoring/treatment are a mainstay. A review (Brestan & Eyberg 1998) entitled "Effective psychosocial treatments for conduct-disordered children and adolescents: 29 years, 82 studies and 5,272 kids" found two interventions that met criteria as having well-established efficacy, parent training programs based on Patterson & Guillon's manual *Living with Children* (1968) and videotaped modeling parent training (Webster-Stratton 1984). Parent management training focuses upon training parents to both develop and implement contingency management programs. Such programs involve establishing clear behavioral goals, reinforcing steps in the direction of the goals and providing consequences for inappropriate behavior. Parent management training programs also seek to improve the quality (and sometimes the quantity) of parent child interaction, supervision and monitoring. As seen in Table 12.4, much of the practical advice for conduct disorder management in primary care settings (Searight et al. 2001) reflects contingency management and parent education.

Subsequent review of more than 500 programs designed to treat and prevent youth antisocial behavior found just 3 that reduced adolescent criminal behavior (Mihalic et al. 2001). All three are manualized family-based ecological

TABLE 12.4
PRACTICAL INTERVENTIONS FOR MANAGEMENT OF PATIENTS WITH CONDUCT DISORDER IN PRIMARY CARE

Assess severity and refer for treatment with a subspecialist as needed.

Describe the likely longterm prognosis without intervention to caregiver.

Structure children's activities and implement consistent behavior guidelines.

Emphasize parental monitoring of children's activities (where they are, who they are with). Encourage the enforcement of curfews.

Encourage children's involvement in structured and supervised peer activities (e.g., organized sports, Scouting).

Discuss and demonstrate clear and specific parental communication techniques.

Help caregivers establish appropriate rewards for desirable behavior.

Help establish realistic, clearly communicated consequences for noncompliance.

Help establish daily routine of child-directed play activity with parent(s).

Source: Adapted from Searight et al, 2001.

TABLE 12.5

COMMON PROPERTIES OF 3 TREATMENTS WHICH DECREASED CRIMINAL BEHAVIOR IN ADOLESCENCE

—Treatment planning is informed by the science base about risk factors and tailored to the youth and family's social ecology. E.g. All seek to limit contact with antisocial peers, to increase family monitoring, to use behavioral techniques to structure home and school settings and to increase prosocial contact and activities.
—Engaging the family in treatment is a necessary step
—Once engagement has occurred, parent training and behavioral techniques are utilized to push behavioral change
—Generalization is a later step which seeks to integrate indigenous resources
—Manualized treatment delivered by trained therapists accompanied by quality assurance and treatment fidelity methodology

Source: Adapted from Henggeler & Sheidow,

models: multisystemic therapy (MST) (Henggeler et al. 1998); functional family therapy (Alexander et al. 1998) and mutidimensional treatment foster care (Chamberlain & Mihalic 1998). Elements common to the three treatments are outlined in Table 12.5.

Supervision, monitoring and behavioral management interventions for youth with CD can involve systems or settings beyond a parental home. Levels of intervention have been outlined for the treatment of acute psychiatric illness and follow a general principal of "least restrictive" setting ranging from general outpatient treatment up to hospitalization (APA & AACAP 1997). Some recent data support the least restrictive concept. A trial comparing traditional inpatient hospitalization to multisystemic therapy (MST) for youth referred for psychiatric hospitalization found MST was more effective at decreasing youths' externalizing symptoms and improving their family functioning and school attendance four months after randomization (Henggeler et al. 1999). However, even with intensive treatment and commitment to family collaboration, hospitalization, or therapeutic foster care may be needed (Henggeler et al. 1999). Therapeutic foster care involves placement of youth in homes with foster parents trained to provide a structured environment that supports the child learning social and emotional skills. Some data suggest therapeutic foster care can reduce violence by chronically delinquent adolescents (Hahn et al. 2004). One randomized controlled trial assessed the effects of therapeutic foster care, which included active collaboration with program personnel on a daily basis, with group home placement using reported felony assaults as an outcome measure (Chamberlain & Reid 1998). Program intensive therapeutic foster care reduced felony assaults by 73%. Subsequent analysis of data from that study found that family management skills (discipline, supervision, and a positive adult child relationship) and deviant peer association explained 32% of the variance in outcome (Eddy & Chamberlain 2000).

Analyses of the ecological family-based treatments for juvenile delinquents discussed above are very encouraging in terms of cost effectiveness (Aos et al. 2001; Miller and Levy 2000). However, caveats exist. One limitation is that many studies involve conduct *problems* rather than address those individuals meeting full criteria for CD. Only 28% of studies Brestan & Eyberg (1998) reviewed included subjects meeting DSM criteria for *CD or oppositional defiant disorder*. There are studies that include clinically severe "real world" samples. For example, the Multisystemic Treatment (MST) studies of Henggeler et al. (1999, 2002) treat substance abusing delinquents or youth presenting for psychiatric hospitalization. Results of MST are encouraging and consistent with the Surgeon General's recommended treatment emphases (i.e., family-focused, attending to multiple determinants of problems, and strength based) (USPHS 2001). Four randomized trials demonstrated the capacity of MST to achieve improved longterm (> 2 year) outcomes (Henggeler et al. 2003). However, assuming the results generalize to those with the DSM-IV conduct disorder diagnosis or to predominantly mental health populations is likely to be unfair. In the study of MST as an alternative to hospitalization, 33 of 109 subjects had caregiver DISC interviews meeting criteria for conduct disorder (Henggeler et al. 1999). Thus, the bulk of subjects in that study did not meet CD criteria.

Treatment of comorbid conditions is a logical part of conduct disorder/aggression treatment algorithms (Kruesi & Lelio 1996; Pappadopulous et al. 2003; Kutcher et al. 2004), but may or may not impact CD symptoms. For example, a controlled trial of cognitive behavioral therapy (CBT) for depression in 93 adolescents with depression and conduct disorder found that CBT improved Beck depression scores post treatment but did not improve CD (Rohde et al. 2004). In contrast, 11 of 13 prepubertal boys with comorbid CD and depression had improvement in their conduct disorders when their depression went into remission (Puig-Antich et al. 1982). Although there is some uncertainty about the degree to which treatment of comorbid conditions impacts conduct disorder, there is a definite deleterious impact of psychiatric comorbidity upon the treatment of delinquents. The lasting results seen in the juvenile justice based samples treated with MST were not found to persist in a psychiatric population (Henggeler et al. 2003).

Psychopharmacologic Interventions

Currently, there are no United States Food and Drug Administration (FDA) approved medication indications for conduct disorder. Despite the salience of violence and the suffering it causes, there is comparatively little investigation of pharmacologic intervention for aggression and inquiry has often been limited by meager financial support and stalled by political concerns (Enserink, 2000, Kruesi, in press). However, many readers may be surprised to note that chlorpromazine carries a long-standing FDA indication for "the treatment of severe behavioral problems in children (1 to 12 years of age) marked by combativeness and/or explosive hyperexcitable behavior" (FDA Web-site, www.fda.gov). Traditionally, pharmacological approaches to conduct disorder have focused on comorbid conditions, such as ADHD or affective disorders, or on specific target symptoms that mimic symptomatology of other disorders. The most well-studied classes of medications for use in CD include the mood stabilizers, neuroleptics, and stimulants.

Mood Stabilizers

Evidence for the utility of mood stabilizers in aggression/conduct disorder is gradually growing. Lithium has been a treatment for adult bipolar disorder for several decades. Since manic aggression responds to lithium, it has been proposed that aggression associated with conduct disorder may also respond to this medication. Thus far, three placebo-controlled trials, including a combined total of 151 subjects, have yielded positive results (Campbell et al. 1984; Campbell et al. 1995, Malone et al. 2000). However, Rifkin and colleagues observed no separation from placebo for lithium among 33 adolescent inpatients with CD (1997). Additionally, problems with compliance as well as the potential for significant adverse effects and toxicity may limit lithium's use among youths with CD.

Donovan and colleagues have investigated the use of divalproex among children with disruptive behaviors. An open trial among ten subjects (1997) and a double blind, placebo-controlled study among twenty youths (2000) revealed positive results. Steiner and colleagues conducted a seven-week randomized, controlled trial of divalproex in seventy-one youths with CD, noting significant symptom improvement among those receiving a dose usually associated with the therapeutic range for anticonvulsant usage (2003). Divalproex was well tolerated by the subjects in these studies. While these initial results are encouraging, further study must be undertaken to further elucidate the role of divalproex in treating CD.

Carbamazepine appeared effective in an open study among subjects with temper outbursts (Mattes 1990) and in controlled trials among youths with aggression and impulsivity (Groh 1976; Puente 1976), but was not superior to placebo in a double-blind study of twenty-two children with aggressive CD (Cueva et al. 1996).

Neuroleptics

Neuroleptics are considered a treatment of later resort in patients with CD because of their potential side effects (Pappadopoulos et al. 2003; Schur et al. 2003; Kruesi & Lelio 1996). However, available evidence suggests neuroleptics will decrease some aggression. Pimozide, a neuroleptic, was effective in a study of ten children with antisocial behavior (Broche 1980). The typical neuroleptics haloperidol, thioridazine, and molindone were superior to placebo among inpatient CD patients (Campbell et al. 1984; Greenhill et al. 1985), though the potential for adverse events, including movement disorders, limits the use of typical neuroleptics among youths. Recent investigation of risperidone, an atypical neuroleptic, in CD (Buitelaar et al. 2001; Ercan et al. 2003; Findling et al. 2000) and in disruptive behavior among youth with subaverage intelligence (Aman et al. 2002; Snyder et al. 2002) have yielded positive results. Risperidone was generally well tolerated and likely poses less risk for movement disorders than typical neuroleptics. An open trial of olanzapine, another atypical neuroleptic, yielded improvement among six aggressive youths (Soderstrom et al. 2002). Further study of atypical neuroleptics may elucidate their role in treatment of CD. At present, risperidone appears particularly promising given its expanding evidence base. Caution is indicated, though, as atypical neuroleptics have increased risk for obesity, diabetes and dyslipidemia (American Diabetes Association 2004).

Stimulants and atomoxetine

Stimulants and atomoxetine have FDA approved indications for ADHD. Given the frequent comorbidity of conduct or oppositional defiant disorders with ADHD (which may be as high as 80% in clinical samples (Abikoff & Klein 1992), stimulants have been investigated in youths with both diagnoses, with generally positive results (Gadow et al. 1990; Hinshaw et al. 1992; Kaplan et al. 1990; Klein et al. 1997; Kolko et al. 1999). Of note, one third of the subjects in the study conducted by Klein and colleagues met criteria for CD but not ADHD. Interestingly, these subjects exhibited positive effects, which may indicate a role for stimulant treatment in CD without ADHD. Similarly encouraging are the results of a meta-analysis of stimulant effects on aggressive behaviors in ADHD, which revealed effect sizes similar to those for the core symptoms of ADHD (Connor et al. 2002). But, a recent trial of pemoline in conduct disorder youth found that although ADHD symptoms improved, CD did not (Riggs et al. 2004).

Other agents

Controlled studies with other agents are lacking. Antidepressants may play a role in treatment, given the frequent comorbidity between CD and affective disorders. An open trial of fluoxetine in eight adolescents with major depression, CD, and substance use disorder yielded positive results (Riggs et al. 1997). Some children have had uncomfortable side effects with fluoxetine (Riddle et al. 1991). Safety and tolerability in children is reflected in both its FDA approval for treatment of childhood depression and its FDA public health advisory about the possibility of increased suicidality (http://www.fda.gov/cder/drug/antidepressants/AntidepressanstPHA.htm). Open trials of trazodone among aggressive inpatient youths also revealed symptom improvement (Ghaziuddin and Alessi 1992; Zubieta and Alessi 1992). Clonidine, and alpha-adrenergic agonist often used as an adjunctive agent in ADHD, was effective in reducing aggression in open studies (Hunt et al. 1986; Jaselskis et al. 1992; Kemph et al. 1993). Additionally, a pilot study investigated clonidine and methylphenidate, each alone or in combination, among three randomized groups of eight male children with ADHD and comorbid aggressive oppositional defiant or conduct disorder, revealing significant improvements in oppositional and conduct disordered symptoms (Connor et al. 2000).

Summary and Conclusions

Our neuropsychiatric understanding and appreciation of conduct disorder grows and the time to cease confusing conduct disorder, psychopathy, delinquency and aggression has arrived. The disorder appears to involve frontal and temporal brain regions and may also be expressed in structural, autonomic, and reproductive features.

Recognition of the enormous impact of conduct disorder/sociopathy is in its beginning stages. Knowledge of the evolutionary fit of the disorder is primitive. But as a society, we need to recognize that mistreatment of children (e.g. abuse, neglect, and prenatal malnutrition) increases the risk for and perhaps the prevalence of conduct disorder/ASP (Jaffee et al. 2004). Genetic influences are present whether conduct disorder/sociopathy, delinquency/crime, aggression, and/or psychopathy are the behavioral outcomes of interest. Interactions of the environment and genes as well as gene–gene interactions are receiving increasing recognition for their relevance to conduct disorder/sociopathy. But, the mechanisms remain elusive.

Conduct disorders are heterogeneous. Evidence mounts that parsing psychopathy, particularly the callous-unemotional dimension from CD, will be useful in increasing our understanding and in designing better interventions.

REFERENCES

Abikoff H, Klein RG. Attention-deficit hyperactivity and conduct disorder: co-morbidity and implications for treatment. J Consult Clin Psychol 1992; 60:881–92.

Achenbach, TM, and Edelbrock, CS. Manual for the Child Behavior Checklist and Revised Child Behavior Profile. Burlington, VT: University of Vermont, 1983.

Alexander RC, Breslin N, Molnar C, Richter J, et al. Counterclockwise scalp hair whorl in schizophrenia. Biol Psychiatry 1992 32:842–5.

Alexander JF, Parsons BV. Short-term behavioral intervention with delinquent families: impact on family process and recidivism. J Abnorm Psychol 1973; 81:219–225.

Aman MG, De Smedt G, Derivan A, et al. Double-blind, placebo-controlled study of risperidone for the treatment of disruptive behaviors in children with subaverage intelligence. Am J Psychiatry 2002; 159:1337–46.

American Academy of Child and Adolescent Psychiatry. Practice parameters for the assessment and treatment of children and adolescents with conduct disorder. J Am Acad Child Adolesc Psychiatry. 1997;36(suppl):122–39.

Ary DV, Duncan TE, Biglan A, Metzler CW, Noell JW, Smolkowski K. Development of adolescent problem behavior. J Abnorm Child Psychol 1999; 27:141–50.

Awad IA, Johnson PC, Spetzler RF, Hodak JA. Incidental subcortical lesions identified on magnetic resonance imaging in the elderly. II. Postmortem pathological correlations. Stroke 1986 17:1090–1097.

Bagley C, Bolitho F, Bertrand L. Mental health profiles, suicidal behavior, and community sexual assault in 2112 Canadian adolescents. Crisis 1995;16:126–31.

Bardone AM, Moffitt T, Caspi A, Dickson N. Adult mental health and social outcomes of adolescent girls with depression and conduct disorder. Dev Psychopathol 1996; 8:811–29.

Bardone AM, Moffitt TE, Caspi A, Dickson N, Stanton WR, Silva PA. Adult physical health outcomes of adolescent girls with conduct disorder, depression, and anxiety. J Am Acad Child Adolesc Psychiatry 1998; 37:594–601.

Barratt ES, Stanford MS, Dowdy, L, Liebman, MJ, Kent, TA. Impulsive and premeditated aggression: a factor analysis of self-reported acts. Psychiatry Res 1999; 86:163–173.

Bauer LO, Hesselbrock VM. Brain maturation and subtypes of conduct disorder: interactive effects on p300 amplitude and topography in make adolescents. J Am Acad Child Adolesc Psychiatry 2003; 42:106–15.

Bear DM, and Fedio P. Quantitative analysis of interictal behavior in temporal lobe epilepsy. Arch. Neural 34: 454–467.

Bennett KJ, Brown KS, Boyle M, Racine Y, Offord D. Does low reading achievement at school entry cause conduct problems? Soc Sci Med 2003; 56:2443–8.

Blair RJR. Neurobiological basis of psychopathy. Brit J Psychiatry 2003; 182:5–7.

Blonigen DM, Carlson SR, Krueger RF, Patrick CJ. A twin study of self-reported psychopathic personality traits. Pers Individ Diff 2003; 35:179–197.

Brennan PA, Gretkin ER, Mednick SA. Maternal smoking during pregnancy and adult male criminal outcomes. Arch Gen Psychiatry 1999; 56:215–9.

Brestan EV, Eyberg SM. Effective Psychosocial Treatments of Conduct-Disordered Children and Adolescents: 29 Years, 82 Studies, and 5,272 Kids. J Clin Child Psychol 1998; 27:180–189.

Breteler MM, van Amerongen NM, van Swieten JC, Claus JJ, Grobbee DE, can Gijn J, et al. Cognitive correlates of ventricular enlargement and cerebral white matter lesions on magnetic resonance imaging. The Rotterdam Study. Stroke 1994;25:1109–1115.

Breton JJ, Bergeron L, Valla JP, et al. Quebec child mental health survey: prevalence of DSM-III-R mental health disorders. J Child Psychol Psychiatry 1999; 40:375–84.

Broche JP. Use of pimozide (ORAP) in child psychiatry. Acta Psychiatr Belg 1980; 80:341–6.

Buitelaar JK, van der Gaag RJ, Cohen-Kettenis P, Melman CTM. A randomized controlled trial of risperidone in the treatment of aggression in hospitalized adolescents with subaverage cognitive abilities. J Clin Psychiatry 2001; 62:239–48.

Cadoret RJ, Yates WR, Troughton E, et al. Genetic-environmental interaction in the genesis of aggressivity and conduct disorders. Arch Gen Psychiatry 1995; 52:916–24.

Campbell M, Adams PB, Small AM, et al. Lithium in hospitalized aggressive children with conduct disorder: a double-blind and placebo-controlled study. J Am Acad Child Adolesc Psychiatry. 1995; 34:445–53.

Campbell M, Small AM, Green WH, et al. Behavioral efficacy of haloperidol and lithium carbonate: a comparison in hospitalized aggressive children with conduct disorder. Arch Gen Psychiatry 1984; 41:650–6.

Castellanos FX, Elia J, Kruesi MJ, Gulotta CS, Mefford IN, Potter WZ, Ritchie GF, and Rapoport JL. Cerebrospinal fluid monoamine metabolites in boys with attention-deficit hyperactivity disorder. Psychiatry Res 1994; 52:305–316.

Chilcoat HD, Breslau N. Pathways from ADHD to Early Drug Use. 1999; J Am Acad ChildAdolesc Psychiatry 1999; 38:1347–1354.

Cohen P, Cohen J, Kasen S, et al. An epidemiological study of disorders in late childhood and adolescence, I: age and gender-specific prevalence. J Child Psychol Psychiatry 1993; 34:851–67.

Comings DE, Gade-Andavolu R, Gonzales N et al. Comparison of the role of dopamine, serotonin, and noradrenaline genes in ADHD, ODD and conduct disorder: multivariate regression analysis of 20 genes. Clin Gene 2000a; 57:178–196.

Comings DE, Gade-Andavolu R, Gonzales N et al. Multivariate analysis of associations of 42 genes in ADHD, ODD, and conduct disorder. Clin Gene 2000b; 58:31–40.

Compton WM, Cottler LB, Shillington AM, Price RK. Is antisocial personality disorder associated with increased HIV risk behaviors in cocaine users? Drug Alcohol Depend 1995; 37:34–43.

Connor DF, Barkley RA, Davis HT. A pilot study of methylphenidate, clonidine, or the combination in ADHD comorbid with aggressive oppositional defiant or conduct disorder. Clin Pediatr 2000; 39:15–25.

Critchley HD, Simmons A, Daly EM, Russell A, van Amelsvoort T, Robertson DM, Glover A, and Murphy DGM. Prefrontal and medial temporal correlates of repetitive violence to self and others. Biol Psychiatry 2000.

Cueva JE, Overall JE, Small AM, et al. Carbamazepine in aggressive children with conduct disorder: a double-blind and placebo-controlled study. J Am Acad Child Adolesc Psychiatry 1996; 35: 480–90.

Damasio H, Grabowski T, Frank R, Galaburda A, Damasio AR. The return of Phineas Gage: clues about the brain from a skull of a patient. Science 1994;264:1102–1105.

Dishion TJ, McCord J, Poulin F. When Interventions harm. Peer groups and problem behavior. Am Psychol 1999; 54:755–64.

Dmitrieva TN, Oades RD, Hauffa BP, Eggers C. Dehydroepiandrosterone sulphate and corticotropin levels are high in young male patients with conduct disorder: comparisons for growth factors, thyroid and gonadal hormones. Neuropsychobiology 2001; 43:134–40.

Dodge KA, and Coie JD. 1987: Social information processing factors in reactive and proactive aggression in children's peer groups. J Pers Soc Psychol 1987; 53:1146–1158.

Dolan, M. Psychopathy—A neurobiological perspective. Br J Psychiatry 1994; 165:151–159.

Dolan MC, Anderson IM. The relationship between serotonergic function and the Psychopathy Checklist: Screening Verson. J Psychopharmacol 2003; 17:216–22.

Donovan S, Stewart J, Nunes EV, et al. Divalproex treatment for youth with explosive temper and mood lability: a double-blind, placebo-controlled crossover design. Am J Psychiatry 2000; 157:818–20.

Donovan SJ, Susser ES, Nunes EV, et al. Divalproex treatment of disruptive adolescents: a report of 10 cases. J Clin Psychiatry 1997; 58:12–15.

Douglas JWB. The school progress of nervous and troublesome children. Br J Psychiatry 1966; 112:1115–6.

Enserink, M. Searching for the mark of Cain. Science 2000; 289:575–579.

Ensminger ME, Kellam SG, Rubin BR. School and family origins of delinquency: comparison by sex. In: van Dusen, K, Mednick, S, eds. Prospective Studies of Crime and Delinquency. The Hague, Netherlands: Kluwer-Niehoff, 1983, pp. 73–97.

Epps P, Parnell R. Physique and temperament of women delinquents compared with women undergraduates. Br J Med Psychol 1952; 25:249–55.

Ercan ES, Kutlu A, Cikoglu S, et al. Risperidone in children and adolescents with conduct disorder: a single-center, open-label study. Curr Ther Res 2003; 64:55–64.

Esser G, Schmidt MH, Woerner W. Epidemiology and course of psychiatric disorders in schoolage children: results of a longitudinal study. J Child Psychol Psychiatry 1990; 31:243–63.

Fabiani M, Gratton G, Coles MGH. Event-related brain potentials. Methods, theory and application. In: Cacioppo JT, Tassinary LG and Bernston GG, eds. Handbook of Psychophysiology. 2nd Ed. Cambridge, UK: Cambridge University Press, 2000.

Farrington DP. Childhood aggression and adult violence: early precursors and later-life outcomes. In: Pepler DJ, Rubin KH, eds. The Development and Treatment of Childhood Aggression. Hillsdale, NJ: Lawrence Erlbaum, 1991, pp 189–197.

Farrington DP. Early predictors of adolescent aggression and adult violence. Violence Vict 1989; 4:79–100.

Feehan M, McGee R, Raja SN, Williams SM. DSM-III-R disorders in New Zealand 18-year-olds. Aust N Z J Psychiatry 1994; 28:87–99.

Feldhusen JF, Aversano FM, Thurston JR. Prediction of youth contacts with law enforcement agencies. Crim Justice Behav 1976; 2:235–53.

Fergusson DM and Lynskey MT. Early reading difficulties and later conduct problems. J Child Psychol Psychiatry 1997; 38:899–907.

Fergusson DM, Horwood J, Lynskey MT. Maternal smoking before and after pregnancy: effects on behavioral outcomes in middle childhood. Pediatrics 1993; 92:815–22.

Fergusson DM, Woodward LJ, Horwood J. Maternal smoking during pregnancy and psychiatric adjustment in late adolescence. Arch Gen Psychiatry 1998; 55:721–7.

Findling RL, McNamara NK, Braniky LA, et al. A double-blind pilot study of risperidone in the treatment of conduct disorder. J Am Acad Child Psychiatry 2000; 39:509–16.

Frick PJ, Cornell AH, Barry CT, Bodin SD, Dane HE. Callous-unemotional traits and conduct problems in the prediction of conduct proble severity, aggression, and self-report of delinquency. J Abnorm Child Psychol 2003; 31:457–70.

Furlow B, Gangestad SW, Armijo-Prewitt T. Developmental stability and human violence. Proc R Soc of Lond B Biol Sci 1998; 265:1–6.

Gadow KC, Nolan EE, Sverd J, et al. Methylphenidate in aggressive-hyperactive boys: I. Effects on peer aggression in public school settings. J Am Acad Child Adolesc Psychiatry 1990; 29:710–718.

Galli V, McElroy SL, Soutullo CA, Kizer D, Raute N, Keck PE Jr, McConville BJ. The psychiatric diagnoses of twenty-two adolescents who have sexually molested other children.Compr Psychiatry 1999; 40(11):85–8.

Gangestad SW, Yeo RA. Parental handedness and relative hand skill: a test of the developmental instability hypothesis. Neuropsychology 1994; 8:572–578.

Ghaziuddin N, Alessi N. An open clinical trial of trazodone in aggressive children. J Child Adolesc Psychopharmacol. 1992; 2:291–8.

Ghodesian-Carpey, J, Baker LA. Genetic and environmental influences on aggression in 4- to 7-year-old twins. Aggressive Beh 1987; 13:173.

Gill K, Nolimal D, Crowley TJ. Antisocial personality disorder, HIV risk behavior and retention in methadone maintenance therapy. Drug Alcohol Depend 30:247–252, 1992.

Glueck S, Glueck E. Physique and Delinquency. New York: Harper, 1956.

Greenhill LL, Solomon M, Pleak R, Ambrosini P. Molindone hydrochloride treatment of hospitalized children with conduct disorder. J Clin Psychiatry 1985; 46:20–25.

Groh C. The psychotropic effect of Tegretol in nonepileptic children, with particular reference to the drug's indications. In: Birkmayer W, ed. Epileptic Seizures-Behavior-Pain. Bern, Switzerland: Hans Huber, 1976, pp 259–263.

Hare RD. Without conscience: The disturbing world of the psychopaths among us. New York: Pocket Books 1993.

Hart SD, Hare RD. Psychopathy and antisocial personality disorder. 1996; Curr Opin Psychiatry 9:129–132

Harpending HC, Sobus J. Sociopathy as an adaptation. Ethol Sociobiol 1987; 8:63S–72S.

Henggeler SW, Rowland MD, Halliday-Boykins C, Sheidow AJ, Ward DM, Randall J, Pickrel SG, Cunningham PB, & Edwards J. One-year follow-up of multisystemic therapy as an alternative to the hospitalization of youths in psychiatric crisis. J Am Acad Child Adolesc Psychiatry, 2003; 42, 543–551.

Henggeler SW, Schoenwald SK, Borduin CM, Rowland MD, Cunningham PB. Multisystemic treatment of antisocial behavior in children and adolescents. New York: The Guildford Press, 1998.

Hinshaw SP. Externalizing behaviour problems and academic underachievement in childhood and adolescence: causal relationships and underlying mechanisms. Psychol Bull 1992; 111:127–155.

Hinshaw SP, Heller T, McHale JP. Covert antisocial behavior in boys with attention-deficit hyperactivity disorder: external validation and effects of methylphenidate. J Consult Clin Psychol 1992; 60: 274–81.

Huessmann LR, Eron LD. Cognitive processes and the persistence of aggressive behavior. Aggressive Beh 1984; 10:243–51.

Hunt R, Minderaa R, Cohen D. The therapeutic effect of clonidine in attention deficit disorder with hyperactivity: a comparison with placebo and methylphenidate. Psychopharmacol Bull. 1986; 22: 229–36.

Ishikawa SS, Raine A, Lencz T, Bihrle S, LaCasse L. Increased height and bulk in antisocial personality disorder and its subtypes. Psychiatry Res 2001; 105:211–19.

Jaffee SR, Caspi A, Moffitt TE, Taylor A. Physical maltreatment victim to antisocial child: evidence of an environmentally mediated process. J Abnorm Psychol 2004;113:44–55.

Jaselskis C, Cook E, Fletcher K, et al. Clonidine treatment of hyperactive and impulsive children with autistic disorder. J Clin Psychopharmacol 1992; 12:322–7.

Kaplan SL, Busner J, Kupietz S, et al. Effects of methylphenidate on adolescents with aggressive conduct disorder and ADHD: a preliminary report. J Am Acad Child Adolesc Psychiatry. 1990; 29:719–23.

Keenan K, Wakschlag LS. Can a valid diagnosis of disruptive behavior disorder be made in preschool children? Am J Psychiatry 2002; 159:351–358.

Kemph J, DeVane C, Levin G, et al. Treatment of aggressive children with clonidine: results of an open pilot study. J Am Acad Child Adolesc Psychiatry 1993; 33:35–44.

Kessler RC, Berglund PA, Foster CL, Saunders WB, Stang PE, Walters EE. Social consequences of psychiatric disorders, II: Teenage parenthood. Am J Psychiatry 1997;154:1405–11.

Kiehl, KA, Smith AM, Hare RD, Mendrek A, Forster BB, Brink J, Liddle PF. Limbic abnormalities in affective processing by criminal psychopaths as revealed by functional magnetic resonance imaging. Biol Psychiatry 2001; 50: 677–684.

Klein RG, Abikoff H, Klass E, et al. Clinical efficacy of methylphenidate in conduct disorder with and without attention deficit hyperactivity disorder. Arch Gen Psychiatry 1997; 54:1073–80.

Kolko DJ, Bukstein OG, Barron J. Methylphenidate and behavior modification in children with ADHD and comorbid ODD or CD: main and incremental effects across settings. J Am Acad Child Adolesc Psychiatry 1999; 38:578–86.

Kovacs M, Krol RSM, Voti L. Early onset psychopathology and the risk for teenage pregnancy among clinically referred girls. J Am Acad Child Adolesc Psychiatry 1994; 33:106–113.

Krueger RF, Moffitt TE, Caspi A, Bleske A, Silva PA. Assortative mating for antisocial behavior: developmental and methodological implications.: Behav Genet 1998;28:173–86.

Kruesi MJP, Swedo SE, Leonard HL, et al. CSF somatostatin in childhood psychiatric disorders: a preliminary investigation. Psychiatry Res 1990; 33:277–84.

Kruesi, MJP, Rapoport, JL, Hamburger, S, Hibbs, E, Potter, WZ, Lenane, M, and Brown, GL. Cerebrospinal fluid monoamine metabolites, aggression, and impulsivity in disruptive behavior disorders of children and adolescents. Arch. Gen. Psychiatry 1990; 47:419–426.

Kruesi MJP, Hibbs ED, Zahn TP, Keysor CS, Hamburger SD, Bartko JJ, and Rapoport JL. A 2-year prospective follow-up study of children and adolescents with disruptive behavior disorders: prediction by cerebrospinal fluid 5-hydroxyindoleacetic acid, homovanillic acid, and autonomic measures. Arch. Gen. Psychiatry 1992; 49:429–435.

Kruesi MJP, Jacobsen T. Serontonin and human violence: do environmental mediators exist? In: Raine A, Farrington D, Brennan P, Mednick SA, eds. Biosocial Bases of Violence. New York: Plenum, 1997, pp 189–205.

Kruesi MJP, Keller S, Wagner MW. Neurobiology of aggression. In: Martin A, Scahill L, Charney DS, Leckman JF, eds. Pediatric Psychopharmacology: Principles and Practice. New York: Oxford University Press, 2003, pp 210–223.

Kruesi MJP, Casanova MF, Mannheim G, Johnson-Bilder A. Reduced temporal volume in early onset conduct disorder. Psychiatry Research: Neuroimaging, 2004.

Kruesi MJP and Lelio DF. Disorders of conduct and behavior. In: Weiner J, ed. Diagnosis and Psychopharmacology of Childhood and Adolescent Disorders. 2nd Ed. New York: John Wiley and Sons, 1996, pp 401–447.

Kruesi MJP, Hibbs ED, Hamburger SD, Rapoport JL, Keysor CS, Elia J. Measurement of Aggression in Children with Disruptive Behavior Disorders. Journal of Offender Rehabilitation 1994; 21: 159–172.

Kruesi MJP and Schowalter IE. Conduct Disorder and Evolutionary Biology. In: Jensen A, Knapp P, Mrazek D, eds. Beyond DSM-IV. New York, Guilford Publications (in press).

Kruesi MJP. Psychopharmacology of Violence. In: Waldman I, Flannery DJ, Vazsony A, eds. Cambridge Handbook of Violent Behavior. Cambridge. (in press).

Laasko MP, Vaurio O, Koivisto E, Savolainen L, Eronen M, Aronen H, Hakola, Repo, E, Soininen H, Tiihonen. Psychopathy and the posterior hippocampus. Behav Brain Res 2001; 118: 187–193.

Lahey BB, Loeber R, Burke J, Rathouz PJ, McBurnett K. Waxing and waning in concert: dynamic comorbidity of conduct disorder with other disruptive and emotional problems over 7 years among clinic-referred boys. J Abnorm Psychol 2002; 111:556–567.

Lahey BB, Miller TL, Gordon RA, Riley AW. Developmental epidemiology of the disruptive behavior disorders. In: Quay HC, Hogan A, eds. Handbook of the Disruptive Behavior Disorders. New York: Plenum, 1999, pp 23–48.

Lalumiere ML, Harris GT, Rice ME. Psychopathy and developmental instability. Evol Hum Behav 2001; 22:75–92.

LaPierre D, Braun CMJ, and Hodgins S. Ventral front deficits in psychopathy: neuropsychological test findings. Neuropsychologia 1995; 131:39–151.

Lester D. The concentration of neurotransmitter metabolites in the cerebrospinal fluid of suicidal individuals: a meta-analysis. Pharmacopsychiatry 1995; 28:45–50.

Lewinsohn PM, Hops M, Robert RE, Seeley JR, Andrews JA. Adolescent psychopathology, I: prevalence and incidence of depression and other DSM-III-R disorders in high school students. J Abnorm Psychol 1993; 102:133–44.

Liu RSN, Lemieux L, Shorvon SD, Sisodiya SM, Duncan JS. Association between brain size and abstinence from alcohol. Lancet 2000; 355:1969–1970.

Loeber R. Antisocial behavior: more enduring than changeable? J Am Acad Child Adolesc Psychiatry 1991; 30:393–7.

Loney J, Kramer J, Milich RS. The hyperactive child grows up: predictors of symptoms, delinquency and achievement at follow-up. In: Gadow KD, Loney J, eds. Psychosocial Aspects of Drug Treatment for Hyperactivity (AAAS Selected Symposium, vol 44). Boulder, CO: Westview, 1981, pp 381–416.

Lyons MJ, True WR, Elsen SA, et al. Differential heritability of adult and juvenile antisocial traits. Arch Gen Psychiatry 1995; 52:906–915.

Lyoo IK, Lee HK, Jung JH, Noam GG, Renshaw PF. White Matter Hyperintensities on Magnetic Resonance Imaging of the Brain in Children With Psychiatric Disorders. Compr Psychiatry 2002; 43:361–368.

MacMillan J, Kofoed L. Sociobiology and Antisocial Personality Disorder. J Nerv Ment Dis 1984; 172:701–706.

Malone RP, Delaney MA, Luebbert JF, et al. A double-blind placebo-controlled study of lithium in hospitalized aggressive children and adolescents with conduct disorder. Arch Gen Psychiatry 2000; 57:649–54.

Manfred HM, Grotevant HD, Dunbar N, et al. Connecting national survey data with DSM-IV criteria. J Adolesc Health 2002; 31:475–81.

Manning JT, Wood D. Fluctuating asymmetry and aggression in boys. Human Nature 1998; 9:53–65.

Manuck SB, Flory JD, Ferrell RE, Dent KM, Mann JJ, Muldoon MF. Aggression and anger-related traits associated with polymorphism of the tryptophan hydroxylase gene. Biol Psychiatry 1999; 45:603–14.

Mattes JA. Comparative effectiveness of carbamazepine and propranolol for rage outbursts. J Neuropsychiatry Clin Neurosci 1990; 2:159–64.

Maughan B, Pickles A, Hagell A, Rutter M, Yule W. Reading problems and antisocial behaviour: developmental trends in comorbidity. J Child Psychol Psychiatry 1996; 37:405–418.

Maughan B, Taylor C, Taylor A. Pregnancy smoking and childhood conduct problems: a causal association? J Child Psychol Psychiatry 2001; 42:1021–1028.

McBurnett K, Lahey BB, Rathouz PJ, Loeber R. Low salivary cortisol and persistent aggression in boys referred for disruptive behavior. Arch Gen Psychiatry 2000; Jan 57:38–43.

McGee R, Feehan H, Williams S, et al. DSM-III disorders from age 11 to age 15. J Am Acad Child Adolesc Psychiatry 1992; 31:50–59.

Mealey L. The sociobiology of psychopathy: an integrated evolutionary model. Behav Brain Sci 1995; 18:523–599.

Meyer-Bahlburg HF, Dolezal CL, Wasserman GA, Jaramillo BM. Prepubertal boys' sexual behavior and behavior problems. AIDS Educ Prev 1999; 11:174–86.

Moffitt TE. Adolescence-limited and life-course persistent antisocial behavior: a developmental taxonomy. Psychol Rev 1993;100: 674–701.

Moore TM, Scarpa A, Raine A. A Meta-Analysis of Serontonin Metabolite 5-HIAA and Antisocial Behavior. Aggressive Beh 2002; 28:299–316.

Moran P. The epidemiology of antisocial personality disorder. Soc Psychiatry Psychiat Epidemiol 1999; 34:231–242.

Morgan AB, Lilienfield SO. A meta-analytic review of the relation between antisocial behavior and neuropsychological measures of executive functions. Clin Psychol Rev 2000; 20:113–136.

Morris HH, Escoll PJ, Wexler MSW. Aggressive behavior disorders in children: a follow-up study. Am J Psychiatry 1956; 112:991–7.

Muller JL, Sommer M, Wagner V, Lange K, Taschler H, Roder CH, Schuierer G, Klein HE, Hajak G. Abnormalities in emotion processing within cortical and subcortical regions in criminal psychopaths. Biol Psychiatry 2003; 54:152–162.

Neiderhiser JM, Reiss D, Hetherington EM, Plomin R. Relationships between parenting and adolescent adjustment over time: genetic and environmental contributions. Dev Psychol 1999; 35: 680–92.

Neugebauer R, Hoek HW, Susser E. Prenatal exposure to wartime famine and development of antisocial personality disorder in early adulthood. JAMA 1999; 282:455–62.

Noble EP, Ozkaragoz TZ, Ritchie TL, Zhang X, Belin TR, Sparkes RS. D2 and D4 dopamine receptor polymorphisms and personality. Am J Med Geneti (Neuropsychiatr Genet) 1998; 81:257–67.

Nolan EE, Gadow KD, Sprafkin J. Teacher reports of DSM-IV ADHD, ODD, and CD symptoms in schoolchildren. J Am Acad Child Adolesc Psychiatry 2001; 40:241–9.

Offord DR, Boyle MH, Szatmari P, et al. Ontario Child Health Study, II: six-month prevalence of disorder and rates of service utilization. Arch Gen Psychiatry 1987; 44:832–6.

Offord DR, Bennett KJ. Conduct disorder: long-term outcomes and intervention effectiveness. J Am Acad Child Adolesc Psychiatry 1994; 33:1069–77.

Offord DR, Boyle MH, Racine YA, et al. Outcome, prognosis and risk in a longitudinal follow-up study. J Am Acad Child Adolesc Psychiatry 1992; 31:916–23.

Olweus S. Stability of aggressive reaction patterns in males: a review. Psychol Bull 1979; 36:852–75.

Ono Y, Manki H, Yoshimura K, Muramatsu T, Mizushima H, Higuchi S, Yagi G, Kanba S, Asai M. Association between dopamine D4 receptor (D4DR) exon III polymorphism and novelty seeking in Japanese subjects. Am J Med Genet (Neuropsychiatr Genet). 1997; 74:501–3.

Orlebeke JF, Knol DL, Verhulst FC. Increase in child behavior problems resulting from maternal smoking during pregnancy. Arch Environ Health 1997; 52:317–21.

Ortiz J, Raine A. Heart rate level and antisocial behavior in children and adolescents: a meta-analysis. J Am Acad Child Adolesc Psychiatry 2004; 43:154–162.

Pajer K, Gardner W, Rubin RT, Perel J, Neal S. Decreased cortisol levels in adolescent girls with conduct disorder. Arch Gen Psychiatry 2001; 58:297–302.

Pappadopulos E, Macintyre Ii JC, Crismon ML, Findling RL, Malone RP, Derivan A, Schooler N, Sikich L, Greenhill L, Schur SB, Felton CJ, Kranzler H, Rube DM, Sverd J, Finnerty M, Ketner S, Siennick SE, Jensen PS. Treatment recommendations for the use of antipsychotics for aggressive youth (TRAAY). Part II. J Am Acad Child Adolesc Psychiatry 2003; 42:145–61.

Patterson GR, Gullion ME. Living with children: new methods for parents and teachers. Champaign, IL: Research Press, 1968.

Patterson GR, DeBaryshe BD, Ramsey E. A developmental perspective on antisocial behavior. Am Psychol 1989; 44:329–35.

Pfeffer CR, Plutchik R, Mizruchi MS. Predictors of assaultiveness in latency age children. Am J Psychiatry 1983; 140:31–35.

Pine DS, Cohen P, Brook J, Coplan JD. Psychiatric symptoms in adolescence as predictors of obesity in early adulthood: a longitudinal study. Am J Public Health 1997; 87:1303–1310.

Puente R. The use of carbamazepine in the treatment of behavioral disorders in children. In: Birkmayer W, ed. Epileptic Seizures-Behavior-Pain. Bern, Switzerland: Hans Huber, 1976, pp 244-247.

Puri BK, El-Dosoky A, Cheema S, Lekh SK, et al. Parietal scalp hair whorl patterns in schizophrenia. Biol Psychiatry 1995; 37:278–9.

Quay HC. Classification. In: Quay HC and Werry JC, eds. Psychopathological Disorders of Childhood. 2nd Ed. New York: John Wiley and Sons, 1979.

Raine A, Reynolds C, Venables PH, Mednick SA, Farrington DP. Fearlessness, stimulation-seeking, and large body size at age 3 years as early predispositions to childhood aggression at age 11 years. Arch Gen Psychiatry 1998; 55:745–51.

Raine A, Brennan M, Mednick SA. Birth complications with early maternal rejection at age 1 year predispose to violent crime at age 18 years. Arch Gen Psychiatry 1994; 51:984–8.

Raine A, Mellingen K, Liu J, et al. Effects of environmental enrichment at ages 3–5 years on schizotypal personality and antisocial behavior at ages 17 and 23 years. Am J Psychiatry 2003; 160:1627–1635.

Raine A, Lencz T, Taylor K, Hellige JB, Bihrle S, Lacasse L, Lee M, Ishikawa S, Colletti P. Corpus Callosum Abnormalities in Psychopathic Antisocial Individuals. Arch Gen Psychiatry 2003; 60:1134–1142.

Raine A, Lencz T, Bihrle S, LaCasse L, and Colletti P. Reduced prefrontal gray matter volume and reduced autonomic activity in antisocial personality disorder. Arch Gen Psychiatry 2000; 57: 119–127.

Raine A, Meloy JR, Bihrl, S, Stoddard J, LaCasse L, Buchsbaum MS. Reduced prefrontal and increased subcortical brain functioning assessed using positron emission tomography in predatory and affective murderers. Beh Sci and the Law 1998; 16:319–332.

Raine A, Ishikawa SS, Arce E, Lencz T, Knuth T, Knuth KH, Bihrle S, LaCasse L, Colletti P. Hippocampal Structural Asymmetry in Unsuccessful Psychopaths. Biol Psychiatry 2004; 55:185–1191

Ramrakha S, Caspi A, Dickson N, Moffitt TE, Paul C. Psychiatric disorders and risky sexual behaviour in young adulthood: cross sectional study in birth cohort. BMJ 2000; 321:263–6.

Rantakallio P, Laara E, Isohanni M, Moilanen I. Maternal smoking during pregnancy and delinquency of offspring: an association without causation? Int J Epidemiol 1992; 21:1106–13.

Reiss D, Hetherington EM, Plomin R, et al. Genetic questions for environmental studies: differential parenting and psychopathology in adolescence. Arc Gen Psychiatry 1995; 52:925–936.

Riddle M, King R, Hardin M, et al. Behavioral side effects with fluoxetine in children and adolescents. J Child Adolesc Psychopharmacol 1990/1991; 4:31–41.

Rifkin A, Karajgi B, Dicker R, et al. Lithium treatment of conduct disorders in adolescents. Am J Psychiatry 1997; 154:554–5.

Riggs PD, Mikulich SK, Coffman LM, Crowley TJ. Fluoxetine in drug-dependent delinquents with major depression: an open trial. J Child Adolesc Psychopharmacol 1997; 7:87–95.

Riggs PD, Hall SK, Mikulich-Gilbertson SK, Lohman M, Kayser A. A randomized controlled trial of pemoline for attention-deficit/ hyperactivity disorder in substance-abusing adolescents. J Am Acad Child Adolesc Psychiatry 2004;43:420–429.

Robins LN. Deviant Children Grown Up. Baltimore, MD: William and Wilkins, 1966.

Robins LN. Sturdy childhood predictors of adult antisocial behavior: replications from longitudinal studies. Psychol Med 1978; 8:611–22.

Robins LN, Tipp J, McEvoy L. Antisocial personality. In: Robins LN, Regier D, eds. Psychiatric Disorders in America. New York: Free Press, 1991, pp. 258–290.

Roff JD, Wirt RD. Childhood aggression and social adjustment as antecedents of delinquency. J Abnorm Child Psychol 1984; 12: 111–126.

disorder: Findings from the Great Smoky Mountains Study. J Child Psychol Psychiatry 2002; 40:365–373.

Rubinow DR, and Schmidt PJ. Androgens, brain and behavior. Am J Psychiatry 1996; 153:974–984.

Rutter M, Cox A, Tupling C, et al. Attainment and adjustment in two geographical areas, I: prevalence of psychiatric disorder. Br J Psychiatry 1975; 126:493–509.

Rutter M, Tizard J, Whitmore K. Education, Health and Behavior. London: Longmans, 1970.

Rutter M. Pathways from childhood to adult life. J Child Psychol Psychiatry. 1989; 30:23–51.

Rutter M, Giller H, Hagell A. Antisocial Behavior by Young People. Cambridge, UK: Cambridge University Press, 1998.

Scarpa A, and Raine A. Psychophysiology of anger and violent behavior. Psychiatr Clin North Am 1997; 20:375–394.

Schur SB, Sikich L, Findling R, Malone RP, Crismon ML, Derivan A, Macintyre JC, Pappadopulos E, Greenhill L, Schooler N, Van Orden K, Jensen PS. Treatment Recommendations for the Use of Antipsychotics for Aggressive Youth (TRAAY). J Am Acad Child Adoles Psychiatry 2003; 42:132–144.

Sheldon WH. Varieties of Delinquent Youth: An Introduction to Constitutional Psychiatry. New York: Harper, 1949.

Silberg JL, Parr T, Neale MC, et al. Maternal smoking during pregnancy and risk to boys' conduct disturbance: an examination of the causal hypothesis. Biol Psychiatry 2003; 53:130–135.

Simonoff E, Pickles A, Meyer J, Silberg J, Maes H. Genetic and environmental influences on subtypes of conduct disorder behavior in boys. J Abnorm Child Psychol 1998; 26:495–509.

Slutske WE, Heath AC, Dinwiddie SH, Madden PA, Bucholz KK, Dunne MP, Statham DJ, Martin NG. Modeling genetic and environmental influences in the etiology of conduct disorder: a study of 2682 adult twin pairs. J Abnorm Psychol. 1997; 106:266–79.

Snyder R, Turgay A, Aman M, et al. Effects of risperidone on conduct and disruptive behavior disorders in children with subaverage IQs. J Am Acad Child Adolesc Psychiatry 2002; 41:1026–36.

Soderstrom H, Rastam M, Gillberg C. A clinical case series of six extremely aggressive youths treated with olanzapine. Eur Child Adolesc Psychiatry 2002; 11:138–41.

Soderstrom H, Hultin L, Tullberg M, Wikkelso, C, Ekholm Forsman A. Reduced frontotemporal perfusion in psychopathic personality. Psychiatry Research Neuroimaging 114; 2002:81–94.

Soderstrom H, Blennow K, Manhem A, Forsman A. CSF studies in violent offenders I. 5-HIAA as a negataive and HVA as a positive predictor of psychopathy. J Neural Transm 2001; 108:869–878.

Soloff PH, Lynch KG, Moss HB. Serotonin, impulsivity, and alcohol use disorders in the older adolescent: a psychobiological study. Alcohol Clin Exp Res 2000; 24:1609–19.

Stanger C, McConaughy SH, Achenbach TM. Three-year course of behavioral/emotional problems in a national sample of 4- to 16-year-olds, II: predictors of syndromes. J Am Acad Child Adolesc Psychiatry 1992; 31:941–50.

Stattin H, Magnusson D. The role of early aggressive behavior in the frequency, seriousness, and types of later crime. J Consult Clin Psychol 1989; 57:710–8.

Steiner H, Petersen ML, Saxena K, et al. Divalproex sodium for the treatment of conduct disorder: a randomized controlled clinical trial. J Clin Psychiatry 2003; 64:1183–91.

Stoff DM, Pasatiempo AP, Yeung J, Cooper TB, Bridger WH, and Rabinovich H. (1992) Neuroendocrine responses to challenge with dl-fenfluramine and aggression in disruptive behavior disorders of children and adolescents. Psychiatry Res 43:263–276.

Takeuchi Y, Houpt K. Behavior genetics. Vet Clin Small Anim 2003; 33:345–63.

Taylor J, Loney BR, Bobadilla L, Iacono WG, McGue M. Genetic and Environmental Influences on Psychopathy Trait Dimensions in a Community Sample of Mail Twins. J of Abnormal Psychiatry. 2003; 31:633–645.

Tolan PH, Henry D. Patterns of psychopathology among urban-poor children: comorbidity and aggression effects. J Consult Clin Psychol 1996; 64:1094–9.

Tremblay RE, Schaal B, Boulerice B, et al. Testosterone, physical aggression, dominance, and physical development in early adolescence. Int J Behav Dev 1998; 22:753–777.

United States Food and Drug Administration Web site "www.fda.gov".

van den Oord EJCG, Boomsma DI, and Verhulst, FC. A study of problem behaviors in 10- to 15-year-old biologically related and unrelated international adoptees. Behav Genet 1994; 24:193–205.

Van Goozen SHM, Matthys W, Cohen-Kettenis PT, Thijssen JHH, van Engeland H. Society of Biological Psychiatry 1998:156–158.

Veit, R, Flor H, Erb M, Hermann C, Lotze M, Grodd W, Birbaumer N. Brain circuits involved in emotional learning in antisocial behavior and social phobia in humans. Neuroscience Letter 2002; 328:233–236.

Velez CN, Johnson J, Cohen P. A longitudinal analysis of selected risk factors for childhood psychopathology. J Am Acad Child Adolesc Psychiatry 1989; 28:861–4.

Vitiello B, Behar D, Hunt J, Stoff D, Ricciuti A. Subtyping Aggression in children and adolescents. J Neuropsychiatry Clin Neurosci 1990; 2:189–192.

Volavka J. Electroencephalogram among criminals. In: Mednick SA, Moffit EE, Stack SA, eds. Causes of Crime. Cambridge, UK: Cambridge University Press, 1987.

Wakschlag LS, Lahey BB, Loeber R, et al. Maternal smoking during pregnancy and the risk of conduct disorder in boys. Arch Gen Psychiatry 1997; 54:670–76.

Webster-Stratton C. Randomized trial of two parent-training program for families with conduct-disordered children. J Consult Clin Psychol 1984; 51:666–678.

Weissman MM, Warner V, Wickramaratne PJ, Kandel DB. Maternal smoking during pregnancy and psychopathology in offspring followed to adulthood. J Am Acad Child Adolesc Psychiatry 1999; 38:892–899.

Williams GM, O'Callaghan M, Najman JM, et al. Maternal cigarette smoking and child psychiatric morbidity: a longitudinal study. Pediatrics 1998; 102:E111–E118.

Woermann FG, van Elst LT, Koepp MJ, Free SL, Thompson PJ, Trimble MR, Duncan JS. Reduction of frontal neocortical grey matter associated with affective aggression in patients with temporal lobe epilepsy: an objective voxel by voxel analysis of automatically segmented MRI. J Neurol Neurosurg Psychiatry 2000; 68:162–9.

Wong MTH, Lumsden J, Fenton GW, and Fenwick PBC. Electroencephalography, computer tomography and violence rating of male patients in a maximum-security mental hospital. Acta Psychiatr Scand 1994; 90:97–101.

Zahn TP, Kruesi MJP: Autonomic Activity in Boys with Disruptive Behavior Disorders. Psychophysiology 1993; 30:605–14.

Zoccolillo M, Rogers K. Characteristics and outcome of hospitalized adolescent girls with conduct disorder. J Am Acad Child Adolesc Psychiatry 1991; 30:973–81.

Zubieta J, Alessi N. Acute and chronic administration of trazodone in the treatment of disruptive behavior disorders in children. J Clin Psychopharmacol 1992; 12:346–51.

Pediatric Mood Disorders

13

Robert A. Kowatch, MD   **Melissa P. DelBello, MD**   **Taryn Mayes, MS**

Beth D. Kennard, PsyD   **Graham J. Emslie, MD**

Pediatric mood disorders include depressive disorders (major depression and dysthymia) and bipolar disorders (bipolar I and II disorder, and cyclothymia). These are prevalent disorders in children and adolescents which cause significant morbidity and mortality. The course of illness for children and adolescents with mood disorders is generally chronic and most will continue to have mood disorders into adulthood. In this chapter, we examine mood disorders in the pediatric population from a neuropsychiatric perspective. In this context, we emphasize the use of established criteria for diagnosis and the neurobiology of these disorders. Specifically, we (1) discuss the diagnosis, epidemiology, and course of mood disorders; (2) review the neurobiology of mood disorders; and (3) describe how pediatric mood disorders are treated. These areas are examined as they relate to children and adolescents with mood disorders, with reference to adult information where relevant.

DIAGNOSIS

The diagnosis of a mood disorder in a child or adolescent requires careful and systematic interviewing of the child, the parent, or the guardian. Other sources of information about the child (e.g., school personnel) are often useful as well. A number of instruments are available for assessing mood disorders in children and adolescents. Structured and semistructured interviews are used to elicit symptoms and to establish whether a child meets certain diagnostic criteria. Items from the diagnostic interviews have also been used as clinical-severity measures (the Kiddie Schedule for Affective Disorders and Schizophrenia [K-SADS]. Diagnostic interviews vary in the degree of clinical experience required for their administration, whether or not they are computerized, and which mood disorders they target. These instruments are not restricted to research applications; the availability of computerized interviews can assist clinicians in ascertaining that all diagnostic domains are covered. Structured psychiatric interviews require continual modifications as diagnostic criteria change. Clinician-rated and self-report measures of clinical symptom severity can be a useful addition to ongoing clinical management, even though the unreliability of self-report measures in pediatric and adolescent populations is well documented. Self-report measures have been used to screen large populations. Kandel and Davies (1986) reported on 1,004 adolescents identified as having depressive symptoms on a self-report scale. When followed to adulthood, subjects with depressive symptoms showed a poorer outcome compared with those without depressive symptoms, a finding that supports the partial validity of these measures.

Depressive disorders are generally characterized as either major depressive disorder or dysthymic disorder. Major depressive disorder (MDD) and dysthymic disorder differ with regard to the prominent and persistent nature of the mood disturbance or pervasive anhedonia and the number and intensity of associated symptoms. Dysthymic disorder is long-standing (greater than 1 year's duration), with depressive moods and feelings and variable vegetative symptoms that fluctuate with no prolonged stable (well) states. Patients with dysthymic disorder have a significantly elevated risk of experiencing a superimposed major depressive episode. Criteria for MDD are the same in children and adolescents as in adulthood, except that youth may present with irritable mood, even in the absence of depressed mood. The presentation or dysthymia is consistent across the life span, but may be present for only 1 year in youth, rather than the required 2 years for adults. Age-related and gender-related differences in depressive symptom presentation are difficult to detect, if they do indeed exist. Eliciting symptoms from children and adolescents is somewhat difficult, particularly in younger children, as they are often not cognitively developed enough to express their experiences. Kovacs (1996) suggested children might have less hypersomnia, more appetite and weight changes, and delusions as compared to adolescents. Luby et al. (2003) concluded that depressed preschool children show less "masked" symptoms (e.g., sleep problems, appetite changes) and more typical symptoms (e.g., anhedonia, sadness/irritability).

Many children and adolescents are labeled "bipolar" without careful consideration of the diagnostic complexities and subtypes of this disorder. The symptoms of bipolarity in children and adolescents can be difficult to establish because of the variability of symptom expression depending on the context and phase of the illness, the effects of development upon symptom expression, and the mood and behavioral effects of the various psychotropic medications that the patient is taking. Children and adolescents with a bipolar disorder (BPD) often present with a mixed or "dysphoric" picture characterized by frequent short periods of intense mood liability and irritability rather than classic euphoric mania. Clinicians who evaluate children with pediatric bipolar disorders often try to fit them into the DSM-IV "rapid cycling" subtype and find that this subtype does not fit bipolar children well, as these children often do not have clear episodes of mania. Rather, researchers are reporting that bipolar children cycle far more frequently than four episodes per year. In 81% of a well-defined group of patients, continuous daily cycling from mania or hypomania to euthymia or depression was reported. Findling et al. (2001) reported that in a sample of 90 bipolar I subjects with a mean age of 10.8 years that the age of the first manic episode was 6.7 years with 50% of these patients categorized as "rapid cycling." The picture that emerges from several independent research groups is that prepubertal bipolar children typically have multiple daily mood swings and that irritability is much more common than euphoria.

There are also a number of medications and medical disorders that may exacerbate or mimic bipolar symptoms, and it is important to assess these potential confounds before initiating treatment. Potential medical disorders and medications that should be evaluated before making the diagnosis of a pediatric BPD are listed in Table 13.1.

A complete evaluation of children and adolescents with a mood disorder should include a detailed family history of psychiatric illnesses that includes first-degree, second-

TABLE 13.1

MEDICAL CONDITIONS THAT MAY MIMIC MANIA IN CHILDREN AND ADOLESCENTS

Hyperthyroidism
Temporal lobe epilepsy
Closed or open head injury
Multiple sclerosis
Systemic lupus erythematosus (SLE)
Wilson's disease

Medications That May Increase Mood Cycling in Children and Adolescents

Antidepressants
Tricyclic antidepressants
Serotonin-specific reuptake inhibitors
Serotonin and norepinephrine reuptake inhibitors

Oral or IV Corticosteroids
Aminophylline
Sympathomimetic amines (e.g., pseudoephedrine)
Antibiotics (e.g., clarithromycin, erythromycin, and amoxicillin)

degree, and third-degree relatives. The offspring of adults with affective illness show a high rate of depression and bipolar disorder. Conversely, the first-degree and second-degree relatives of children with major depressive disorder have a high aggregation of depression, alcoholism, anxiety, and other psychiatric diagnoses. It has been noted that children and adolescents with a mood disorder have a family history of mood disorders in 50 to 60% of cases, depending on which criteria are used (i.e., treated versus untreated, definite versus possible) and whether first-degree or second-degree relatives are evaluated.

In summary, as advised by the American Academy of Child and Adolescent Psychiatry (AACAP), a complete evaluation for a mood disorder is essential in developing an appropriate treatment plan. The assessment involves systematic interviewing of the child and the parent(s) independently to ascertain the presence (or absence) of specific symptoms of depressive and other psychiatric disorders. Family history, course of illness, number of episodes, presence of comorbid diagnoses, and psychosocial stressors may impact outcome, and need to be carefully evaluated to adequately diagnose and treat this population.

COMORBIDITY

The most common comorbid diagnoses in children with major depression are anxiety disorders (30 to 80%), disruptive disorders (10 to 80%), and substance use disorders (20 to 30%).

Anxiety disorders commonly co-occur in children with major depression (41%) and typically persist even after the depressive episode remits. Furthermore, the presence of social anxiety disorder in adolescence predicts major depression in young adulthood. Half of children diagnosed with dysthymic disorder have a co-occurring disorder. Anxiety disorders are commonly comorbid in children and adolescents with dysthymic disorder, especially separation anxiety disorder in children (33%) and generalized anxiety disorder in adolescents (67%). Conduct disorder (30%), attention deficit hyperactivity disorder (ADHD) (24%), and enuresis or encopresis (15%) are also commonly present in children with dysthymic disorder.

The most common comorbid diagnosis among bipolar youth is ADHD. Despite the high co-occurrence of juvenile mania and ADHD that has been reported in several studies, the relationship between these disorders remains unclear. Several studies have determined that ADHD is more common in prepubertal onset bipolar disorder than in adolescent onset bipolar disorder.

Another disorder that is frequently comorbid in children with bipolar disorder is conduct disorder. Kovacs and Pollock (1995) found a 69% rate of conduct disorder among 26 bipolar children and adolescents. Several studies report that conduct disorder in youth with bipolar disorder predicts a worse clinical course. Moreover, adolescents with bipolar disorder are five times more likely to develop a substance use disorder than those without bipolar disorder. Children and adolescents with pervasive developmental disorders may be at increased risk for developing mania.

EPIDEMIOLOGY OF MOOD DISORDERS

The prevalence of depressive disorders in children and adolescents ranges from 0.4 to 8.3% and is greater in adolescents than in children. Dysthymic disorder is reported in 0.6 to 8.0% of children and adolescents. This prevalence compares with that in adults, in whom the 12-month prevalence of major depressive disorder is reported to be 10.3% ± 0.8% (12.9 ± 0.8% in women and 7.7 ± 0.8% in men). This finding also highlights the gender differences in prevalence; whereas major depressive disorder in children appears to occur at about the same rate in girls and boys, the approximately 2:1 adult female:male ratio becomes evident in adolescents. Of particular relevance to children and adolescents is the suggestion of a secular trend in the onset of depressive disorders, which has been reported in both referred and nonreferred samples of children and adolescents. Ryan et al. (1992b) reported on siblings of prepubertal depressed and normal children and demonstrated that affective disorders are more frequent in siblings born more recently. Similarly, in a psychiatric referred depressed school-age sample, Kovacs and Gatsonis (1994) noted that the successive birth cohorts were younger when they first developed MDD. Thus,

the rate of depression in youth is likely increasing, and patients are presenting more frequently for treatment for these disorders.

In a large and well-designed population study of the incidence of mood disorders in adolescents, Lewinsohn et al. (1995) reported an overall lifetime prevalence of 1% for bipolar spectrum disorders which included bipolar I disorder, bipolar II disorder and cyclothymia. In this study, the largest groups of adolescent subjects were what Lewinsohn et al. (1995) called the "core-positive" group. These adolescent subjects reported a distinct period of elevated, expensive or irritable mood and best fit the DSM-IV criteria of bipolar disorder, not otherwise specified (NOS). These subjects had an overall prevalence of 5.7% and accounted for 84% of Lewinsohn's bipolar sample. These bipolar NOS subjects also had high rates of psychosocial impairment and mental health service utilization like the bipolar type I subjects.

Wozniak et al. (1995) reported that of 262 consecutively referred children to a specialty pediatric psychopharmacology clinic, 16% met DSM-III-R criteria for mania. Isaac (1992) reported that eight out of 12 students in a special education class met DSM-IIIR criteria for a bipolar disorder. In more specialized psychiatric settings like a pediatric psychopharmacology clinic, the occurrence of pediatric bipolar disorder is expected to be much greater than that found in the general population.

E. COURSE/NATURAL HISTORY

The developmental course of mood disorders suggests that there is a continuum of pathology from childhood to adults. Similar to adults with depressive disorder, depressed children and adolescents often have a chronic course. Most studies report the average length of a major depressive episode in children and adolescents is 7 to 9 months. In a study of 42 child outpatients with MDD, Kovacs et al. (1984) found that 59% had recovered (asymptomatic for 2 months) by 1 year, 92% had recovered by 18 months. Strober et al. (1993) found that 81% of 58 adolescent inpatients with MDD had recovered by 1 year and 98% by 2 years from the time of admission, with the average time to recovery of 27.5 weeks from admission. They also reported that 28% of those with psychotic depression developed mania over the 2-year follow-up period. Similarly, McCauley et al. (1993) found that 80% of predominately outpatient children with major depression had recovered by 1 year.

While most children and adolescents recover from the depressive episode, recurrence is common, possibly even more so than in adult depression. Recurrence (i.e., a new episode of depression) has been reported in 54 to 72% of depressed children and adolescents followed for 3 to 8 years, with similar rates seen in inpatients and outpatients.

Poznanski et al. (1976) report that 50% of a sample of depressed adolescent outpatients were depressed when contacted 6.5 years later. Eastgate and Gilmour (1984) contacted 19 of 36 child inpatients with depression 7 to 8 years after their episode and reported that 42% were psychiatrically ill, 21% with major depression. These rates are based on naturalistic follow-up studies, which do not take into account whether or not patients are on medication at the time of the recurrence or the length of time on medication prior to the recurrence. One study of relapse prevention in children and adolescents demonstrated that continued treatment with fluoxetine reduced relapse rates and delayed time to relapse over placebo. Factors contributing to recurrence of depression include comorbidity, severity of depression, hopelessness, low self-esteem, family dysfunction, stressful life events, and suicidality at baseline. In a longitudinal study investigating recurrence of MDD during adulthood (19 to 23 years of age) in formerly treated depressed adolescents, Lewinsohn et al. (2001) found that recurrence was predicted by multiple episodes of depression, family history of recurrence of major depression, borderline personality disorder symptoms, and increased conflict with parents (for females only).

Early onset depression often continues into adulthood for most (70%) children and adolescents. Kandel and Davies (1986) described poor adult outcomes in a large sample of adolescents (n = 1,004) identified as having depressive symptoms using a self-report scale. Similarly, in a retrospective, longterm follow-up study of 80 depressed and 80 nondepressed outpatient adolescents, Harrington et al. (1990) reported that depressed adolescents were more likely than nondepressed adolescents to have depression in adulthood; however, they noted that most adult depressions are not preceded by adolescent depression. Weissman et al. (1980) studied 73 patients with adolescent onset depression into adulthood and found that while 37% survived without an episode of major depression in adulthood, there was substantial increased risk of suicide and adult major depressive disorder in adulthood than those without adolescent major depressive disorder.

Although there are few investigations of the outcome of childhood onset dysthymic disorder, children with dysthymic disorder are more likely to develop depressive disorders and recurrent affective illnesses. Moreover, co-occurring externalizing disorders predict worse outcome in children with dysthymia. Mean episode length is typically 4 years and children with dysthymia usually develop their first episode of major depression within 2 to 3 years after the onset of dysthymic disorder.

The outcome of bipolar disorder in children and adolescents has received little study. McGlashen (1979) interviewed 62 adult patients who met DSM-III criteria for mania and divided them into two groups: 35 with adolescent onset mania and 31 with adult onset mania. He reported that the adolescent-onset group had more hospitalizations, displayed more psychotic symptoms, and were more frequently misdiagnosed as having schizoaffective disorder than the adult-onset group. Surprisingly, the adolescent-onset group had outcomes superior to those of the adult-onset group in terms of social relationships and their ability to work. In contrast, Geller et al. (2004) reported diagnostic stability in 93 prepubescent and early adolescent subjects. At 4-year follow-up, 86 of the patients were assessed and rate of recovery was 87%. However, rate of relapse after recovery was 64%. In these studies recovery was defined as no mania or hypomania for at least 2 weeks and relapse was defined as having full DSM-IV criteria for mania or hypomania and a Childhood Global Assessment Scale score of less than or equal to 60 for at least 2 weeks.

NEUROBIOLOGY OF MOOD DISORDERS

There are several excellent reviews of the neurobiology of mood disorders, but the majority of this information is from adult studies as there have been relatively few investigations of the neurobiology of childhood and adolescent mood disorders. Biologic studies in children are difficult to implement since they often require several blood draws, subjects remaining still more long periods of time, and the overall cooperation of the children and adolescents.

Neurotransmitter and Neuroendocrine Studies

Studies of neurotransmitters in depressed adults have focused on norepinephrine, serotonin, and acetylcholine. Serotonin (5-hydroxytryptamine) regulation has also been studied in adults with depression. Ryan et al. (1992a) reported that in response to L-5-hydroxytryptophan (5-HT) in 37 prepubertal depressed children secreted less cortisol and more prolactin than age-matched and gender-matched normal controls, suggesting a dysregulation of central serotonergic systems in childhood depression. Abnormalities of the hypothalamic-pituitary adrenal (HPA) axis, the hypothalamic pituitary-thyroid (HPT) axis, and the hypothalamic pituitary-growth hormone (HPGH) axis have been reported in depression in adults. However, cortisol hypersecretion, as measured by repeated samples over a 24-hour period or by nocturnal sampling, has not been identified in depressed children and adolescents although depressed adolescents showed a cortisol elevation at the approximate time of sleep onset. In one study (Rao et al., 1996) there was a trend toward elevated cortisol levels near sleep onset in adolescents with a course of recurrent depression as compared to those with no further episodes of major depression. De-Bellis et al. (1996) found that prepubertal depressed children had lower cortisol levels during the first 4 hours of sleep than healthy controls.

Birmaher et al. (1996) found no significant difference between prepubertal children with major depression and normal controls in baseline or postcorticotropin releasing hormone (CRH) stimulation values of cortisol or adreno-corticotropin releasing hormone (ACTH). PostCRH ACTH may be increased in depressed children who have been abused as compared to depressed children who have no history of abuse. Nonsuppression of cortisol by dexamethasone has been found in many studies in depressed children and adolescents.

Molecular Genetic Studies

There have been few molecular genetic studies of children with mood disorders, despite the fact that familial risk studies have suggested that early-onset major depression may be a more familial form of the illness than adult onset major depression. Two molecular genetic studies in children with bipolar disorders by Geller et al. (1999) have been reported. In the first study of a sample of bipolar children, the serotonin transporter linked promoter region (HTTLPR) short and long alleles were studied and the transmission disequilibrium test was negative in the children with bipolar disorder. The second study examined the linkage disequilibrium of catechol-O-methyltransferase (l-COMT) in bipolar children and transmission and the disequilibrium tests were not significant for preferential transmission of l-COMT in this sample. The brain-derived neurotrophic factor (BDNF) belongs to a family of so-called neurotrophic factors, which were suggested to play an important role in modulating neuronal development, growth, survival, and synaptic plasticity of a broad variety of CNS neurons—processes nowadays believed to play important role in the neuropathogenesis of mood disorders. The BDNF gene was first reported to be localized on the short arm of chromosome 11 (11p13) and was later mapped at the boundary of 11p13 and 11p14. Findings of some linkage and association studies, including the studies of two samples from the NIMH Genetics Initiative bipolar pedigrees, provide evidence that the BDNF gene is located in a locus where other genes, contributing to the pathophysiology of BPD are located (11p13-p15). Two family-based association studies provided evidence that one or more sequence variants within or near the brain-derived neurotrophic factor (BDNF) gene show an association with susceptibility to BPD in adults. Geller et al. (2004) reported preferential transmission of the Val66 allele in 53 children with bipolar disorder indicating possible involvement of BDNF in prepubetal BPD.

It is still early in our knowledge about the molecular genetics of psychiatric disorders, and it is likely that multiple genes are involved that interact with each other and are expressed differentially during development. It is unlikely that a single genetic locus will be identified that causes either depressive or bipolar disorders in children or adolescents.

NEUROIMAGING STUDIES

Major Depressive Disorders

There have been few structural neuroimaging studies of children and adolescents with MDD. Steingard et al. (1996) retrospectively evaluated the magnetic resonance imaging (MRI) scans of children with MDD or dysthymia (n = 65) and found that frontal lobe volume was decreased and lateral ventricular volume was increased as compared to hospitalized psychiatric controls (n = 18). No group difference was found in total cerebral volume. In contrast, in a more recent study, the same authors reported whole brain volumes were significantly smaller in depressed adolescents compared with the healthy comparison subjects. Additionally, in the latter study they found significantly smaller frontal white matter volumes and significantly larger frontal gray matter volumes in the depressed adolescents after controlling for age and whole brain volume. These results are similar to findings from MRI studies of adults with MDD that suggest prefrontal abnormalities. Similarly, in another study, Nolan et al. (2002) reported patients with nonfamilial MDD had larger left-sided prefrontal cortical volumes than patents with familial MDD and controls. Moreover, in a positron-emission tomography (PET) study of familial bipolar and MDD depressed subjects, Drevets et al. (1997) reported decreased activity and grey matter volume in the subgenual prefrontal cortex, indicating that nature of prefrontal abnormalities may be different depending on the presence of family history of affective illness. Together, these studies suggest the importance of considering family history in neuroimaging studies. Additionally, other studies have reported structural abnormalities in the subgenual prefrontal cortex in young women with adolescent onset MDD, suggesting that this prefrontal region may be particularly important in the neurophysiology of early onset and familial MDD.

In general, structural MRI studies of adults with MDD have found decreased subcortical volumes. There have been relatively few morphometric investigations that have examined structures other than the frontal cortex in MDD youth. In one study, MDD adolescents had 25% increased pituitary gland volumes, suggesting pediatric MDD may involve neuroendocrine dysfunction. Frodl et al. (2002) found enlarged amygdala volumes compared to patients with recurrent MDD and healthy controls, suggesting this finding may be a marker for MDD early in illness course. Indeed, increased amygdala: hippocampal volume ratios that were associated with severity of anxiety and not depression were observed in pediatric MDD patients prior to treatment as compared to healthy controls. This study suggests the importance of considering comorbid illnesses in imaging studies of pediatric patients with affective disorders. Similarly, the presence of prior suicide attempts has been associated with increased number of white matter hyperintensities (WMH) in MDD youth. However, the temporal relationship between suicide attempts and WMH remains unclear.

To our knowledge, there have been four published functional neuroimaging studies in children or adolescents with MDD. Kowatch et al. (1999) used technetium-99m hexamethylpropylene amine oxime (99mTc-HM-PAO) single photon emission tomography (SPECT) to compare relative rCBF between unmedicated MDD adolescents (n = 7) and healthy controls (n = 7) and described relative increases in rCBF in the mesial, right superior-anterior and left infero-lateral temporal lobe and decreases in the left parietal lobe, anterior thalamus, and right caudate in MDD adolescents. These findings suggest that adolescents with MDD exhibit rCBF abnormalities similar to those found in adults with MDD with involvement of the limbic-thalamic-cortical circuit and portions of the basal ganglia.

In another 99mTc-HMPAO SPECT study, evaluating untreated MDD adolescents (n = 14) and age-matched normal controls (n = 11), Tutus et al. (1998) calculated a relative perfusion index (PI) as the ratio of regional cortical activity to the whole brain activity and reported significant reduced PI in the left anterior frontal and left temporal cortical regions of untreated MDD adolescents. SPECT scans repeated after MDD adolescents were treated and their depression remitted demonstrated a return toward normal. This study suggests that adolescents with MDD may have state-dependent regional cerebral blood flow deficits in frontal and temporal regions and right-left perfusion asymmetry compared with normal subjects, similar to results in studies of MDD adults.

In a more recent study, Dahlstrom et al. (2000) used SPECT to study serotonin and dopamine transporter levels in drug-naive children and adolescents with MDD (n = 31) and children and adolescents without depression (n = 10). They found significantly higher serotonin transporter availability in MDD children in the hypothalamic/midbrain region, suggesting that abnormalities in serotonin might play a role in the physiology of pediatric MDD. In a small study using functional magnetic resonance imaging (fMRI), children with anxiety disorders showed an exaggerated amygdala response to fearful faces compared with healthy children, whereas depressed children showed a blunted amygdala response to these faces. In addition, the magnitude of the amygdala's signal change between fearful and neutral faces was positively correlated with the severity of everyday anxiety symptoms, suggesting that amygdala dysfunction is present in youth with anxiety disorders and those with MDD, although the nature of the dysfunction may differ between disorders.

There have been several MRS studies of MDD youth. Reduced anterior cingulate glutamine/glutamate/GABA concentrations associated with severity of functional impairment was reported in one study of MDD youth.

MRS studies of adults with MDD also suggest reduced anterior cingulate Glx peaks. Another study reported increased levels of orbitofrontal choline in depressed adolescents, suggesting abnormalities in cell membrane metabolism may underlie the neurophysiology of MDD in youth. Similarly, Farchione et al. (2002) demonstrated elevated choline in the left dorsolateral prefrontal cortex (DLPFC) of MDD youth. Increased thalamic choline specific to youth with obsessive-compulsive disorder (OCD) and not MDD youth or healthy controls was reported by Smith et al. (2003), suggesting that this finding may be useful as a diagnostically specific biological marker for pediatric OCD.

Bipolar Disorders

Structural magnetic resonance imaging (MRI) studies of adults with bipolar disorder have revealed several abnormalities including decreased prefrontal cortex volumes, increases in the volume of the amygdala and putamen, and atrophy of the V3 vermal area and larger lateral ventricles. Additionally, increased white matter hyperintensities are commonly identified in adults with bipolar disorder, although their significance is unknown. Structural MRI studies of children and adolescents with bipolar disorder have also revealed several neuroanatomical abnormalities, including an increased incidence of subcortical white matter hyperintensities, reduced intracranial volumes, increased frontal and temporal sulcal size, reduced thalamic area, reduced amygdala volumes, and increased putamen volumes.

The results of SPECT and PET studies of bipolar adults suggest rCBF abnormalities in both the frontal and temporal cortex. In general, investigators report increased rCBF in patients during mania and decreased rCBF during depression in adults with bipolar disorder. However, many of the SPECT and PET studies failed to report whether subjects and healthy comparison groups were diagnosed using standardized diagnostic interviews as well as the effects of confounding variables, such as medications. To our knowledge, there have been no published SPECT or PET studies in children or adolescents with bipolar disorder.

fMRI is a noninvasive imaging technique that does not involve exposure to ionizing radiation and has the advantage of better spatial and temporal resolution than PET or SPECT. The ability to recognize unique identities and forms of affect in human faces is an essential component of human social behavior, and the use of neurobehavioral probes, such as human facial affect recognition, with fMRI allows greater sensitivity and specificity in identifying the neural systems involved in mood disorders. There have been several fMRI studies in children where faces were used as neurobehavioral probes, and the Ekman facial recognition paradigm with the Ekman face set is most often used. Thomas et al. (2001) studied a group of

12 normal children with a mean age of 11 years with fMRI. In this experiment, the subjects passively viewed fearful and neutral Ekman faces. They reported predominantly increased left amygdala and substantia innominata brain activation during the presentation of nonmasked fearful faces relative to fixation and a decrease in activation in these regions with repeated exposure to the faces. In a similar fMRI study with the Ekman faces, Thomas et al. (2001) studied 12 children with generalized anxiety or panic disorder, 12 healthy controls, and five girls with major depressive disorder. In this experiment, children with anxiety disorders showed an exaggerated amygdala response to fearful faces compared with healthy children, whereas depressed children showed a blunted amygdala response to these faces.

There are few published fMRI studies in patients with bipolar disorder. Yergelun-Todd et al. (2000) found increased left amygdala and decreased dorsolateral prefrontal cortex activation in adults with bipolar disorder as compared to normal controls using the Ekman fearful and happy faces as visual stimuli. However, the differences observed may have been due to group differences in performance since all of the normal controls and only 10 of 14 (71%) bipolar patients were able to correctly identify the fearful Ekman faces. Blumberg et al. (2003a) evaluated regional brain activation in adults and adolescents with bipolar disorder using a Stroop task. They reported dorsal anterior cingulate and prefrontal cortical activation in controls and bipolar adults. Right ventral prefrontal activation was decreased in the manic bipolar adults, and left ventral prefrontal cortical activation was increased in depressed bipolar adults compared with euthymic bipolar adults. Rostral left ventral prefrontal cortical activation was decreased in bipolar adults as compared to the healthy controls, independent of mood state, suggesting that adults with bipolar disorder exhibit a trait abnormality in left ventral prefrontal cortex and that additional ventral prefrontal abnormalities may be associated with specific acute mood states. In a similar fMRI study, adolescents with bipolar disorder demonstrated an increase in activation in left putamen and thalamus compared with healthy adolescents. Age was positively correlated with signal increases in the bilateral rostroventral prefrontal cortex and the striatum in the healthy adolescents but not in the bipolar adolescents, suggesting that a developmental disturbance in prefrontal function may emerge in bipolar disorder over the course of adolescence.

Magnetic resonance spectroscopy (MRS) is a noninvasive neuroimaging technique that provides in vivo information regarding the concentration of specific biochemicals in localized brain regions. A benefit of MRS is that no ionizing radiation is used, thereby allowing serial studies to be performed on a subject. Typical isotopes evaluated with MRS include hydrogen or proton (^{1}H), lithium (^{7}Li), carbon (^{13}C), fluorine (^{19}F), sodium (^{23}Na), and phosphorus (^{31}P). Most of the studies of neurochemical changes in patients with bipolar disorder have used ^{1}H spectroscopy. There have been several studies of bipolar patients using magnetic resonance spectroscopy (MRS).

In general, ^{1}H studies of adults with bipolar disorder report abnormalities in choline concentrations in the basal ganglia, suggesting abnormal cell membrane phospholipids metabolism. Additionally, decreased N-acetyl aspartate (NAA) has been reported in the dorsolateral prefrontal cortex (DLPFC), prefrontal gray matter, hippocampus, and lenticular nuclei of adults with bipolar disorder, suggesting neuronal loss or dysfunction or mitochondrial dysfunction may be present in these brain regions. In contrast, increased NAA has been reported in the thalamus of male adults with bipolar disorder, suggesting neuronal hypertrophy or hyperplasia or abnormal synaptic or dendritic pruning is present in this brain region. Decreased NAA is also found in the cerebellar vermis and DLPFC and of bipolar children with familial bipolar disorder, indicating that neuronal dysfunction or loss in these brain regions occurs early in the course of illness. Castillo et al. (2000) found increased prefrontal and temporal Glx concentrations in children with bipolar disorder, suggesting that in addition to structural abnormalities, neurochemical dysfunction may be present in these brain regions. The Glx resonance is composed of glutamate, glutamine, and GABA, and elevated Glx may be a sign of neurotoxicity.

MRS can also be useful to identify the neurochemical effects and predictors of response to medications commonly used to treat bipolar disorder. The *myo*-inositol (mI) peak is of particular interest when evaluating the effects of lithium. The phosphainositide cycle is a major second messenger system by which lithium is thought to exert its therapeutic role in bipolar disorder. Lithium inhibits *myo*-inositol monophosphatase, thereby increasing inositol monophosphate (I-1-P) levels and decreasing *myo*-inositol levels in the brain. Lithium, by depleting *myo*-inositol, may slow down the phosphoinositide cycle in overactive synapses of bipolar patients. To evaluate the in vivo effects of lithium on brain *myo*-inositol, Moore et al. (2002) used ^{1}H MRS to assess mI levels in depressed bipolar patients at baseline prior to receiving any medications, after 5 to 7 days of acute lithium treatment, and following 3 to 4 weeks of lithium treatment. A significant decrease in right frontal mI was observed as early as 5 to 7 weeks following lithium treatment. Since the reduction was detected prior to the onset of observed clinical improvement, the authors concluded that decreased mI may be an early marker for a more downstream second messenger mechanism by which lithium may exert its mood stabilization effects. In a similar study in bipolar youth, Davanzo et al. (2001) used ^{1}H MRS to examine the anterior cingulate of 11 children and adolescents with bipolar disorder and 11 healthy adolescents and reported an elevation in *myo*-inositol/Cr in patients. Additionally, the authors report a significant reduction in mI following acute lithium treatment in lithium responders, suggesting a reduction in mI may also be an early marker of lithium response in bipolar youth. However, this study is limited by most of the patients receiving concomitant medications. Future MRS studies evaluating the effects of lithium monotherapy, as well as the effects of other medications commonly used to treat bipolar disorder may facilitate targeted treatment intervention by identifying neurochemical predictors of treatment response.

In summary, neuroimaging studies of MDD youth suggest structural, function and neurochemical deficits in prefrontal regions. Additionally, abnormalities in amygdala structure and function have been observed, but seem to be associated with anxiety in MDD youth. Future studies examining other brain regions, including the striatum, are necessary.

MOOD DISORDERS DUE TO GENERAL MEDICAL CONDITIONS

DSM-IV defines a mood disorder due to a general medical condition as a prominent and persistent disturbance of mood (depressed mood; markedly diminished interest or pleasure; or elevated, expansive, or irritable mood) that is judged to be due to the direct physiological effects of a general medical condition. Implicit in this definition is the assumption that treating the medical condition would result in elimination of the mood symptoms. Several general questions arise with regard to secondary mood disorders in the context of medical illness. First, are all mood symptoms and disabilities a consequence of the medical problem? Second, are there symptoms of both a primary mood disorder and a medical condition? Third, is the primary mood disorder causing increased morbidity in a known medical disorder? For example, in chronic infectious mononucleosis or chronic fatigue syndrome with depressive symptoms, is the disability a consequence of the infection, or does a primary mood disorder interact with the infection to cause a more protracted course?

Thyroid disease and infectious mononucleosis with an indolent course are commonly associated with mood disorders, and whether to routinely screen for these common or other rare disorders in children with mood disturbance remains a clinical decision based on history and physical examination. Laboratory testing rarely identifies occult medical disorders that are not evident from history and examination in child psychiatric populations. In this context, no routine laboratory evaluation studies are indicated. In children and adolescents presenting with mood disorders, features suggestive of an occult medical cause include atypical presentation of mood symptoms and poor or idiosyncratic responses to psychiatric treatment. In adults, the most frequent secondary causes of mania are corticosteroid use, human immunodeficiency virus (HIV) infection, and temporal lobe epilepsy.

SUBSTANCE-INDUCED MOOD DISORDERS

Substance Abuse/Dependence

Mood disorders can occur in association with acute intoxication with alcohol, amphetamines, cocaine, hallucinogens, inhalants, or other drugs of abuse. Also, mood symptoms can be associated with withdrawal from such drugs. Again, as with medical conditions, the assumption is that the substance is etiologically related to the mood symptoms. Mood symptoms in substance-abusing adolescents present significant clinical and diagnostic challenges. Although both primary and secondary mood disorders are common in substance-abusing patients, clinical treatment must initially focus on abstinence from continuing substance abuse, as evaluation and appropriate treatment of the primary mood disorder (if it is present) cannot take place while an individual is actively abusing substances.

Mood Disorders Associated with Neurological Conditions

Studies have identified a high rate of psychiatric disorders in children and adolescents with various neurological conditions. The neurological disorders most commonly associated with psychiatric symptoms are brain injuries, epilepsy, migraine headaches, and learning disabilities.

Brain Injury
Although emotional and behavioral symptoms often associated with psychiatric disorders are frequently observed after brain injury, such symptoms are usually interpreted as either a direct effect of the injury or a normative reaction to the injury. Several groups have found increased rates of psychiatric disorders including depressive disorders in children following a head injury.

Epilepsy
The association between epilepsy and depression has received extensive study. Suicide has been reported to occur at a higher rate in patients with epilepsy than in those without epilepsy. Rutter et al. (1976), in the Isle of Wight study, found psychiatric disturbance in 58% of the 8-year-old to 10-year-old children with epilepsy. In adults with epilepsy, depression is common but mania appears to be rare. The association between epilepsy and depression is important for several reasons. First, in some patients with epilepsy, comorbid depression is associated with poor seizure control. One study has suggested that treatment with fluoxetine can reduce seizure frequency in patients with resistant epilepsy. Ojemann et al. (1987) also reported that seizure control and general functioning were improved when psychotropic medications were added to the subjects' anticonvulsant regimens. Second, an unrecognized depression can lead to

increased morbidity that often is wrongly attributed to the epilepsy. Third, some medications for epilepsy can cause a worsening of mood. Children and adolescents with epilepsy who continue to function poorly despite having adequate seizure control should be examined for mood disorders.

Migraine

One of the first criteria for identifying depression in pre-pubertal children was suggested from a study of children manifesting severe headache. Of the 25 children presenting with headache, 4 of 16 (25%) with migraine headaches were depressed and 6 of 9 (64%) with nonmigraine headaches were depressed. Some of these children manifested classic migraine. Couch and Hassanein (1979) subsequently demonstrated that TCAs were efficacious in preventing migraine headaches in adults, regardless of the presence of depression. This finding raises the question of whether a common etiological mechanism may be operating in migraine and depression. Clinically, children and adolescents with frequent, incapacitating headaches (migraine or nonmigraine) often manifest depression. Treatment of the depression resolves both the frequent headaches and the depression. Commonly used medications for the prevention of migraine include beta-adrenergic blockers and periactin; these agents do not benefit depression.

Learning Disabilities

The relationship between learning disabilities and affective disorders is a complex one. Children doing poorly in school often present with both learning disability symptoms and emotional/behavioral problems. It is an over-simplification to say either that the learning disability leads to the emotional problems or that the emotional problems are the only cause of the school failure. Initially it is helpful to assess both dimensions separately rather than assuming causation from an association. Affective disorder is the comorbid condition most commonly seen with learning disability.

The prevalence of mood disorders is higher in learning-disabled than in nonlearning disabled populations. The reasons for this difference in prevalence are not clear. It is possible that learning disabilities and the difficulties they cause induce mood disorders in susceptible individuals. Also, chronic mood disorders can, over time, interfere with school adaptation. There is evidence that neuropsychological deficits may accompany altered mood states, which in the developing individual could lead to delays in learning. However, for clinicians the association between learning disabilities and mood disorders is a familiar one, because a learning-disabled child with a mood disorder is more likely to be referred for evaluation than one without a comorbid affective illness.

TREATMENT

General Management

The treatment of children and adolescents with mood disorders is ideally multimodal. Family, school, and social environments are affected by these disorders and in turn may play a role in precipitating episodes of illness. Children, parents, and schools must all participate in treatment. The primary aim of treatment is to shorten the mood disorder episode, to prevent recurrence, and to decrease the negative consequences of depressive or manic episodes.

Education about mood disorders is essential for parents and affected children. Such information decreases self-blame and the tendency to blame others. It is common for schools to blame parents and parents to blame schools for a child's deteriorating behavior, and this can lead to inappropriate solutions to the problem, such as changing schools. Parents need to know that mood disorders represent biological conditions and not personality flaws. Coping with a mood disorder is a daily struggle. Specific therapies can be beneficial as an adjunct to management. Treatment should be individualized and based on need, resources, and assessment of stressors involved in a particular case.

In addition to eliciting the family's participation in managing the individual's symptoms, a family assessment is conducted to evaluate the premorbid level of family functioning, the parents' marital relationship, the impact of the mood disorder on the family, the family's understanding of the disorder, and their attempts to manage it. The family should assist in developing a treatment plan, including the identification of problem areas for change. Studies have found that at the time of treatment, 30 to 50% of depressed adolescents have a parent who is affectively ill. Thus, appropriate identification of parents who need treatment is important in the management of these patients.

As previously mentioned, the school setting is extremely important in the treatment process. Often, treatment includes adapting the patient's school setting in order to reduce stress. This strategy could take the form of shortening the school day; limiting the amount of schoolwork assigned, developing assignment-completion checklists, or arranging a more structured classroom setting; or using bypass compensatory strategies such as computers, calculators, and books on tape. For learning-disabled children, a continual focus on deficits can lead to worsening mood symptoms. Developing a positive school environment is essential for these children.

Many children with mood disorders have interpersonal problems resulting from social deficits. These deficits compound the depression and often contribute to feelings of worthlessness, hopelessness, and alienation. It is important for therapists, parents, and teachers to clarify reality for these patients. Group-therapy approaches that help build skills through role play, problem-solving techniques, communication and assertiveness training, and strategies for self-control and conflict resolution can be effective.

Psychotherapy of Depressive Disorders

Several studies indicated that specific psychotherapies are effective treatments for depression in adolescent populations. The most extensive research has been with cognitive-behavior group therapy, individual cognitive behavioral therapy and interpersonal psychotherapy (IPT) in adolescent populations. Individual psychotherapy for depression has been strongly influenced by earlier work in adults that primarily focused on cognitive therapy and interpersonal therapy. Modifications of these therapies for adolescents have been found to be effective and have resulted in the development of treatment manuals.

Cognitive behavioral therapy (CBT) is the most commonly used specific psychotherapy for children and adolescents with depression, and the most widely studied. As with adult populations, it is generally time limited and focused on identifying thought patterns and behaviors that contribute to the child's depression. Behavioral activation and problem-solving strategies are emphasized, as well as skill development. Several studies have demonstrated the effectiveness of child and adolescent CBT. For example, a study by Brent et al. (1997) compared CBT, systematic-behavioral family therapy (SBFT), and individual nondirective supportive therapy (NST) and found rates of remission to be 60%, 37%, and 39%, respectively. A meta-analysis of six controlled CBT studies in depressed adolescents yielded a reasonably robust overall posttreatment effect size of 1.02, whereas the overall effect size at 5 weeks to 3 months posttreatment was 0.61. Group CBT for adolescents has also been found to be effective with a response rate of 66.7% of subjects assigned to a CBT group, compared to only 48.1% of the waitlist controls.

Interpersonal therapy (IPT) is based on the premise that depressive illness operates in an interpersonal context. In particular, this treatment focuses on the resolution of four possible problem areas, including grief, interpersonal role disputes, role transitions, and interpersonal deficits. Thus, the goal of IPT when treating depression is to understand current relationships and renegotiate interpersonal problems occurring at the onset of depressive symptoms. IPT has demonstrated some effectiveness in the treatment of depressive symptoms in adolescents. In a controlled, single-blind study of clinical-referred depressed adolescents, IPT was found to be more effective than clinical monitoring for depressive symptom reduction and social functioning improvement. Similarly, in a 12-week open study of IPT for 25 moderately to severely depressed adolescents, 84% meet criteria for remission by the end of the treatment. In addition, IPT has also been show to be effective in Puerto Rican populations.

Another potential treatment for severe depression, particularly in patients with a history of suicide attempts, is dialectical behavior therapy (DBT). DBT was originally developed for adult chronically parasuicidal women diagnosed with borderline personality disorder (BPD) and was found to significantly reduce anger, suicide attempts, parasuicidal acts, and the number of inpatient psychiatric days. DBT has also been shown to improve social adjustment, treatment compliance, and dropout rates. The efficacy of DBT was reported in an open study of 27 14-year-old to 19-year-old suicidal adolescents diagnosed with BPD or borderline features. Improvement was reported in areas of confusion about self, impulsivity, emotional instability, and interpersonal problems. The most helpful DBT skills were identified as mindfulness and distress tolerance.

Pharmacotherapy of Depressive Disorders

Several factors should be considered prior to initiating medication treatments in children and adolescents. These factors include history, course, and severity of illness, family history of psychiatric illness, and environmental and psychosocial factors. It is imperative to get an accurate diagnosis, and the use of structured interviews can greatly facilitate this process. Understanding the family's view of the illness and their beliefs about medications is also critical.

To date, limited guidelines are available for treatment of pediatric depression. In 1998, the AACAP published treatment guidelines for pediatric depression. At that time, only two trials of selective serotonin reuptake inhibitors (SSRIs) had been reported: one positive and one negative. Limited data were available on specific psychotherapy trials, as well. In that guideline, psychotherapy was indicated as the first line of treatment for mild to moderate depression. Medication (specifically, SSRIs) was recommended for psychotic depression, bipolar depression, and severe depression. The Texas Children's Medication Algorithm Project (CMAP) project also provided guidelines specifically for medication treatment. This algorithm, which was published in 1999 was also based on limited available data. However, with regard to medication treatment for pediatric depression, the later research supports the CMAP recommendations of SSRIs as first-line treatment.

Since these guidelines were published, we now have reports of many other treatment trials for both therapy and psychopharmacology. We also now have a trial with a head-to-head comparison of the two treatments (TADS). Although these guidelines provide a good framework, new guidelines to include the more recent data are warranted. For example, should single modality treatments be used versus combination treatments? The APA Practice Guidelines for adults state that combination treatment is suggested for individuals with significant psychosocial problems, a history of partial response to pharmacotherapy or psychotherapy alone, or poor adherence to a single mode of treatment. While medications often work quickly to reduce symptoms, the failure rate of medication alone is about 40%. Combination treatment may enhance the probability of response, as well as the magnitude of response. In other words, two treatments may be more robust than one, and if one method is not helpful in reducing symptoms, the other one may be.

The first study to demonstrate an antidepressant medication treatment to be superior to placebo in treating early-onset depression was by Emslie et al. (1997a). In this study of 96 children and adolescents (ages 8 to 18) with MDD, 56% of those randomized to fluoxetine versus 33% of those randomized to placebo were considered much or very much improved following 8 weeks of treatment. A large multisite trial replicating the design of this first trial was then conducted with 219 children and adolescents (ages 8 to 17). Subjects were randomized to 9 weeks of treatment with fluoxetine or placebo. Similar to the initial study, 52% versus 37%, respectively, were considered much or very much improved (Emslie et al., 2002). As mentioned, a 12-week trial comparing fluoxetine, CBT, combination treatment, and placebo (sponsored by the National Institutes of Health [NIH]) also supported the use of fluoxetine, both alone and in combination treatment. Sixty-one percent of those on fluoxetine alone and 71% of those on fluoxetine plus CBT were considered responders, while only 35% of subjects on placebo responded. Thus, fluoxetine has shown efficacy over placebo in three controlled trials to date. Fluoxetine is the only antidepressant approved for treatment of pediatric depression. In addition, both the British Medicine and Healthcare Products Regulatory Agency (MHRA) and the U.S. Federal Drug Administratioin (FDA) stated that the risk–benefit ratio for using fluoxetine to treat pediatric depression was satisfactory.

In another large, multisite industry-funded study, 275 adolescents (ages 12 to 18) with MDD were randomized to paroxetine, imipramine, or placebo for an 8-week acute trial. Paroxetine was superior in efficacy to placebo (66% versus 48%), but imipramine (52%) was not. This study demonstrates additional support for the efficacy of SSRIs, while also reinforcing that TCAs may not be effective treatments for depressed youth, although they may have a role in specific individuals. Two other studies have been conducted with paroxetine, but have had negative results. In both cases, the placebo rate was quite high, suggesting methodological issues may have contributed to the negative outcome (GSK Website).

Two multisite trials of sertraline versus placebo have also been conducted, and the data were pooled for analyses. In this study, 376 children and adolescents (ages 6 to 17) with MDD were randomized to sertraline or placebo for 10 weeks. Sixty-three percent of subjects randomized to sertraline were considered much or very much improved, compared to 53% on placebo. Finally, Wagner et al. (2001) report on a multisite, double-blind, placebo-controlled study of citalopram in 174 children and adolescents (ages 7 to 17) with MDD. In this study, a significant difference was seen between the active treatment group and the placebo group beginning after 1 week of treatment. Rates of response were not as high as in other studies (36% for

citalopram versus 24% for placebo; $p < .05$); however, this is due to the definition of response defined in this trial. In this study response was defined as CDRS-R$\leq$28, which is generally used to define remission (symptom-free or "well") in other trials.

A treatment algorithm was developed for the pharmacological management of pediatric depression. The Texas Children's Medication Algorithm Project (CMAP) developed a medication algorithm that provides initial strategies of single medications that have been found to be safe and effective. Treatment follows a stage approach where patients progress to the next strategy or medication based on lack of sufficient symptom improvement or medication intolerance. The algorithm and increasing evidence from controlled trials support the use of selective serotonin reuptake inhibitors (SSRIs) as the first-line of treatment. This recommendation is based on lack of efficacy of tricyclic antidepressants and positive trials in four of the SSRI medications, including fluoxetine, paroxetine, sertraline, and citalolpram. To date, only fluoxetine is approved by the FDA for the treatment of pediatric depression.

Despite the several trials showing significant improvement of depression in SSRIs over placebo, controversies about SSRIs being used in children and adolescents have surfaced. In June 2003, Great Britain's Department of Health (under the direction of the country's Medicines and Healthcare Products Regulatory Agency (MHRA)) stated that paroxetine was contraindicated in children and adolescents with depression due to lack of efficacy and increased risk of suicidal behavior in this population. The FDA followed suit, stating that paroxetine should not be used in children under 18. In October 2003, the FDA reported that they would be conducting analyses on all antidepressant data to determine the risk–benefit profile of the SSRIs and other newer antidepressants. Finally, in March 2004, the FDA has requested that the manufacturers of many of the newer antidepressants, including SSRIs, include a warning in the label recommending that health care providers closely monitor all patients taking these medications for worsening of depression and emergence of suicidal behavior.

It is important to note that in 2,885 depressed patients reviewed (who participated in clinical controlled trials), there were no completed suicides. In a reanalysis and reclassification of all the suicide-related events in pediatric controlled trials of antidepressants (for any disorder), there were 95 clear suicide-related behaviors in 4,250 youth studied. Combining all antidepressants for all disorders showed a risk ratio of 1.78 (Confidence Interval [CI]: 1.14 to 2.77), which is significantly greater than placebo. For SSRI MDD trials, the risk ration was 1.41 (CI: 0.84 to 2.37; not significant). Most individual antidepressants were not associated with increased risk of suicidal behavior. However, paroxetine and venlafaxine did show significantly higher risk of suicidal behavior over placebo 2.65 (CI: 1.00 to 7.02) for paroxetine, 4.97 (CI: 1.09 to 22.72) for venlafaxine.

Although SSRIs are currently under scrutiny, these medications continue to be used in this population, and, as a group, remain the pharmacological treatment of choice for depression in this age group. Unfortunately, alternative treatments, such as CBT, have limited data and are simply not readily available in most communities. In a trial, which was sponsored by NIH and not funded through pharmaceutical agencies, adolescents were randomized to fluoxetine alone, CBT alone, combination fluoxetine and CBT, or placebo. Combination treatment and fluoxetine alone were significantly more effective than CBT alone and placebo. Seventy-one percent of those on combination treatment responded well to treatment, compared with 61% on fluoxetine alone, 43% on CBT, and 35% on placebo. Thus, this single trial suggests that treatment with an antidepressant is more effective than CBT or no treatment for moderate to severe depression in teens. Addition of a specific psychotherapy such as CBT may further enhance response.

Thus, despite the controversies facing SSRIs, several trials have demonstrated positive effect of SSRIs. There are no data in adults suggesting that the individual SSRIs are different (e.g., widely different mechanisms of action), so it is expected that the pediatric age group would be no different. To state it more clearly, the different rates of response to placebo does not cause people to think that the placebos are different across trials. Rather, it is more likely that the methodologies across trials are the primary cause of different response outcomes. Thus, it has been clearly established that SSRIs are effective in treating children and adolescents with MDD, and due to the relatively low side effects profile and safety in overdose, these medications are considered the first-line of treatment in this population.

Unfortunately, up to 40% of depressed youth do not respond to initial antidepressant treatments. To date, no trials have been reported on second-line treatment. The CMAP algorithm suggests that an alternative SSRI be used next, followed by one of the other new antidepressants, such as venlafaxine. Two placebo-controlled trials have been conducted with venlafaxine (ages 7 to 17). The studies were pooled for analyses, and results indicated that there was no significant difference between venlafaxine and placebo. However, when age groups were separated out, venlafaxine was more effective than placebo in adolescents in relieving depressive symptoms ($P = .02$). Wyeth Ayerst Pharmaceuticals, manufacturers of venlafaxine, have stated that venlafaxine should not be used to treat depression in youth under 18, as the company states there is an increased chance of suicidal behavior in youth taking this medication (2 versus 0%; not significant). Other medication options for second-line and third-line treatments are nefazodone, mirtazapine, and bupropion. A study of adolescents (ages 12 to 17) treated with either nefazodone or placebo demonstrated greater response in teens treated with nefazodone (65 versus 46%, respectively; $P = .005$). Two controlled-studies have been conducted in mirtazapine, but they have not yet been published. Communication with the sponsor indicates these trials were negative due to a high placebo response rate. No controlled studies have been reported on depression treatment with bupropion. Thus, although these medications are optional treatments for pediatric depression, substantially less positive results have been reported with these medications. To date, no studies have assessed which second-line treatments are most effective in youth who do not improve during acute treatment. Therefore, in youth who do not improve with initial SSRI treatment, a second SSRI trial or switching to an alternative type of medication such as these may be viable options. Finally, augmenting with a mood stabilizer (i.e., lithium) or electroconvulsive therapy (ECT) are treatment options for severely refractory depression, though these alternatives have not received adequate investigation in this population. All of these recommendations are based mainly on adult data and need further study in the pediatric population.

Bipolar Disorders

There is increasing information about the effectiveness of psychosocial treatments that complement and support medication treatment in children and adolescents with bipolar disorders. Several trials have been conducted, suggesting support for psychotherapeutic intervention as an intervention to augment medication in reducing the symptoms of bipolar disorder and in improving adherence to the medication regime. There is some evidence that the most beneficial of multifamily psychoeducational treatments, is that which provides education about bipolar illness in a group discussion format, along with skills training for both parents and children.

The clinical use of mood stabilizers and atypical antipsychotic agents in children and adolescents with bipolar disorders (BPD) has increased significantly over the past few years, despite the fact that there are few controlled trials in this population. Many of the same psychotropic medications used to treat adults with bipolar disorders are also used for children and adolescents. To date, there have been only two double-blind placebo controlled studies of the treatment for acute mania in children and adolescents with bipolar disorder and one uncontrolled maintenance treatment study.

Lithium is the most studied medication for children and adolescents with bipolar disorder and is the only medication approved by the Food and Drug Administration for the treatment of acute mania and bipolar disorder in adolescents or children (ages 12 to 18 years). Approximately 40 to 50% of children and adolescents with mania or hypomania will respond to lithium monotherapy. In general, lithium should be titrated to a dose of 30 mg/kg/day in two to three divided doses, which typically results in a therapeutic serum level of 0.8 to 1.2 mEq per L. Common side effects of lithium in children and adolescents include hypothyroidism, nausea, polyuria, polydipsia, tremor, acne, and weight gain. Lithium levels and thyroid function tests should be monitored as in adults.

In the only prospective, placebo-controlled, investigation of lithium in children and adolescents with bipolar disorders (n = 25), Geller et al. (1998) found that after 6 weeks of treatment, subjects treated with lithium showed a statistically significant decrease in positive urine toxicology screens and a significant improvement in global assessment of functioning (46% in the lithium treated group versus 8% in the placebo group). This study demonstrated the efficacy of lithium carbonate for the treatment of bipolar adolescents with comorbid substance use disorders, but it did not measure the effect of lithium on mood in these adolescents. Risk factors for poor lithium response in children and adolescents with bipolar disorder include prepubertal-onset and the presence of co-occurring ADHD.

Surprisingly, despite their wide use, there are no published placebo controlled studies of antiepileptic medication for the treatment of pediatric bipolar disorder. Open label studies of divalproex in manic adolescents have reported response rates ranging from 53 to 82%. There have also been several case reports and series describing the successful use of carbamazepine as monotherapy and adjunctive treatment in children and adolescents with bipolar disorder. Kowatch et al. are currently completing an NIMH sponsored clinical trial of the efficacy of lithium and valproate in children and adolescents with BP I disorder. This trial will provide much needed data about the efficacy and safety of these widely used two-mood stabilizers.

In general, divalproex is initiated at a dose of 20 mg/kg/day, which will typically produce a serum level of 80 to 120 ug per ml, and carbamazepine is usually titrated to a dose of 15 mg/kg/day to produce a serum level of 7 to 10 ug per ml. Common side effects of divalproex in children are weight gain, nausea, sedation, and tremor. There has been much debate regarding the possible association between divalproex and polycystic ovarian syndrome (PCOS). The initial reports of PCOS were in women with epilepsy who were treated with divalproex. The hypothesized mechanism for divalproex induced PCOS is that obesity secondary to divalproex results in elevated insulin levels, which leads to increased androgen levels and ultimately PCOS. Further investigations of the risk of developing PCOS for female bipolar adolescents are necessary. Until this issue is settled, clinicians should monitor female patients treated with divalproex for any signs of PCOS that include weight, menstrual abnormalities, hirsutism, or acne.

Carbamazepine is used widely for seizure management but less commonly than divalproex in children and adolescents with bipolar disorder. This anticonvulsant must be titrated slowly and requires frequent monitoring of blood levels because of CYP450 drug interactions. Its most common side effects are sedation, rash, nausea, and hyponatremia. Aplastic anemia and severe dermatologic reactions such as Stevens-Johnson syndrome occur uncommonly. Side effects of carbamazepine include developing aplastic anemia and severe dermatological reactions, such as Stevens-Johnson's syndrome, hyponatremia, nausea, and sedation, and it is therefore, less commonly used in children and adolescents with bipolar disorder. Oxcarbazepine, an analog of carbamazepine, is a promising agent for acute mania in adults, but no pediatric data are available.

Several new antiepileptic agents have been developed for the treatment of epilepsy that may have mood stabilizing properties. Data are presently limited regarding the efficacy and tolerability of these agents for the treatment of pediatric bipolar disorder. However, they may be useful as adjuncts for the treatment of manic and hypomanic episodes. There have been several case reports of lamotrigine as adjunctive treatment for children and adolescents with bipolar disorder. However, its use for pediatric bipolar disorder has been limited due to the risk of potentially lethal cutaneous reactions, such as Stevens-Johnson syndrome and toxic epidermal necrolysis. The risk of a serious rash is approximately two to three times greater in children and adolescents younger than 16 years old compared with adults, but a more conservative dosing schedule appears to have substantially reduced the rate of serious rashes. Double-blind placebo controlled studies of gabapentin have demonstrated that gabapentin is no more effective than placebo for the treatment of acute mania in adults. However, gabapentin may be effective for the treatment of anxiety disorders in adults and is generally well tolerated in children and adolescents. Therefore, gabapentin may be particularly useful for treating children and adolescents with bipolar disorder who are also diagnosed with a comorbid anxiety disorder. Preliminary data from open studies suggest that topiramate may be effective as an adjunctive treatment for pediatric bipolar disorder, although more recent double-blind placebo controlled studies in adults with mania suggest that as monotherapy it is no more effective than placebo. Word finding difficulties have been reported in up to one third of adult patients treated with topiramate. Topiramate is associated with anorexia and weight loss, and therefore it may be useful as adjunctive treatment for children and adolescents with bipolar disorder who have gained weight as a result of treatment with other psychotropic medications.

The atypical antipsychotics are powerful psychotropic agents that have been found to be efficacious in the treatment of adults with schizophrenia and acute bipolar mania. These atypical agents not only have antipsychotic activity but may also possess thymoleptic properties with favorable effects on the depressive and manic symptoms of patients with bipolar disorders. To date, there have been three large controlled studies of olanzapine, two controlled trials of risperidone, and one controlled trial of ziprasidone in the treatment of adults with acute mania.

Several case series and open-label reports suggest that atypical antipsychotics clozapine, risperidone, olanzapine, and quetiapine are effective in the treatment of pediatric mania. However, there may be significant weight gain associated with olanzapine and risperidone. Ziprasidone can cause QTc prolongation and there are limited safety data in children and adolescents. Therefore, ziprasidone should be used with caution in children and adolescents with bipolar disorder and electrocardiograms should be monitored at baselines and when significant dosage increases are made. In the only double-blind placebo-controlled study of an atypical antipsychotic for the treatment of bipolar adolescents, quetiapine in combination with divalproex (n = 15) resulted in a greater reduction of manic symptoms than divalproex monotherapy (n = 15), suggesting that the combination of a mood stabilizer and atypical antipsychotic is more effective than a mood stabilizer alone for the treatment of adolescent mania. In this study, quetiapine was titrated to a dose of 450 mg per day in 7 days and was well tolerated.

If a child or adolescent has euphoric mania without psychotic symptoms, then a trial of lithium is many times helpful. Adult patients with dysphoric mania appear to respond better to divalproex than to lithium. But if psychotic symptoms are present as part of the child or adolescent's mania, then treatment with an atypical antipsychotic agent is indicated. If a patient does not respond to monotherapy with either a traditional mood stabilizer like lithium or valproate, or an atypical antipsychotic, then a combination of a traditional mood stabilizer and any atypical antipsychotic may be effective.

Most children with BPD will have comorbid ADHD, and mood stabilization with mood stabilizers or atypical antipsychotics is a necessary prerequisite prior to initiating stimulant medications. A randomized controlled trial of 40 bipolar children and adolescents with ADHD demonstrated that low-dose Dexedrine can be safely and effectively used for treatment of comorbid ADHD symptoms after the child's BPD symptoms are stabilized with divalproex. Sustained release psychostimulants may be more effective at reducing rebound symptoms in bipolar children and adolescents. A typical dose of such stimulants for a child with BPD and ADHD would be 36 mg per day of Concerta or Adderall XR, 10 to 20 mg per day.

Many agents used to treat children and adolescents with bipolar disorder are associated with weight gain. A series of general medical, metabolic problems may occur as a result of increases in weight. These include type II (noninsulin dependent) diabetes mellitus, and changes in lipid levels, and transaminase elevation. Children who experience significant weight gain should be monitored especially closely for these possibilities and should be referred for exercise and nutritional counseling. The American Diabetes Association, in collaboration with the American Psychiatric Association, published a monitoring protocol for all patients prior to initiating treatment with an atypical antipsychotic. This protocol includes inquiring about a personal and family history of obesity, diabetes, dyslipidemia, hypertension, or cardiovascular disease; weight and height, so that body mass index (BMI) can be calculated; measurement of waist circumference (at the level of the umbilicus); blood pressure; fasting plasma glucose; and a fasting lipid profile. This group recommended that the patient's weight should be reassessed at 4, 8, and 12 weeks after initiating or changing therapy with an atypical antipsychotic and quarterly thereafter at the time of routine visits. If a patient gains more than 5% of his or her initial weight at any time during therapy, the patient should be switched to an alternative agent. These guidelines should be followed in all children and adolescents treated with atypical antipsychotics. It should be also be recognized that although these guidelines are extremely helpful, they were not written for a pediatric population, and the 5% weight gain threshold may not be sensitive enough for children and adolescents.

CONCLUSION

Despite increased awareness of the occurrence of mood disorders in children and adolescents, pediatric mood disorders frequently go undiagnosed and untreated. Misdiagnosis is particularly likely when clinicians attempt to differentiate primary mood disorders from mood disorders due to general medical conditions or to substance-induced mood disorders. It is important that these disorders are recognized and appropriately treated as they can cause significant suffering, morbidity, and suicide.

REFERENCES

Achamallah NS, Decker DH: Mania induced by fluoxetine in an adolescent patient (letter). Am J Psychiatry 148:1404, 1991.

Adams M, Kutcher S, Antoniw E, et al.: Diagnostic utility of endocrine and neuroimaging screening tests in first-onset adolescent psychosis. J Am Acad Child Adolesc Psychiatry 35:67–73, 1996.

Agren H: Symptom patterns in unipolar and bipolar depression correlating with monoamine metabolites in cerebrospinal fluid, I: general patterns. Psychiatry Res 3:211–223, 1980.

Akiskal HS, Downs J, Jordan P, et al.: Affective disorders in referred children and younger siblings of manic-depressives: mode of onset and prospective course. Arch Gen Psychiatry 42:996–1003, 1985.

Altman EG, Hedeker DR, Janicak PG, et al.: The Clinician Administered Rating Scale for Mania (CARS-M): development, reliability, and validity. Biol Psychiatry 36:124–134, 1994.

Altshuler LL, Bartzokis G, Grieder T, Curran J, Mintz, J: Amygdala enlargement in bipolar disorder and hippocampal reduction in schizophrenia: an MRI study demonstrating neuroanatomic specificity [letter]. Arch Gen Psychiatry 55:663–664, 1998.

Altshuler LL, Curran JG, Hauser P, et al.: T2 hyperintensities in bipolar disorder: magnetic resonance imaging comparison and literature meta-analysis. Am J Psychiatry 152:1139–1144, 1995.

Ambrosini PJ, Emslie GJ, Greenhill LL, et al.: Selecting a sequence of antidepressants for treating depression in youth. J Child Adolesc Psychopharmacol 5:233–240, 1995.

American Diabetes Association and American Psychiatric Association: Consensus development conference on antipsychotic drugs and obesity and diabetes. Diabetes Care 27:596–601, 2004.

American Psychiatric Association: Diagnostic and Statistical Manual of Mental Disorders, 3rd Edition. Washington, DC: American Psychiatric Association, 1980.

American Psychiatric Association: Diagnostic and Statistical Manual of Mental Disorders, 3rd Ed., Revised. Washington, DC: American Psychiatric Association, 1987.

American Psychiatric Association: Diagnostic and Statistical Manual of Mental Disorders, 4th Ed. Washington, DC: American Psychiatric Association, 1994.

Anthony J, Scott P: Manic-depressive psychosis in childhood. J Child Psychol Psychiatry 4:53–72, 1960.

Asarnow JR, Goldstein MJ, Carlson GA, et al.: Childhood-onset depressive disorders: a follow-up study of rates of rehospitalization and out-of-home placement among child psychiatric inpatients. J Affect Disord 15:245–253, 1988.

Baldessarini RJ: Current status of antidepressants: clinical pharmacology and therapy. J Clin Psychiatry 50:117–126, 1989.

Barczak P, Edmunds E, Belts T: Hypomania following complex partial seizures: a report of three cases. Br J Psychiatry 152:137–139, 1988.

Barraclough B: Suicide and epilepsy, in *Epilepsy and Psychiatry*. Edited by Reynolds EH, Trimble MR. Edinburgh, Scotland, Churchill Livingstone, pp. 72–76, 1981.

Baxter LR: PET studies of cerebral function in major depression and obsessive-compulsive disorder: the emerging prefrontal cortex consensus. Ann Clin Psychiatry 3:103–109, 1991.

Bear DM: Hemispheric specialization and neurology of emotion. Arch Neurol 40:195–202, 1983.

Belsher G, Wilkes TCR: An open multi-site pilot study of cognitive therapy for depressed adolescents. J Psychother Pract Res 4:52–66, 1995.

Berk M., Ichim L, Brook S: Olanzapine compared to lithium in mania: a double-blind randomized controlled trial. Int Clin Psychopharmacol 14(Nov):339–343, 1999.

Biederman J, Faraone SV, Keenan K, et al.: Evidence of familial association between attention deficit disorder and major affective disorders. Arch Gen Psychiatry 48:633–642, 1991.

Biederman J, Mick E, Prince J, Bostic JQ, Wilens TE, Spencer T, Wozniak J, Faraone SV: Systematic chart review of the pharmacologic treatment of comorbid attention deficit hyperactivity disorder in youth with bipolar disorder. J Child Adolesc Psychopharmacol 9:247–256, 1999.

Biederman J, Munir K, Knee D, Armentano M, Autor S, Waternaux C, Tsuang M: High rate of affective disorders in probands with attention deficit disorder and in their relatives: a controlled family study. Am J Psychiatry 144:330–333, 1987.

Birleson P, Hudson I, Buchanan DG, et al.: Clinical evaluation of a self-rating scale for depressive disorder in childhood (Depression Self-Rating Scale). JAMA 28:43–60, 1987.

Birmaher B, Ryan N, Williamson D, Brent D, Kaufman J: Childhood and adolescent depression: a review of the past 10 years. Part II. J Am Acad Child Adolesc Psychiatry 35(Dec):1575–183, 1996a.

Birmaher B, Ryan N, Williamson D, Brent D, Kaufman J, Dahl R, Perel J, Nelson B: Childhood and adolescent depression: a review of the past 10 years. Part I. J Am Acad Child Adolesc Psychiatry 35(Nov):1427–1439, 1996b.

Birmaher B, Dahl RE, Perel J, Williamson DE, Nelson B, Stull S, Kaufman J, Waterman GS, Rao U, Nguyen N, Puig-Antich J, Ryan ND: Corticotropin-releasing hormone challenge in prepubertal major depression. Biol Psychiatry 39: 267–277, 1996c.

Black IB, Hendry IA, Iverser LL: Trans-synaptic regulation of growth and development of adrenergic neurons in a mouse sympathetic ganglion. Brain Res 24:229–240, 1971.

Blumberg HP, Leung HC, Skudlarski P, Lacadie CM, Fredericks CA, Harris BC, Charney DS, Gore JC, Krystal JH, Peterson BS: A functional magnetic resonance imaging study of bipolar disorder: state- and trait-related dysfunction in ventral prefrontal cortices. Arch Gen Psychiatry 60:601–609, 2003a.

Blumberg HP, Martin A, Kaufman J, Leung HC, Skudlarski P, Lacadie C, Fulbright RK, Gore JC, Charney DS, Krystal JH, Peterson BS: Frontostriatal abnormalities in adolescents with bipolar disorder: preliminary observations from functional MRI. Am J Psychiatry 160:1345–1347, 2003b.

Blumberg SH, Izard CE: Affective and cognitive characteristics of depression in 10- and 11-year-old children. J Pers Soc Psychol 49: 194–202, 1985.

Botteron KN, Vannier MW Geller B, et al.: Preliminary study of magnetic resonance imaging characteristics in 8- to 16-year-olds with mania. J Am Acad Child Adolesc Psychiatry 34:742–749, 1995.

Boulos C, Kutcher S, Gardner D, et al.: An open naturalistic trial of fluoxetine in adolescents and young adults with treatment-resistant major depression. J Child Adolesc Psychopharmacol 2:103–111, 1992.

Bowden CL: Predictors of response to divalproex and lithium. J Clin Psychiatry 56 (sup 3):25–30, 1995.

Bowden CL, Brugger AM, Swann AC, et al.: Efficacy of divalproex vs. lithium and placebo in the treatment of mania: the Depakote Mania Study Group. JAMA 271:918–924, 1994 (published erratum appears in JAMA 271:1830, 1994 [see comments]).

Bowring MA, Kovacs M: Difficulties in diagnosing manic disorders among children and adolescents. J Am Acad Child Adolesc Psychiatry 31:611–614, 1992.

Breiter HC, Etcoff NL, Whalen PJ, Kennedy WA, Rauch SL, Buckner RL, Strauss MM, Hyman SE, Rosen BR: Response and habituation of the human amygdala during visual processing of facial expression. Neuron 17:875–887, 1996.

Brent DA: Correlates of the medical lethality of suicide attempts in children and adolescents. J Am Acad Child Adolesc Psychiatry 26:87–91, 1987a.

Brent DA, Birmaher B, Holder D, et al.: A clinical psychotherapy trial for adolescent major depression. Paper presented at the 42nd Annual Meeting of the American Academy of Child and Adolescent Psychiatry, New Orleans, LA, October 1995.

Brent DA, Crumrine PK, Varma RR, et al.: Phenobarbital treatment and major depressive disorder in children with epilepsy. Pediatrics 80:909–917, 1987b.

Brent DA, Holder D, Kolko D, et al.: A clinical psychotherapy trial for adolescent depression comparing cognitive, family, and supportive therapy. Arch Gen Psychiatry 54:877–885, 1997.

Brumback RA: Childhood depression and medically treatable learning disability, in Brain Lateralization in Children. Edited by Molfese DL, Segalowitz SJ. New York, Guilford, pp. 463–505, 1988.

Brumback RA, Deitz-Schmidt SG, Weinberg WA: Depression in children referred to an educational diagnostic center: diagnosis and treatment and analysis of criteria and literature review. Dis Nerv Syst 38:529–535, 1977.

Brumback RA, Staton RD, Wilson H: Neuropsychological study of children during and after remission of endogenous depressive episodes. Percept Mot Skills 50:1163–1167, 1980.

Brumback RA, Staton RD, Wilson H: Right cerebral hemisphere dysfunction. Archives of General Neurology 41:248–249, 1984.

Brumback RA, Weinberg WA: Mania in childhood, It: therapeutic trial of lithium carbonate and further description of manic-depressive illness in children. Am J Dis Child 131:1122–1126, 1977.

Brumback RA, Weinberg WA: Pediatric behavioral neurology: an update on the neurological aspects of depression, hyperactivity, and learning disabilities. Neurol Clin 8:677–703, 1990.

Bunney WE Jr, Davis JM: Norepinephrine in depressive reactions: a review. Arch Gen Psychiatry 13:483–494, 1965.

Burke KC, Burke JD, Rae DS, et al.: Comparing age at onset of major depression and other psychiatric disorders by birth cohorts in five US community populations. Arch Gen Psychiatry 48:789–795, 1991.

Campbell JD: Manic depressive psychosis in children: report of 18 cases. J Nerv Ment Dis 116:424–439, 1952.

Campbell JD: Manic depressive disease in children. JAMA 158:154–157, 1953.

Cantwell D, Baker L: Academic failures in children with communication disorders. J Am Acad Child Psychiatry 19:579–591, 1980.

Carlson GA, Kashani JH: Manic symptoms in a nonreferred adolescent population. J Affect Disord 15:219–226, 1988.

Castillo M, Kwock L, Courvoisie H, Hooper SR: Proton MR spectroscopy in children with bipolar affective disorder: preliminary observations. AJNR Am J Neuroradiol 21: 832–838, 2000.

Chambers WJ, Puig-Antich J, Hirsch M, et al.: The assessment of affective disorders in children and adolescents by semistructured interview: test-retest reliability of the Schedule for Affective Disorders and Schizophrenia for School-Age Children, Present Episode Version. Arch Gen Psychiatry 42:696–702, 1985.

Chang K, Ketter T: Mood stabilizer augmentation with olanzapine in acutely manic children. J Child Adolesc Psychopharmacol 10: 45–49, 2000.

Clark C, Burge MR: Diabetes mellitus associated with atypical anti-psychotic medications. Diabetes Technol Ther 5:669–683, 2003.

Clarke GN, Hawkins W Murphy M, et al.: Targeted prevention of unipolar depressive disorder in an at-risk sample of high school adolescents: a randomized trial of a group cognitive intervention. J Am Acad Child Adolesc Psychiatry 34:312–321, 1995.

Coffey CE: Cerebral laterality and emotion: the neurology of depression. Compr Psychiatry 28:197–219, 1987.

Coffey CE, Figiel GS: Neuropsychiatric significance of subcortical encephalomalacia, in *Psychopathology and the Brain*. Edited by Barrett JE, Carroll BJ. New York, Raven, pp. 243–264, 1991.

Coffey CE, Wilkinson WE, Weiner RD, et al.: Quantitative cerebral anatomy in depression: a controlled resonance imaging study. Arch Gen Psychiatry 50:7–16, 1993.

Copeland JRM: Psychotic and neurotic depression: discriminant function analysis and five-year outcome. Psychol Med 13:373–383, 1983.

Coryell W Akiskal HS, Leon AC, et al.: The time course of nonchronic major depressive disorder: uniformity across episodes and samples. Arch Gen Psychiatry 51:405–410, 1994.

Costello AJ, Edelbrock C, Dulcan MM, et al.: Report of the NIMH Diagnostic Interview Schedule for Children (DISC). Washington, DC: National Institute of Mental Health, 1985.

Couch JR, Hassanein RS: Amitriptyline in migraine prophylaxis. Arch Neurol 36:695–699, 1979.

Coyle JT: Biochemical development of the brain: neurotransmitters and child psychiatry, in *Psychiatric Pharmacosciences of Children and Adolescents*. Edited by Popper C. Washington, DC: American Psychiatric Press, pp. 1–26, 1987.

Crawford, P: An audit of topiramate use in a general neurology clinic. Seizure 7(Jun):207–211, 1998.

Curry JF: Specific psychotherapies for childhood and adolescent depression. Biol Psychiatry 49:1091–1100, 2001.

Dahl RE, Puig-Antich J, Ryan N, et al.: Cortisol secretion in adolescents with major depressive disorder. Acta Psychiatr Scand 80:18–26, 1989.

Dahl RE, Puig-Antich J, Ryan ND, et al.: EEG sleep in adolescents with major depression: the role of suicidality and inpatient status. J Affect Disord 19:63–75, 1990.

Dahl RE, Ryan ND, Matty MA, et al.: Sleep onset abnormalities in depressed adolescents. Biol Psychiatry 39:400–410, 1996.

Dahlstrom M, Ahonen A, Ebeling H, Torniainen P, Heikkila J, Moilanen I: Elevated hypothalamic/midbrain serotonin (monoamine) transporter availability in depressive drug-naive children and adolescents. Mol Psychiatry 5: 514–522, 2000.

Dasari M, Friedman L, Jesberger J, Stuve TA, Findling RL, Swales TP, Schulz, SC: A magnetic resonance imaging study of thalamic area in adolescent patients with either schizophrenia or bipolar disorder as compared to healthy controls. Psychiatry Res 91:155–162, 1999.

Davanzo P, Thomas MA, Yue K, Oshiro T, Belin T, Strober M, McCracken J: Decreased anterior cingulate myo-inositol/creatine spectroscopy resonance with lithium treatment in children with bipolar disorder. Neuropsychopharmacology 24: 359–369, 2001.

DeBellis MD, Dahl RE, Perel JM, Birmaher B, al-Shabbout M, Williamson DE, Nelson B, Ryan ND: Nocturnal ACTH, cortisol, growth hormone, and prolactin secretion in prepubertal depression. J Am Acad Child Adolesc Psychiatry 35: 1130–1138, 1996.

DelBello M, Kowatch R, Warner J, Strakowski S: Topiramate treatment for pediatric bipolar disorder: a retrospective chart review. J Child and Adol Psychopharmacol 12:323–330, 2002a.

DelBello M, Schwiers M, Rosenberg H, Strakowski S: Quetiapine as adjunctive treatment for adolescent mania associated with bipolar disorder. J Am Acad Child Adolesc Psychiatry 41:1216–1223, 2002b.

DelBello MP, Strakowski SM, Zimmerman ME, Hawkins JM, Sax KW: MRI analysis of the cerebellum in bipolar disorder: a pilot study. Neuropsychopharmacology 21:63–68, 1999.

DeLong GR, Aldershof AL: Long-term experience with lithium treatment in childhood: correlation with clinical diagnosis. J Am Acad Child Adolesc Psychiatry 26:389–394, 1987.

Depression Guideline Panel: *Depression in Primary Care, Vol 1: Detection and Diagnosis* (Clinical Practice Guideline No 5; AHCPR Publ No 93–0550). Rockville, MD: U.S. Department of Health and Human Services, Public Health Service, Agency for Health Care Policy and Research, 1993.

DeVilliers AS, Russell VA, Carstens ME, et al.: Noradrenergic function and hypothalamic-pituitary-adrenal axis activity in adolescents with major depressive disorder. Psychiatry Res 27:101–109, 1989.

Doherty MB, Madansky D, Kraft J, et al.: Cortisol dynamics and test performance of the dexamethasone suppression test in 97 psychiatrically hospitalized children aged 3–16 years. J Am Acad Child Psychiatry 25:400–408, 1986.

Drevets WC, Price JL, Simpson JR Jr., Todd RD, Reich T, Vannier M, Raichle ME: Subgenual prefrontal cortex abnormalities in mood disorders. Nature 386:824–827, 1997.

Drevets WC, Videen TO, Price JL, et al.: A functional anatomical study of unipolar depression. J Neurosci 12:3628–3641, 1992.

Eastgate J, Gilmour L: Long-term outcome of depressed children: a follow-up study. Dev Med Child Neurol 26:68–72, 1984.

Ekman P, Oster H: Facial expressions of emotion. Annu Rev Psychology 30:527–554, 1979.

Emslie GJ, Heiligenstein JH, Wagner KD, et al.: Fluoxetine for acute treatment of depression in children and adolescents: A placebo-controlled, randomized clinical trial. J Am Acad Child Adolesc Psychiatry 41:1205–1215, 2002.

Emslie GJ, Hughes CW, Crismon ML, et al.: A Feasibility Study of the Childhood Depression Medication Algorithm: The Texas Children's Medication Algorithm Project (CMAP). J Am Acad Child Adolesc Psychiatry. 43:519–527, 2004.

Emslie GJ, Kennard BD, Kowatch RA: Affective disorders in children: diagnosis and management. J Child Neurol 10 (sup 1):S42–S49, 1995.

Emslie, GJ, Mayes, TL. Mood disorders in children and adolescents: psychopharmacological treatment. Biol Psychiatry 49:1082–1090, 2001.

Emslie GJ, Rush AJ, Weinberg WA, et al.: Children with major depression show reduced rapid eye movement latencies. Arch Gen Psychiatry 47:119–124, 1990a.

Emslie G, Rush AJ, Weinberg WA, et al.: Double-blind, randomized placebo-controlled trial of fluoxetine in depressed children and adolescents. Arch Gen Psychiatry 54:1031–1037, 1997a.

Emslie GJ, Rush AJ, Weinberg WA, et al.: Recurrence of major depressive disorder in hospitalized children and adolescents. J Am Acad Child Adolesc Psychiatry 36:785–792, 1997b.

Emslie GJ, Rush AJ, Weinberg WA, et al.: Sleep EEG features of adolescents with major depression. Biol Psychiatry 36:573–581, 1994.

Emslie GJ, Weinberg WA, Rush AJ, et al.: Depression and dexamethasone suppression testing in children and adolescents. J Child Neurol 2:31–37, 1987.

Emslie GJ, Weinberg WA, Rush AJ, et al.: Depressive symptoms by self report in adolescence: phase I of the development of a questionnaire for depression by self-report. J Child Neurol 3:114–121, 1990b.

Evans RW, Clay TH, Gualtieri CT: Carbamazepine in pediatric psychiatry. J Am Acad Child Adolesc Psychiatry 26:2–8, 1987.

Extein I, Rosenberg G, Pottash A, et al.: The dexamethasone suppression test in depressed adolescents. Am J Psychiatry 139:1617–1619, 1982.

Faedda GL, Baldessarini RJ, Suppes T, et al.: Pediatriconset bipolar disorder: a neglected clinical and public health problem. Harv Rev Psychiatry 3:171–195, 1995.

Farchione TR, Moore GJ, Rosenberg DR: Proton magnetic resonance spectroscopic imaging in pediatric major depression. Biol Psychiatry 52: 86–92, 2002.

Favale E, Rubina V Mainardi P, et al.: Anticonvulsant effect of fluoxetine in humans. Neurology 45:1926–1927, 1995.

Findling RL, Gracious EL, McNamara NK, Youngstrom EA, Demeter CA, Branicky LA, Calabrese JR: Rapid, continuous cycling and psychiatric co-morbidity in pediatric bipolar I disorder. Bipolar Disord 3(Aug):202–210, 2001.

Findling RL, McNamara NK, Gracious BL, Youngstrom EA, Stansbrey RJ, Reed MD, Demeter CA, Branicky LA, Fisher KE, Calabrese JR. Combination lithium and divalproex sodium in pediatric bipolarity. J Am Acad Child Adolesc Psychiatry 42:895–901, 2003.

Fleming JE, Boyle MH, Offord DR: The outcome of adolescent depression in the Ontario Child Health Study follow-up. J Am Acad Child Adolesc Psychiatry 32:28–33, 1993.

Fleming JE, Offord DR: Epidemiology of childhood depressive disorders: a critical review. J Am Acad Child Adolesc Psychiatry 29: 571–580, 1990.

Flor-Henry P: On certain aspects of the localization of the cerebral systems regulating and determining emotion. Biol Psychiatry 14:677–698, 1979.

Frank E, Kupfer DJ, Perel JM, et al.: Three-year outcomes for maintenance therapies in recurrent depression. Arch Gen Psychiatry 47:1093–1099, 1990.

Frazier J, Meyer M, Biederman J, Wozniak J, Wilens T, Spencer T, Kim G, Shapiro S: Risperidone treatment for juvenile bipolar disorder: a retrospective chart review. J Am Acad Child Adolesc Psychiatry 38(Aug):960–965, 1999.

Freeman RL, Galaburda AM, Cabal RD, et al.: The neurology of depression: cognitive and behavioral deficits with focal findings in depression and resolution after electroconvulsive therapy. Arch Neurol 42:289–291, 1985.

Friedman L, Findling RL, Kenny JT, Swales TP, Stuve TA, Jesberger JA, Lewin JS, Schulz SC: An MRI study of adolescent patients with either schizophrenia or bipolar disorder as compared to healthy control subjects. Biol Psychiatry 46:78–88, 1999.

Fristad MA, Gavazzi SM, Mackinaw-Koons B: Family psychoeducation: An adjunctive intervention for children with bipolar disorder. Biol Psychiatry 53:1000–1008, 2003.

Fristad MA, Gavazzi SM, Soldano KW: Multi-family psychoeducation groups for childhood mood disorders: A program description and preliminary efficacy data. Contemporary Family Therapy 20:385–402, 1998.

Fristad MA, Weller EB, Weller RA: The Mania Rating Scale: can it be used in children? A preliminary report. J Am Acad Child Adolesc Psychiatry 31:252–257, 1992.

Fristad MA, Weller RA, Weller EB: The Mania Rating Scale (MRS): further reliability and validity studies with children. Ann Clin Psychiatry 7:127–132, 1995.

Fristad MA, Goldberg-Arnold JS, Gavazzi SM: Multifamily psychoeducation groups (MFPG) for families of children with bipolar disorder. Bipolar Disord 4:254–262, 2002.

Frodl T, Meisenzahl EM, Zetzsche T, Born C, Jager M, Groll C, Bottlender R, Leinsinger G, Moller HJ: Larger amygdala volumes in first depressive episode as compared to recurrent major depression and healthy control subjects. Biol Psychiatry 53: 338–344, 2003.

Fromm D, Schopflocher D: Neuropsychological test performance in depressed patients before and after drug therapy. Biol Psychiatry 19:55–72, 1984.

Garber J, Kriss MR, Koch M, et al.: Recurrent depression in adolescents: a follow-up study J Am Acad Child Adolesc Psychiatry 27:49–54, 1988.

Geller B, Cook EH Jr.: Serotonin transporter gene (HTTLPR) is not in linkage disequilibrium with prepubertal and early adolescent bipolarity. Biol Psychiatry 45:1230–1233, 1999.

Geller B, Cook EH Jr.: Ultradian rapid cycling in prepubertal and early adolescent bipolarity is not in transmission disequilibrium with val/met COMT alleles. Biol Psychiatry 47:605–609, 2000.

Geller B, Cooper TB, Sun K, Zimerman MA, Frazier J, Williams M, Heath J: Double-blind and placebo-controlled study of lithium for adolescent bipolar disorders with secondary substance dependency. J Am Acad Child Adolesc Psychiatry 37:171–178, 1998.

Geller B, Fox LW Clark KA: Rate and predictors of prepubertal bipolarity during follow-up of 6- to 12-year-old depressed children [see comments]. J Am Acad Child Adolesc Psychiatry 33:461–468, 1994.

Geller B, Fox LW, Fletcher M: Effect of tricyclic antidepressants on switching to mania and on the onset of bipolarity in depressed 6- to 12-year-olds. J Am Acad Child Adolesc Psychiatry 32:43–50, 1993.

Geller B, Luby J: Child and adolescent bipolar disorder: a review of the past 10 years. J Am Acad Child Adolesc Psychiatry 36: 1168–1176, 1997.

Geller B, Tillman R, Craney JL, Bolhofner K: Four-year prospective outcome and natural history of mania in children with a prepubertal and early adolescent bipolar disorder phenotype. Arch Gen Psychiatry 61:459–467, 2004.

Geller B, Zimerman B, Williams M, Bolhofner K, Craney J, Delbello M, Soutullo C: Diagnostic characteristics of 93 cases of a prepubertal and early adolescent bipolar disorder phenotype by gender, puberty and comorbid attention deficit hyperactivity disorder. J Child Adolesc Psychopharmacol 10:157–164, 2000.

Geller BK, Sun K, Zimerman J, et al.: Complex and rapid cycling in bipolar children and adolescents: a preliminary study. J Affect Disord 34:259–268, 1995.

George MS, Ketter TA, Post RM: SPECT and PET imaging in mood disorders. J Clin Psychiatry 54:6–13, 1993.

Geschwind N, Galaburda AM: Cerebral lateralization: biological mechanisms, associations, and pathology, a hypothesis and a program for research. Arch Neurol 42:428–459, 521–522, 634–654, 1985.

Ghazuiddin N, Naylor MW, King CA: Fluoxetine in tricyclic refractory depression in adolescents. Depression 2:287–291, 1995.

Glennon RA: Central serotonin receptors as targets for drug research. J Med Chem 30:1–12, 1987.

Glick I, Murray S, Vasudevan P, Marder S, Hu R: Treatment with atypical antipsychotics: new indications and new populations. J Psychiatr Res 35:187–191, 2001.

Goetz RR, Puig-Antich J, Ryan N, et al.: Electroencephalographic sleep of adolescents with major depression and normal controls. Arch Gen Psychiatry 44:61–68, 1987.

Gold PW, Goodwin FK, Chrousos GP: Clinical and biochemical manifestations of depression: relation to the neurobiology of stress. N Engl J Med 319:348–353, 413–420, 1988.

Golden RM, Potter WZ: Neurochemical and neuroendocrine dysregulation in affective disorders. Psychiatr Clin North Am 9:313–327, 1986.

Goldman-Rakic PS, Brown RM: Postnatal development of monoamine content and synthesis in the cerebral cortex of rhesus monkeys. Developmental Brain Research 4:339–349, 1982.

Gonzales LR, Lewinsohn PM, Clarke GN: Longitudinal follow-up of unipolar depressives: an investigation of predictors of relapse. J Consult Clin Psychol 53:461–469, 1985.

Goodwin FK, Jamison KR: *Manic-Depressive Illness.* New York: Oxford University Press, 1990.

Goodyer I, Germany E, Gowrusankur J, et al.: Social influences on the course of anxious and depressive disorders in school-age children. Br J Psychiatry 158:676–684, 1991.

Gray JW, Dean RS, D'Amato RC, et al.: Differential diagnosis of primary affective depression using the HalsteadReitan Neuropsychological Battery. Int J Neurosci 35:43–49, 1987.

Gur RC, Erwin RJ, Gur RE: Neurobehavioral probes for physiologic neuroimaging studies. Arch Gen Psychiatry 49:409–414, 1992.

Guy W (ed.): Clinical Global Impressions (CGI), in *ECDEU Assessment Manual for Psychopharmacology*, Revised (DREW Publ No ADM 76–388). Rockville, MD: U.S. Department of Health, Education and Welfare, pp. 218–222, 1976.

Hanna GL: Assessment of mood disorders. Child and Adolescent Psychiatric Clinics of North America 1:73–88, 1992.

Harrington R, Fudge H, Rutter M, et al.: Adult outcomes of childhood and adolescent depression. Arch Gen Psychiatry 47:465–473, 1990.

Hazell P, O'Connell D, Heathcote D, et al.: Efficacy of tricyclic drugs in treating child and adolescent depression: a meta-analysis. BMJ 310:897–901, 1995.

Heilman KM, Bowers D, Valenstein E: Emotional disorders associated with neurological diseases, in *Neuropsychology.* Edited by Heilman KM, Valenstein E. New York: Oxford University Press, pp. 377–402, 1983.

Heilman KM, Watson RT, Valenstein E: Neglect and related disorders, in *Clinical Neuropsychology.* Edited by Heilman KM, Valenstein E. New York, Oxford University Press, pp. 234–294, 1985.

Hendren RL, Hodde-Vargas JE, Vargas LA, et al.: Magnetic resonance imaging of severely disturbed children: a preliminary study. J Am Acad Child Adolesc Psychiatry 30:466–470, 1991.

Herjanic B, Reich W: Development of a structured psychiatric interview for children: agreement between child and parent on individual symptoms. J Abnorm Child Psychol 10:307–324, 1982.

Hirschfeld RMA: American Psychiatric Association practice guidelines for the treatment of patients with bipolar disorder. Am J Psychiatry 151 (suppl 12) :1–36, 1994.

Hodges K, Kline J, Stern L, et al.: The development of a child assessment interview for research and clinical use. J Abnorm Child Psychol 10:173–189,1982.

Hughes CW, Emslie GJ, Crismon ML, et al.: The Texas Children's Medication Algorithm Project: Report of the Texas Consensus Conference Panel on medication treatment of childhood major depressive disorder. J Am Acad Child Adolesc Psychiatry 38:1442–1454, 1999.

Hummel B, Stampfer R, Grunze H, Schlosser S, Amann B, Frye M, Walden J: Acute antimanic afficacy and safety of oxcarbazepine in and open trial with on-off-on design. Bipolar Disord 3(suppl 1):43, 2001.

Isaac G: Is bipolar disorder the most common diagnostic entity in hospitalized adolescents and children? Adolescence 30:273–276, 1995.

Isaac G: Misdiagnosed bipolar disorder in adolescents in a special educational school and treatment program. J Clinical Psychiatry 53:133–136 1992.

Isojarvi JI, Laatikainen TJ, Pakarinen AJ, Juntunen KT, Myllyla VV: Polycystic ovaries and hyperandrogenism in women taking valproate for epilepsy. N Engl J Med 329:1383–1388, 1993.

Jain U, Birmaher B, Garcia M, et al.: Fluoxetine in children and adolescents with mood disorders: a chart review of efficacy and adverse effects. J Child Adolesc Psychopharmacol 2:259–265, 1992.

Janicak PG, Davis JM, Preskorn SH, et al.: *Principles and practice of psychopharmacology.* Baltimore, MD: Williams & Wilkins, 1993.

Kafantaris V: Treatment of bipolar disorder in children and adolescents. J Am Acad Child Adolesc Psychiatry 34:732–741, 1995.

Kahn JS, Kehle TJ, Jenson WR, et al.: Comparison of cognitive-behavioral, relaxation, and self-modelling interventions for depression among middle-school students. School Psychol Rev 19:195–210, 1990.

Kandel DB, Davies M: Adult sequela of adolescent depressive symptoms. Arch Gen Psychiatry 43:255–262, 1986.

Kanner L. *Child psychiatry.* Springfield, IL: Charles C Thomas, 1957.

Kapur S, Remington G:Atypical antipsychotics: new directions and new challenges in the treatment of schizophrenia. Annu Rev Medicine 52:503–517, 2001.

Kashani JH, Beck NC, Hoeper E, et al. Psychiatric disorders in a community sample of adolescents. Am J Psychiatry 144:584–589, 1987a.

Kashani JH, Carlson GA, Beck NC, et al.: Depression, depressive symptoms, and depressed mood among a community sample of adolescents. Am J Psychiatry 144:931–934, 1987b.

Kaslow NJ, Rehm LP, Siegel AW Social-cognitive and cognitive correlates of depression in children. J Abnorm Child Psychol 12:605–620, 1984.

Kaslow NJ, Tanenbaum RL, Abramson LY, et al.: Problemsolving deficits and depressive symptoms among children. J Abnorm Child Psychol 11:497–501, 1983.

Kazdin AE: Child Depression Scale. J Child Psychol Psychiatry 28:29–41, 1987.

Kazdin AE, French NH, Unis AS, et al.: Assessment of childhood depression: correspondence of child and parent ratings. J Am Acad Child Adolesc Psychiatry 22:157–164, 1983.

Keck PE Jr., Versiani M, Potkin S, West SA, Giller E, Ice K: Ziprasidone in the treatment of acute bipolar mania: a three-week, placebo-controlled, double-blind, randomized trial. Am J Psychiatry 160:741–748, 2003.

Keck PJ, McElroy S, Arnold L: Bipolar disorder. Medical Clinics of North America 85(May):ix, 645–661, 2001.

Keller MB, Beardslee W Lavori P, et al.: Course of major depression in nonreferred adolescents: a retrospective study. J Affect Disord 15:235–243, 1988.

Keller MB, Lavori PW, Beardslee WR, et al.: Depression in children and adolescents: new data on "undertreatment" and a literature review on the efficacy of available treatments. J Affect Disord 21:163–171, 1991.

Keller MB, Lavori PW, Endicott J, et al.: Double depression: two-year follow-up. Am J Psychiatry 140:689–694, 1983.

Keller MB, Lavori PW, Mueller TI, et al.: Time to recovery, chronicity, and levels of psychopathology in major depression: a 5-year prospective follow-up of 431 subjects. Arch Gen Psychiatry 49:809–816, 1992.

Keller MB, Ryan N, Strober M, et al.: Efficacy of paroxetine in the treatment of adolescent major depression: A randomized, controlled trial. J Am Acad Child Adolesc Psychiatry 40:762–772, 2001.

Keller MB, Shapiro RW, Lavori PW, et al.: Relapse in major depressive disorder: analysis with the life table. Arch Gen Psychiatry 39:911–915, 1982.

Kelsoe JR: Arguments for the genetic basis of the bipolar spectrum. J Affect Disord 73:183–197, 2003.

Kessler RC, McGonagle KA, Nelson CB, et al.: Sex and depression in the national comorbidity survey, II: cohort effects. J Affect Disord 30:15–26, 1994.

Khouzam H, and E.-G. F:Treatment of bipolar I disorder in an adolescent with olanzapine. J Child Adolesc Psychopharmacol 10: 147–151, 2000.

Kolb B, Whishaw IQ: *Fundamentals of Human Neuropsychology.* San Francisco, CA: WH Freeman, 1980.

Kovacs M: Affective disorders in children and adolescents. Am Psychol 44:209–215, 1989.

Kovacs M: Children's Depression Inventory (CDI). Psychopharmacol Bull 21:995–998, 1985a.

Kovacs M: Interview Schedule for Children (ISC). Psychopharmacol Bull 21:991–994, 1985b.

Kovacs M: Presentation and course of major depressive disorder during childhood and later years of the life span. J Am Acad Child Adolesc Psychiatry 35:705–715, 1996.

Kovacs M, Gatsonis C: Secular trends in age at onset of major depressive disorder in a sample of children. J Psychiatr Res 28:319–329, 1994.

Kovacs M, Feinberg TL, Crouse-Novak MA: Depressive disorders in childhood, I: a longitudinal prospective study of characteristics and recovery. Arch Gen Psychiatry 41:229–237, 1984a.

Kovacs M, Feinberg TL, Crouse-Novak MA: Depressive disorders in childhood, II: a longitudinal study of the risk for a subsequent major depression. Arch Gen Psychiatry 41:643–649, 1984b.

Kovacs M, Goldston D: Cognitive and social cognitive development of depressed children and adolescents. J Am Acad Child Adolesc Psychiatry 30:388–392, 1991.

Kovacs M, Goldston D, Gatsonis C: Suicidal behaviors and childhood-onset depressive disorders: a longitudinal investigation. J Am Acad Child Adolesc Psychiatry 32:8–20, 1993.

Kovacs M, Pollock M: Bipolar disorder and comorbid conduct disorder in childhood and adolescence. J Am Acad Child Adolesc Psychiatry 34:715–723, 1995.

Kowatch RA, Devous MD, Sr., Harvey DC, Mayes TL, Trivedi MH, Emslie GJ, Weinberg WA: A SPECT HMPAO study of regional cerebral blood flow in depressed adolescents and normal controls. Prog Neuropsychopharmacol Biol Psychiatry 23: 643–656, 1999.

Kraepelin E: Mixed states in manic-depressive insanity and paranoia, in *Psychiatrische Klinik Vlerte Auflage Band 11 Allgemeine Ubersicht.* Edited by Edinburgh E, Livingston S. Leipzig, Germany: Druck von Breitkopf & Härtel, pp. 14–35, 1921.

Kron L, Decina P, Kestenbaum CJ, et al.: The offspring of bipolar manic-depressives: clinical features. Adolesc Psychiatry 10:273–298, 1982.

Kutcher S, Marton P, Korenblum M, et al.: Relationship between psychiatric illness and conduct disorder in adolescents. Can J Psychiatry 34:526–529, 1989.

Kutcher S, Malkin D, Silverberg J, et al.: Nocturnal cortisol, thyroid stimulating hormone, and growth hormone secretory profiles in depressed adolescents. J Am Acad Child Adolesc Psychiatry 30:407–414, 1991.

Kutcher S, Papatheodorou G, Reiter S, et al.: The successful pharmacological treatment of adolescents and young adults with borderline personality disorder: a preliminary open trial of flupenthixol. J Psychiatry Neurosci 20:113–118, 1995.

Lahmeyer HW Poznanski EO, Bellur SN: Sleep in depressed adolescents. Am J Psychiatry 140:1150–1153, 1983.

Lang M, Tisher M: *Children's Depression Scale.* Victoria, Australia: Australian Council for Educational Research, 1978.

Lenhart RE, Katlin ES: Psychophysiological evidence for cerebral laterality effects in a high risk sample of students with subsyndromal bipolar depressive disorder. Am J Psychiatry 143:602–607, 1986.

Levy IIB, Harper CR, Weinberg WA: A practical approach to children failing in school. Pediatr Clin North Am 39:895–928, 1992.

Lewinsohn PM, Duncan EM, Stanton AK, et al.: Age at onset for first unipolar depression. J Abnorm Psychol 95:378–383,1986.

Lewinsohn PM, Clarke GN, Hops H, et al.: Cognitive-behavioral treatment for depressed adolescents. Behavior Therapy 21:385–401, 1990.

Lewinsohn PM, Clarke GN, Rhode P, et al.: A course in coping: a cognitive-behavioral approach to the treatment of adolescent depression, in *Psychosocial Treatments for Children and Adolescent Disorders: Empirically Based Strategies for Clinical Practice.* Edited by Hibb ED, Jensen PS. Washington, DC: American Psychiatric Press, pp. 109–135, 1996.

Lewinsohn PM, Clarke GN, Seeley JR, et al.: Major depression in community adolescents: age at onset, episode duration, and time to recurrence. J Am Acad Child Adolesc Psychiatry 33:809–818, 1994.

Lewinsohn PM, Hops H, Roberts RE, et al.: Adolescent psychopathology, I: prevalence and incidence of depression and other DSM-III-R disorders in high school students. J Abnorm Psychol 102:133–144, 1993.

Lewinsohn PM, Klein DN, Seeley JR: Bipolar disorders in a community sample of older adolescents: prevalence, phenomenology, comorbidity, and course. J Am Acad Child Adolesc Psychiatry 34:454–463, 1995.

Lewinsohn PM, Rohde P, Seeley JR, Klein DN, Gotlib IH: Natural course of adolescent major depressive disorder in a community sample: predictors of recurrence in young adults. Am J Psychiatry 157:1584–1591, 2000.

Lewinsohn PM, Seeley JR, Buckley ME, and Klein DN: Bipolar disorder in adolescence and young adulthood. Child Adolesc Psychiatr Clin N Am 11:vii, 461–475, 2002.

Ling W, Oftedal G, Weinberg W: Depressive illness in childhood presenting as severe headache. Am J Dis Child 120:122–124, 1970.

Livingston R: Depressive illness and learning difficulties: research needs and practical implications. J Learn Disabil 18:518–520, 1985.

Maas JW, Fawcett J, Dekirmenjian H: 3-Methoxy-4-hydroxyphenylglycol (MHPG) excretion in depressed states: a pilot study. Arch Gen Psychiatry 19:129–134, 1968.

Maj M, Veltro F, Pirozzi R, et al.: Pattern of recurrence of illness after recovery from an episode of major depression: a prospective study. Am J Psychiatry 149:795–800, 1992.

Manji HK, Zarate CA: Molecular and cellular mechanisms underlying mood stabilization in bipolar disorder: implications for the development of improved therapeutics. Mol Psychiatry 7 Suppl 1:S1-7, 2002.

McCauley E, Myers K, Mitchell J, et al.: Depression in young people: initial presentation and clinical course. J Am Acad ChildAdolesc Psychiatry 32:714–722, 1993.

McClellan J: Practice parameters for the assessment and treatment of children and adolescents with bipolar disorder. J Am Acad Child Adolesc Psychiatry 36 (suppl):157S–176S, 1997.

McCracken JT, Poland RE, Lutchmansingh P et al.: Sleep electroencephalographic abnormalities in adolescent depressives: effects of scopolamine. Biol Psychiatry 42:577–584, 1997.

McCracken JT, Rubin RT, Poland RE: Neuroendocrine aspects of primary endogenous depression, VI: receiver operating characteristic analysis of the cortisol suppression index versus the dexamethasone suppression test in patients and matched controls. Psychiatry Res 26:69–78, 1988.

McElroy SL, Keck PE Jr.: Pharmacologic agents for the treatment of acute bipolar mania. Biol Psychiatry 48:539–557, 2000.

McElroy SL, Suppes T, Keck PE, Frye MA, Denicoff KD, Altshuler LL, Brown ES, Nolen WA, Kupka RW, Rochussen J, Leverich GS, Post RM: Open-label adjunctive topiramate in the treatment of bipolar disorders. Biol Psychiatry 47:1025–1033, 2000.

McGee R, Williams S: A longitudinal study of depression in nine-year-old children. J Am Acad Child Adolesc Psychiatry 27:342–348, 1988.

McGlashan TH: Adolescent versus adult onset of mania. Am J Psychiatry 145:221–223, 1988.

McKnew DH, Cytryn L, Buchsbaum MS, et al.: Lithium in children of lithium-responding parents. Psychiatry Res 4:171–180, 1981.

McKnew D, Cytryn L, Efron A, et al.: Offspring of patients with affective disorders. Br J Psychiatry 134:148–152, 1979.

Mendelson WB, Jacobs LS, Sitaram N, et al.: Methoscopolamine inhibition of sleep-related growth hormone secretion. J Clin Invest 61:1683–1690, 1978.

Messenheimer, J: Efficacy and safety of lamotrigine in pediatric patients. J Child Neurology 17 Suppl 2(Feb):2S34–2S42, 2002.

Messenheimer JA, Guberman AH: Rash with lamotrigine: dosing guidelines. Epilepsia 41(Apr):488, 2000.

Mesulam MM: *Principles of Behavioral Neurology.* Philadelphia, PA: FA Davis, 1985.

Miklowitz DJ, Goldstein MJ: Behavioral family treatment for patients with bipolar affective disorder. Behav Modif 14:457–489, 1990 .

Miller AL, Wyman SE, Huppert JD, et al.: Analysis of behavioral skills utilized by suicidal adolescents receiving dialectical behavioral therapy. Cognitive and Behavioral Practice 7:183–187, 2000.

Moore GJ, Galloway MP: Magnetic resonance spectroscopy: neurochemistry and treatment effects in affective disorders. Psychopharmacol Bull 36:5–23, 2002.

Mufson L, Moreau D, Weissman MM, et al.: *Interpersonal Psychotherapy for Depressed Adolescents.* New York: Guilford, 1993.

Mufson L, Moreau D, Weissman MM, et al.: Modification of interpersonal psychotherapy with depressed adolescents (IPT-A): phase I and II studies. J Am Acad Child Adolesc Psychiatry 33:695–705, 1994.

Mufson L, Weissman MM, Moreau D, Garfinkel R: Efficacy of interpersonal psychotherapy for depressed adolescents. Arch Gen Psychiatry 56:573–579, 1999.

Mullins LJ, Siegel LJ, Hodges K: Cognitive problemsolving and life event correlates of depressive symptoms in children. J Abnorm Child Psychol 13:305–314, 1985.

Naylor MW Greden JF, Alessi NE: Plasma dexamethasone levels in children given the dexamethasone suppression test. Biol Psychiatry 27:592–600, 1990.

Newman PJ, Silverstein ML: Neuropsychological test performance among major clinical subtypes of depression. Arch Clin Neuropsychol 2:115–125, 1987.

Newman PJ, Sweet JJ: The effects of clinical depression on the Luria-Nebraska Neuropsychological Battery. Int J Clin Neuropsychol 8:109–114, 1986.

Nolan CL, Moore GJ, Madden R, Farchione T, Bartoi M, Lorch E, Stewart CM, Rosenberg DR: Prefrontal cortical volume in childhood-onset major depression: preliminary findings. Arch Gen Psychiatry 59: 173–179, 2002.

Ojemann LM, Baugh-Bookman C, Dudley DL: Effect of psychotropic medications on seizure control in patients with epilepsy. Neurology 37:1525–1527, 1987.

Papatheodorou G, Kutcher SP: Divalproex sodium treatment in late adolescent and young adult acute mania. Psychopharmacol Bull 29:213–219, 1993.

Papez JW: A proposed mechanism of emotion. Arch Neurol Psych 38:725–743, 1937.

Petti TA: Scales of potential use in the psychopharmacological treatment of depressed children and adolescents. Psychopharmacol Bull 21:951–955, 1985.

Pfeffer CR, Klerman GL, Hurt SW, et al.: Suicidal children grow up: demographic and clinical risk factors for adolescent suicide attempts. J Am Acad Child Adolesc Psychiatry 30:609–616, 1991.

Post RM: Issues in the long-term management of bipolar affective illness. Psychiatric Annals 23:86–93, 1993.

Post RM, Rubinow DR, Uhde TW, et al.: Dysphoric mania: clinical and biological correlates. Arch Gen Psychiatry 46:353–358, 1989.

Poznanski EO, Carroll VJ, Banegas ME, et al.: The dexamethasone suppression test in prepubertal depressed children. Am J Psychiatry 139:321–324, 1982.

Poznanski EO, Freeman LN, Mokros HB: Children's Depression Rating Scale—Revised. Psychopharmacol Bull 21:979–989, 1985.

Poznanski EO, Krahenbuhl V, Zrull JP: Childhood depression. J Am Acad Child Adolesc Psychiatry 15:491–501, 1976.

Prange AJ, Wilson IC, Lynn CW, et al.: L-tryptophan in mania: contribution to a permissive hypothesis of affective disorders. Arch Gen Psychiatry 30:56–62, 1974.

Prien RF, Potter WZ: NIMH workshop report on treatment of bipolar disorder. Psychopharmacol Bull 26:409–427, 1990.

Puig-Antich J, Dahl R, Ryan N, et al.: Cortisol secretion in prepubertal children with major depressive disorder. Arch Gen Psychiatry 46:801–809, 1989.

Puig-Antich J, Goetz R, Hanlon C, et al.: Sleep architecture and REM sleep measures in prepubertal children with major depression: a controlled study. Arch Gen Psychiatry 39:932–939, 1982.

Rao U, Dahl RE, Ryan ND, Birmaher B, Williamson DE, Giles DE, Rao R, Kaufman J, Nelson B: The relationship between longitudinal clinical course and sleep and cortisol changes in adolescent depression. Biol Psychiatry 40:474–484, 1996.

Rao U, Ryan ND, Birmaher B, et al.: Unipolar depression in adolescents: clinical outcome in adulthood. J Am Acad Child Adolesc Psychiatry 34:566–578, 1995.

Rao U, Weissman MM, Martin JA, et al.: Childhood depression and risk of suicide: a preliminary report of a longitudinal study. J Am Acad Child Adolesc Psychiatry 31:21–27, 1993.

Rathus JH, Miller AL: Dialectical behavarioal therapy adapted for suicidal adolescents. Suicide Life-Threat Behav 32:146–157, 2002 .

Reinecke MA, Ryan NE, DuBois DL: Cognitive-behavioral therapy of depression and depressive symptoms during adolescence: A review and meta-analysis. J Am Acad Child Adolesc Psychiatry 37:26–34, 1998.

Reynolds WM, Coats KI: A comparison of cognitivebehavioral therapy and relaxation training for the treatment of depression in adolescents. J Consult Clin Psychol 54:653–660, 1986.

Ring HA, Trimble MR: Depression in epilepsy, in *Depression in Neurological Disease*. Edited by Starkstein SE, Robinson RG. Baltimore, MD: Johns Hopkins University Press, pp. 63–83, 1993.

Robbins DR, Alessi NE, Yanchyshyn GW et al.: Preliminary report on the dexamethasone suppression test in adolescents. Am J Psychiatry 139:942–943, 1982.

Robertson MM: The organic contribution to depressive illness in patients with epilepsy. J Epilepsy 2:189–230, 1989.

Robertson MM, Trimble MR, Townsend HRA: Phenomenology of depression in epilepsy. Epilepsia 28:364–372, 1987.

Robinson RG, Boston JD, Starkstein SE, et al. Comparison of mania and depression after brain injury: causal factors. Am J Psychiatry 145:172–178, 1988.

Robinson RG, Starkstein SE: Current research in affective disorders following stroke. J Neuropsychiatry Clin Neurosci 2:1–14, 1990.

Rosenberg DR, Johnson K, Sahl R: Evolving mania in an adolescent treated with low-dose fluoxetine. J Child Adolesc Psychopharmacol 2:299–306, 1992.

Ross ED: The aprosodias: functional-anatomic organization of the affective components of language in the right hemisphere. Arch Neurol 36:144–148, 1981.

Ross ED, Homan RW Buck R: Differential lateralization of primary and social emotions. Neuropsychiatry Neuropsychol Behav Neurol 7:1–19, 1994.

Ross ED, Rush AJ: Diagnosis and neuroanatomical correlates of depression in brain-damaged patients. Arch Gen Psychiatry 38:1344–1354, 1981.

Rosello J, Bernal G: The efficacy of cognitive-behavioral and interpersonal treatments for depression in Puerto Rican adolescents. J Consul Clin Psychol 67:734–745, 1999.

Rundell JR, Wise MG: Causes of organic mood disorders. J Neuropsychiatry Clin Neurosci 1:398–400, 1989.

Rutter M, Graham P, Yule W: *A neuropsychiatric study in childhood, in Clinics in Developmental Medicine, Nos 35–36*. London: Spastics Society/Heinemann Medical, 1970.

Rutter M, Tizard J, Yule W et al.: Isle of Wight studies, 1964–1974. Psychol Med 6:313–332, 1976.

Ryan ND, Dahl RE, Birmaher B, et al.: Stimulatory tests of grown hormone secretion in prepubertal major depression: depressed versus normal children. J Am Acad Child Adolesc Psychiatry 33:824–833, 1994.

Ryan ND, Birmaher B, Perel JM, et al.: Neuroendocrine response to L-5-hydroxytryptophan challenge in prepubertal major depression: depressed versus normal children. Arch Gen Psychiatry 49: 843–851, 1992a.

Ryan ND, Williamson DE, Iyengar S, et al.: A secular increase in child and adolescent onset affective disorder. J Am Acad Child Adolesc Psychiatry 31:600–605, 1992b.

Sackeim JA, Prohovnik I, Moeller JR, et al.: Regional cerebral blood flow in mood disorders. Arch Gen Psychiatry 47:60–70, 1990.

Santor DA, Kusumakar V: Open trial of interpersonal therapy in adolescents with moderate to severe major depression: Effectiveness of novice IPT therapists. J Am Acad Child Adolesc Psychiatry 40:236–240, 2001.

Schatzberg A, Orsulak P, Rosenbaum A, et al.: Toward a biochemical classification of depressive disorders, V: heterogeneity of unipolar depression. Am J Psychiatry 139:471–475, 1982.

Schatzberg AF, Rothschild AJ: Psychotic (delusional) major depression: should it be included as a distinct syndrome in DSM-IV? Am J Psychiatry 149:733–745, 1992.

Schneekloth T, Rummans T, Logan K: Electroconvulsive therapy in adolescents. Convuls Ther 9:158–166, 1993.

Shaffer D, Fisher P, Dulcan MK, et al.: The NIMH Diagnostic Interview Schedule for Children, version 2.3 (DISC-2.3): description, acceptability, prevalence rates, and performance in the Methods for the Epidemiology of Child and Adolescent Mental Disorders (MECA) Study. J Am Acad Child Adolesc Psychiatry 35:865–877, 1996.

Shea MT, Elkin I, Imber SD, et al.: Course of depressive symptoms over follow-up. Arch Gen Psychiatry 49:782–787, 1992.

Silver JM, Hales RE, Yudofsky SC: Psychopharmacology of depression in neurological disorders. J Clin Psychiatry 51 (suppl 1):33–34, 1990.

Silver JM, Yudofsky SC, Hales RE: Depression in traumatic brain injury. Neuropsychiatry Neuropsychol Behav Neurol 4:12–23, 1991.

Silverstein ML, Strauss BS, Fogg L: A cluster analysis approach for deriving neuropsychologically based subtypes of psychiatric disorders. Int J Clin Neuropsychol 12:7–13, 1990.

Simeon JE, Dinicola VF, Ferguson JB, et al.: Adolescent depression: a placebo-controlled fluoxetine study and follow-up. Prog Neuropsychopharmacol Biol Psychiatry 14:791–795, 1990.

Smith EA, Russell A, Lorch E, Banerjee SP, Rose M, Ivey J, Bhandari R, Moore GJ, Rosenberg DR: Increased medial thalamic choline found in pediatric patients with obsessive-compulsive disorder versus major depression or healthy control subjects: a magnetic resonance spectroscopy study. Biol Psychiatry 54:1399–1405, 2003.

Solomon DA, Keitner GI, Miller 1W et al.: Course of illness and maintenance treatments for patients with bipolar disorder. J Clin Psychiatry 56:5–13, 1995.

Starkstein SE, Mayberg HS, Berthier ML, et al.: Mania after brain injury: neuroradiological and metabolic findings. Ann Neurol 27:652–659, 1990.

Starkstein SE, Robinson RG: Cerebral lateralization in depression. Am J Psychiatry 143:1631–1632, 1986.

Steingard RJ, Renshaw PF, Yurgelun-Todd D, et al.: Structural abnormalities in brain magnetic resonance images of depressed children. J Am Acad Child Adolesc Psychiatry 35:307–311, 1996.

Strober M, Lampert C, Schmidt S, et al.: The course of major depressive disorder in adolescents, I: recovery and risk of manic switching in a follow-up of psychotic and nonpsychotic subtypes. J Am Acad Child Adolesc Psychiatry 32:34–42, 1993.

Strober M, Morrell W, Lampert C, et al.: Relapse following discontinuation of lithium maintenance therapy in adolescents with bipolar I illness: a naturalistic study. Am J Psychiatry 147:457–461, 1990.

Strober M, Schmidt-Lackner S, Freeman R, et al.: Recovery and relapse in adolescents with bipolar affective illness: a five-year naturalistic, prospective follow-up. J Am Acad Child Adolesc Psychiatry 34:724–731, 1995.

Swayze VWD, Andreasen NC, Alliger RJ, et al.: Subcortical and temporal structures in affective disorder and schizophrenia: a magnetic resonance imaging study. Biol Psychiatry 31:221–240, 1992.

Taylor DO, Miklowitz DJ, George EL, et al.: *Modifying focused family therapy for adolescents with bipolar disorder*. Presented at the 5th International Conference on Bipolar Disorder. Pittsburgh, PA, June 12–14, 2003.

Thase MW, Trivedi MH, Rush AJ: MAOIs in the contemporary treatment of depression. Neuropsychopharmacology 12:185–219, 1995.

Thomas KM, Drevets WC, Dahl RE, Ryan ND, Birmaher B, Eccard CH, Axelson D, Whalen PJ, Casey BJ: Amygdala response to fearful faces in anxious and depressed children. Arch Gen Psychiatry 58:1057–1063, 2001.

Tierney E, Joshi PT, Minas JF, et al.: Sertraline for major depression in children and adolescents: preliminary clinical experience. J Child Adolesc Psychopharmacol 5:13–27, 1995.

Tramontana MG, Hooper SR: Neuropsychology of child psychopathology, in *Handbook of Clinical Child Neuropsychology*. Edited by Reynolds CR, Fletcher-Janzen E. New York: Plenum, pp. 87–106, 1989.

Treatment for Adolescents with Depression Study Team; Treatment for Adolescents with Depression Study Team Duke University Medical Ctr Duke Clinical Research Inst; Deptartment of Psychiatry and Behavior Science Durham NC US: Treatment for Adolescents with Depression Study (TADS): Rationale, design, and methods. J Am Acad Child Adolesc Psychiatry 42:531–542, 2003.

Trimble MR, Cull CA: Antiepileptic drugs, cognitive function and behavior in children. Cleve Clin J Med 56 (suppl):140–146, 1989.

Tutus A, Kibar M, Sofuoglu S, Basturk M, Gonul AS: A technetium-99m hexamethylpropylene amine oxime brain single-photon emission tomography study in adolescent patients with major depressive disorder. Eur J Nucl Med 25: 601–606, 1998.

Vankataraman S, Naylor MW, King CA: Mania associated with fluoxetine treatment in adolescents. J Am Acad Child Adolesc Psychiatry 31:276–281, 1992.

Van Praag HM: Depression and schizophrenia: a contribution on their chemical pathologies. New York, Spectrum, 1977.

Wagner KD, Ambrosini PJ, Rynn M, et al.: Efficacy of sertraline in the treatment of children and adolescents with major depressive disorder. J Am Med Assoc 290:1033–1041, 2003.

Wagner KD, Robb AS, Findling RL, Jin J, Gutierrez MM, Heydorn WE: A randomized, placebo-controlled trial of citalopram for the treatment of major depression in children and adolescents. Am J Psychiatry 161: 1079–1083, 2004.

Weinberg WA: Epilepsy and interictal behavioral disorders. International Pediatrics 2:196–204, 1987.

Weinberg WA, Brumback RA: Mania in childhood: case studies and literature review. Am J Dis Child 130:380–385, 1976.

Weinberg WA, Brumback RA: The myth of attention deficit hyperactivity disorders: symptoms resulting from multiple causes. J Child Neurol 7:431–445, 1992.

Weinberg WA, Emslie GJ: Adolescents and school problems: depression, suicide and learning disorders, in *Advances in Adolescent Mental Health, Vol 3: Depression and Suicide.* Edited by Feldman RA, Stiffman AR. Greenwich, CT: JAI Press, pp. 181–205, 1988a.

Weinberg WA, Emslie GJ: Weinberg Screening Affective Scales (WSAS and WSAS-SF). J Child Neuro13:294–296, 1988b.

Weinberg WA, Harper CR, Brumback RA: Neuroanatomic substrate of developmental specific learning disabilities and select behavioral syndromes. J Child Neurol 10 (suppl):S78–S80, 1995.

Weinberg WA, McLean A: A diagnostic approach to developmental specific learning disorders. J Child Neurol 1:158–172, 1986.

Weinberg WA, Rehmet A: Childhood affective disorder and school problems, in *Affective Disorders in Childhood and Adolescence: An Update.* Edited by Cantwell DP, Carlson GA. Jamaica, NY: Spectrum, pp. 109–128, 1983.

Weinberg WA, Rutman J, Sullivan L, et al.: Depression in children referred to an educational diagnostic center: diagnosis and treatment. J Pediatr 83:1065–1072, 1973.

Weinberg WA, Harper CR, Emslie GJ: The effect of depression and learning disabilities on school behavior problems. Directions in Clinical Psychology 4:1–21, 1994.

Weissman MM, Orvaschel H, Padian N: Children's symptoms and social functioning self-report scales. J Nerv Ment Dis 168:736–740, 1980.

Weller EB, Weller RA, Fristad MA: Bipolar disorders in children: misdiagnosis, under-diagnosis, and future directions. J Am Acad Child Adolesc Psychiatry 34:709–714, 1995.

Weller EB, Weller RA, Fristad MA: Lithium dosage guide for prepubertal children: a preliminary report. J Am Acad Child Psychiatry 25:92–95, 1986.

West SA, Keck PEJ, McElroy SL, et al.: Open trial of valproate in the treatment of adolescent mania. J Child Adolesc Psychopharmacol 4:263–267, 1994.

Wilkes TCR, Belsher G, Rush AJ, et al.: *Cognitive Therapy for Depressed Adolescents.* New York: Guilford, 1994.

Wilkes TCR, Rush AJ: Case study: Adaptations of cognitive therapy for depressed adolescents. J Am Acad Child Adolesc Psychiatry 27:381–386, 1988.

Williams D: The structure of emotions reflected in epileptic experiences. Brain 79:29–67, 1956.

Willner P: *Depression: A Psychobiological Synthesis.* New York: Wiley, 1985.

Wolf P: Acute behavioral symptomatology at disappearance of epileptiform EEG abnormality: paradoxical or "forced" normalization. Adv Neurol 55:127–142, 1991.

Wozniak J, Biederman J: Childhood mania: insights into diagnostic and treatment issues. J Assoc Acad Minor Phys 8:78–84, 1997.

Wozniak J, Biederman J, Kiely K, et al.: Mania-like symptoms suggestive of childhood-onset bipolar disorder in clinically referred children. J Am Acad Child Adolesc Psychiatry 34:867–876, 1995.

Young RC, Biggs JT, Ziegler VE, et al.: A rating scale for mania: reliability, validity, and sensitivity. Br J Psychiatry 133:429–435, 1978.

Yurgelun-Todd D, Gruber S, Kanayama W, Baird A, Young A: fMRI during affect discrimination in bipolar affective disorder. Bipolar Disorders 2:237–248, 2000.

Zubenko GS, Moossy J, Kopp U: Neurochemical correlates of major depression in primary dementia. Arch Neurol 47:209–214, 1990.

Anxiety Disorders

Sanjeev Pathak, MD   **Bruce D. Perry, MD, PhD**

14

ANXIETY

Anxiety can be defined as the apprehensive anticipation of future danger or misfortune accompanied by a feeling of dysphoria or somatic symptoms of tension. The focus of anticipated danger may be internal or external (DSM-III-R, 1987). It is the uneasiness associated with the anticipation of danger or perceived rejection and loss of love. Anxiety, an emotion, is the subjective sensation that accompanies the body's response to real or perceived threat. All individuals experience some degree of real or perceived threat, and, therefore, we all have had the sensation of anxiety. Fears and anxieties of a mild and transient nature are part of normal development, though this expectation may mask the presence of emerging or existing anxiety disorder (Zahn-Waxler et al., 2000). For some individuals, however, the frequency, duration, intensity, or context of the anxiety is extreme and can interfere with normal development and functioning. These individuals are considered to have anxiety disorders.

Anxiety disorders are the most common psychiatric syndromes in children and adolescents, with estimated point prevalence of 3 to 13% (Kashani and Orvaschel, 1988, 1990). There is a much higher prevalence of anxiety disorders in medical and psychiatric settings. The disability and impairment in health-related quality of life due to anxiety disorders can be severe (Beidel et al., 1991; Francis et al., 1992; Strauss et al., 1988). Feelings of worthlessness, low self-esteem, and difficulties with concentration and motivation are common in anxiety disorders, and these symptoms along with core symptoms of fear and anxiety impair school performance. These symptoms also strain relationships with peers and family members leading to poor social life. In addition, anxiety disorders may interrupt educational attainment and thus affect human capital accumulation and future earnings. Longitudinal data of children with anxiety conditions indicate that anxiety disorders can be chronic and disabling, and they can increase risk of comorbid disorders (Pine et al., 1998). Reports in the adult literature

also demonstrate the risk for lifelong impairment, reduced quality of life, and increased rates of suicidality (Katzelnick et al., 2001). Rates of anxiety increase as children move into adolescence, which can adversely affect their development.

Scientific efforts to classify abnormal anxiety symptoms resulted in the clustering of similar clinical presentations of anxiety symptoms into anxiety disorders. The *Diagnostic and Statistical Manual of Mental Disorders*, Third Edition, Revised (DSR-III-R) recognized two child-specific anxiety disorders: separation anxiety of childhood and overanxious disorder of childhood (DSM-III-R, 1987). It also recognized that anxiety disorders occur in both children and adults, such as panic disorder, agoraphobia, specific phobias (e.g., social phobia), posttraumatic stress disorder (PTSD), and obsessive-compulsive disorder (OCD). Although each of these disorders had distinguishing clinical phenomenology, profound anxiety was the core symptom common to all. With DSM-IV (American Psychiatric Association, 1994) and DSM-IV-TR, there has been a refinement of this phenomenology.

PHENOMENOLOGY, CLASSIFICATION, AND DIAGNOSIS

Anxiety is a universal feeling experienced by all. It is thought to be a safety mechanism designed to prepare an individual for flight or fight in reaction to perceived risk or damage. At mild to moderate levels, anxiety may be a useful and adaptive mechanism. At extreme levels, however, it is usually maladaptive and debilitating. One means of judging whether a patient has an anxiety disorder is whether the response of an individual is proportionate to the presenting stressor or anxiety-provoking stimulus.

Numerous physiological changes take place in association with anxiety. These changes may present as many signs and symptoms of anxiety disorders involving many organ systems. A sense of palpitations, tachycardia, increased blood pressure, and flushing or pallor may be seen. A subjective sense of shortness of breath and an increased respiratory rate can be seen. Blotching of the skin, rashes, changes in skin temperature, and increased perspiration may be noted. Patients may demonstrate tremulousness, muscle tension, and cramping. Patients may have gastrointestinal symptoms such as by diarrhea, nausea, bloating, and abdominal pain. Additional nonspecific physical symptoms such as headache, chest pain, insomnia, dizziness, fainting, and urinary frequency may be observed.

Patients may also present with psychological and cognitive symptoms such as worrying and reports of feeling scared, feeling tense, nervous, or stressed. In states of panic, patients may express a fear of dying, a fear of imminent disaster, or the feeling that one is going crazy. Patients may be easily startled or hyperaroused and may show behavioral symptoms with significant social impact, such as appearing dependent, needy, clingy, shy, withdrawn, and uneasy in social situations. Individuals with anxiety disorders may appear nervous and high strung.

Children and adolescents with anxiety disorders can have a clinical picture that is somewhat different from those seen in adults. For instance, children may not report any worries or anxieties but may have pronounced physical symptoms. Severe tantrums may be their only manifestation of anxiety problems and thus can be confused with mood disorders or oppositional behavior. Anxiety-related tantrums may occur in children who may be generally compliant and cooperative but then unexpectedly have a severe tantrum. These tantrums can be extraordinarily long and involve the child demanding that the guardian help her or him to avoid an anxiety-provoking situation or stimuli. Examples of such tantrums include a child with social phobia (SP) having a temper tantrum to avoid school or children with obsessive-compulsive disorder (OCD) having a tantrum to avoid breaking a ritual or seek parental assistance with cleaning up. Some children present to the pediatrician with physical symptoms such as nausea, stomachache, or headache occurring on Monday morning or Sunday night, which may represent separation anxiety disorder. Children with generalized anxiety disorder (GAD) may feel sick after the news of a thunderstorm or natural disaster.

The diagnosis of normal versus abnormal anxiety largely depends on the degree of distress and its effect on a child's functioning in life. The degree of abnormality must be gauged within the context of the child's age and developmental level (Table 14.1). The following section delineates the diagnostic rubrics utilized to describe anxiety disorders.

SEPARATION ANXIETY DISORDER (SAD)

Separation anxiety is characterized by excessive anxiety or fear concerning separation from home or from those to whom the child is attached. By definition, it begins before age 18 (DSM-IV-TR, 2000). The disorder usually manifests

TABLE 14.1

NORMAL DEVELOPMENTAL ANXIETY AND ITS COMMON CAUSES

0–6 Months	Loud noises, rapid position changes, rapidly approaching unfamiliar objects
7–12 Months	Strangers, unfamiliar objects, confrontation with unfamiliar people
1–5 Years	Strangers, storms, animals, dark, loud noises, toilet, monsters, ghosts, insects, bodily injury, separation from parents
6–12 Years	Bodily injury, disease, ghosts, supernatural beings, staying alone, criticism, punishment, failure
12–18 Years	Tests and examinations, school performance, bodily injury, appearance, peer scrutiny and rejection, social embarrassment

to the clinician with somatic complaints that the child experiences when there is impending separation from home or the parents, such as going to school. The child can have difficulty when left with relatives, day care providers, babysitters, and other caregivers. This disorder also frequently involves refusal to attend sleepovers or outings requiring a separation from parents. Children who have severe symptoms may refuse to sleep in their own rooms or refuse to go to school, leading to significant impairment. Sunday night and Monday morning illnesses are typical in these children, who may feel great on Fridays and weekends. These children have a difficult time going back to school after holiday breaks and especially after summer vacations. Separation anxiety should be distinguished from social phobia, in which the child avoids school because of a fear of being scrutinized by peers.

Separation anxiety disorder is associated with the development of subsequent depression and panic disorder (McCauley et al., 1993; Mitchell et al., 1988). As it may be an antecedent to subsequent pathology and causes significant distress, appropriate diagnosis and treatment is necessary (Labellarte et al., 1999).

GENERALIZED ANXIETY DISORDER (GAD)

This disorder was referred to as "overanxious disorder of childhood" in previous versions of the *Diagnostic and Statistical Manual of Mental Disorders* (DSM). Generalized anxiety disorder can be defined as excessive worry, apprehension, and anxiety occurring most days for a period of 6 months or more that involves concern over a number of activities or events (DSM-IV-TR, 2000). The focus of the worry and fear is not a specific stimulus as it is in other anxiety disorders such as the extreme anxiety in social situations in social phobia. The person has difficulty controlling the anxiety, which is associated with at least one of the following: restlessness, feeling "keyed up" or on edge; being easily fatigued; difficulty concentrating or having the mind go blank; irritability; muscle tension; or difficulty falling asleep or staying asleep, or restless sleep. The anxiety causes significant distress and impairs functioning.

PANIC DISORDER

Panic disorder is different from panic attacks; panic attacks are defined as sudden, discrete episodes of intense fear or discomfort accompanied by 4 out of 13 bodily or cognitive symptoms, often manifesting with an intense desire to escape, feeling of doom or dread, and impending danger (DSM-IV-TR, 2000). These symptoms peak within 10 minutes and often subside within 20 to 30 minutes. The 13 symptoms are heart palpitations or fast heart rate; sweating; trembling or shaking; shortness of breath or smothering; choking sensation; chest discomfort or pain; nausea or abdominal distress; feeling dizzy, lightheaded, faint, or unsteady; feelings of unreality or being detached from oneself; fear of losing control or going crazy; fear of dying; numbness or tingling sensations; and chills or hot flashes. Panic disorder consists of recurrent unexpected panic attacks with interepisode worry about having others; the panic attacks lead to marked changes in behavior related to the attacks. Panic attacks are frequently associated with agoraphobia (the fear of the marketplace or public places and avoidance of situations from which escape might be difficult or help might not be available and often experienced as a fear of leaving the home). Although agoraphobia can occur alone, it most often occurs in the presence of panic disorder.

OBSESSIVE-COMPULSIVE DISORDER (OCD)

This disorder is defined by persistent obsessions (intrusive, unwanted thoughts, images, ideas, or urges) or compulsions (intense, uncontrollable repetitive behaviors or mental acts related to the obsessions) that are noted to be unreasonable and excessive (DSM-IV-TR, 2000). These obsessions and compulsions cause notable distress and impairment and are time consuming (more than 1 hour a day). The most common obsessions concern dirt and contamination, repeated doubts, need to have things arranged in a specific way, fearful aggressive or murderous impulses, and disturbing sexual imagery. The most frequent compulsions involve repetitive washing of hands or using handkerchief/tissue to touch things; checking drawers, locks, windows, and doors; counting rituals; repeating actions; and requesting reassurance. Eighty percent of subjects suffering from OCD have both obsessions and compulsions.

Young children with OCD may not recognize their obsessive thoughts or the compulsions and rituals as problematic or unusual. Therefore children between 4 and 10 may frequently have severe tantrums with atypical precipitants as the chief complaint. A child might be usually very compliant, but have a tantrum if asked to speed up his or her cleaning. Young children may also be unable to verbalize their obsessions, but parents can describe avoidance behaviors, compulsions, and rituals.

Pediatric autoimmune neuropsychiatric disorders associated with streptococcal infection (PANDAS) are a group of disorders that are believed to be the result of an autoimmune response to group A beta-hemolytic streptococcal infections (Swedo et al., 1998). These disorders can present with tics and obsessions and compulsions. The onset of OCD symptoms is typically more abrupt if associated with PANDAS.

POSTTRAUMATIC STRESS DISORDER (PTSD)

In this disorder, a person experiences, witnesses, or is confronted by a traumatic event or events that involve an actual or perceived threat of death or serious bodily injury, and the person's response involves intense fear, helplessness, or horror. In children, probably the most common traumatic event is abuse. The traumatic event is continually re-experienced in the following ways: recurrent and intrusive distressing remembrances of the event involving images, thoughts, or perceptions; distressing dreams of the event; acting or believing that the traumatic event is recurring; intense anxiety and distress to exposure to situations that resemble the traumatic event; or bodily reactivity on exposure situations that resemble the traumatic event (DSM-IV-TR, 2000). The person avoids situations that are associated with and remind him or her of the traumatic event, leading to avoidance of thoughts, feelings, or conversations associated with the trauma; activities, places, or people that remind him or her of the traumatic event; an inability to remember details of the event; markedly diminished participation and interest in usual activities; feeling detached and estranged from others; restricted range of emotional expression; sense of a foreshortened future or life span; persistent signs of physiologic arousal, such as difficulty falling asleep or staying asleep, irritability or anger outbursts, difficulty concentrating, excessive vigilance, and exaggerated startle response. These symptoms persist for more than 1 month and cause significant distress and impairment of functioning.

ACUTE STRESS DISORDER

A person is exposed to a traumatic event in which he or she experiences, witnesses, or is confronted by an event or events that involve an actual or perceived threat of death or serious bodily injury, and the person's response involves intense fear, helplessness, or horror. The traumatic event is continually re-experienced in the following ways: recurrent and intrusive distressing remembrances of the event involving images, thoughts, or perceptions; distressing dreams of the event; acting or believing that the traumatic event is recurring; intense anxiety and distress to exposure to situations that resemble the traumatic event; bodily reactivity on exposure situations that resemble the traumatic event. The person avoids situations that are associated with and remind him or her of the traumatic event, leading to avoidance of thoughts, feelings, or conversations associated with the trauma; activities, places, or people that remind the person of the traumatic event; inability to remember details of the event; markedly diminished participation and interest in usual activities; feeling detached and estranged from others; restricted range of emotional expression; sense of a foreshortened future or life span; persistent signs of physiologic arousal, such as difficulty falling asleep or staying asleep, irritability or anger outbursts, difficulty concentrating, excessive vigilance, and exaggerated startle response. This disorder differs from PTSD in that the symptoms persist for less than 1 month.

SOCIAL PHOBIA (SP)

This disorder is characterized by a persistent and significant fear of one of more social situations in which a person is exposed to unfamiliar persons or scrutiny by others and feels he or she will behave in a way that will be embarrassing or humiliating (DSM-IV-TR, 2000). Exposure to the feared social situations almost always causes significant anxiety, even a panic attack, despite the fact that the anxiety is seen as excessive and unreasonable. This belief may lead to avoidance of such situations or endurance under extreme distress, leading to marked interference in the person's functioning and routine. In children and adolescents, the symptoms must be present for a minimum of 6 months and cause significant impairment in functioning or marked distress in order to warrant the diagnosis. The DSM-III-R diagnosis of avoidant disorder of childhood has been subsumed under this rubric in DSM-IV-TR. Children and adolescents with social phobia usually have few friends and tend to avoid group activity and report feeling lonely. They are also fearful of social situations such as reading aloud in class, asking the teacher for help, eating in the cafeteria, unstructured activities with peers, and so on (DSM-IV-TR, 2000).

SELECTIVE MUTISM

Selective mutism is the failure to speak in social situations when there is no underlying language problem and the child has the capacity to speak (DSM-III-R, 1987). The onset of this disorder is in childhood. The child usually speaks normally in the company of familiar adults or family and familiar settings. At school or in other public settings, the child may be silent. The disorder is considered by some to be a severe form of social phobia as these youth are often painfully shy. The disorder cannot otherwise be explained by a developmental abnormality. There is a high rate of family history of anxiety disorders in these children.

SPECIFIC PHOBIA

This disorder is characterized by persistent and significant fear that is recognized as unreasonable and excessive and that is triggered by the presence or perception of a specific feared situation or object; exposure to this situation or object immediately provokes an anxiety reaction (DSM-IV-TR, 2000). The distress, avoidance, and anxious anticipation of the feared situation or object significantly interfere with a person's normal functioning or routine. This disorder may present as one of many types: the animal type is manifested as a fear of animals or insects; the natural environmental type is manifested as a fear of storms, heights, water, and the like; the blood-injection-injury type is manifested as a fear of getting injections, seeing blood, seeing injuries, or watching or having invasive medical procedures; the situational type is manifested as a fear of elevators, flying, driving, bridges, escalators, trains, tunnels, closets, and so on. In children, specific phobia may be expressed as anxiety or by symptoms such as crying, temper tantrums, or a marked increase in clinging behavior.

ADJUSTMENT DISORDER WITH ANXIETY (WITH OR WITHOUT DEPRESSED MOOD)

This disorder can be diagnosed when the development of emotional or behavioral symptoms occur within 3 months in response to an identifiable stressor (DSM-III-R, 1987). These symptoms and behaviors cause marked distress in excess of that which could be expected and results in significant occupational, social, or academic performance. Once the initiating stressor has ceased, the disturbance does not last longer than 6 months.

ANXIETY DISORDER DUE TO A GENERAL MEDICAL CONDITION

This disorder may result when the physiologic consequences of a distinct medical condition is judged to be the cause of prominent anxiety symptoms.

DRUG-INDUCED ANXIETY DISORDER

This disorder may result when the physiologic consequences of the use of a drug or medication is judged to be the cause of prominent anxiety symptoms.

ANXIETY DISORDER NOT OTHERWISE SPECIFIED

This disorder may result when the prominent symptoms of anxiety and avoidance exist but do not fully meet the preceding diagnostic criteria.

DIAGNOSTIC ISSUES IN ANXIETY DISORDERS

As more than 50% of individuals who meet criteria for one anxiety disorder also meet criteria for a second anxiety disorder, an underlying vulnerability to anxiety is probably common to all anxiety disorders (Kashani and Orvaschel, 1990; Last et al., 1992). However, it is not clear whether there is a specific inheritance related to a particular anxiety disorder or whether a broader genetic predisposition toward problems with overarousal and reactivity to stimuli may be responsible. In addition, the categorical DSM-IV-TR nomenclature may result in artificially carving various anxiety disorders into discrete categories.

COMORBIDITY

Childhood anxiety disorders have astounding comorbidity with other childhood neuropsychiatric disorders (Last et al., 1987a; Leckman et al., 1983). Attention-deficit/hyperactivity disorder (ADHD) co-occurs with anxiety disorders with high frequency (Biederman et al., 1991). In some studies, more than 60% of the children with affective disorders also had an anxiety disorder, and 70% of children with school refusal had comorbid affective disorders (Bernstein et al., 1996).

The presence of anxiety disorders in childhood appears to confer risk for the development of affective and anxiety disorders in adolescence and adulthood (Reinherz et al., 1989). In turn, depressive symptoms in childhood apparently play a role in vulnerability to anxiety disorders throughout the life cycle (Kovacs et al., 1989; Kovacs and Goldston, 1991). In addition, adolescents with anxiety disorders who develop major depression are at a high risk for attempting suicide (Pawlak et al., 1999). That many disorders co-occur with anxiety disorders and that vulnerability to anxiety disorders also confers vulnerability to affective disorders, and vice versa, should not be surprising, considering that the brainstem monoamines (e.g., norepinephrine, serotonin, dopamine) are common mediators of both arousal and affect. Primary "anxiety" symptoms induced by abnormal regulation of these brainstem monoamine systems would likely be accompanied by affective symptoms, and vice versa.

Other neuropsychiatric conditions in which anxiety is a prominent symptom include psychotic disorders, mental retardation, traumatic head injury, developmental delay, profound neglect, and physical abuse. The common thread in all of these disorders is a compromised capacity to effectively and efficiently interpret experience. Regardless of which specific capacity (processing, storing, or recalling stored information) is affected by the cortical and subcortical impairments in these disorders, the effect is the same—every experience is too "new." Any condition that alters the brain's capacity to make associations in response to an event, store them, and then generalize from that event to a future event causes the affected individual to experience each moment as novel. Novel cues are interpreted by the brain as threat related until proven otherwise. To a psychotic child in whom abnormal pairing of sensory information is taking place, the environment is ever-changing from moment to moment, with all experience continually being processed and perceived as "novel."

Although anxiety plays a major role in the clinical presentation of all of these neuropsychiatric disorders, no single neuropathological process has been found that is specific to a given diagnostic category or to specific anxiety-related symptoms. The threat-response systems in the human brain are redundant and widely distributed, and there are many mechanisms and sites in which dysregulation may occur.

ANXIETY DISORDER SECONDARY TO NEUROLOGICAL ILLNESS

One of the best described neurological disorders that presents with symptoms of anxiety is pediatric autoimmune neuropsychiatric disorders associated with streptococcal (group A β-hemolytic streptococcal [GABHS]) infections (PANDAS) (Swedo et al., 1998). Swedo et al. described the clinical characteristics of 50 pediatric patients diagnosed with PANDAS, OCD, and tic disorders with a prepubertal onset in association with GABHS. The children's symptom onset was acute and dramatic, typically triggered by GABHS infections at a very early age (mean = 6.3 years, SD = 2.7, for tics; mean = 7.4 years, SD = 2.7, for OCD). The PANDAS clinical course was characterized by a relapsing-remitting symptom pattern with significant psychiatric comorbidity accompanying the exacerbations; emotional lability, separation anxiety, nighttime fears and bedtime rituals, cognitive deficits, oppositional behaviors, and motoric hyperactivity were particularly common. Giedd et al. used computer-assisted morphometric techniques to analyze the cerebral magnetic resonance images of 34 children with PANDAS and 82 healthy comparison children who were matched for age and sex (Giedd et al., 2000). The average sizes of the caudate, putamen, and globus pallidus, but not of the thalamus or total cerebrum, were significantly greater in the group of children with streptococcus-associated OCD or tics than in the healthy children. The basal ganglia enlargements were consistent with a hypothesis of a selective cross-reactive antibody-mediated inflammation of the basal ganglia underlying the development of poststreptococcal OCD or tics in some individuals. However, there was a lack of correlation between basal ganglia size and symptom severity, indicating that the relationship between basal ganglia size and pathophysiology is not direct. In addition, because of poor sensitivity and specificity of the MRI findings, an MRI scan is not warranted for the diagnosis or clinical monitoring of children with poststreptococcal OCD or tics.

Apart from PANDAS, there are limited descriptions of pediatric anxiety disorders secondary to neurological illness. Gamazo-Garran et al. described a 16-year-old-boy who had a midline germinal tumor affecting the caudate nuclei; left lenticular, right internal capsule's genu; and bilateral involvement of the interventricular septum close to the interventricular foramina. He developed OCD symptoms and elevated tumor markers when he had a tumor relapse, and fluorodeoxyglucose positron emission tomography showed caudate nuclei involvement. He responded to treatment with 80 mg of citalopram. As noted in this case report, the treatment for anxiety secondary to neurological/infectious causes is the same as that for primary anxiety disorders (Storch et al., 2004).

EPIDEMIOLOGY

Although quite common, anxiety disorders in children often are overlooked or misjudged, even though they are treatable conditions with good, persistent medical care. What does seem to be developing in the medical literature is the consensus that many "adult" psychiatric disorders likely have their first (although perhaps subtle or ignored) manifestations in childhood, and that if left untreated these anxiety disorders in children likely progress to adult versions.

Epidemiological studies that used DSM-III-R diagnostic criteria have demonstrated that over 10% of all children meet criteria for some anxiety disorder (Kashani and Orvaschel, 1988; King et al., 1995; Milne et al., 1995). In two cross-sectional epidemiological studies, 21% of the sampled children reported symptoms meeting DSM anxiety disorder diagnostic criteria (Kashani and Orvaschel, 1988; Kashani et al., 1989). In these samples, the prevalence rates for separation anxiety disorder were 12.9%, 12.4% for over-anxious disorder, 3.3% for specific phobia, and 1.1% for social phobia. The National Institute of Mental Health (NIMH) adolescent OCD study showed a lifetime prevalence of 1.9% for the general adolescent population (Flament et al., 1988). Valleni-Basile et al. reported a higher rate of 3% of clinical OCD and 19% for subclinical OCD symptoms in their community sample of 3,283 adolescents (Valleni-Basile et al., 1994). A few studies have investigated the epidemiology of panic disorder. These studies have found a lifetime prevalence ranging from 0.3 to 1% in adolescence (Lewinsohn et al., 1993; Verhulst et al., 1997;

Whitaker et al., 1990). Warren et al., in a sample of 388 adolescents reported a higher (4.7%) prevalence of panic disorder. Unfortunately, because of controversies regarding the occurrence of panic disorder in the pediatric age group, panic disorder was not mentioned in the most widely cited epidemiological studies of panic disorder in youth (Anderson et al., 1987; Kashani and Orvaschel, 1988)

COURSE

Understanding the course of anxiety disorders is critical to planning treatment and assessing future medical need. In addition, knowledge about the course of various anxiety disorders will answer parental concerns about how long the child will need treatment and when the child might be free from impairment. Emerging evidence is suggesting that several anxiety disorders begin early in childhood, increase the risk for developing other comorbid disorders, and if untreated may result in a chronic course (Achenbach et al., 1995; Pine et al., 1998b; Spence et al., 2001).

Separation anxiety disorder (SAD) can have an early and acute onset following a significant stressor, such as move to a new neighborhood, death of a parent, or a period of developmental change (Last et al., 1987a). SAD tends to have a variable course with remission and periods of recurrence during periods of increased stress and sometimes seems to come out of the blue. Moreover, SAD increases the risk for subsequent depression and social phobia, and girls with SAD are at increased risk for panic disorder and agoraphobia (Black and Robbins, 1990). Simple phobia also seems to be chronic for a significant proportion of children and adolescents, though there have been reports of spontaneous remission also (Agras et al., 1972; Essau et al., 2000).

OCD has a chronic fluctuating course marked by remissions and recurrences (Swedo et al., 1989). In a 2-year follow-up of adolescents who had a lifetime diagnosis of OCD, Berg et al. found that 31% of subjects received a diagnosis of OCD at follow-up (Berg et al., 1989). Wewetzer et al., in a long-term follow-up study, assessed 55 patients whose mean age of onset of OCD was 12.5 years and the mean follow-up time was 11.2 years. At the follow-up investigation, 71% of the patients met the criteria for some form of psychiatric disorder, while 36% were still suffering from OCD.

Patients with social phobia are at increased risk of developing major depression, as well as substance abuse and dependence (Kessler et al., 1994; Last et al., 1992). There are little data available on the course of GAD. However, the minimal data suggest that GAD is unstable over time, with the majority of the patients having a different diagnosis at follow-up in addition to increased risk for alcohol abuse (Cantwell and Baker, 1989; Kaplow et al., 2001). Though data are lacking in children for the course of panic disorder, the data from adults suggests that this is a chronic and recurrent diagnosis (Breier et al., 1986).

Genetic Factors

Systematic study of the temperament of infants has suggested that certain properties of the sensitivity of the arousal system may be constitutional (Kagan et al., 1987). The rudimentary organization and sensitivity of the arousal systems appear to be present at birth. Differential internal states of anxiety seem to be associated with distinct behaviors, such as initiation of social contact, exploration, and the capacity to form and maintain peer attachments (Last et al., 1987b; Waldron et al., 1975). Panic disorder, generalized anxiety disorder, phobias, and OCD all have significant familial aggregation (Hettema et al., 2001). Furthermore, twin studies have established that genes account for a significant variance in anxiety measures. In a large twin study, Torgersen considered 32 monozygotic (MZ) and 53 dizygotic (DZ) adult same-sexed twins (Torgersen, 1983). The frequency of anxiety disorders was twice as high in MZ as in DZ twins of the total proband group, alike in the MZ and DZ co-twins of the generalized anxiety disorder proband group, and three times as high in MZ as in DZ co-twins of the other proband groups. Anxiety disorders with panic attacks were more than five times as frequent in MZ as in DZ co-twins in a combined group of probands with panic disorders and agoraphobia with panic attacks. Thus, for generalized anxiety disorder, heritability was not apparent, while genetic factors seemed significant in other anxiety disorders, especially panic disorder and agoraphobia with panic attacks. Stevenson et al. studied 319 same-gender twin pair and showed that around 29% of the variance for fear and phobic symptoms was heritable (Stevenson et al., 1992).

With advances in molecular genetic techniques and high throughput genotyping methodology (see Chapter 29), scientists have conducted genetic association and linkage studies in an effort to identify specific genes and genetic regions that may increase susceptibility for anxiety disorders. (See Table 14.2 for commonly cited genetic studies). Because the animal literature has supported a role for serotonin in anxiety and fear, the usual focus of the studies has been candidate genes that code for neurotransmitters in the serotonin pathway including monoamine oxidase A (MAO-A), catechol-O-methyl-transferase (COMT), serotonin transporter (SLC6A4), receptors involved in serotonin transduction (such as 5HT1B), and GABA-A (Lesch, 2001). As is the case with genetics of complex diseases, findings from linkage and association studies have been inconsistent and conflicting, and therefore need further replication. Thus, several human studies have reported findings of association of polymorphisms in the promoter region of the serotonin transporter gene with anxiety, though other studies have been negative (Battaglia et al., 2005; Katsuragi et al., 1999; Lesch et al., 1996; Nakamura et al., 1997). In association studies of COMT genes in patients with OCD, two studies found an association in males (Karayiorgou et al., 1997, 1999), one found an

association for females (Alsobrook et al., 2002), and another found no association in any gender (Ohara et al., 1998). In one study, Samochowiec et al. looked at association studies of MAO-A, COMT, and serotonin transporter genes polymorphisms in patients with anxiety disorders of the phobic spectrum (Samochowiec et al., 2004). While there were no significant differences between controls (n = 202) and patients (n = 101) in the allele and genotype frequencies of the serotonin and COMT gene polymorphisms, the frequency of >3 repeat alleles of the MAO-A gene polymorphism was significantly higher in female patients suffering from anxiety disorders, specifically panic attacks and generalized anxiety disorder.

NEUROBIOLOGY

Overview: Neurobiological Correlates of Anxiety

The prime directive of the human brain is to promote survival and procreation. When potentially threatening cues are present in these environments, the brain activates a complex set of neurophysiological, neuroendocrinological, and neuroimmunological responses to optimize the survival of the individual. In humans, activation of these threat-response systems is accompanied by the subjective perception of anxiety or fear.

An anxiety-inducing or fear-inducing stimulus generates sensory information that is transmitted from the peripheral sensory receptors to the dorsal thalamus. However, sensory information from the olfactory system is not relayed through the thalamus and is relayed to the amygdala and the entorhinal cortex (Turner et al., 1978). Visceral afferent pathways relay information to the amygdala and locus ceruleus directly or through the nucleus paragigantocellularis and nucleus tractus solitarius (Elam et al., 1986; Nauta and Whitlock, 1956; Saper, 1982). The thalamus relays sensory information to the primary sensory receptive areas of the cortex. These primary sensory regions project to adjacent cortical association areas. The visual, auditory and somatosensory cortical association areas send projections to the amygdala, orbitofrontal cortex, entorhinal cortex, cingulate gyrus, and other brain structures.

The hippocampus and amygdala are sites of convergent reciprocal projections form cortical association areas. These interconnections help a single sensory stimulus such as a smell, sight, or sound to elicit a specific memory or flashback along with symptoms of anxiety and fear (in case the smell, sight, or sound was associated with a traumatic event). We examine the possible neurobiological correlates of anxiety disorders in the following section by considering the abnormal organization, regulation, or development of neurobiological systems and subsystems within various brain regions that appear to be involved in sensing, processing, and responding to threat.

TABLE 14.2
GENETIC STUDIES

Candidate Gene	Diagnosis/Trait or Symptom	Results	Reference/Lead Authors
5-HTTLPR (promoter region of the serotonin transporter gene)	Harm avoidance	Association with S allele	(Katsuragi et al., 1999)
	Harm avoidance, neuroticism	Association with S allele	(Lesch et al., 1996)
	Anticipatory worry	Linkage with SLC6A4*C, no association	(Mazzanti et al., 1998)
	Harm avoidance, neuroticism	No association with S allele	(Nakamura et al., 1997)
	Harm avoidance, neuroticism	No association with S allele	(Stoltenberg et al., 2002)
	OCD	No association with S allele	(Cavallini et al., 2002)
	OCD	No association with S allele	(Billett et al., 1997)
	Panic	No association with S allele	(Deckert et al., 1997)
	Panic	No association with S allele	(Hamilton et al., 1999)
	Social phobia	No association with S allele	(Stein et al., 1998)
Catechol-O-methyltransferase (COMT)	GAD	No association with COMT allele	(Ohara et al., 1998)
	OCD	Association with low activity allele, 22q11 microdeletions, low/low genotype in males only	(Karayiorgou et al., 1997)
	OCD	Association with low activity allele in males	(Karayiorgou et al., 1999)
	OCD	Association with the low-activity allele in females probands ($P = 0.049$)	(Alsobrook et al., 2002)
	OCD	No association with COMT allele	(Ohara et al., 1998)
	Panic	Association with marker D22S944	(Hamilton et al., 2002)
	Panic	No association with COMT allele	(Ohara et al., 1998)
	Phobia	No association with COMT allele	(Ohara et al., 1998)
Monoamine oxidase-A (MOA-A)	OCD	Association with MAO-A*297CGG allele	(Karayiorgou et al., 1999)
HTR1B (Serotonin 1B receptor)	GAD	No association with HTR1B 861G>C polymorphism	(Fehr et al., 2000)
	Panic	No association with HTR1B 861G>C polymorphism	(Fehr et al., 2000)
5HT1Dβ	OCD	No association with a silent G-to-C substitution at nucleotide 861	(Di Bella et al., 2002)

(continued)

TABLE 14.2
(continued)

Candidate Gene	Diagnosis/Trait or Symptom	Results	Reference/Lead Authors
5HTR2A (Serotonin 2A receptor)	Social phobia	No linkage	(Stein et al., 1998)
Genome Wide Scans	Panic	Linkage at 7p15, LOD = 2.2 (469 markers)	(Crowe et al., 2001)
	Harm avoidance	LOD = 3.2, Linkage with locus on 8p21–23, epistasis with 8p21–23 (291 markers studied)	(Cloninger et al., 1998)
	OCD	LOD = 2.25 on 9p (349 markers studied)	(Hanna et al., 2002)

OCD, obsessive-compulsive disorder; GAD, generalized anxiety disorder.

THREAT-RESPONSE NEUROBIOLOGY IN THE MATURE CENTRAL NERVOUS SYSTEM

Reticular Activating System: Arousal and Alarm

The reticular activating system is a network of ascending, arousal-related neural systems in the brain that consists of locus ceruleus noradrenergic neurons, dorsal raphe serotonergic neurons, cholinergic neurons from the lateral dorsal tegmentum, and mesolimbic and mesocortical dopaminergic neurons, among others. Much of the original research on arousal, fear, and response to stress and threat was conducted using various lesion models of the reticular activating system (Moore and Bloom, 1979). With the advent of more sophisticated neuropharmacological techniques that allowed precise manipulation and lesioning of individual neurochemical systems, the concept of the reticular activating system as a functional unit lost popularity. Recently, however, interest has been rekindled in the reticular activating system as an integrated neurophysiological system involved in arousal, anxiety, and modulation of limbic and cortical processing (Munk et al., 1996). Working together, the brainstem monoamine systems in the reticular activating system provide the flexible and diverse functions necessary to modulate the variety of functions responsible for anxiety regulation.

Locus Coeruleus: Regulation of Arousal

The locus coeruleus is involved in initiating, maintaining, and mobilizing the total body response to threat (Aston-Jones et al., 1986). A bilateral grouping of norepinephrine-containing neurons originating in the pons, the locus coeruleus sends diverse axonal projections to virtually all major brain regions and thus functions as a general regulator of noradrenergic tone and activity (Foote et al., 1983). The locus coeruleus plays a major role in determining the "valence," or value, of incoming sensory information; in response to novel or potentially threatening information, it increases its activity (Abercrombie and Jacobs, 1987a, 1987b). The ventral tegmental nucleus also plays a part in regulating the sympathetic nuclei in the pons/medulla (Moore and Bloom, 1979). Acute stress results in an increase in locus coeruleus and ventral tegmental nucleus activity and the release of catecholamines throughout the brain and the rest of the body. These brainstem catecholamine systems (locus coeruleus and ventral tegmental nucleus) play a critical role in regulating arousal, vigilance, affect, behavioral irritability, locomotion, attention, and sleep, as well as the startle response and the response to stress (Levine et al., 1990; Morilak et al., 1987a, 1987b, 1987c).

A number of other neurotransmitters and neuropeptides play a role in modulating locus coeruleus activity, thus influencing the sensitivity of the threat response. Serotonin (Adell et al., 1988), enkephalins (Abercrombie and Jacobs, 1988), corticotrophin releasing hormone (CRH) (Butler et al., 1990), and epinephrine (Perry et al., 1983; Vantini et al., 1984) all can alter locus coeruleus sensitivity.

Dopaminergic Systems: Sensitization

Dopaminergic systems play a critical role in the response to threat. In animal models, various stress paradigms have demonstrated alterations in dopamine metabolism and dopamine-receptor densities and sensitivity (Kalivas and Duffy, 1989; Kalivas et al., 1988). Dopaminergic systems originating in the mesencephalon send projections to key limbic and cortical areas involved in the afferent and efferent wings of the threat response. These systems are very important in sensation, perception, and interpretation of stress-related and threat-related cues.

Studies of psychostimulant-induced and stress-induced sensitization of dopaminergic systems provide important clues to the neurophysiological mechanisms that may underlie the development of a sensitized anxiety response (Kalivas et al., 1988). Sensitization—an increased sensitivity to a constant stimulus—occurs in response to specific patterns of activation of these dopaminergic systems. In rats (Kleven et al., 1990), primates (Farfel et al., 1992), and humans (Post et al., 1988), psychostimulants (e.g., methamphetamine, cocaine) administered in moderate dosages can induce dramatic sensitization syndromes that include agitation, impulsivity, autonomic arousal, and even seizures (see case example below). Stress can induce similar sensitization in animal models (Antelman et al., 1980; Kalivas and Duffy, 1989).

CASE EXAMPLE: PSYCHOSTIMULANT-INDUCED PANIC ATTACKS

S., a 16-year-old, was admitted to the emergency room with diaphoresis, tachycardia, a sense of impending doom, and profound anxiety. He had no previous history of psychiatric disorder and denied previous anxiety or panic attacks. S. described a 4-month history of cocaine use characterized by binge nasal use. His last binge was 5 days prior to the admission. Since that time, he had been experiencing an escalating "sensitivity" to stress, with increased irritability and difficulty sleeping. Following an extensive medical and neuropsychiatric workup, S.'s episodes were formulated as reflecting a psychostimulant-induced panic disorder related to a sensitizing pattern of cocaine use. After discharge, S. experienced more panic attacks (approximately two per week) and elected to pursue recommended outpatient treatment. Successful drug rehabilitation and pharmacotherapy with a benzodiazepine anxiolytic for 6 weeks resulted in disappearance of the panic attacks.

Sensitization involves a cascade of cellular and molecular processes that are probably related to longterm potentiation (Brown et al., 1988; Kandel, 1989; Kandel and Schwartz, 1982; Madison et al., 1991). It has been hypothesized that sensitization of the biogenic amines (norepinephrine, epinephrine, and dopamine) in the reticular activating system and related systems plays a key role in the development of seizure disorders (Kalivas et al., 1988), affective disorders (Post, 1992), anxiety disorders (Post et al., 1988), and PTSD in both adults and children.

Organization of the developing brain occurs in a use-dependent fashion (see Chapter 1), and this organization may be affected by hypervigilance or anxiety that is pervasive, out of context, and extreme in reaction to neutral or minor threatening cues (Adell et al., 1988; Konarska et al., 1989). Therefore, many anxiety syndromes may reflect a maladaptive generalized activation of the alarm response (i.e., a sensitization), with symptoms representing exaggerations of originally adaptive and appropriate functions; for example, hypervigilance instead of appropriate prediction and early detection of future danger, and avoidance and reenactment rather than adaptation and survival.

Hypothalamic/Thalamic Nuclei: Sensory Integration

Sensory thalamic areas receive input from various afferent sensory systems, and at this level, "feeling" begins. Although thalamic nuclei are important in the stress response, these regions have been studied primarily as way stations that transmit important arousal information from the reticular activating system neurons (e.g., locus coeruleus noradrenergic neurons) to key limbic, subcortical, and cortical areas involved in sensory integration and perception of threat-related information (Castro-Alamancos and Connors, 1996). The neuroendocrinological—and likely neuroimmunological—afferent and efferent wings of the threat response are mediated by hypothalamic and other anatomically related nuclei. Animal studies have demonstrated important roles for various hypothalamic nuclei and hypothalamic neuropeptides in the stress response (Bartanusz et al., 1993; Miaskowski et al., 1988); (Rosenbaum et al., 1988), and this suggests that future studies in humans may demonstrate a key role of hypothalamic nuclei in anxiety disorders (Young and Lightman, 1992).

Limbic System: Emotion Processing

The central role of the subcortical network of brain structures in emotion was hypothesized by Papez (Papez, 1937). In 1949, MacLean coined the term *limbic system*, a name that integrated Papez's circuit (hypothalamus, anterior thalamus, cingulate gyrus, and hippocampus) with other anatomically and functionally related areas (amygdala, septum, orbitofrontal cortex). Over the years, various regions have been added to or removed from this "emotion"-processing circuit.

Amygdala: Perception of Threat and Emotional Memory

The amygdala has emerged as the key brain region responsible for the processing, interpretation, and integration of emotional functioning (Clugnet and LeDoux, 1990). Just as the locus coeruleus plays the central role in orchestrating arousal, the amygdala plays the central role in the brain in processing afferent and efferent connections related to emotional functioning (LeDoux et al., 1988; Pavlides et al., 1993; Phillips and LeDoux, 1992). The amygdala receives input directly from the sensory thalamus, the hippocampus (via multiple projections), the entorhinal cortex, and the sensory association and polymodal sensory association areas of the cortex as well as from various brainstem arousal systems via the reticular activating system (Selden et al., 1991). The amygdala processes and determines the emotional valence of simple sensory input, complex multisensory perceptions, and complex cognitive abstractions, even responding specifically to complex socially relevant stimuli. In turn, the amygdala orchestrates the organism's response to this emotional information by sending projections to brain areas involved in motor (behavioral), autonomic nervous system, and neuroendocrine areas of the CNS (Davis, 1992a, 1992b; LeDoux et al., 1988). In a series of landmark studies, LeDoux and colleagues demonstrated the key role of the amygdala in "emotional" memory (LeDoux et al., 1990). Animals, including humans, store emotional as well as cognitive information, and the storage of emotional information is critically important in both normal and abnormal regulation of anxiety. The site at which anxiety is perceived is the amygdala (Davis, 1992a). It is in these limbic areas that the patterns of neuronal activity associated with threat—and mediated by the monoamine neurotransmitter systems of the reticular activating system—become an emotion.

Hippocampus: Association, Generalization, and Storage of Threat-Related Cues

A key neuroanatomic region in memory and learning is the hippocampus. This brain area is involved in the storage of various kinds of sensory information and is very sensitive to stress activation (Pavlides et al., 1993; Phillips and LeDoux, 1992; Sapolsky et al., 1984). The hippocampus appears to be critical in the storage and recall of cognitive and emotional memory (Selden et al., 1991). Any emotional state related to arousal or threat may alter hippocampal functioning, changing the efficiency and nature of hippocampal storage and retrieval. These state-dependent memory and learning functions are vital for understanding various clinical aspects of childhood anxiety disorders. Threat alters the ability of the hippocampus and connected cortical areas to "store" certain types of cognitive information (e.g., verbal) but does not affect the storage of other types (e.g., nonverbal). Many of the cognitive distortions that appear to be associated with the development of anxiety disorders (e.g., agoraphobia) may be related to anxiety-related alterations in the "tone" of hippocampal and cortical association areas.

Neuronal systems are capable of making remarkably strong associations between paired cues (e.g., the growl of a tiger and threat). Although associations between patterns of neuronal activity and specific sensory stimuli occur in many brain areas, the most complex associations involving the integration of multiple sensory modalities are made in the more complex brain areas (i.e., the amygdala and cortex). Under ideal conditions, this threat-response capacity for association allows rapid identification of threat-related sensory information in the environment, enabling the organism to act quickly to protect its own survival. Yet this remarkable capacity of the brain to generalize from a specific event renders humans vulnerable to the development of false associations and overgeneralizations from specific threat situations to other nonthreatening situations.

In anxiety disorders, specific complex cues (e.g., snakes) may become linked with limbic-mediated emotions (e.g., anxiety). Limbic activation may result from cortically

mediated images (e.g., interpreting a specific event as potentially threatening or imagining a specific fear-inducing object such as a snake). Once these limbic areas have been activated, however, it is the sensitivity of the individual's stress-response systems that determines whether the afferent and efferent wings of the alarm response will be activated.

Cortical Systems: Interpretation of Threat

The quality and intensity of any emotional response, including anxiety, depend on subjective interpretation or cognitive appraisal of the specific situation eliciting the response (Maunsell, 1995; Singer, 1995). Most theories addressing the etiology of anxiety disorders focus on the process by which stimuli are "mislabeled" as being "threat" related, thereby inducing a fear response and anxiety in situations where no true threat exists. How individuals "cortically interpret" the limbic-mediated activity (i.e., their internal state) associated with arousal plays a major role in their subjective sense of anxiety (Gorman et al., 1989). Klüver-Bucy syndrome, which results from damage to or surgical ablation of the temporal lobes, is characterized by absence of fear in response to current and previously threatening cues (Kluver and Bucy, 1937). The general disinhibition characteristic of this syndrome suggests a loss of the capacity to recall cortically stored information related to previous threat or to efficiently store threat-related cues from new experience.

Other areas of the cortex play a role in threat. Primary among these are the multimodal association areas, which have direct connections to the amygdala. Important neurotransmitters in cortical as well as other regions involved in threat are gamma-aminobutyric acid (GABA) and glycine. The capacity of benzodiazepines to alter arousal and sensitivity to threat has long been known. Benzodiazepines target the GABA receptor complexes. Although GABA binding sites are ubiquitous in the CNS, the specific brain site at which the benzodiazepines exert their therapeutic effects is unknown. It is likely that the therapeutic effects of these agents are the result of action in multiple areas of the brain, including the cortex.

> **CASE EXAMPLE: ANXIETY AFTER FRONTAL LOBE DAMAGE**
>
> X., an 8-year-old boy, presented to a neuropsychiatric clinic 8 months after a car accident in which he suffered a traumatic head injury. He had sustained significant frontotemporal injury with resulting loss of fluent speech and of motor and complex integrated sensory processing capabilities. Rehabilitative progress was being impeded by symptoms of profound anxiety, unwillingness to travel to the hospital for rehabilitation services, and a combative and "frightened animal"–like reaction when X. was forced to leave the house. All novel situations appeared to trigger his fearful, regressive, and combative tantrums. Once

an episode started, it was nearly impossible to stop, and it took almost a whole day for him to calm down and return to his baseline state.

After extensive neuropsychiatric evaluation, X.'s episodes were conceptualized as being fear equivalents complicated by—and related to—(1) difficulty in processing complex, novel stimuli and (2) failure of previously intact cortical modulatory mechanisms to contain his arousal and impulsivity once they were activated.

Neuropeptides

Hormonal signals affect heterogeneous corticosteroid nuclear receptors; that is, type 1 (mineralocorticoid) or type 2 (glucocorticoid) in the hypothalamic-pituitary-adrenal (HPA) axis. Stressful life events such as isolation increase HPA axis activity (McEwen, 2001). The hippocampus, amygdala, and mPFC are limbic structures that are targets for and also modulate adrenal steroids. Glucocorticoids can result in neurotoxic damage to the hippocampus with suppression of neurogenesis (McEwen, 2001; Sapolsky, 2000). Exposure to stress results in release of corticotrophin releasing hormone (CRH), adrenocorticotropic hormone (ACTH), and cortisol via activation of the HPA axis. During periods of stress there is partial resistance to feedback inhibition of cortisol release and increase in plasma cortisol levels, in addition to a decrease in glucocorticoid receptors (Sapolsky and Plotsky, 1990). Glucocorticoid receptors are present in the brain in high density in areas relevant to stress and anxiety such as the hypothalamus, hippocampus, serotonergic, and noradrenergic cell bodies on both eneurons and glia. Based on animal studies, mineralocorticoid expression is high in limbic regions such as hippocampus, septum, and amygdala (Reul and de Kloet, 1985; Veldhuis and de Kloet, 1982). Animal studies suggest that stress experienced during critical years of development can have long-lasting effects on HPA axis. For instance, rats that experience in utero stress or early maternal deprivation have increased corticosterone concentrations when exposed to stress. Early postnatal stress is associated with changes in basal concentrations of hypothalamic CRH, mRNA, hippocampal glucocorticoid receptor mRNA, and median eminence CRH, in addition to the stress-induced CRH, cortocosterone, and ACTH release (Levine et al., 1993a, 1993b; Stanton et al., 1988). Adults with PTSD and nonhuman primates with early adverse experiences have elevated CRH concentrations and decreased cortisol levels in the cerebrospinal fluid (Coplan et al., 1996).

The CRH1 and CRH2 receptors have a reciprocal role in anxiety and stress (Koob and Heinrichs, 1999). While CRH1-deficient mice exhibit diminished anxiety related behaviors, CRH2-deficient mice have heightened anxiety (Bale et al., 2000; Smith et al., 1998; Timpl et al., 1998).

Cholecystokinin (CCK) is an octapeptide that has been implicated in anxiety as well. It is found in high concentrations in the cerebral cortex, amygdala, and hippocampus in mammals (Woodruff et al., 1991). Studies in healthy human subjects suggest that CCK induces anxiety and panic, which can be reduced by lorazepam (de Montigny, 1989). In addition, CCK antagonists seem to have an anxiolytic effect (Bradwejn, 1992).

Neuropeptide Y is another neuropeptide which when administered intraventricularly has anxiolytic effects (Heilig et al., 1989). Thus, disturbance in its regulation may be involved in pathophysiology of anxiety disorders (Heilig et al., 1994).

Perinatal Factors

At birth, infants are capable of exhibiting distress (anxiety) when exposed to loud noises, pain, heights, and strangers (Ball and Tronick, 1971; Bronson, 1972). While it is unwise to presume that what they are feeling is anxiety, it is certainly reasonable to hypothesize that they are experiencing subjective sensations of distress. Distress may be due to feeling cold, having low blood sugar, or hearing loud noises. Any simple set of sensory cues, internal or external, that threatens the integrity of the organism can activate the threat-response apparatus in infants.

A variety of in utero experiences may influence the sensitivity of the threat-response neurobiology in children. For example, prenatal exposure to psychoactive drugs may disrupt normal development of the brainstem catecholamines (Perry, 1988). In animal models, prenatal and perinatal stress can cause altered development of hippocampal organization and the hypothalamic-pituitary-adrenal axis (Plotsky and Meaney, 1993; Shors et al., 1990).

Whether temperament is related to genetic or to intrauterine factors is unknown. As is true of all complex human behavioral phenomena, it is likely that temperament is the result of a combination of genetic and intrauterine factors and that there is significant individual variation as to which factors are primary.

Developmental Experience

Whereas the brainstem nuclei essential in the reticular activating system and the threat response are intact at birth, thalamic, limbic, and cortical systems are not yet fully developed and organized. The human brain develops sequentially, organizing in a use-dependent fashion and altering neuronal migration, differentiation, synaptogenesis, apoptosis, and other processes of neurophysiological organization in response to a host of external molecular cues (e.g., nerve growth factor, cellular adhesion molecules, pattern, and quantity of neurotransmitter receptor stimulation) (Thoenen, 1995). Therefore, as the child matures, limbic (emotional) and cortical (cognitive) development is very experience sensitive. What is different in the young child compared with the adult may not be the subjective emotion related to the threat so much as the response of the still-developing CNS to the internal state of distress (Perry and Pollard, 1998) and the capacity of the immature cortex to make complex interpretations of the associations between paired stimuli (Singer, 1995).

Response to Threat

The immature threat-response systems have developmentally appropriate precursors of the mature systems but are quite sensitive to experience. Because the brain organizes and develops in a "use-dependent" manner (Perry and Pollard, 1998), the presence and pattern of threat experienced during childhood play a major role in determining the sensitivity and final organization of the individual's threat-response apparatus. Thus, children who are exposed to traumatic experiences develop anxiety-regulation problems with remarkable consistency (Perry and Pollard, 1998).

The classic adult response to impending threat is fight or flight (Cannon, 1914). Clearly, infants are incapable of effectively fighting or fleeing. Therefore, in response to the same internal state of anxiety and sense of impending doom experienced by the adult, infants will display a different behavior set; they will cry and thrash, and if these are unsuccessful in eliciting a response from the caregiver, they will typically use a very primitive adaptive response comparable to the defeat reaction observed in animals that are subjected to inescapable stress (Henry et al., 1986). When they are extremely anxious, infants and young children typically freeze and may dissociate as opposed to fighting or fleeing (Perry and Pollard, 1998). As children get older, their actions and reactions begin to change (although they may experience the same subjective sensation of anxiety that they did when younger), demonstrating a more "adult-like" efferent wing of the threat response.

Use-Dependent Development

Before developing a mature internal stress-response capacity, the infant has an external stress-response apparatus, the primary caregiver (Bowlby, 1982; Erickson et al., 1985). When feeling internal distress associated with hunger, cold, or fear, the infant cries and the parent responds. If the caregiver responds in a reliable and consistent manner, there occurs over time a "building in" of the neurobiology that allows the infant to carry around, or internalize, what once was an external stress-response capacity (Bowlby, 1969).

Abnormal stress-response capacities and anxiety result when there are anomalies in these early experiences (Lee and Bates, 1985; Schneider-Rosen et al., 1985). These experiences may involve inconsistent or absent soothing by a caretaker or persistent "overmothering", a situation in which a child's behavior is excessively restricted (allegedly for the child's own protection), such that he or she never has the opportunity to build in and organize (in a use-dependent way) a healthy stress-response apparatus. When such a child reaches school age, he or she has the

stress-response apparatus of a much younger child. This mismatch between the developmental maturity of the stress response and the increasing demands of the child's environment can lead to significant school-based anxiety.

As children get older, they develop fears in reaction to specific situations and objects. These fears are common, and some may even involve genetic "fixed-action" patterns developed over eons of evolution (e.g., fear of snakes or of dogs). Most of these specific fears, however, are related to the paired (or mispaired) internalization of cues with anxiety from previous experience. During infancy and childhood, children mirror their caretakers' responses when interpreting internal states of pain, arousal, or anxiety (Ainsworth, 1969; Bowlby, 1969). The child who falls on the playground and hurts her knee will look over to her father to see how to interpret her internal state. She can receive either a calm, reassuring look or an anxious, frightened response. Over time, then, the child will come to label a host of external cues as potentially threatening and certain internal sensations as fearful. This labeling process has been hypothesized to be an etiology of specific phobias and generalized anxiety disorders in children. Another illustration of these principles is seen in the offspring of adults with PTSD; such children often develop PTSD-like symptoms in response to the same cues that trigger PTSD symptoms in their parents.

CLINICAL IMPLICATIONS

Conceptualizing Anxiety as Related to the Neurobiology of Threat

Diverse areas of brain appear to be involved in the response to threat. For example, the subjective symptom of anxiety may result from either cortically-originated signals (e.g., a thought) or brainstem-originated signals (e.g., tachycardia, hypoxia). In each of these situations, a different primary pathophysiology can produce the same subjective sense of anxiety. The specific phenomenology and treatment issues associated with anxiety disorders and anxiety symptoms in other neuropsychiatric disorders reflect this diverse pathophysiology. The current classifications of childhood anxiety disorders depend on the phenotypic manifestations of emotional and behavioral functioning. Similar phenotypic manifestations, however, are likely to result from a variety of etiologies. The anxiety that manifests as the predominant symptom in any given disorder may be related to dysregulation within any of the key threat-response systems previously described or any combination of these systems. In addition, the principal "deficit" in any given system (e.g., locus coeruleus) may be attributable to dysfunction within any single neurobiological process or combination of processes (e.g., altered adrenergic receptor/effector coupling, abnormal neurotransmitter reuptake or release, inefficiencies in membrane transduction). Clearly, complex neurobiology underlies anxiety regulation.

ASSESSMENT AND TREATMENT

The assessment of anxiety in children and adolescents is based on a thorough neuropsychiatric history and examination. Semistructured interviews are usually used in research settings for diagnosis such as the Anxiety Disorders Interview for Children (Silverman and Nelles, 1988), the Schedule for Affective Disorder and Schizophrenia for School-Age Children (K-SADS) (Kaufman et al., 1997), and the Diagnostic Interview for Children and Adolescents (Welner et al., 1987). A thorough diagnostic interview is usually sufficient in a clinical setting to confirm a diagnosis of anxiety disorders. Anxiety disorders should be considered in cases (even though anxiety may not be the primary complaint) with recurrent complaints of gastrointestinal symptoms, headaches, especially if these tend to resolve on weekends or vacations and present in anticipation of an anxiety-provoking stimulus. Frequent primary care visits for a variety of somatic complaints could also be a manifestation of anxiety disorders (Beidel et al., 1991). Inattentiveness in school could be secondary to anxiety, as anxious children can be preoccupied with anxiety provoking cognitions and appear distractible. It is also important to evaluate the intensity of symptoms, whether they cause functional impairment and evaluate their existence in a number of different contexts such as school or social gatherings. In addition, it is important to take a good history of concomitant medications as some medications may induce anxiety symptoms, such as St. John's wort, ephedra preparations, caffeine containing preparations, sympathomimetics, and asthma medicines.

A family history of anxiety disorders can assist with clinical diagnosis. In addition, it is helpful to ascertain the family history of response to treatment interventions as this has the potential to inform treatment.

Children often are not good historians; therefore, it is important to interview caregivers separately in addition to interviewing the patient in a developmentally sensitive manner. Young children can convey with gestures whether anxiety is a great big problem or a little problem. Older children can use a scale of 0 to 10 with 0 being never worried and 10 being intense fear or worry about many things. Children respond well to questions asking whether they worry or are fearful of things more than other kids. Children and parental ratings of each symptom (on a scale of 1 to 10) and examples of functional impairment (hours of rituals, missing school, avoidance of parties) can be written down at each visit to monitor progress. Patient rated, subjective scales such as the Supervised Children Manifest Anxiety Scale (Reynolds and Richmond, 1997) and the Multi-Dimensional Anxiety Scale (MASC) (March et al., 1997) can also be used to monitor progress. Clinician rated instruments that have utility in clinical and research settings include the Hamilton Anxiety Rating Scale (HAM-A)(Hamilton, 1959), the Children's Yale Brown Obsessive Compulsive Scale (CY-BOCS) (Scahill et al., 1997), and the Screen for Child Anxiety Related Emotional Disorders (SCARED) (Birmaher et al., 1999).

Laboratory studies are obtained only if indicated by the history or examination. Thyroid screening (thyroid stimulating hormone levels) should be considered, unless anxiety symptoms are clearly contextual, such as in specific phobia or social phobia. Neuroimaging studies are not used for diagnostics because of poor sensitivity and specificity in anxiety disorders.

Among the most effective treatments of childhood anxiety disorders are cognitive-behavioral interventions (CBT) (Compton et al., 2004; Pediatric OCD Treatment Study (POTS) Team, 2004). CBT includes a diverse collection of complex interventions including cognitive restructuring and exposure-based interventions that promote habituation or extinction of inappropriate fears (Graziano et al., 1979). CBT also emphasizes psychoeducation as it can enhance compliance, family participation, and treatment success. Information resources for families are provided in Table 14.3. CBT also fits well into the current medical practice environment that encourages and values empirically supported, brief, problem-focused treatments.

The practice parameters for the assessment and treatment of pediatric anxiety disorders developed by the American Academy of Child and Adolescent Psychiatry recommend that pharmacotherapy should not be used as the sole intervention but as an adjunct to behavioral or psychotherapeutic interventions (Bernstein and Shaw, 1997). This is because of persuasive empirical support for CBT and the belief that benefits from CBT may be more enduring than pharmacotherapy (Bernstein and Shaw, 1997). Though these parameters were published in 1997, this treatment approach has been supported by subsequent comparative research where CBT appears at least as effective as pharmacotherapy (Pediatric OCD Treatment Study (POTS) Team, 2004). In addition, concerns about safety of antidepressants make CBT the first-line intervention (Newman, 2004). Utilization of pharmacotherapy is recommended when there is inadequate improvement with CBT (Bernstein and Shaw, 1997).

Although, data supporting the efficacy of anxiolytic pharmacotherapy in children are limited, progress has been made with publication of large multisite controlled trials using selective serotonin reuptake inhibitors (SSRIs). SSRIs are the first-line pharmacological interventions for pediatric anxiety disorders. Table 14.4 presents an overview of SSRIs.

The first large pediatric OCD trial utilized fluvoxamine, an SSRI, in a controlled trial of 120 subjects, ages 8 to 17 years (Riddle et al., 2001). This double-blind, placebo-controlled study utilized 10 weeks of core treatment, followed by a 1-year extension phase. The average daily dose of fluvoxamine was approximately 150 mg/d, and the dose range was between 50 and 200 mg/d. Significant improvement of OCD symptoms began at week 1 and continued over the course of the study. Improvement was

TABLE 14.3
RESOURCES FOR FAMILIES AND PATIENTS

Books

Helping Your Anxious Child: A Step-by-Step Guide for Parents by Ronald M. Rapee (Editor), New Harbinger Publications
Your Anxious Child: How Parents and Teachers Can Relieve Anxiety in Children by John S. Dacey, Lisa B. Fiore, Jossey-Bass
The OCD Workbook: Your Guide to Breaking Free From Obsessive-Compulsive Disorder by Bruce M. Hyman PhD, Cherry Pedrick RN,
    New Harbinger Publications
Freeing Your Child from Obsessive-Compulsive Disorder : A Powerful, Practical Program for Parents of Children and Adolescents by
    Tamar E. Chansky, Three Rivers Press

Support Organizations and Their Web Sites

www.ocfoundation.org (Obsessive Compulsive Foundation)
www.nimh.nih.gov/publicat/anxiety.cfm (National Institute of Mental Health)
www.athealth.com/consumer/newsletter (Athealth.com is a provider of Mental Health Information)
www.nmha.org/children (National Mental Health Association)
www.nami.org (National Alliance for the Mentally Ill)
www.adaa.org (Anxiety Disorders Association of America)

noted on three outcome measures: the Children's Yale-Brown Obsessive-Compulsive Scale (CY-BOCS), the National Institute of Mental Health Obsessive-Compulsive Scale (NIMH-OCS), and the Clinical Global Impressions-Improvement Scale (CGI). Fluvoxamine was well tolerated and few subjects dropped out due to lack of efficacy (9%) or untoward effects (3%). These data resulted in an FDA indication for fluvoxamine for treatment of OCD in children and adolescents ages 8 to 17 years old. This trial was followed by another large controlled SSRI trial for OCD was a sertraline study of 187 children and adolescents, ages 6 to 17 years old (March et al., 1998). Patients were treated with sertraline during a 4-week titration up to 200 mg/d, followed by 8 weeks at a stable dose. Significant differences between sertraline and placebo emerged at week 3 and persisted for the duration of the study. In intent-to-treat analyses, patients treated with sertraline showed significantly greater improvement than did placebo-treated patients on the CY-BOCS (adjusted mean, -6.8 versus -3.4, respectively; $P = .005$), the NIMH OCS (-2.2 versus -1.3,

respectively; $P = .02$), and the CGI-I (2.7 versus 3.3, respectively; $P = .002$) scales. Significant differences in efficacy between sertraline and placebo emerged as early as 3 weeks and persisted for the duration of the study. These data earned an Federal Drug Administration (FDA) indication for sertraline treatment of OCD in children and adolescents ages 6 to 17 years old. This study was followed up by a randomized controlled trial of sertraline, cognitive behavioral psychotherapy (CBT), and a combination of CBT and sertraline in 112 children and adolescents diagnosed with OCD (Pediatric OCD Treatment Study [POTS] Team, 2004). Intent-to-treat random regression analyses indicated a statistically significant advantage for sertraline alone ($P = .007$), and combined treatment ($P = .001$) compared with placebo. Combined treatment also proved superior to CBT alone ($P = .008$) and to sertraline alone ($P = .006$), which did not differ from each other. The rate of clinical remission for combined treatment was 53.6% (95% confidence interval [CI], 36% to 0%); and for sertraline alone.

TABLE 14.4
SELECTIVE SEROTONIN REUPTAKE INHIBITORS

Agent	FDA Pediatric Labeling	Clinical Use	Dose-Mg/d	Schedule	Adverse Effects
Fluoxetine	OCD (7–17 years)	OCD, GAD, SP, SAD, PD	5–60	QD	Suicidality, irritability, insomnia akathesia, GI disturbance
Paroxetine	N/A		10–30	QD	Headache
Sertraline	>6 years for OCD		25–200	QD	Rash, fluelike symptoms on rapid discontinuation, CYP inhibition
Fluvoxamine	>8 years for OCD		12.5–200	QD	
Citalopram	N/A		10–40	QD	
Escitalopram	N/A		5–30	QD	

OCD, obsessive-compulsive disorder; GAD, generalized anxiety disorder; SP, social phobia; SAD, separation anxiety disorder; PD, panic disorder.

Rosenberg et al. utilized paroxetine (10 to 20 mg) in a 12-week, open-label trial with 20 patients diagnosed with OCD, ages 8 to 17 years. Paroxetine was effective in this small sample as mean CY-BOCS scores decreased significantly (z = 3.49, P = .0005) from 30.6 +/− 3.5 to 21.6 +/− 6.8. Another psychotropic agent with controlled safety and efficacy data for pediatric OCD is clomipramine (DeVeaugh-Geiss et al., 1992; Flament et al., 1985; Leonard et al., 1989), a tricyclic antidepressant with potent serotonin (5-HT) reuptake inhibitor and noradrenergic activity. DeVeaugh-Geiss et al. enrolled 60 children, ages 10 to 17 years old and diagnosed with OCD, and demonstrated significant improvements in OCD symptoms (DeVeaugh-Geiss et al., 1992). The side effects from clomipramine were those seen typically with tricyclic antidepressant such as tachycardia, decreased systolic blood pressure, dry mouth, somnolence, dizziness, fatigue, tremor, and constipation. In a meta-analysis, Geller et al. demonstrated that clomipramine was statistically superior to SSRIs in reducing OCD symptoms but did not recommend it as a first-line treatment due to its side effect profile (Geller et al., 2003). The SSRIs examined in this meta-analysis had equivalent efficacy in this population (Geller et al., 2003).

Data are also emerging on the efficacy of SSRIs in anxiety disorders such as social phobia (SP), separation anxiety disorder (SAD), and generalized anxiety disorder (GAD). However, no pharmaceutical agent is currently approved by the FDA for treatment of these disorders in children and adolescents. The Research Unit on Pediatric Psychopharmacology Anxiety Study Group (RUPP, 2001) studied 128 children who were 6 to 17 years of age; who met the criteria for social phobia, separation anxiety disorder, or generalized anxiety disorder; and who had received psychological treatment for three weeks without improvement. The children were randomly assigned to receive fluvoxamine (at a maximum of 300 mg per day) or placebo for 8 weeks. Subjects in the fluvoxamine group had a mean (+/−SD) decrease of 9.7+/−6.9 points in symptoms of anxiety on the Pediatric Anxiety Rating Scale (range of possible scores, 0 to 25, with higher scores indicating greater anxiety), as compared with a decrease of 3.1+/−4.8 points among children in the placebo group (P ≤ 0.001). On the Clinical Global Impressions-Improvement scale, 48 of 63 children in the fluvoxamine group (76%) responded to the treatment, as indicated by a score of less than 4, as compared with 19 of 65 children in the placebo group (29%, P ≤ 0.001) (RUPP, 2001).

Birmaher et al. evaluated the efficacy of fluoxetine for the acute treatment of pediatric GAD, SAD, or SP by randomizing youths (7 to 17 years old) who had significant functional impairment due to the above diagnoses to fluoxetine (20 mg/day) (n = 37) or placebo (n = 37) for 12 weeks (Birmaher et al., 2003). Using intent-to-treat analysis, 61% of patients taking fluoxetine and 35% taking placebo showed much to very much improvement. Youths with social phobia and generalized anxiety disorder

responded better to fluoxetine than placebo, but only social phobia moderated the clinical and functional response. Severity of the anxiety at intake and positive family history for anxiety was a predictor of poorer functioning at the end of the study (Birmaher et al., 2003).

In a multicenter, 16-week, randomized, double-blind, placebo-controlled trial with flexible-dose paroxetine, Wagner et al. enrolled 322 children (8 to 11 years of age) and adolescents (12 to 17 years of age) with social anxiety disorder as their predominant psychiatric illness (Wagner et al., 2004). Patients were randomized to receive paroxetine (10 to 50 mg/d) or placebo. At the week 16 last observation carried forward end point, the odds of responding (Clinical Global Impression-Improvement score of 1 or 2) were statistically significantly greater for paroxetine (77.6% response than for placebo 38.3% response [59/154]; adjusted odds ratio, 7.02; 95% confidence interval, 4.07 to 12.11; P ≤ 001). The proportion of patients who were "very much" improved (Clinical Global Impression-Improvement score of 1) was 47.8% (77/161) for paroxetine compared with 14.9% (23/154) for placebo.

Based on these data, SSRIs are a useful intervention for pediatric anxiety disorder. While prescribing SSRIs, it would be prudent to weigh the risks against the benefits of prescribing these agents. SSRIs may produce stomachache, nausea, vomiting, diarrhea, and anorexia (Birmaher et al., 2003; Scharko, 2004). According to a joint advisory committee for the Food and Drug Administration, antidepressants can increase the risk of suicidal behavior in the pediatric age group. On September 14, 2004, the advisory committee voted in favor of a "black box warning" stating the risk of suicidality with antidepressants in acute treatment trials. This warning was based on a pooled analysis of short-term (4 to 16 weeks) placebo-controlled trials of nine antidepressant drugs (SSRIs and others) in children and adolescents with MDD and other anxiety disorders including OCD. This analysis included 24 trials with approximately 4,400 patients, and it revealed a greater risk of adverse events representing suicidal thinking or behavior (suicidality) across all antidepressants and almost all trials during the first few months of treatment in those receiving antidepressants. The average risk of such events on drug was 4%, twice the placebo risk of 2%. No suicides occurred in these trials.

FUTURE DIRECTIONS

The completion of a working draft of the human genome sequence promises to provide unprecedented opportunities to explore the genetic basis of individual differences in anxiety disorders, in addition to vulnerability to fear and anxiety (Hariri and Weinberger, 2003). Functional neuroimaging, because of its unique ability to assay information processing at the level of brain, will be a powerful approach that will supplement functional genomics.

Published fMRI studies are already beginning to established important physiological links between functional genetic polymorphisms and differences in information processing within specific brain regions (Hariri et al., 2005). Further utilization of such technical advancements is likely to improve understanding of the biological basis of anxiety disorders, which could lead to novel and more effective treatments for these disorders. Since the mid-1990s, results of several large clinical trials have been published or presented in scientific conferences. These trials demonstrate that often the best available treatments fail to produce full symptom remission. Therefore advancement in scientific knowledge is sorely needed to aid development of new and better treatments.

REFERENCES

Abercrombie ED, Jacobs BL (1987a). Microinjected clonidine inhibits noradrenergic neurons of the locus coeruleus in freely moving cats. *Neurosci Lett* 76: 203–8.

Abercrombie ED, Jacobs BL (1987b). Single-unit response of noradrenergic neurons in the locus coeruleus of freely moving cats. II. Adaptation to chronically presented stressful stimuli. *J Neurosci* 7: 2844–8.

Abercrombie ED, Jacobs BL (1988). Systemic naloxone administration potentiates locus coeruleus noradrenergic neuronal activity under stressful but not non-stressful conditions. *Brain Res* 441: 362–6.

Achenbach TM, Howell CT, McConaughy SH, Stanger C (1995). Six-year predictors of problems in a national sample: III. Transitions to young adult syndromes. *J Am Acad Child Adolesc Psychiatry* 34: 658–69.

Adell A, Garcia-Marquez C, Armario A, Gelpi E (1988). Chronic stress increases serotonin and noradrenaline in rat brain and sensitizes their responses to a further acute stress. *J Neurochem* 50: 1678–81.

Agras WS, Chapin HN, Oliveau DC (1972). The natural history of phobia. Course and prognosis. *Arch Gen Psychiatry* 26: 315–7.

Ainsworth MD (1969). Object relations, dependency, and attachment: a theoretical review of the infant-mother relationship. *Child Dev* 40: 969–1025.

Alsobrook JP, 2nd, Zohar AH, Leboyer M, Chabane N, Ebstein RP, Pauls DL (2002). Association between the COMT locus and obsessive-compulsive disorder in females but not males. *Am J Med Genet* 114: 116–20.

Anderson JC, Williams S, McGee R, Silva PA (1987). DSM-III disorders in preadolescent children. Prevalence in a large sample from the general population. *Arch Gen Psychiatry* 44: 69–76.

Antelman SM, Eichler AJ, Black CA, Kocan D (1980). Interchangeability of stress and amphetamine in sensitization. *Science* 207: 329–31.

Aston-Jones G, Ennis M, Pieribone VA, Nickell WT, Shipley MT (1986). The brain nucleus locus coeruleus: restricted afferent control of a broad efferent network. *Science* 234: 734–7.

Bale TL, Contarino A, Smith GW, Chan R, Gold LH, Sawchenko PE, Koob GF, Vale WW, Lee KF (2000). Mice deficient for corticotropin-releasing hormone receptor-2 display anxiety-like behaviour and are hypersensitive to stress. *Nat Genet* 24: 410–4.

Ball W, Tronick E (1971). Infant responses to impending collision: optical and real. *Science* 171: 818–20.

Bartanusz V, Jezova D, Bertini LT, Tilders FJ, Aubry JM, Kiss JZ (1993). Stress-induced increase in vasopressin and corticotropin-releasing factor expression in hypophysiotrophic paraventricular neurons. *Endocrinology* 132: 895–902.

Battaglia M, Ogliari A, Zanoni A, Citterio A, Pozzoli U, Giorda R, Maffei C, Marino C (2005). Influence of the serotonin transporter promoter gene and shyness on children's cerebral responses to facial expressions. *Arch Gen Psychiatry* 62: 85–94.

Beidel DC, Christ MG, Long PJ (1991). Somatic complaints in anxious children. *J Abnorm Child Psychol* 19: 659–70.

Berg CZ, Rapoport JL, Whitaker A, Davies M, Leonard H, Swedo SE, Braiman S, Lenane M (1989). Childhood obsessive compulsive disorder: a two-year prospective follow-up of a community sample. *J Am Acad Child Adolesc Psychiatry* 28: 528–33.

Bernstein GA, Borchardt CM, Perwien AR (1996). Anxiety disorders in children and adolescents: a review of the past 10 years. *J Am Acad Child Adolesc Psychiatry* 35: 1110–9.

Bernstein GA, Shaw K (1997). Practice parameters for the assessment and treatment of children and adolescents with anxiety disorders. American Academy of Child and Adolescent Psychiatry. *J Am Acad Child Adolesc Psychiatry* 36: 69S–84S.

Biederman J, Newcorn J, Sprich S (1991). Comorbidity of attention deficit hyperactivity disorder with conduct, depressive, anxiety, and other disorders. *Am J Psychiatry* 148: 564–77.

Billett EA, Richter MA, King N, Heils A, Lesch KP, Kennedy JL (1997). Obsessive compulsive disorder, response to serotonin reuptake inhibitors and the serotonin transporter gene. *Mol Psychiatry* 2: 403–6.

Birmaher B, Axelson DA, Monk K, Kalas C, Clark DB, Ehmann M, Bridge J, Heo J, Brent DA (2003). Fluoxetine for the treatment of childhood anxiety disorders. *J Am Acad Child Adolesc Psychiatry* 42: 415–23.

Birmaher B, Brent DA, Chiappetta L, Bridge J, Monga S, Baugher M (1999). Psychometric properties of the Screen for Child Anxiety Related Emotional Disorders (SCARED): a replication study. *J Am Acad Child Adolesc Psychiatry* 38: 1230–6.

Black B, Robbins DR (1990). Panic disorder in children and adolescents. *J Am Acad Child Adolesc Psychiatry* 29: 36–44.

Bowlby J (1969). *Attachment and Loss.* New York: Basic Books.

Bowlby J (1982). Attachment and loss: retrospect and prospect. *Am J Orthopsychiatry* 52: 664–78.

Bradwejn J (1992). CCK agonists and antagonists in clinical studies of panic and anxiety. *Clin Neuropharmacol* 15 Suppl 1 Pt A: 481A–482A.

Breier A, Charney DS, Heninger GR (1986). Agoraphobia with panic attacks. Development, diagnostic stability, and course of illness. *Arch Gen Psychiatry* 43: 1029–36.

Bronson GW (1972). Infants' reactions to unfamiliar persons and novel objects. *Monogr Soc Res Child Dev* 37: 1–46.

Brown TH, Chapman PF, Kairiss EW, Keenan CL (1988). Long-term synaptic potentiation. *Science* 242: 724–8.

Butler PD, Weiss JM, Stout JC, Nemeroff CB (1990). Corticotropin-releasing factor produces fear-enhancing and behavioral activating effects following infusion into the locus coeruleus. *J Neurosci* 10: 176–83.

Cannon WB (1914). The emergency function of the adrenal medulla in pain and the major emotions. *Am J Physiol* 33: 356–72.

Cantwell DP, Baker L (1989). Stability and natural history of DSM-III childhood diagnoses. *J Am Acad Child Adolesc Psychiatry* 28: 691–700.

Castro-Alamancos MA, Connors BW (1996). Short-term plasticity of a thalamocortical pathway dynamically modulated by behavioral state. *Science* 272: 274–7.

Cavallini MC, Di Bella D, Siliprandi F, Malchiodi F, Bellodi L (2002). Exploratory factor analysis of obsessive-compulsive patients and association with 5-HTTLPR polymorphism. *Am J Med Genet* 114: 347–53.

Cloninger CR, Van Eerdewegh P, Goate A, Edenberg HJ, Blangero J, Hesselbrock V, Reich T, Nurnberger J, Jr., Schuckit M, Porjesz B, Crowe R, Rice JP, Foroud T, Przybeck TR, Almasy L, Bucholz K, Wu W, Shears S, Carr K, Crose C, Willig C, Zhao J, Tischfield JA, Li TK, Conneally PM, et al. (1998). Anxiety proneness linked to epistatic loci in genome scan of human personality traits. *Am J Med Genet* 81: 313–7.

Clugnet MC, LeDoux JE (1990). Synaptic plasticity in fear conditioning circuits: induction of LTP in the lateral nucleus of the amygdala by stimulation of the medial geniculate body. *J Neurosci* 10: 2818–24.

Compton SN, March JS, Brent D, Albano AMT, Weersing R, Curry J (2004). Cognitive-behavioral psychotherapy for anxiety and depressive disorders in children and adolescents: an evidence-based medicine review. *J Am Acad Child Adolesc Psychiatry* 43: 930–59.

Coplan JD, Andrews MW, Rosenblum LA, Owens MJ, Friedman S, Gorman JM, Nemeroff CB (1996). Persistent elevations of cerebrospinal fluid concentrations of corticotropin-releasing factor in adult nonhuman primates exposed to early-life stressors: implications for the pathophysiology of mood and anxiety disorders. *Proc Natl Acad Sci USA* 93: 1619–23.

Crowe RR, Goedken R, Samuelson S, Wilson R, Nelson J, Noyes R, Jr. (2001). Genomewide survey of panic disorder. *Am J Med Genet* 105: 105–9.

Davis M (1992a). The role of the amygdala in fear and anxiety. *Annu Rev Neurosci* 15: 353–75.

Davis M (1992b). The role of the amygdala in fear-potentiated startle: implications for animal models of anxiety. *Trends Pharmacol Sci* 13: 35–41.

de Montigny C (1989). Cholecystokinin tetrapeptide induces panic-like attacks in healthy volunteers. Preliminary findings. *Arch Gen Psychiatry* 46: 511–7.

Deckert J, Catalano M, Heils A, Di Bella D, Friess F, Politi E, Franke P, Nothen MM, Maier W, Bellodi L, Lesch KP (1997). Functional promoter polymorphism of the human serotonin transporter: lack of association with panic disorder. *Psychiatr Genet* 7: 45–7.

DeVeaugh-Geiss J, Moroz G, Biederman J, Cantwell D, Fontaine R, Greist JH, Reichler R, Katz R, Landau P (1992). Clomipramine hydrochloride in childhood and adolescent obsessive-compulsive disorder—a multicenter trial. *J Am Acad Child Adolesc Psychiatry* 31: 45–9.

Di Bella D, Cavallini MC, Bellodi L (2002). No association between obsessive-compulsive disorder and the 5-HT (1Dbeta) receptor gene. *Am J Psychiatry* 159: 1783–5.

DSM-III-R (1987). *Diagnostic and Statistical Manual of Mental Disorders,* 3rd ed. Washington, DC: American Psychiatric Association.

DSM-IV-TR (2000). *Diagnostic and Statistical Manual of Mental Disorders,* 4th ed. Washington, DC: American Psychiatric Association.

Elam M, Thoren P, Svensson TH (1986). Locus coeruleus neurons and sympathetic nerves: activation by visceral afferents. *Brain Res* 375: 117–25.

Erickson MF, Sroufe LA, Egeland B (1985). The relationship between quality of attachment and behavior problems in preschool in a high-risk sample. *Monogr Soc Res Child Dev* 50: 147–66.

Essau CA, Conradt J, Petermann F (2000). Frequency, comorbidity, and psychosocial impairment of specific phobia in adolescents. *J Clin Child Psychol* 29: 221–31.

Farfel GM, Kleven MS, Woolverton WL, Seiden LS, Perry BD (1992). Effects of repeated injections of cocaine on catecholamine receptor binding sites, dopamine transporter binding sites and behavior in rhesus monkey. *Brain Res* 578: 235–43.

Fehr C, Grintschuk N, Szegedi A, Anghelescu I, Klawe C, Singer P, Hiemke C, Dahmen N (2000). The HTR1B 861G>C receptor polymorphism among patients suffering from alcoholism, major depression, anxiety disorders and narcolepsy. *Psychiatry Res* 97: 1–10.

Flament MF, Rapoport JL, Kilts C (1985). A controlled trial of clomipramine in childhood obsessive compulsive disorder. *Psychopharmacol Bull* 21: 150–2.

Flament MF, Whitaker A, Rapoport JL, Davies M, Berg CZ, Kalikow K, Sceery W, Shaffer D (1988). Obsessive compulsive disorder in adolescence: an epidemiological study. *J Am Acad Child Adolesc Psychiatry* 27: 764–71.

Foote SL, Bloom FE, Aston-Jones G (1983). Nucleus locus ceruleus: new evidence of anatomical and physiological specificity. *Physiol Rev* 63: 844–914.

Francis G, Last CG, Strauss CC (1992). Avoidant disorder and social phobia in children and adolescents. *J Am Acad Child Adolesc Psychiatry* 31: 1086–9.

Geller DA, Biederman J, Stewart SE, Mullin B, Martin A, Spencer T, Faraone SV (2003). Which SSRI? A meta-analysis of pharmacotherapy trials in pediatric obsessive-compulsive disorder. *Am J Psychiatry* 160: 1919–28.

Giedd JN, Rapoport JL, Garvey MA, Perlmutter S, Swedo SE (2000). MRI Assessment of Children With Obsessive-Compulsive Disorder or Tics Associated With Streptococcal Infection. *Am J Psychiatry* 157: 281–283.

Gorman JM, Liebowitz MR, Fyer AJ, Stein J (1989). A neuroanatomical hypothesis for panic disorder. *Am J Psychiatry* 146: 148–61.

Graziano AM, DeGiovanni IS, Garcia KA (1979). Behavioral treatment of children's fears: a review. *Psychol Bull* 86: 804–30.

Hamilton M (1959). The assessment of anxiety states by rating. *Br J Med Psychol* 32: 50–5.

Hamilton SP, Heiman GA, Haghighi F, Mick S, Klein DF, Hodge SE, Weissman MM, Fyer AJ, Knowles JA (1999). Lack of genetic linkage or association between a functional serotonin transporter polymorphism and panic disorder. *Psychiatr Genet* 9: 1–6.

Hamilton SP, Slager SL, Heiman GA, Deng Z, Haghighi F, Klein DF, Hodge SE, Weissman MM, Fyer AJ, Knowles JA (2002). Evidence for a susceptibility locus for panic disorder near the catechol-O-methyltransferase gene on chromosome 22. *Biol Psychiatry* 51: 591–601.

Hanna GL, Veenstra-VanderWeele J, Cox NJ, Boehnke M, Himle JA, Curtis GC, Leventhal BL, Cook EH, Jr. (2002). Genome-wide linkage analysis of families with obsessive-compulsive disorder ascertained through pediatric probands. *Am J Med Genet* 114: 541–52.

Hariri AR, Drabant EM, Munoz KE, Kolachana BS, Mattay VS, Egan MF, Weinberger DR (2005). A susceptibility gene for affective disorders and the response of the human amygdala. *Arch Gen Psychiatry* 62: 146–52.

Hariri AR, Weinberger DR (2003). Imaging genomics. *Br Med Bull* 65: 259–70.

Heilig M, Koob GF, Ekman R, Britton KT (1994). Corticotropin-releasing factor and neuropeptide Y: role in emotional integration. *Trends Neurosci* 17: 80–5.

Heilig M, Soderpalm B, Engel JA, Widerlov E (1989). Centrally administered neuropeptide Y (NPY) produces anxiolytic-like effects in animal anxiety models. *Psychopharmacology (Berl)* 98: 524–9.

Henry JP, Stephens PM, Ely DL (1986). Psychosocial hypertension and the defence and defeat reactions. *J Hypertens* 4: 687–97.

Hettema JM, Neale MC, Kendler KS (2001). A Review and Meta-Analysis of the Genetic Epidemiology of Anxiety Disorders. *Am J Psychiatry* 158: 1568–78.

Kagan J, Reznick JS, Snidman N (1987). The physiology and psychology of behavioral inhibition in children. *Child Dev* 58: 1459–73.

Kalivas PW, Duffy P (1989). Similar effects of daily cocaine and stress on mesocorticolimbic dopamine neurotransmission in the rat. *Biol Psychiatry* 25: 913–28.

Kalivas PW, Duffy P, DuMars LA, Skinner C (1988). Behavioral and neurochemical effects of acute and daily cocaine administration in rats. *J Pharmacol Exp Ther* 245: 485–92.

Kandel ER (1989). Genes, nerve cells, and the remembrance of things past. *J Neuropsychiatry Clin Neurosci* 1: 103–25.

Kandel ER, Schwartz JH (1982). Molecular biology of learning: modulation of transmitter release. *Science* 218: 433–43.

Kaplow JB, Curran PJ, Angold A, Costello EJ (2001). The prospective relation between dimensions of anxiety and the initiation of adolescent alcohol use. *J Clin Child Psychol* 30: 316–26.

Karayiorgou M, Altemus M, Galke BL, Goldman D, Murphy DL, Ott J, Gogos JA (1997). Genotype determining low catechol-O-methyltransferase activity as a risk factor for obsessive-compulsive disorder. *Proc Natl Acad Sci USA* 94: 4572–5.

Karayiorgou M, Sobin C, Blundell ML, Galke BL, Malinova L, Goldberg P, Ott J, Gogos JA (1999). Family-based association studies support a sexually dimorphic effect of COMT and MAOA on genetic susceptibility to obsessive-compulsive disorder. *Biol Psychiatry* 45: 1178–89.

Kashani JH, Orvaschel H (1988). Anxiety disorders in mid-adolescence: a community sample. *Am J Psychiatry* 145: 960–4.

Kashani JH, Orvaschel H (1990). A community study of anxiety in children and adolescents. *Am J Psychiatry* 147: 313–8.

Kashani JH, Orvaschel H, Rosenberg TK, Reid JC (1989). Psychopathology in a community sample of children and adolescents: a developmental perspective. *J Am Acad Child Adolesc Psychiatry* 28: 701–6.

Katsuragi S, Kunugi H, Sano A, Tsutsumi T, Isogawa K, Nanko S, Akiyoshi J (1999). Association between serotonin transporter gene polymorphism and anxiety-related traits. *Biol Psychiatry* 45: 368–70.

Katzelnick DJ, Kobak KA, DeLeire T, Henk HJ, Greist JH, Davidson JR, Schneier FR, Stein MB, Helstad CP (2001). Impact of generalized social anxiety disorder in managed care. *Am J Psychiatry* 158: 1999–2007.

Kaufman J, Birmaher B, Brent D, Rao U, Flynn C, Moreci P, Williamson D, Ryan N (1997). Schedule for Affective Disorders and Schizophrenia for School-Age Children-Present and Lifetime Version (K-SADS-PL): initial reliability and validity data. *J Am Acad Child Adolesc Psychiatry* 36: 980–8.

Kessler RC, McGonagle KA, Zhao S, Nelson CB, Hughes M, Eshleman S, Wittchen HU, Kendler KS (1994). Lifetime and 12-month prevalence of DSM-III-R psychiatric disorders in the United States. Results from the National Comorbidity Survey. *Arch Gen Psychiatry* 51: 8–19.

King N, Ollendick T, Heyne D, Tonge B (1995). Treatment of school refusal. Strategies for the family physician. *Aust Fam Physician* 24: 1250–3.

Kleven MS, Perry BD, Woolverton WL, Seiden LS (1990). Effects of repeated injections of cocaine on D1 and D2 dopamine receptors in rat brain. *Brain Res* 532: 265–70.

Kluver H, Bucy PC (1937). "Psychic blindness" and other symptoms following bilateral temporal lobectomy in rhesus monkeys. *Am J Physiol* 119: 352–3.

Konarska M, Stewart RE, McCarty R (1989). Sensitization of sympathetic-adrenal medullary responses to a novel stressor in chronically stressed laboratory rats. *Physiol Behav* 46: 129–35.

Koob GF, Heinrichs SC (1999). A role for corticotropin releasing factor and urocortin in behavioral responses to stressors. *Brain Res* 848: 141–52.

Kovacs M, Gatsonis C, Paulauskas SL, Richards C (1989). Depressive disorders in childhood. IV. A longitudinal study of comorbidity with and risk for anxiety disorders. *Arch Gen Psychiatry* 46: 776–82.

Kovacs M, Goldston D (1991). Cognitive and social cognitive development of depressed children and adolescents. *J Am Acad Child Adolesc Psychiatry* 30: 388–92.

Labellarte MJ, Ginsburg GS, Walkup JT, Riddle MA (1999). The treatment of anxiety disorders in children and adolescents. *Biol Psychiatry* 46: 567–78.

Last CG, Francis G, Hersen M, Kazdin AE, Strauss CC (1987a). Separation anxiety and school phobia: a comparison using DSM-III criteria. *Am J Psychiatry* 144: 653–7.

Last CG, Perrin S, Hersen M, Kazdin AE (1992). DSM-III-R anxiety disorders in children: sociodemographic and clinical characteristics. *J Am Acad Child Adolesc Psychiatry* 31: 1070–6.

Last CG, Phillips JE, Statfeld A (1987b). Childhood anxiety disorders in mothers and their children. *Child Psychiatry Hum Dev* 18: 103–12.

Leckman JF, Weissman MM, Merikangas KR, Pauls DL, Prusoff BA (1983). Panic disorder and major depression. Increased risk of depression, alcoholism, panic, and phobic disorders in families of depressed probands with panic disorder. *Arch Gen Psychiatry* 40: 1055–60.

LeDoux JE, Cicchetti P, Xagoraris A, Romanski LM (1990). The lateral amygdaloid nucleus: sensory interface of the amygdala in fear conditioning. *J Neurosci* 10: 1062–9.

LeDoux JE, Iwata J, Cicchetti P, Reis DJ (1988). Different projections of the central amygdaloid nucleus mediate autonomic and behavioral correlates of conditioned fear. *J Neurosci* 8: 2517–29.

Lee CL, Bates JE (1985). Mother-child interaction at age two years and perceived difficult temperament. *Child Dev* 56: 1314–25.

Leonard HL, Swedo SE, Rapoport JL, Koby EV, Lenane MC, Cheslow DL, Hamburger SD (1989). Treatment of obsessive-compulsive disorder with clomipramine and desipramine in children and adolescents. A double-blind crossover comparison. *Arch Gen Psychiatry* 46: 1088–92.

Lesch KP (2001). Molecular foundation of anxiety disorders. *J Neural Transm* 108: 717–46.

Lesch KP, Bengel D, Heils A, Sabol SZ, Greenberg BD, Petri S, Benjamin J, Muller CR, Hamer DH, Murphy DL (1996). Association of anxiety-related traits with a polymorphism in the serotonin transporter gene regulatory region. *Science* 274: 1527–31.

Levine ES, Litto WJ, Jacobs BL (1990). Activity of cat locus coeruleus noradrenergic neurons during the defense reaction. *Brain Res* 531: 189–95.

Levine S, Atha K, Wiener SG (1993a). Early experience effects on the development of fear in the squirrel monkey. *Behav Neural Biol* 60: 225–33.

Levine S, Wiener SG, Coe CL (1993b). Temporal and social factors influencing behavioral and hormonal responses to separation in mother and infant squirrel monkeys. *Psychoneuroendocrinology* 18: 297–306.

Lewinsohn PM, Hops H, Roberts RE, Seeley JR, Andrews JA (1993). Adolescent psychopathology: I. Prevalence and incidence of depression and other DSM-III-R disorders in high school students. *J Abnorm Psychol* 102: 133–44.

Madison DV, Malenka RC, Nicoll RA (1991). Mechanisms underlying long-term potentiation of synaptic transmission. *Annu Rev Neurosci* 14: 379–97.

March JS, Biederman J, Wolkow R, Safferman A, Mardekian J, Cook EH, Cutler NR, Dominguez R, Ferguson J, Muller B, Riesenberg R, Rosenthal M, Sallee FR, Wagner KD, Steiner H (1998). Sertraline in children and adolescents with obsessive-compulsive disorder: a multicenter randomized controlled trial. *JAMA* 280: 1752–6.

March JS, Parker JD, Sullivan K, Stallings P, Conners CK (1997). The Multidimensional Anxiety Scale for Children (MASC): factor structure, reliability, and validity. *J Am Acad Child Adolesc Psychiatry* 36: 554–65.

Maunsell JH (1995). The brain's visual world: representation of visual targets in cerebral cortex. *Science* 270: 764–9.

Mazzanti CM, Lappalainen J, Long JC, Bengel D, Naukkarinen H, Eggert M, Virkkunen M, Linnoila M, Goldman D (1998). Role of the serotonin transporter promoter polymorphism in anxiety-related traits. *Arch Gen Psychiatry* 55: 936–40.

McCauley E, Myers K, Mitchell J, Calderon R, Schloredt K, Treder R (1993). Depression in young people: initial presentation and clinical course. *J Am Acad Child Adolesc Psychiatry* 32: 714–22.

McEwen BS (2001). From molecules to mind. Stress, individual differences, and the social environment. *Ann NY Acad Sci* 935: 42–9.

Miaskowski C, Ong GL, Lukic D, Haldar J (1988). Immobilization stress affects oxytocin and vasopressin levels in hypothalamic and extrahypothalamic sites. *Brain Res* 458: 137–41.

Milne JM, Garrison CZ, Addy CL, McKeown RE, Jackson KL, Cuffe SP, Waller JL (1995). Frequency of phobic disorder in a community sample of young adolescents. *J Am Acad Child Adolesc Psychiatry* 34: 1202–11.

Mitchell J, McCauley E, Burke PM, Moss SJ (1988). Phenomenology of depression in children and adolescents. *J Am Acad Child Adolesc Psychiatry* 27: 12–20.

Moore RY, Bloom FE (1979). Central catecholamine neuron systems: anatomy and physiology of the norepinephrine and epinephrine systems. *Annu Rev Neurosci* 2: 113–68.

Morilak DA, Fornal CA, Jacobs BL (1987a). Effects of physiological manipulations on locus coeruleus neuronal activity in freely moving cats. I. Thermoregulatory challenge. *Brain Res* 422: 17–23.

Morilak DA, Fornal CA, Jacobs BL (1987b). Effects of physiological manipulations on locus coeruleus neuronal activity in freely moving cats. II. Cardiovascular challenge. *Brain Res* 422: 24–31.

Morilak DA, Fornal CA, Jacobs BL (1987c). Effects of physiological manipulations on locus coeruleus neuronal activity in freely moving cats. III. Glucoregulatory challenge. *Brain Res* 422: 32–9.

Munk MH, Roelfsema PR, Konig P, Engel AK, Singer W (1996). Role of reticular activation in the modulation of intracortical synchronization. *Science* 272: 271–4.

Nakamura T, Muramatsu T, Ono Y, Matsushita S, Higuchi S, Mizushima H, Yoshimura K, Kanba S, Asai M (1997). Serotonin transporter gene regulatory region polymorphism and anxiety-related traits in the Japanese. *Am J Med Genet* 74: 544–5.

Nauta WJ, Whitlock DG (1956). Subcortical projections from the temporal neocortex in Macaca mulatta. *J Comp Neurol* 106: 183–212.

Newman TB (2004). A black-box warning for antidepressants in children? *N Engl J Med* 351: 1595–8.

Ohara K, Nagai M, Suzuki Y, Ochiai M (1998). No association between anxiety disorders and catechol-O-methyltransferase polymorphism. *Psychiatry Res* 80: 145–8.

Papez JW (1937). A proposed mechanism of emotion. *Arch of Neurology and Psychiatry* 38: 725–40.

Pavlides C, Watanabe Y, McEwen BS (1993). Effects of glucocorticoids on hippocampal long-term potentiation. *Hippocampus* 3: 183–92.

Pawlak C, Pascual-Sanchez T, Rae P, Fischer W, Ladame F (1999). Anxiety disorders, comorbidity, and suicide attempts in adolescence: a preliminary investigation. *Eur Psychiatry* 14: 132–6.

Pediatric OCD Treatment Study (POTS) Team (2004). Cognitive-Behavior Therapy, Sertraline, and Their Combination for Children and Adolescents With Obsessive-Compulsive Disorder: The Pediatric OCD Treatment Study (POTS) Randomized Controlled Trial. *JAMA* 292: 1969–76.

Perry BD (1988). Placental and blood element neurotransmitter receptor regulation in humans: potential models for studying neurochemical mechanisms underlying behavioral teratology. *Prog Brain Res* 73: 189–205.

Perry BD, Pollard R (1998). Homeostasis, stress, trauma, and adaptation. A neurodevelopmental view of childhood trauma. *Child Adolesc Psychiatr Clin N Am* 7: viii, 33–51.

Perry BD, Stolk JM, Vantini G, Guchhait RB, U'Prichard DC (1983). Strain differences in rat brain epinephrine synthesis: regulation of alpha-adrenergic receptor number by epinephrine. *Science* 221: 1297–9.

Phillips RG, LeDoux JE (1992). Differential contribution of amygdala and hippocampus to cued and contextual fear conditioning. *Behav Neurosci* 106: 274–85.

Pine DS, Cohen P, Gurley D, Brook J, Ma Y (1998). The risk for early-adulthood anxiety and depressive disorders in adolescents with anxiety and depressive disorders. *Arch Gen Psychiatry* 55: 56–64.

Plotsky PM, Meaney MJ (1993). Early, postnatal experience alters hypothalamic corticotropin-releasing factor (CRF) mRNA, median eminence CRF content and stress-induced release in adult rats. *Brain Res Mol Brain Res* 18: 195–200.

Post RM (1992). Transduction of psychosocial stress into the neurobiology of recurrent affective disorder. *Am J Psychiatry* 149: 999–1010.

Post RM, Weiss SR, Pert A (1988). Cocaine-induced behavioral sensitization and kindling: implications for the emergence of psychopathology and seizures. *Ann NY Acad Sci* 537: 292–308.

Reinherz HZ, Stewart-Berghauer G, Pakiz B, Frost AK, Moeykens BA, Holmes WM (1989). The relationship of early risk and current mediators to depressive symptomatology in adolescence. *J Am Acad Child Adolesc Psychiatry* 28: 942–7.

Reul JM, de Kloet ER (1985). Two receptor systems for corticosterone in rat brain: microdistribution and differential occupation. *Endocrinology* 117: 2505–11.

Reynolds CR, Richmond BO (1997). What I Think and Feel: a revised measure of Children's Manifest Anxiety. *J Abnorm Child Psychol* 25: 15–20.

Riddle MA, Reeve EA, Yaryura-Tobias JA, Yang HM, Claghorn JL, Gaffney G, Greist JH, Holland D, McConville BJ, Pigott T, Walkup JT (2001). Fluvoxamine for children and adolescents with obsessive-compulsive disorder: a randomized, controlled, multicenter trial. *J Am Acad Child Adolesc Psychiatry* 40: 222–9.

Rosenbaum JF, Biederman J, Gersten M, Hirshfeld DR, Meminger SR, Herman JB, Kagan J, Reznick JS, Snidman N (1988). Behavioral inhibition in children of parents with panic disorder and agoraphobia. A controlled study. *Arch Gen Psychiatry* 45: 463–70.

RUPP (2001). Fluvoxamine for the treatment of anxiety disorders in children and adolescents. The Research Unit on Pediatric Psychopharmacology Anxiety Study Group. *N Engl J Med* 344: 1279–85.

Samochowiec J, Hajduk A, Samochowiec A, Horodnicki J, Stepien G, Grzywacz A, Kucharska-Mazur J (2004). Association studies of MAO-A, COMT, and 5-HTT genes polymorphisms in patients with anxiety disorders of the phobic spectrum. *Psychiatry Res* 128: 21–6.

Saper CB (1982). Convergence of autonomic and limbic connections in the insular cortex of the rat. *J Comp Neurol* 210: 163–73.

Sapolsky RM (2000). Glucocorticoids and hippocampal atrophy in neuropsychiatric disorders. *Arch Gen Psychiatry* 57: 925–35.

Sapolsky RM, Krey LC, McEwen BS (1984). Glucocorticoid-sensitive hippocampal neurons are involved in terminating the adrenocortical stress response. *Proc Natl Acad Sci USA* 81: 6174–7.

Sapolsky RM, Plotsky PM (1990). Hypercortisolism and its possible neural bases. *Biol Psychiatry* 27: 937–52.

Scahill L, Riddle MA, McSwiggin-Hardin M, Ort SI, King RA, Goodman WK, Cicchetti D, Leckman JF (1997). Children's Yale-Brown Obsessive Compulsive Scale: reliability and validity. *J Am Acad Child Adolesc Psychiatry* 36: 844–52.

Scharko A (2004). Selective serotonin reuptake inhibitor-induced sexual dysfunction in adolescents: a review [In Process Citation]. *J Am Acad Child Adolesc Psychiatry* 43: 1071–9.

Schneider-Rosen K, Braunwald KG, Carlson V, Cicchetti D (1985). Current perspectives in attachment theory: illustration from the study of maltreated infants. *Monogr Soc Res Child Dev* 50: 194–210.

Selden NR, Everitt BJ, Jarrard LE, Robbins TW (1991). Complementary roles for the amygdala and hippocampus in aversive conditioning to explicit and contextual cues. *Neuroscience* 42: 335–50.

Shors TJ, Foy MR, Levine S, Thompson RF (1990). Unpredictable and uncontrollable stress impairs neuronal plasticity in the rat hippocampus. *Brain Res Bull* 24 663–7.

Silverman WK, Nelles WB (1988). The Anxiety Disorders Interview Schedule for Children. *J Am Acad Child Adolesc Psychiatry* 27: 772–8.

Singer W (1995). Development and plasticity of cortical processing architectures. *Science*, Vol 270: 758–64.

Smith GW, Aubry JM, Dellu F, Contarino A, Bilezikjian LM, Gold LH, Chen R, Marchuk Y, Hauser C, Bentley CA, Sawchenko PE, Koob GF, Vale W, Lee KF (1998). Corticotropin releasing factor receptor 1-deficient mice display decreased anxiety, impaired stress response, and aberrant neuroendocrine development. *Neuron* 20: 1093–102.

Spence SH, Rapee R, McDonald C, Ingram M (2001). The structure of anxiety symptoms among preschoolers. *Behav Res Ther* 39: 1293–316.

Stanton ME, Gutierrez YR, Levine S (1988). Maternal deprivation potentiates pituitary-adrenal stress responses in infant rats. *Behav Neurosci* 102: 692–700.

Stein DJ, Mendelsohn I, Potocnik F, Van Kradenberg J, Wessels C (1998). Use of the selective serotonin reuptake inhibitor citalopram in a possible animal analogue of obsessive-compulsive disorder. *Depress Anxiety* 8: 39–42.

Stevenson J, Batten N, Cherner M (1992). Fears and fearfulness in children and adolescents: a genetic analysis of twin data. *J Child Psychol Psychiatry* 33: 977–85.

Stoltenberg SF, Twitchell GR, Hanna GL, Cook EH, Fitzgerald HE, Zucker RA, Little KY (2002). Serotonin transporter promoter polymorphism, peripheral indexes of serotonin function, and personality measures in families with alcoholism. *Am J Med Genet* 114: 230–4.

Storch EA, Gerdes AC, Adkins JW, Geffken GR, Star J, Murphy T (2004). Behavioral treatment of a child with PANDAS. *J Am Acad Child Adolesc Psychiatry* 43: 510–1.

Strauss CC, Lahey BB, Frick P, Frame CL, Hynd GW (1988). Peer social status of children with anxiety disorders. *J Consult Clin Psychol* 56: 137–41.

Swedo SE, Leonard HL, Garvey M, Mittleman B, Allen AJ, Perlmutter S, Lougee L, Dow S, Zamkoff J, Dubbert BK (1998). Pediatric autoimmune neuropsychiatric disorders associated with streptococcal infections: clinical description of the first 50 cases. *Am J Psychiatry* 155: 264–71.

Swedo SE, Rapoport JL, Leonard H, Lenane M, Cheslow D (1989). Obsessive-compulsive disorder in children and adolescents. Clinical phenomenology of 70 consecutive cases. *Arch Gen Psychiatry* 46: 335–41.

Thoenen H (1995). Neurotrophins and neuronal plasticity. *Science* 270: 593–8.

Timpl P, Spanagel R, Sillaber I, Kresse A, Reul JM, Stalla GK, Blanquet V, Steckler T, Holsboer F, Wurst W (1998). Impaired stress response and reduced anxiety in mice lacking a functional corticotropin-releasing hormone receptor 1. *Nat Genet* 19: 162–6.

Torgersen S (1983). Genetic factors in anxiety disorders. *Arch Gen Psychiatry* 40: 1085–9.

Turner BH, Gupta KC, Mishkin M (1978). The locus and cytoarchitecture of the projection areas of the olfactory bulb in Macaca mulatta. *J Comp Neurol* 177: 381–96.

Valleni-Basile LA, Garrison CZ, Jackson KL, Waller JL, McKeown RE, Addy CL, Cuffe SP (1994). Frequency of obsessive-compulsive disorder in a community sample of young adolescents. *J Am Acad Child Adolesc Psychiatry* 33: 782–91.

Vantini G, Perry BD, Guchhait RB, U'Prichard DC, Stolk JM (1984). Brain epinephrine systems: detailed comparison of adrenergic and noradrenergic metabolism, receptor number and in vitro regulation, in two inbred rat strains. *Brain Res* 296: 49–65.

Veldhuis HD, de Kloet ER (1982). Significance of ACTH4–10 in the control of hippocampal corticosterone receptor capacity of hypophysectomized rats. *Neuroendocrinology* 34: 374–80.

Verhulst FC, van der Ende J, Ferdinand RF, Kasius MC (1997). The prevalence of DSM-III-R diagnoses in a national sample of Dutch adolescents. *Arch Gen Psychiatry* 54: 329–36.

Wagner K, Berard R, Stein M, Wetherhold E, Carpenter D, Perera P, Gee M, Davy K, Machin A (2004). A Multicenter, Randomized, Double-blind, Placebo-Controlled Trial of Paroxetine in Children and Adolescents With Social Anxiety Disorder [In Process Citation]. *Arch Gen Psychiatry* 61: 1153–62.

Waldron S, Jr., Shrier DK, Stone B, Tobin F (1975). School phobia and other childhood neuroses: a systematic study of the children and their families. *Am J Psychiatry* 132: 802–8.

Welner Z, Reich W, Herjanic B, Jung KG, Amado H (1987). Reliability, validity, and parent-child agreement studies of the Diagnostic Interview for Children and Adolescents (DICA). *J Am Acad Child Adolesc Psychiatry* 26: 649–53.

Whitaker A, Johnson J, Shaffer D, Rapoport JL, Kalikow K, Walsh BT, Davies M, Braiman S, Dolinsky A (1990). Uncommon troubles in young people: prevalence estimates of selected psychiatric disorders in a nonreferred adolescent population. *Arch Gen Psychiatry* 47: 487–96.

Woodruff GN, Hill DR, Boden P, Pinnock R, Singh L, Hughes J (1991). Functional role of brain CCK receptors. *Neuropeptides* 19 Suppl: 45–56.

Young WS, 3rd, Lightman SL (1992). Chronic stress elevates enkephalin expression in the rat paraventricular and supraoptic nuclei. *Brain Res Mol Brain Res* 13: 111–7.

Zahn-Waxler C, Klimes-Dougan B, Slattery MJ (2000). Internalizing problems of childhood and adolescence: prospects, pitfalls, and progress in understanding the development of anxiety and depression. *Dev Psychopathol* 12: 443–66.

Eating Disorders

15

David C. Jimerson, MD *Barbara E. Wolfe, PhD, RN, CS*
Silke Naab, Dr Med

There has been increasing awareness of the prevalence of anorexia nervosa and bulimia nervosa and of the need for intensified clinical investigation of the pathophysiology of these neuropsychiatric disorders. Much has been learned regarding etiological factors and new treatment approaches. For both anorexia nervosa and bulimia nervosa, distinguishing clinical features involve abnormalities in eating patterns, with related alterations in perceptions regarding body weight and appearance. In this chapter, we provide a clinical overview of these disorders from a neuropsychiatric perspective.

NEUROBIOLOGY OF EATING BEHAVIOR

Patterns of ingestive behavior result from a complex interaction of neurobiological substrate with social, cultural, and psychological influences. Neurochemicals that influence eating behavior include a wide range of endogenous central nervous system (CNS) monoamine neurotransmitters, neuropeptides, and hormones. For many of these chemical messengers, neuronal receptors mediating effects on eating behavior are localized in the hypothalamus. Thus, lesions of the hypothalamus may disrupt normal patterns of eating behavior.

Laboratory methods have been developed to identify selective effects of endogenous neurochemical pathways on hunger, satiety, and food preferences (1, 2). Important variables for describing eating patterns include meal size, rate of food intake during initial and later phases of the meal, interval between meals, and timing of meals over the course of the day. Hunger is associated with initiation of eating and a rapid initial rate of food ingestion. Satiety reflects the slowing of food intake that normally takes place during a meal, with subsequent termination of the meal. Eating patterns are influenced by palatability of the meal and food reward (i.e., the feeling of pleasure associated with a meal). These characteristics can be assessed by evaluating food selection, including relative preferences for protein, carbohydrate, and fat.

The influence of the monoamine neurotransmitters on eating behavior has been studied in detail (3). Serotonergic pathways arising from cell bodies in the raphe nuclei and terminating in the medial basal hypothalamus contribute to postingestive satiety (4). Thus, serotonin (5-hydroxytryptamine [5-HT]) antagonists increase food intake, as do drugs that inhibit serotonin release by stimulating inhibitory 5-HT_{1A} somatodendritic autoreceptors. Pharmacological studies, and observations in mutant mice (5), suggest that postsynaptic 5-HT_2 receptors are particularly important in the satiety produced by serotonergic drugs. Clinically, serotonin-active medications (e.g., sibutramine) have been used to facilitate weight loss in the treatment of obesity (6).

The catecholamines act at several sites in the CNS to influence food intake. In the paraventricular nucleus of the hypothalamus, norepinephrine acts at α_2-adrenoceptors to augment feeding behavior (7). Systemic administration of noradrenergic drugs is typically associated with decreased food intake, however, reflecting activation of β- and α_1-adrenoceptors (3). Research in rodents suggests that β_3-adrenoceptor agonists may facilitate weight loss by increasing energy metabolism in peripheral fat stores (8). Dopamine acts at receptors in the lateral hypothalamus to suppress food intake (7), while dopamine release in mesolimbic pathways appears to contribute to the hedonic/reward responses that sustain food intake (9).

A wide range of hypothalamic neuropeptides, gut-related peptides, and adipokines are active in modulating food intake, and may play a role in symptom patterns in the eating disorders (Table 15.1) (10). Interest has focused

Acknowledgments: Supported in part by USPHS Grants R01 MH45466 (DCJ) and R01 MH57395 (BEW) from the National Institute of Mental Health.

TABLE 15.1
NEUROTRANSMITTERS, NEUROPEPTIDES, AND ADIPOCYTOKINES COMMONLY ASSOCIATED WITH ALTERED EATING PATTERNS

Increased Food Intake	Decreased Food Intake
Neuropeptide Y	Serotonin
Ghrelin	Cholecystokinin
Opioid peptides	Leptin
Galanin	alpha-Melanocyte stimulating hormone
Orexins	Corticotrophin-releasing hormone

on the role of neuropeptide Y, galanin and ghrelin in increasing food intake, and on the effects of cholecystokinin (CCK), corticotrophin-releasing hormone (CRH), and the melanocortins in terminating feeding behavior (11, 12). Additional research is needed to map the interactions among the neurochemical regulators of eating behavior. For example, studies have shown that serotonin interacts with CCK and melanocortin pathways in postingestive satiety (13, 14).

Body weight regulation reflects a balance between energy intake and energy expenditure. The major components of energy expenditure include resting metabolic rate, physical activity, and the thermic effect of food. The sympathetic nervous system and the hypothalamic-pituitary-thyroid axis modulate metabolic rate. Research has shown that leptin, the protein product of the *obese* gene, is important in body weight regulation. Defects in leptin function have been implicated in several rodent models of obesity (15, 16). In that leptin may act at specific hypothalamic receptors to decrease eating behavior, the leptin system provides a potential target site for new pharmacological agents for the treatment of eating disorders and obesity.

ANOREXIA NERVOSA

Diagnostic Features

Anorexia nervosa is an eating disorder characterized by "refusal to maintain body weight at or above a minimally normal weight for age and height" (Table 15.2). Additional criteria for the diagnosis of anorexia nervosa include intense fear of excessive weight gain, markedly abnormal attitudes and perceptions regarding body shape and weight, and amenorrhea (in postmenarcheal women). In DSM-IV (17), anorexia nervosa is designated as "binge-eating/purging type" or "restricting type," based on presence or absence of regular binge–purge behaviors. There is relatively limited information regarding physiological or neuropsychiatric differences between "binge-eating/purging" and "restricting" subtypes of anorexic patients, although the latter group may gain weight more slowly during initial treatment and may have a lower rate of recovery (18, 19). Clinical and family studies in individuals with anorexia nervosa have shown significant co-occurrence of several Axis I disorders, particularly major depression and anxiety disorders (20). Studies of eating behavior in patients with anorexia nervosa have demonstrated a variety of patterns in premeal and postprandial hunger and satiety (21). In general, eating patterns in patients with this disorder do not appear to reflect loss of appetite or abnormality in taste perception.

Epidemiology and Etiology

Epidemiological studies indicate that the prevalence of anorexia nervosa is approximately 0.2 to 0.5% among adolescent and young adult females, with a lifetime prevalence rate of 0.5 to 3.7% (22–25). The clinical syndrome of anorexia nervosa has been recognized in the medical

TABLE 15.2
DSM-IV DIAGNOSTIC CRITERIA FOR ANOREXIA NERVOSA

A. Refusal to maintain body weight at or above a minimally normal weight for age and height (e.g., weight loss leading to maintenance of body weight less than 85% of that expected or failure to make expected weight gain during period of growth, leading to body weight less than 85% of that expected).

B. Intense fear of gaining weight or becoming fat, even though underweight.

C. Disturbance in the way in which one's body weight or shape is experienced, undue influence of body shape and weight on self-evaluation, or denial of the seriousness of current low body weight.

D. In postmenarcheal females, amenorrhea—that is, the absence of at least three consecutive menstrual cycles. (A woman is considered to have amenorrhea if her periods occur only following hormone, e.g., estrogen, administration.)

Specify Type

Restricting Type: During the episode of anorexia nervosa, the person has not regularly engaged in binge-eating or purging behavior (i.e., self-induced vomiting or the misuse of laxatives, diuretics, or enemas).

Binge-Eating/Purging Type: During the current episode of anorexia nervosa, the person has regularly engaged in binge-eating or purging behavior (i.e., self-induced vomiting or the misuse of laxatives, diuretics or enemas).

Source: Reprinted with permission from the Diagnostic and Statistical Manual of Mental Disorders, 4th ed., Text Revision. Copyright 2000. American Psychiatric Association.

literature since the nineteenth century (26). Although some studies have suggested that the prevalence of the disorder has increased in recent decades, this has not been a consistent finding (27). The female-to-male ratio for anorexia nervosa is approximately 10 to 1. Among patients with early onset of the disorder, however, boys may represent up to 30% of all cases (28).

Specific etiological factors have not been identified for anorexia nervosa, although psychosocial, cultural, and occupational factors that contribute to preoccupation with body shape and weight have been implicated. Family and twin studies point to a combination of psychosocial and genetic factors in the etiology of the disorder (24, 29–31).

Neurobiology

Neurotransmitter Studies

A central focus of neurotransmitter studies in anorexia nervosa has been the serotonin system (32). Studies of cerebrospinal fluid (CSF) concentrations of the major serotonin metabolite 5-hydroxyindoleacetic acid (5-HIAA) have demonstrated low concentrations in patients with anorexia nervosa, with recovery toward normal values as patients regain weight (33). Pharmacological challenge studies have assessed neuroendocrine and behavioral responses to serotonin agonist medications as a probe for responsiveness in CNS serotonergic pathways. In general, these studies have shown blunting of serotonin-stimulated neuroendocrine responses in low-weight patients, with restoration toward normal responses as patients regain weight (34–37).

It is not known whether changes observed in the low-weight state are strictly secondary to nutritional deprivation and weight loss or whether they have a specific association with the disorder. In anorexic patients evaluated after long-term weight restoration, there is a return to normal neuroendocrine responses. Trait-related changes in serotonin function appear to persist, however, as reflected in abnormally elevated CSF 5-HIAA values and abnormal behavioral responses to a serotonergic drug (38–40). Consistent with this hypothesis, brain imaging studies have shown that the decreased 5-HT$_{2A}$ receptor binding that is found in low-weight patients is also seen in individuals studied following long-term weight recovery (41–43).

From a clinical perspective, in that serotonin is thought to play an important role in postingestive satiety responses, excessive serotonin function could contribute to the small meal sizes and weight loss presaging the onset of anorexia nervosa (44). Additionally, dysregulation of serotonin function could contribute to comorbidity with other psychiatric disorders, particularly major depression and obsessive-compulsive disorder (32, 45).

Other neurotransmitter abnormalities that have been demonstrated in low-weight patients with anorexia nervosa include low CSF concentrations of norepinephrine and the dopamine metabolite homovanillic acid (46). Additionally, as recently reviewed, alterations in CSF concentrations of neuropeptide immunoreactivity have been demonstrated in low-weight patients with anorexia nervosa, including low levels of opiate-related peptides, low thyroid-releasing hormone, and elevated neuropeptide Y (10).

Neuroendocrine Function

Anorexia nervosa is characterized by dysregulation of hypothalamic-pituitary neuroendocrine systems (47). Amenorrhea in female patients with anorexia nervosa is associated with decreased circulating levels of follicle stimulating hormone and luteinizing hormone (48). Elevated serum cortisol levels reflect increased activity in the hypothalamic-pituitary-adrenal axis (49, 50). The hypothalamic-pituitary-thyroid axis is down-regulated, consistent with an energy-conserving metabolic state. Low serum levels of triiodothyronine (T$_3$), usually with normal thyrotropin levels, reflect a "sick euthyroid" syndrome (51).

The neuroendocrine abnormalities of anorexia nervosa are generally thought to be a consequence of changes in nutritional status and weight loss. Hormone levels return toward normal as the recovering patient regains body weight, although delays may be experienced; for example, in the restoration of normal menstrual cycles. The physiological signals involved in the neuroendocrine changes of weight loss are not fully understood, although laboratory data suggest a possible role for decreased circulating levels of leptin, an adipokine that reflects body fat stores (52, 53). The clinician should be alert to the possibility that neuroendocrine abnormalities may also reflect factors other than weight loss. Hypercortisolemia may reflect comorbid major depression, for example. For a patient with primary amenorrhea associated with hypogonadotropic hypogonadism and atypical symptoms of anorexia nervosa, the possibility of the rarely occurring Kallmann's syndrome should be considered (54).

Clinical studies have suggested that in some children with tics and obsessive-compulsive behaviors, these symptoms could be associated with a syndrome known as "pediatric autoimmune neuropsychiatric disorders associated with streptococcal infection" (PANDAS) (55). Initial reports suggest that some patients with anorexia nervosa have laboratory findings consistent with the PANDAS syndrome (56). Until additional studies are published, however, the nature of this possible association remains uncertain.

Morphometric Brain-Imaging Studies

In that neuropsychiatric consultation for anorexia nervosa may include questions regarding alterations in brain morphology reported in imaging studies, results of investigations in this area are outlined in some detail. Initial studies in anorexia nervosa based on radiograph-computed tomographic (CT) data showed abnormal enlargement of cortical sulci and the interhemispheric fissures (57–59). Subsequent controlled CT studies provided further evidence for cortical sulcal atrophy in anorexic subjects, as reflected in enlargement of subarachnoid spaces (60–65). Additionally, cerebral ventricular enlargement has been demonstrated in a number of these studies (61–64).

Investigations using magnetic resonance imaging (MRI) have also shown increased ventricular size and enlarged cortical sulci in patients with anorexia nervosa compared with control subjects (62, 66–71). One study reported localized decreases in the size of the thalamus and midbrain regions (72), and several studies have reported reduced pituitary gland height (62, 69, 73).

Data indicate that structural brain changes in anorexia nervosa may particularly involve white matter regions (74). This study showed that in comparison to controls, low-weight patients had significant decrements in frontal, parietal, temporal, and total white matter, with less prominent decreases in gray matter. It is of interest that studies using proton magnetic resonance spectroscopy (MRS) have shown significant changes in white matter composition in anorexic patients (75, 76).

In general, patients with the greatest weight loss have the most pronounced enlargements of the ventricles and cortical sulci on brain-imaging studies (60, 63, 64, 66, 68, 69, 77, 78), although this correlation has not been observed in all investigations (61, 62). Physiological factors that may contribute to alterations in low-weight anorexia include malnutrition, fluid and electrolyte abnormalities, and hormonal influences; for example, hypercortisolemia or decreased insulin-like growth factor-1 (74, 79). In some patients the abnormalities could be associated with developmental insults or other preexisting alterations (57, 65). One study reported that chronic self-induced vomiting was associated with abnormal brain ventricular enlargement (67).

It is noteworthy that although brain imaging studies have consistently shown structural abnormalities in low-weight patients compared with matched control subjects, the magnitude of these changes has typically not been large enough to be identified as "clinically abnormal" in a nonresearch setting (69). Although significant cognitive impairments have been found in anorexic patients, there is limited evidence for an association between structural abnormalities and measures of cognitive function (64, 65, 69, 70, 80).

Longitudinal studies suggest that enlargement of cortical sulci and brain ventricles and decreased total brain volume observed at low weight tend to return toward normal following weight gain (57, 59, 61–64, 66, 69, 71). There are, however, some data to suggest that individuals who have achieved stable weight recovery from anorexia nervosa have persistent increases in ventricular volume and decreased gray matter volume in comparison to controls (81, 82). One study indicated that there is an enduring selective decrease in volume in the hippocampus-amygdala area in weight-recovered individuals (83). Additional studies are needed to evaluate the potential clinical implications of these findings.

Functional Brain-Imaging Studies

Studies to assess resting regional brain activity in anorexia nervosa have utilized [^{18}F]-2-deoxyglucose positron-emission tomography (PET) to measure glucose metabolism and single-photon emission computed tomography (SPECT) and functional magnetic resonance imaging (fMRI) to measure regional cerebral blood flow (rCBF). PET imaging showed global hypometabolism in anorexic patients, particularly prominent in the frontal and parietal cortices (84). Absolute hypometabolism was also found in low-weight depressed patients, suggesting the importance of weight loss per se (85). A notable finding was relative hypermetabolism in the caudate nuclei and inferior frontal cortex (86, 87). The investigators postulated that this finding could be associated with symptoms of increased vigilance and attention to detail, consistent with brain imaging findings in patients with obsessive-compulsive disorder (88, 89). Following weight recovery, differences between patients and controls were no longer significant (87), although there was a persistent trend toward relative parietal hypometabolism and inferior frontal hypermetabolism (86).

Comparison of resting rCBF in patients with anorexia nervosa and controls based on SPECT have generally shown decreased blood flow in areas of the cerebral cortex. Most, but not all studies (90), have shown decreases in areas including the parietal, frontal, and temporal regions (91–94). A series of 21 subjects with adolescent-onset disorder, many studied following stable weight recovery, showed hypoperfusion of temporal, parietal, and orbitofrontal regions that appeared to persist following recovery (95). In contrast to these findings, a recent ^{15}O-PET study showed bilateral elevation of rCBF within medial temporal lobes in anorexic patients compared to healthy controls, although data were averaged across baseline and provocation conditions (96). Differences in specific regional findings across these studies are likely to reflect sample size constraints, heterogeneity of the patient groups, and limitations in the availability of satisfactory control data.

From a pediatric perspective, a finding of interest was that in 15 children and adolescents with anorexia nervosa, 87% had asymmetric temporal lobe hypoperfusion (97). A follow-up study of an additional 15 patients, with a mean age of approximately 15 years, found consistent evidence for blood flow asymmetry (hypoperfusion) in 11 of the subjects, including asymmetrical temporal lobe perfusion in 9 subjects (98). In that scans from control subjects were not available for these studies because of concerns related to radiation exposure, follow-up studies using fMRI will be of interest.

Imaging studies in association with symptom provocation paradigms provide another approach to identification of regional alterations of cerebral function in anorexia nervosa. Initial studies have employed paradigms including ingestion of a test meal, visualization of high-calorie and low-calorie foods, and visualization of distorted body images. Areas of differences in response between patients and controls have included the left inferior frontal region (91); the right inferior prefrontal, superior prefrontal, and parietal regions (99); the left insula, anterior cingulate gyrus, and left amygdala-hippocampal region (100); the left occipital cortex and right temporo-occipital cortex (96); and the inferior parietal region (101). Additional studies will be useful in clarifying the extent to which these paradigms result in reproducible emotional, cognitive, and physiological responses in anorexia nervosa, paving the way for future replication studies with independent patient samples.

Course and Prognosis

The typical age of onset of anorexia nervosa is in late adolescence, with an average age of 18 to 21 years at the time of diagnosis (24, 102). Reviews of anorexia nervosa with early onset (between 8 and 14 years of age) point to similarities in symptom patterns and clinical course when compared with later onset illness (28, 103–107).

Estimates of long-term outcome of anorexia nervosa are complicated by limitations in sample size and methodological differences across studies. Studies suggest, however, that 40 to 75% of patients are recovered at 10-year to 21-year follow-up, with 10 to 20% of patients having significant persisting symptomatology (108–112). However, a comprehensive review of follow-up studies of more than 5,000 patients with anorexia nervosa suggests that fewer than half actually achieve full recovery (106). Although at 7.5 years follow-up, 30% of patients with the disorder were found to be in full remission, 40% would relapse (113). Poor prognosis has been associated with duration of illness, binge-eating and purging behaviors, and obsessive-compulsive personality symptoms (106). Risk for relapse is associated with low weight at presentation and at time of discharge from inpatient hospitalization (113–115).

Anorexia nervosa is among the neuropsychiatric conditions having the highest mortality rate (116). Based on a review of outcome studies, the aggregate mortality rate has been estimated to be approximately 5.6% per decade (117). Clinical characteristics such as prolonged duration of illness, bingeing and purging behavior, and comorbid substance abuse and affective disorder have been associated with death in patients with the disorder (118).

There are insufficient data to detect differential patterns of longterm outcome for early-onset and later-onset cases (28, 119, 120). Potential physiological consequences of prolonged malnutrition associated with premenarcheal-onset anorexia nervosa have been described (121).

Clinical Features and Assessment

A "Practice Guideline" for the assessment and treatment of patients with anorexia nervosa has been published by the American Psychiatric Association (122). As this manual outlines, the clinical assessment of cachectic patients with symptoms suggestive of anorexia nervosa entails a comprehensive neuropsychiatric and general medical history and physical examination. Evaluation of current symptomatology includes a detailed review of eating patterns, exercise patterns, and attitudes toward body shape and weight. It is often useful for the clinician to inquire about specifics of meal content and schedule. The clinician should assess whether the patient is engaging in binge-eating and purging behaviors, including possible use of laxatives, diuretics, appetite suppressants, or syrup of ipecac. Patterns of body weight during development, including previous high and low weights in relationship to height, should be noted, as well as details regarding the initial onset of weight loss.

Comorbid psychiatric disorders in patients with anorexia nervosa include mood and anxiety disorders (123, 124), particularly obsessive-compulsive disorder (125, 126). Thus, the clinician should be particularly alert to symptoms suggestive of current or past depression, anxiety disorders, obsessive-compulsive disorder, and substance abuse disorders.

The psychosocial history includes a review of recent personal stresses and family/social tensions (127) and evidence for previous physical or sexual abuse. The family history obtains information on the presence of eating disorders or other neuropsychiatric disorders or obesity in family members (128). A family assessment may be useful to evaluate the residential environment for younger patients living at home.

When performing the medical history and review of symptoms, the clinician should be alert to history of fainting related to dehydration, symptoms of anemia, cold intolerance, and disrupted sleep patterns. Symptoms suggestive of medical illness that could contribute to unexplained weight loss, such as tumors or infectious illness, should be evaluated. For adolescent and adult females, information is obtained on age at menarche, regularity of menstrual periods, and episodes of secondary amenorrhea.

In the context of a complete mental status examination, the clinician should be alert to symptoms such as delusions or psychotic thought processes, which could signal the presence of another primary psychiatric disorder. Assessment of current mood includes questions about suicidal, destructive, or impulsive ideation. Cognitive function is evaluated for changes suggestive of a neurological or metabolic disorder. Impaired cognitive performance in patients with anorexia nervosa has been noted by some investigators (129–133), but not by others (65, 134). In anorexic patients studied longitudinally, there is evidence that cognitive function improves with weight restoration (59).

The initial evaluation of a patient with apparent anorexia nervosa generally includes a physical examination, laboratory studies, and an electrocardiogram (122, 135, 136). Bradycardia and postural hypotension are common findings in patients with severe weight loss. A dental examination, if not recently performed, can indicate whether self-induced vomiting has resulted in erosion of the dental enamel. Selection of laboratory tests depends on the severity of symptoms and results of the medical history and physical examination; such testing often includes a complete blood count, serum electrolytes, blood urea nitrogen (BUN), serum creatinine, blood levels of thyroid hormones, and urinalysis. For cachectic patients, additional laboratory studies include liver function tests and blood levels of calcium, magnesium, and phosphorus. In some situations, bone mineral densitometry may be considered to evaluate the risk of fracture from osteoporosis related to malnutrition and possibly to low estrogen levels (137, 138). Data suggest that following longterm remission (11 years), bone mineral density is inversely associated with duration of anorexia nervosa; thus, duration of illness may be predictive of risk for osteopenia in this patient population (139).

In general, brain-imaging studies and electroencephalography are not routinely obtained in the assessment of the patient with anorexia nervosa. More extensive laboratory or imaging studies may be appropriate when atypical history or initial findings suggest the possibility of medical or neurological illness. Brain tumors in the area of the hypothalamus or brainstem, for example, may manifest as anorexic behavior prior to the appearance of other neurological symptoms (140, 141). Case reports of patients with eating disorders have described a broad spectrum of neurological symptoms, ranging from disorientation, motor ataxia, and stupor to seizures, bulbar paresis, and coma (142–144). Brain-imaging studies, particularly MRI, may be helpful in identifying any associated anatomical lesions (144, 145). Although not a routine component of the clinical assessment, sleep electroencephalographic studies have shown decreased sleep time and decreased time in stage 1 sleep in low-weight patients compared with control subjects (146, 147).

Patients with anorexia nervosa may have significant disturbances of serum electrolytes, such as hypokalemia associated with laxative abuse. In rare cases, neuropsychiatric symptoms have been associated with osmotic demyelination syndrome (or central pontine myelinolysis) in patients with severe hyponatremia and hypokalemia (145, 148, 149). Excessively rapid repletion of electrolytes may play a role in the pathophysiology of this syndrome, resulting in damage to myelin in the ventral region of the pons.

Treatment

Guidelines for the treatment of anorexia nervosa have been summarized (122). When medical problems such as electrolyte abnormalities, hypoglycemia, anemia, bradycardia, or hypotension reach a critical threshold, acute hospitalization is required (135). Indications for hospitalization include progressive weight loss, chronic persistence of extremely low weight in spite of intensive outpatient treatment, and symptoms of severe depression with suicidal ideation. Cachectic patients with anorexia nervosa can suffer serious cardiac arrhythmias, possibly resulting in

sudden death (150). After medical stabilization, psychiatric treatment for the anorexic patient in an inpatient or day treatment setting typically involves a behaviorally oriented weight-restoration program, usually including individual and group psychotherapy (151).

Outpatient psychotherapeutic approaches for patients with anorexia nervosa include a range of shortterm and longterm individual, group, and family therapies (122, 152–157). Family therapy is particularly likely to be a helpful component of treatment for adolescent patients (158). This randomized, controlled 1-year trial showed that in patients with onset of illness prior to age 19 years, family therapy was more effective than individual supportive therapy provided as the control condition. Adjunctive treatments include psychoeducational interventions and nutritional counseling.

In general, controlled studies in low-weight patients have not demonstrated significant advantages for medication treatment compared with psychotherapeutic interventions alone, including studies with the selective serotonin reuptake inhibitor (SSRI) fluoxetine (159–161). A randomized, controlled study did show that cyproheptadine administration was associated with a small but statistically significant enhancement in the rate of weight gain for hospitalized patients with the restricting subtype of anorexia nervosa (162). Psychotropic medications may be useful in alleviating comorbid conditions, such as major depression or severe anxiety disorder, although the clinician needs to remain alert to possible risks (e.g., the potential risk of increased suicidal behavior) associated with medication treatment. In the low-weight patient, considerations related to medical stability (e.g., sensitivity to orthostatic hypotension) often dictate a cautious approach with medication intervention. There are preliminary data from a randomized, controlled 1-year trial in 35 patients with restricting-type anorexia nervosa suggesting that fluoxetine may be helpful in stabilizing mood and possibly in preventing relapse to low weight after weight restoration (163).

BULIMIA NERVOSA

Diagnostic Features

Bulimia nervosa is characterized by recurrent binge-eating episodes that are associated with inappropriate compensatory behaviors used to avoid weight gain (Table 15.3). These behaviors occur with an average frequency of two or more episodes per week over a period of 3 months, at a time during which the individual does not meet criteria for anorexia nervosa. Additionally, the individual's self-evaluation is overly dependent on perception of body weight and shape. In DSM-IV, bulimia nervosa is subclassified as either "purging type" or "nonpurging type" based on the presence or absence of regular self-induced vomiting or misuse of laxatives, diuretics, or enemas (17).

TABLE 15.3
DSM-IV DIAGNOSTIC CRITERIA FOR BULIMIA NERVOSA

A. Recurrent episodes of binge eating. An episode of binge eating is characterized by both of the following:
  (1) Eating, in a discrete period of time (e.g., within any 2-hour period) an amount of food that is definitely larger than most people would eat during a similar period of time and under similar circumstances
  (2) A sense of lack of control over eating during the episode (e.g., a feeling that one cannot stop eating or control what or how much one is eating)
B. Recurrent inappropriate compensatory behavior in order to prevent weight gain, such as self-induced vomiting; misuse of laxatives, diuretics, enemas, or other medications; fasting; or excessive exercise.
C. The binge eating and inappropriate compensatory behaviors both occur, on average, at least twice a week for 3 months.
D. Self-evaluation is unduly influenced by body shape and weight.
E. The disturbance does not occur exclusively during episodes of anorexia nervosa.

Specify Type

Purging Type: During the current episode of bulimia nervosa, the person has regularly engaged in self-induced vomiting or the misuse of laxatives, diuretics, or enemas.
Nonpurging Type: During the current episode of bulimia nervosa, the person has used other inappropriate compensatory behaviors, such as fasting or excessive exercise, but has not regularly engaged in self-induced vomiting or the misuse of laxatives, diuretics, or enemas.

Source: Reprinted with permission from the Diagnostic and Statistical Manual of Disorders, 4th ed., Text Revision. Copyright 2000. American Psychiatric Association.

Up to 30% of overweight individuals in treatment for weight loss have symptoms of binge-eating disorder, a provisionally defined syndrome manifested by recurrent binge eating associated with prominent symptoms of psychological distress (164). Preliminary criteria for binge-eating disorder are listed in Appendix B of DSM-IV ("Criteria Sets and Axes Provided for Further Study"). In overweight individuals, careful review of symptom patterns may be required to differentiate nonpurging bulimia nervosa from binge-eating disorder.

Epidemiology and Etiology

The prevalence of bulimia nervosa in young women is 1 to 2% (27, 165, 166). The female-to-male ratio is approximately 10 to 1. Historically, it had been recognized that up to half of patients with anorexia nervosa reported symptoms of binge eating and purging. During the 1970s, a number of reports describe individuals in a normal weight range with symptoms of binge eating and purging (167), leading to the inclusion the syndrome of "bulimia" in DSM-III (168).

In bulimia nervosa, as in anorexia nervosa, psychosocial, cultural, and occupational factors are thought to contribute to preoccupation with body shape and weight. Family and twin studies have demonstrated a role for genetic factors in the etiology of the disorder (29, 124, 169).

NEUROBIOLOGY

Neurotransmitter Studies

Laboratory studies of eating behavior suggest that patients with bulimia nervosa have impaired postingestive satiety (170). Thus, binge-eating episodes may in part result from absence of normal feelings of satiety following a meal, a possibility that has prompted clinical investigations of the satiety-related neurotransmitter serotonin and the neuropeptide CCK. CSF concentration of the serotonin metabolite 5-HIAA is abnormally low in bulimic patients with frequent binge-eating behavior (171). Additionally, pharmacological challenge studies with serotonin-active medications have shown blunted neuroendocrine responses in patients with bulimia nervosa in comparison to control subjects (172–176). Initial results from brain imaging studies have shown decreased availability of the serotonin transporter in the hypothalamus and thalamus (177). In individuals who have recovered from bulimia nervosa, serotonin-related neuroendocrine abnormalities are no longer observed (178, 179). Similar to findings in anorexia nervosa, however, individuals who have recovered from bulimia nervosa appear to have persistent, trait-related alterations in serotonin function as reflected in elevated levels of CSF 5-HIAA (178), abnormalities in 5-HT_{2A} receptor binding (180), and recurrence of symptoms during acute tryptophan depletion testing (181). It has been postulated that persistent changes in serotonin function may contribute to the recurrence of bulimic symptoms and episodes of depression in many of these individuals.

As noted earlier, findings of diminished satiety responses in bulimia nervosa have prompted studies of the gut-related satiety peptide CCK. Serum CCK response after a test meal is blunted in bulimic patients (182–184), and CSF concentration of CCK-octapeptide is abnormally low (185). As recently reviewed, abnormalities in other CNS neurotransmitter and neuropeptide systems have also been identified in symptomatic patients with bulimia nervosa

(10, 46). Follow-up studies in symptom-recovered patients should help to differentiate state-related versus trait-related aspects of these alterations.

Neuroendocrine Function

Alterations in neuroendocrine function in normal-weight patients with bulimia nervosa are much less prominent than those in patients with anorexia nervosa. When abnormalities do appear, they are often thought to reflect recent weight loss, low weight relative to weight "set point," or the presence of comorbid psychiatric disorder. Thus, low serum thyroid hormone levels with normal thyrotropin levels have been reported in patients with bulimia nervosa (186), consistent with evidence for slightly reduced metabolic rate in comparison to age-matched control subjects (187).

Abnormalities in menstrual cycle patterns may occur in as many as 50% of patients with bulimia nervosa, with evidence for an association between relatively low body weight and disturbances in luteal phase gonadal hormone patterns (188, 189). Small but statistically significant decreases in serum prolactin levels relative to healthy controls have also been reported (173). In studies of the hypothalamic-pituitary-adrenal axis, most patients with bulimia nervosa have normal serum cortisol levels and show normal cortisol suppression following the administration of dexamethasone, although abnormalities in adrenocorticotropic hormone (ACTH) secretion have been reported (50, 190). Circulating levels of the adipokine leptin are decreased in patients with bulimia in comparison to weight-matched controls (191–193), possibly contributing to the reduced resting metabolic rate and menstrual cycle alterations associated with the disorder.

Morphometric Brain-Imaging Studies

Brain-imaging studies in patients with bulimia nervosa reveal less prominent and consistent changes than in patients with anorexia nervosa. Thus, studies with CT reported modest cerebral ventricular enlargement and sulcal widening, with increased ventricular/brain ratio, in patients with bulimia nervosa compared to control subjects (194–196). A study using MRI found a significant reduction in the sagittal cerebral/cranial ratio but no difference in the ventricular/brain ratio in bulimic patients compared with control subjects (197). A subsequent study found no significant differences between patients with bulimia nervosa and control subjects in size of the thalamus, midbrain, pons, corpus callosum, septum pellucidum, or fourth ventricle (72). Reductions in the MRI proton longitudinal relaxation time (T1) in the inferior frontal gray matter have been demonstrated in a small group of patients with bulimia nervosa compared with control subjects (198).

Imaging studies in bulimia nervosa have generally not shown significant correlations between brain morphology and clinical characteristics such as alcohol use, duration of illness, cognitive performance, or symptom severity (80, 194, 196, 199). One study did find an inverse relationship between the ventricular/brain ratio and plasma thyroid hormone concentrations (196), and another found a correlation between frequency of binge eating and the ventricle/brain ratio (67). It is of interest that structural alterations in the prefrontal area have been associated with impulsive behaviors and excessive appetite (200).

Functional Brain-Imaging Studies

Several studies have used PET to evaluate regional brain metabolic activity in bulimia nervosa. Women with bulimia nervosa studied during standardized cognitive tasks exhibited higher cortical metabolic activity in the left hemisphere than in the right hemisphere, in contrast to the reverse asymmetry observed in healthy control subjects (201, 202). Measurement of rCBF in patients with bulimia nervosa with SPECT imaging also showed abnormalities in left-right asymmetries (92). This laterality in rCBF in bulimic patients may be a state-dependent variable, which can be influenced by binge eating (92, 203, 204).

Patients with bulimia nervosa appear to have significant bilateral elevations in metabolic rate/rCBF in the inferior temporal area in comparison with control subjects (92, 202). Consistent with findings in patients with depression, an association was found between left anterior lateral prefrontal cortex hypometabolism in bulimia nervosa and the severity of depressive symptoms (202). Elevated rCBF was also found bilaterally in the inferior frontal region in one study (92). Data from patients during a resting baseline condition showed a significant decrease in relative glucose metabolic rate in the parietal cortex for the bulimic patients in comparison to the controls, paralleling results in anorexia nervosa (205, 206).

In contrast to the findings described earlier, a study of women who had achieved stable recovery from bulimia nervosa found that rCBF values did not differ from results for age-matched control women (207). This finding indicates that underlying trait-related neurobiological risk factors for bulimia nervosa are apparently not reflected in abnormalities in resting rCBF.

Course and Prognosis

As is the case for anorexia nervosa, the symptoms of bulimia nervosa typically begin in late adolescence. The average age at diagnosis has been reported as 20 to 23 years (124, 166, 208). Premenarcheal onset of bulimia nervosa is thought to be uncommon (28). Patients with early onset (age 15 years or younger) resemble older patients in terms of eating-disorder symptomatology but appear to have a history of increased exposure to psychosocial stressors (209).

As summarized later, controlled treatment trials have shown substantial rates of response both to psychotherapy and to pharmacotherapy in individuals with bulimia nervosa. However, relatively high relapse rates have been noted; for example, a rate of 31% over 2 years for patients treated in an intensive day-hospital program (210). Naturalistic follow-up studies ranging from 3 to 10 years in duration indicate that whereas 50 to 60% of patients achieve recovery, 10 to 20% are likely to still meet full criteria for the disorder at the end of the study period (211–214). It is also important to note that presence of an eating disorder during adolescence has been linked to increased risk during early adulthood for anxiety disorders, depressive disorders, and suicide attempts, as well as range of medical and neurological symptoms, including cardiovascular symptoms and infectious diseases (215).

Clinical Features and Assessment

As noted earlier, a "Practice Guideline" for the assessment and treatment of patients with eating disorders has been published by the American Psychiatric Association (122). As this manual outlines, the evaluation of a patient with bulimia nervosa requires a comprehensive neuropsychiatric evaluation and careful medical assessment, with particular attention to detailed assessment of eating patterns, exercise patterns, and attitudes toward body shape and weight. Differentiation between the patient's subjective assessment and the interviewer's objective assessment of binge-eating episodes is frequently useful (216). Patterns of weight fluctuation and previous low and high weight relative to age should be noted, with specific attention to a history of low weight suggestive of past anorexia nervosa. Current and past use of diet pills, laxatives or enemas, diuretics, or syrup of ipecac should be noted.

Current or past symptoms of other psychiatric disorders should be evaluated, particularly mood disorders, anxiety disorders, and substance abuse disorders. The most common comorbid Axis I disorders among patients with bulimia nervosa include major depression, substance use disorders, and anxiety disorders (20, 128).

Of particular importance in the psychosocial history is an evaluation of recent stressful events at school or home, evidence of previous physical or sexual abuse, and illness-related impairments in social and school/occupational settings. The family history includes information on eating disorders, other psychiatric disorders, or obesity in family members.

During the medical history and review of systems, specific attention should be paid to symptoms of orthostatic hypotension, persistent lethargy, evidence of blood in emesis, and history of excessive dental caries associated with erosion of dental enamel. For adolescent and adult females, additional pertinent history includes age of menarche, regularity of menstrual periods, changes in eating patterns observed premenstrually, and episodes of secondary amenorrhea. Details of previous treatment response should be elicited.

The mental status examination includes an assessment of mood and cognition and any evidence of suicidal, impulsive, or destructive ideation. Specifics regarding physical examination and laboratory studies for evaluation of the patient with bulimia nervosa are individualized based on the clinical setting (122). Laboratory tests commonly include a complete blood count, serum electrolytes, BUN, serum creatinine levels, and urinalysis. Anemia associated with abnormal nutrition is not uncommon in bulimia nervosa. Electrolyte abnormalities, particularly hypokalemia and hypochloremia, are associated with recurrent self-induced vomiting or use of laxatives or diuretics (217) and tend to occur in patients with more frequent bulimia episodes (218). Serum total amylase concentrations are frequently elevated in bulimic patients, reflecting increased levels of the salivary amylase isoenzyme (219). An electrocardiogram is helpful in identifying arrhythmias associated with electrolyte disturbances. In general, sleep electroencephalographic studies have not demonstrated significant differences between nondepressed patients with bulimia nervosa and control subjects (147, 220).

Brain-imaging studies are not routinely performed in the assessment of bulimia nervosa. However, brain lesions associated with unexplained vomiting or appetite changes could cause symptoms that initially resemble those of bulimia nervosa. The clinician should also be alert to the possibility of the relatively rare Kleine-Levin syndrome (221). This syndrome, which is of unknown etiology, characteristically appears during adolescence and is more common in men than women. Patients with this condition experience recurrent episodes of hypersomnia (thought to average two to four episodes per year) that may be associated with hyperphagia, mood changes, and other psychiatric symptoms.

Treatment

As described in a recent practice guideline, based on controlled trials, a trial of short-term outpatient psychotherapy in an individual or group setting is often the first treatment approach recommended for bulimia nervosa (122, 222). However, hospitalization may be indicated if medical instability or comorbid neuropsychiatric disorders (e.g., severe depression) are present. Controlled trials have demonstrated the efficacy of cognitive-behavior therapy and interpersonal psychotherapy in the treatment of bulimia nervosa (223–225). Cognitive-behavior therapy focuses on symptom control and the restructuring of beliefs, attitudes, and values that maintain the condition. Components of restructuring include the use of dietary monitors, journal records, behavioral contracts, and patient education. Stimulus control, positive and negative reinforcement, self-monitoring, response prevention, and relaxation training may be incorporated into the treatment plan. Other treatment approaches used with bulimic patients include psychoeducation and psychodynamic therapies, although fewer controlled data regarding outcome are available for these modalities.

Placebo-controlled trials with a range of antidepressant medications have demonstrated significant decreases in frequency of binge-eating and purging episodes in bulimia nervosa (122, 160, 226). Only a minority of the patients studied, however, achieved complete cessation of binge-eating behavior. In general, these trials used medication doses similar to those used in depressed patients, although the SSRI fluoxetine was more effective in bulimic patients at a higher dose than that used in depression (227). Based on the results of clinical trials, the Food and Drug Administration approved fluoxetine for the treatment of bulimia nervosa in adults (122). As noted earlier, the clinician needs to remain alert to possible risks (e.g., the potential risk of increased suicidal behavior) associated with medication treatment. Preliminary results suggest that continued fluoxetine treatment over the course of a year may help to prevent relapse in patients who recover from bulimia nervosa, although follow-up studies are needed to replicate this finding (228).

Randomized studies comparing psychotherapy alone versus medication alone versus combined treatment in patients with bulimia nervosa tend to favor psychotherapy. Initial results have been interpreted cautiously, however, because of limited sample size and unique characteristics of the treatment setting (225, 229, 230). Combined treatment with psychotherapy and medication may be particularly helpful in alleviating symptoms of anxiety and depression.

SUMMARY

Anorexia nervosa and bulimia nervosa appear to develop as a result of interactions between predisposing psychosocial and biological influences. Nutritional alterations appear to contribute to many of the metabolic, hormonal, and other neurobiological changes observed in these disorders. Additional research is needed to differentiate state-related versus trait-related aspects of abnormalities revealed in brain-imaging studies and neurotransmitter/neuropeptide investigations. Initial psychiatric assessment and subsequent treatment planning include careful attention to medical and neuropsychiatric features of the disorders. The evaluation and treatment of patients with an eating disorder may involve extensive consultation and collaboration among members of a clinical team, frequently including a primary mental health care provider, a medical primary care provider, a nutritionist, and an eating disorders specialist.

REFERENCES

1. Blundell JE. Serotonin manipulations and the structure of feeding behaviour. Appetite 1986; 7 Suppl:39–56.
2. Saper CB, Chou TC, Elmquist JK. The need to feed: homeostatic and hedonic control of eating. Neuron 2002; 36:199–211.
3. Samanin R, Garattini S. Pharmacology of ingestive behaviour. Therapie 1996; 51:107–115.
4. Leibowitz SF, Alexander JT, Cheung WK, et al. Effects of serotonin and the serotonin blocker metergoline on meal patterns and macronutrient selection. Pharmacol Biochem Behav 1993; 45:185–194.
5. Tecott LH, Sun LM, Akana SF, et al. Eating disorder and epilepsy in mice lacking 5-HT2c serotonin receptors. Nature 1995; 374:542–546.
6. Appolinario JC, Bacaltchuk J, Sichieri R, et al. A randomized, double-blind, placebo-controlled study of sibutramine in the treatment of binge-eating disorder. Arch Gen Psychiatry 2003; 60:1109–1116.
7. Leibowitz SF. Brain monoamines and peptides: role in the control of eating behavior. Fed Proc 1986; 45:1396–1403.
8. Lowell BB, Flier JS. Brown adipose tissue, beta 3-adrenergic receptors, and obesity. Annu Rev Med 1997; 48:307–316.
9. Blackburn JR, Phillips AG, Jakubovic A, et al. Increased dopamine metabolism in the nucleus accumbens and striatum following consumption of a nutritive meal but not a palatable non-nutritive saccharin solution. Pharmacol Biochem Behav 1986; 25:1095–1100.
10. Jimerson DC, Wolfe BE. *Neuropeptides in Eating Disorders.* CNS Spectr 2004; 9:516–522.
11. Neary NM, Small CJ, Bloom SR. Gut and mind. Gut 2003; 52:918–921.
12. Zigman JM, Elmquist JK. Minireview: From anorexia to obesity—the yin and yang of body weight control. Endocrinology 2003; 144:3749–3756.
13. Poeschla B, Gibbs J, Simansky KJ, et al. Cholecystokinin-induced satiety depends on activation of 5-HT1C receptors. Am J Physiol 1993; 264:R62–R64.
14. Heisler LK, Cowley MA, Tecott LH, et al. Activation of central melanocortin pathways by fenfluramine. Science 2002; 297:609–611.
15. Halaas JL, Gjiwala KS, Maffei M, et al. Weight-reducing effects of the plasma protein encoded by the obese gene. Science 1995; 269:543–546.
16. Schwartz MW, Baskin DG, Kaiyala KJ, et al. Model for the regulation of energy balance and adiposity by the central nervous system. Am J Clin Nutr 1999; 69:584–596.
17. American Psychiatric Association. *Diagnostic and Statistical Manual of Mental Disorders*, 4th Ed., Text Revision. Washington, DC, American Psychiatric Association, 2000.
18. Herzog DB, Field AE, Keller MB, et al. Subtyping eating disorders: is it justified? J Am Acad Child Adolesc Psychiatry 1996; 35:928–936.
19. Neuberger SK, Rao R, Weltzin TE, et al. Differences in weight gain between restrictor and bulimic anorectics. Int J Eat Disord 1995; 17:331–335.
20. Braun DL, Sunday SR, Halmi KA. Psychiatric comorbidity in patients with eating disorders. Psychol Med 1994; 24:859–867.
21. Sunday SR, Halmi KA. Micro- and macroanalyses of patterns within a meal in anorexia and bulimia nervosa. Appetite 1996; 26:21–36.
22. Hsu LK. Epidemiology of the eating disorders. Psychiatr Clin North Am 1996; 19:681–700.
23. Lucas AR, Beard CM, O'Fallon WM, et al. 50-year trends in the incidence of anorexia nervosa in Rochester, Minn.: a population-based study. Am J Psychiatry 1991; 148:917–922.
24. Walters EE, Kendler KS. Anorexia nervosa and anorexic-like syndromes in a population-based female twin sample. Am J Psychiatry 1995; 152:64–71.
25. Whitaker A, Johnson J, Shaffer D, et al. Uncommon troubles in young people: prevalence estimates of selected psychiatric disorders in a nonreferred adolescent population. Arch Gen Psychiatry 1990; 47:487–496.
26. Silverman JA. Sir William Gull (1819–1890). Limner of anorexia nervosa and myxoedema. An historical essay and encomium. Eat Weight Disord 1997; 2:111–116.
27. Hoek HW, van Hoeken D. Review of the prevalence and incidence of eating disorders. Int J Eat Disord 2003; 34:383–396.
28. Lask B, Bryant-Waugh R. Early-onset anorexia nervosa and related eating disorders. J Child Psychol Psychiatry 1992; 33:281–300.

29. Bulik CM, Sullivan PF, Wade TD, et al. Twin studies of eating disorders: a review. Int J Eat Disord 2000; 27:1–20.

30. Holland AJ, Sicotte N, Treasure J. Anorexia nervosa: evidence for a genetic basis. J Psychosom Res 1988; 32:561–571.

31. Strober M, Lampert C, Morrell W, et al. A controlled family study of anorexia nervosa: evidence of familial aggregation and lack of shared transmission with affective disorders. Int J Eat Disord 1990; 9:239–253.

32. Wolfe BE, Metzger E, Jimerson DC. Research update on serotonin function in bulimia nervosa and anorexia nervosa. Psychopharmacol Bull 1997; 33:345–354.

33. Kaye WH, Ebert MH, Raleigh M, et al. Abnormalities in CNS monoamine metabolism in anorexia nervosa. Arch Gen Psychiatry 1984; 41:350–355.

34. Brewerton TD, Jimerson DC. Studies of serotonin function in anorexia nervosa. Psychiatry Res 1996; 62:31–42.

35. Goodwin GM, Shapiro CM, Bennie J, et al. The neuroendocrine responses and psychological effects of infusion of L-tryptophan in anorexia nervosa. Psychol Med 1989; 19:857–864.

36. Hadigan CM, Walsh BT, Buttinger C, et al. Behavioral and neuroendocrine responses to metaCPP in anorexia nervosa. Biol Psychiatry 1995; 37:504–511.

37. Monteleone P, Brambilla F, Bortolotti F, et al. Prolactin response to d-fenfluramine is blunted in people with anorexia nervosa. Br J Psychiatry 1998; 172:439–442.

38. Kaye WH, Gwirtsman HE, George DT, et al. Altered serotonin activity in anorexia nervosa after long-term weight restoration. Does elevated cerebrospinal fluid 5-hydroxyindoleacetic acid level correlate with rigid and obsessive behavior? Arch Gen Psychiatry 1991; 48:556–562.

39. O'Dwyer AM, Lucey JV, Russell GF. Serotonin activity in anorexia nervosa after long-term weight restoration: response to D-fenfluramine challenge. Psychol Med 1996; 26:353–359.

40. Ward A, Brown N, Lightman S, et al. Neuroendocrine, appetitive and behavioural responses to d-fenfluramine in women recovered from anorexia nervosa. Br J Psychiatry 1998; 172:351–358.

41. Audenaert K, Van Laere K, Dumont F, et al. Decreased 5-HT2a receptor binding in patients with anorexia nervosa. J Nucl Med 2003; 44:163–169.

42. Frank GK, Kaye WH, Meltzer CC, et al. Reduced 5-HT2A receptor binding after recovery from anorexia nervosa. Biol Psychiatry 2002; 52:896–906.

43. Bailer UF, Price JC, Meltzer CC, et al. Altered 5-HT(2A) receptor binding after recovery from bulimia-type anorexia nervosa: relationships to harm avoidance and drive for thinness. Neuropsychopharmacology 2004;24:1143–1155.

44. Jimerson DC, Lesem MD, Hegg AP, et al. Serotonin in human eating disorders. Ann NY Acad Sci 1990; 600:532–544.

45. Kaye WH. Anorexia nervosa, obsessional behavior, and serotonin. Psychopharmacol Bull 1997; 33:335–344.

46. Kaye WH, Strober M, Jimerson DC. The neurobiology of eating disorders. In Charney DS, Nestler EJ (eds.), *The Neurobiology of Mental Illness*. Oxford, Oxford University Press, 2004, 1112–1128.

47. Stoving RK, Hangaard J, Hansen-Nord M, et al. A review of endocrine changes in anorexia nervosa. J Psychiatr Res 1999; 33:139–152.

48. Weiner H. The physiology of eating disorders. Int J Eat Disord 1985; 4:347–388.

49. Licinio J, Wong ML, Gold PW. The hypothalamic-pituitary-adrenal axis in anorexia nervosa. Psychiatry Res 1996; 62:75–83.

50. Walsh BT, Roose SP, Katz JL, et al. Hypothalamic-pituitary-adrenal-cortical activity in anorexia nervosa and bulimia. Psychoneuroendocrinology 1987; 12:131–140.

51. Tamai H, Mori K, Matsubayashi S, et al. Hypothalamic-pituitary-thyroidal dysfunctions in anorexia nervosa. Psychother Psychosom 1986; 46:127–131.

52. Ahima RS, Prabakaran D, Mantzoros C, et al. Role of leptin in the neuroendocrine response to fasting. Nature 1996; 382:250–252.

53. Mantzoros C, Flier JS, Lesem MD, et al. Cerebrospinal fluid leptin in anorexia nervosa: correlation with nutritional status and potential role in resistance to weight gain. J Clin Endocrinol Metab 1997; 82:1845–1851.

54. White REB, Mccluskey SE, Varma TR, et al. Kallmann's syndrome and anorexia nervosa: a diagnostic dilemma. Int J Eat Disord 1993; 13:415–419.

55. Kurlan R, Kaplan EL. The pediatric autoimmune neuropsychiatric disorders associated with streptococcal infection (PANDAS) etiology for tics and obsessive-compulsive symptoms: hypothesis or entity? Practical considerations for the clinician. Pediatrics 2004; 113:883–886.

56. Sokol MS, Ward PE, Tamiya H, et al. D8/17 expression on B lymphocytes in anorexia nervosa. Am J Psychiatry 2002; 159:1430–1432.

57. Artmann H, Grau H, Adelmann M, et al. Reversible and non-reversible enlargement of cerebrospinal fluid spaces in anorexia nervosa. Neuroradiology 1985; 27:304–312.

58. Enzmann DR, Lane B. Cranial computed tomography findings in anorexia nervosa. J Comput Assist Tomogr 1977; 1:410–414.

59. Kohlmeyer K, Lehmkuhl G, Poutska F. Computed tomography of anorexia nervosa. AJNR Am J Neuroradiol 1983; 4:437–438.

60. Datlof S, Coleman PD, Forbes GB, et al. Ventricular dilation on CAT scans of patients with anorexia nervosa. Am J Psychiatry 1986; 143:96–98.

61. Dolan RJ, Mitchell J, Wakeling A. Structural brain changes in patients with anorexia nervosa. Psychol Med 1988; 18:349–353.

62. Kornreich L, Shapira A, Horev G, et al. CT and MR evaluation of the brain in patients with anorexia nervosa. AJNR Am J Neuroradiol 1991; 12:1213–1216.

63. Krieg JC, Pirke KM, Lauer C, et al. Endocrine, metabolic, and cranial computed tomographic findings in anorexia nervosa. Biol Psychiatry 1988; 23:377–387.

64. Lankenau H, Swigar ME, Bhimani S, et al. Cranial CT scans in eating disorder patients and controls. Compr Psychiatry 1985; 26:136–147.

65. Palazidou E, Robinson P, Lishman WA. Neuroradiological and neuropsychological assessment in anorexia nervosa. Psychol Med 1990; 20:521–527.

66. Golden NH, Ashtari M, Kohn MR, et al. Reversibility of cerebral ventricular enlargement in anorexia nervosa, demonstrated by quantitative magnetic resonance imaging. J Pediatr 1996; 128:296–301.

67. Hoffman GW, Jr., Ellinwood EH, Jr., Rockwell WJ, et al. Cerebral atrophy in anorexia nervosa: a pilot study. Biol Psychiatry 1989; 26:321–324.

68. Katzman DK, Lambe EK, Mikulis DJ, et al. Cerebral gray matter and white matter volume deficits in adolescent girls with anorexia nervosa. J Pediatr 1996; 129:794–803.

69. Kingston K, Szmukler G, Andrewes D, et al. Neuropsychological and structural brain changes in anorexia nervosa before and after refeeding. Psychol Med 1996; 26:15–28.

70. Neumärker KJ, Bzufka WM, Dudeck U, et al. Are there specific disabilities of number processing in adolescent patients with Anorexia nervosa? Evidence from clinical and neuropsychological data when compared to morphometric measures from magnetic resonance imaging. Eur Child Adolesc Psychiatry 2000; 9 Suppl 2:II111–II121.

71. Swayze VW, Andersen A, Arndt S, et al. Reversibility of brain tissue loss in anorexia nervosa assessed with a computerized Talairach 3-D proportional grid. Psychol Med 1996; 26:381–390.

72. Husain MM, Black KJ, Doraiswamy PM, et al. Subcortical brain anatomy in anorexia and bulimia. Biol Psychiatry 1992; 31:735–738.

73. Doraiswamy PM, Krishnan KR, Figiel GS, et al. A brain magnetic resonance imaging study of pituitary gland morphology in anorexia nervosa and bulimia. Biol Psychiatry 1990; 28:110–116.

74. Swayze VW, Andersen AE, Andreasen NC, et al. Brain tissue volume segmentation in patients with anorexia nervosa before and after weight normalization. Int J Eat Disord 2003; 33:33–44.

75. Roser W, Bubl R, Buergin D, et al. Metabolic changes in the brain of patients with anorexia and bulimia nervosa as detected by proton magnetic resonance spectroscopy. Int J Eat Disord 1999; 26:119–136.

76. Schlemmer HP, Mockel R, Marcus A, et al. Proton magnetic resonance spectroscopy in acute, juvenile anorexia nervosa. Psychiatry Res 1998; 82:171–179.

77. Kohn MR, Ashtari M, Golden NH, et al. Structural brain changes and malnutrition in anorexia nervosa. Ann NY Acad Sci 1997; 817:398–399.

78. Nussbaum M, Shenker IR, Marc J, et al. Cerebral atrophy in anorexia nervosa. J Pediatr 1980; 96:867–869.

79. Gold PW, Kaye W, Robertson GL, et al. Abnormalities in plasma and cerebrospinal-fluid arginine vasopression in patients with anorexia nervosa. N Engl J Med 1983; 308:1117–1123.

80. Laessle RG, Krieg JC, Fichter MM, et al. Cerebral atrophy and vigilance performance in patients with anorexia nervosa and bulimia nervosa. Neuropsychobiology 1989; 21:187–191.

81. Katzman DK, Zipursky RB, Lambe EK, et al. A longitudinal magnetic resonance imaging study of brain changes in adolescents with anorexia nervosa. Arch Pediatr Adolesc Med 1997; 151:793–797.

82. Lambe EK, Katzman DK, Mikulis DJ, et al. Cerebral gray matter volume deficits after weight recovery from anorexia nervosa. Arch Gen Psychiatry 1997; 54:537–542.

83. Giordano GD, Renzetti P, Parodi RC, et al. Volume measurement with magnetic resonance imaging of hippocampus-amygdala formation in patients with anorexia nervosa. J Endocrinol Invest 2001; 24:510–514.

84. Delvenne V, Lotstra F, Goldman S, et al. Brain hypometabolism of glucose in anorexia nervosa: a PET scan study. Biol Psychiatry 1995; 37:161–169.

85. Delvenne V, Goldman S, De Maertelaer V, et al. Brain glucose metabolism in anorexia nervosa and affective disorders: influence of weight loss or depressive symptomatology. Psychiatry Res 1997; 74:83–92.

86. Delvenne V, Goldman S, De Maertelaer V, et al. Brain hypometabolism of glucose in anorexia nervosa: normalization after weight gain. Biol Psychiatry 1996; 40:761–768.

87. Herholz K, Krieg JC, Emrich HM, et al. Regional cerebral glucose metabolism in anorexia nervosa measured by positron emission tomography. Biol Psychiatry 1987; 22:43–51.

88. Baxter LR, Jr., Phelps ME, Mazziotta JC, et al. Local cerebral glucose metabolic rates in obsessive-compulsive disorder. A comparison with rates in unipolar depression and in normal controls. Arch Gen Psychiatry 1987; 44:211–218.

89. Breiter HC, Rauch SL, Kwong KK, et al. Functional magnetic resonance imaging of symptom provocation in obsessive-compulsive disorder. Arch Gen Psychiatry 1996; 53:595–606.

90. Krieg JC, Lauer C, Leinsinger G, et al. Brain morphology and regional cerebral blood flow in anorexia nervosa. Biol Psychiatry 1989; 25:1041–1048.

91. Nozoe S, Naruo T, Nakabeppu Y, et al. Changes in regional cerebral blood flow in patients with anorexia nervosa detected through single photon emission tomography imaging. Biol Psychiatry 1993; 34:578–580.

92. Nozoe S, Naruo T, Yonekura R, et al. Comparison of regional cerebral blood flow in patients with eating disorders. Brain Res Bull 1995; 36:251–255.

93. Kuruoglu AC, Kapucu O, Atasever T, et al. Technetium-99m-HMPAO brain SPECT in anorexia nervosa. J Nucl Med 1998; 39:304–306.

94. Naruo T, Nakabeppu Y, Deguchi D, et al. Decreases in blood perfusion of the anterior cingulate gyri in Anorexia Nervosa Restricters assessed by SPECT image analysis. BMC Psychiatry 2001; 1:2.

95. Rastam M, Bjure J, Vestergren E, et al. Regional cerebral blood flow in weight-restored anorexia nervosa: a preliminary study. Dev Med Child Neurol 2001; 43:239–242.

96. Gordon CM, Dougherty DD, Fischman AJ, et al. Neural substrates of anorexia nervosa: a behavioral challenge study with positron emission tomography. J Pediatr 2001; 139:51–57.

97. Gordon I, Lask B, Bryant-Waugh R, et al. Childhood-onset anorexia nervosa: towards identifying a biological substrate. Int J Eat Disord 1997; 22:159–165.

98. Chowdhury U, Gordon I, Lask B, et al. Early-onset anorexia nervosa: is there evidence of limbic system imbalance? Int J Eat Disord 2003; 33:388–396.

99. Naruo T, Nakabeppu Y, Sagiyama K, et al. Characteristic regional cerebral blood flow patterns in anorexia nervosa patients with binge/purge behavior. Am J Psychiatry 2000; 157:1520–1522.

100. Ellison Z, Foong J, Howard R, et al. Functional anatomy of calorie fear in anorexia nervosa [letter]. Lancet 1998; 352:1192.

101. Wagner A, Ruf M, Braus DF, et al. Neuronal activity changes and body image distortion in anorexia nervosa. Neuroreport 2003; 14:2193–2197.

102. Lucas AR, Crowson CS, O'Fallon WM, et al. The ups and downs of anorexia nervosa. Int J Eat Disord 1999; 26:397–405.

103. Cooper PJ, Watkins B, Bryant-Waugh R, et al. The nosological status of early onset anorexia nervosa. Psychol Med 2002; 32:873–880.

104. Gowers SG, Crisp AH, Joughin N, et al. Premenarcheal anorexia nervosa. J Child Psychol Psychiatry 1991; 32:515–524.

105. Heebink DM, Sunday SR, Halmi KA. Anorexia nervosa and bulimia nervosa in adolescence: effects of age and menstrual status on psychological variables. J Am Acad Child Adolesc Psychiatry 1995; 34:378–382.

106. Steinhausen HC. The outcome of anorexia nervosa in the 20th century. Am J Psychiatry 2002; 159:1284–1293.

107. Warren W. A study of anorexia nervosa in young girls. J Child Psychol Psychiatry 1968; 9:27–40.

108. Deter HC, Herzog W. Anorexia nervosa in a long-term perspective: results of the Heidelberg-Mannheim Study. Psychosom Med 1994; 56:20–27.

109. Eckert ED, Halmi KA, Marchi P, et al. Ten-year follow-up of anorexia nervosa: clinical course and outcome. Psychol Med 1995; 25:143–156.

110. Gillberg IC, Rastam M, Gillberg C. Anorexia nervosa outcome: six-year controlled longitudinal study of 51 cases including a population cohort. J Am Acad Child Adolesc Psychiatry 1994; 33:729–739.

111. Herpertz-Dahlmann BM, Wewetzer C, Remschmidt H. The predictive value of depression in anorexia nervosa. Results of a seven-year follow-up study. Acta Psychiatr Scand 1995; 91:114–119.

112. Strober M, Freeman R, Morrell W. The long-term course of severe anorexia nervosa in adolescents: survival analysis of recovery, relapse, and outcome predictors over 10–15 years in a prospective study. Int J Eat Disord 1997; 22:339–360.

113. Herzog DB, Dorer DJ, Keel PK, et al. Recovery and relapse in anorexia and bulimia nervosa: a 7.5-year follow-up study. J Am Acad Child Adolesc Psychiatry 1999; 38:829–837.

114. Baran SA, Weltzin TE, Kaye WH. Low discharge weight and outcome in anorexia nervosa. Am J Psychiatry 1995; 152:1070–1072.

115. Hebebrand J, Himmelmann GW, Herzog W, et al. Prediction of low body weight at long-term follow-up in acute anorexia nervosa by low body weight at referral. Am J Psychiatry 1997; 154:566–569.

116. Harris EC, Barraclough B. Excess mortality of mental disorder. Br J Psychiatry 1998; 173:11–53.

117. Sullivan PF. Mortality in anorexia nervosa. Am J Psychiatry 1995; 152:1073–1074.

118. Herzog DB, Greenwood DN, Dorer DJ, et al. Mortality in eating disorders: A descriptive study. Int J Eat Disord 2000; 28:20–26.

119. Swift WJ. The long-term outcome of early onset anorexia nervosa. J Am Acad Child Psychiatry 1982; 21:38–46.

120. Walford G, McCune N. Long-term outcome in early-onset anorexia nervosa. Br J Psychiatry 1991; 159:383–389.

121. Russell GFM. Premenarchal anorexia nervosa and its sequelae. J Psychiatr Res 1985; 19:363–369.

122. American Psychiatric Association Workgroup on Eating Disorders. Practice guideline for the treatment of patients with eating disorders (revision). Am J Psychiatry 2000; 157:1–39.

123. Halmi KA, Eckert E, Marchi P, et al. Comorbidity of psychiatric diagnoses in anorexia nervosa. Arch Gen Psychiatry 1991; 48:712–718.

124. Kendler KS, MacLean C, Neale M, et al. The genetic epidemiology of bulimia nervosa. Am J Psychiatry 1991; 148:1627–1637.

125. Halmi KA, Sunday SR, Klump KL, et al. Obsessions and compulsions in anorexia nervosa subtypes. Int J Eat Disord 2003; 33:308–319.

126. Milos G, Spindler A, Ruggiero G, et al. Comorbidity of obsessive-compulsive disorders and duration of eating disorders. Int J Eat Disord 2002; 31:284–289.

127. North C, Gowers S, Byram V. Family functioning in adolescent anorexia nervosa. Br J Psychiatry 1995; 167:673–678.

128. Lilenfeld LR, Kaye WH, Greeno CG, et al. A controlled family study of anorexia nervosa and bulimia nervosa: psychiatric disorders in first-degree relatives and effects of proband comorbidity. Arch Gen Psychiatry 1998; 55:603–610.

129. Green MW, Elliman NA, Wakeling A, et al. Cognitive functioning, weight change and therapy in anorexia nervosa. J Psychiatr Res 1996; 30:401–410.

130. Hamsher KDS, Halmi KA, Benton AL. Prediction of outcome in anorexia nervosa from neuropsychological status. Psychiatry Res 1981; 4:79–88.

131. Laessle RG, Fischer M, Fichter MM, et al. Cortisol levels and vigilance in eating disorder patients. Psychoneuroendocrinology 1992; 17:475–484.

132. Lauer CJ, Gorzewski B, Gerlinghoff M, et al. Neuropsychological assessments before and after treatment in patients with anorexia nervosa and bulimia nervosa. J Psychiatr Res 1999; 33:129–138.

133. Mathias JL, Kent PS. Neuropsychological consequences of extreme weight loss and dietary restriction in patients with anorexia nervosa. J Clin Exp Neuropsychol 1998; 20:548–564.

134. Touyz SW, Beumont PJV, Johnstone LC. Neuropsychological correlates of dieting disorders. Int J Eat Disord 1986; 5:1025–1034.

135. Palla B, Litt IF. Medical complications of eating disorders in adolescents. Pediatrics 1988; 81:613–623.

136. Sharp CW, Freeman CPL. The medical complications of anorexia nervosa. Br J Psychiatry 1993; 162:452–462.

137. Grinspoon S, Thomas E, Pitts S, et al. Prevalence and predictive factors for regional osteopenia in women with anorexia nervosa. Ann Intern Med 2000; 133:790–794.

138. Ward A, Brown N, Treasure J. Persistent osteopenia after recovery from anorexia nervosa. Int J Eat Disord 1997; 22:71–75.

139. Wentz E, Mellstrom D, Gillberg C, et al. Bone density 11 years after anorexia nervosa onset in a controlled study of 39 cases. Int J Eat Disord 2003; 34:314–318.

140. Chipkevitch E. Brain tumours and anorexia nervosa syndrome. Brain Dev 1994; 16:175–179.

141. DeVile CJ, Sufraz R, Lask BD, et al. Occult intracranial tumours masquerading as early onset anorexia nervosa. BMJ 1995; 311: 1359–1360.

142. Copeland PM. Diuretic abuse and central pontine myelinolysis. Psychother Psychosom 1989; 52:101–105.

143. Greenberg WM, Shah PJ, Vakharia M. Anorexia nervosa/bulimia and central pontine myelinolysis [letter]. Gen Hosp Psychiatry 1992; 14:357–358.

144. Steckler TL. Central pontine myelinolysis in a patient with bulimia. South Med J 1995; 88:858–859.

145. Sterns RH, Riggs JE, Schochet SS, Jr. Osmotic demyelination syndrome following correction of hyponatremia. N Engl J Med 1986; 314:1535–1542.

146. Lacey JH, Crisp AH, Kalucy RS, et al. Weight gain and the sleeping electroencephalogram: study of 10 patients with anorexia nervosa. BMJ 1975; 4:556–558.

147. Walsh BT, Goetz R, Roose SP, et al. EEG-monitored sleep in anorexia nervosa and bulimia. Biol Psychiatry 1985; 20:947–956.

148. Lohr JW. Osmotic demyelination syndrome following correction of hyponatremia: association with hypokalemia. Am J Med 1994; 96:408–413.

149. Sugimoto T, Murata T, Omori M, et al. Central pontine myelinolysis associated with hypokalaemia in anorexia nervosa. J Neurol Neurosurg Psychiatry 2003; 74:353–355.

150. Brotman AW, Rigotti NA, Herzog DB. Medical complications of eating disorders. Compr Psychiatry 1985; 26:258–272.

151. Andersen AE, Morse CL, Santmyer KS. Inpatient treatment for anorexia nervosa. In Garner DM, Garfinkel PE (eds.), *Anorexia Nervosa & Bulimia.* New York, Guilford Press, 1985, 311–343.

152. Channon S, de Silva P, Hemsley D, et al. A controlled trial of cognitive-behavioural and behavioural treatment of anorexia nervosa. Behav Res Ther 1989; 27:529–535.

153. Crisp AH, Callender JS, Halek C, et al. Long-term mortality in anorexia nervosa. A 20-year follow-up of the St George's and Aberdeen cohorts. Br J Psychiatry 1992; 161:104–107.

154. Crisp AH, Norton K, Gowers S, et al. A controlled study of the effect of therapies aimed at adolescent and family psychopathology in anorexia nervosa. Br J Psychiatry 1991; 159:325–333.

155. Hall A, Crisp AH. Brief psychotherapy in the treatment of anorexia nervosa. Outcome at one year. Br J Psychiatry 1987; 151:185–191.

156. le Grange D, Lock J. The dearth of psychological treatment studies for anorexia nervosa. Int J Eat Disord 2005; 37:79–91.

157. Treasure J, Todd G, Brolly M, et al. A pilot study of a randomised trial of cognitive analytical therapy vs educational behavioral therapy for adult anorexia nervosa. Behav Res Ther 1995; 33: 363–367.

158. Russell GF, Szmukler GI, Dare C, et al. An evaluation of family therapy in anorexia nervosa and bulimia nervosa. Arch Gen Psychiatry 1987; 44:1047–1056.

159. Attia E, Haiman C, Walsh BT, et al. Does fluoxetine augment the inpatient treatment of anorexia nervosa? Am J Psychiatry 1998; 155:548–551.

160. Jimerson DC, Wolfe BE, Brotman AW, et al. Medications in the treatment of eating disorders. Psychiatr Clin North Am 1996; 19: 739–754.

161. Strober M, Pataki C, Freeman R, et al. No effect of adjunctive fluoxetine on eating behavior or weight phobia during the inpatient treatment of anorexia nervosa: an historical case-control study. J Child Adolesc Psychopharmacol 1999; 9:195–201.

162. Halmi KA, Eckert E, LaDu TJ, et al. Anorexia nervosa. Treatment efficacy of cyproheptadine and amitriptyline. Arch Gen Psychiatry 1986; 43:177–181.

163. Kaye WH, Nagata T, Weltzin TE, et al. Double-blind placebo-controlled administration of fluoxetine in restricting- and restricting-purging-type anorexia nervosa. Biol Psychiatry 2001; 49:644–652.

164. Devlin MJ. Assessment and treatment of binge-eating disorder. Psychiatr Clin North Am 1996; 19:761–772.

165. Fairburn CG, Beglin SJ. Studies of the epidemiology of bulimia nervosa. Am J Psychiatry 1990; 147:401–408.

166. Garfinkel PE, Lin E, Goering P, et al. Bulimia nervosa in a Canadian community sample: prevalence and comparison of subgroups. Am J Psychiatry 1995; 152:1052–1058.

167. Russell G. Bulimia nervosa: An ominous variant of anorexia nervosa. Psychol Med 1979; 9:429–448.

168. American Psychiatric Association. *Diagnostic and Statistical Manual of Mental Disorders,* 3rd Ed. Washington, DC, American Psychiatric Press, 1980.

169. Kassett JA, Gershon ES, Maxwell ME, et al. Psychiatric disorders in the first-degree relatives of probands with bulimia nervosa. Am J Psychiatry 1989; 146:1468–1471.

170. Kissileff HR, Wentzlaff TH, Guss JL, et al. A direct measure of satiety disturbance in patients with bulimia nervosa. Physiol Behav 1996; 60:1077–1085.

171. Jimerson DC, Lesem MD, Kaye WH, et al. Low serotonin and dopamine metabolite concentrations in cerebrospinal fluid from bulimic patients with frequent binge episodes. Arch Gen Psychiatry 1992; 49:132–138.

172. Brewerton TD, Mueller EA, Lesem MD, et al. Neuroendocrine responses to m-chlorophenylpiperazine and L-tryptophan in bulimia. Arch Gen Psychiatry 1992; 49:852–861.

173. Jimerson DC, Wolfe BE, Metzger ED, et al. Decreased serotonin function in bulimia nervosa. Arch Gen Psychiatry 1997; 54:529–534.

174. Levitan RD, Kaplan AS, Joffe RT, et al. Hormonal and subjective responses to intravenous meta-chlorophenylpiperazine in bulimia nervosa. Arch Gen Psychiatry 1997; 54:521–527.

175. Monteleone P, Brambilla F, Bortolotti F, et al. Plasma prolactin response to D-fenfluramine is blunted in bulimic patients with frequent binge episodes. Psychol Med 1998; 28:975–983.

176. Steiger H, Young SN, Kin NM, et al. Implications of impulsive and affective symptoms for serotonin function in bulimia nervosa. Psychol Med 2001; 31:85–95.

177. Tauscher J, Pirker W, Willeit M, et al. [123I] b-CIT and single photon emission computed tomography reveal reduced brain serotonin transporter availability in bulimia nervosa. Biol Psychiatry 2001; 49:326–332.

178. Kaye WH, Greeno CG, Moss H, et al. Alterations in serotonin activity and psychiatric symptoms after recovery from bulimia nervosa. Arch Gen Psychiatry 1998; 55:927–935.

179. Wolfe BE, Metzger ED, Levine JM, et al. Serotonin function following remission from bulimia nervosa. Neuropsychopharmacology 2000; 22:257–263.

180. Kaye WH, Frank GK, Meltzer CC, et al. Altered serotonin 2A receptor activity in women who have recovered from bulimia nervosa. Am J Psychiatry 2001; 158:1152–1155.

181. Smith KA, Fairburn CG, Cowen PJ. Symptomatic relapse in bulimia nervosa following acute tryptophan depletion. Arch Gen Psychiatry 1999; 56:171–176.

182. Devlin MJ, Walsh BT, Guss JL, et al. Postprandial cholecystokinin release and gastric emptying in patients with bulimia nervosa. Am J Clin Nutr 1997; 65:114–120.

183. Geracioti TD, Jr., Liddle RA, Altemus M, et al. Regulation of appetite and cholecystokinin secretion in anorexia nervosa. Am J Psychiatry 1992; 149:958–961.

184. Pirke KM, Kellner MB, Friess E, et al. Satiety and cholecystokinin. Int J Eat Disord 1993; 15:63–69.

185. Lydiard RB, Brewerton TD, Fossey MD, et al. CSF cholecystokinin octapeptide in patients with bulimia nervosa and in normal comparison subjects. Am J Psychiatry 1993; 150:1099–1101.

186. Altemus M, Hetherington M, Kennedy B, et al. Thyroid function in bulimia nervosa. Psychoneuroendocrinology 1996; 21:249–261.

187. Obarzanek E, Lesem MD, Goldstein DS, et al. Reduced resting metabolic rate in patients with bulimia nervosa. Arch Gen Psychiatry 1991; 48:456–462.

188. Devlin MJ, Walsh BT, Katz JL, et al. Hypothalamic-pituitary-gonadal function in anorexia nervosa and bulimia. Psychiatry Res 1989; 28:11–24.

189. Pirke KM, Fichter MM, Chlond C, et al. Disturbances of the menstrual cycle in bulimia nervosa. Clin Endocrinol (Oxf) 1987; 27:245–251.

190. Mortola JF, Rasmussen DD, Yen SS. Alterations of the adrenocorticotropin-cortisol axis in normal weight bulimic women: evidence for a central mechanism. J Clin Endocrinol Metab 1989; 68:517–522.

191. Brewerton TD, Lesem MD, Kennedy A, et al. Reduced plasma leptin concentrations in bulimia nervosa. Psychoneuroendocrinology 2000; 25:649–658.

192. Jimerson DC, Mantzoros C, Wolfe BE, et al. Decreased serum leptin in bulimia nervosa. J Clin Endocrinol Metab 2000; 85:4511–4514.

193. Monteleone P, Di Lieto A, Tortorella A, et al. Circulating leptin in patients with anorexia nervosa, bulimia nervosa or binge-eating disorder: relationship to body weight, eating patterns, psychopathology and endocrine changes. Psychiatry Res 2000; 94: 121–129.

194. Kiriike N, Nishiwaki S, Nagata T, et al. Ventricular enlargement in normal weight bulimia. Acta Psychiatr Scand 1990; 82:264–266.

195. Krieg JC, Backmund H, Pirke KM. Cranial computed tomography findings in bulimia. Acta Psychiatr Scand 1987; 75:144–149.

196. Krieg JC, Lauer C, Pirke KM. Structural brain abnormalities in patients with bulimia nervosa. Psychiatry Res 1989; 27:39–48.

197. Hoffman GW, Ellinwood EH, Jr., Rockwell WJ, et al. Cerebral atrophy in bulimia. Biol Psychiatry 1989; 25:894–902.

198. Hoffman GW, Ellinwood EH, Jr., Rockwell WJ, et al. Brain T1 measured by magnetic resonance imaging in bulimia. Biol Psychiatry 1990; 27:116–119.

199. Lauer CJ, Lässle RG, Fichter MM, et al. Structural brain alterations and bingeing and vomiting behavior in eating disorder patients. Int J Eat Disord 1990; 9:161–166.

200. Fuster JM. *The Prefrontal Cortex: Anatomy, Physiology and Neuropsychology of the Frontal Lobe.* New York, Raven Press, 1989.

201. Wu JC, Hagman J, Buchsbaum MS, et al. Greater left cerebral hemispheric metabolism in bulimia assessed by positron emission tomography. Am J Psychiatry 1990; 147:309–312.

202. Andreason PJ, Altemus M, Zametkin AJ, et al. Regional cerebral glucose metabolism in bulimia nervosa. Am J Psychiatry 1992; 149:1506–1513.

203. Hirano H, Tomura N, Okane K, et al. Changes in cerebral blood flow in bulimia nervosa. J Comput Assist Tomogr 1999; 23:280–282.

204. Karhunen LJ, Vanninen EJ, Kuikka JT, et al. Regional cerebral blood flow during exposure to food in obese binge eating women. Psychiatry Res 2000; 99:29–42.

205. Delvenne V, Goldman S, Simon Y, et al. Brain hypometabolism of glucose in bulimia nervosa. Int J Eat Disord 1997; 21:313–320.

206. Delvenne V, Goldman S, De Maertelaer V, et al. Brain glucose metabolism in eating disorders assessed by positron emission tomography. Int J Eat Disord 1999; 25:29–37.

207. Frank GK, Kaye WH, Greer P, et al. Regional cerebral blood flow after recovery from bulimia nervosa. Psychiatry Res 2000; 100: 31–39.

208. Soundy TJ, Lucas AR, Suman VJ, et al. Bulimia nervosa in Rochester, Minnesota from 1980 to 1990. Psychol Med 1995; 25:1065–1071.

209. Schmidt U, Hodes M, Treasure J. Early onset bulimia nervosa: Who is at risk? A retrospective case-control study. Psychol Med 1992; 22:623–628.

210. Olmsted MP, Kaplan AS, Rockert W. Rate and prediction of relapse in bulimia nervosa. Am J Psychiatry 1994; 151:738–743.

211. Collings S, King M. Ten-year follow-up of 50 patients with bulimia nervosa. Br J Psychiatry 1994; 164:80–87.

212. Herzog DB, Nussbaum KM, Marmor AK. Comorbidity and outcome in eating disorders. Psychiatr Clin North Am 1996; 19: 843–859.

213. Hsu LKG, Sobkiewicz TA. Bulimia nervosa: a four- to six-year follow-up study. Psychol Med 1989; 19:1035–1038.

214. Keel PK, Mitchell JE. Outcome in bulimia nervosa. Am J Psychiatry 1997; 154:313–321.

215. Johnson JG, Cohen P, Kasen S, et al. Eating disorders during adolescence and the risk for physical and mental disorders during early adulthood. Arch Gen Psychiatry 2002; 59:545–552.

216. Fairburn CG, Cooper Z. The Eating Disorder Examination, 12th Ed. In Fairburn CG, Wilson GT (eds.), *Binge Eating: Nature, Assessment, and Treatment.* New York, Guilford Press, 1993, 317–360.

217. Mitchell JE, Specker SM, de Zwaan M. Comorbidity and medical complications of bulimia nervosa. J Clin Psychiatry 1991; 52 Suppl:13–20.

218. Wolfe BE, Metzger ED, Levine JM, et al. Laboratory screening for electrolyte abnormalities and anemia in bulimia nervosa: a controlled study. Int J Eat Disord 2001; 30:288–293.

219. Metzger ED, Levine JM, McArdle CR, et al. Salivary gland enlargement and elevated serum amylase in bulimia nervosa. Biol Psychiatry 1999; 45:1520–1522.

220. Hudson JI, Pope HG, Jr., Jonas JM, et al. Sleep EEG in bulimia. Biol Psychiatry 1987; 22:820–828.

221. Gillberg C. Kleine-Levin Syndrome: unrecognized diagnosis in adolescent psychiatry. J Am Acad Child Adolesc Psychiatry 1987; 26:793–794.

222. Fairburn CG, Peveler RC. Bulimia nervosa and a stepped care approach to management. Gut 1990; 31:1220–1222.

223. Fairburn CG, Norman PA, Welch SL, et al. A prospective study of outcome in bulimia nervosa and the long-term effects of three psychological treatments. Arch Gen Psychiatry 1995; 52:304–312.

224. Mitchell JE, Raymond N, Specker S. A review of the controlled trials of pharmacotherapy and psychotherapy in the treatment of bulimia nervosa. Int J Eat Disord 1993; 14:229–247.

225. Walsh BT, Wilson GT, Loeb KL, et al. Medication and psychotherapy in the treatment of bulimia nervosa. Am J Psychiatry 1997; 154:523–531.

226. Zhu AJ, Walsh BT. Pharmacologic treatment of eating disorders. Can J Psychiatry 2002; 47:227–234.

227. Fluoxetine Bulimia Nervosa Collaborative Study Group. Fluoxetine in the treatment of bulimia nervosa. A multicenter, placebo-controlled, double-blind trial. Arch Gen Psychiatry 1992; 49: 139–147.

228. Romano SJ, Halmi KA, Sarkar NP, et al. A placebo-controlled study of fluoxetine in continued treatment of bulimia nervosa after successful acute fluoxetine treatment. Am J Psychiatry 2002; 159:96–102.

229. Agras WS, Rossiter EM, Arnow B, et al. One-year follow-up of psychosocial and pharmacologic treatments for bulimia nervosa. J Clin Psychiatry 1994; 55:179–183.

230. Mitchell JE, de Zwaan M, Roerig JL. Drug therapy for patients with eating disorders. Curr Drug Target CNS Neurol Disord 2003; 2:17–29.

Substance Use Disorders

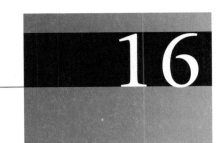

Oscar G. Bukstein, MD   *Ralph E. Tarter, MD*

Substance use by adolescents is a common behavior. According to an annual survey of high school students, the lifetime prevalence of alcohol use among twelfth graders in 2003 was 76.6%, while the lifetime prevalence of use of substances other than alcohol and tobacco was 51.1% (1; see Table 16.1). At some time during their teenage years, an overwhelming majority of adolescents use alcohol, and a substantial proportion use other drugs. Unfortunately, a significant percentage of adolescents also use substances on a regular basis. In 2003, 27.9% and 11.9% of twelfth and eighth graders, respectively, reported drinking at least five drinks on a single occasion within the preceding 2 weeks. Similarly, 24.1% of twelfth graders and 9.7% of eighth graders reported using an illicit substance other than alcohol or tobacco within the previous 30 days. Recent trends in lifetime and daily substance use are found in Table 16.1.

In community studies, lifetime diagnosis of alcohol use disorder (AUD) ranges from 0.4 (2) to 9.6% (3). Lifetime diagnoses of alcohol dependence ranged from 0.6 (2) to 4.3% (4). The lifetime prevalence of substance use disorder (SUD) (abuse or dependence) ranges from 3.3 in 15-year-olds to 9.8% in 17- to 19-year-olds (5, 6). The predicted cumulative prevalence of any SUD by age 16 is 12.2% (7).

When substance use induces problems, the individual qualifies for the diagnosis of SUD. The core feature of a SUD is persistent pattern of use despite negative consequences. To qualify for a diagnosis of SUD (*abuse*) based on DSM-IV (8) criteria, an individual must display a maladaptive pattern of substance use that leads to clinically significant impairment or distress. This maladaptive pattern may manifest as use that results in failure to fulfill major role obligations or use that continues despite causing or exacerbating social or interpersonal problems (see subsequent discussion). The neuropsychiatric sequelae of habitual substance use may exacerbate these problems. To quality for a diagnosis of SUD (*dependence*), maladaptive behaviors continue despite knowledge of having persistent or recurrent physical or psychological problems due to substance use. Neuropsychiatric disturbance may be among these problems.

In this chapter, we review the neuropsychiatric aspects of substance abuse among adolescents. In addition, we discuss the neuropsychiatric factors that amplify the risk for development and maintenance of substance use disorders.

DEVELOPMENT OF SUBSTANCE USE AND USE DISORDERS

Substance use behavior does not proceed in random fashion. Rather, consumption typically begins with legal readily available compounds (e.g., beer, wine), and a subset of the adolescent population progresses to hard liquor and tobacco that in turn may lead to "soft" drugs (marijuana) and ultimately, in a smaller segment, to "hard" illicit drugs. Conceptualized as "stages" within the Gateway Hypothesis (9), it has been speculated that each stage is associated with a specific complement of risk factors that promote subsequent drug use (10). The putative risk factors encompass, for the most part, the interaction between individual and environmental (peer and parent-related) characteristics (see Table 16.2). For example, quality of peer relationships and minor delinquent activities both predict initiation into the earliest stages of use whereas poor relationship with parents and deviant attitudes and behavior are theorized to be more important in the later stages. Furthermore, while

TABLE 16.1

TRENDS IN LIFETIME AND 30–DAY PREVALENCE OF DAILY USE OF VARIOUS DRUGS FOR EIGHTH AND TWELFTH GRADERS

		1991		1996		2000		2003	
		Life-time	Daily use	Life-time	Daily use	Life-time	Daily use	Life-time	Daily use
Any illicit drug	8th grade	18.7	—	31.2	—	26.8	—	22.8	—
	12th grade	44.1	—	50.8	—	53.9	—	51.1	—
Marijuana	8th grade	10.2	0.2	23.1	1.5	20.3	1.3	17.5	1.0
	12th grade	36.7	2.0	44.9	4.9	48.8	6.0	46.1	6.0
Hallucinogens	8th grade	3.2	—	5.9	—	4.6	—	4.0	0.1
	12th grade	9.6	0.1	14.0	0.1	13.0	0.2	10.6	0.1
MDMA (ecstasy)	8th grade	—		3.4		4.3		3.2	
	12th grade	—		6.1		11.0	<.05	8.3	0.1
Inhalants	8th grade	17.6		21.2		17.9		15.8	
	12th grade	17.6	0.5	16.6	0.4	14.2	0.3	11.2	0.4
Cocaine	8th grade	2.3		4.5		4.5		3.6	
	12th grade	7.8	0.1	7.1	0.2	8.6	0.2	7.7	0.2
Heroin	8th grade	1.2		2.4		1.9		1.6	
	12th grade	0.9	<.05	1.8	0.2	2.4	0.1	1.5	0.1
Amphetamines	8th grade	10.5		13.5		9.9		8.4	
	12th grade	15.4	0.2	15.3	0.3	15.6	0.5	14.4	0.5
Metamphetamine	8th grade	—		—		4.2		3.9	
	12th grade	—	0.1	—	0.1	7.9	0.1	6.2	0.1
Alcohol	8th grade	70.1	0.5	55.3	1.0	51.7	0.8	45.6	0.8
	12th grade	88.0	3.6	79.2	3.7	80.3	2.9	76.6	3.2
Cigarettes	8th grade	44.0	7.2	49.2	10.4	40.5	7.4	28.4	4.5
	12th grade	63.1	18.5	63.5	22.2	62.5	20.6	53.7	15.8
Steroids	8th grade	1.9		1.8		3.0		2.5	
	12th grade	2.1	0.1	1.9	0.3	2.5	0.2	3.5	0.2

Source: Monitoring the Future Study, University of Michigan.

the notion of stage-specific characteristics is intuitively appealing, the bulk of the evidence points to the presence of common factors (11). In effect, the likelihood of progressing from abstinence to illicit drug use is a function of the severity of the common liability (12, 13).

Neuropsychiatric Risk Factors for Substance Use/Abuse

Neuropsychiatric disturbance appears to represent an important risk factor that predisposes to substance use. Although there is no evidence linking risk for substance abuse with a focal brain lesion, several neurobehavioral factors have been identified that can increase the risk for substance abuse. We review the literature on these factors next.

Electrophysiological Abnormalities

Event-related potentials (ERPs) measure the neurophysiological substrates of information processing (14). The P300 component of the brainstem auditory-evoked responses or potential waveform has been investigated as an electrophysiological indicator of cognitive processing in subjects at known high risk for alcoholism (15, 16). This waveform component has been shown to reflect complex cognitive functions such as stimulus updating, short-term memory, and working memory. In studying ERPs, and particularly the P300 component, researchers recognize that both amplitude and latency may vary with maturation of the central nervous system (CNS) (17, 18).

Several laboratories have found decreased P300 amplitudes and increased latencies among youth at high risk for substance use or abuse (19). Other investigators have noted that high-risk young people manifest P300 deviations as well as deviations in the N1 and N2 components of the ERP (20). The N1 and N2 waveform components are thought to reflect attentional processes. The investigations conducted to date have ascertained subjects on the basis of a familial history of alcoholism, which through genetic loading confers on these subjects a higher degree of risk for substance abuse than that in the general population. Although many studies have reported ERP differences between high- and low-risk subjects, it is important to note that many investigations have also failed to detect such differences (15). ERP potentials are not established biological markers for substance abuse and may be more important in

TABLE 16.2
RISK FACTORS FOR ADOLESCENT SUBSTANCE USE DISORDERS

Individual risk factors
Early childhood characteristics
Early conduct problems, aggression
Poor academic performance/school failure
Early onset of substance use
Adolescent's attitudes and beliefs about substance use
Risk-taking behaviors
Neuropsychiatric deficits
    Executive function deficits–attention, short-term memory, verbal processing
    Temperamental traits–hyperactivity, impulsivity, mood instability

Peer-related risk factors
Peer substance use
Peer attitudes about substance use
Greater orientation (attachment) to peers
Perception(s) of peer substance use/attitudes

Parent/family risk factors
Parental substance use
Parental beliefs/attitudes about substance use
Parental tolerance of substance use/deviant behavior
Lack of closeness/attachment with parents
Lack of parental involvement in youth's life
Lack of appropriate supervision/discipline

identifying risk to a range of persistent deviant behaviors (21). The ultimate value of any putative differences between high- and low-risk subjects resides in the capacity of these variables to predict which children will eventually develop alcohol or drug problems.

Several investigators have studied high-risk youth to examine ERPs and their relationship to deviant behavior and SUD risk. In a follow-up study of high- and low-risk children, Berman and associates (22) found that the children with the lowest P300 amplitudes at baseline were more likely to be using substances four years later. In an 8-year follow-up study, Hill and colleagues (23) obtained ERPs at baseline and follow-up for a group of 20 children (including 11 high-risk children). Differences in P300 amplitude between high- and low-risk subjects persisted from baseline to follow-up. Four of the 11 high-risk children met criteria for a substance use disorder at follow-up, and all four had lower P300 amplitudes than did the nonaffected high-risk subjects. The fact that P300 amplitudes did not differ between subjects having versus those not having externalizing disorders indicates that abnormalities in this waveform may not be merely a general correlate of behavioral deviancy.

In a study of high-risk children from families of alcoholics, developmental trajectories of P3b amplitude (a highly heritable variant of the P300 component) obtained over the ages 9 to 14 years were related to the child's familial risk for developing alcohol dependence in combination with the presence or absence of the child's specific psychopathol-

ogy (24). Among high-risk children, those with the highest risk for developing a childhood disorder could be predicted based on membership in the class 3 P3b developmental trajectory pattern. Risk status confers a greater likelihood of having lower P3b at the youngest ages studied, and a slower rate of change in amplitude during childhood and adolescence, especially in high-risk male children. High-risk female children exhibit this pattern but only in the presence of a childhood psychiatric diagnosis (25). These findings have relevance to recent suggestions that reduced amplitude of P3b seen in association with familial risk for developing alcoholism is actually due to the greater likelihood that youth with a family history of alcoholism will have externalizing psychopathology, namely, conduct disorder (26). This suggestion is part of a continuing dialogue concerning the overlap between antisocial personality disorder, alcohol dependence, and P300. Based on cross-sectional data obtained from youth who were assessed for presence of conduct symptoms and family history of alcohol dependence, Bauer and Hesselbrock (26) concluded that reduced amplitude of P300 was seen in association with conduct disorder symptoms (subjects did not meet DSM-IV criteria for conduct disorder) and no evidence had been found that the family history variable was responsible for the reduction in amplitude. In the Hill and associates (24) study, because persons in the "any diagnosis" category were as likely to have an internalizing disorder as an externalizing disorder, the presence of an externalizing disorder alone does not appear to explain the increased likelihood of membership in the lower P300 amplitude, slower developmental change group.

Neurological Dysfunction
A few investigators have found differences in the ability to "stand without swaying" between both adult and adolescent individuals with a family history versus those without a family history of substance abuse (31–33). The neurological mechanisms underlying these postural sway differences are not known; whether such ataxic symptoms reflect dorsal column or cerebellar disturbance has not, for example, been investigated. Also, it is not known whether standing steadiness among offspring of alcoholic individuals reflects a facet of generalized neurological disinhibition. Thus, although these findings suggest that neurological dysfunction may be a component of susceptibility to substance abuse, further research is needed to clarify the mechanisms and implications of such motor disturbances.

Neuropsychological Deficits
Adolescents with alcoholic or addicted parent(s) demonstrate impairments on tests measuring attention, short-term memory, and verbal information processing compared with offspring of nonalcoholic, non–drug-dependent parents (34). Theoretical reviews of the emerging literature on neuropsychological risk suggest that this pattern of deficits is consistent with a functional disorder of neural systems in the prefrontal cortex (35). The impairments in "executive"

cognitive processes that accompany the behavioral and emotional dyscontrol point to the possible presence of neuromaturational deficits in high-risk adolescent subjects who are ascertained on the basis of a familial history of substance use disorders (see subsequent discussion).

Individual Pharmacological Variation

Several studies have demonstrated that high-risk adult males with alcoholic fathers experience lower subjective levels of intoxication in response to an alcohol challenge compared with low-risk males (36, 37). Similar findings appear to be present for female offspring (38). This diminished reaction is likely a specific effect of alcohol rather than a general response to CNS depressants such as diazepam (39). These findings suggest that neurochemical variation in the population may be associated with differences in drug reinforcement effects, and hence with differences in propensity to habitually consume abusable compounds.

Temperamental Traits

Temperamental traits are behavioral, affective, and cognitive characteristics that manifest in an individual soon after birth. Temperamental disposition, although modifiable, tends to be relatively stable from birth throughout childhood. The particular expression of a temperamental trait is the product of gene–environment interactions (40, 41). Temperamental deviations are associated with an increased risk for psychopathology and substance abuse (42–44). For example, compared with children whose temperaments are normative, children having "difficult" temperaments more commonly manifest externalizing and internalizing behavior problems by middle childhood (45) and during adolescence (42, 43). The following temperamental traits have been shown to be especially salient risk factors for substance abuse:

- *High behavioral activity level*—Tarter and colleagues (46) reported that male offspring of alcoholic individuals were rated higher on dimensions of behavioral activity compared with sons of nonalcoholic controls. Similarly, adolescents who abuse substances scored higher on ratings of behavioral activity level than nonabusing control subjects (47). In addition, the magnitude of activity level has been shown to co-vary with the severity of substance use, psychiatric disorder, and psychosocial maladjustment (47).
- *Low attention span persistence*—Adolescent sons of alcoholic individuals have been found to perform less well on neuropsychological tests measuring attention capacity compared with sons of nonalcoholic controls (48). In addition, adults with a family history of alcoholism exhibited poorer performance on tests of abstracting, problem solving, and perceptual motor capacity (49) compared to subjects without a family history of alcoholism.
- *High impulsivity*—Poor impulse control differentiates children at high risk for alcoholism from those at low

risk (50, 51). Poor impulse control in childhood also predicts marijuana use at age 18 (52).
- *Mood instability*—Children described as irritable and prone to temper tantrums were more likely to use drugs as adolescents (53) compared with those not displaying such traits. Shyness in early childhood is another predictive factor for adolescent substance use (54). Recent studies have reported an association between early age–onset substance use and emotional reactivity (55, 56). Tarter and associates (57) reported that irritability may be a component of vulnerability to substance use disorders; by early adolescence, irritability is associated with use of alcohol and drugs as a coping response. Deviations in affective dimensions of temperament (e.g., soothability, emotionality), which may underlie instability in arousal regulatory processes, may also constitute risk factors for subsequent substance use disorders (35).

The traits of high activity level, low attention span persistence, and high impulsivity converge to confirm the categorical diagnosis of attention deficit hyperactivity disorder (ADHD) as a risk factor for substance abuse. A number of studies have reported an elevated rate of paternal alcoholism in children diagnosed with hyperactivity (58–60). Retrospective reports of alcoholic adults also suggest an increased frequency of childhood hyperactivity in individuals who subsequently become alcoholic (61, 62). Similarly, the results of prospective studies indicate that childhood hyperactivity increases the risk for alcoholism (58, 63–65). However, substance use disorders among individuals with a history of ADHD may be mediated largely by a history of conduct disorder, although the presence of both ADHD and conduct disorder may confer a level of risk beyond that conferred by either disorder alone (58). Martin and colleagues (66) found that the primary components of ADHD—namely, impulsivity, hyperactivity, and inattention, in addition to aggressivity—distinguished preadolescent sons of substance-abusing fathers from sons of non–substance-abusing fathers.

Many of these temperamental deviations are associated with other nonnormative traits; thus, children and adolescents at risk for substance use/abuse often have multiple risk characteristics (67). In addition, temperamental deviations can be associated with more complex patterns of behavior such as aggression, or with categorical psychiatric diagnoses such as ADHD, conduct disorder, or mood disorders. These diagnoses are all associated with increased risk for substance abuse. The point to be made, however, is that the matrix of risk factors is multifaceted, spanning the dimensional as well as the categorical neuropsychiatric processes that encompass cognition, affect, and behavior.

Several investigators have attempted to define specific temperamental subtypes that may help distinguish subgroups of individuals with substance use disorder. Tarter and colleagues (68) classified alcoholic adolescents into two broad clusters. One subgroup consisted of youth who demonstrated behavioral dyscontrol and hypophoria; a smaller subgroup consisted of individuals with primarily negative affect. These subgroups differed with respect to age at first drug use and age at first substance use disorder diagnosis, as well as with regard to the severity of their substance use disorder, behavioral disturbance, or psychiatric disorder. Adolescents classified as having "difficult" temperaments loaded on the negative-affect factor. On the basis of the distribution of various risk factors, Zucker and coworkers (69) hypothesized the existence of three subtypes of alcoholism: antisocial alcoholism, negative-affect alcoholism, and developmentally limited alcoholism. Cloninger (70) proposed two subtypes of alcoholism—type I (milieu-limited) and type II (male-limited)—defined according to gender, family history of alcoholism, presence of antisocial behavior, age at alcoholism onset, and personality traits. To date, Cloninger's subtypes have not been validated and have been subjected to much criticism (71, 72). Thus, the number of putative subtypes in the literature reinforces the heterogeneity of early-onset alcohol use disorder and illustrates the multiplicity of pathways to this outcome.

Many of the temperamental traits reported to place youth at risk for substance use disorders can be subsumed within the larger construct of impaired executive self-regulation of goal-directed behavior. Executive cognitive functioning encompasses attention, self-monitoring, motor control, abstract reasoning, and cognitive flexibility (73). Deficits in these capacities are generally accepted to reflect prefrontal cortex dysfunction (73, 74). Significantly, preadolescents at risk for substance use disorders have been shown to perform poorly on measures of executive cognitive functioning (34, 75). Executive cognitive functioning is also associated with aggression, another risk factor for substance use disorders (76–78). From these findings, considered in total, it is plausible to conclude that deviations in temperament—reflecting poor regulation of affect and behavior—and deficits in executive cognitive functioning place youth at risk for conduct disorder and substance use disorders. Executive cognitive deficits are noted after head injury and in conditions such as ADHD and conduct disorder, which are also associated with early or adolescent onset of substance use problems (79).

Changes in executive cognitive functioning may also be the result of acute or chronic substance use. Acute alcohol intoxication results in decreases in prefrontal glucose metabolism and disrupts a number of executive cognitive functioning processes (79).

Neuropsychological and Neurobiological Factors in the Development of Substance Dependence

Psychoactive substance consumption is primarily motivated by the reinforcing consequences of substance use (80). In effect, these substances are consumed either to induce a state of euphoria (i.e., positive reinforcement) or to relieve the

person from an aversive mood state (i.e., negative reinforcement). The dependence liability of a psychoactive compound is identified by the propensity of laboratory animals to self-administer that substance (81). Some abusable drugs have no primary reinforcing effects (e.g., hallucinogens, anabolic steroids); for these substances, consumption is regulated primarily by secondary (learned) reinforcers. All abusable compounds have specific neuropsychiatric effects; that is, they change behavior, mood, and cognition. Thus, used as positive reinforcers, drugs enhance mood, cognition, or behavior. Used as negative reinforcers, drugs ameliorate deficiencies in one or more of these processes. In addition to their behavioral effects, abusable drugs have both acute and long-term effects that manifest as neuropsychiatric disturbances (i.e., symptoms or disorders).

Neurobiological Substrates of Drug Reward

Drug reinforcement involves activation of the dopaminergic system subserving reward centers of the brain (80–83). Different substances may have different mechanisms for activating or influencing dopaminergic systems. During drug intoxication, increases in striatal dopamine are associated with a drug's reinforcing effects only if dopamine changes occur rapidly (84). Increases in extracellular dopamine are achieved by blocking dopamine transporters (DAT) (85). The faster the DAT blockade, the stronger the "high"; whereas the rate of clearance from DAT modulates the frequency at which these drugs are self-administered (84). Craving may be related to dopamine-induced activation of the orbitofrontal cortex. In a study of functional magnetic resonance imaging (fMRI) comparing adolescents with AUDs with infrequent drinkers, adolescents with AUDs showed greater brain activation of left anterior, limbic, and visual systems in response to pictures of alcohol beverages. These findings demonstrate an association between the urge to drink and activation of brain areas linked to reward, positive affect, and episodic recall (86).

The orbitofrontal cortex and the anterior cingulated gyrus, which are connected to other limbic structures, are activated in addicted subjects during intoxication, craving, and binging and deactivated during withdrawal (87). These frontal cortical regions are also involved in higher-order cognitive and motivational functions, particularly in determining the salience of a reinforcer. Addiction results from the overvaluation of drug reinforcers (i.e., substances of abuse) and undervaluing alternative reinforcers (e.g., going to work and earning a living, doing well in school, or eating in a sensible manner) in addition to the presence of deficits in inhibitory control for drug and other deviant behavioral responses (87). In a review of the literature underlying motivation, impulsivity, and addiction, Chambers, Taylor, and Potenza (88) speculate that immature inhibitory substrates (e.g., impulsivity) in frontal cortical and subcortical monoaminergic systems promote greater motivational drives for novel experiences, including substance use. Not only are "normal" adolescents vulnerable due to

TABLE 16.3

SITES AND PHARMACOLOGICAL ACTIONS OF COMMON DRUGS OF ABUSE

Substance	Proposed Action	Brain Site
Alcohol	Facilitation	GABA receptors
	Inhibition	NMDA (glutamate) receptors
Cannabis/Marijuana	Agonist	Cannabinoid receptors
Hallucinogens (e.g., LSD)	Partial agonist	5-HT2 receptors
Opiates	Agonist	Opioid receptors
Cocaine	Inhibition	Monoamine reuptake systems (dopamine, norepinephrine, serotonin)
Nicotine	Agonist	Nicotinic acetylcholine receptors

Note: 5-HT2 = 5-hydroxytryptamine (serotonin); GABA = gamma-aminobutyric acid; LSD = lysergic acid diethylamide; NMDA = N-methyl-d-aspartate.

the incomplete development of this neurocircuitry but those with comorbid psychiatric disorders such as ADHD with chronic deficiencies in impulsivity and motivational neurocircuitry are even more vulnerable to substance use and subsequent SUDs.

Other neurotransmitter systems (serotonergic, adrenergic, and gamma-aminobutyric acid [GABAergic]) are also involved in regulating motivated behavior and thus are also linked to the reinforcement effects of drugs (80). For example, serotonin may inhibit many of the systems that activate drug response and reinforcement. Substances of abuse act on many types of neurotransmitters and receptors (see Table 16.3).

Conditioned responses concomitant to drug use develop in relation to environmental cues such as certain people, places, or objects. Activation of conditioned responses produces *craving*. The mechanisms regulating craving are not well understood but are thought to entail an association between reward centers and memory centers located in the hippocampus (80, 83). In effect, the user comes to associate specific cues or stimuli with prior experiences of drug-induced positive or negative reinforcement. Craving ensues as an emotional-motivational anticipatory response to potential reinforcement. Craving as a phenomenon in adolescents has received little research attention; however, it is a central component of the dependence syndrome (89). A significant percentage of adolescents who meet criteria for alcohol dependence report craving (90).

Activation of brain reward centers that results in motivation to continue ingestion explains only one facet of substance dependence behavior. *Physical dependence*, manifesting as chronic tolerance or as onset of withdrawal upon cessation of use, is also a major factor in the progressive increase and maintenance of substance use. Tolerance results when the CNS adapts to the substance in an attempt to promote homeostasis. *Withdrawal*, a related phenomenon, is a rebound condition caused by substance-induced CNS alteration; that is, readaptation of the CNS occurs consequent to the absence of the substance. A sustained period of regular

drug use is required for both development of tolerance to a substance and termination of withdrawal symptoms after discontinuing its use, and their presence and severity vary according to the frequency of use and the amount of the substance consumed. The more variable pattern of substance use in adolescents compared with adults might explain the relatively infrequent occurrence (in less than 10% of adolescents with SUDs) of withdrawal syndromes or of high levels of tolerance in this population (90–92). Among heavy adolescent alcohol users (drinking five or more drinks 16 or more times a month), 18.6% met DSM-III-R criteria for alcohol withdrawal syndrome and reported an average of 2.72 withdrawal symptoms, most commonly nausea and vomiting, depression/irritability, muscle aches, and course tremor (91). Recent reports have found a high rate of withdrawal symptoms for adolescents with higher levels of cannabis and amphetamine use (91, 93) as well as with marijuana users in the community (94). Polysubstance use and cigarette use predicted a higher level of withdrawal symptoms.

Because of their disruptive physiological effects and the aversive state associated with drug withdrawal, abusable substances act as negative reinforcers (i.e., by promoting substance use behaviors). Concomitantly, as tolerance increases with continued drug use, the reinforcing effects become progressively more difficult to obtain and the abstinence syndrome becomes more severe (95). This dilemma results in a motivational spiral of progressively larger amounts of drugs being consumed both to achieve a reinforcing effect and to forestall the onset of withdrawal. At this stage, dependence is recognized to be severe.

Neuropsychological factors may not be important at all stages in the development of a substance use disorder. The factors that lead to initial and experimental use of psychoactive substances by children or adolescents are likely very different from those that lead to persistent or pathological use (96). The onset of substance use in youth is usually socially based and is linked to preexisting dispositional traits such as behavioral deviancy (97). Numerous factors that predispose to drug use have been identified. Social influences, including the need for peer approval, may be sufficient to produce levels of use high enough to cause psychosocial impairment or negative consequences that meet diagnostic criteria for substance abuse. At later stages of use, neuropsychological and conditioning factors become more important as the adolescent begins to display a pattern of dependence manifested by craving, compulsions to use, and preoccupation with procuring and consuming the substance. The diagnostic criteria for dependence are most often met when the substance-induced effects are themselves reinforcing.

Genetic Influences on Adolescent Substance Use

Researchers have long observed that alcohol and other substance use run in families (98, 99). The familial risk for substance use and substance use problems does not assume a genetic basis because both genetic and environmental factors within a family can influence substance use outcomes (100). Using twin or adoption studies to disentangle environmental versus genetic risk, there is substantial evidence for genetic influences on adolescent substance use, although the magnitude of the influences is moderated by such factors as specific environmental contexts, gender, specific substances, age, and regional influences (101).

Genetic factors appear to play a greater role in individual differences in the persistence of serious drug problems than in social or experimental use of substances (102–105). Genetic influences play a role when environments allow for the expression of the genetic risk. The genetic risk, as well as the shared environmental risk, appears to be nonspecific (106, 107), although some groups have reported substance-specific risk (108). Shared environment, particularly sibling interactions, have a large influence on adolescent alcohol use, smoking, and other substance use (101). Shared environment may have a more substantial impact in early adolescence or upon initiation into substance use, although genetic influences may be stronger for older adolescents (109). Genetic variation in personality dimensions such as impulsivity or disinhibition (see previous discussion) or in liability to externalizing disorders (e.g., conduct disorder) may influence the risk for SUDs for most substances (110). Genetic variation may also exist in systems such as the dopaminergic reward system, which are activated by most substances of abuse (111).

The recent increase in knowledge about the human genome has allowed identification of chromosomes, regions of chromosomes, and specific regions that may contribute to the complex behaviors of AUDs. As research has not identified a single gene responsible for substance use or SUDs, studies have centered on the search for genes that contribute the largest percentage of risk for developing SUDs. A specific form of a gene (i.e., polymorphism) may be only one of several genetic mechanisms for the development of AUDs. Given the significance of dopamine in the reward pathway, most studies have focused on dopamine gene polymorphisms. Variation at the dopamine D2 receptor gene (i.e., DRD2) has been extensively studied in relation to the risk for AUDs and SUDs (104). As with much of the genetic literature, although some studies report an association between SUDs and D2, others have failed to find this association. Other evidence suggests that the DRD2 gene may be nonspecific in conferring risk for various addictive, compulsive, and impulsive disorders. Several genes have been associated with other deviant behaviors associated with the risk for SUDs, such as aggression and impulsive behavior (Monoamine oxidase A (MAOI-A); serotonin 5-HT-1B), ADHD (e.g., DRDR, dopamine transporter–1 [DAT-1]), sensation-seeking (DRD4) (104).

NEUROPSYCHIATRIC EFFECTS OF SUBSTANCE USE

Acute Effects

The acute effects of substance use pertain to level of intoxication and pharmacological recovery from a single exposure. There are numerous factors however that can modify both the effect of the substance and the experience of the user. Compared with adults, adolescents are more likely to be novice or inexperienced in the use of specific substances and their simultaneous combinations (e.g., alcohol and tobacco). Adolescents may not be knowledgeable about what constitutes a safe dose, nor about the level of change or impairment produced by specific substances. In part because of this inexperience, the manifestation of pronounced effects may precipitate in the adolescent user an extreme level of distress, particularly agitation and anxiety. These reactive, dysphoric states may compound the direct neuropharmacological effects of a drug use episode.

Expectations regarding use and the social context of use are also important mediators of the pharmacological actions (112) that culminate in mood, cognitive, and behavioral changes. Adolescents' expectations of the effects of substance consumption are different from those of adults. These expectations may influence an adolescent's decision to initiate consumption. Importantly, in the absence of knowledge or experience, expectations can be both incorrect and maladaptive. With respect to inaccuracy, young people may believe that alcohol is an aphrodisiac or an analgesic. Furthermore, expectations regarding substance use can impose personal risk. Among adolescents, disinhibition—for example, getting "falling down drunk"—may be seen as a goal of drinking rather than a negative consequence to avoid. Deviant social behavior while under drug influence (e.g., aggressive behavior) may also be more acceptable in certain adolescent populations than in adults in general. Thus, users' expectations about the effects of drugs, and the resulting behaviors while under acute influence, moderate the neuropharmacological effects of drug use.

Drug dose, of course, is an important determinant of a drug's acute effects. Dose is a multifaceted parameter that is often difficult to ascertain in naturalistic settings. Quantity and purity synergistically determine the individual's response from both a pharmacological and a neuropsychiatric perspective. Intoxication is thus a graded effect, albeit one that is reversible and substance specific (113). Very little is known about intoxication sequelae in youth however, because laboratory research on the response of human subjects to pharmacological challenge is ethically unjustifiable.

Not every intoxication episode is pathological (i.e., producing maladaptive changes). Among adolescents, many such episodes do not appear to be accompanied by negative consequences (or at least not by negative neuropsychiatric sequelae). Nonetheless, it is important for clinicians to be cognizant of the paucity of empirical research on this topic.

Adolescents commonly display a pattern of substance use behavior different from that of adults. Alcohol consumption is typically expressed as a binge pattern rather than as persistent and continuous drinking (114). Intoxication, depending on the specific substance, produces an array of neuropsychiatric effects involving alteration of perception, thought processes, mood/affect, and behavior. Table 16.4 summarizes the acute neuropsychiatric effects of drugs commonly used by adolescents.

TABLE 16.4
ACUTE NEUROPSYCHIATRIC EFFECTS OF DRUGS COMMONLY USED BY ADOLESCENTS

Substance	Perception	Thought processes	Mood/affect	Behavior
Alcohol				
Low dose	• Impaired visual-motor abilities (e.g., judging distances) • Dulling of pain perception	• Impaired judgment, concentration, recent memory	• Initial excitement, relaxation, joviality • Occasional irritability • Later depression	• Increased motor activity • Disinhibition • Impaired reaction time, fine motor dexterity • Slurred speech
High dose	• More of the above	• Disorganized thinking, confusion • Stupor, coma	• Low frustration tolerance • Mood swings • Depression	• Impaired motor control • Socially unacceptable behavior
Cannabis (marijuana)				
Low dose	• Greater sensitivity to stimuli	• Impaired judgment, short-term memory, attention span, information processing	• Euphoria • Sense of well-being • Relaxation	• Sedation • Impaired motor coordination (balance, standing) • Disinhibition • Spontaneous laughter • Impaired ability to perform complex motor tasks
High dose	• Altered self-image (depersonalization) • Anesthesia (pseudohallucination) • Hallucination	• Rapid, fragmented thoughts • Confusion • Delusions, paranoia, psychosis, delirium	• Anxiety, panic	• Impaired ability to perform simple motor tasks; impaired reaction time • Agitation
Cocaine/stimulants				
Low dose		• Improved concentration, attention, task persistence • Flight of ideas	• "Rush," euphoria, increased energy • Grandiosity • Dysphoria (irritability), anxiety	• Restlessness, excitement, activation • Decreased appetite • Insomnia
High dose	• Hallucinations • Perceptual distortions • Pseudohallucinations, including tactile	• Psychosis • Paranoia • Coma	• Panic, dysphoria	• Excitation, agitation, impulsivity, aggression

Postuse			• "Crash"
			  – Dysphoria
			  – Depression
			  – Irritability
				• Agitation

(continued)

TABLE 16.4
(continued)

Substance	Perception	Thought processes	Mood/affect	Behavior
Opiates				
Low dose	• Analgesia (reduced sensitivity and emotional response to pain)	• Mental clouding • Impaired concentration and attention	• Euphoria • Relaxation • Rush • Giddiness	• Sedation • Decreased physical activity • Apathy • Motor incoordination, slurred speech
High dose		• Stupor, coma		• Sleep
Sedatives/hypnotics				
Low dose	• Impaired perception • Blurred vision	• Impairment in attention, memory, concentration	• Relaxation, calm • Occasional euphoria	• Sedation • Motor incoordination • Disinhibition • Slurred speech
High dose		• Confusion • Stupor • Coma	• Mood swings • Depression	• Deep sleep
Hallucinogens				
Low dose	• Visual hallucinations • Perceptual (time, space) distortions • Sensory overflow (anesthesia)	• Impaired short-term memory, concentration • Pseudoinsight	• Labile mood • Tension • Fearfulness	• Variable withdrawal • Hypervigilance
High dose	• Depersonalization • Derealization		• Depression • Anxiety • Panic • "Bad trip"	

Postuse	• "Flashbacks"
	  – Intensification of perceived stimuli
	  – Perception of motion of fixed objects
	  – Geometric patterns superimposed on field of vision			

Phencyclidine (PCP)				
Low dose	• Distortion (time, body image, space, visual, auditory, perception)	• Impaired attention, concentration • Preoccupation with trivial matters	• Euphoria • Relaxation • Lability	• Sedation • Motor incoordination • Restlessness • Incoherence
High dose	• Derealization • Depersonalization • Decreased pain awareness	• Disorganization • Confusion • Paranoia • Psychosis • Stupor • Amnesia	• Anxiety • Panic • Depression	• Agitation • Aggression, violence • Mutism • Catatonia (rigidity) • Erratic/bizarre behavior
Inhalants				
Low dose	• Dizziness • Anesthesia (numbness) • Disassociation • Perceptual distortions (size, shapes, time) • Pseudohallucinations • Abnormal sensitivity to light • Double vision • Ringing in ears	• Impaired judgment	• Euphoria	• Disinhibition • Motor incoordination • Slurred speech

(continued)

TABLE 16.4
(continued)

Substance	Perception	Thought processes	Mood/affect	Behavior
High dose	• Hallucinations	• Temporary delusions • Toxic psychosis • Delirium	• Depression	• Impulsive, bizarre behavior • Aggression
Tobacco (nicotine)				
		• Impaired vigilance, information processing, attention	• Relaxation	• Improved reaction time

A compound's neuropsychiatric effects are determined largely by its neuropharmacological properties. Amphetamines and other stimulants exert their action by releasing dopamine and norepinephrine from the presynaptic neuron and by blocking their reuptake by the presynaptic neuron. The net result is greater availability of neurotransmitter in the synapse. Thus, stimulant action on dopaminergic neurons in the mesolimbic area produces mood changes, whereas action in the mesocortical cortex affects higher cognitive processes.

Lysergic acid diethylamide (LSD) acts primarily on the serotonergic system, where it exerts both inhibitory and excitatory effects. Alcohol and other sedative/hypnotic compounds affect several neurotransmitter systems. Effects on GABA (a major inhibitory neurotransmitter) receptors and the associated calcium channel complex may be involved in alcohol-induced anxiolytic responses. Alcohol's effects on the dopaminergic and serotonergic systems probably influence its reinforcing properties (115, 116). Opiates stimulate endogenous opiate receptors, inducing permanent changes in receptor function (117). Marijuana exerts its action by way of is primary psychoactive ingredient, delta-9-tetrahydrocannabinol (THC), which acts through activation of the CB1 cannabinod receptor (118). CB1 is a G protein–linked receptor located in the central and peripheral nervous systems and located presynaptically. CB1 reduces the uptake of GABA and dopamine, thus potentiating their action.

With respect to specific acute neuropsychiatric disturbances, an interesting phenomenon is the *blackout*, a form of anterograde amnesia during which the individual loses memory for all or part of the events taking place during a drinking episode (119, 120). A blackout is most likely to occur when a large volume of alcohol is consumed within a short time. Although usually associated with alcohol, blackouts can also occur with other depressant substances, such as benzodiazepines and barbiturates (121, 122). Blackouts may be an important warning sign of the development of alcohol dependence (123). Blackouts are common among adolescents with alcohol use disorders, although they occur at a somewhat lower frequency in youth

than in adults (48 versus 84) with these disorders (124). *Alcohol idiosyncratic intoxication*, or pathological intoxication, is a condition characterized by maladaptive behavioral changes (e.g., aggressive or assaultive behavior) induced by the ingestion of amounts of alcohol insufficient to produce intoxication in most people. Although listed in DSM-III-R (8), idiosyncratic intoxication was omitted as a separate diagnosis from DSM-IV because supporting evidence was lacking that the condition is distinct from intoxication or that it exists under experimental conditions.

Chronic Effects

There is considerable literature on the neuropsychiatric sequelae of alcohol and other substance use among adults (125, 126) (see Table 16.5). In contrast, there is a dearth of research directed at the chronic or long-term neuropsychiatric sequelae of substance use and abuse among adolescents. This lack of attention is rather remarkable, given these substances' strong neuropharmacological effects and the fact that adolescents are still undergoing brain maturation in tandem with physical, psychological, and endocrinological maturation (127, 128).

The available evidence indicates for example, that mild deficits in Wechsler Verbal IQ or poor academic language performance distinguish alcoholic adolescents from nonalcoholic control subjects (129). It is possible, however, that these deficits may not be attributable solely to chronic exposure to alcohol but partially antedate substance involvement, especially in adolescents displaying other forms of deviant social behavior (130, 131). Female adolescent substance abusers have also been shown to have mild intellectual deficits (132).

Protracted substance abuse in adolescents over 4 years of follow-up was associated with significantly poorer subsequent functioning on tests of attention (133). In addition, alcohol and drug withdrawal accounted for significant variance in visual-spatial functioning, above and beyond demographic, educational, and health variables in detoxified late adolescents and young adults. These results suggest that

TABLE 16.5
LONGTERM NEUROPSYCHIATRIC SEQUELAE OF SUBSTANCES OF ABUSE

Substance	Potential chronic effects/sequelae
Alcohol	Confusion, apathy, memory loss Wernicke-Korsakoff syndrome
Marijuana/Cannabis	Anxiety, panic episodes, paranoia chronic fatigue, lethargy, psychosis
Hallucinogens	Flashbacks (persistent perception disorder), paranoia
Opiates	Dependence syndrome Mood symptoms
Cocaine	Mood symptoms (depression/mania) Anxiety Psychosis, paranoia Insomnia, anorexia
Stimulants/ amphetamines	Mood symptoms (depression/mania) Anxiety Psychosis Insomnia, anorexia
Sedative/hypnotics	Dependence syndrome
Inhalants	Cognitive dysfunction (memory, concentration deficits), encephalopathy, confusion, depression, psychosis, paranoia
Anabolic steroids	Mood symptoms (depression/mania) Aggression

alcohol and drug withdrawal may be a more powerful marker of protracted neuropsychological impairments than other indices of youthful alcohol and drug involvement. After controlling for recent use, age, education, practice effects, and baseline neuropsychological functioning, substance use over the 8-year follow-up period significantly predicted performances on tests of memory and attention at Year 8 in youths with histories of substance use disorders and comparable youths with no such lifetime histories (134). Additionally, withdrawal symptoms during the follow-up predicted visuospatial and attention scores at Year 8.

An interesting example of a chronic, substance-induced cognitive-sensory effect is the "flashback." Flashbacks from LSD or other hallucinogens spontaneously occur weeks or months following an episode of use and may be precipitated by stress, fatigue, or ingestion of other substances such as marijuana (135). This experience is more common in frequent users. Examples of flashback phenomena include intensification of stimuli, apparent motion of fixed objects, and superimposition of geometric shapes on the field of vision (136).

Psychiatric Disorders
Despite ample evidence demonstrating the neuropsychiatric effects of substance use (and associated transient neuropsychiatric symptoms) and acute intoxication, little evidence exists that substance use or abuse directly causes persistent neuropsychiatric syndromes (137). With respect

to externalizing or disruptive-behavior disorders (i.e., ADHD, conduct disorder, oppositional defiant disorder) or delinquency, for example, it has been consistently found that these conditions almost always precede substance use, although conduct disorder can worsen or be more persistent in adolescents with SUDs (110). A relation appears to exist between substance use/abuse and mood disorders. Marijuana may worsen depressive symptoms in depressed patients (138). Cross-sectional studies have shown an association between cannabis use and depressive symptoms in a community sample of adolescents (139, 140). Marijuana use increases the risk of later depression (141) and of both depression and anxiety (142).

Depressive disorders among adolescents have been shown to emerge after the onset of a SUD; however, the natural history of comorbid mood–substance use disorders in adolescents appears to be different from that in adults (143, 144). Whereas depressive symptoms in adults with SUDs usually remit rapidly with abstinence, a substantial proportion of adolescents with comorbidity continue to display depressive symptoms after several weeks of abstinence. This finding suggests that these adolescents may have a predisposition toward affective disorders such that these disorders, once manifest, are less responsive to abstinence or treatment. Thus, whereas in adults the rapid amelioration of depressive symptoms indicates that psychoactive substances have a direct etiological effect on mood (145), the lack of a similar response in adolescents suggests that the etiological mechanisms leading to depressive symptoms in this age group may be different from those in adults.

Anxiety disorders are frequently present in adolescents with SUDs (146, 147). Generalized anxiety disorder and panic disorder may be consequences of chronic use (148). Similar to the findings in adults, adolescents in treatment for SUDs and in the community manifest high rates of social phobia and posttraumatic stress disorder (146, 147). However, panic disorder and generalized anxiety disorder appear to be rare among adolescents seeking treatment for alcohol abuse or dependence (146), a finding which suggests that social phobia likely precedes alcohol dependence and that initiation of alcohol use may represent an attempt to self-medicate this disorder. Children and adolescents with posttraumatic stress disorder (PTSD) are also at increased risk for the development or morbidity of SUDs in adolescence and adulthood (149, 150).

Substance use disorder among adolescents is a risk factor for suicidal behavior, including ideation, attempts, and completed suicide (151). Marijuana use for example is associated with an increase in suicidal behavior (152). Possible mechanisms underlying this relationship include the acute and chronic effects of psychoactive substances. Adolescents who commit suicide are frequently found to have been using alcohol or other drugs at the time of the suicide (153, 154). Acute effects of substances include a transient and intense dysphoric state, disinhibition, impaired judgment, and an increased level of impulsivity. Drug use may also exacerbate preexisting psychopathology, including depression or anxiety disorders (145, 155). In adolescents, substance use disorders are often seen concurrently with other neuropsychiatric conditions, including mood, anxiety, eating, and conduct disorders (137). Each of these disorders confers an increased risk of suicidal behavior in adolescents (156) as well as an increased risk of substance use disorders (137). Comorbidity, especially that of mood disorders with other nonmood conditions such as substance use disorders, is one of several putative risk factors for completed suicide (157, 158).

Many adolescents with substance use disorders manifest aggressive behavior (155, 159). Consumption of abusable substances such as alcohol, amphetamines, or phencyclidine increases the likelihood of aggressive behavior (160). The direct pharmacological effects of drugs may be exacerbated by the presence of preexisting psychopathology, the use of multiple agents simultaneously, or other factors having to do with the relative inexperience of the adolescent substance user. Chronic aggressive behavior among adolescents is often associated with a diagnosis of conduct disorder, and this diagnosis almost always precedes the substance use (161–163). Aggressive behavior at an early age predicts subsequent substance abuse (10, 164). Severely aggressive behavior precedes serious involvement with drugs (165).

Individuals with suicidal or aggressive behavior share certain biochemical characteristics, such as deficits in noradrenergic, serotonergic, and GABA/ benzodiazepine systems (166). Psychoactive substances can affect each of these neurotransmitter systems, and each has a role in the pathogenesis of several neuropsychiatric disorders. For example, Ballanger and colleagues (167) reported that chronic alcohol use may result in serotonergic depletion, although this finding is complicated by the possibility that these states preceded alcohol use. Research has linked low serotonergic states with suicidal and aggressive behavior in adults (168). Among aggressive and impulsive adult offenders, investigators have found very high rates of suicidal behavior and early onset substance abuse that correlate with low levels of serotonin metabolites (169, 170).

In addition to the acute and chronic effects of psychoactive substances on neurotransmitter systems, abnormalities of these neurotransmitter systems may precede the development of SUDs. Such biochemical abnormalities may contribute to increased risk by means of a number of possible mechanisms. For example, serotonergic deficits may underlie impulsive and aggressive behavior and poor mood regulation, as well as predispose an individual to specific psychiatric diagnoses. These psychiatric problems may lead to an increased risk for the development of substance use disorders. In addition to problems with aggression, impulsivity, and mood, neurotransmitter abnormalities may manifest as sensitized brain reinforcement produced in response to various psychoactive substances, thus promoting the risk for a behavioral pattern that leads to substance dependence.

Psychiatric disorders in childhood, primarily disruptive-behavior disorders as well as mood or anxiety disorders, confer an increased risk for the development of substance use disorders in adolescence (110, 137). The etiological mechanisms underlying this effect have not, however, been systematically researched. Within a general pattern of deviancy, alcohol and drug consumption can be considered as part of the nonnormative lifestyle. In an individual with an internalizing type of disorder (e.g., anxiety or depression), substances have the obvious short-term benefit of reducing negative or aversive mood states. Hence, there are many factors, including classical conditioning principles, that interact to predispose an individual to initiation and maintenance of substance use. The literature on the risk for adolescent substance use disorders has recently been reviewed within an epigenetic framework (68) in which a substance abuse outcome is viewed as the culmination of ongoing gene--environment interactions. Conceptualizing substance abuse in this way—as the end point of a succession of ontogenetic processes rather than the result of a single isolated event—has the potential to yield new perspectives on and possibly more effective approaches to prevention.

Brain Changes

Both cross-sectional and longitudinal imaging studies have suggested greater brain shrinkage in adults with alcohol dependence relative to comparison subjects. Volumetric magnetic resonance imaging (MRI) comparisons between alcohol-dependent subjects and healthy subjects have reported that individuals diagnosed with alcohol dependence show greater age-related brain atrophy (171, 172). Morphometric characteristics of adult cocaine abusers, including blunted age-related increases in frontal and temporal white matter (173) and accelerated age-related reductions in temporal lobe gray matter (174), are similar to characteristics seen in adult subjects with alcohol dependence atrophy. Comorbid cocaine and alcohol use disorders (but not marijuana use disorder alone) may accelerate white matter shrinkage with age relative to alcohol dependence alone (175).

Two studies in adolescents show consistent findings. De-Bellis and associates (176) used MRI to measure the hippocampal volumes and volumes of comparison brain regions in 12 subjects with alcohol use disorders and 24 comparison subjects matched on age, gender, and handedness. Both left and right hippocampal volumes were significantly smaller in subjects with alcohol use disorders than in comparison subjects. Total hippocampal volume correlated positively with the age at onset and negatively with the duration of the alcohol use disorder. There were no group differences in intracranial, cerebral, and cortical gray and white matter volumes and midsagittal area of the corpus callosum. Hill and colleagues (177) used MRI to measure cerebral, amygdala, and hippocampal volumes in 17 high-risk adolescent and young adult offspring from multiplex alcoholism families and 17 matched control subjects without a family history for alcoholism or other substance dependence. As 22 of the subjects were part of a longitudinal prospective study examining P300 ERPs, this study was able to relate developmental trajectories in ERPs to structural brain volumes. High-risk adolescents and young adults showed reduced right amygdala volume in comparison with control subjects. Right amygdala volume was significantly correlated with visual P300 amplitude. These results suggest that high-risk offspring from high-density alcoholic families differ in both neurophysiological and neuroanatomical characteristics that could not be explained by personal drinking history or particular childhood and adolescent psychopathology. Because amygdala volume tends to increase during childhood and adolescence, the smaller volumes in high-risk children may indicate a developmental marker for alcoholism risk that parallels the association between risk and delays seen in visual P300 amplitude (24).

Effects of Maternal Drug Use on Offspring

Establishing links between prenatal drug exposure and subsequent developmental, neurological, and neuropsychiatric outcomes is problematic because it is difficult to determine the dose or extent of the exposure (i.e., the type[s] of substances used by the mother, the frequency and quantity used, and the pregnancy stage[s] during which the use occurred) and to separate the effects of the exposure from those of other forces in the prenatal and postnatal environment. Additional influences include poor maternal nutrition, stress, and psychiatric illness (178).

Fetal alcohol syndrome occurs in approximately 1.9 live births per 1,000 worldwide, between 2.8 and 4.8/1,000 in the United States, and among 2 to 10% of alcoholic mothers (179, 180). In addition to intrauterine growth retardation and distinctive facial and other minor physical abnormalities, fetal alcohol syndrome is characterized by microcephaly, delayed development (including intellectual delays), attentional deficits, learning disabilities, and hyperactivity (181–183). Non–fetal alcohol syndrome offspring of alcoholic mothers show an increased incidence of intellectual impairment (184). Several reports have documented lower intellectual ability, poorer academic achievement, and greater problems with attention and hyperactivity (185, 186) in these offspring of alcoholic mothers.

For infants prenatally exposed to *cannabis* (*marijuana*), investigators reported a variety of neurobehavioral abnormalities, including decreased visual responsiveness, tremors, increased startle response, and changes in sleep patterns in the postpartum period (187–191). Long-term studies of children with intrauterine marijuana exposure are few and provide no consistent findings of neuropsychiatric sequelae (192).

Studies of prenatal *cocaine* exposure suggest that these infants exhibit impaired startle responsivity, habituation,

recognition, and reactivity to novel stimuli in the postpartum period (193–195). Postnatal irritability and poor recognition memory may persist into the early years of the child's life (194, 196). Serious language delays, especially in receptive language abilities, may be present in preschool children exposed in utero to cocaine, although their general development is similar to that of nonexposed peers in comparisons at 24 months of age (197, 198). Although a few studies show significant, unequivocal negative associations between toddler's developmental scores and prenatal exposure to cocaine, most of the results from controlled, large-scale prospective studies of cocaine exposure show more equivocal results after controlling for prenatal exposure to other drugs, gestational age and size at birth, and caretaker and maternal characteristics (199, 200).

In several studies, *opiate*-exposed neonates appeared to be more irritable and easily aroused, to have more active (versus quiet) sleep, and to spend more time in states of diminished alertness compared with nonexposed neonates (178, 201). Children prenatally exposed to opiates have been found to display poor motor coordination, hyperactivity, impulsivity, and difficulty with focused attention (202, 203, 198).

Although the prenatal drug exposure literature strongly suggests real but fairly modest effects on growth and development, it is extremely difficult to disentangle the effects of other concurrent drug use (such as alcohol and particularly tobacco), socioeconomic deprivation, and maternal psychopathology and genetic risk of the very outcomes prenatal exposure is supposed to cause. These modest effects are certainly not the perception of clinicians and the public that "crack babies" are forever grossly impaired. This exaggerated perception stigmatizes mothers and their offspring who are affected by cocaine or other substance use (200).

In summary, prenatal exposure to many agents of abuse may contribute to impairments in arousal modulation, activity level, and attention in the infant (178, 192, 204). While each of these impairments may significantly affect the child's functioning, the effects of the environment—including parental psychopathology, addiction, violence, abuse and neglect, and poverty—may greatly influence the ultimate manifestation of any neuropsychiatric sequelae of intrauterine exposure.

RELEVANCE OF NEUROPSYCHIATRIC FACTORS TO INTERVENTION AND CLINICAL PRACTICE

Assessment

Regardless of whether neuropsychiatric factors are viewed as causes or as effects of substance use, a number of clinical issues are especially relevant to the assessment of adolescents presenting to health care settings. It is essential for clinicians working with adolescents to be knowledgeable about common psychoactive substances and their acute effects on perception, behavior, mood, and thought processes. Adolescents often come to the attention of the health care system as a result of the acute psychoactive effects of substances that can affect perception, judgment, and coordination. Accidents and trauma (including head trauma and brain injury) can result, necessitating emergency evaluation and treatment. The percentage of medically treated injuries among adolescents ages 15 to 19 years who abuse drugs and alcohol or alcohol alone is similar to the rate of medically treated injuries among older patients (57%) and 10% higher than their similar age cohorts who are not drug or alcohol abusers (205).

Accidents involving adolescents and substance use commonly occur during activities such as bicycling or skateboarding (206), swimming (as many as 40% of cases of drowning may involve alcohol) (207), or driving motor vehicles (208). Despite drinking less than adults, adolescents who drink alcohol are at higher risk of being involved in an accident (209). Also increasing adolescents' risk for brain or other injury is their propensity to speed, run red lights, not use seat belts, drink after marijuana use, and ride with intoxicated drivers (210). Given this association between trauma and substance use in adolescents, health care workers should have strong suspicion of substance use among adolescents presenting to trauma centers or emergency departments.

Similarly, the common co-occurrence of psychiatric disorders with SUDs among adolescents should prompt the use of comprehensive evaluation processes and multimodal treatment interventions. Given the multiple risk factors, frequent comorbidity, and many potential areas of dysfunction, including neuropsychiatric sequelae, in youth who use substances, the comprehensive assessment of adolescent SUDs requires evaluation of multiple areas or domains in areas of the adolescent's life (211). Prominent among these domains for assessment are psychiatric and behavioral problems. Other potential domains, including substance use behavior, school or vocational functioning, family functioning, social competency/peer relations, and leisure/recreation, can be influenced by either preexisting neuropsychiatric factors or substance-induced neuropsychiatric effects.

In summary, as recommended by the Substance Abuse and Mental Health Services Administration (SAMHSA) "screening for adolescent substance use should be conducted by health care delivery systems, juvenile justice and family court systems, and community organizations such as schools, vocational rehabilitation, and religious organizations. Those who should be screened include all teens who receive mental health assessments, enter the child welfare system, drop out of school, or stay at homeless shelters. Adolescents arrested or detained within juvenile justice and family court systems also should be screened."

Prevention

Primary prevention is generally thought of as preventing the onset—or early onset of substance use or SUDs, themselves. A broader view also considers identification of the temperamental traits and psychiatric disorders presaging substance use and aggressive treatment focused on ameliorating or modifying these disturbances. Early identification of high-risk traits and disorders in children and adolescents with a family history of substance use disorders should be routine practice in both adult and child/adolescent clinical settings. In this manner, interventions can be directed toward reducing the liability conferred by these risk factors.

Targeting neuropsychiatric risk factors applies to preventive interventions with high-risk adolescents as well as to intervention or treatment with youth affected by SUDs. Most prevention efforts are based on various theoretical models of adolescent substance use/abuse development. Prevention efforts primarily involve strengthening resilience factors and reducing risk factors for the development of SUDs (212). Because use or experimentation of substances such as alcohol or even marijuana may be considered normative, prevention efforts might also serve to delay the experimental use of these agents, which would make progression to SUDs less likely. The National Institute on Drug Abuse has published an evidenced-based guide on preventing drug use among youths for parents, educators, and community leaders (NIDA. Preventing drug use among children and adolescents, 2nd Ed. Bethesda, MD: US Department of Health and Human Services, 2003).

Early intervention for psychopathology in youth at risk for SUDs or secondary prevention is also critical to prevent early onset substance use and SUDs. For example, the use of stimulant medication to treat ADHD in youth appears to decrease the risk for later substance use and SUDs (213).

Treatment

Acute Detoxification

Although withdrawal syndromes occur infrequently in adolescents, treatment of these syndromes should follow the same procedures used in adults (214). Unless the clinician can obtain a history of withdrawal symptoms or substance use patterns (e.g., specific agents used in sufficient quantity and frequency), a conservative approach should be taken, with careful monitoring of emergent symptoms before using medications for withdrawal. For more details on specific withdrawal management, the reader is referred to reviews and guidelines for withdrawal management in adults (214).

Adolescents with opiate addiction present the largest single group having a need for detoxification. While the use of opiate agonists such as methadone for substitution withdrawal therapy is common in inpatient settings, the use of buprenorphine, a partial opiate agonist is increasing in both inpatient and ambulatory settings (215). For adolescents, the most common detoxification medication is clonidine.

For alcohol and sedatives, benzodiazepines remain the treatment of choice (216). Unless the adolescent has a history of significant withdrawal problems, the best approach is a symptom-triggered therapy, in which the medication is given only after withdrawal symptom exceed a threshold of severity. The symptom-triggered approach is as effective but usually requires less medication than a fixed dose regimen. Because it requires regular monitoring and the use of a validated withdrawal scale, its use is limited to inpatient detoxification.

Substance Use Rehabilitation

Specific pharmacologic treatment of substance use behavior includes drug substitution (e.g., methadone maintenance), antagonist therapy (e.g., naltrexone), aversive agents (e.g., disulfiram), or agents theoretically directed toward brain neurotransmitter systems that may underlie neuroadaptation to the particular substance, craving, or other substance use-reinforcement mechanisms. Particularly promising is the use of buprenorphine for opiate dependence. Because there are no controlled studies of the use of medications in the treatment or withdrawal or in substitution, antagonist or adverse therapy, the reader is referred to the adult literature for guidelines (see previous citations).

Psychosocial modalities are the cornerstone of addiction treatment for adolescents. Reviews of the literature of adolescent treatment outcome have concluded that treatment is better than no treatment (220, 223). In the Drug Abuse Treatment Study for Adolescents (DATOS-A), adolescents reported decreased heavy drinking, marijuana and other illicit drug use, and criminal involvement, as well as improved psychological adjustment and school performance in the year following treatment (224, 225). Longer duration of treatment is associated with several favorable outcomes. Pretreatment factors associated with poorer outcomes (usually substance use and relapse to use) are nonWhite race, increased seriousness of substance use, criminality, and lower educational status. The intreatment factors predictive of outcome are time in treatment, involvement of family, use of practical problem-solving, and provision of comprehensive services such as housing, academic assistance, and recreation. Posttreatment variables that are thought to be the most important determinants of outcome include association with non-using peers and involvement in leisure time activities, work, and school. Variables reported to be most consistently related to successful outcome are treatment completion, low pretreatment use, and peer and parent social support and nonuse of substances (222, 223).

Most adolescents return to some level of substance use following treatment (226, 227). Currently, empirical support exists for family-based interventions such as Strategic Family Therapy, Muti-Dimensional Family Therapy (MDFT), and Multi-Systemic Therapy (MST), as well as

cognitive behavioral therapies for the treatment of adolescents with SUDs. Promising, but with less support, are Motivational Interviewing and Enhancement and specific behavioral interventions such as contingency contracting and community reinforcement. Although many clinicians use 12-step based treatment and self-support groups such as Alcoholic or Narcotics Anonymous (e.g., AA or NA), there are no published controlled treatment studies that have examined their efficacy. Cohort studies of adolescents having received SUD treatment have found that attendance in aftercare treatment or self-support groups is related to positive outcomes such as higher rates of abstinence (228–230).

Based on the combination of empirical research and current clinical consensus, the clinician dealing with adolescents with SUDs should develop a treatment plan that uses modalities that target motivation and engagement; family involvement to improve supervision, monitoring, and communication between parents and adolescent; skills to improve problem solving, social skills, and for relapse prevention; comorbid psychiatric disorders through psychosocial and/or medication treatments; and social ecology in terms of increasing prosocial behaviors and peer relationships, and academic functioning. Self-support groups can be encouraged as adjuncts to the previous modalities. Table 16.6 presents examples of treatment targets and suggested intervention modalities for adolescents with SUDs.

TABLE 16.6

INTERVENTIONS DIRECTED TOWARD NEUROPSYCHIATRIC RISK FACTORS FOR ADOLESCENT SUBSTANCE USE DISORDER

Risk Factor(s)	Intervention
ADHD (including relevant temperamental traits)	Pharmacological agents • norepinephrine reuptake inhibitors • CNS stimulants • TCAs • bupropion • adrenergic agents Behavioral interventions
Information-processing deficits (may be part of ADHD or LD)	As per ADHD
Aggressive behavior	Behavioral interventions Pharmacological agents • CNS stimulants • Atypical neuroleptics • Mood stabilizers
Depression/other mood disorders	Cogntive behavioral interventions Pharmacological agents • Serontonergic reuptake inhibitors
Social skills deficits	Social skills training

ADHD = attention deficit hyperactivity disorder; CNS = central nervous system; LD = learning disability; TCAs = tricyclic antidepressants.

Pharmacotherapy of Comorbid Psychiatric Disorders

The most common use of pharmacotherapy in adolescents with substance use disorders is for treatment of coexisting psychiatric disorders. Potential treatment targets include mood disorders, anxiety disorders, ADHD, and aggression. Open trials with pemoline and bupropion for ADHD and fluoxetine for depression in a population of drug-dependent delinquents have shown promise (217–219). More recently, a double-blind placebo-controlled trial of a stimulant medication demonstrated the efficacy of medication improving ADHD symptoms in adolescents with co-morbid ADHD and SUD. This study also demonstrated that medication treatment of ADHD alone, without specific SUD or other psychosocial treatment, did not decrease substance use (220). Lithium, in a randomized controlled trial (221), and serotonergic reuptake inhibitors, in open trials (217, 219), have produced significant improvements in adolescents with SUDs and comorbid mood disorders.

Persistence of symptoms beyond several weeks of abstinence should prompt consideration of pharmacotherapy. Factors that may indicate a need to consider more aggressive use of pharmacotherapy include psychiatric symptoms that predate the substance abuse or that present during periods of abstinence, a family history of the psychiatric disorder, past treatment failure (i.e., nonresponse to pharmacotherapy) and multiple relapses, and past successful treatment with pharmacotherapy. Two critical concerns in using pharmacotherapy with adolescents with substance use disorders are the abuse potential of the prescribed pharmacological treatment and the possibility of interactions between this treatment and potential substances of abuse.

Treatment of Neuropsychiatric Sequelae

In adults, many of the chronic neuropsychiatric sequelae of substance (such as alcohol) use, result from nutritional deficiencies or longterm damage of organ systems. In adolescents, with rare exceptions, the duration or amounts of use are insufficient to lead to such results. The most appropriate approach is abstinence or a substantial reduction of use, patience, and time. For example, postperceptual disturbances due to hallucinogens often resolve after short or extended periods (a year or more) without pharmacotherapy. Gross psychotic phenomenon may require antipsychotic agents. Even when mood or anxiety symptoms can be tied specifically to substance use, the clinician should consider targeting the specific symptoms with appropriate medications.

CONCLUSION

Acute substance use and substance use disorders can produce a wide variety of adverse effects on perception, thought processes, mood, and behavior. These effects are usually transient but may place adolescents at risk for a wide range of outcomes such as accidents, interpersonal/family conflict, and academic/vocational failure. Largely because of their variable pattern of substance use, children and adolescents rarely experience signs and symptoms of physical dependence (i.e., abstinence syndrome). While social and peer factors may be more important in the initiation and early stages of substance use, neurobiological mechanisms become increasingly important in the progression to substance dependence. Certain neurobiological characteristics increase an individual's risk of developing a substance use disorder, including information-processing deficits and temperamental traits such as high activity level and mood instability. Overall, research findings indicate that syndromes involving general dysregulation or disinhibition of cognitive, affective, and behavioral processes predispose an individual to substance abuse. Genetic factors appear to be partially responsible for these psychiatric syndromes, which by the time of adolescence, is featured by substantial comorbidity. A substantial and growing literature points to a number of interventions that are effective in preventing and treating substance use and substance use disorders in children and adolescents. Elucidating the neurobiological factors underlying the risk for substance use disorders and acute and chronic neuropsychiatric sequelae paves the way for a more complete understanding of etiology that in turn will lead to more effective prevention and treatment.

REFERENCES

1. University of Michigan, Institute for Social Research: "Monitoring the Future" Survey (press release). Ann Arbor, MI, 2003.
2. Costello JE, Angold A, Burns, BJ, Stangl DK, Tweed DL, Erkanli A, Worthman CM: The great smoky mountains study of youth: goals, design, methods, and the prevalence of DSM-III-R disorders. Arch Gen Psychiatry 53:1129–1136, 1996.
3. Kessler RC, McGonagle KA, Zhao S, Nelsen CB, Hughes M, Eshleman S, Wittchen HU: Lifetime and 12-month prevalence of DSM-III-R psychiatric disorders in the United States: Results from the National Comorbidity Study. Arch Gen Psychiatry 51:8–19, 1994.
4. Lewinsohn PM, Rohde P, Seeley JR: Alcohol consumption in high school adolescents: frequency of use and dimensional structure of associated problems. Addiction 91:375–390, 1996.
5. Kashani JH, Beck NC, Hoeper EW, Fallahi C, Corcoran CM, McAllister JA, Rosenberg TK, Reid JC: Psychiatric disorders in a community sample of adolescents. Am J Psychiatry 144:584–589, 1987.
6. Reinherz HZ, Giaconia RM, Lefkowitz ES, et al: Prevalence of psychiatric disorders in a community population of older adolescents. J Am Acad Child Adolesc Psychiatry 32:369–377, 1993.
7. Costello EJ, Mustillo S, Erkanli A, Keeler G, et al: Prevalence and development of psychiatric disorders in childhood and adolescence. Arch Gen Psychiatry 60:837–844, 2003.
8. American Psychiatric Association: Diagnostic and Statistical Manual of Mental Disorders, 3rd Edition, Revised. Washington, DC: American Psychiatric Association, 1987.
9. Kandel D: Stages in adolescent involvement in drug use. Science 190:92–914, 1975
10. Kandel DB, Kessler RC, Margulies RZ: Antecedents of adolescent initiation into stages of drug use: a developmental analysis, in Longitudinal Research on Drug Use: Empirical Findings and Methodological Issues. Edited by Kandel DB. Washington, D.C.: Hemisphere (Halstead-Wiley), 1978, pp. 73–99.

11. Jessor R, Jessor S: Problem Behavior and Psychosocial Development–A Longitudinal Study of Youth. New York: Academic Press, 1977.

12. Vanyukov M, Tarter R, Kirisci L, Kirillova G, Maher B, Clark D: Liabilty to substance use disorders: 1. Common mechanisms and manifestations. Neurosci Biobehav Rev 27:507–515, 2003a.

13. Vanyukov M, Kirisci L, Tarter R, Simkevitz H, Kirillova G, Maher B, Clark D: Liabilty to substance use disorders: 2. A measurement approach. Neurosci Biobehav Rev 27:517–526, 2003b.

14. Donchin E: Event-related potentials: a toll in the study of human information processing, in Evoked Brain Potentials and Behavior, vol 2. Edited by Begleiter H. New York: Plenum, 1979, pp. 13–88.

15. Begleiter H, Porjesz B: Neurophysiological phenotypic factors in the development of alcoholism, in The Genetics of Alcoholism. Edited by Begleiter H, Kissin B. New York: Oxford University Press, 1995, pp. 269–293.

16. Porjesz B, Begleiter H, Reich T, Van Eerdewegh P, Edenberg HJ, Foroud T, Goate A, Litke A, Chorlian DB, Stimus A, Rice J, Blangero J, Almasy L, Sorbell J, Bauer LO, Kuperman S, O'Connor SJ, Rohrbaugh J: Amplitude of visual P3 event-related potential as a phenotypic marker for a predisposition to alcoholism: preliminary results from the COGA project Alcoholism. Clin Exp Res 22:1317–1323, 1998.

17. Hill SY, Steinhauer S: Assessment of prepubertal and post pubertal boys and girls at risk for developing alcoholism with p300 from a visual discrimination task. J Stud Alcohol 54:350–358, 1993a.

18. Steinhauer S, Hill SY: Auditory event-related potentials in children at high risk for alcoholism. J Stud Alcohol 54: 408–421, 1993.

19. Polich J, Pollack V Bloom FE: Meta-analysis of p300 amplitude from individuals at risk for alcoholism. Psychol Bull 115:55–73, 1994.

20. Brigham J, Herning RI, Moss HB: Event-related potentials and alpha synchronization in preadolescent boys at risk for psychoactive substance use. Biol Psychiatry 37:834–846, 1995.

21. Iacono WG, Carlson SR, Malone SM, McGue M: P3 event-related potential amplitude and the risk for disinhibitory disorders in adolescent boys. Arch Gen Psychiatry 59:750–757, 2003.

22. Berman SM, Whipple SC, Fitch RJ, et al: P3 in young boys as a predictor of adolescent substance use. Alcohol 10:69–76, 1993.

23. Hill SY, Steinhauer S, Lowers L, et al: Eight-year longitudinal follow-up of P300 and clinical outcome in children from high risk for alcoholism families. Biol Psychiatry 37:823–827, 1995.

24. Hill SY, Shen S: Neurodevelopmental patterns of visual P3b in association with familial risk for alcohol dependence and childhood diagnosis. Biol Psychiatry 51:621–631, 2002.

25. Hill SY, Shen S, Locke J, Steinhauer SR, Konicky C, Lowers L, Connolly J: Developmental delay in P300 production in children at high risk for developing alcohol-related disorders. Biol Psychiatry 46:970—981, 1999.

26. Bauer LO, Hesselbrock VM: P300 decrements in teenagers with conduct problems: Implications for substance abuse risk and brain development. Biol Psychiatry 46:263–272, 1999.

27. Bauer LO, Hesselbrock VM: Brain maturation and subtypes of conduct disorder; interactive effects on P300 amplitude and topography in male adolescents. J Am Acad Child Adolesc Psychiatry 42:106–115, 2003.

28. Tarter R, Vanyukov M, Dawes M, Blackson T, Mezzich A, Clark DB: Etiology of early onset substance use disorder: A maturational perspective. Dev Psychopathol 11:657–683, 1999.

29. Bauer LO: Frontal P300 decrements, childhood conduct disorder, family history, and the prediction of relapse among abstinent cocaine abusers. Drug Alcohol Depend 44:1–10, 1997.

30. Costa L, Bauer LO, Kuperman S et al: Frontal P300 decrements, alcohol dependence, and antisocial personality disorder. Biol Psychiatry 47:1064–1071, 2000.

31. Hegedus A, Alterman A, Tarter R: Learning achievement in sons of alcoholics. Alcohol Clin Exp Res 8:330–333, 1984.

32. Hill SY, Steinhauer S: Postural sway in children from pedigrees exhibiting a high density of alcoholism. Biol Psychiatry 33:313–325, 1993b.

33. Schuckit MA: Ethanol induced changes in body sway in men at high alcoholism risk. Arch Gen Psychiatry 42: 375–379, 1985.

34. Tarter RE, Jacob T, Breme DA: Cognitive status of sons of alcoholic men. Alcohol Clin Exp Res 13:232–235, 1989.

35. Tarter RE, Moss HB, Vanyukov MM: Behavioral genetics and the etiology of alcoholism, in The Genetics of Alcoholism. Edited by Begleiter H, Kissin B. New York, Oxford University Press, 1995c, pp. 294–326.

36. Schuckit MA: Self-rating of alcohol intoxication by young men with and without family histories of alcoholism. J Stud Alcohol 41:242–249, 1980.

37. Schuckit MA: Subjective responses to alcohol in sons of alcoholics and control subjects. Arch Gen Psychiatry 41: 879–884, 1984.

38. Schuckit MA, Smith TL, Kalmijn J, Tsuang, J, Hesselbrock V, Bucholz K: Response to alcohol in daughters of alcoholics: a pilot study and a comparison with sons of alcoholics. Alcohol & Alcoholism 35:242–248, 2000.

39. Pollack VE: Meta-analysis of subjective sensitivity to alcohol in sons of alcoholics. Am J Psychiatry 149:1534–1538, 1992.

40. Bouchard T, Lykken D, McGue M, et al: Sources of human psychological differences: the Minnesota study of twins reared apart. Science 250:223–228, 1990.

41. Plomin R, Petersen N, McClearn G, et al: EAS temperament during the last half of the life span: twins reared apart and twins reared together. Psychol Aging 3:43–50, 1988.

42. Maziade M, Caron C, Cote R, et al: Psychiatric status of adolescents who had extreme temperaments at age 7. Am J Psychiatry 147:1531–1537, 1990a.

43. Maziade M, Caron C, Cote P, et al: Extreme temperament and diagnosis: a study in a psychiatric sample of consecutive children. Arch Gen Psychiatry 47:477–484, 1990b.

44. Reich W, Earls F, Frankel O, et al: Psychopathology in children of alcoholics. J Am Acad Child Adolesc Psychiatry 32:995–1002, 1993.

45. Earls F, Jung K: Temperament and home environment characteristics in the early development of child psychopathology. J Am Acad Child Psychiatry 26:491–498, 1987.

46. Tarter R, Kabene M, Escallier E, et al: Temperament deviation and risk for alcoholism. Alcohol Clin Exp Res 14:380–382, 1990a.

47. Tarter R, Laird S, Kabene M, et al: Drug abuse severity in adolescents is associated with magnitude of deviation in temperament traits. Br J Addiction 85: 1501–1504,1990b.

48. Tarter RE, Hegedus A, Goldstein G, et al: Adolescent sons of alcoholics: neuropsychological and personality characteristics. Alcohol Clin Exp Res 46:259–261, 1984.

49. Schaeffer K, Parsons O, Yohman J: Neuropsychological differences between male familial alcoholics and nonalcoholics. Alcohol Clin Exp Res 8:347–351, 1984.

50. Fitzgerald HE, Sullivan LA, Ham HP, et al: Predictors of behavioral problems in 3-year-old sons of alcoholics: early evidence for the onset of risk. Child Dev 64:110–123, 1993.

51. Noll RB, Zucker RA, Fitzgerald HE, et al: Cognitive and motoric functioning of sons of alcoholic fathers and controls: the early childhood years. Dev Psychol 28: 665–675, 1992.

52. Shedler J, Block J: Adolescent drug use and psychological health: a longitudinal inquiry. Am Psychol 45:612–630, 1990.

53. Brook JS, Whiteman M, Gordon AS, et al: The psychosocial etiology of adolescent drug use: a family interactional approach. Genet Soc Gen Psychol Monogr 116: 111–267, 1990.

54. Kellam SG, Brown CH, Rubin BR, et al: Paths leading to teenage psychiatric symptoms and substance use: development epidemiological studies in Woodlawn, in Childhood Psychopathology and Development. Edited by Guze SB, Earles FJ, Barrett JE. New York: Norton, 1983, pp 17–52.

55. Blackson TC: Temperament: a salient correlate of risk factors for alcohol and drug abuse. Drug Alcohol Depend 36:205–214, 1994.

56. Chassin L, Pillow D, Curran P, et al: Relation of parental alcoholism to early adolescent substance use: a test of three mediating mechanisms. J Abnorm Psychol 102: 3–19, 1993.

57. Tarter RE, Blackson T, Brigham J, et al: The association between childhood irritability and ability to substance use in early adolescence: a 2-year follow-up study of boys at risk for substance abuse. Drug Alcohol Depend 39:253–261, 1995a.

58. Barkley RA, Fischer M, Edelbrock C S, et al: The adolescent outcome of hyperactive children diagnosed by research criteria, I: an 8-year prospective follow-up study. J Am Acad Child Adolesc Psychiatry 29:546–557, 1990.

59. Cantwell D: Psychiatric illness in the families of hyperactive children. Arch Gen Psychiatry 27:414–417, 1972.

60. Morrison JR, Stewart MA: A family study of the hyperactive child syndrome. Biol Psychiatry 3:189–195, 1971.

61. DeObaldia R, Oarsons O, Yohman R: Minimal brain dysfunction symptoms claimed by primary and secondary alcoholics: relation to cognitive functioning. J Neurosci 20:173–181, 1983.

62. Tarter R, McBride H, Buonpane N, et al: Differentiation of alcoholics: childhood history of minimal brain dysfunction, family history, and drinking pattern. Arch Gen Psychiatry 34:761–768, 1977.

63. Hechtman L, Weiss G, Perlman T: Hyperactive as young adults: past and current antisocial behavior and moral development. Am J Orthopsychiatry 54:415–425, 1984.

64. McCord W McCord J: Origins of Alcoholism. Stanford, CA: Stanford University Press, 1960.

65. Milberger, S, Biederman J, Faraone SV, Wilens T, Chu MP: Associations between ADHD and psychoactive substance use disorders: Findings from a longitudinal study of high-risk siblings of ADHD children. Am J Addictions 6:318–329, 1997.

66. Martin CS, Earlywine M, Blackson TC, et al: Aggressivity, inattention, hyperactivity and impulsivity in boys at high and low risk for substance abuse. J Abnorm Child Psychol 22:177–203, 1994.

67. Tarter RE: Etiology of adolescent substance abuse: A developmental perspective. Am J Addictions 11:171–191, 2002.

68. Tarter R, Kirisci L, Hegedus A, et al: Heterogeneity of adolescent alcoholism. Ann NY Acad Sci 708:172–180, 1994.

69. Zucker RA, Ellis DA, Fitzgerald HE: Developmental evidence for at least two alcoholism, I: biopsychosocial variation among pathways into symptomatic difficulty. Ann NY Acad Sci 708:134–146, 1994.

70. Cloninger CR: Neurogenetic adaptive mechanisms in alcoholism. Science 236:410–416, 1987.

71. Irwin M, Schuckit MA, Smith TL: Clinical importance of age at onset in type 1 and type 2 primary alcoholics. Arch Gen Psychiatry 47:481–487, 1990.

72. Schuckit MA, Irwin M: Analysis of the clinical relevance of type 1 and type 2 alcoholics. Br J Addiction 84:869–876, 1989.

73. Foster J, Eskes G, Stuss D: The cognitive neuropsychology of attention: a frontal lobe perspective. Cognitive Neuropsychology 11:133–147, 1994.

74. Mega MS, Cumings JL: Frontal-subcortical circuits and neuropsychiatric disorders. J Neuropsychiatry Clin Neurosci 6:358–370, 1994.

75. Giancola PR, Tarter RE: Executive cognitive functioning and risk for substance abuse. Psychol Sci 10: 203–205, 1999.

76. Giancola PR, Martin CS, Tarter RE, et al: Executive cognitive functioning and aggressive behavior in preadolescent boys at high risk for substance abuse/dependence. J Stud Alcohol 57:352–359, 1996a.

77. Giancola PR, Moss HB, Martin CS, et al: Executive cognitive functioning predicts reactive but not proactive aggression in young boys at high risk for substance abuse: a prospective study. Alcohol Clin Exp Res 20: 740–744, 1996b.

78. Giancola, PR, Shoal GD, Mezzich AC: Constructive thinking, executive functioning, antisocial behavior, and drug use involvement in adolescent females with a substance use disorder. Exp Clin Psychopharmacol 9:215–227, 2001.

79. Giancola, PR Moss HB: Executive cognitive functioning in alcohol use disorders, in Recent Developments in Alcoholism. Edited by Galanter M. New York: Plenum Press, 1998.

80. Gardner EL: Brain reward mechanisms, in Substance Abuse: A Comprehensive Text Book. Edited by Lowinson JH, Ruiz P, Millman RB. Baltimore, MD: Williams & Wilkins, 1992, pp. 70–99.

81. Brady, JV Lucas SE: Testing drugs for physical dependence potential and abuse liability (NIDA Research Monograph Series, No 52). Washington, DC: US Government Printing Office, 1984.

82. Wise RA: The dopamine synapse and the notion of "pleasure centers" in the brain. Trends Neurosci 3:91–95, 1980.

83. Wise RA, Rompre P-P: Brain dopamine and reward. Annu Rev Psychol 40:191–225, 1989.

84. Volkow ND, Fowler JS, Wang G-J: Role of dopamine in drug reinforcement and addiction in humans: results from imaging studies. Behav Pharmacol 13:355–366, 2002.

85. Ritz, MC, Lamb, RJ, Goldberg, SR, Kuhar, MJ: Cocaine receptors on dopamine transporters are related to self-administration of cocaine. Science 237: 1219–1223, 1987.

86. Tapert SF, Cheung EH, Brown, GG, Frank LR, et al: Neural response to alcohol stimuli in adolescents with alcohol use disorder. Arch Gen Psychiatry 60:727–735, 2003.

87. Goldstein RZ, Volkow ND: Drug addiction and its underlying neurological basis: Neuroimaging evidence for the involvement of the frontal cortex. Am J Psychiatry 159:1642–1652, 2002.

88. Chambers RA, Taylor JR, Potenza, MN Developmental neurocircuitry of motivation in adolescence: a critical period of addiction vulnerability. Am J Psychiatry 160: 1041–1052, 2003.

89. Edwards G, Gross MM: Alcohol dependence: provisional description of a clinical syndrome. BMJ 1:1058–1061, 1976.

90. Martin CS, Kaczynski NA, Maisto SA, et al: Patterns of DSM-IV alcohol abuse and dependence symptoms in adolescent drinkers. J Stud Alcohol 56:672–680, 1995.

91. Stewart, DG, Brown, SA: Withdrawal and dependency symptoms among adolescent alcohol and drug abusers. Addiction 90:627–635, 1995.

92. Winters KC, Stinchfield R: Current issues in future needs in the assessment of adolescent drug abuse, in Adolescent Drug Abuse: Clinical Assessment and Therapeutic Interventions (NIDA Res Monogr 156; NIH Publ No 95–3908). Edited by Rahdert E, Czechowicz D. Washington, DC: US Government Printing Office, 1995.

93. Crowley TJ, Macdonald MJ, Whitmore EA, Mikulick SK: Cannabis dependence, withdrawal and reinforcing effects among adolescents with conduct symptoms and substance use disorders. Drug Alcohol Depend 50:27–37, 1998.

94. Coffey C, Carlin JB, Lynskey M et al.: Adolescent precursors of cannabis dependence: findings from the Victorian Adoelscent Health Cohort Study. Br J Psychiatry 182: 330–337, 2003.

95. Koop GF, Stinus L, LeMoal M, et al: Opponent process theory of motivation: neurobiological evidence from studies of opiate dependence. Neurosci Biobehav Rev 13: 135–140, 1989.

96. Bukstein OG: Adolescent Substance Abuse: Assessment, Prevention and Treatment. New York: Wiley, 1995.

97. Hawkins JD, Catalano RF, Miller JY: Risk and protective factors for alcohol and other drug problems in adolescence and early adulthood: implications for substance abuse prevention. Psychol Bull 112: 64–105, 1992.

98. Brook JS, Whiteman M, Brook DW, Gordon AS: Sibling influences on adolescent drug use: older brothers on younger brothers. J Am Acad Child Adolesc Psychiatry 30:958–966, 1991.

99. Hopfer CJ, Stallings M C, Hewitt, JK, Crowley, TJ: Family transmission of marijuana use, abuse, and dependence. J Am Acad Child Adolesc Psychiatry 42:834–841, 2003.

100. Goldman D, Bergen A: General and specific inheritance of substance abuse and alcoholism. Arch Gen Psychiatry 55:964–965, 1998.

101. Hopfer CJ, Crowley TJ, Hewitt JK: Review of twin and adoption studies of adolescent substance use. J Am Acad Child Adolesc Psychiatry 42:710–719, 2003.

102. Kendler KS, Karkowski L, Neale MC, Prescott CA: Illicit psychoactive substance use, heavy use, abuse, and dependence in a US population-based sample of male twins. Arch Gen Psychiatry 57:261–269, 2000.

103. Koopmans JR, Slutske WS, Heath AC, Neale MC, Boomsma DI: The genetics of smoking initiation and quantity smoked in Dutch adolescent and young adult twins. Behav Genet 29:383–393, 1999.

104. Vanyukov NN, Tarter RE: Genetic studies of substance abuse. Drug Alcohol Depend 59:101–123, 2000.

105. Viken RJ, Kaprio J, Koskenvuo M, Rose RJ: Longitudinal analyses of the determinants of drinking and of drinking to intoxication in adolescent twins. Behav Genet 29:455–460, 1999.

106. Kendler K S, Jacobson K C, Prescott, CA, Neale, MC: Specificity of genetic and environmental risk factors for use and abuse/dependence of cannabis, cocaine, hallucinogens, sedatives, stimulants, and opiates in male twins. Am J Psychiatry 160:687–695, 2003.

107. Tsuang MT, Lyons MJ, Meyer JM, Doyle T, Eisen SA, Goldberg J, True W, Lin N, Toomey R, Eaves L: Co-occurrence of abuse of different drugs in men. Arch Gen Psychiatry 55:967–972, 1998.

108. Bierut LJ, Dinwiddie SH, Begleiter H, Crowe RR, Hesselbrock V, Nurnberger JI, Porjesz B, Schuckit M, Reich T: Familial transmission of substance dependence: alcohol, marijuana, cocaine, and habitual smoking. Arch Gen Psychiatry 55:982–988, 1998.

109. Koopmans JR, van Doornen LJ, Boomsma DI: Association between alcohol use and smoking in adolescent and young adult twins: a bivariate genetic analysis. Alcohol Clin Exp Res 21: 537–546, 1997.

110. Loeber R: Natural histories of conduct problems, delinquency and associated substance use, in Advances in Clinical Child Psychology, Vol 11. Edited by Lahey BB, Kazdin AE. New York: Plenum, 1988, pp. 73–124.

111. Koob GF, Le Moral M: Drug abuse: hedonic homeostatic dysregulation. Science 278:52–57, 1997.

112. Christiansen BA, Goldman MS, Inn A: Development of alcohol-related expectancies in adolescents: separating pharmacological from social learning influences. J Consult Clin Psychol 50:336–344, 1982.

113. American Psychiatric Association: Diagnostic and Statistical Manual of Mental Disorders-Text Revision, 4th Edition (DSM-IV-TR). Washington, DC: American Psychiatric Association, 2002.

114. Martin CS, Arria AM, Mezzich AC, et al: Patterns of polydrug use in adolescent alcohol abusers. Am J Drug Alcohol Abuse 19:511–522, 1993.

115. Tabakoff B, Hoffman PL: Biochemical pharmacology of alcohol, in Psychopharmacology: The Third Generation of Progress. Edited by Meltzer HY. New York: Raven, 1987, pp. 1521–1526.

116. Tabakoff B, Hoffman PL: Alcohol: neurobiology, in Substance Abuse: A Comprehensive Text Book. Edited by Lowinson JH, Ruiz P, Millman RB. Baltimore, MD: Williams & Wilkins, 1992, pp. 152–185.

117. Koop GF, Bloom FE: Cellular and molecular mechanisms of drug dependence. Science 242:715–723, 1988.

118. Wiley JL, Martin BR: Cannabinoid pharmacology: implications for additional cannabinoid receptor subtypes. Chem Phys Lipids 121: 57–63, 2002.

119. Goodwin DW, Crane JB, Guze SB: Phenomenological aspects of the alcoholic "blackout." Br J Psychiatry 115: 1033–1038, 1969.

120. Goodwin DW, Othmer E, Halikas JA, et al: Loss of short-term memory as a predictor of the alcoholic "blackout." Nature 27:201–202, 1970.

121. Anthenelli RM, Klein JL, Tsuang JW et al: The prognostic importance of blackouts in young men. J Stud Alcohol 55:290–295, 1994.

122. Vinson DC: Acute transient memory loss. Am Fam Physician 39: 249–254, 1989.

123. Newlin DB, Pretorious MB: Sons of alcoholics report greater hangover symptoms than sons of nonalcoholics: a pilot study. Alcohol Clin Exp Res 14:713–719, 1990.

124. Deas D, Riggs P, Langenbucher, J, Goldman M, Brown S: Adolescents are not adults: developmental considerations in alcohol users. Alcoholism Clin Exp Res 24:232–237, 2000.

125. Fals-Stewart W Schafer J, Luccente S, et al: Neurobehavioral consequences of prolonged alcohol and substance abuse: a review of findings and treatment implications. Clin Psychol Rev 14:755–778, 1994.

126. Parsons OA: Impaired neuropsychological cognitive functioning in sober alcoholics, in Alcohol-Induced Brain Damage (Monograph 22). Edited by Hunt WA, Nixon SJ. Rockville, MD: National Institute on Alcohol Abuse and Alcoholism, 1993.

127. Lewis M, Volkmar F: Clinical Aspects of Child and Adolescent Development. Philadelphia: Lea & Febinger, 1990.

128. Rutter M, Rutter M: Developing Minds. New York: Basic Books, 1993.

129. Moss HB, Kirisci L, Gordon HW, et al: A neuropsychological profile of adolescent alcoholics. Alcohol Clin Exp Res 18:159–163, 1994.

130. Schonfeld JS, Shaffer D, O'Connor P, et al: Conduct disorder and cognitive functioning: testing three causal hypotheses. Child Dev 59:993–1007, 1988.

131. Yeudell LT, Fromm-Auch D, Davies P: Neuropsychological impairment of persistent delinquency. J Nerv Ment Dis 170: 257–265, 1982.

132. Tarter RE, Mezzich AC, Hsieh Y, et al: Cognitive capacity in female adolescent substance abusers. Drug Alcohol Depend 39:15–21, 1995b.

133. Tapert SF, Brown SA: Neuropsychological correlates of adolescent substance abuse: four year outcomes. J Int Neuropsychol Soc 5:481–493, 1999.

134. Brown SA, Tapert SF, Granholm E, Delis DC: Neurocognitive functioning of adolescents: effects of protracted alcohol use. Alcohol Clin Exp Res 24:164–17, 2000.

135. Smith DE, Seymour RB: LSD: History and toxicity. Psychiatr Ann 24:145–147, 1994.

136. Shick JF, Smith DE: Analysis of the LSD flashback. J Psychedelic Drugs 3:13–19, 1970.

137. Bukstein OG, Brent DA, Kaminer Y: Comorbidity of substance abuse and other psychiatric disorders in adolescents. Am J Psychiatry 146:1131–1141, 1989.

138. Gruber AJ, Pope HG, Brown ME: Do patients use marijuana as an antidepressant? Depression 4: 77–80, 1996.

139. Degenhardt L, Hall, W, Lynskey M: The relationship between cannabis use, depression and anxiety among Australian adults: findings from the National Survey of Mental Health and Wellbeing. Soc Psychiat Epidemiol 36:219–227, 2001.

140. Rey JM, Sawyer MG, Raphael B, et al: The mental health of teenagers who use marijuana: results of an Australian survey. Br J Psychiatry 180:222–226, 2002.

141. Brook DW, Brook JS, Zhang C et al: Drug use and the risk of major depressive disorder, alcohol dependence, and substance use disorders. J Am Acad Child Adolesc Psychiatry 42:485–492, 2002.

142. Patton GC, Coffey C, Cartlin JB, et al: Cannabis use and mental health in young people: A cohort study. BMJ 325:1195–1198, 2002.

143. Bukstein OG, Glancy LJ, Kaminer Y: Patterns of affective comorbidity in a clinical population of dually diagnosed adolescent substance abusers. J Am Acad Child Adolesc Psychiatry 31: 1041–1045, 1992.

144. Riggs PD, Baker S, Mikulich SK, et al: Depression in substance-dependent delinquents. J Am Acad Child Adolesc Psychiatry 34:764–771, 1995.

145. Schuckit MA: Genetic and clinical implications of alcoholism and affective disorder. Am J Psychiatry 143:140–147, 1986.

146. Clark DB, Bukstein OG, Smith MG, et al: Identifying anxiety disorders in adolescents hospitalized for alcohol abuse or dependence. Psychiatr Serv 46:618–620, 1995.

147. Zimmermann P, Wittchen HU, Hofler M, Pfister H, Kessler RC, Lieb R: Primary anxiety disorders and the development of subsequent alcohol use disorders: A 4-year community study of adolescents and young adults. Psychol Med 33:1211–1222, 2003.

148. Kushner MG, Sher KJ, Beitman, BD: The relation between alcohol problems and anxiety disorders. Am J Psychiatry 147, 685–695, 1990.

149. De Bellis, MD: Developmental traumatology: A contributory mechanism for alcohol and substance use disorders. Psychoneuroendocrinology 27(1):155–170, 2002.

150. Giaconia RM, Reinherz HZ, Paradis AD, Stashwick CK: Comorbidity of substance use disorders and posttraumatic stress disorder in adolescents in Trauma and Substance Abuse: Causes, Consequences, and Treatment of Comorbid Disorders. Edited by Ouimette P, Brown PJ. Washington, DC: American Psychological Association, 2003.

151. Crumley FE: Substance abuse and adolescent suicidal behavior. JAMA 263:3051–3056, 1990.

152. Ferguson DM, Horwood LJ, Swain-Campbell N: Cannabis use and psychosocial adjustment in adolescence and young adulthood. Addiction 97:1123–1135, 2002.

153. Brent DA, Perper JA, Allman C: Alcohol, firearms and suicide among youth: temporal trends in Allegheny County, Pennsylvania, 1960 to 1983. JAMA 257:3369–3372, 1987.

154. Friedman IM: Alcohol and unnatural deaths in San Francisco youths. Pediatrics 76:191–193, 1985.

155. Bukstein OG: Substance abuse, in Handbook of Aggressive and Destructive Behavior in Psychiatric Patients. Edited by Hersen M, Ammerman RT, Sisson LA. New York: Plenum, 1994, pp. 445–468.

156. Brent DA, Kolko DJ: The assessment and treatment of children and adolescents at risk for suicide, in Suicide Over the Life Cycle. Edited by Blumenthal SJ, Kupfer DJ. Washington, DC: American Psychiatric Press, 1990, pp. 253–302.

157. Brent DA, Perper JA, Goldstein CE, et al: Risk factors for adolescent suicide: a comparison of adolescent suicide victims with suicidal inpatients. Arch Gen Psychiatry 45:581–588, 1988.

158. Bukstein OG, Brent DB, Perper JA, et al: Risk factors for completed suicide among adolescents with a lifetime history of substance abuse: a case control study. Acta Psychiatr Scand 88:403–408, 1993.

159. Milan R, Halikas JA, Meller JE, et al: Psychopathology among substance abusing juvenile offenders. J Am Acad Child Adolesc Psychiatry 30:569–574, 1991.

160. Moss HB, Tarter RE: Substance abuse, aggression and violence: what are the connections? Am J on Addictions 2:149–160, 1993.

161. Giancola PR, Mezzich AC, Tarter RE: Disruptive, delinquent and aggressive behavior in female adolescents with a psychoactive substance use disorder: Relation to executive cognitive functioning. J Studies Alcohol 59:560–567, 1998.

162. Loeber R: Development and risk factors of juvenile antisocial behavior and delinquency. Clin Psychol Rev 10:1–41, 1990.

163. Loeber R: Antisocial behavior: more enduring than changeable? J Am Acad Child Adolesc Psychiatry 30: 393–397, 1991.

164. Robins L: Deviant Children Grown Up. Baltimore, MD: Williams & Wilkins, 1966.

165. Johnston LD, O'Malley P, Eveland L: Drugs and delinquency: a search for causal connections, in Longitudinal Research on Drug Use: Empirical Findings and Methodological Issues. Edited by Kandel DB. Washington, DC: Hemisphere-Wiley, 1978, pp. 137–156.

166. Eichelman B: Neurochemical and pharmacological aspects of aggressive behavior, in Psychopharmacology: The Third Generation of Progress. Edited by Melzer HY New York: Raven, 1987, pp. 697–706.

167. Ballanger JC, Goodwin FK, Major FL, et al: Alcohol and central serotonin metabolism in man. Arch Gen Psychiatry 36:224–227, 1979.

168. Roy A, Linnoila M: Alcoholism and suicide. Suicide Life Threat Behav 16:244–273, 1986.

169. Buydens-Branchey L, Branchey M, Noumair D, et al: Age of alcoholism onset, II: relationship to susceptibility to serotonin precursor availability. Arch Gen Psychiatry 46:231–236, 1989.

170. Linnoila M, DeJong J, Virkkunen M: Family history of alcoholism in violent offenders and impulsive fire setters. Arch Gen Psychiatry 46:613–616, 1989.

171. Fadda F, Rossetti ZL: Chronic ethanol consumption: from neuroadaptation to neurodegeneration. Prog Neurobiol 56:385–431, 1998.

172. Pfefferbaum A, Lim KO, Zipursky RB, Mathalon DH, Rosenbloom MJ, Lane B, Ha CN, Sullivan EV: Brain gray and white matter volume loss accelerates with aging in chronic alcohol-dependent subjects: a quantitative MRI study. Alcohol Clin Exp Res 16:1078–1089, 1992.

173. Bartzokis G, Beckson M, Lu PH, Edwards N, Bridge P, Mintz J: Brain maturation may be arrested in chronic cocaine addicts. Biol Psychiatry 51:605–611, 2002.

174. Bartzokis G, Beckson M, Lu PH, Edwards N, Rapoport R, Wiseman E, Bridge P: Age-related brain volume reductions in amphetamine and cocaine addicts and normal controls: implications for addiction research. Psychiatry Res 98:93–102, 2000.

175. Bjork JM, Grant SJ, Hommer DW: Cross-Sectional Volumetric analysis of brain atrophy in alcohol dependence: effects of drinking history and comorbid substance use disorder. Am J Psychiatry 160: 2038–2045, 2003.

176. DeBellis MD, Clark DB, Beers SR, Soloff PH, et al: Hippocampal volume in adolescent-onset alcohol use disorders. Am J Psychiatry 157:737–744, 2000.

177. Hill SY, DeBellis, MD, Keshavan MS, Lowers L, Shen S, Hall J, Pitts T: Right amygdala volume in adolescent and young adult offspring from families at high risk for developing alcoholism. Biol Psychiatry 49: 894–905, 2001.

178. Mayes LC, Granger RH: Teratologic and developmental effects of prenatal drug exposure: alcohol, heroin, marijuana and cocaine, in Child and Adolescent Psychiatry. Edited by Lewis M. Baltimore, MD: Williams & Wilkins, 1996, pp. 374–382.

179. Sampson PD, Stresissguth AP, Bookstein FL, et al: Incidence of fetal alcohol syndrome and prevalence of alcohol-related neurodevelopmental disorder. Tetrology 56:317–326, 1997.

180. Sokol RJ, Miller S, Reed G: Alcohol use during pregnancy: an epidemiological study. Alcohol Clin Exp Res 4:135–145, 1980.

181. Larkby C and Day N: The effects of prenatal alcohol exposure. Alcohol Health Res World 21:192–198, 1997.

182. Smith I, Coles C, Lancaster J, et al: The effect of volume and duration of prenatal ethanol exposure on neonatal physical and behavioral development. Neurobehav Toxicol Teratol 14:375–381, 1986.

183. Testa M, Quigley BM, Das ER: The effects of prenatal alcohol exposure on infant mental development: A meta-analytic review. Alcohol Alcoholism 38:295–304, 2003.

184. Day NL: Effects of prenatal alcohol exposure, in Maternal Substance Abuse and the Developing Nervous System. Edited by Zagon IS, Slotkin TA. Boston, MA: Academic Press, 1992, pp. 27–44.

185. Aronson M, Kyllerman M, Sabel KG, et al: Children of alcoholic mothers: developmental, perceptual, and behavioral characteristics as compared to matched controls. Acta Paediatr Scand 74:27–35, 1985.

186. Coles C, Brown R, Smith I, et al: Effects of prenatal exposure at school age, I: physical and cognitive development. Neurotoxicol Teratol 13:357–367, 1991.

187. Day NL, Richardson GA: Prenatal marijuana use: epidemiology, methodologic issues and infant outcome. Clin Perinatol 18:77, 1991.

188. Fried PA: Marijuana use by pregnant women: neurobehavioral effects in neonates. Drug Alcohol Depend 6:415–454, 1980.

189. Fried PA, Innes KS, Barnes MV: Soft use prior to and during pregnancy: a comparison of sample over a four year period. Drug Alcohol Depend 10:161–176, 1984.

190. Levy M, Koren G: Clinical toxicology of the neonate. Semin Perinatol 16:63–75, 1992.

191. Scher MS, Richardson GA, Coble PA, et al: The effects of prenatal alcohol and marijuana exposure: disturbances in neonatal sleep cycling and arousal. Pediatr Res 24:101–105, 1988.

192. Chirboga CA: Fetal alcohol and drug effects. Neurologist 9:267–279, 2003.

193. Anday H, Cohen ME, Kelley NE, et al: Effect of in utero cocaine exposure on startle and its modification. Dev Pharmacol Ther 12:137–145, 1989.

194. Mayes LC, Granger RH, Frank MA, et al: Neurobehavioral profiles of infants exposed to cocaine prenatally. Pediatrics 95:539–783, 1993.

195. Tronick EZ, Frank DA, Bateman DA et al: Late doe response effects of prenatal cocaine exposure on newborn neurobehavioral performance. Pediatrics 98:76–83, 1996.

196. Struthers JM, Hansen RL: Visual recognition in drug-exposed infants. J Dev Behav Pediatr 13:108–111, 1992.

197. Chasnoff IJ, Griffith DR, Freier C: Cocaine/polydrug use in pregnancy: 2-year follow-up. Pediatrics 89:284–289, 1992.

198. Richardson, GA: Prenatal cocaine exposure: A longitudinal study of development. Ann NY Acad Sci. 846:144–152, 1998.

199. Frank D, Augustyn M, Grant-Knight W, Pell T, Zuckerman B Growth, development, and behavior in early childhood following prenatal exposure: a systematic review. JAMA 285:1613–1625, 2001.

200. Zuckerman B, Frank DA, Mayes L: Cocaine-exposed infants and developmental outcomes. JAMA 287: 1990–1991, 2002.

201. Jeremy RJ, Hans SL: Behavior of neonates exposed in utero to methadone as assessed on the Brazelton scale. Infant Behav Dev 8:323–336, 1985.

202. Hans SL: Maternal opiate use and child development, in Maternal Substance Abuse and the Developing Nervous System. Edited by Zagon IS, Slotkin TA. Boston, MA: Academic Press, 1992, pp. 177–214.

203. Oloffson M, Buckley W Andersen GE, et al: Investigation of 89 children born by drug-dependent mothers: follow-up 1–10 years after birth. Acta Paediatr Scand 72:407–410, 1983.

204. Noland JS, Singer LT, Arendt RE, Minnes S, Short EJ, Bearer CF: Executive functioning in preschool-age children prenatally exposed to alcohol, cocaine, and marijuana. Alcoholism: Clinical and Experimental Research 27:647–656, 2003.

205. Miller TR, Lestina DC, Smith GS: Injury risk among medically identified alcohol and drug abusers. Alcoholism: Clinical and Experimental Research 25:54–59, 2001.

206. Milstein SG, Irwin CE: Accident-related behaviors in adolescents: a biopsychosocial view. Alcohol Drugs Driving 4:21–29, 1987.

207. Howland J, Hingson R: Alcohol as a risk factor for drownings: a review of the literature (1950–1985). Accid Anal Prev 20:19–20, 1988.

208. National Center for Health Statistics: Advance Reports of Final Mortality Statistics, 1990. Monthly Vital Statistics Reports 41:1–52, 1992.

209. Runyan CW Gerken EA: Epidemiology and prevention of adolescent injury: a review and research agenda. JAMA 262:2273–2279, 1989.

210. Hingson R, Howland J: Promoting safety in adolescents, in Promoting the Health of Adolescents: New Directions for the Twenty-First Century. Edited by Milstein SG, Peterson AC, Nightengale EO. London: Oxford University Press, 1993, pp. 305–327.

211. Tarter RE: Evaluation and treatment of adolescent substance abuse: a decision tree method. Am J Alcohol Abuse 16:1–46, 1990.

212. National Institute on Drug Abuse (NIDA): Preventing Drug Use Among Children and Adolescents: A Research-Based Guide. Rockville, MD: NIDA/NIH, 2001.

213. Wilens TE, Faraone SV, Biederman J, Gunawardene S: Does stimulant therapy of attention-deficit/hyperactivity disorder beget later substance abuse? A meta-analytic review of the literature. Pediatrics 111:179–85, 2003.

214. Kosten TR, O'Conner PG: Current Concepts: management of drug and alcohol withdrawal. N Engl J Med 348: 1786–1795, 2003.

215. O'Connor PG, Fiellin DA: Pharmacologic treatment of heroin-dependent patients. Ann Intern Med 133: 40–54, 2000.

216. Mayo-Smith MF: Pharmacologic management of alcohol withdrawal: a meta-analysis and evidence-based practice guideline. JAMA 278:144–151, 1997.

217. Riggs PD, Mikovich SK, Coffman LM, Crowley, TJ: Fluoxetine in drug-dependent delinquents with major depression: an open trial. J Child Adolesc Psychopharm 7: 87–95,1997.

218. Riggs PD, Leon SL, Mikulich SK, Pottle LC: An open trial of bupropion for ADHD in adolescents with substance use disorders and conduct disorder. J Am Acad Child Adolesc Psychiatry 37:1271–1278, 1998.

219. Cornelius JR, Bukstein OG, Birmaher B, Sallum IM, Pollock NK, Gershon S, Clark DB: Open label fluoxetine in depressed substance-abusing adolescents. Addic Behav 26:735–739, 2001.

220. Riggs PD, Mikulich SK, Hall S: Effects of pemoline on ADHD, antisocial behaviors, and substance use in adolescents with conduct disorder and substance use disorder. J Am Acad Child Adoles Psychiatry.

221. Geller B, Cooper TB, Sun K, Zimermann B, Frazier J, Williams M, Heath J: Double-blind and placebo-controlled study of lithium for adolescent bipolar disorders with secondary substance dependency. J Am Acad Child Adolesc Psychiatry 37:171–178, 1998.

222. Williams RJ, Chang SY: A comprehensive and comparative review of adolescent substance abuse treatment outcome. Clin Psychol: Sci Pract 7:38–166, 2000.

223. Deas D, Thomas SE: An overview of controlled studies of adolescent substance abuse treatment. Am J Addictions 10:178–189, 2001.

224. Hser Y, Grella CE, Hubbard RL, Hsieh S, Fletcher BW, Brown BS, Anglin M: An evaluation of drug treatments for adolescents in 4 US cities. Arch Gen Psychiatry 58:689–695, 2001.

225. Grella CE, Hser Y, Joshi V, Rounds-Bryant J: Drug treatment outcomes for adolescents with comorbid mental and substance use disorders. J Nerv Ment Dis 189:384–392, 2001.

226. Brown SA, Vik PN, Creamer VA: Characteristics of relapse following adolescent substance abuse treatment. Addict Behav 14:291–300, 1989.

227. Brown SA, Vik PW, McQuaid JR, et al: Severity of psychosocial stress and outcome of alcoholism treatment. J Abnorm Psycho 99:344–348, 1990.

228. Alford GS, Koehler RA, Leonard J: Alcoholics anonymous-narcotics anonymous model inpatient treatment of chemically dependent adolescents: A 2-year outcome study. J Stud Alcohol 52:118–126, 1991.

229. Brown SA, Myers MG, Mott MA, Vik PW: Correlates of success following treatment for adolescent substance abuse. Appl Prev Psychol 3:61–73, 1994.

230. Winters KC, Stinchfield RD, Opland E: The effectiveness of the Minnesota Model approach in the treatment of adolescent drug abusers. Addiction 95:601–612, 2000.

Neuropsychiatric Aspects of Neurologic Disorders of Children and Adolescents

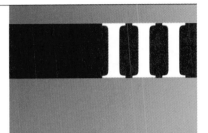

Dyslexia

17

Kytja K.S. Voeller, MD

Dyslexia is the most common learning disability, accounting for 80% of all learning disabilities and, depending on the way it is defined, affecting approximately 5 to 20% of children and adults (1, 2). There are a number of relatively synonymous terms—reading disability, specific reading retardation, reading backwardness, and in some contexts, illiteracy or the more general term "learning disability" is used to mean dyslexia. In the United Kingdom, the term dyslexia is often applied to adults who have acquired lesions that impair reading—a group of patients that are described as alexic in the United States.

The definition of dyslexia, developed by the Orton Dyslexia Society Research Committee is as follows: ". . . a specific language-based disorder of constitutional origin characterized by difficulties in single word decoding, usually reflecting insufficient phonological processing"(3). Important features of this definition include the emphasis on *language* rather than the visual processing of written text and the focus on the mechanics of the reading process ("difficulties in *single word decoding*") rather than on comprehending what is read.

Many of the essential behavioral characteristics of dyslexia were described with great accuracy in the late 1800s. In an article in the British Medical Journal, published in1896, W. Pringle Morgan described a 14-year-old boy who was "always bright. . .quick at games, and in no way inferior to others of his age" but had been unable to learn to read, despite having been tutored since the age of 7 years. His instructors described him "as the smartest lad in the school if the instruction were. . .oral." In addition to providing examples of the boy's difficulty reading, Morgan also noted that when he attempted to write his own name, "Percy", he spelled it "Precy" and seemed unaware of the error. Morgan used Kussmaul's term to describe the child's diagnosis—*caecitas syllabaris et verbalis*—word-blindness. (Kussmaul had coined this term in 1877 to describe acquired word-blindness in adults following a lesion in the left angular gyrus in right-handed people.). He

also called it *congenital* word blindness, noting that it was "due most probably to defective development of that region of the brain, disease of which in adults produces practically the same symptoms—that is. . .the angular gyrus" (4) (p. 1378).

In 1900, in an article in Lancet (nestled between one article describing surgical treatment of open sinuses in the pre-antibiotic era, and another discussing the incubation period of plague), Hinshelwood described four children with "congenital word-blindness" (5). His classical description of a dyslexic child could be applied to any dyslexic child 105 years later.

"A boy, aged 11 years, was at school for four and a half years, but was finally sent away because he could not be taught to read. His father informed me that he was a considerable time at school before the defect was noted. He had such an excellent memory that he learned his lessons by heart; in fact, his first little reading-book he knew by heart, so that whenever it came to his turn he could from memory repeat his lesson, although he could not read the words. His father also informed me that in every respect, unless in his ability to learn to read, the boy seemed quite as intelligent as any of his brothers and sisters. His auditory memory was excellent and better than that of any of other members of the family. When a passage was repeated to him aloud he could commit it to memory very rapidly. . . . When I examined the boy first on March 4th, 1900. . . he seemed a smart and intelligent lad for his years. He knew the alphabet by heart, repeating it rapidly and correctly. He could recognize by sight, however, only a very few letters and those not with any degree of certainty. He could spell correctly most simple words of one syllable, such as "cat," "dog," "man," "boys," etc., but he could not recognize by sight the simplest and commonest words, such as "the," "of," "in," etc. He had no difficulty in recognizing all other visual objects, such as faces, places, and pictures. On each page of the little primer in which I tested him there was a picture of some object. . . He at once recognized each picture—e.g., a cat. I would then ask him to spell the word which he nearly always did quite correctly. On asking him to pick out the word "cat" on the page he was unable to do it. . . On testing him with figures I found that he could repeat from memory fluently and correctly numbers up to 100. He could also perform mentally simple sums of addition. He could not, however, recognize all the figures by sight, but he knew them better than the letters and recognized a greater number of them. . . (pp. 1506–1507).

The second case described a 10-year-old boy who, although he had learned to recognize many words, was still a very poor reader. Hinshelwood noted another important feature of the clinical profile:

Another very significant fact about this boy, who was otherwise very intelligent, was the fact, told to us by his father, that he never read for amusement. As his father expressed it, "reading seemed to take a good deal out of him" (p. 1507).

By 1904, Hinshelwood was well aware that congenital word-blindness ran in families. A family of 11 children had been referred to him by a teacher. The first seven children had posed no particular educational challenges, but the last four boys (numbers eight through 11) had great difficulty learning to read. The children's teacher noted that ". . .he had never before met with anything like the difficulties encountered in attempting to teach these four boys to read. . ." (6) (p. 1230). Hinshelwood further noted in his 1911 paper that ". . .

it is evident that the abnormal condition of the visual memory centre is a matter of faulty development, and it is probable that in most cases of congenital work-blindness the condition is the result neither of disease nor injury at birth, but of defective development of this definite cerebral area occurring in the early stages of embryonic growth. This view, that congenital word-blindness is the result of faulty development and not of disease or injury, derives considerable further support from the fact that homonymous hemianopsia, which is so frequently associated with acquired word-blindness, has never been met in any case of congenital word-blindness" (7) (p. 609).

Hinshelwood was also interested in approaches to the treatment of congenital word blindness.

I have. . . insisted on the fact that all these children should be taught alone and not in a class along with other children with normally developed brains. The contrast between their own difficulty and the comparative ease with which other children learn to read is a constant source of discouragement both to themselves and to their teachers. The task is abandoned as hopeless, and such children often leave school without being able to read. . . I always advocate a number of short reading lessons every day rather than one long one. It is only the very frequent repetition of the visual impressions that we can hope for the retention of the visual word memories in the brains of these patients. Hence the best method is to give them short and frequent reading lessons during the day without anything leading to exhaustion. At the outset I have often found great assistance in teaching these patients to read by building up the words with block letters, and thus deepening the visual impressions by associating them with the tactile ones (p. 1232).

His report of J, an 18 year old, identifies another important feature of dyslexics:

The most interesting point in J.'s career was that any progress made in reading had been accomplished during the last four years, after he had left school. He has thus practically taught himself. He is a great football enthusiast and. . . since leaving school he has got the Referee every Monday and Friday, which gives detailed accounts of all the football matches. Every night. . . after his work, he would spend a large part of the evening in poring over this newspaper and attempting with the help of others to spell out the results of the matches in which he was interested. At first he could do this only very imperfectly and laboriously with the help of others, but now he can do this without help. On testing his power of reading with a child's first primer I found that he could only read about one half of the words, without spelling them, the other half he could read if allowed to spell them out letter by letter, so that he could not read fluently even the child's primer. . . . with an ordinary book. . . he recognized by sight very few words of more than one syllable. . . When I examined his ability to read football news, I found he could do this much better, as he could recognize by sight a much greater number of words. . .") (7) (pp. 1230–1231).

J's 16-year-old brother dropped out of school at the age of 14 years and was working as a miner. He did not make any attempt to learn to read and never looks at any written material. He refused to let Dr. Hinshelwood examine him.

These descriptions are remarkably accurate in that they capture the characteristic features of the dyslexic individual and the dyslexic's attempts at reading. There is often a striking discrepancy between the dyslexic's intellectual ability (normal or above-average) and ability to read. They can often grasp arithmetical computations with relative ease, and some have great expertise in this area. Hinshelwood recognized that the deficit not so much related to the visual system as it was to a specific segment of associational cortex. Although dyslexic children often have great difficulty recognizing letters and words they are quite able to recognize objects and other aspects of the environment. Many, but not all young dyslexic children, show a tendency to reverse letters, and although the absence of letter reversal does not rule out the diagnosis in any way. It is, however, unusual to observe reversals in a 14-year-old. Another similarity, which sadly persists to the present day, is the fact that the child described above by Hinshelwood was not recognized as having difficulty reading until the age of 11 years. Even now, a child who is able to use a series of clever compensatory strategies and does not pose behavioral problems in the classroom may not be identified as having a reading problem until third or fourth grade. Hinshelwood was fully aware of the fact that dyslexic children readily grasp the difference between their struggles with reading and that of their normally reading peers. Most children are aware of this by the time they are in first grade, although they usually do not volunteer the information. However, it is important for the clinician to be aware of this fact, because it contributes to the young child's sense of defeat and inadequacy. The risk in the dyslexic children population for psychiatric disability is significant. Hinshelwood also noted that reading was extremely effortful and attention-demanding for these children. As the 10-year-old's father astutely noted, "reading seemed to take a good deal out of him" (p. 1507). Moreover, he recognized how this sense of frustration and defeat can lead to abandoning school in favor of a job as a laborer.

Hinshelwood also clearly recognized that these children could be taught to read, but that they required a high level of repetition at frequent intervals. He also understood that with enough motivation and repetition, a dyslexic can master a relatively specialized reading vocabulary but this did not generalize to global improvement in reading skills. The fact that with a lot of motivation the 18-year-old essentially developed relatively functional reading skills specific to football is quite characteristic.

Moreover, Hinshelwood also suggested that dyslexia involved some sort of anomalous development of the parietal-occipital region. Dejerine had published his paper describing acquired alexia in an adult with a lesion in the angular gyrus 10 years ealier (8). The main difference between these dyslexic children, who lived over a century ago, and those who attend school at present, is that they would not be currently banished from school because of reading backwardness.

In the 1920s, Samuel Orton (9, 10) suggested that dyslexia was the result of some sort of incomplete or delayed development of left hemisphere language processing functions. He coined the term strephosymbolia, "twisted symbols." In the 1950s and 1960s, the features of dyslexia were blended into other behavioral disorders of childhood, such as hyperkinetic syndrome of childhood, and the terms minimal brain damage or minimal brain dysfunction came into vogue and often overlapped in an unclear way with dyslexia. At the time, there was considerable controversy about the etiology of dyslexia and many educators and clinicians viewed dyslexia as the result of some sort of visual disturbance. Rutter and Yule observed that the concept of reading retardation suffered from a "vagueness of definitions and a general looseness in the use of words. . ." but even more so "from fundamental disputes about the nature of reading problems" (11) (p. 181).

Norman Geschwind and his colleagues played a crucial role in refocusing attention on the neural features of dyslexia. In 1976, Denckla and Rudel made the significant observation that dyslexic children did not perform as well as normally reading peers on a confrontation naming test and thus appeared to be relatively anomic (12). An additional extremely important contribution was that they were much slower than controls in their performance on rapid automatized naming tasks (13, 14). These tasks required that the child rapidly generate names for common, over-learned items, such as primary colors (generally mastered at the latest by kindergarten), numbers, letters, or common

objects. This series of tasks involved presenting the child a page of the same six targets (e.g., six primary colors, or six letters) arranged in random order. The child was asked to "read" these items aloud while being timed by a stop watch. In addition to a relatively rapid increase in rate across the early childhood years, there was also a highly significant difference between dyslexic children and controls. This simple task continues to be studied by dyslexia researchers and is one of the fundamental components of the diagnostic workup of a dyslexic child.

Although Hinshelwood had postulated the presence of some sort of anomalous neuronal development involving the angular gyrus, this concept had been largely lost in the focus on the visual impairments of dyslexics. In 1979, Galaburda and Kemper (15) described neuronal migration anomalies in the brain of a young man who had a well-documented history of severe dyslexia. Galaburda subsequently defined many of the cytoarchitectonic features of a series of dyslexic brains (16). The development of magnetic resonance imaging (MRI), positron emission tomography (PET), and functional MRI (fMRI) techniques has also contributed immensely to the understanding of normal reading and dyslexia. Many of these studies were conducted with support from the Learning Disability Centers that were funded by NICHD grants under the leadership of David Gray, Reid Lyon, and Duane Alexander.

EPIDEMIOLOGY

Estimates of prevalence of dyslexia are dependent on the diagnostic and definitional criteria that are used, and, to some extent, the population that is sampled. Yule and colleagues (17) noted that there were large regional variations in the prevalence of dyslexia (e.g., two times as frequent in London as on the Isle of Wight). In general, fewer children are identified as reading disabled when disability is defined in terms of a discrepancy between cognitive ability (IQ) and reading level. The magnitude of the discrepancy that is used in identifying cases will also affect prevalence estimates. Using discrepancy criteria, prevalence estimates ranged from 3.5 to 6% when reading disability was defined as a reading level falling -2 S.D. below the level predicted by IQ. In an epidemiologic sample in the Connecticut public schools, the prevalence estimate when research criteria were used was 7.6%, which is slightly higher than the prevalence figures based on school identification procedures. When an absolute measure, such as single word reading or phonological awareness tasks are used, the incidence of the dyslexic trait is much closer to 20% (1, 18).

GENDER DIFFERENCES

Early studies reported that more boys than girls have reading disability (male: female ratios ranging from 2:1 to 5:1

have been reported) (19, 20). However, based on their epidemiologic study in the Connecticut public school system, Shaywitz and colleagues observed that school systems tended to identify many more boys than girls; in a sample of 414 children, aged 7 to 8 years, reading disability was noted in 8.7% of boys versus 6.9% of girls and a year later (mean age 8.7 years), there were 9.0% boys and 6.0% girls (2). Shaywitz and colleagues suggested that identification of a reading disability might in part be colored by the presence of comorbid disruptive behavior problems in the boys, which would bring the boys to the attention of the school authorities. Dyslexic girls without behavior problems would be much less likely to be identified, and thus the prevalence of dyslexia in females would likely be underestimated in this context.

However, based on a review of several of large epidemiological studies, Rutter and colleagues concluded that there is, indeed, a male preponderance (21). This was based on two large epidemiological studies conducted in the United States; the National Collaborative Perinatal Project, which involved 32,223 women and their children (22), and a survey encompassing 5,718 children in Rochester, Minnesota (1). In addition, data from four large epidemiological studies totaling 9,799 subjects were drawn from New Zealand (the Dunedin Multidisciplinary Health and Development Study and Christchurch Health and Development Study), England (Office for National Statistics Study), and the Environmental Risk Longitudinal Twin Study from England and Wales. These studies varied in terms of definitional criteria as some involved IQ and others did not, but all the studies used standardized testing and did not involve samples with a referral bias. Moreover, although there was considerable variation in the magnitude of the differences between boys and girls, the authors concluded that in New Zealand, the United Kingdom, and the United States, dyslexia was much more likely in boys than in girls. In two family aggregation studies in which members of entire families were evaluated for the presence of language impairment, articulatory deficits, and dyslexia there were more affected males than females. Although much smaller in scope, this is nonetheless instructive as it included entire families (23).

LINGUISTIC AND COGNITIVE FEATURES OF DYSLEXIA

The characteristic feature of dyslexia is the inability to learn to read efficiently. For the normal reader, reading is an easy, pleasurable, and efficient process. For the dyslexic, it is an effortful, frustrating, and time-consuming undertaking. The core deficit in dyslexia involves impaired phonological processing. Wagner and colleagues defined phonological processing as having three components: phonological awareness, phonological memory, and rapid naming (24). Numerous studies have demonstrated that these various

aspects of phonological processing are strongly correlated with the ability to learn to read (25, 26). In kindergarten and first grade, performance on phonological awareness tasks predicts later reading and spelling skills in both normal children and future dyslexics (27, 28). Elbrow, in a study of Danish children, noted that letter naming, phoneme awareness, and distinctness of phonological representation (defined as the quality of unstressed vowels in phonologically complex words) were statistically highly significant contributors to a future dyslexic profile (29).

Phonological Awareness and the Motor Theory of Speech

Phonological awareness is the ability to segment and manipulate the phonemes in one's native language and is the deficit that affects most dyslexics. Lack of phonological awareness makes it impossible for the young dyslexic child to sort out the phonologic structure of his native language. For example, if one tests an English-speaking dyslexic child (and many adults), the /p/ in the word "top" is not easily recognized as the same /p/ as in the word "pansy" or "pot." When asked to perform an elision task (e.g., "say tiger without saying /r/") the word generated might be "tie." Or, when asked to segment (that is, to say each sound separately), a word like "beast" the child might say "b-ee-st" or "bee-st," being unable to develop a representation of the four different phonemes in that word. This ability to represent the phonemic structure of one's native language is what is referred to as "the alphabetic principle" (30). The alphabetic principle also involves understanding that words are composed of phonemes and the phonemes are represented in a relatively systematic way by letters.

An important contribution to the understanding of phonological awareness came from Liberman and Mattingly at Haskin's Laboratory, who put forth "the motor theory of speech," which, in simplified terms, means that to decode the speech signal in language, the listener uses the articulatory gestures which create the speech signal to perceive the signal as well. Essentially, they postulated that there is a speech module and that speech production and speech perception are computationally similar. Liberman and colleagues also suggested that it is not so much the acoustic signal which is involved in the perception of phonemes, but rather the articulatory motor movements which are somehow "run backwards" and thus used in the process of perceiving or decoding the acoustic signal. This is the basis for the "McGurk effect" in which an observer will "hear" a different vocal signal than the one actually presented if they are observing a face making a different articulatory gesture (31). Moreover, Liberman and Mattingly point out that there is an innateness in this process. Very young infants show a distinct preference for looking at faces that are articulating sounds that match the sound they are hearing and are much less interested in faces in which there is a mismatch between the vocal signal and the articulated gesture (32, 33). This was a very significant observation, because it provided a way of understanding at least some of the deficits in dyslexia and, more importantly, providing an effective approach for treatment.

If the articulatory motor theory of speech perception is correct, then one would expect that individuals who had weak phonological awareness might also have an imprecise awareness of the position of the articulatory structures that generate specific phonemes. Montgomery described an experiment in which adult dyslexics were asked to select pictures of the articulatory gestures associated with the production of English phonemes. The performance of the dyslexics was significantly impaired relative to that of controls (34). A decade later, Zatorre conducted a PET scan study on normal adults who were asked to attend to specific aspects of the speech signal. When the subjects were asked to discriminate between specific phonemes, increased activity was noted in Broca's area (the motor speech area), rather than in areas involved in the perception of auditory signal (35). An fMRI study employed a first sound-matching task (the task required subjects to view pictures of objects, compare the first sounds of the name, and indicate if they are the same or different). Control tasks involved baseline matching tasks and a visual matching task that controlled for the visual complexity of the stimuli. The inferior and superior frontal gyrus was selectively activated in response to the phonological comparison task, a finding in agreement with Zatorre's study and additional support for the articulatory motor theory of speech (36). Ruff and colleagues compared dyslexics and controls on a pseudopassive listening task to /pa/ and /ta/ syllables. In response to categorically deviant stimuli, activations of the left angular gyrus, right inferior frontal gyrus, and the right superior cingulate cortex occurred. These regions were not activated in the dyslexic group (37). In another study in which articulatory gestures were observed under fMRI monitoring, subjects activated left primary somatosensory cortex SI when viewing another individual speaking (38).

Thus, it would appear that, in comparison to normal subjects, dyslexics are impaired in their ability to develop accurate internal representations of the motor gestures associated with speech production (39). As a result, the ability of dyslexics to isolate and sequence phonologic information is impaired and phonological awareness is affected. Functional neuroimaging studies suggest that they do not activate critical areas like the left inferior frontal gyrus that appears to be the fundamental site for phonological processing.

A possible mechanism involves anomalous development of mirror neurons. Mirror neurons are located in the rostral part of monkey ventral premotor cortex (area F5) in the area homologous to Broca's area (the inferior frontal gyrus) in the human. These neurons fire when the animal performs a goal-directed hand action and when it observes another individual performing the same or a similar action. Mirror neurons also fire during mouth movements (40). They underlie the ability to learn motor behaviors by observation and it would make sense that they underlie the acquisition of speech, given the fact that speech involves motor articulatory movements. The infant's preference to observing a moving mouth which is uttering sounds that are correctly synchronized with the verbalizations may underlie the acquisition of language and likely involve minor neurosis.

Phonological Memory

Phonological memory or working auditory memory (or Baddeley's "phonological loop") is the ability to keep verbal information "in mind" for a few seconds (41). A weak phonological memory has also been shown to predict difficulty in phonologically encoding verbal material. Children with phonological memory weakness have difficulty sounding out words (which requires being able to keep the first part of the word in mind while generating the last sounds). They also perform poorly when asked to learn verbal sequences; the rate at which they learn new words is impaired (42, 43).

Rapid Naming

Rapid naming is essentially a measure of "eye-to-mouth" time, the ability to rapidly encode visual information into oral articulatory sequences. In the young child as well as older individuals, rapid naming speed, particularly the speed of naming letters, rather than objects, is a strong predictor of later reading fluency (44–46). Because rapid automatized naming involves two neural processes—seeing and speaking—one important question is the extent to which rapid naming is related to the visual system versus the oral language system. Compton devised several different versions of a rapid automatized letter naming task. In one condition, letters were phonologically similar; in the other they were visually similar. Dyslexics performed more poorly than controls only on the task that demanded a greater level of phonological decoding skill (49).

Not all dyslexic children have deficits in all three areas. Some children, however, are impaired in both phonological awareness and rapid automatized naming. These children are described as having a "double deficit," and appear to have greater difficulty learning to read than those with deficits restricted to either phonological awareness or rapid naming (45, 50).

THE DYSLEXIC CHILD ENTERS SCHOOL

Even before the dyslexic child enters kindergarten, he lags behind peers in his ability to recognize and name letters. By the time dyslexics are ready to move on to first grade, there is considerable variability: some future dyslexics know most of their letter names, others remain confused through first grade. However, to a trained observer, it is apparent that letter recognition is not an automatic, fluent process. These children do not seem to grasp the alphabetic principle; that is they do not understand the process of "sounding out" words. This skill is essential for a beginning reader because every day, the child is confronted with unknown words. Many of these words are known to the child who uses them in daily life, words such as mother, ball, and dog. Although they are part of the child's oral vocabulary, if the child cannot apply a phonic strategy to decode the word, it is impossible to match the word to his internal vocabulary (51–53). The only other solution (besides guessing) is to attempt to store the word in visual memory. This, however, is a limited resource.

By second grade, most normal readers have acquired a workable sight-word vocabulary and have some skill in tackling the decoding of words that they do not know by sight. Given anything that is remotely interesting to read, they are quite willing to undertake the task of decoding unknown words as they are usually successful even when working independently. Compared to normally reading peers, the dyslexic has a much more restricted repertoire of sight words and lacks age- and grade-appropriate strategies for applying phonic strategies for decoding unknown words. Most dyslexic children grow tired of attempting the decoding process and arrive at the strategy of guessing what a word is based on the first letter or two, or if they are really thinking strategically, trying to make an informed guess based on context. These are, obviously, strategies that will not work out well because their attempts at decoding are fraught with errors. On the other hand, a good reader can make a reasonably informed guess if she can decode at least part of a word correctly. Regardless of the strategy that is used, the dyslexic child does not have fluent word recognition. It should be apparent that this situation does not improve by itself, and every day the dyslexic child loses a little ground. This inexorable failure to keep up with peers is subtle and if one sees a child on a day-to-day basis, it is not apparent that he or she is steadily losing ground. Because even the most dyslexic child makes a little progress, these small gains are encouraging, and allow parents and teachers to overlook the fact that the rate at which the child is learning to read is much slower than that of peers. Parents of young children who are still denying the child's difficulty in reading can state blithely that "Billy is making good progress."

In first and second grades, normal readers practice analyzing and decoding more complex sound structures, such as the representations of long vowel sounds, consonant and vowel digraphs, word endings, root words, prefixes, and suffixes to gain information about the meaning of words. A normal reader in second grade routinely performs the following processes: when encountering an unfamiliar word, decoding it, matching it to the internal lexicon, and repeating this process until the word becomes a "sight word" that can be recognized rapidly and effortlessly. This requires consistent, accurate decoding and a great deal of

repetition (54). In addition, the child needs to be able to remember the components of the word while attempting to decode it, which requires the ability to store the sounds in working memory. Children who do not have an adequate working memory buffer find this process quite difficult. The young dyslexic child finds reading so difficult that she tends to avoid it and thus not acquire a "sight word" vocabulary. This sets up a vicious cycle: the fewer sight words the child learns, the more difficult it is to read, particularly because the teacher's expectations for reading fluency are increasing, not remaining the same. Thus, by the time a dyslexic child is in third grade, there is usually a significant gap between the sight words that he has compared to those of normally reading peers.

An important aspect of the difference between the young normal reader and the dyslexic is the fact that except for the word-length effect, the second grader's performance does not differ qualitatively from that of the older normal reader. Word familiarity effects are apparent by second grade which indicates that the rapid visual recognition of previously encountered words is occurring. Until the fifth to sixth grade, normal children can get bogged down attempting to decode long words. Experience essentially decreases processing speed (55). By 11 to 12 years of age, the normal reader differs from the adult only in needing to take time to decode unknown words. The normal adult reader is able to process text at an extremely rapid rate. Less than 250 milliseconds after viewing a written word, the visual system extracts the information necessary for the computations in the language system. This occurs regardless of the size of the letters, the number of letters that compose the word (that is, in the range of three to six letters) the font, or the viewing angle (56). Letters are identified more efficiently when they are embedded in words than when they occur outside of words (57).

DYSLEXIC INFANTS, TODDLERS, AND PRESCHOOLERS

What are dyslexics like *before* they enter kindergarten? Are there are any characteristic features in the young child which would make it possible to identify them very early and initiate treatment before they start to lose ground in the reading process?

There is a considerable body of research that suggests that children at risk for dyslexia can be identified long before they enter kindergarten. Molfese described a study in which 186 full-term newborns were tested within 36 hours of birth and then retested each year. At age 8 years, they underwent an IQ test and a reading screening test. The newborns who are later diagnosed with dyslexia could be identified at birth (and distinguished from the newborns who later were normal readers) by their response to speech and nonspeech sounds using auditory event-related potentials (58). A longitudinal study of Finnish infants born into dyslexic families and those from nondyslexic families also demonstrated differences in the way the at-risk infants processed speech sounds (59). At 6 months of age, the babies from dyslexic families continue to manifest differences in processing speech sounds (60). In addition to these very early differences in sound-processing, the children at risk for dyslexia began to manifest subtle differences in development by the time they are 2 years of age. Up to that point, they did not differ from the control population in motor or early language development, or cognitive ability. However, around 2 years of age, subtle deficits in language began to be apparent. These consisted mainly in slightly shorter length of sentences. Any mild delay in language did not persist, unless the child came from a dyslexic family. By the time the children were 40 months old, the performance of those from dyslexic families began to differ significantly from that of the controls on phonological and naming tasks (61). Between 18 and 24 months, the investigators were able to identify two groups of children: those with relatively slow motor development and those with fast motor development. The children at risk for dyslexia who also had slow motor development had a smaller vocabulary and generated shorter sentences than all the other children (62). Gallagher and colleagues followed a group of children identified as genetically at risk for dyslexia and a control group who did not have a family history of dyslexia. At the age of 6 years, 57% of the at-risk group was delayed in reading acquisition, compared to 12% of controls. The children in the literacy-delayed group also manifested delays in speech and language development (63).

By age 4 to 5 years, it becomes possible to identify children who are likely to evolve into future dyslexics as differences between the "at risk" group and normal controls becomes more striking. In the study by Gallagher and colleagues, described previously, letter knowledge at 45 months was the strongest predictor of reading at age 6 years. Children at risk performed more poorly on tasks assessing letter-sound knowledge, naming, and phonemic awareness (29, 64–67).

As these dyslexic children move through school, the gap between the rate at which the normal reader and the dyslexic acquire new sight words and develop fluency widens with each passing month. School-based special education interventions, which cannot deliver phonological training at a level of sufficient intensity or repetition, do not substantially improve the child's reading or decrease the magnitude of the gap. At best the rate at which the gap widens may be slowed (68, 69).

A factor that likely contributes to the widening gap in fluency between the dyslexic child and peers is the fact that dyslexic children do not practice reading to the extent that their normal peers do. This lack of exposure to print may also increase the degree to which the neural connections are not maintained. It is a "use it or lose it" proposition. This concept has considerable support from a PET study performed on the oldest daughter in Portuguese house-

holds. The custom in the past was that the oldest daughter remained at home to raise her younger siblings, who went to school and learned to read and write. The illiterate older sisters did not. When these women were tested on a phonological awareness task, it was apparent, both from the activation patterns and from their test performance, that they had a marked deficit in phonological awareness and also a much reduced pattern of activation compared to their younger literate siblings (70). There is no reason to believe that this group of women represented a cluster of adult dyslexics, as their younger siblings were efficient readers. Thus, it would appear that even a brain that would have little difficulty learning to read may not do so if appropriate stimulation is not present.

THE DYSLEXIC ADOLESCENT AND ADULT

As the dyslexic child moves into adolescence and young adulthood, many begin to acquire some degree of reading skill, but they are often not very efficient in reading and may take twice as long to read as nondyslexic peers. One bright dyslexic college student commented that his friends could read a chapter in an hour and it took him the entire afternoon. However, deficits in spelling and writing continue to impair their academic performance. In the older student, spelling is often a more sensitive indication of dyslexia than reading (71).

These deficits also do not go away with maturation, but persist, to a greater or lesser extent, into adulthood. Although many dyslexic adults ultimately learn to read, many do not read for pleasure, describe themselves as "terrible spellers," and have difficulty trying to learn a foreign language. (The process of learning a foreign language is hard because it often requires applying the alphabetic principle to a new set of phonemes.) Some dyslexic adults have managed to acquire relatively good reading skills, but even these "compensated" dyslexics continue to exhibit both the phonological deficits and the characteristic pattern of brain activation compared to nondyslexic controls (72, 73) (*Paulesu 1996*).

It is important for professionals who work with dyslexic children to understand the persistence into adulthood and the potential long-term impact on function in adulthood. In one longterm study, subjects who were re-evaluated in their thirties, had lower grades in high school, completed fewer years of formal education, and tended to gravitate to unskilled or semiskilled jobs (*Felsenfeld 1994*) (74).

SUCCESSFUL ADULT DYSLEXICS

A few dyslexics go on to become quite successful, even in careers that demand a high level of reading and writing. Fink described an extremely productive and well-published scientist who was a distinguished professor and a member of the National Academy of Sciences. He had consented to being examined Dr. Fink using many of the same tests that are administered to dyslexic children. The characteristic dyslexic profile was still present; he continued to have significant deficits in sight-word reading and phonological decoding strategies. However, he had mastered the vocabulary in his field of work well enough to produce numerous scientific articles (75). This is not an isolated case. The author had the experience of administering the Lindamood Auditory Conceptualization Test (76) (a phonological awareness assessment) to a successful MD/PhD researcher whose score fell at an elementary school level. These cases are similar to that of the young man, described by Hinshelwood, who acquired a specialized vocabulary so that he could follow local football games.

Adult dyslexics, particularly those who are successful, seem to gravitate to specific occupations. They are likely to become architects, movie stars, electrical and mechanical engineers, high-ranking managers, accountants, and finance officers. Many CEOs of large corporations are self-described dyslexics. *The Sunday Times* (London), reportedly ran a story about this group: "You don't have to be dyslexic, but it helps. A study has revealed that millionaires are significantly more likely to suffer from the condition than the rest of the population. . . . About 40 percent of the 300 studied had been diagnosed with the condition. . ." (77, 78). In the medical field, dyslexics often gravitate to radiology, psychiatry, pathology, and surgery. A number of dentists are dyslexic. The fact that an individual has successfully negotiated high school and, in some cases, college, does not eliminate the possibility that he or she is dyslexic. One successful 40-year-old architect, whose son was evaluated for dyslexia and attention deficit–hyperactivity disorder (ADHD), presented himself for an evaluation, which revealed that he was indeed dyslexic and also had ADHD. He reported that he had worked with a psychotherapist who told him that he could not possibly be dyslexic because he had successfully graduated from college. The architect reported that he had gotten through college in a high state of anxiety, studying all the time. He had also been advised by his high school counselor that he was not college material.

DEVELOPMENTAL LANGUAGE DISORDER AND DYSLEXIA

A substantial percentage of children with these phonological processing deficits also have a language disorder. The extent of the overlap between these two entities is not precisely worked out, but there is little doubt, based on numerous studies on somewhat different populations, that many children with phonological processing deficits also have a language disorder. The risk for later reading dis-

ability conferred by deficits in phonological awareness is well established and has been reviewed previously. Phonological awareness deficits are associated with language disorder. There is also an extensive literature indicating that language disorders identified in the toddler confer a high risk for future reading disability (23, 63, 65–67, 79–83). Some of the difficulty arises from the fact that although all of these disorders lie on the same developmental pathway, they emerge at different times in a child's life. In addition, at certain points in development, the range of "normal" is very broad and only children at the very severe end would be identified with confidence. The definitive diagnosis of language disorder in the young child is difficult and there is considerable examiner disagreement (84, 85). The normal range of language development is so broad and there are so few well-standardized test instruments that making a firm diagnosis at the age of 2 or 3 years is difficult and only children who manifest very severe expressive or receptive language deficits can be identified with certainty. By the age of 4 to 5 years, the diagnosis of a language disorder is easier, in part, because some standardized tests are available. However, children do not read at this age, so that it is technically not possible to apply a label of dyslexia. During the first two grades of elementary school, although some formal test instruments are available, the variance is again quite large, and only children at the very severe end of the spectrum can be identified with certainty. As a result, defining a developmental pathway that starts with atypical responses to phonemes in a laboratory in the newborn period and linking that to a child with a reading disability at age 10 years is not yet possible. However, if one considers the longitudinal studies that cover segments of this developmental trajectory, the suggestion that phonological awareness deficits is linked to early language disorder and both predict later reading disability with great consistency is easier to accept. However, at best, one can only use an "at risk" modifier to the diagnosis; that is, "this four year-old is *at risk* for dyslexia in the future."

There is one other factor that will increase the certainty of this diagnosis and that is knowing with some certainty that other family members have a language disorder and/or dyslexia. The results of two family aggregation studies that assessed the co-occurrence of oral language impairment and reading impairment in children with developmental language disorder concluded that affected members were more likely to have both oral language and reading impairment than either impairment alone (23). For any individual child, this increases the probability that he or she is at risk, but it lacks the certainty of a categorical diagnosis. However, this approach would have some appeal for clinicians and educators who are interested in preventing future dysfunction in a young child. At the point that the genetic markers for these disorders are known, the identification of the young child who is at risk will be somewhat easier.

DYSLEXIA AND PSYCHIATRIC COMORBIDITY

In the previous discussion, the close relationship between phonological awareness deficits, language disorder, and dyslexia was reviewed. The next question is the degree to which early language disorder and/or reading disorder are associated with comorbid psychiatric disorders. There are a number of studies that support the concept that language disorder and dyslexia confer a risk for subsequent emotional problems. The psychiatric diagnoses described as most frequently associated with dyslexia include ADHD, oppositional defiant disorder, conduct disorder, depression, and anxiety disorder.

There is a significant overlap between ADHD and dyslexia, regardless of whether one examines dyslexic children for ADHD or children with ADHD for dyslexia (86–88). In some of these studies the investigation focused on whether the hyperactive/impulsive type or the inattentive type of ADHD was most closely associated with dyslexia. Wilcutt and colleagues reported that common genetic influences explained 95% of the phenotypic covariance between dyslexia and symptoms of inattention, whereas there was only a 21% of phenotypic overlap between dyslexia and hyperactivity/impulsivity (89). Maughan and colleagues, in a large epidemiologic longitudinal study of boys, found that reading disability was strongly associated with ADHD inattentive type, but not with hyperactivity/impulsivity (90). In the reading remediation study in which severely dyslexic children were closely monitored for impairing symptoms of ADHD, 80% of the subjects were inattentive and/or hyperactive/impulsive (91, 92). Wilcutt and colleagues conducted a comprehensive neuropsychological test battery on groups of children with dyslexia, those with ADHD and ADHD plus dyslexia. They noted that the group of children with comorbid ADHD and dyslexia showed a combination of the deficits associated with ADHD and dyslexia. Slow and variable processing speed was present in all three groups (89). Ghelani and colleagues compared reading strategies in children with dyslexia, ADHD, ADHD plus dyslexia, and normal controls. The subjects with ADHD performed adequately on single word reading tasks with evidence of subtle (but average-range) impairment in rate, accuracy, and comprehension. Those with dyslexia had difficulty on the mechanical aspects of reading but had average-range performance in comprehension. The group with combined ADHD and dyslexia also had deficits in rate and accuracy but had greatest difficulty on tasks requiring comprehension of text during silent reading (93).

There is evidence that the overlap between ADHD and dyslexia is possibly due to shared linkage to certain genes. Several different candidate genes have been identified that are linked to ADHD and dyslexia. These include 6p (94, 95), 2p, 8p, 15q, 16p, and 17q (96).

Older children and adolescents should be assessed for depression. As many as one third of dyslexic patients evaluated in an inpatient setting were depressed (97). In the study described by Maughan and colleagues, the incidence of depressed mood was greater in the poor readers (23%) compared to those who were not defined as having reading problems (9.6%) in the first- and fourth-grade samples, but depressed mood dropped substantially in the seventh-grade subjects (74, 98). The investigators further noted that although low reading achievement was linked to depressed mood at all three time points, there was no increased risk for depression beyond the presence of depression at the first evaluation. An evaluation of other factors that might contribute to depression (such as family environment, other comorbid disruptive behavior disorders). These factors had a minor effect, but the most robust effect remained the association in the first time period between low reading achievement and depression. However, the childhood depression did not always persist: adult dyslexics were reported to be functioning at a level comparable to controls, although they continued to have reading and spelling problems, ADHD, and were more likely to report symptoms of anxiety and depression (99).

It is not unusual for dyslexic children, particularly girls, to become depressed and anxious in response to the effects of their reading disability (81, 100). There was also a higher incidence of somatic complaints in this group. Dyslexic children often complain of stomachaches or some other somatic symptoms that serve to keep them out of school.

It is sometimes difficult for parents, teachers, and mental health professionals to consider the possibility that a child may have both a learning disability and a psychiatric disorder. There tends to be an "either/or" conceptualization. It is important for parents to be aware of the significant comorbidity between dyslexia and psychiatric disorders. The management of both entities should be monitored closely. Although schools may have classrooms for children with externalizing behavior problems, comorbid learning disabilities are rarely effectively addressed in those settings. In one study, children were retested 3 years later and there was essentially no change in the number that met diagnostic criteria for learning disability (68) (p. 1460).

NEUROBIOLOGY OF DYSLEXIA

Neuropathology

Galaburda and colleagues have examined a number of brains of dyslexics using thin-serial section technique, and have demonstrated focal areas of microdysgenesias maximal in the temporoparietal region, coupled with "brain warts" (15, 16, 101, 102). Similar lesions are in NBZ mice, used as models for autoimmune disorders (Sherman 1987) (103). Such lesions can also be induced experimentally by freezing cortex during the period of cortical development during which neurons are migrating (104). Fitch and colleagues reported that mice with this type of lesion had much the same difficulty processing rapid acoustic transients as children with specific language impairment (105, 106).

Neuroimaging Studies

MRI-morphometric studies have also shown substantial differences between dyslexics and normal children in brain morphology. Many dyslexics show a reversal of the usual left greater than right asymmetry (107). The ratio of parietal to temporal plana in the left and right hemispheres is also reversed (108, 109). In an MRI study using diffusion tensor imaging to examine white matter in children with dyslexia, anomalies of the temporoparietal pathways were observed, which were significantly correlated with performance on reading, spelling, and rapid naming tasks (110). In an MRI study, Casanova et al. noted that the brains of dyslexics were significantly smaller than those of controls and had a reduced gyrification index. There were no changes in cortical thickness (111). Gray matter anomalies have also been noted in dyslexics. Brambati and colleagues noted abnormalities in gray matter volume bilaterally in the planum temporale, inferior temporal cortex, and cerebellar nuclei (112). Similarly, Vinkenbosch observed decreased gray matter density in the middle and inferior temporal lobe with reduced gray matter density in the middle and inferior temporal gyri. Increased gray matter density was found in the precentral gyri (113).

Neuroimaging studies have indicated that phonological processing tasks and reading in normal readers relies heavily on a network that involves visual cortex, angular gyrus, fusiform gyrus (specifically the visual word form area). These neuroimaging studies must be interpreted in the context of a number of methodological issues, such as diagnostic criteria used to select subjects, type of reading task, selection of stimuli and duration of exposure to word stimuli, and the statistical analysis that is used. Phonological processing appears to be subserved by the left inferior frontal regions (114). However, some of the processes involved can be dissociated. In one fMRI study, there appeared to be different components of phonological processing. Gelfand and Bookheimer concluded that sequential operations (both sequencing phonemes and sequencing hummed notes) were instantiated in posterior Broca's area, whereas the left supramarginal gyrus was more specifically activated by phoneme sequencing (115).

Normal efficient adult readers have a characteristic pattern of activation that has been demonstrated in multiple PET and fMRI studies. Normal readers demonstrate functional connectivity in the left hemisphere between occipital cortex, angular gyrus, and temporal lobe. There is some activation of prefrontal cortex right hemisphere structures. In contrast, studies in dyslexic readers have revealed a disruption in functional connectivity between the occipital lobe, angular gyrus, and temporal lobe, which is most strikingly apparent when the task requires assembling phonological information. There is also increased activation of inferior prefrontal cortex and of posterior cortex in the right hemisphere which are likely compensatory responses (73, 116–125).

Shaywitz and colleagues conducted an fMRI study on a group of adult dyslexics and controls using five tasks that varied with the degree of phonological processing that was required. The analysis involved a within-subjects hierarchical design so that each subject served as his or her own control. There was no difference between the normal and dyslexic readers on a purely visuospatial task. However, on a task requiring phonological analysis, the control subjects manifested a systematic increase in activation in striate cortex (Broca's area 17), angular gyrus (Broca's Area 39) and Wernicke's area (Broca's Area 22) in response to increasing phonological demands, which was not seen in the dyslexic reader. In the normal readers, there was a preponderance of left-hemisphere activation, whereas the dyslexics manifested some degree of right hemisphere activation. The inferior frontal gyrus (Broca's Area 46/47) was activated in dyslexic subjects more than in controls in response to increasing demand for phonological processing. A gender difference was seen in that men showed greater activation of left inferior frontal gyrus and women showed a greater right hemisphere activation. These findings suggested a functional disruption in the extensive neural system involved in reading. These fMRI findings are substantially supported by the report from a large multisite diverse sample of dyslexics demonstrating altered density of the left arcuate fasciculus, the white matter pathway connecting posterior temporoparietal cortex (Wernicke's area) to Broca's area, coupled with increased grey matter density in the left middle and inferior temporal gyri (126). In adults, lesions disrupting the arcuate fasciculus are described as resulting in conduction aphasia, characterized by impaired repetition. This is not the picture that would come to mind in the dyslexic. However, it is also true that not all acquired lesions of the arcuate fasciculus lesions are associated with deficient repetition (127).

Another important component of the system subserving reading is the visual word form area, which has been proposed as the part of the system responsible for the efficient processing of visual stimuli (i.e., words). The visual word form area is a small area, located in the left fusiform gyrus. Acquired lesions of this area result in a form of alexia ("word form" or "pure" alexia) in which the patient loses the ability to read words but must hear the word spelled out or have it presented through tactual channels (128). There is a body of evidence that suggests that this area is highly specialized in extracting salient visual information from words. The fusiform face area is in proximity and is involved in the "expert" recognition of faces. Other populations of neurons in the same area are involved in the processing of other classes of objects. McCandliss and colleagues have postulated that the visual word form area contains a population of neurons, functioning as an ensemble that is "tuned to invariant stimulus properties and structural regularities characteristic of written words" (p. 294) (129). Visual presentation of words activates this particular area in a reliable fashion, more so than other areas, and words activate it more consistently than similar control stimuli. The spatial localization is well defined, with a significant peak of activation in the area in over 90% of individual subject scans, and a narrow standard deviation, on the order of 5 mm. Activation occurs approximately 150 to 200 milliseconds after stimulus presentation. The area can be activated subliminally (that is, without conscious awareness), indicating some degree of automaticity. It is also the area that has been linked in other studies to perceptual expertise (130, 131).

A direct demonstration of the role of the visual word form area in phonological processing of words involved a fMRI study in which there were four conditions: word type (pseudo and real) by response modality (silent and aloud reading). Somewhat different patterns of activation were noted in each condition. Activation of the bilateral motor, auditory, and extrastriate cortex was greater when words were read aloud than when they were read silently. Only the posterior segment of the fusiform cortex (Brodman's area 19) was the only one modulated by different phonological processing demands. The investigators concluded that once a word form is recognized as an alphabetic stimulus, it is then subjected to phonological analysis (132).

The neural signature of reading disability persists, even in older adolescents and adults who appear to have developed reasonably adequate reading skills. Shaywitz and colleagues described a study that involved three groups of young adults (18 to 22.5 years of age). The groups consisted of normal readers; compensated dyslexics, who had a history of difficulty learning to read but had compensated to the point that they were accurate but not fluent readers; and a group of poor readers who read slowly and inaccurately. The compensated dyslexics, manifested relative underactivation of the left parietotemporal and occipitotemporal regions. The poor readers activated posterior reading systems but the pattern was quite different from that of the unimpaired readers, suggesting that they were relying more on reading strategies that relied on memory (133).

A sequential developmental model for acquiring reading skill has been proposed by Shaywitz and associates. This model fits well with observations described previously about the acquisition of reading skill in the young child. Initially, the dorsal circuit, involving the angular gyrus is predominant as the beginning reader learns to map the orthographic features of text onto phonological and lexical-semantic information. With increasing exposure and practice, this process is shifted to the ventral area, the main node of which is the visual word form area, which is adapted for rapid, automatic processing of visual information (134). Turkeltaub and colleagues studied children and young adults ranging in age from 6 to 22 years. In the youngest readers, activation of the left-posterior superior temporal sulcus was prominent and related to increasing skill in phonological processing. Additional changes in reading pattern with maturation were associated with increased activity in the left-hemisphere middle temporal and inferior frontal gyri and decreased activity in right inferotemporal cortical areas (135).

Visual Deficits

Although Hinshelwood's description of dyslexia emphasized the visual aspects of the problem ("word-blindness"), he identified angular gyrus/associational cortex as the site of the dysfunction. Reading unquestionably involves a visual process, yet there is ample evidence that it is the underlying difficulty in phonological awareness and the impaired ability to link visual information with phonemes that is the major problem in dyslexia. The difficulty seems more associational than visual and may involve some early dysfunction of the mirror neuron system.

Having said that, it is also true that reading involves a visual process. Effective reading requires maintaining fixation on a small segment of text, systematically shifting gaze and then attending to another segment of text. This depends not so much the size of the perceptual span as the ability to rapidly integrate phonological and semantic information (136). In addition, attentional factors are also involved (137). Proponents of the visual deficits associated with reading point to the fact that dyslexics frequently transpose letters and complain that words move around on the page.

A number of studies have demonstrated visual and oculomotor dysfunction in dyslexics (138–140); but these results are often hotly contested, and have not been replicated (141–144). Lovegrove demonstrated that as a group dyslexics have mildly reduced contrast sensitivity at low spatial frequencies and low luminance levels, particularly during flicker fusion. In contrast, at higher spatial frequencies contrast sensitivity is intact (145). Flicker fusion rate is slow (146) and impaired vergence amplitudes are noted, compared to controls (147). Cornelissen and colleagues demonstrated that dyslexics had impaired visual motion sensitivity even when high contrast and illumination levels were present (148). This observation was supported in a visual-evoked potential study that used a binocularly presented checkerboard pattern at low and high contrasts. At high contrast, the groups did not differ. Examining steady-state visual-evoked potentials at a variety of contrast levels, they found that at high contrast there was no difference, but at 15 Hz using low-contrast stimuli, the responses of normal subjects were slightly reduced, but were virtually absent in the dyslexic subjects. The investigators interpreted this early negative wave as reflecting activity in layer 4C of primary visual cortex (V1) in response to thalamic projections (149).

Many of the deficits in visual processing during reading in dyslexics have been interpreted as associated with the difficulties in processing phonological information. Eden and colleagues conducted a series of studies on dyslexics, "backward readers," and controls that involved visual tasks (measures of fixation, vergence amplitude, saccade, and smooth pursuit) that did not involve phonological processing. Results indicate that fixation instability at the end of saccades, poor smooth pursuit (particularly left to right), and vergence amplitudes were lower in the dyslexic group. All dyslexics with small vergence amplitudes were also impaired in phonemic awareness (as assessed by pig Latin). The "backward reading" group showed a similar profile (the question here is whether this group was biologically different from the dyslexics). Eye movement abnormalities were not correlated with attention deficit, gender, IQ, or handedness. The conclusion was that the oculomotor abnormalities appeared unrelated to the phonemic awareness deficit (150). In an fMRI study of visual motion processing in dyslexic men and controls, there were no group differences in activation pattern visual cortex, or extrastriate cortex, or stationary visual stimuli were presented, but the dyslexics did not activate the middle temporal area (V5/MT) to the same extent as controls when moving stimuli were presented (151). These findings have been interpreted as showing an abnormality in the magnocellular pathway at the level of primary visual cortex (area 17;V1) or earlier, indicating that the magnocellular system of dyslexics can respond to low-contrast stimuli, but the response is slow. These findings were further supported by neuropathological studies of the lateral geniculate nucleus that revealed disorganized, shrunken magnocellular layers without any changes in the parvocellular layers in the dyslexics in comparison to controls.

A subsequent visual evoked potential study in which low- and high-spatial frequency targets were presented in either a steady or flickering background showed no differences in the high spatial condition between dyslexics and controls, but when low spatial frequencies were used, there were longer latencies of early components of the visual-evoked potential in the dyslexics. However, Victor and colleagues attempted unsuccessfully to replicate these findings (152).

Although, as this brief review indicates, there is some evidence suggesting that visual deficits are present in some dyslexics, there is little reason to believe that visual processing is the underlying deficit. Some dyslexics have been shown to have associated motor, timing, praxis, and/or coordination deficits; some have more complex auditory processing deficits. However, these might be considered to be "add-ons," distinct from the primary pathophysiology. In a well-constructed and executed study by Ramus, young adult dyslexics and controls underwent extensive psychometric, phonological, auditory, visual and cerebellar testing. One hundred percent of the dyslexics had a phonological deficit, 63% an auditory deficit, 25% a motor deficit, and 12.5% a visual magnocellular deficit. Thus, a phono-

logical processing deficit is a sufficient explanation for dyslexia and has much theoretical and empirical support. In addition, the phonological processing deficit model has given rise to effective treatment strategies that have demonstrated efficacy.

GENETIC ASPECTS

The familial nature of dyslexia has been known for over a century. In 1907, Stephenson described a family with six cases in three generations (153). The first formal genetic study was published in 1950 (154). Rutter and Yule, using data from the Isle of Wight study, noted that a family history of reading disability occurred in approximately one third of the children with reading disability compared to 9% of the controls. They cautioned that this did not eliminate the possibility that environmental factors were also involved.

Twin studies also have supported the genetic etiology of dyslexia, although there has been considerable variability from study to study. Bakwin reported that the probandwise concordance rate in twin pairs, in which at least one twin was reading disabled, was two times higher in monozygotic twins (91%) than in dizygotic twins (45%) (155). In a study of 13-year-old monozygotic and dizygotic twins, Stevenson noted that the genetic contribution was relatively modest if only reading scores were used. When spelling was added, heritability increased to 0.75 (71). Data from the large number of twin pairs that have been studied in the Colorado Family Reading Study provide particularly convincing support for the heritability of dyslexia (156, 157). These investigators employed a multiple regression analysis which made it possible to use an alternative test of genetic etiology of reading disability. They concluded that about half of the impairment in reading performance of the probands was the result of heritable influences, and 40% could be attributed to shared environmental influences. Even more importantly, these investigators were able to show that IQ was not a factor in either genetic etiology of reading disability or twin resemblance. Moreover, a comparison of the phonological and orthographic coding scores of the twins supported the concept that reading-disabled children have a deficit in phonological coding and that individual differences in word recognition are largely the result of heritable variation in phonological coding ability (158, 159).

Genetic linkage analyses on large families of subjects with reading disability have identified a number of candidate genes at different loci. It is not clear at this point if there are several different genes that lead to the dyslexic phenotype, if there are specific dyslexic phenotypes (which, at this point have not been definitively identified), or how a specific gene affects brain development and function to produce the dyslexic cognitive profile. The manner in which the diagnosis of dyslexia is made is of great importance in this type of study because of the variability in clinical presentation and the age-related changes in reading skill. Moreover, large sample sizes are required in this type of work.

The chromosome region that has been most consistently linked to dyslexia is in the region 6p23–p21.3 (160, 161). A possible association with deficits in phonological awareness was suggested by Grigorenko and colleagues (162). However, investigators have not been particularly successful in targeting the specific gene locus responsible for the linkage in the 575-kb region under scrutiny on chromosome 6p22. The myelin oligodendrocyte glycoprotein (MOG) gene, which maps to 6p21.3, appeared to be a possible candidate but this has not been substantiated on closer inspection (165, 166). Francks and colleagues found an association with this area in three samples, two from the United Kingdom and an independent sample from Colorado (167). In a family-based and case-control study, Cope et al. identified two single nucleotide polymorphisms in the KIAA0319 gene on 6p.22 that best explained the linkage to dyslexia. Thus KIAA0319 is a strong candidate for a susceptibility gene: it is expressed in the brain, but its function is currently unknown (168, 167).

The first study reported linkage of reading disability to chromosome 15 in 84 individuals from nine families in which reading disability appeared to be transmitted in autosomal dominant manner (169). However, in only one of the nine families was there a high lod score. A later study based on a much larger sample indicated that approximately 20% of families with reading-disabled children showed linkage to chromosome 15 (170). In a Finnish study, a gene (DYX1C1 near the DYX1 locus on chromosome 15q21), disrupted by a translocation, was found to coincidentally segregate with dyslexia (171, 172). Subsequently, in a large study (898 individuals in 111 families), this gene has been found to be linked to single word reading (173). However, this association was not supported in a large sample from the United Kingdom (174, 175), and investigators have not been particularly successful in narrowing down the area and identifying any specific gene (176). In another study by the Toronto group, the gene in the region of the translocation was found to be associated with phonological awareness, word identification, decoding, rapid automatized naming, language ability, and verbal short-term memory but involved different alleles and haplotypes than was reported in the Finnish sample (177). Chromosome 15 has also been reported to be associated with ADHD in a sample of Dutch children (94).

The region on chromosome 1p34–p36 has also been considered as the site of a possible susceptibility gene for dyslexia (178, 179). Grigorenko and colleagues studied eight dyslexic families and suggested the possibility of a two-locus interaction with 1 p and 6 p (180). In a sample of 100 dyslexic Canadian families, assessed using phonological awareness, phonological coding, spelling, and rapid automatized naming speed, further confirmation of a possible linkage on 1p34–36 was found (181).

Kaminen and colleagues reported that they had confirmed a site on chromosome 2p11 (DYX3) that was associated with dyslexia (182). Chromosome 3 has also been identified as a possible candidate. In a study of a large pedigree, dyslexia was found to segregate with an autosomal dominant locus in the pericentromeric region of chromosome 3 (183).

A quantitative trait locus on 18p11.2 that was significantly associated with single-word reading was identified. The investigators felt that this might constitute a "general risk factor for dyslexia, influencing several reading-related processes" (184).

A locus on the X chromosome between markers DXS1227 and DXS8091 was described in a single large Dutch family. Males were predictably more severely affected, whereas females had a somewhat milder presentation but could still be diagnosed as dyslexic on the basis of the composite score (185).

Kaminen and colleagues noted that there was a possible linkage to chromosome 7q32, but did not observe any specific mutations when they sequenced the FOXP2 (forkhead box P2) coding region in six of their Finnish subjects with dyslexia (182).

Nonetheless, the FOXP2 gene remains an interesting candidate for a specific subtype of dyslexia. There is a compelling confluence of structural, functional, and neurodevelopmental information which suggests that FOXP2 may be related to dyslexia associated with severe speech/language dysfunction. The association of severe dyspraxia of speech, as a possible marker for dysfunction of the mirror neuron system (the result of anomalous neurodevelopmental processes), and subsequent difficulty acquiring adequate phonological awareness is intriguing (186). A mutation in exon 14 of the FOXP2 gene has been linked to severe speech/language disorders in the KE kindred, a large, three-generation family that has been extensively studied. A morphometric MRI study revealed bilateral reduction of grey matter in the caudate, the cerebellum, and left and right inferior frontal gyrus in affected family members with increased grey matter density in the planum temporale. A fMRI study involving silent and spoken verb generation and repetition was conducted on family members with the FOXP2 mutation and unaffected members from the same family. Those with the FOXP2 mutation showed significant underactivation of a variety of cortical language areas, including Broca's area, its right homolog, and the putamen (187). FOXP2 is involved in the development of corticostriatal and olivocerebellar circuits, which are critically involved in motor control. Moreover, a study in songbirds suggests that it may be related to neural plasticity underlying vocalization (188).

However, studies of other subjects with speech-language disorders and/or verbal apraxia have not consistently revealed association with this locus. In a study of 96 subjects with speech-language impairment, a mutation in FOXP2 was not identified but an association with a marker adjacent to FOXP2 was observed (189). A heterozygous nonsense mutation resulting in a truncated protein product that cosegregates with severe verbal apraxia and concomitant language disability has been identified in three of 49 subjects with apraxia of speech (190).

APPROACHES TO THE EVALUATION OF DYSLEXIA

An adequate assessment of the child with dyslexia requires a multidisciplinary approach. A detailed history is used to elucidate any obstetrical or medical problems that might contribute to the problem, such as prematurity, hyperbilirubinemia, or a history of chronic otitis media, or significant medical illness or surgical problems. The child's language and motor development should be reviewed in great detail: was he an interactive pleasant baby who cooed responsively? When did babbling commence? When did the child start uttering words with communicative intent? When did he start using words to communicate effectively? At what point was the child intelligible to persons outside the family? Was he able to follow simple directions? Or was it necessary to use a lot of gesturing? Did the child engage in symbolic play activities? What about chewing and swallowing food? Is he a messy eater? Can the child swallow pills?

The family history should also be carefully reviewed. This should include asking about the educational and professional status of the parents and their siblings, and the grandparents. In addition, one should find out if the parents (and if possible other family members) read for pleasure, can master foreign languages, and are able to spell. In families from lower socioeconomic groups, dropping out of school, and finding work as a laborer are highly suggestive. However, because some dyslexic adults can be quite successful, it is important to review their educational history and past and present reading and spelling skills.

All children being evaluated for dyslexia should also be screened for ADHD. Given the extremely high comorbidity of reading disability and ADHD, it is important to be aware of attentional problems, which make it even more difficult for the child to perform adequately. In addition, screening for depression, anxiety, oppositional defiant disorder, and conduct disorder are warranted. Some anxious dyslexic children who perform well despite their handicap have a rather obsessive approach to school work.

The history should also inquire in detail about the child's school performance: what kind of school does the child attend? Has the child had any previous evaluations? How did the child fare in kindergarten and first grade? Was he able to recognize letters? How about spelling and writing and arithmetic? Is the child independent in homework skills (this depends, to some extent, on the child's grade level). One expects a child in second grade to require some supervision. However, a child in fifth grade who requires constant supervision by parents and teachers to keep track of, finish,

and turn in homework should be closely scrutinized for reading disability and ADHD. The amount of effort that a parent must put in at home around completing homework is also an important aspect of the history. The child whose parents describe time-consuming, nightly battles surrounding homework should be considered at high risk for dyslexia.

The formal assessment should involve a standardized IQ test. Examination of reading skills should include assessing the child's ability to read single sight-words and decode nonwords. An assessment of phonological awareness, phonological memory, and rapid naming should be carried out (Comprehensive Test of Phonological Processing) (24). The Lindamood Auditory Conceptualization Test-3 not only assesses phonemic awareness but also a child's ability to conceptualize syllables and phoneme-syllable relationships. (190a) The Test of Word Reading Efficiency is well-normed and measures not only accuracy but also decoding speed (190b). Oral reading fluency and reading comprehension, as measured on the Gray Oral Reading Test-4, is particularly helpful because it sometimes highlights an obvious a discrepancy between poor mechanical reading skills and above-average reading comprehension (190c).

Spelling should be evaluated. The child's ability to write, both in terms of the motor mechanics and legibility, as well as speed should be assessed. In addition, the child's ability to organize a story or a report should be assessed. Arithmetic should be evaluated. Many dyslexics have relative strengths in arithmetic and in terms of managing psychosocial issues and school curricula, this is an important piece of information.

An assessment for dyslexia should also include a thorough examination of language. In addition to assessing the child's lexical, semantic, and syntactic processing through a formal language assessment, confrontation naming, verbal fluency, and short- and longterm verbal memory should be evaluated. An assessment of frontal executive function and visuospatial skills should also be conducted. These are often areas of strength.

The child should also be carefully evaluated for ADHD as well as any other psychiatric comorbidities. An interview with the parents, teacher, and child should focus on screening for ADHD, other disruptive behavior disorders, anxiety, and depression. Simply asking the child what part of their school day they like best can be very informative (an answer such as "lunch" or "recess" tells one a great deal). Some children will be quite clear about their dislike for certain school subjects. A diagnostic screening questionnaire completed by the parents and teachers is helpful. The child's level of attention, arousal, impulsivity, and restlessness as well as his or her ability to express ideas in language should be monitored during the interview and assessments. A continuous performance task is often helpful. This evaluation is obviously considerably more extensive than is typically administered in a school setting. However, because dyslexia is not simply a "learning disability" it is important to have a clear idea of what one is dealing with. Understanding the child's self-image, coping strategies, and insight is particularly helpful. It is also important to understand how the parents view the situation. Some parents deny the child's difficulty and may see the school's concerns as unjustified and intrusive. Other parents see the child's struggles as mirroring their own experience in school and feel guilty.

Many bright dyslexic children are able to cope with school work, not because they can read well, but rather because they can understand what they are reading without actually having read it. This may not pose a problem in terms of classroom performance, but in situations in which there is a high level of pressure to perform, or a high stakes test, the child may decompensate. In many school systems, informal teacher-conducted reading assessments are heavily weighted toward reading comprehension rather than mechanical reading skills.

TREATMENT/MANAGEMENT OF DYSLEXIA

Reading disability has a pervasive effect on a child's academic success and may cast a shadow on accomplishment and self-esteem throughout adult life. Treatment of dyslexia has therefore been a focus of attention for parents, teachers, and professionals who seek effective strategies for treating the disorder. Many methods have been devised, ranging from the teaching of explicit reading strategies, using a multisensory approach (such as the Orton-Gillingham method) (191) or the commercial programs that are based on the Orton-Gillingham, such as Alphabetic Phonics, Project Read, the Herman Approach, Slingerland Approach, the Spalding Approach, the Wilson Approach, or LANGUAGE! Other therapies include vision training, colored lenses, craniosacral therapy, motor treatments designed to address cerebellar deficits, and so on.

There are two general approaches to the treatment of dyslexia. One is a "top-down," whole language approach that uses semantic or syntactic clues for word reading but does not train phonologic awareness in an explicit, sequential fashion. The other is a "bottom up" approach that addresses phonological awareness in a direct, explicit fashion. An example of this direct approach using explicit training of phonological awareness is the program, developed by the Lindamoods, initially called Auditory Discrimination in Depth (ADD) (192). This program has undergone some revision and was renamed LiPS (Lindamood Phoneme Sequencing program) (193). The treatment approach needs to be adjusted to the age of the child. Very different strategies need to be used if one is dealing with an at-risk 4-year-old child with a language disorder or working with a 20-year-old college student. In addition, the treatment needs to be delivered in an intensive fashion with close monitoring, feedback, and an orderly, sequential approach. For example, in the treatment study reported by Eden and colleagues, dyslexic adults received 3-hour daily sessions in a small group setting for 8 weeks, an average of 112.5 hours of training. It is interesting that Hinshelwood,

a century ago, recognized the importance of frequent training. Lacking intensity, treatment can go on for many years and in severely dyslexic individuals, may result in only minimal gains (Lyon 1985, Snowling and Hulme 1989).

There is a relative paucity of well-designed peer-reviewed studies that support these various methods. The reader is referred to the review by Alexander and Slinger-Constant, which discusses in depth various current strategies for treating dyslexia and critically reviews the supporting research (194).

There are now a number of studies that indicate that appropriate, intensive, treatment designed to enhance phonologic awareness will result in a shift in the pattern of brain activity to a pattern resembling that of the normal reader. This suggests that the brain has sufficient plasticity to respond to appropriate explicit intensive treatment by modifying neuronal connectivity. These studies, which have been reported out of several different research centers, using somewhat different programs, are quite encouraging (195–198). However, this treatment approach is based on neurorehabilitation. It is important that once a child has completed the intensive program that they continue to practice the skills that they have acquired until they become automatic and self-sustaining. For a moderately severe dyslexic, intensive treatment will significantly improve decoding accuracy but fluency will follow much more slowly. The child will need continued support or there is a risk of return to the previous state. In adults, the response to intensive treatment is somewhat different, involving more right hemisphere activity (199). The fact that such changes can be made in the activation pattern suggests that it should be possible to effectively help children and adults with dyslexia, given how valuable reading is in our society.

In addition to the direct treatment of the underlying phonological awareness deficit, other issues must be incorporated into the management of the dyslexic patient. After chronic failure in school, older children and adults need work with a sensitive psychotherapist to help them reframe their perceptions of themselves. Therapy directed at helping them acquire a realistic view of their cognitive strengths and weaknesses, and coaching them on how to bypass areas of deficit, can be extremely helpful. A substantial number of dyslexics also have significant attention deficits, which may not be at all clinically obvious. They benefit from psychostimulant treatment. Books on Tape are often very helpful for the dyslexic with a heavy reading load. Effective text-reading and voice-recognition software packages are now available. Learning to touch-type and use a spell-checker also helps these students function effectively.

REFERENCES

1. Katusic SK; Colligan RC, Barbaresi WJ, et al. Incidence of reading disability in a population-based birth cohort, 1976–1982, Rochester, Minn. Mayo Clin Proc 2001;76:1081–1092.
2. Shaywitz SE, Shaywitz BA, Fletcher JM, et al. Prevalence of reading disability in boys and girls: Results of the Connecticut longitudinal study. JAMA 1990;264:998–1002.

3. Lyons GR. Toward a definition of dyslexia. Ann Dyslexia 1995; 45:3–30.
4. Morgan WP. A case of congenital word blindness. BMJ 1896;2: 1378.
5. Hinshelwood J. Congenital word blindness. Lancet 1900;1: 1506–1508.
6. Hinshelwood J. Four cases of congenital word-blindness occurring in the same family. BMJ 1907;2:1229–1232.
7. Hinshelwood J. Two cases of hereditary word-blindness. BMJ 1911;1:608–609.
8. Dejerine, J. Sur un cas de cécité verbal avec agraphie suivi d'autopsie. Memoires de la Societe Biologique 1891;3:197–201.
9. Orton ST. "Word-blindness" in school children. Arch Neurol Psychiatry 1925;14:581–615.
10. Orton S. Specific reading disability—strephosymbolia. JAMA 1928;90:1095–1099.
11. Rutter M, Yule W. The concept of specific reading retardation. J Child Psychol Psychiatry 1975;16:181–197.
12. Denckla MB, Rudel RG. Naming of object-drawings by dyslexic and other learning disabled children. Brain Language 1976;3: 1–15.
13. Denckla MB, Rudel R. Rapid "Automatized" naming of pictured objects, colors,letters and numbers by normal children. Cortex 1974;10:186–202.
14. Denckla MB, Rudel R. Rapid automatized naming (R.A.N.): dyslexia differentiated from other learning disabilities. Neuropsychologia 1976;14:471–479.
15. Galaburda AM, Kemper TL. Cytoarchitectonic abnormalities in developmental dyslexia: a case study. Ann Neurol 1979;6: 94–100.
16. Galaburda AM, Sherman GF, Rosen GD, et al. Developmental dyslexia: four consecutive patients with cortical anomalies. Ann Neurol 1985;18:222–233.
17. Yule W, Rutter M, Berger M, et al. Over- and under-achievement in reading: distribution in the general population. Br J Ed Psychol 1974;44:1–12.
18. Fletcher JM, Shaywitz SE, Shankweiler DP, et al. Cognitive profiles of reading disability: comparisons of discrepancy and low achievement definitions. J Ed Psychol 1994;86:6–23.
19. Finucci JM, Childs B. Are there really more dyslexic boys than girls? In: Ansara A, Geschwind N, Galaburda A, Albert M, Gartrell N, eds. Gender Differences in Dyslexia. Towson, MD: Orton Dyslexia Society, 1981:1–9.
20. Critchley M. The Dyslexic Child. Springfield, Illinois: Thomas, 1970.
21. Rutter M, Caspi A, Fergusson D, et al. Sex differences in developmental reading disability: new findings from 4 epidemiological studies. JAMA 2004;291:2007–2012.
22. Flannery, KA, Liederman J, Daly L, et al. Male prevalence for reading disability is found in a large sample of black and white children free from ascertainment bias. J Int Neuropsychol Soc 2000;6:433–442.
23. Flax JF, Realpe-Bonilla T, Hirsch LS, et al. Specific language impairment in families: evidence for co-occurrence with reading impairments. J Speech Lang Hear Res 2003;46:530–543.
24. Wagner RK, Torgesen JK, Rashotte CA. Examiner's Manual: The Comprehensive Test of Phonological Processing. Austin: Pro-Ed, 1999.
25. Torgesen JK, Wagner RK. The nature of phonological processing and its causal role in acquisition of reading skills. Psychol Bull 1987;101:192–212
26. Torgesen JK, Wagner R, Rashotte C, et al. Contributions of phonological awareness and rapid automatic naming ability to the growth of word-reading skills in second to fifth grade. Scientific Studies of Reading 1997;1:161–185.
27. Torgesen JK, Wagner RK, Rashotte CA. Longitudinal studies of phonological processing and reading. J Learn Disabil 1994; 27:276–286; discussion 287–291.
28. Wagner RK, Torgesen JK, Rashotte CA, et al. Changing relations between phonological processing abilities and word-level reading as children develop from beginning to skilled readers: a 5-year longitudinal study. Dev Psychol 1997;33:468–479.
29. Elbro C, Borstrom I, Peterson DK. Predicting dyslexia from kindergarten: the importance of distinctness of phonological representations of lexical items. Reading Res Q 1998;33:36–60.

30. Liberman I, Shankweiler D, Liberman A. The alphabetic principle in learning to read. In: Shankweiler D, Liberman I, ed. Phonology and Reading Disability. Ann Arbor, MI: University of Michigan Press, 1989: 1–33.
31. McGurk M, MacDonald J. Hearing lips and seeing voices. Nature 1976;264:746–748.
32. Kuhl PK, Meltzoff AN. The bimodal perception of speech in infancy. Science 1982;218:1138–1141.
33. MacKain K, Studdert-Kennedy M, Spieker S, et al. Infant intermodal speech perception is a left-hemisphere function. Science 1983;219:1347–1349.
34. Montgomery D. Do dyslexics have difficulty accessing articulatory information? Psychol Res 1981;43:235–243.
35. Zatorre RJ, Evans AC, Meyer E, et al. Lateralization of phonetic and pitch discrimination in speech processing. Science 1992; 256:846–849.
36. Katzir T, Misra M, Poldrack RA. Imaging phonology without print: Assessing the neural correlates of phonemic awareness using fMRI. Neuroimage 2005; 27:106–115.
37. Ruff S, Marie N, Celsis P, et al. Neural substrates of impaired categorical perception of phonemes in adult dyslexics: an fMRI study. Brain Cogn 2003;53:331–334.
38. Mottonen R, Jarvelainen J, Sams M, et al. Viewing speech modulates activity in the left SI mouth cortex. Neuroimage 2005; 24:731–737.
39. Heilman KM, Voeller K, Alexander AW. Developmental dyslexia: A motor-articulatory feedback hypothesis. Ann Neurol 1996; 39:407–412.
40. Rizzolatti G, Craighero L. The mirror-neuron system. Annu Rev Neurosci 2004;27:169–192.
41. Baddeley A. Working Memory. Oxford: Oxford University Press, 1986.
42. Gathercole SE, Baddeley AD. Working memory and language. Hove, UK: Lawrence Erlbaum Associates, 1993.
43. Torgesen JK. Studies of children with learning disabilities who perform poorly on memory span tasks. J Learn Disabil 1988; 21:605–612.
44. Bowers PG. Exploration of the basis for rapid naming's relationship to reading. In: Wolf M, ed. Dyslexia, Fluency, and the Brain. Parkton, MD: Yorkton Press, 2001: 41–63.
45. Bowers PG, Wolf M. Theoretical links between naming speed, precise timing mechanisms and orthographic skill in dyslexia. Reading and Writing: An Interdisciplinary Journal 1993; 5:69–85.
46. Wolf M. Rapid alternating stimulus naming in the developmental dyslexias. Brain Lang 1986;27:360–379.
47. Wolf M, Baily H, Morris R. Automaticity, retrieval processes, and reading: a longitudinal study in average and impaired readers. Child Development 1986;57:988–1000.
48. Denckla MB. Color-naming defects in dyslexic boys. Cortex 1972;8:164–176.
49. Compton DL. The influence of item composition on RAN letter performance in first grade children. J Special Educ 2004; 37:81–94.
50. Lovett MW, Steinbach KA, Frijters JC. Remediating the core deficits of developmental reading disability: a double-deficit perspective. J Learn Disabil 2000;33:334–358.
51. Ehri, L. Phases of development in learning to read words. In: Oakhill J, and Beard R, ed. Reading Development and the Teaching of Reading: A Psychological Perspective. Oxford UK: Blackwell, 1990:79–108.
52. Ehri L. Phases of acquisition in learning to read words and implications for teaching. In: Stainthorp R, and Tomlinson, P, ed. Learning and Teaching Reading. 2. London: British Journal of Educational Psychology Monograph Series, 2002.
53. Share DL, Stanovich K, Share DL, Stanovich KE. Cognitive processes in early reading development: Accommodating individual differences into a model of acquisition. Issues in Education: Contributions from Educational Psychology 1995;1:1–57.
54. Reitsma P. Printed word learning in beginning readers. J Exp Child Psychol 1983;36:321–339.
55. Aghababian V, Nazir TA. Developing normal reading skills: aspects of the visual processes underlying word recognition. J Exp Child Psychol 2000;76:123–150.

56. Rayner K, Pollatsek A. *The Psychology of Reading*. New York: Prentice-Hall, 1980.
57. Reicher GM. Perceptual recognition as a function of meaningfulness of stimulus material. J Exp Psychol 1969;81:275–280.
58. Molfese DL. Predicting dyslexia at 8 years of age using neonatal brain responses. Brain Lang 2000;72:238–245.
59. Leppanen PH, Pihko E, Eklund KM, et al. Cortical responses of infants with and without a genetic risk for dyslexia: II. Group effects. Neuroreport 1999;10:969–973.
60. Richardson U, Leppanen PH, Leiwo M, et al. Speech perception of infants with high familial risk for dyslexia differ at the age of 6 months. Dev Neuropsychol 2003;23:385–397.
61. Lyytinen H, Ahonen T, Eklund K, et al. Developmental pathways of children with and without familial risk for dyslexia during the first years of life. Dev Neuropsychol 2001;20:535–554.
62. Viholainen H, Ahonen T, Cantell M, et al. Development of early motor skills and language in children at risk for familial dyslexia. Dev Med Child Neurol 2002;44:761–769.
63. Gallagher A, Frith U, Snowling MJ. Precursors of literacy delay among children at genetic risk of dyslexia. J Child Psychol Psychiatry All Disc 2000;41:203–213.
64. Catts H. Early identification of dyslexia: evidence of a follow-up study of speech-language impaired children. Ann Dyslexia 1991;41:163–177.
65. Scarborough H. Very early language deficits in dyslexic children. Child Dev 1990;61:1728–1743.
66. Scarborough H. Early syntactic development of dyslexic children. Ann of Dyslexia 1991;41:207–220.
67. Scarborough H. Early identification of children at risk for reading disabilities: Phonological awareness and some other promising predictors. In: Shapiro/Accardo PJ, and Capute AJ BK, eds. *Specific Reading Disability: A View of the Spectrum*. Hillsdale, NJ: Erlbaum, 1998: 77–121.
68. Mattison RE, Hooper SR, Glassberg LA. Three-year course of learning disorders in special education students classified as behavioral disorder. J Am Acad Child Adolesc Psychiatry 2002; 41:1454–1461.
69. Vaughn SR, Moody SW, Schumm JS. Broken promises: reading instruction in the resource room. Except Child 1998;64: 211–225.
70. Castro-Caldas A, Petersson KM, Reis A, et al. The illiterate brain. Learning to read and write during childhood influences the functional organization of the adult brain. Brain 1998;121 Pt 6: 1053–1063.
71. Stevenson J, Graham P, Fredman G, et al. A twin study of genetic influences on reading and spelling ability and disability. J Child Psychol Psychiatry 1987;28:229–247.
72. Felton RH, Naylor CE, Wood FB. Neuropsychological profile of adult dyslexics. Brain Lang 1990;39:485–497.
73. Flowers L, Wood FB, Naylor CE. Regional cerebral blood flow correlates of language processes in reading disabilities. Arch Neurol 1991;48:637–643
74. Maughan, B, Rowe R, Loeber R, et al. Reading problems and depressed mood. J Abnorm Child Psychol 2003;31:219–229.
75. Fink RP Resilience and success. A surprising path to the National Academy. Presented at the annual meeting of the International Academy for Research in Learning Disabilities, July 2004, Ann Arbor, MI.
76. Lindamood CH. Lindamood Auditory Conceptualization Test. Austin: Pro-Ed. 1979.
77. Dowell B. Secret of the super successful...they're dyslexic. The Sunday Times, October 5, 2003;1.
78. West TG. Secret of the super successful. . .they're dyslexic. Thalamus 2003;21:48–52.
79. Aram DM, Ekelman BL, Nation JE. Preschoolers with language disorders: 10 years later. J Speech Hear Res 1984;27:232–244.
80. Baker L, Cantwell DP. A prospective psychiatric follow-up of children with speech/language disorders. J Am Acad Child Adolesc Psychiatry 1987;26:546–553.
81. Beitchman JH, Young AR. Learning disorders with a special emphasis on reading disorders: A review of the past ten years. J Am Acad Child Adolesc Psychiatry 1997;36:1020–1032.
82. Silva PA, Williams S, McGee R. A longitudinal study of children with developmental language delay at age three: later intelligence, reading and behaviour problems. Dev Med Child Neurol 1987;29:630–640.
83. Stark RE, Bernstein LE, Condino R, et al. Four-year follow-up study of language impaired children. Ann Dyslexia 1984;34: 49–68.
84. Aram DM, Morris R, Hall NE. Clinical and research congruence in identifying children with specific language impairment. J Speech Hearing Res 1993;36:580–591.
85. Stark RE, Tallal P. Selection of children with specific language deficits. J Speech Hear Disord 1981;46:114–122.
86. Frick PJ, Kamphaus RW, Lahey BB, et al. Academic underachievement and the disruptive behavior disorders. J Consulting Clin Psychol 1991;59:289–294.
87. Sanson A, Prior M, Smart D. Reading disabilities with and without behaviour problems at 7–8 years: prediction from longitudinal data from infancy to 6 years. J Child Psychol Psychiatry 1996;37:529–541.
88. Semrud-Clikeman M, Biederman J, Sprich-Buckminster S, et al. Comorbidity between ADDH and learning disability: a review and report in a clinically referred sample. J Am Acad Child Adolesc Psychiatry 1992;31:439–448.
89. Willcutt EG, Pennington BF, Olson RK, et al. Neuropsychological analyses of comorbidity between reading disability and attention deficit hyperactivity disorder: in search of the common deficit. Dev Neuropsychol 2005;27:35–78.
90. Maughan B, Pickles A, Hagell A, et al. Reading problems and antisocial behavior: developmental trends in comorbidity. J Child Psychol Psychiatry 1996;37:405–418.
91. Torgesen JK, Alexander AW, Wahner RK, et al. Intensive remedial instruction for children with severe reading disabilities: immediate and long-term outcomes from two instructional approaches. J Learning Disabil 2001;34:33–58.
92. Voeller KKS. Neurological factors underlying the comorbidity of attentional dysfunction and dyslexia. In: Duane DD, ed. *Reading and Attention Disorders: Neurobiological Correlates*. Baltimore, MD: York Press, 1999:185–212.
93. Ghelani K, Sidhu R, Jain U, et al. Reading comprehension and reading related abilities in adolescents with reading disabilities and attention-deficit/hyperactivity disorder. Dyslexia 2004;10: 364–384.
94. Bakker SC, van der Meulen EM, Buitelaar JK, et al. A whole-genome scan in 164 Dutch sib pairs with attention-deficit/hyperactivity disorder: suggestive evidence for linkage on chromosomes 7p and 15q. Am J Hum Genet 2003;72:1251–1260.
95. Willcutt EG, Pennington BF, Smith SD, et al. Quantitative trait locus for reading disability on chromosome 6p is pleiotropic for attention-deficit/hyperactivity disorder. Am J Med Genet 2002; 114:260–268.
96. Loo SK, Fisher SE, Francks C, et al. Genome-wide scan of reading ability in affected sibling pairs with attention-deficit/hyperactivity disorder: unique and shared genetic effects. Mol Psychiatry 2004;9:485–493.
97. Horwitz SM, Irwin JR, Briggs-Gowan MJ, et al. Language delay in a community cohort of young children. J Am Acad Child Adolesc Psychiatry 2003;42:932–940.
98. Cohen NJ, Davine M, Meloche-Kelly M. Prevalence of unsuspected language disorders in a child psychiatric population. J Am Acad Child Adolesc Psychiatry 1989;28:107–111.
99. Feldman E, Levin BE, Lubs H, et al. Adult familial dyslexia: a retrospective developmental and psychosocial profile. J Neuropsychiatry Clin Neurosci 1993;5:195–199.
100. Willcutt E, Pennington B, DeFries J. Twin study of the etiology of comorbidity between reading disability and attention-deficit/hyperactivity disorder. Am J Med Genet 2000;96: 293–301.
101. Galaburda AM. Ordinary and extraordinary brain development: anatomical variation in developmental dyslexia. Ann Dyslexia 1989;39:67–80.
102. Humphreys P, Kaufman WE, Galaburda AM. Developmental dyslexia in women: neuropathological findings in three patients. Ann Neurol 1990;28:727–738.
103. Sherman GF, Galaburda AM, Geschwind N. Cortical anomalies in brains of New Zealand mice: a neuropathologic model of dyslexia? Proc Natl Acad Sci USA 1985;82:8072–8074.
104. Dvorak K, Feit J, Jurankova Z. Experimentally induced focal microgyria and status verrucosus deformis in rats—pathogenesis

and interrelation histological and autoradiographical study. Acta Neuropathol 1978;44:121–129.

105. Fitch RH, Tallal P, Brown CP, et al. Induced microgyria and auditory temporal processing in rats: a model for language impairment? Cereb Cortex 1994;4:260–270.

106. Tallal P, Piercy M. Developmental aphasia: rate of auditory processing and selective impairment of consonant perception. Neuropsychologia 1974;12:83–93.

107. Hynd GW, Semrud-Clikeman M, Lorys AR, et al. Brain morphology in developmental dyslexia and attention deficit disorder/hyperactivity. Arch Neurol 1990;47:919–926.

108. Leonard CM, Eckert MA, Lombardino LJ, et al. Anatomical risk factors for phonological dyslexia. Cereb Cortex 2001;11:148–157.

109. Leonard CM, Voeller KKS, Lombardino LJ, et al. Anomalous cerebral structure in dyslexia revealed with magnetic resonance imaging. Arch Neurol 1993;50:461–469.

110. Deutsch GK, Dougherty RF, Bammer R, et al. Children's reading performance is correlated with white matter structure measured by diffusion tensor imaging. Cortex 2005;41:354–363.

111. Casanova MF, Araque J, Giedd J, et al. Reduced brain size and gyrification in the brains of dyslexic patients. J Child Neurol 2004;19:275–281.

112. Brambati SM, Termine C, Ruffino M, et al. Regional reductions of gray matter volume in familial dyslexia. Neurology 2004;63:742–745.

113. Vinckenbosch E, Robichon F, Eliez S. Gray matter alteration in dyslexia: converging evidence from volumetric and voxel-by-voxel MRI analyses. Neuropsychologia 2005;43:324–331.

114. Poldrack RA, Temple E, Protopapas A, et al. Relations between the neural bases of dynamic auditory processing and phonological processing: evidence from fMRI. J Cogn Neurosci 2001;13:687–697.

115. Gelfand JR, Bookheimer SY. Dissociating neural mechanisms of temporal sequencing and processing phonemes. Neuron 2003;38:831–842.

116. Demonet JF, Chollet F, Ramsay S, et al. The anatomy of phonological and semantic processing in normal subjects. Brain 1992;115:1753–1768.

117. Fiez JA, Petersen SE. Neuroimaging studies of word reading. Proc Natl Acad Sci U S A 1998;95:914–921.

118. Horwitz B, Rumsey JM, Donohue BC. Functional connectivity of the angular gyrus in normal reading and dyslexia. Proc Natl Acad Sci U S A 1998;95:8939–8944.

119. Paulesu E, Frith U, Snowling M, et al. Is developmental dyslexia a disconnection syndrome? Evidence from PET scanning. Brain 1996;119:143–158.

120. Pugh KR, Shaywitz BA, Shaywitz SE, et al. Cerebral organization of component processes in reading. Brain 1996;119:1221–1238.

121. Rumsey JM, Andreason P, Zametkin AJ, et al. Failure to activate the left temporoparietal cortex in dyslexia: an oxygen 15 positron emission tomographic study [published erratum appears in Arch Neurol 1994;51:2437]. Arch Neurol 1992;49: 527–534.

122. Rumsey JM, Berman KF, Denckla MB, et al. Regional cerebral blood flow in severe developmental dyslexia. Arch Neurol 1987;44:1144–1150.

123. Rumsey JM, Horwitz B, Donohue BC, et al. Phonologic and orthographic components of word recognition: a PET-rCBF study. Brain 1997;120:739–759.

124. Shaywitz SE, Shaywitz BA, Pugh KR, et al. Functional disruption in the organization of the brain for reading in dyslexia. Proc Natl Acad Sci USA 1998;95:2636–2641.

125. Turkeltaub PE, Eden GF, Jones KM, et al. Meta-analysis of the functional neuroanatomy of single-word reading: method and validation. Neuroimage 2002;16:765–780.

126. Silani G, Frith U, Demonet JF, et al. Brain abnormalities underlying altered activation in dyslexia: a voxel based morphometry study. Brain 2005.

127. Shuren JE, Schefft BK, Yeh HS, et al. Repetition and the arcuate fasciculus. J Neurol 1995;242:596–598.

128. Warrington EK, Shallice T. Word-form dyslexia. Brain 1980;103:99–112.

129. McCandliss BD, Cohen L, Dehaene S. The visual word form area: expertise for reading in the fusiform gyrus. Trends Cogn Sci 2003;7:293–299.

130. Gauthier I, Tarr MJ. Becoming a "Greeble" expert: exploring mechanisms for face recognition. Vision Res 1997;37:1673–1682.

131. Gauthier I, Skudlarski P, Gore JC, et al. Expertise for cars and birds recruits brain areas involved in face recognition. Nat Neurosci 2000;3:191–197.

132. Dietz NA, Jones KM, Gareau L, et al. Phonological decoding involves left posterior fusiform gyrus. Hum Brain Mapp 2005.

133. Shaywitz SE, Shaywitz BA, Fulbright RK, et al. Neural systems for compensation and persistence: young adult outcome of childhood reading disability. Biol Psychiatry 2003;54:25–33.

134. Pugh, KR, Mencl WE, Shaywitz BA, et al. The angular gyrus in developmental dyslexia: task-specific differences in functional connectivity within posterior cortex. Psychol Sci 2000;11:51–56

135. Turkeltaub PE, Gareau L, Flowers DL, et al. Development of neural mechanisms for reading. Nat Neurosci 2003;6:767–773.

136. Pollatsek A, Lesch M, Morris RK, et al. Phonological codes are used in integrating information across saccades in word identification and reading. J Exp Psychol [Hum Percept] 1992;18:147–162.

137. Blanchard HE, Pollatsek A, Rayner K. The acquisition of parafoveal word information in reading. Percept Psychophy 1989;46:85–94.

138. Martos FJ, Vila J. Differences in eye movement control amongst dyslexic, retarded and normal readers in the Spanish population. Reading and Writing: An Interdisciplinary Journal 1990;2:175–188.

139. Pavlidis GT. Do eye movements hold the key to dyslexia? Neuropsychologia 1981;18:57–64.

140. Zangwill O, Blakemore C. Dyslexia: Reversal of eye movements during reading. Neuropsychologia 1972;10:371–373.

141. Black JL, Collins DWK, DeRoach JN, et al. A detailed study of sequential saccadic eye movements for normal and poor reading children. Percept Mot Skills 1984;59:423–434.

142. Brown B, Haegerstrom-Portnoy G, Adams A. Predictive eye movements do not discriminate between dyslexic and control children. Neuropsychologia 1983;21:112–128.

143. Olson RK, Kliegl R, Davidson BJ. Dyslexic and normal readers' eye movements. J Exp Psychol [Hum Percept] 1983;9:816–825.

144. Stanley G, Smith GA, Howell EA. Eye-movements and sequential tracking in dyslexic and control children. Br J Psychol 1983;74:181–187.

145. Lovegrove WJ, Bowling A, Badcock D, et al. Specific reading disability: differences in contrast sensitivity as a function of spatial frequency. Science 1980;210:439–440.

146. Martin F, Lovegrove W. Flicker contrast sensitivity in normal and specifically disabled readers. Perception 1987;16:215–221.

147. Stein JF, Fowler MS. Visual dyslexia. Trends Neurosci 1981;4:77–80.

148. Cornelissen PL, Richardson AJ, Mason AJ, et al. Contrast sensitivity and coherent motion detection measured at photopic luminance levels in dyslexics and controls. Vision Res 1995;35:1483–1494.

149. Livingstone MS, Rosen GD, Drislane FW, et al. Physiological and anatomical evidence for a magnocellular defect in developmental dyslexia. Proc Natl Acad Sci USA 1991;88:7943–7947.

150. Eden GF, Stein JF, Wood HM, et al. Differences in eye movements and reading problems in dyslexic and normal children. Vision Res 1994;34:1345–1358.

151. Eden GF, VanMeter JW, Rumsey JM, et al. Abnormal processing of visual motion in dyslexia revealed by functional brain imaging. Nature 1996;382:66–69.

152. Victor JD, Conte MM, Burton L, et al. Visual evoked potentials in dyslexics and normals: failure to find a difference in transient or steady-state responses. Vis Neurosci 1993;10:939–946.

153. Stephenson S. Six cases of congenital word-blindness affecting three generations of one family. Ophalmoscope 1907;5:482–484.

154. Hallgren B. Specific dyslexia "congenital word blindness": a clinical and genetic study. Acta Psychiatr Neurol Scand 1950;Suppl-65:1–287.

155. Bakwin H. Reading disability in twins. Dev Med Child Neurol 1973;15:184–187.

156. DeFries JC, Fulker DW. Multiple regression analysis of twin data: etiology of deviant scores versus individual differences. Acta Genet Med Gemellol 1985;37:205–216.

157. DeFries J, Alarcon M. Genetics of specific reading disabilities. Ment Retard Dev Dis Res Rev 1996;2:39–49.

158. Olson R, Wise B, Conners F, et al. Specific deficits in component reading and language skills: genetic and environmental influences. J Learning Disabil 1989;22:339–348.

159. Olson R, Gillis JJ, Rack JP, et al. Confirmatory factor analysis of word recognition and process measures in the Colorado Reading Project. Reading and Writing: An Interdisciplinary Journal 1991;3:235–248.

160. Cardon LR, Smith SD, Fulker DW, et al. Quantitative trait locus for reading disability on chromosome 6. Science 1994;266: 276–279.

161. Grigorenko EL, Wood FB, Golovyan L, et al. Continuing the search for dyslexia genes on 6p. Am J Med Genet 2003;118B:89–98.

162. Grigorenko EL, Wood FB, Meyer MS, et al. Susceptibility loci for distinct components of developmental dyslexia on chromosomes 6 and 15. Am J Hum Gen 1997;60:27–39.

163. Grigorenko EL, Wood FB, Meyer MS, et al. Chromosome 6p influences on different dyslexia-related cognitive processes: further confirmation. Am J Hum Genet 2000;66:715–723.

164. Turic D, Robinson L, Duke M, et al. Linkage disequilibrium mapping provides further evidence of a gene for reading disability on chromosome 6p21.3–22. Mol Psychiatry 2003;8:176–185.

165. Smith SD, Kelley PM, Askew JW, et al. Reading disability and chromosome 6p21.3: evaluation of MOG as a candidate gene. J Learn Disabil 2001;34:512–519.

166. Deffenbacher KE, Kenyon JB, Hoover DM, et al. Refinement of the 6p21.3 quantitative trait locus influencing dyslexia: linkage and association analyses. Hum Genet 2004;115:128–138.

167. Francks C, Paracchini S, Smith SD, et al. A 77-kilobase region of chromosome 6p22.2 is associated with dyslexia in families from the United Kingdom and from the United States. Am J Hum Genet 2004;75:1046–1058.

168. Cope N, Harold D, Hill G, et al. Strong evidence that KIAA0319 on chromosome 6p is a susceptibility gene for developmental dyslexia. Am J Hum Genet 2005;76:581–591.

169. Smith SD, Kimberling WJ, Pennington BF, et al. Specific reading disability: identification of an inherited form through linkage analysis. Science 1983;219:1345–1347.

170. Smith SD, Pennington BF, Kimberling WJ, et al. Familial dyslexia: use of genetic linkage data to define subtypes. J Am Acad Child Adolesc Psychiatry 1990;29:204–213.

171. Nopola-Hemii J, Taipale M, Haltia T, et al. Two translocations of chromosome 15q associated with dyslexia. J Med Genet 2000;37:771–775.

172. Taipale M, Kaminen N, Nopola-Hemmi J, et al. A candidate gene for developmental dyslexia encodes a nuclear tetratricopeptide repeat domain protein dynamically regulated in brain. Proc Natl Acad Sci USA 2003;100:11553–11558.

173. Chapman NH, Igo RP, Thomson JB, et al. Linkage analyses of four regions previously implicated in dyslexia: confirmation of a locus on chromosome 15q. Am J Med Genet B Neuropsychiatr Genet 2004;131:67–75.

174. Scerri TS, Fisher SE, Francks C, et al. Putative functional alleles of DYX1C1 are not associated with dyslexia susceptibility in a large sample of sibling pairs from the UK. J Med Genet 2004;41: 853–857.

175. Marino C, Giorda R, Luisa Lorusso M, et al. A family-based association study does not support DYX1C1 on 15q21.3 as a candidate gene in developmental dyslexia. Eur J Hum Genet 2005;13:491–499.

176. Morris DW, Ivanov D, Robinson L, et al. Association analysis of two candidate phospholipase genes that map to the chromosome 15q15.1–15.3 region associated with reading disability. Am J Med Genet B Neuropsychiatr Genet 2004;129:97–103.

177. Wigg KG, Couto JM, Feng Y, et al. Support for EKN1 as the susceptibility locus for dyslexia on 15q21. Mol Psychiatry 2004;9: 1111–1121.

178. Rabin M, Wen XL, Hepburn M, et al. Suggestive linkage of developmental dyslexia to chromosome 1p34–36. Lancet 1993;342: 178.

179. Froster U, Schulte-Korne G, Hebebrand J, et al. Cosegregation of balanced translocation (1;2) with retarded speech development and dyslexia. Lancet 1993;342:178–179.

180. Grigorenko EL, Wood FB, Meyer MS, et al. Linkage studies suggest a possible locus for developmental dyslexia on chromosome 1p. Am J Med Genet 2001;105:120–129.

181. Tzenova J, Kaplan BJ, Petryshen TL, et al. Confirmation of a dyslexia susceptibility locus on chromosome 1p34-p36 in a set of 100 Canadian families. Am J Med Genet B Neuropsychiatr Genet 2004;127:117–124.

182. Kaminen N, Hannula-Jouppi K, Kestila M, et al. A genome scan for developmental dyslexia confirms linkage to chromosome 2p11 and suggests a new locus on 7q32. J Med Genet 2003;40: 340–345.

183. Nopola-Hemmi J, Myllyluoma B, Haltia T, et al. A dominant gene for developmental dyslexia on chromosome 3. J Med Genet 2001;38:658–664.

184. Fisher SE, Francks C, Marlow AJ, et al. Independent genome-wide scans identify a chromosome 18 quantitative-trait locus influencing dyslexia. Nat Genet 2002;30:86–91.

185. de Kovel CG, Hol FA, Heister JG, et al. Genomewide scan identifies susceptibility locus for dyslexia on Xq27 in an extended Dutch family. J Med Genet 2004;41:652–657.

186. Corballis MC. FOXP2 and the mirror system. Trends Cogn Sci 2004;8:95–96.

187. Liegeois F, Baldeweg T, Connelly A, et al. Language fMRI abnormalities associated with FOXP2 gene mutation. Nat Neurosci 2003;6:1230–1237.

188. Haesler S, Wada K, Nshdejan A, et al. FoxP2 expression in avian vocal learners and non-learners. J Neurosci 2004;24:3164–3175.

189. O'Brien EK, Zhang X, Nishimura C, et al. Association of specific language impairment SLI to the region of 7q31. Am J Hum Genet 2003;72:1536–1543.

190. Macdermot KD, Bonora E, Sykes N, et al. Identification of FOXP2 truncation as a novel cause of developmental speech and language deficits. Am J Hum Genet 2005;76:1074–1080.

190a. Lindamood C, Lindamood P. *Lindamood Auditory Conceptualization Test.* Austin, TX: Pro-Ed, 1979.

190b. Torgesen JK, Wagner RK, Rashotte CA. *Test of Word Reading Efficiency (TOWRE).* Austin, TX: Pro-Ed, 1999.

190c. Weiderholt JL, Bryant RB. *Gray Oral Reading Test, 4th edition.* Austin, TX: Pro-Ed, 2001.

191. Orton J. The Orton-Gillingham Approach. In: Money J, ed. *The Disabled Reader: Education of the Dyslexic Child.* Baltimore, MD: The Johns Hopkins Press, 1966.

192. Lindamood CH, Lindamood P. *Auditory Discrimination in Depth.* Allen, TX: DLM/Teaching Resources, 1975.

193. Lindamood PH, Lindamood P. *The Lindamood Phoneme Sequencing Program for Reading, Spelling and Speech.* Austin, TX: Pro-Ed, 2004d.

194. Alexander AW, Slinger-Constant A-M. Current status of treatments for dyslexia: Critical Review. J Child Neurol 2004;19: 744–758.

195. Aylward EH, Richards TL, Berninger VW, et al. Instructional treatment associated with changes in brain activation in children with dyslexia. Neurology 2003;61:212–219.

196. Richards TL, Corina D, Serafini S, et al. Effects of a phonologically driven treatment for dyslexia on lactate levels measured by proton MR spectroscopic imaging. Am J Neuroradiol 2000; 21:916–922.

197. Shaywitz BA, Shaywitz SE, Blachman BA, et al. Development of left occipitotemporal systems for skilled reading in children after a phonologically-based intervention. Biol Psychiatry 2004;55: 926–933.

198. Simos PG, Fletcher JM, Bergman E, et al. Dyslexia-specific brain activation profile becomes normal following successful remedial training. Neurology 2002;58:1203–1213.

199. Eden GF, Jones KM, Cappell K, et al. Neural changes following remediation in adult developmental dyslexia. Neuron 2004;44: 411–422.

18

Sleep Disorders in Children

Rafael Pelayo, MD   Kin Yuen, MD   James Winde, MD   Maria-Cecilia Lopes, MD

Sleep disorders in children are relatively common and readily treatable. This chapter will review the various sleep disorders common in children and the management of these sleep disorders. Perhaps nowhere else in this text does modern neurology and psychiatry merge as naturally as in a discussion of sleep disorders. Sleep and dreams are at the core of the mystery (and wonderment) of the relationship between the brain and the mind. Seeking an understanding of sleep has been influential in the development of our culture. In prehistoric societies, attempts to understand the imagery of nighttime dreams and nightmares might have given rise to concepts of the spiritual world and religion. In medieval times, the phenomena of sleep paralysis, night terrors, and sleepwalking may have been interpreted as manifestations of demons.

Three hundred years ago the recurring nighttime afflictions of restless leg syndrome were thought to be a curse until Willis (of Circle of Willis fame) accurately described it as a neurological disease. In the late 19th century, sleep was viewed as a passive state that occurred in the absence of brain stimulation. Thomas Edison thought that the invention of the light bulb would allow us to avoid sleeping. The interest of a young neurologist named Sigmund Freud in sleep and dreams opened a new chapter in psychiatry. Years later a medical student, William Dement, became interested in finding a neurological basis to understand Freud's dream theories (1). In 1952, he helped discover the relationship between electroencephalographically measured rapid eye movements in sleep and dream recall. Infants and small children were an early part of Dement's research into rapid eye movement (REM) sleep. This research led to worldwide studies of the basic physiology of sleep.

Dement became a psychiatrist and initially studied the relationship of sleep and dreams to mental illness. In 1972,

he hired a young neurologist, Christian Guilleminault, and together they established the first medical clinic devoted exclusively to the treatment of patients with sleep disorders within the department of psychiatry at Stanford University. Guilleminault, as a student, had studied child development with Jean Piaget in France. Not surprisingly, children were among the first patients seen at the new clinic. This landmark clinic served as a model for the comprehensive multidisciplinary care of patients with sleep disorders. It also contributed to the recognition of sleep disorders medicine as a recognized medical specialty. The synergy of neurology and psychiatry, which was essential in establishing this new field, should continue for it to progress. The study of normal sleep and sleep disorders in children is an integral part of the development of modern sleep medicine.

It was probably not a coincidence that these researchers were relatively young when they embarked on their studies on sleep. The young seem to be particularly curious about sleep and dreams. Listening to children talk about their sleep can be fascinating. The REMs associated with dreaming are more easily seen in infants and young children than in adults and do not require sophisticated instrumentation. Dement has speculated that perhaps the discovery of REM sleep would have been made earlier if we had only paid closer attention to children when they were asleep (1). This tendency to not pay attention to children while sleeping has persisted. The author (RP) recalls being told as a pediatric intern to advise his patients' parents not to watch their children sleep as they would only return with too many unanswerable questions! Current knowledge of sleep disorders in children has not been incorporated into most medical training programs. This reality is hard to reconcile with the high prevalence of sleep disorders in children. Infant's sleep problems represent one of the most frequent complaints of parents consulting a pediatrician (2). The National Commission on Sleep Disorders concluded that 25% of parents had some concerns about their children's sleep. One survey estimated that 38% of children had experienced parasomnias such as sleep walking or night terrors, 14% had excessive daytime sleepiness, and 11% had sleep disordered breathing (3). When a child comes in for an evaluation of a possible sleep problem, the first concern of the parents or caretakers is whether the problem is due to a behavioral or physical cause. Often, the sleep problem is neither purely behavioral nor purely physical, but rather represents a combination of these factors.

The most common question asked about a child's normal sleep is, "how much time does my child need to sleep?" When a child has trouble sleeping, parents will often turn to a variety of paperback advice books on the market. The quality of advice offered is quite variable and conflicting. Clinicians should be aware of the advice put forth by the more popular of these books since parents may quote or have specific questions about the material as it applies to their child. Also parents are unlikely to seek a clinician's opinion if the advice book has solved the problem, so the questions that do arise are sometimes the result of frustration or confusion about what the parents have read. Often these books do not provide any longterm longitudinal data about the amount of time that a normal child spends sleeping at different ages.

NORMAL SLEEP

The basic principles of normal sleep are the same for children and adults. Normal sleep can be simply described as the ability to fall asleep easily, sleep through the night, and wake up feeling refreshed. What does this require? When adults with chronic insomnia describe their sleep difficulty, they initially say it has been a lifelong pattern. However, if you ask them specifically if they had insomnia when they were 8 or 9 years old they will often answer either "no" or "I don't remember." The insomnia problems often emerge in adolescence or even later. When insomnia is present at an early age, fear of sleeping alone is often a component.

Long-term longitudinal data has been published by Iglowstein and colleagues to illustrate the developmental course and age-specific variability of sleep patterns (4). As part of the Zurich Longitudinal Studies, they followed 493 children for 16 years. The study used structured sleep related questionnaires at 1, 3, 6, 9, 12, 18, and 24 months after birth and then at annual intervals until 16 years of age. Total sleep duration decreased from an average of 14.2 hours (SD: 1.9 hours) at 6 months of age to an average of 8.1 hours (SD: 0.8 hours) at 16 years of age. Total sleep duration decreased across the studied cohorts (1974–1993) as a result of later bedtime, but wake time remained essentially unchanged. Between 1.5 years and 4 years of age, there was a prominent decline in napping habits. At age 1.5

years, 96.4% of children had naps; by 4 years of age, only 35.4% napped. This is consistent with a prior study of napping patterns by Weissbluth (5).

Napping patterns were monitored in a cohort of 172 children followed from 6 months to 7 years of age. There were no differences in the number of naps at 6 months of age or the pattern of napping based on gender, birth order, and whether naps disappeared spontaneously or were stopped by the parents. Total daytime sleep remained a stable individual characteristic between 6 and 18 months of age. A pattern of two naps per day was well established by 9 to 12 months of age and one afternoon nap by 15 to 24 months. The duration of naps from 2 to 6 years was 2 hours. During the third and fourth years, napping occurred in the majority of children, but at decreasing rates. A minority of children were napping by 5 to 6 years and naps usually disappeared by age 7. If a child continues to nap by the age of 7 years, it is possible that a sleep disorder may be present. In 2004, Watamuran and colleagues showed changes in cortisol activity in infants who took frequent short naps (6). However, nap behavior can be put into a cultural context; it would be less of a concern if napping or "siestas" are part of the cultural environment. However, it is important to ask about the child's behavior in the afternoon. Naps may not be called naps but rather reported as falling asleep while riding home from school. This overall normative data can serve as a guide to determine if a problem is due to an inadequate amount of sleep.

To determine if a problem is due to an inadequate quality of sleep, more detailed measurements of sleep and the underlying physiology may be needed. Sleep physiology begins with an understanding that sleep is not a homogenous state, but is instead a mixture of rhythms associated with different states and stages. The brain seems to have three basic states or modes: awake, dreaming, or sleeping without dreaming. Evaluating these states and stages requires three electrophysiological measurements: the electrical activity of the brain during the sleep states, the muscle tone, and eye movements. These parameters are measured with an electroencephalogram (EEG), a chin electromyogram (EMG), and an electrooculogram (EOG), respectively. The patterning of these measures (electrical activity of the brain, muscle tone, and eye movements) divides sleep into two broad categories: REM sleep and non-REM sleep. REM sleep is referred to as paradoxical sleep because the brain waves are similar to those of the awake state but the body seemed paralyzed. REM sleep accounts for approximately 20% of total sleep time after age 3 years. At birth, REM sleep takes up 50% of the total sleep time. Dreaming is associated closely with REM sleep. REM sleep is characterized by loss of muscle tone (atonia), which results in absent or greatly diminished deep tendon reflexes. When a person is awakened from REM sleep, wakefulness returns quickly. REM periods occur in cycles of approximately 90 minutes throughout the night, with the longest and most intense REM periods occurring just after the body temperature reaches a minimum (approximately 2 hours before waking up). At the end of every REM cycle, there is usually an arousal or brief awakening. In infants, REM cycles are shorter (approximately 40 to 60 minutes). Parents may be concerned that their infant seems to "wake up every hour." These brief awakenings may be part of the child's normal rhythm, but an overly attentive parent may inadvertently reinforce and prolonged the awakenings. On the other hand, it is possible that the awakenings are due to a condition that is exacerbated by REM sleep, such as obstructive sleep apnea.

NonREM sleep is subdivided into stages 1, 2, 3, and 4. Stage 1 is the lightest sleep and is typically a transition from awake to drowsiness to sleep. Stage 1 occupies less than 10% of the total sleep time. In stage 1, people may not realize they are asleep and think they were awake. They may also have fragments of auditory or dreamlike imagery called *hypnagogic* hallucinations. Similar episodes upon awakening are called *hypnopompic* hallucinations. These episodes occur more commonly with sleep deprivation and in conditions such as narcolepsy. They should not be confused with psychosis. Stage 2 is an intermediate state that can be over half of the total sleep time. Stages 3 and 4 (also called delta or slow-wave sleep) represent the deepest sleep as measured by the amount of stimulation needed to wake up. This stimulation is called the arousal threshold. It is called delta sleep because the EEG is dominated by slow waves in the delta range (<4 Hz). Delta sleep has homeostatic properties: it increases in duration and intensity in response to sleep deprivation. The amount of delta sleep is at least 10 % of the total sleep time in children and decreases after adolescence. Delta sleep clusters in the first third of the night. During delta, it is extremely difficult to arouse children. If aroused, they often appear disoriented and cognitively slowed. Parasomnias, such as sleepwalking and sleep terrors, usually emerge from slow-wave sleep and are common in the first third of the night.

A discussion of normal sleep would be incomplete without reviewing the role of circadian rhythm and the biological clock (7–11). The circadian modulation of alertness and sleepiness is an important part of sleep physiology. A successful terrestrial animal must be able to predict dawn and dusk and anticipate the change in seasons. Humans are, in general, diurnal. We have excellent color vision in the daytime but our night vision is not as good as that of many of our potential predators. Part of our circadian physiology is our tendency to have decreased alertness in the afternoon and to have a surge of alertness ("second wind") in the evenings. This process is modulated by the suprachiasmatic nucleus and is referred to as clock-dependent alerting (12, 13). If a person is having trouble falling asleep, then an earlier bedtime may make the problem worse by creating greater frustration. Dramatic shifts in wake-up times on school days compared to nonschool days can alter the circadian patterns and lead to sleep problems.

GENERAL CLINICAL GUIDELINES

Sleep disorders should be considered whenever a child is being evaluated for a behavioral problem. Insufficient quality or quantity of sleep may be associated with learning difficulties and attention problems. When a child does not sleep well, it can disrupt the entire household and lead to significant stress for the family. Unrecognized and undertreated sleep disturbances can carry over into adulthood.

In pediatrics, a medical history usually starts with the history of the pregnancy and delivery. However, an adequate history of a child's sleep disorder should begin with a history of the sleep patterns of the parents/caretakers before the child was born. For example, if an infant sleeps continuously for 7 hours at night and the mother was in the habit of sleeping 6.5 hours before the pregnancy she might be pleased with the way the child is sleeping. However, if the mother usually slept 8 or 9 hours she might complain that the child is not sleeping enough at night. The family's cultural background must also be taken into account when evaluating a complaint of poor sleep. Also, the influence of other family members, such as grandparents, in shaping the family's views should be considered. The parents need to be in agreement about their expectations of the child's sleep, especially if the parents come from different cultural backgrounds. The parent's own experience in childhood should be explored. The mother and father may view the infant's sleep pattern from quite different perspectives. However, studies have included both parents to analyze parent-child interactions (14). Particularly in the early years, a child's life is centered at home. If a parent had a history of occasional insomnia before the infant was born, he or she might be overly sensitized to interruptions of sleep by the infant, whereas the other parent might find the disruption more tolerable. A parent who has a history of snoring or mild obstructive sleep apnea might be less able to tolerate what would otherwise be considered normal interruptions of sleep.

When taking a history it is important to keep in mind that the need for sleep is biological; however, the way someone sleeps is learned. Sleep clearly fulfills some biological needs and has homeostatic properties (15), and the longer you stay awake, the more intense the desire to sleep; the better you sleep, the better you are able to stay awake. At the same time, in theory, a person is more vulnerable and could be attacked while sleeping, so there must be mechanisms present that allow us to sleep and be safe at the same time. Like other animals, we sleep differently depending on the particular circumstances in which we find ourselves. A woman late in her pregnancy will have very fragmented sleep due to multiple factors. Will she then be able to regularly sleep soundly for 8 hours in a row after she becomes a mother? Certainly not, if she has to nurse her newborn every 2 to 4 hours! All of us sleep best when we go to sleep feeling safe and comfortable. We learn to feel this way by forming associations with our sleeping environment and these associations are formed starting from infancy. Infant and children, like adults, may develop maladaptive associations that result in sleep difficulties. When evaluating school age children for a sleep problem, it is important to ask the child directly if he is scared of the dark or of being alone. The parents may minimize these concerns and the children may be too embarrassed to volunteer the information. In any evaluation, it is crucial to keep in mind the interaction between the physiological need for sleep and the psychology of sleep.

When evaluating a sleep problem, it is important to recognize that what awakens the patient may not be what keeps the patient awake. For example, you could be awakened at night because of the sudden loud noise coming from a party next door. The fact that you were not invited to the party could bother you and keep you awake! It is not uncommon in a clinical situation to have two or more sleep disorders interacting in the same patient. A child may have an awakening due to difficulty breathing from sleep apnea, but then be unable to return to sleep because she has not learned to settle back down without the parents' intervention. Since patients can not provide us with information about their sleep once they are asleep, it is important to get as much information as possible from other members of the household.

PHARMACOLOGICAL GUIDELINES

There is relatively little information available on the pharmacological management of sleep disorders in children. Most pharmacological guidelines were developed for sleep disorders in adults and must be empirically extrapolated to children. The medications are typically neither US Food and Drug Administration (FDA) approved for the specific sleep disorder nor for the pediatric age range. The physician is often forced to prescribe medications as an "off label" indication. This may result in frustrating insurance reimbursement delays or denials for the family. These reimbursement problems may affect the availability of a specific medication, the family's compliance with the medication, or force the physician to prescribe a less desirable alternative medication. The medication may not be available commercially in an easily administered format. Young children may not be able to swallow pills or ingest chewable tablets, requiring the local pharmacist to compound the medication into a suspension. In addition, due to the natural aversion among both parents and physicians to use medications for pediatric sleep disorders, medications are usually prescribed as a last resort or in the most refractory situations.

At times, a decision to use medication in a child may be made not necessarily to assist the child as much as to help the parents or other family members sleep better. It is not unusual for parents to finally seek help for a child's long-standing sleep problem when they feel they can no longer

put up with interruptions to their own sleep. Further complicating the pharmacological treatment of sleep disorders in children is the general lack of specialized training in sleep disorders available to the health care providers who are working with these children. Failure to consider or properly apply nondrug treatments as part of the comprehensive management of the child may also lead to unsatisfactory results for the patient and the family. Children with sleep disorders may not be properly managed due to either underdosing or overdosing of medication or incorrect medication selection.

There maybe an overreliance on the effects of the medication by both the parents and health care provider without adequate application of behavioral techniques to help improve the child's sleep. A common scenario in clinical practice is a parent's complaint of a child's paradoxical reaction to a hypnotic medication. "It made it worse" or "he became hyper" may be the parent's complaint. This may occur because the timing or the dose provided was incorrect. The parents may expect that once a medication has been finally prescribed to help their child sleep that it will "knockout" the child. It is important that the health care provider advising this family take into account the circadian modulation of alertness. Humans will typically experience enhanced alertness in the evening, which is often referred to as a "second wind." During this circadian phase, it is harder to fall asleep. If the hypnotic medication is given during this circadian time window, the medication may not work or the child may be frightened by hypnagogic hallucinations. If a medication has been shown to shorten sleep latency by only 20 or 30 minutes, giving this medication 2 or 3 hours before the usual falling asleep time could elicit this common scenario. This same medication given at a more appropriate circadian time could be effective. A similar lack of efficacy or paradoxical reaction could occur if the medication dose is inadequate.

This lack of proper management of the sleep problem may be particularly common among children with neurological or psychiatric disabilities. If the child cannot communicate what she feels is causing the sleep difficulty, incorrect assumptions may be made by the family or health care provider. In a case of insomnia, this can result in an escalating cycle of progressively more sedating agents with increasing likelihood of adverse effects. Concomitant daytime sedation may occur, which may interfere with the child's therapeutic program and exacerbate the child's disabilities. In some situations, the fear of addiction may deter the physician or the family from using pharmacotherapy adequately to improve the child's sleep.

SLEEP DISORDERS

There are over 80 recognized sleep disorders, encompassing a wide range of disturbances including parasomnias, sleep-related disordered breathing, (obstructive sleep apnea), restless leg syndrome, and disorders of initiating and maintaining sleep. However, we lack sufficient normative and epidemiological data in the field of pediatric sleep disorders and much more research is needed. There is a paucity of therapeutic clinical trials and health policy outcomes research.

Sleep-Disordered Breathing

Sleep-disordered breathing is a clinical syndrome ranging from simple snoring to potentially life-threatening obstructive sleep apnea syndrome. This clinical spectrum can occur at any age. Charles Dickens provided a classical description of "Pickwickian" snoring with arousals and excessive daytime sleepiness in a boy named Joe (16). The first medical description in English of children with abnormal breathing in sleep is attributed to William Osler in 1892 in his textbook (17).

In the modern medical literature, Guilleminault reported the first series of children with obstructive sleep apnea in 1976 (18). That report describes the essential clinical features of this condition. More recently there has been a realization that patients may be symptomatic in the absence of frank apneas (19, 20). This has led to use of the terms "sleep-disordered breathing" and "sleep-related breathing disorders" to better describe the clinical spectrum, which includes obstructive sleep apnea syndrome, upper airway resistance syndrome, and obstructive hypopnea syndrome.

The most obvious nocturnal symptom is snoring. Snoring is very common in the pediatric population. It can indicate turbulent airflow and is not normal (21–23). While awake, breathing is silent. If a sleeping animal is vulnerable to attack by a predator, why would it make breathing noise when its guard is down? Indeed animals in the wild do not seem to snore; only domestic animals snore. Not all snoring is due to obstructive sleep apnea. It may be due to other forms of obstruction such as nasal allergies or a cold (24, 25). Chervin et al. assessed the frequency of childhood sleep problems in two general pediatric clinics. Parents of 1,038 unselected children (554 boys) aged 2.0 to 13.9 years completed a validated Pediatric Sleep Questionnaire. Habitual snoring was reported in 176 (17%) of the children (26).

While sleep-disordered breathing in children has many important similarities to the adult version of this disorder, there are also marked differences in presentation, diagnosis, and management. Abnormal daytime sleepiness may be recognized more often by school teachers than by parents. Some parents may consider an increase in total sleep time or an extra long nap as normal. Nonspecific behavioral difficulties in children with sleep disorders may be reported to the pediatrician such as abnormal shyness, depression, hyperactivity, developmental delays, or rebellious or aggressive behavior (27). Chervin and associates found conduct problems and hyperactivity are frequently described in children referred for sleep-disordered breath-

ing. They surveyed parents of children aged 2 to 14 years at two general clinics between 1998 and 2000. Parents of 872 children completed the surveys. Bullying and other specific aggressive behaviors were two to three times more frequent among children at high risk for sleep-disordered breathing (28). Other daytime symptoms may include speech defects, poor appetite, or swallowing difficulties (19, 29). Bedwetting accidents should raise suspicion of sleep-disordered breathing. Crabtree et al. found more impairments in quality of life and depressive symptoms in children who snored (30).

Many of these children breathe through their mouths, and regular mouth breathing should always lead to suspicion of sleep-disordered breathing (31). Children with disordered breathing may avoid going to bed at night due to hypnagogic hallucinations. Upon awakening, these children may report morning headaches, dry mouth, confusion, or irritability. As mentioned, depending on the child's age, daytime sleepiness may not be obvious. It may present only as a complaint of daytime tiredness or as a tendency to take naps easily anywhere.

A study from Israel found that children with sleep-disordered breathing had lower scores on neurocognitive testing compared to controls; test performance improved after treatment (32). In this prospective study, 39 children aged 5 to 9 years underwent a battery of neurocognitive tests containing process-oriented intelligence scales. Children with sleep-disordered breathing had lower scores compared with healthy children in some of the Kaufman Assessment Battery for Children (K-ABC) subtests and in the general scale Mental Processing Composite, indicating impaired neurocognitive function. Six to 10 months after adenotonsillectomy, the children with obstructive sleep apnea syndrome demonstrated significant improvement in sleep characteristics, as well as in daytime behavior. Their neurocognitive performance improved considerably, reaching the level of the control group in the following subtests: Gestalt Closure, Triangles, Word Order, and Matrix analogies, as well as in the K-ABC general scales, Sequential and Simultaneous Processing scales, and the Mental Processing Composite scale. The magnitude of the change expressed as effect sizes showed medium and large improvements in all three general scales of the K-ABC tests. The authors concluded that neurocognitive function is impaired in otherwise healthy children with sleep-disordered breathing. Most functions improve to the level of the control group, indicating that the impaired neurocognitive functions are mostly reversible, at least 3 to 10 months following adenotonsillectomy (32). An abrupt and persistent deterioration in grades must also raise the question of abnormal sleep and sleep-disordered breathing (23, 33–36).

In schools, tiredness and sleepiness may be labeled as "inattentive in class," "daydreaming," or "not being there" (37, 38). Concerns about school performance were raised in the original description of obstructive sleep apnea syndrome in children (14). More recently, a number of studies have addressed the possible association between sleep-disordered breathing and attention deficit hyperactivity disorder (ADHD) (39–45). O'Brien et al. examined the hypothesis that certain domains of neurobehavioral function would be selectively affected by sleep-disordered breathing. They conducted a survey of 5,728 children, aged 5 to 7 years old, asking questions about the frequency of various sleep-related problem behaviors, including snoring. The parents were also asked if the child was hyperactive. Children with reported symptoms of hyperactivity were then randomly selected for an overnight polysomnographic assessment and a battery of neurocognitive tests. Controls were selected from the group of children whose parents did not endorse hyperactive symptoms. Parents completed standardized rating scales relating to ADHD. Frequent and loud snoring was reported in 11.7% of the children; 7.3% of the parents viewed their children as being hyperactive or as having received a diagnosis of ADHD. The majority (76.5%) were boys. Eighty-three children with parentally reported symptoms of ADHD had sleep studies together with 34 control children. The Conners' Parent Rating Scale was administered to identify the degree of hyperactivity. Overnight polysomnography revealed that obstructive sleep apnea was present in 5% of those with significant ADHD symptoms, 26% with mild symptoms, and 5% of the nonhyperactive control group. REM latency and the proportion of REM sleep were more likely to be affected in the group with significant symptoms of ADHD. The groups did not differ in any other objective sleep measure. The authors concluded that an unusually high prevalence of snoring was identified among of the children who had mild symptoms of ADHD. Thus, sleep-disordered breathing is associated with mild ADHD-like behaviors that can be misdiagnosed as ADHD and potentially delay diagnosis and appropriate treatment (31).

Clinical signs of sleep-disordered breathing include increased respiratory efforts with nasal flaring, suprasternal or intercostal retractions, abnormal paradoxical inward motion of the chest during inspiration, along with sweating during sleep. Sweating may be limited to only the nuchal region, particularly in infants; it may be severe enough to necessitate changing clothes during the night. The parents may mention the child feeling warm at night or preferring to sleep without a blanket. Parents may also observe that the child stops breathing, then gasps for breath. It is surprising to note how often parents have observed abnormal breathing patterns during sleep but were never questioned about it by pediatricians during regular visits. Information regarding the sleep position is also helpful. Typically, the neck is hyperextended and the mouth is open. Another typical sleeping position is prone with the knee tucked under the chest with the head turned to the side and hyperextended. Rarely the child with sleep-disordered breathing prefers to sleep propped up on several pillows (19).

Ohayon has found that individuals identified with sleep-disordered breathing have a much higher incidence of nightmares, with reports of "drowning," "being buried alive," and "choking" (46). Night-terrors may lead to escape behavior and sleepwalking. If sleep fragmentation induced by the breathing events occurs during slow-wave sleep, night-terrors and sleepwalking may be triggered (47). A physical finding that may be overlooked in a child with sleep-disordered breathing is a narrow and high arched palate (19). Interestingly, the DSM-IV's description of ADHD mentions that minor physical anomalies such as high arched palates may be present (48). The possibility of a sleep disorder being present should be considered in any child being evaluated for ADHD. This is particularly important because treatment of sleep-disordered breathing may improve behavior and academic performance (49, 50).

The diagnostic criteria used for adults with obstructive sleep apnea syndrome cannot be used reliably in children (51–53). The diagnosis of sleep-disordered breathing is based on the history, physical findings, and supportive data. Laboratory testing should be, ideally, tailored to the clinical question. For example, if there are concerns about excessive daytime sleepiness, a multiple sleep latency test (MSLT) may be indicated (54). The MSLT is ideally performed in subjects who are at least 8 years old. The polysomnogram in a child uses the same technology and the same type of information as in adults. Airflow, respiratory effort, and pulse oximetry are the breathing measurements usually monitored. The respiratory effort is measured most accurately in a clinical sleep study using esophageal pressure measurements with a water-filled catheter.

Esophageal pressure measurements are not yet part of the routine polysomnogram in most sleep laboratories. An alternative measurement can be obtained using end-tidal CO_2 monitoring, which can detect important transient episodes of hypercarbia. A more recent technique to measure air flow using a nasal cannula has been introduced. This technique has been replacing nasal thermistors and is less invasive than esophageal manometry (55–58).

In addition to the absence of controlled studies of sleep-disordered breathing in the pediatric age group, there is also a lack of consensus in the definitional criteria. In adults, obstructive sleep apneas are defined as lasting at least 10 seconds. However, because children have faster respiratory rates, the duration is less for clinically significant apneas. Apneas as brief as 3 or 4 seconds may result in oxygen desaturation. There is also no uniform measure of hypopneas in children. The clinician needs to know how apneas and hypopneas are defined and scored when interpreting a polysomnogram report.

The upper airway resistance syndrome is present in individuals with symptoms of sleep-disordered breathing, who on the polysomnogram have evidence of sleep disruption associated with increased work of breathing, without a significant degree of apneas or hypopneas. In children, the work of breathing can be measured by recording esophageal pressure. Calibration is conducted by measuring esophageal pressure while the child is awake. The baseline pressure usually ranges from −10 to −5 cm of water. A repetitive breathing pattern can be identified with increasingly more negative esophageal pressure culminating in a brief arousal (59, 60). Controversy exists over whether a diagnosis of obstructive sleep apnea, or the larger spectrum of sleep-disordered breathing, should routinely be made without a formal polysomnogram. While some have suggested that this diagnosis can be made in patients using either the history and physical, or the history, physical, and an audio or videotape, others have found that the clinical history alone does not distinguish primary snoring from obstructive sleep apnea syndrome in children (61). The situation is further complicated by the description of upper airway resistance syndrome in children, which may have been missed in the studies cited previously. Therefore, a sleep study is the most definitive test for sleep-disordered breathing (62, 63). Currently, some otolaryngologists who treat children with sleep-disordered breathing may make the surgical recommendation based on clinical findings of airway obstruction, sometimes reviewing an audio or videotape (64, 65). Clinicians must be aware of the potential pitfalls of this practice. Certainly, there are individual cases in which a diagnostic sleep study is not available, but ideally, this should be the exception. The challenge we face in sleep medicine is providing easily accessible and cost-effective care working within a multidisciplinary model. We do not know, for certain, how accurate clinical diagnosis is without objective testing. Until we have a better answer, the diagnostic gold standard should not be disregarded particularly in a tertiary care setting. The American Thoracic Society and American Academy of Sleep Medicine and the American Academy of Pediatrics all support the use of sleep studies (66, 67).

Sleep-disordered breathing is not the only sleep disorder a child may have. Clinical impression may have both false-negative and false-positive results, leading to possible misdiagnosis or unnecessary surgery. For example, without confirmatory testing, a child with only "simple snoring" and symptomatic periodic limb movements will inevitably be misdiagnosed with sleep-disordered breathing and may have unnecessary surgery. Periodic limb movements of sleep and restless leg syndrome may not be rare in children (68). However, the history may be vague or hard to elicit.

Sleep-disordered breathing may occur more frequently in special populations. Any condition or syndrome associated with craniofacial anomalies may be associated with sleep-disordered breathing. Pierre-Robin, Apert's, and Crouzon's are among these syndromes. Approximately half of all children with Down syndrome have sleep-disordered breathing (69). Symptoms of daytime sleepiness and sleep disruptions at night may be due to nonneurological factors such as maxillofacial abnormalities, large tonsils or adenoids, hypognathus, large tongues, or other abnormalities.

Such factors often lead to sleep fragmentation and daytime sleepiness. Sleep disorders often occur in patients with neuromuscular disorder associated with weakness in respiratory muscles, which is further exacerbated by hypotonia during sleep. In disorders such as Duchenne's muscular dystrophy, daytime pulmonary function studies do not predict the severity of apneic events during sleep. These patients can have nocturnal oxygen desaturation, significant sleep fragmentation, recurrent hypoventilation, and reduced REM sleep, and are also at risk for aspiration during sleep. Diagnosis and treatment of sleep-disordered breathing in these patients can be an important part of comprehensive management.

There are four treatment options for sleep-disordered breathing in adults. These treatments may be combined. The most common treatment is continuous positive airway pressure (CPAP) to help splint open the upper airway. When CPAP is used correctly, snoring should be absent during sleep. There are several surgical options with a wide range of success. In adults, oral appliances that help re-position the mandible have improved breathing during sleep in selected patients. As a conservative measure, adults with sleep-disordered breathing are advised to sleep off their backs, lose weight, and avoid alcohol before sleeping.

In children, adenotonsillectomy is the most common initial treatment for sleep-disordered breathing; however it does not always cure the sleep disorder. The true cure rate of adenotonsillectomy for sleep-disordered breathing is unknown (70-71). Suen and colleagues designed a prospective study of 69 children, age 1 to 14 years, who were referred to an otolaryngologist. Thirty-five (51%) had a repiratory disturbance index greater than 5 on polysomnography. Of these, 30 underwent adenotonsillectomy and 26 of these children then had follow-up polysomnography. Although all 26 children had a lower respiratory disturbance index after surgery, four still had an index greater than 5. Using a respiratory disturbance index cut-off of 5, the cure rate of the surgery would be 85%. However, three children with a post-operative respiratory disturbance index less than 5 continued to snore. If these children were considered to have residual sleep-disordered breathing, then the cure rate of surgery would only be 73%. All patients improved with adenotonsillectomy but the true cure rate was not clear. The possibility of residual sleep-disordered breathing should always be considered after surgery if the child is symptomatic. Suen and associates concluded history and physical findings were not useful in predicting outcome (72). Different surgical techniques may improve the success of surgery in these children (73).

Some may argue that in clear-cut cases of sleep disordered breathing the sleep study may be skipped. However, the adult experience teaches us that it is precisely these obviously more severe or "clear-cut" cases that will have residual disease. Adenotonsillectomy will not change the relationship of tongue size and shape to the palate. The parents may report that the child is "100 % better"; however, these children can still have residual obstruction. If the child still has trouble paying attention in school, a sleep problem may be overlooked and no longer be considered a possibility. The child may end up labeled as having attention deficit disorder because there was no postoperative sleep test done (74).

If surgery is not a option for the child, then CPAP therapy should be considered (75–77). CPAP uses a small air compressor attached to a mask via a hose. The mask usually only covers the nose but masks are available that cover the nose and mouth. By forcing positive pressure into the airway, the negative pressure of inspiration can be countered to avoid airway narrowing or collapse. CPAP is effective but can be cumbersome to use. Over time, the CPAP devices have become smaller and quieter. The masks have also improved with many more styles and sizes available. Despite these advances, it remains a second choice over surgery in most children, because of the advantage of the surgical option. The main drawbacks of using CPAP are related to getting a properly fitting CPAP mask. If the mask is not fitted correctly, the air pressure may not be maintained causing discomfort and disrupting sleep. If the mask is on too tight, it can cause facial abrasions or bruising. In small children, the possibility of sleeping with the CPAP mask interfering with growth of the maxilla should be considered. As the child grows, the CPAP may require adjustments both in terms of mask size and the amount of pressure delivered to the airway. In addition to a continuous pressure delivery mode, a bi-level mode is available. In this mode, the pressure on expiration is lower than the inspiratory pressure. This may allow the device to be more comfortable and may be preferred in patients with neuromuscular weakness. The most recent advance in positive airway pressure has been the development of machines that can adjust the pressure required to keep the airway open on a breath-by-breath basis. These so-called "smart CPAP" units are promising but are not part of the mainstream treatment of children at this time (75,78).

In summary, it is important for clinicians to be aware that sleep-disordered breathing and snoring are not normal. Difficulty breathing while asleep may impact the daytime behavior of children. Sleep-disordered breathing is readily treatable.

Narcolepsy

Narcolepsy is a chronic neurological disorder in which the boundaries between the awake, sleeping, and dreaming brain are blurred. The awake narcoleptic will feel sleepy. The sleeping narcoleptic will have disturbed sleep due to arousals. Historically, the word "narcolepsy" was first coined by Gélineau in 1880 to designate a pathological condition characterized by irresistible episodes of sleep of short duration recurring at close intervals. In the same article, he noted that the attacks were sometimes accompanied by falls or "astasias." The cardinal features of narcolepsy are daytime somnolence, cataplexy, sleep paralysis, and hypnagogic hallucinations (79). These symptoms were called the "tetrad" of narcolepsy by Yoss and Daly (80,81). The abnormal sleep onset REM sleep periods in narcolepsy were described by Rechtschaffen et al. (82). Since 1975, narcolepsy has been described as a "pentade" of symptoms due to prominent sleep fragmentation in several patients (83).

Narcolepsy is a rare condition; the prevalence of narcolepsy has been calculated at about 1 per 2,000 of the general population (84). Age at onset varies from early childhood to the fifth decade, with a peak in the second decade. It is important to consider narcolepsy, especially in young patients, because it can take up to 20 years between the apperance of the first symptom, commonly sleepiness, and the emergence of the full clinical syndrome. During this time, the patient may be mislabeled with a variety of diagnoses. The patient may be considered lazy or depressed. Before being correctly diagnosed, the patient may turn to illegal drugs, such as "crank" amphetamine, to combat the sleepiness.

Clinical Presentation

Narcolepsy is characterized by abnormal sleep, including excessive daytime sleepiness with often-disturbed nocturnal sleep later in life and pathological manifestations related to REM sleep. REM sleep-related abnormalities include early REM sleep onset and cataplexy (79).

Cataplexy is an abrupt and reversible decrease or loss of muscle tone, most frequently provoked by emotion, particularly laughter. Consciousness typically remains intact. It may involve only certain muscles or the entire voluntary musculature. Most typically, the jaw sags, the head falls forward, the arms drop to the side, and the knees buckle. The severity and extent of cataplectic attacks can range from a state of absolute powerlessness, which seems to involve the entire body, to no more than a fleeting sensation of weakness. Severe cataleptic attacks can involve a complete loss of muscle tone, resulting in a fall with risk of serious injuries, including skull and other bone fractures, but can consist only of a slight buckling of the knees. Patients may perceive this abrupt and short-lasting weakness and may simply sit or stand against a wall. The attacks may be so subtle as not to be noticed by an observer. Although the extraocular muscles are supposedly not involved, the patient may complain of blurred vision. Speech may be slurred owing to intermittent weakness affecting the arytenoid muscles. Respiration may become irregular during an attack, which may be related to weakness of the abdominal muscles.

As seen during nocturnal REM sleep, the abrupt muscle inhibition is interrupted by sudden bursts of returning muscle tone, which at times even seems enhanced. If the weakness involves only the jaw or speech, the subject may present with wide masticatory movement or odd attacks of stuttering. If it involves the upper limbs, the patient

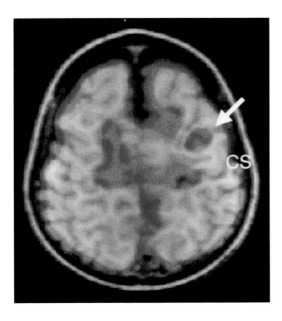

Figure 6.7 Ictal SPECT focus in a 2.5-year-old girl with seizures of left frontal origin. The red area represents the region with highest blood flow increase. Coregistration with high-resolution MRI demonstrated that the focus (arrow) was just in front of the precentral gyrus (CS = central sulcus). Seizure onset on intracranial EEG monitoring colocalized with the SPECT focus.

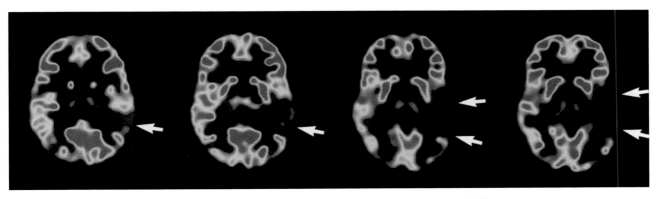

Figure 6.8 PET scan of an infant with medically refractory infantile spasms and with normal MRI. The focus of decreased glucose utilization in the left temporal lobe *(arrows)* corresponded to the interictal and ictal epileptiform activity on the EEG.

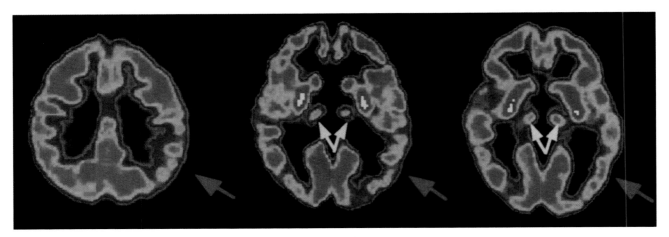

Figure 6.17 PET images from a 4-year-old child with spastic diplegic cerebral palsy associated with premature birth who was evaluated for delayed language skills. MRI revealed irregular contour to the walls of the lateral ventricles and high signal intensity in the periventricular white matter but no abnormalities in the cortex. PET revealed moderate hypometabolism in the left parietal and temporal cortex *(large arrows)*. In addition, there may be mild thalamic hypometabolism bilaterally *(small arrows)*.

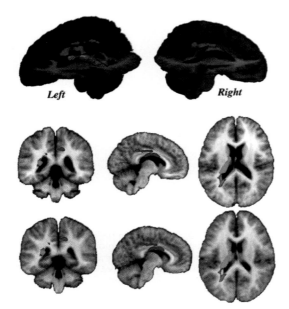

Left   Right

Figure 10.2 Statistical parametric mapping (SPM) results from the UCLA childhood-onset schizophrenia study. The <u>top panel</u> shows the three-dimensional renderings of the significant clusters from the gray matter (blue), white matter (red), and CSF (green). SPMs mapped into the average brain space of the nine subjects with COS. Significant voxels from the gray matter (in blue; voxel threshold $p < .01$, corrected at $p = .05$), white matter (in red; voxel threshold $p < .01$, corrected at $p = .05$), and CSF (in green; voxel threshold $p < .01$, corrected at $p = .10$) SPMs are mapped onto three orthogonal slices from the average schizophrenic brain (<u>middle panel</u>) and over the same three slices of the average control brain (<u>bottom panel</u>). From: Sowell ER, Toga AW, Asarnow R. Brain abnormalities observed in childhood-onset schizophrenia: A review of the structural magnetic resonance imaging literature. *MRDD Res. Rev.* 2000;6:180–185. Copyright @ 2000. Reprinted by permission of Wiley-Liss, Inc., a subsidiary of John Wiley & Sons, Inc.

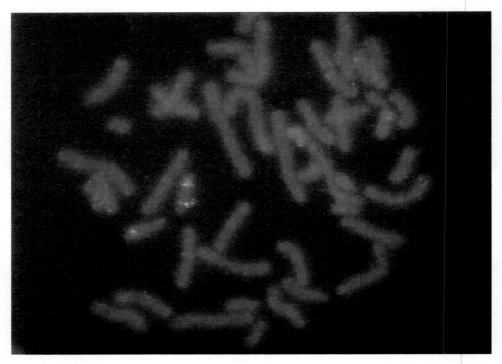

Figure 29.3 A fluorescent in situ hybridization (FISH) study on a metaphase spread. The chromosomes look orange when viewed under the fluorescent microscope. Fluorescein-tagged probes appear yellow. The metaphase preparation has been hybridized with a mixture of two cosmid probes. One identifies 15g11g12, the Prader-Willi syndrome/Angelman's syndrome (PWS/AS) critical region. The other probe hybridizes to the 15q22 area to identify the fact that there are two number-15 chromosomes. The analysis reveals two number-15 homologues but only one copy of the PWS/AS critical region. This microdeletion was not visible on prometaphase spreads.
Source: Figure courtesy of Jolla Gibas, Cytogenetics Laboratory, Division of Medical Genetics, Jefferson Medical College, Philadelphia, PA.

will complain of "clumsiness," and may describe dropping cups or plates or spilling liquids when surprised or laughing. These attacks are short and do not resemble the "classic" full-blown attack of cataplexy; that is, with a complete fall. In early childhood, cataplexy attacks are more often the complete fall type. The child may present with repetitive falls that cannot be easily explained. Atonic seizures or drop attacks are the most common initial misdiagnosis for children less than 5 years old (85). The duration of each cataplectic attack, partial or total, is highly variable. They usually range from a few seconds to 2 minutes and rarely up to 30 minutes. Attacks can be elicited by emotion, stress, fatigue, or heavy meals. Laughter and anger seem to be the most common triggers, but the attacks can also be induced by a feeling of elation while listening to music, reading a book, or watching a movie. Cataplexy may be induced merely by remembering a funny situation, and this may also occur without obvious precipitating acts or emotions. In children, it often occurs while playing with others.

A pathway similar to the one leading to REM atonia is used in cataplexy (86–89). Cataplexy is associated with inhibition of monosynaptic H-reflexes and multi-synaptic tendon reflexes. H-reflex activity is fully suppressed physiologically during REM sleep, emphasizing the relationship between the motor inhibition of REM sleep and the sudden atonia and areflexia seen during a cataplectic attack.

Apart from overwhelming sleepiness, patients may feel abnormally drowsy. They may spend the day at a low level of alertness resulting in poor performance at school, memory lapses, and even gestural, or speech automatisms. This low alertness may persist despite the use of stimulant medication.

Daytime sleepiness may not be obvious to parents in very young children and may be missed before kindergarten. Sleepy behavior is more often recognized by teachers who may complain of apathy in the child while the parents may misinterpret the behavior as normal napping. Prolonged nocturnal sleep, difficulty waking up in the morning, and aggressiveness before being awakened are commonly seen. However, sleepiness can be hidden behind other abnormal behavior such as hyperactivity, or social withdrawal and shyness (89).

Sleep paralysis can be a terrifying experience that occurs when the narcoleptic falls asleep or wakes up (90). Children find themselves suddenly unable to move their limbs, to speak, or even to breathe deeply. This state can be frequently accompanied by hallucinations. During episodes of sleep paralysis, particularly the first occurrence, the patient may experience extreme anxiety and fear of dying. This anxiety is often greatly intensified by the hallucinations, sometimes terrifying, that may accompany the sleep paralysis. Children are often reluctant to talk about these events. These experiences are so frightening that the child may resist going to bed to sleep.

Visual hypnagogic hallucinations usually consist of simple forms (colored circles, parts of objects, and so forth) that are constant or changing in size. The image of an animal or a person may present itself abruptly, in black and white but more often in color. Auditory hallucinations are also common. The auditory hallucinations can range from simple sounds to an elaborate melody. The patient may also be menaced by threatening sentences or harsh invectives. Hypnagogic hallucinations and sleep paralysis do not affect all subjects and can be transitory (91). Disturbed nocturnal sleep seldom occurs early in the course of the disorder and generally worsens during adulthood.

Diagnosis

Unless cataplexy is unequivocally witnessed by the examiner, an objective sleep study will be necessary to obtain an accurate diagnosis of narcolepsy. Unfortunately in children younger than 8 years of age, no objective test has been developed to confirm the diagnosis. In these younger children the diagnosis is made by a process of elimination when there is an otherwise clear history. Clinical EEG and MRI studies are normal. A key finding in this age group is the absence of another sleep disorder such as periodic limb movement disorder as demonstrated on a complete overnight polysomnogram. The polysomnogram should be normal with the possible exception of a short REM sleep latency. Polysomnogram monitoring should include either a nasal cannula or esophageal pressure (PES) in order not to miss a more subtle condition such as upper airway resistance syndrome (30).

In children 8 years or older, objective testing is available to diagnose narcolepsy. After completing a full nocturnal polysomnogram, a multiple sleep latency test (MSLT) is necessary (92). The MSLT was designed to measure physiological sleep tendencies in the absence of alerting factors. The time or latency between lights-out time and sleep onset is calculated for each nap. The type of sleep, REM or nonREM, is also noted. After each nap, the patient must stay awake until the following scheduled nap. The MSLT records the sleep latency for each nap, the mean sleep latency, and the presence or absence of REM sleep in any of the naps. REM sleep that occurs within 15 minutes of sleep onset is considered a sleep onset REM period.

In normal populations, MSLT scores vary with age, puberty being the critical landmark, with prepubertal children between the ages of 8 and 11 years appearing relatively hyperalert. The maximum mean MSLT score obtainable is 20 minutes, which corresponds to a subject staying awake during all naps. Mean MSLT scores under 8 minutes are generally considered to be in the pathological sleepiness range; those over 10 minutes are considered normal in adults. Before puberty, as mentioned above, children are very alert in the daytime and the normal adult MSLT cut off value of 10 minutes may be too low. Even a 12-minute latency in a prepubertal child may be abnormal. In children undergoing an MSLT, the presence of two or more sleep-onset REM periods is always abnormal and consistent with narcolepsy.

Histocompatibility leukocyte antigen (HLA) typing had been recommended as a test for narcolepsy when it was found to have an association with the DR-2 marker in Japan. However, this marker is neither sufficient nor necessary for the diagnosis because it is present in 10 to 15% of the general population. Determination of HLA haplotypes in children suspected of having narcolepsy is usually not helpful in making the diagnosis (79).

An animal model for narcolepsy has been studied using dogs. Recently, using positional cloning, an autosomal recessive mutation responsible for narcolepsy was discovered in this canine model (92, 93). Canine narcolepsy is caused by disruption of the hypocretin (orexin) receptor 2 gene (*Hcrtr2*). Hypocretins appear to be major sleep-modulating neurotransmitters (93,94). Absence of hypocretins is now thought to be critical in the pathophysiology of most human narcoleptics. In the canine model, the receptor is lacking, but in humans, the actual neurotransmitter is usually lacking. The possibility that an autoimmune mechanism is damaging the hypocretin-producing cells in the lateral hypothalamus has been raised (95). Hypocretin can be measured in cerebrospinal fluid. This research tool is useful in diagnostic situations when the diagnosis is uncertain (96, 97). The absence of hypocretin in cerebrospinal fluid is diagnostic of narcolepsy; however this assay is not widely available. A blood serum equivalent test is not yet available. Future treatment of narcoleptic humans may involve hypocretin analogs.

Treatment Strategies

Successful treatment for narcolepsy includes both behavioral and pharmacological treatments. The situation is analogous to juvenile diabetes mellitus where a combination of diet with medication can control the condition. With the recent discovery of a gene responsible for narcolepsy, novel potential therapeutic approaches may be discovered.

Treatment strategies must include conservative behavioral treatment such as short naps, emotional support to parents and child, and education of school authorities. Repetitive 15- to 20-minute naps at 3-hour intervals are helpful in restoring alertness. Behavioral and emotional disturbances are reported in adolescents with narcolepsy (98). Subjects and families should be referred to narcolepsy support groups led by a therapist who can address issues created by this chronic condition.

Narcolepsy is a lifelong illness, and drug therapy must take this into account when considering possible side effects, because patients will have to take medication for years. Tolerance or addiction may occur with some drugs, and it is importance to balance medication side effects with maintenance of an active life. Hypertension, abnormal liver function, depression, irritability, anorexia, insomnia, or psychosis are associated with some medications (79).

No double-blind placebo controlled trials of medication have been specifically conducted for children with narcolepsy. Central nervous system stimulants have been the drugs most widely used (99). Amphetamines were first proposed in 1935. The alerting effect of a single oral dose of amphetamine is at its maximum 2 to 4 hours after administration, and many patients require a single or twice-daily dose. However, a number of side effects, including irritability, anxiety, nervousness, headache, psychosis, tachycardia, hypertension, nocturnal sleep disturbances, tolerance and drug dependence, may arise. The use of methylphenidate was later encouraged because of a shorter half-life and lower incidence of similar side effects. Pemoline, an oxazolidine derivative with a longer half-life and a slower onset of action, is less efficient but well tolerated. Pemoline, previously the first stimulant used in children, should now be discouraged because of the possibility of severe liver damage. The manufacturer has recommended that baseline liver function tests be obtained before starting pemoline and every 2 weeks thereafter.

There are two drugs with different mode of action that have changed our first-line treatment for narcolepsy. The first one, modafinil, is considered more as a "somnolytic" than a non-specific stimulant. The drug, which has been approved in the United States, has been reported to bring substantial improvement in adults (100). The mechanism of action of modafinil is not entirely clear but it is not dopamine mediated in the same way amphetamines are thought to work (101). The neuronal targets for modafinil in the brain include nuclei of the hypothalamus and amygdala. Modafinil should be considered the initial pharmacological agent used to treat the excessive daytime sleepiness of narcolepsy in children (100). Modafinil does not have the typical side effects of amphetamine. Headaches are the most common side effect of modafinil and may be avoided or minimized by gradually increasing the dose (100). The initial dose should be relatively low, 50 to 100 mg, to avoid headaches. The dosage can later be increased to 200 to 400 mg/day divided twice daily. The second dose should ideally be given before 2 PM because of the long half-life.

The second drug is gamma-hydroxybutyrate (GHB), which, after much difficulty was approved for use in the United States by the FDA in July 2002 (101–103). It is the first substance ever approved specifically for cataplexy. The generic name is sodium oxybate (Xyrem). In the media, it has the infamous name of the "date rape drug" (93). Illegal use of this substance for recreational purposes has been of great concern. Important CNS adverse events associated with abuse of sodium oxybate include seizure, respiratory depression, and profound decreases in level of consciousness, with instances of coma and death. When used outside of clinical trials, for recreational purposes, the circumstances surrounding these adverse events are often unclear (e.g., dose of sodium oxybate taken, the nature and amount of alcohol or any concomitant drugs ingested).

Sodium oxybate has powerful CNS depressant effects and can increase slow-wave sleep (103). When given at bedtime, this medication may reduce cataplexy (101). Patients may prefer this medication over other medications used for cataplexy, particularly if insomnia is also present. Sodium oxybate is rapidly but incompletely absorbed after oral administration; absorption is delayed and decreased by a high fat meal. It is eliminated mainly by metabolism with a half-life of 0.5 to 1 hour. Pharmacokinetics are nonlinear with blood levels increasing 3.7-fold as the dose is doubled from 4.5 to 9 g. The pharmacokinetics are not altered with repeat dosing. Sodium oxybate should be taken at bedtime while in bed and again 2.5 to 4 hours later. The recommended starting dose in adults is 4.5 g/day divided into two equal doses of 2.25 g. The starting dosage can then be increased to a maximum of 9 g/day in increments of 1.5 g/day (0.75 g per dose). Two weeks are recommended between dosage increases to evaluate clinical response and minimize adverse effects. Sodium oxybate is effective at doses of 6 to 9 g/day. The efficacy and safety of sodium oxybate at doses higher than 9 g/day has not been investigated, and doses greater than 9 g/day should not ordinarily be administered. The product's package insert does not recommend using the medication in patients younger than age 16 years and dosing guidelines for patients younger than 16 years old have not been established (104). Ironically, unlike most other medications discussed in this text, sodium oxybate is sold as a liquid, thus making it possible to treat young children if clinically indicated.

Cataplexy seems to respond best to medications with noradrenergic reuptake blocking properties (105). There are no systematic trials of anticataplexy drugs on children. Postpubertal teenagers are usually treated as young adults. In this group, two medications have been more commonly used, clomipramine and fluoxetine. Both of these drugs have active noradrenergic reuptake blocking metabolites (desmethylclomipramine and norfluoxetine). It is through these metabolites that the therapeutic effect may be mediated (106). Other compounds have been found to be effective in children with cataplexy, particularly imipramine and desipramine. The anticholinergic side effects of clomipramine and imipramine may be problematic. Treatment with fluoxetine or viloxazine may avoid these side effects (100).

Restless Legs Syndrome/Periodic Limb Movements of Sleep

Restless legs syndrome (RLS) is a chronic autosomal dominant neurological disorder (107, 108). It is characterized by leg discomfort, most common in the evening, that makes the patients want to move their legs. Discomfort is relieved with movement. The sensation may also be present when the patient is sitting still, such as seated on an airplane or in a movie theater. The leg discomfort may be hard to describe and in children may be characterized as "growing pains." In patients with restless legs syndrome, sleep may be disrupted by hundreds of involuntary kicking movements of the legs during sleep, called *periodic limb movements of sleep* (PLMS). The movement in the leg is the extension of the big toe, while at the same time the ankle, knee, and sometimes the hip are partly flexed. These repetitive episodes of muscle contraction last from half a second to 5 seconds with an interval of about 20 to 40 seconds, and may occur in the absence of RLS (108).

The diagnosis of periodic leg movements of sleep requires an overnight sleep study, which demonstrates a PLMS index of over five episodes per hour. Restless legs syndrome/periodic limb movements of sleep can result in significant daytime drowsiness as a result of poor sleep quality, which may lead to daytime behavior that mimics ADHD (109–112). PLMS has also been described in children. However, the clinical presentation differs from that of adults with PLMS. Chervin reported an even higher prevalence rate in a small referred population of children (26%), half of whom also had evidence of sleep-disordered breathing (115). Picchietti and associates reported a retrospective review of 129 children and adolescents who were found to have PLMS in excess of five per hour (115). Sixty-five (50%) had PLMS in the 5 to 10 per hour range, 48 (37%) in the 10 to 25 per hour range, and 16 (12%) had periodic limb movements exceeding 25 per hour. Of the original 129 children, 117 (91%) had been previously diagnosed as having ADHD. Stimulant medication did not seem to play a role in the production of PLMS. In only 25 of the 129 cases did parents note the presence of PLMS of sleep before being specifically asked to look, and in some case, the leg movements of sleep were initially misdiagnosed as seizures. Daytime symptoms improved with dopaminergic medications. Other studies have been confirmed these associations between PLMS and ADHD (112, 113). Children with RLS may present with nonspecific symptom such as growing pains, restless sleep, insomnia, and daytime sleepiness, but most often these issues go unnoticed by their parents. A family history of RLS or PLMS is common (114–117).

A dysregulation of iron metabolism may play a role in the pathophysiology of RLS. Iron is a cofactor in the production of dopamine. Allen reported that decreases in iron concentration in nigrostriatal areas correlated with the severity of RLS (118). Other investigators reported that in individuals with RLS, transferrin receptor expression in neuromelanin cells of the substantia nigra was decreased, suggesting that RLS may result from a defect in iron regulatory protein (119).

Nondrug treatments may temporarily help counteract the sensations of RLS. Patients may find that walking, stretching, taking a hot or cold bath, massaging the affected limb, applying hot or cold packs, using vibration, performing acupressure, and practicing relaxation techniques (such as biofeedback, meditation, or yoga) may help reduce or relieve the symptoms. In addition some find that keeping their mind actively engaged through activities such as reading an interesting novel, or playing video games helps during times that they must be stay seated, such as when traveling.

Dopamine precursors and agonists have been effective in relieving both RLS and PLMS (120). They have been endorsed by the American Academy of Sleep Medicine however specific guidelines for children were not reviewed (121).

Levodopa (L-DOPA), the metabolic precursor of dopamine, is used for treating Parkinson's disease. It is also used to treat RLS/PLMS in both adults and children (122). Levodopa in itself is largely inert. Its therapeutic as well as adverse effects result from the decarboxylation of levodopa to dopamine in the brain (123). Levodopa is almost always administered in combination with a peripherally acting inhibitor of aromatic L-amino acid decarboxylase such as carbidopa. If levodopa is administered alone, the drug is largely decarboxylated by enzymes in the intestinal mucosa and other peripheral sites so that relatively little unchanged drug reaches the cerebral circulation. In addition, dopamine released into the circulation by peripheral conversion of levodopa produces undesirable effects particularly nausea. Inhibition of peripheral decarboxylase markedly increases the fraction of administered levodopa that remains unmetabolized and available to cross the blood-brain barrier and reduces the incidence of gastrointestinal side effects such as nausea (123). The main complication of levodopa therapy for RLS/PLMS is the development of worsening symptoms during the afternoon or early evening, despite adequate control later at night. This phenomenon which has been termed "restless legs augmentation," may occur frequently, sometimes within months after therapy has been instituted. Once augmentation has occurred, levodopa therapy should be discontinued and, if possible, a different agent should be used. Administering additional doses of levodopa earlier during the day usually results in further exacerbation of the augmentation phenomenon. (124, 125). In addition to motor fluctuations and nausea, other adverse effects observed with levodopa therapy include hallucinations, confusion, and orthostatic hypotension.

These other side effects are more typically seen in adult patients with Parkinson's disease using higher dosages than are used in the treatment of PLMS and RLS. In children, nausea is by far the most common side effect. Sensitivity to side effects makes it necessary to initiate therapy at very low doses (one half of a 25/100 levodopa/carbidopa tablet daily) and increase as tolerated every few days. The therapeutic dose for relief of PLMS and RLS symptoms will be lower than that used in Parkinson's disease. The maximal dose is determined by side effects but most adolescents require at least 75 mg carbidopa and up to 1.5 g of L-DOPA.(126). Levodopa is valuable in the treatment of RLS/PLMS, but the mode of action of the drug is unknown. It seems likely that dopaminergic pathways are involved. Walters and Hening have suggested that the site of action is the postsynaptic dopamine receptor, whereas Guilleminault et al. propose a spinal dopaminergic mechanism as

the site of action (128). There may be differences in the mechanism of action of these medications between patients with RLS and those with only PLMS.

Based on the hypothesis that there is a disturbance of iron regulation in the pathophysiology of idiopathic RLS, a trial of iron supplementation was found to result in improvement in these patients (128–132). Some of the most important findings are that children with PLMS have relatively low serum iron and ferritin levels. In addition, most of these patients will respond favorably to a 3-month course of oral iron therapy, as evidenced by a decrease in PLMS index and an improvement in clinical symptoms (133).

Selective dopamine agonists are potent treatments for PLMS and RLS. They tend to have fewer side effects than carbidopa/levodopa. Pramipexole, ropinirole, and pergolide are the most commonly used medications in this category (134). Selective dopaminergic agonists have similar side effects to carbidopa/levodopa but at a lower frequency. These agents are more potent and allow for lower dosages than with carbidopa/levodopa. Of these agents, pramipexole has been particularly effective in our experience.

Montplasir and colleagues have found pramipexole to be effective in a double-blind placebo-controlled study in adults (135). The starting dose in adults in this study was 0.375 mg. In children, the lowest dose available is an empirical starting dose. Pramipexole is available in a 0.125-mg scored tablet, which can be halved if an even lower starting dosage is desired. It is important to make medication changes slowly because the symptoms of PLMS and RLS both seem to fluctuate independently of the medication. In addition, if the dosage is too high, significant side effects may occur. We advise parents to only adjust the medication once a week at most when they first start the medication. Once an effective dose is found it does not typically have to be adjusted except to allow for the child's growth. In adults, the dosage of pramipexole for restless legs syndrome usually does not exceed 1.5 mg, and is often effective at a much lower dose.

Childhood Insomnia

Insomnia in adults is defined as the subjective complaint of nonrestorative sleep associated with difficulty initiating and or maintaining sleep (107). The nonrestorative sleep of insomnia requires a perception of impaired awake function as result of the sleep difficulty. In children, the parents' perception of impairment is just as important as the child's. If an infant does not sleep well at night, the infant may compensate with more naps.

Insomnia characteristics fluctuate with age. With infants, the problem usually involves trouble settling to sleep without the parents' assistance. In toddlers, the problem may also involve inconsistent limit setting with regard to bedtime expectations. By the time children are 8 or 9 years old, they seem to have fewer problems with insomnia. When problems with sleep are present at this age, there may be some unresolved fear of being alone at night. This might be expressed as a "fear of the dark." This fear may not be initially volunteered during the clinical interview but a description of the sleep routine and environment may reveal a need for nightlights or hallway lights to be left on at night. Adolescents have a characteristic insomnia pattern called delayed sleep phase syndrome (DSPS) (107). DSPS will be discussed subsequently. All of these insomnia types may merge in different ways in a given individual. In addition, with clinical heterogeneity, there are children who are described as being lifelong poor sleepers without any apparent cause. This condition is referred to, for lack of a better term, as idiopathic insomnia, and fortunately is rare (107).

Sleep-Onset Association Disorder and Limit-Setting Sleep Disorder

These two disorders are related to the inconsistent enforcement of bedtime routines. In normal infants, brief awakenings throughout the night are common. The child and the parent are unaware of most of these, and unbeknownst to the parents, the child may simply drift back to sleep. It is only when these awakenings become associated with external events that a problem arises. If a brief awakening is followed by a full arousal in an active, alert child, and the child is unable to fall asleep, the child may simply become agitated. The child can return to sleep after being comforted by the caregiver.

Sleep-onset association problems seem to be common. Although the need for sleep has a biological basis, the way we sleep is learned and influenced by the cultural environment. This is analogous to eating. All newborns first drink milk, but the diet of older children is different throughout the world. The child will learn or form associations with regard to sleep. As the child is readied for bed, the child may associate sleep onset with particular events, and may associate this process with increased attention and activity rather than getting ready for bed. If continued, the child may then develop an association with parental activity that requires continuous parental involvement to fall asleep. The awakenings in the middle of night often necessitate similar actions. What initially were brief awakenings may develop into lengthy struggles. What wakes up the child may not be what is keeping the child awake. Now the parental actions became the focus of the problem. If returning the child to sleep requires frequent parental assistance, the parents' sleep may be very disturbed. The entire family may start to dread the nighttime instead of looking forward to going to sleep. The nighttime routines are no longer pleasurable but become a source of frustration. A vicious cycle may form, which is exacerbated by middle-of-the night awakenings. Parents may report that the infant wakes up crying every hour. The normal sleep cycle length in an infant is approximately 1 hour and is followed by a brief arousal before initiating the next sleep cycle. Therefore, when a parent complains of hourly awakenings with prompt return to sleep with the parents' intervention, the

possibility of a sleep-onset association disorder should be considered.

Limit-setting sleep disorder is term used to describe stalling behaviors or refusal to go to bed at the desired time associated with inadequate limit-setting for a child's behaviors. This sleep disorder is usually seen in a child who is sleeping apart from the parents and is old enough to get out of bed or climb out of the crib, go to the parents' bedroom and disrupt their sleep. Usually there is no enforcement of consistent bedtime rules. The same behaviors may occur after nighttime awakenings. When the child does sleep, it is usually of normal quality and duration. The parents may lack an understanding of the importance of setting limits and inadequate knowledge of limit-setting techniques. There may be underlying psychosocial factors limiting the parents' ability to set limits. The limit-setting difficulties may also be manifest in the child's daytime behavior such as tantrums.

These insomnia patterns are of a behavioral nature and usually do not need to be treated with medication (136). Antihistamines and clonidine may be tried in some of these children but there is little evidence to suggest that these preparations provide anything but short-term sedation (137). In particularly difficult situations, medication can be used as part of a comprehensive treatment program with behavior modification at its core. Behavioral techniques have been helpful and applied to a variety of clinical situations (138, 139). The first issue to be addressed in the evaluation of a behavioral sleep problem in an infant or small child is, where do the parents want the child to sleep? The child will typically prefer to sleep with the parents; the question is what the parents prefer. Many variations are possible with regard to such sleeping arrangements. The child might sleep in a crib in a separate room, a crib in the parents' room, in the same bed with the parents, or in the same bed or bedroom with another member of the family. The sleep situation may change based on multiple factors such as new siblings or the size of the home. Cultural issues will also play a part in this situation. Once the parents and caretakers agree, then a plan to teach the child what to expect can be developed.

Perhaps the best known behavioral approach is that popularized by Dr. Richard Ferber at Harvard (140). This approach has not been without some controversy and the clinician needs to be familiar with it since undoubtedly the parents will be. In essence, a "progressive" approach to helping the child fall asleep and stay asleep is advocated. After a bedtime routine such as singing, rocking, or reading a book, the child is put to bed while still awake. Putting the child in bed awake is thought to teach the child to go to sleep on his own. Parents are advised that once the child is in bed, they should leave the room. If the child cries, wait a while before checking in on the child. The suggested waiting time should be based on how comfortable the family is with the situation and can be charted to help track the progress. When the parent returns to the child's room, the child should be soothed verbally but the parents should avoid picking up, rocking, or feeding the child. The time between parental interventions should be gradually increased. The time should be predetermined and not shortened during the night. Ideally within a week, the child will learn to sleep without the parents' help.

This method is not desirable or effective for all families. Alternatives have been published by various authors some that seem diametrically opposed to the above method (141–143). A discussion of different approaches and counter arguments about helping a child sleep at night are beyond the scope of this chapter. Suffice it to say that parents will typically seek professional help only after they have tried one or more of the different popular approaches. The relationship between the parents may suffer due to frustration and sleep deprivation. Given this situation, a pragmatic approach that takes into account the individual situation is appreciated by the family. A judgmental or patronizing attitude from the health care provider will not be appreciated.

The parents may need additional direction to be able to implement firm limits for the child. For example, reassure the parents they have not abandoned the child if they decide to sleep separately or that they are spoiling the infant if they decide to share their bed with the infant. If the child has learned to sleep in the parents' bed and the parents want to change this arrangement, they need to realize the infant has no incentive to change. One approach is for the parents to start the night sleeping in the child's room. The amount of time that the parent spends with the child in bed could be decreased gradually until the child learns to sleep alone. These gradual interventions are not meant to be punitive, and require patience, persistence, and reassurance for both the parents and the child.

A food allergy may occasionally play a role in a child's insomnia (144, 145). This usually occurs between birth and about 2 years of age. The insomnia is often initiated by food allergens causing somatic manifestations after ingestion of food or formula. Manifestations of an allergy, such as a skin rash, would be expected to be present. A young child fed formula may become fussy and irritable shortly after being fed. In a case of cow's milk allergy, IgE levels may be elevated and a radioallergosorbent test positive for cow's milk protein. A change in formula may be curative and a cow's milk challenge would induce the reappearance of insomnia.

Delayed Sleep Phase Syndrome

The sleep patterns of adolescents seem different from those of other children and adults. This may be due to a combination of physiological changes and external societal influences. In the United States, Dr. Mary Carskadon has done extensive research on adolescent sleep (146–148). The most common form of insomnia in adolescents may be delayed sleep phase. Delayed sleep phase syndrome is a circadian disorder characterized by chronic sleep-onset insom-

nia and an inability to arise at an appropriate time in the morning. Once the major sleep episode has been initiated, the individual has the ability to sleep soundly and for a normal duration (149). When not required to maintain a strict sleep schedule (e.g., weekends, vacations, and holiday periods) patients will awaken spontaneously, albeit at a late morning or early afternoon hour. They will have a normal nocturnal total sleep time.

Delayed sleep phase syndrome is associated with depression and should be considered when evaluating adolescents with depression (150–152). A study in Japan attempted to define the psychological features of patients with delayed sleep phase syndrome (153). They administered a series of neuropsychiatric tests including the Minnesota Multiphasic Personality Inventory (MMPI) and Rorschach. Compared to the controls they found that patients with delayed sleep phase syndrome manifested increased nervousness, depression, and difficulty regulating emotional displays. They were defensive, introspective, overly abstract in their thinking, compulsive, and tended to set high standards for intellectual achievement, despite questionable cognitive ability, which made them vulnerable to disappointment. However, they were also impulsive, and sought immediate gratification. The investigators described them as neurotic, hypochondriacal, depressed, and prone to conversion symptomatology. They suggested that these characteristics might increase social withdrawal, decreasing the social cues that might entrain circadian rhythm. Finally, they concluded the phase shift becomes more difficult and a vicious circle is constituted.

Patients with delayed sleep phase syndrome describe themselves as "night owls" and the preference for "eveningness" appears to run in families (154, 155). Several genes have been identified that may play a role in delayed sleep phase syndrome. Mammalian circadian rhythmicity has been shown to be regulated at the genetic level by transcription-translation feedback loops. Key molecular components are proteins, among which are called Clock, Timeless, and Period (Per). A single nucleotide polymorphism of the human *CLOCK* gene has been shown to be related to diurnal preference. Individuals carrying one of the two *CLOCK* alleles showed a strong preference for "eveningness" (154). There are three subtypes of the Per protein. Researchers in the United Kingdom reported that the shorter allele of the Per 3 polymorphism was strongly associated with "eveningness" (75% of the subjects were homozygous for this polymorphism), whereas the longer allele was associated with "morningness" (156–159). A different molecular mechanism for delayed sleep phase syndrome has been reported by investigators in Japan who identified a polymorphism in the gene for a rate-limiting enzyme used in the synthesis of melatonin, arylalkylamine N-acetyltransferase (155). They suggested this could be a susceptibility gene for delayed sleep phase syndrome (156). In general, it may be intrinsically easier for people to go to sleep later than usual (delay) than to go to sleep earlier than usual (advance). People susceptible to delayed sleep phase syndrome may have more difficulty adjusting to an earlier sleep time than others (160–162).

Delayed sleep phase syndrome is not difficult to diagnosis once the clinical suspicion is raised but obtaining satisfactory response to treatment is more difficult. Attempts to correct the sleep schedule will be fruitless unless the adolescent is motivated to alter the lifestyle factors that influenced the late bedtime, particularly on weekends (163). The original treatment for delayed sleep phase was called chronotherapy by Weitzman (149). Chronotherapy resets the patient's sleep cycle by a series of consecutive delayed adjustments of the bedtime, which are made over several days. To maintain the readjusted sleep pattern, the patient is encouraged to keep strictly to the new sleep onset and wake times. This treatment can be impractical because the progressive forward bed time shifts will have the child at one point temporally sleeping in the daytime. The child must be constantly supervised to avoid falling asleep at the wrong time. This treatment, although physiologically sound, has been impractical.

Another treatment technique resets the sleep-wake rhythm by using bright morning light combined with evening light restriction to phase-shift the patient's sleep time (164–166). The term *phototherapy* is used for this treatment (163). The essential principals of phototherapy are that bright light in the morning can phase advance sleep onset and bright light in the evening can phase delay sleep onset. Different phototherapy protocols have been used with various success rates. A pragmatic approach for the individual patient needs to be developed. Our practice is to use light intensity 10,000 lux for 30 to 45 minutes within a few minutes of awakening for several weeks. In addition, bright lights should be minimized in the last 2 hours before the expected sleep time. This includes the use of computer monitors. A practical compromise in adolescents may be to minimize or restrict watching television or using a computer before bedtime but allow their use promptly after awakening. This might serve as an incentive for the adolescent to get up on time or early if this time is available for recreational computer use. Phototherapy should not be used in patients who are bipolar because it may aggravate mania (163).

Treatment with melatonin has been described (151–154). Melatonin is a hormone secreted by the pineal gland and its primary function seems to be to convey information about the changing length of the night in the course of the year. This information is used by photoperiodic animals to ensure the correct timing of seasonally variable functions such as reproduction, coat growth, and probably the duration and organization of sleep. The clinical use of melatonin may be difficult and perhaps its use by the nonspecialist discouraged. Melatonin has been used to treat poor sleep in a variety of conditions including Asperger syndrome (167–169). Melatonin is not regulated as a pharmaceutical in the United States, but rather is classi-

fied as a food additive (170). This lack of regulation may make the quality of over-the-counter melatonin highly variable. The timing of the dose must be individually determined based on the subject's core body temperature rhythm. The patient's motivation to modify their lifestyle is essential for successful treatment. Adolescents may have a variety of social and academic reasons to avoid going to bed at an earlier time. A large difference between the bedtimes and wake-up times from school nights compared to weekends can reinforce the delayed sleep phase.

Parasomnias

According to the International Classification of Sleep Disorders, parasomnias are clinical disorders that are not abnormalities of the processes responsible for sleep and wake states per se but, rather, are undesirable physical phenomena that occur predominantly during sleep (107). This nosology describes over 20 different parasomnias, the majority of which can occur in children. These are divided into four groups: arousal parasomnias, sleep–wake transition parasomnias, parasomnias associated with REM sleep, and other parasomnias.

The arousal parasomnias are more common in children and include the clinical spectrum of confusional arousals, sleep terrors, and sleepwalking. These conditions are thought to arise from impaired arousal from sleep, typically slow-wave sleep. Since slow-wave sleep (stages 3 and 4) dominates in the first third of the night, the arousal parasomnias also occur at that time. Anything that increases the amount of slow-wave sleep, such as recovery from sleep deprivation, may increase the likelihood of these parasomnias occurring in susceptible individuals. If necessary, clonazepam may help decrease these arousal parasomnias but should be avoided in the presence of sleep-disordered breathing (136).

Confusional arousals may be partial manifestations of sleep terrors and sleepwalking events. As the name implies, confusion occurs during and following arousals, usually in the first third of night. The individual is disoriented, speech and mentation are slowed, and response to questioning is confused (107). These behaviors usually last only a few minutes in children and can be precipitated by forced awakenings out of slow-wave sleep. The condition is benign and tends to decrease over time. However, a child with a tendency to have these events may also be at risk for sleepwalking, and parents/caretakers should be warned of this possibility. The events can be minimized by avoiding situations that can increase slow-wave sleep or sleep disruption.

Sleep terrors are characterized by a sudden arousal from slow-wave sleep with a characteristic "blood-curdling" scream accompanied by intense fear. Pronounced autonomic nervous system discharge may occur with tachycardia and sweating. The child may be described as wide-eyed with an intense look of fear staring past the parents. The prevalence of sleep terrors in children is 3% in children and decreases with age to about 2% in adults (46). Arousal is difficult, and if successful, the patient may be confused and disoriented. The child may try to describe fragments of images with poor coherence. These images will not have the rich detail of a nightmare. Waking the child 15 minutes after they have fallen asleep has been a popular treatment. Awakening the child at the point that they would be expected to be entering slow-wave sleep seems somehow to decrease the tendency for these parasomnias to occur. When the child returns to sleep, the homeostatic mechanism driving slow-wave sleep may raise the arousal threshold and decrease the likelihood of the recurrence of the sleep terror. The parents should be warned that the child with sleep terrors might also sleepwalk.

Sleepwalking is also called somnambulism (107). The term sleepwalking may be a misnomer, perhaps "sleep fleeing" would better characterize the dramatic behaviors. The range of behaviors witnessed may range from simply sitting up in bed to running out of the home and driving an automobile. During the sleepwalking episode, pain thresholds are elevated (171). The child will be hard to awaken and may be confused and disoriented. Motor activity may terminate spontaneously or the child may simply return to bed without reaching alertness. Sleeptalking may occur during this event. The treatments mentioned previously for the other arousal parasomnias may be helpful. Safety precautions should always be taken. Specifically the child should sleep on a ground floor if possible to avoid injury while negotiating stairs. If the child has a bunk bed, he should use the lower bunk. Drapery should be kept over the bedroom windows to protect the hands of the child in case the child tries to punch a window. A door alarm is helpful to warn the parents if the child walks out of the home. Weapons should be kept away from adults who may sleepwalk. It is helpful to keep precipitants of sleepwalking at a minimum. Thus, sleep deprivation should be avoided. Obstructive sleep apnea may be an occult aggravator, and should be treated if present (47).

Parasomnias such as sleepwalking and sleep terrors need to be distinguished from nocturnal seizures. The timing of seizures is different from sleepwalking and sleep terrors. Nocturnal seizures do not cluster during slow-wave sleep in the first third of the night. The motor activity of generalized tonic–clonic seizures is very different from these parasomnias. Tongue biting and urinary incontinence are not characteristically seen in sleepwalking and night terrors. Patients with generalized nocturnal seizures have a low risk of daytime seizures (172). The motor activity of a partial complex seizure may be more difficult to distinguish from parasomnias and may resemble a confusional arousal (173). Usually the overall clinical picture can help with the diagnosis. If a patient has been injured during an apparent parasomnia, a comprehensive neurological evaluation should be considered including a sleep-deprived electroencephalogram.

Some forms of epilepsy may be misidentified as a benign parasomnia (174) or as narcolepsy in children (159). Frontal lobe epilepsy is poorly understood and often unrecognized by health care workers dealing with children. Age of onset varies from infancy to adolescence. Seizures are typically brief (30 seconds to 2 minutes), stereotypic, nocturnal, and can occur several times during the night. They have an explosive onset, characterized by screaming, agitation, stiffening, kicking or bicycling of the legs, and incontinence. The interictal electroencephalogram is usually normal. Longterm video electroencephalographic monitoring is required to demonstrate the frontal epileptic discharges. This condition may be misdiagnosed as a sleep disorder or psychiatric problem. Nocturnal paroxysmal dystonia is a sleep disturbance that may be misidentified as a pseudo-seizure (176–178). It appears to be a form of frontal lobe epilepsy with motor attacks characterized by complex behavior, with dystonic–dyskinetic or ballistic movements arising from non-REM sleep. The movements are not symmetrical. Seizure control is difficult and may require epilepsy surgery (179).

CONCLUSION

Sleep disorders are very common in children and are often associated with daytime behavioral problems. Most sleep disorders will improve when correctly addressed. It is important for children and their caretakers to give sleep the same priority as exercise and nutrition. We cannot continue to punish our children by sending them to bed early and reward them by permitting them to go to bed late and expecting them to grow up valuing a full night of sleep. There is a need for greater information on the pharmacological management of sleep disorders in children. Health care providers need to have a comprehensive understanding of clinical sleep disorders in children. Training programs should play a lead role in enhancing knowledge of sleep disorders in children.

REFERENCES

1. Dement WC, Vaughan C. The Promise of Sleep. New York City: Delacorte Press, 1999.
2. Ferber R. Assement of sleep disorders in the child. In Ferber R, Kryger M, eds. Principles and Practice of Sleep Medicine in the Child. Philadelphia: WB Saunders, 1995:45–53.
3. Archbold KH, Pituch KJ, Panahi P, Chervin RD. Symptoms of sleep disturbances among children at two general pediatric clinics. J Pediatr 2002;140:97–102.
4. Iglowstein I, Jenni OG, Molinari L, Largo RH. Sleep duration from infancy to adolescence: reference values and generational trends. Pediatrics 2003;111:302–307.
5. Weissbluth M. Naps in children: 6 months-7 years. Sleep 1995; 18:82–87.
6. Watamura S, Donzella B, Kertes DA, Gunnar MR. Developmental changes in baseline cortisol activity in early childhood : relations with napping and effortful control. Dev Psyhcobiol 2004; 45:125–133.
7. Panda S, Hogenesch JB, Kay SA. Circadian rhythms from flies to human. Nature 2002;417:329–335.

8. Mirmiran M, Maas YG, Ariagno RL. Development of fetal and neonatal sleep and circadian rhythms. Sleep Med Rev 2003;7(4): 321–334.

9. Monk TH, Welsh DK. The role of chronobiology in sleep disorders medicine. Sleep Med Rev 2003;7:455–473.

10. Wolfson AR, Carskadon MA. Understanding adolescents' sleep patterns and school performance: a critical appraisal. Sleep Med Rev 2003;7:491–506.

11. Grigg-Damberger M. Neurologic disorders masquerading as pediatric sleep problems. Pediatr Clin North Am 2004;51(1):89– 115.

12. Edgar DM, Dement WC, Fuller CA. Effect of SCN lesions on sleep in squirrel monkeys: evidence for opponent processes in sleep-wake regulation. J Neurosci 1993;13:1065–1079.

13. Wurts SW, Edgar DM. Circadian and homeostatic control of rapid eye movement (REM) sleep: promotion of REM tendency by the suprachiasmatic nucleus. J Neurosci 2000;20(11):4300– 4310.

14. Ferber R. Introduction: Pediatric Sleep Disorders Medicine. In Ferber R, Kryger M, eds. Principles and Practice of Sleep Medicine in the Child. Philadelphia: WB Saunders; 1995:45–53.

15. Borbely AA. A two process model of sleep regulation. Hum Neurobiol. 1982;1:195–204.

16. Dickens C. The Posthumous Papers of the Pickwick Club. London: Chapman & Hall, published in serial form; 1836–1837.

17. Osler W. Chronic tonsillitis. In: The Principles and Practice of Medicine. New York: Appleton, 1892:335–339.

18. Guilleminault C, Eldridge FL, Simmons FB, Dement WC. Sleep apnea in eight children. Pediatrics 1976;58(1):23–30.

19. Guilleminault C, Pelayo R, Leger D, Clerk A, Bocian RC. Recognition of sleep-disordered breathing in children. Pediatrics 1996; 98(5):871–882.

20. Downey R, 3rd, Perkin RM, MacQuarrie J. Upper airway resistance syndrome: sick, symptomatic but underrecognized. Sleep 1993;16(7):620–623.

21. Gozal D, O'Brien L, Row BW. Consequences of snoring and sleep disordered breathing in children. Pediatr Pulmonol Suppl 2004; 26:166–168.

22. Gozal D, O'Brien LM. Snoring and obstructive sleep apnoea in children: why should we treat? Paediatr Respir Rev 2004;5 Suppl A:S371–S376.

23. Archbold KH, Giordani B, Ruzicka DL, Chervin RD. Cognitive executive dysfunction in children with mild sleep-disordered breathing. Biol Res Nurs 2004;5(3):168–176.

24. Montgomery-Downs HE, O'Brien LM, Holbrook CR, Gozal D. Snoring and sleep-disordered breathing in young children: subjective and objective correlates. Sleep 2004;27(1):87–94.

25. Tauman R, O'Brien LM, Holbrook CR, Gozal D. Sleep pressure score: a new index of sleep disruption in snoring children. Sleep 2004;27(2):274–278.

26. Chervin RD, Archbold KH, Panahi P, Pituch KJ. Sleep problems seldom addressed at two general pediatric clinics. Pediatrics 2001;107(6):1375–1380.

27. Ivanenko A, Crabtree VM, Gozal D. Sleep in children with psychiatric disorders. Pediatr Clin North Am 2004;51(1):51–68.

28. Chervin RD, Dillon JE, Archbold KH, Ruzicka DL. Conduct problems and symptoms of sleep disorders in children. J Am Acad Child Adolesc Psychiatry 2003;42(2):201–208.

29. Sterni LM, Tunkel DE. Obstructive sleep apnea in children: an update. Pediatr Clin North Am 2003;50(2):427–443.

30. Crabtree VM, Varni JW, Gozal D. Health-related quality of life and depressive symptoms in children with suspected sleep-disordered breathing. Sleep 2004;27(6):1131–1138.

31. Guilleminault C, Li K, Khramtsov A, Palombini L, Pelayo R. Breathing patterns in prepubertal children with sleep-related breathing disorders. Arch Pediatr Adolesc Med 2004;158(2): 153–161.

32. Friedman BC, Hendeles-Amitai A, Kozminsky E, et al. Adenotonsillectomy improves neurocognitive function in children with obstructive sleep apnea syndrome. Sleep 2003;26(8):999–1005.

33. O'Brien LM, Gozal D. Neurocognitive dysfunction and sleep in children: from human to rodent. Pediatr Clin North Am 2004;51 (1):187–202.

34. Chervin RD, Clarke DF, Huffman JL, et al. School performance, race, and other correlates of sleep-disordered breathing in children. Sleep Med 2003;4(1):21–27.

35. Kennedy JD, Blunden S, Hirte C, et al. Reduced neurocognition in children who snore. Pediatr Pulmonol 2004;37(4):330–337.

36. Montgomery-Downs HE, Crabtree VM, Gozal D. Cognition, sleep and respiration in at-risk children treated for obstructive sleep apnoea. Eur Respir J 2005; 25: 336–342.

37. O'Brien LM, Holbrook CR, Mervis CB, et al. Sleep and neurobehavioral characteristics of 5- to 7-year-old children with parentally reported symptoms of attention-deficit/hyperactivity disorder. Pediatrics 2003;111(3):554–563.

38. O'Brien LM, Ivanenko A, Crabtree VM, et al. Sleep disturbances in children with attention deficit hyperactivity disorder. Pediatr Res 2003;54(2):237–243.

39. Kirov R, Kinkelbur J, Heipke S, et al. Is there a specific polysomnographic sleep pattern in children with attention deficit/hyperactivity disorder? J Sleep Res 2004;13(1):87–93.

40. Kaemingk KL, Pasvogel AE, Goodwin JL, et al. Learning in children and sleep disordered breathing: findings of the Tucson Children's Assessment of Sleep Apnea (tuCASA) prospective cohort study. J Int Neuropsychol Soc 2003;9(7): 1016–1026.

41. Gottlieb DJ, Vezina RM, Chase C, et al. Symptoms of sleep-disordered breathing in 5-year-old children are associated with sleepiness and problem behaviors. Pediatrics 2003;112(4):870–877.

42. Crabtree VM, Ivanenko A, Gozal D. Clinical and parental assessment of sleep in children with attention-deficit/hyperactivity disorder referred to a pediatric sleep medicine center. Clin Pediatr (Phila) 2003;42(9):807–813.

43. Chervin RD, Archbold KH, Dillon JE, et al. Inattention, hyperactivity, and symptoms of sleep-disordered breathing. Pediatrics 2002;109(3):449–456.

44. Chervin RD, Archbold KH, Dillon JE, et al. Associations between symptoms of inattention, hyperactivity, restless legs, and periodic leg movements. Sleep 2002;25(2):213–218.

45. Stein MA. Unravelling sleep problems in treated and untreated children with ADHD. J Child Adolesc Psychopharmacol 1999;9 (3):157–168.

46. Ohayon MM, Guilleminault C, Priest RG. Night terrors, sleep-walking, and confusional arousals in the general population: their frequency and relationship to other sleep and mental disorders. J Clin Psychiatry 1999;60(4):268–276.

47. Guilleminault C, Palombini L, Pelayo R, Chervin RD. Sleep-walking and sleep terrors in prepubertal children: what triggers them? Pediatrics 2003;111(1):e17–25.

48. Association AP. Diagnostic and Statistical Manual of Mental Disorders: DSM-IV. Washington, DC: American Psychiatric Press, 1994.

49. Gozal D. Sleep-disordered breathing and school performance in children. Pediatrics 1998;102(3 Pt 1):616–620.

50. Guilleminault C, Rosekind M. The arousal threshold: sleep deprivation, sleep fragmentation, and obstructive sleep apnea syndrome. Bull Eur Physiopathol Respir 1981;17(3):341–349.

51. Carroll JL. Obstructive sleep-disordered breathing in children: new controversies, new directions. Clin Chest Med 2003;24(2): 261–282.

52. Uliel S, Tauman R, Greenfeld M, Sivan Y. Normal polysomnographic respiratory values in children and adolescents. Chest 2004;125(3):872–878.

53. Rosen CL. Obstructive sleep apnea syndrome in children: controversies in diagnosis and treatment. Pediatr Clin North Am 2004;51(1):153–167, vii.

54. Carskadon MA, Dement WC, Mitler MM. Guidelines for the multiple sleep latency test (MSLT): a standard measure of sleepiness. Sleep 1986;9(4): 519–524.

55. Norman RG, Ahmed MM, Walsleben JA, Rapoport DM. Detection of respiratory events during NPSG: nasal cannula/pressure sensor versus thermistor. Sleep 1997;20(12):1175–1184.

56. Hosselet J, Ayappa I, Norman RG, Krieger AC, Rapoport DM. Classification of sleep-disordered breathing. Am J Respir Crit Care Med 2001;163(2):398–405.

57. Ayappa I, Norman RG, Krieger AC, Rosen A, O'Malley R L, Rapoport DM. Non-invasive detection of respiratory effort-related arousals (RERas) by a nasal cannula/pressure transducer system. Sleep 2000;23(6):763–771.

58. Johnson PL, Natalie Edwards N, Burgess KB, Sullivan CE. Detection of increased upper airway resistance during overnight polysomnography. Sleep 2005:28(1):85–90.

59. Messner AH, Pelayo R. Pediatric sleep-related breathing disorders. Am J Otolaryngol 2000;21(2):98–107.

60. Guilleminault C, Pelayo R. Sleep-disordered breathing in children. Ann Med 1998;30(4):350–356.

61. Carroll JL, McColley SA, Marcus CL, Curtis S, Loughlin GM. Inability of clinical history to distinguish primary snoring from obstructive sleep apnea syndrome in children. Chest 1995;108(3):610–618.

62. Farber JM. Clinical practice guideline: diagnosis and management of childhood obstructive sleep apnea syndrome. Pediatrics 2002;110(6):1255–1257; author reply 1257.

63. Schechter MS. Technical report: diagnosis and management of childhood obstructive sleep apnea syndrome. Pediatrics 2002;109(4):e69.

64. Guilleminault C, Pelayo R. . . .And if the polysomnogram was faulty? Pediatr Pulmonol 1998;26(1):1–3.

65. Messner AH. Treating pediatric patients with obstructive sleep disorders: an update. Otolaryngol Clin North Am 2003;36(3):519–530.

65. Standards and indications for cardiopulmonary sleep studies in children. American Thoracic Society. Am J Respir Crit Care Med 1996;153(2):866–878.

66. Chesson AL, Jr., Ferber RA, Fry JM, et al. The indications for polysomnography and related procedures. Sleep 1997;20(6):423–487.

67. Allen RP, Picchietti D, Hening WA, Trenkwalder C, Walters AS, Montplaisi J. Restless legs syndrome: diagnostic criteria, special considerations, and epidemiology. A report from the restless legs syndrome diagnosis and epidemiology workshop at the National Institutes of Health. Sleep Med 2003;4(2):101–119.

69. de Miguel-Díez J, Villa-Asensi JR, Álvarez-Sala JL. Prevalence of sleep-disordered breathing in children with down syndrome: polygraphic findings in 108 children. Sleep 2003;26(8):1006–1009.

70. Tarasiuk A, Simon T, Tal A, Reuveni H. Adenotonsillectomy in children with obstructive sleep apnea syndrome reduces health care utilization. Pediatrics 2004;113(2):351–356.

71. Guilleminault C, Li KK, Khramtsov A, Pelayo R, Martinez S. Sleep disordered breathing: surgical outcomes in prepubertal children. Laryngoscope 2004;114(1):132–137.

72. Suen JS, Arnold JE, Brooks LJ. Adenotonsillectomy for treatment of obstructive sleep apnea in children. Arch Otolaryngol Head Neck Surg 1995;121(5):525–530.

73. Guilleminault C, Li K, Quo S, Inouye RN. A prospective study on the surgical outcomes of children with sleep-disordered breathing. Sleep 2004;27(1):95–100.

74. Pelayo R, Powell N. Evaluation of obstructive sleep apnea by polysomnography prior to pediatric adenotonsillectomy. Arch Otolaryngol Head Neck Surg 1999;125(11):1282–1283.

75. Palombini L, Pelayo R, Guilleminault C. Efficacy of automated continuous positive airway pressure in children with sleep-related breathing disorders in an attended setting. Pediatrics 2004;113(5):e412–417.

76. Marcus CL, Ward SL, Mallory GB, et al. Use of nasal continuous positive airway pressure as treatment of childhood obstructive sleep apnea. J Pediatr 1995;127(1):88–94.

77. Malow BA, Weatherwax KJ, Chervin RD, et al. Identification and treatment of obstructive sleep apnea in adults and children with epilepsy: a prospective pilot study. Sleep Med 2003;4(6):509–515.

78. Littner M, Hirshkowitz M, Davila D, et al. Practice parameters for the use of auto-titrating continuous positive airway pressure devices for titrating pressures and treating adult patients with obstructive sleep apnea syndrome. An American Academy of Sleep Medicine report. Sleep 2002;25(2):143–147.

79. Guilleminault C, Pelayo R. Narcolepsy in children: a practical guide to its diagnosis, treatment and follow-up. Paediatr Drugs 2000;2(1):1–9.

80. Yoss RE, Daly DD. On the treatment of narcolepsy. Med Clin North Am 1968;52(4):781–787.

81. Yoss RE, Daly DD. Narcolepsy in children. Pediatrics 1960;25:1025–1033.

82. Rechtschaffen A, Dement W. Studies on the relation of narcolepsy, cataplexy, and sleep with low voltage random EEG activity. Res Publ Assoc Res Nerv Ment Dis 1967;45:488–505.

83. Fromherz S, Mignot E. Narcolepsy research: past, present, and future perspectives. Arch Ital Biol. 2004;142(4):479–486.

84. Silber MH, Krahn LE, Olson EJ, Pankratz VS. The epidemiology of narcolepsy in Olmsted County, Minnesota: a population-based study. Sleep 2002;25(2):197–202.

85. Guilleminault C, Pelayo R. Narcolepsy in prepubertal children. Ann Neurol 1998;43(1):135–142.

86. Wu MF, Gulyani SA, Yau E, Mignot E, Phan B, Siegel JM. Locus coeruleus neurons: cessation of activity during cataplexy. Neuroscience 1999;91(4):1389–1399.

87. Fujiki N, Morris L, Mignot E, Nishino S. Analysis of onset location, laterality and propagation of cataplexy in canine narcolepsy. Psychiatry Clin Neurosci 2002;56(3):275–276.

88. Okura M, Riehl J, Mignot E, Nishino S. Sulpiride, a D2/D3 blocker, reduces cataplexy but not REM sleep in canine narcolepsy. Neuropsychopharmacology 2000;23(5):528–538.

89. Rieger M, Mayer G, Gauggel S. Attention deficits in patients with narcolepsy. Sleep 2003;26(1):36–43.

90. Cheyne JA. Situational factors affecting sleep paralysis and associated hallucinations: position and timing effects. J Sleep Res 2002;11:169–177.

91. Aldrich MS, Chervin RD, Malow BA. Value of the multiple sleep latency test (MSLT) for the diagnosis of narcolepsy. Sleep 1997;20:620–29.

92. Lin L, Faraco J, Li R, et al. The sleep disorder canine narcolepsy is caused by a mutation in the hypocretin (orexin) receptor 2 gene. Cell 1999;98(3):365–376.

93. Mignot E, Lammers GJ, Ripley B, et al. The role of cerebrospinal fluid hypocretin measurement in the diagnosis of narcolepsy and other hypersomnias. Arch Neurol 2002;59(10):1553–1562.

94. Mignot E, Chen W, Black J. On the value of measuring CSF hypocretin-1 in diagnosing narcolepsy. Sleep 2003;26(6):646–649.

95. Hecht M, Lin L, Kushida CA, et al. Report of a case of immuno-suppression with prednisone in an 8-year-old boy with an acute onset of hypocretin-deficiency narcolepsy. Sleep 2003;26(7):809–810.

96. Dahl RE, Holttum J, Trubnick L. A clinical picture of child and adolescent narcolepsy. J Am Acad Child Adolesc Psychiatry 1994;33(6):834–841.

97. Mitler MM, Hayduk R. Benefits and risks of pharmacotherapy for narcolepsy. Drug Saf 2002;25(11):791–809.

98. Tafti M, Dauvilliers Y. Pharmacogenomics in the treatment of narcolepsy. Pharmacogenomics 2003;4(1):23–33.

99. Littner M, Johnson SF, McCall WV, et al. Practice parameters for the treatment of narcolepsy: an update for 2000. Sleep 2001;24(4):451–466.

100. Schwartz JRL. Modafinil: new indications for wake promotion. Expert Opin Pharmacother 2005; 6(1):115–129.

101. A 12-month, open-label, multicenter extension trial of orally administered sodium oxybate for the treatment of narcolepsy. Sleep 2003;26(1):31–5.

102. Borgen LA, Cook HN, Hornfeldt CS, Fuller DE. Sodium oxybate (GHB) for treatment of cataplexy. Pharmacotherapy 2002;22(6):798–799; discussion 9.

103. A randomized, double blind, placebo-controlled multicenter trial comparing the effects of three doses of orally administered sodium oxybate with placebo for the treatment of narcolepsy. Sleep 2002;25(1):42–49.

104. Scharf MB, Lai AA, Branigan B, Stover R, Berkowitz DB. Pharmacokinetics of gammahydroxybutyrate (GHB) in narcoleptic patients. Sleep 1998;21(5):507–514.

105. Mignot E, Renaud A, Nishino S, Arrigoni J, Guilleminault C, Dement WC. Canine cataplexy is preferentially controlled by adrenergic mechanisms: evidence using monoamine selective uptake inhibitors and release enhancers. Psychopharmacology 1993;113(1):76–82.

106. Nishino S, Fruhstorfer B, Arrigoni J, Guilleminault C, Dement WC, Mignot E. Further characterization of the alpha-1 receptor subtype involved in the control of cataplexy in canine narcolepsy. J Pharmacol Exp Ther 1993;264(3):1079–1084.

107. Thorpy M. The International Classification of Sleep Disorders, Revised: Diagnostic and Coding Manual. Chicago: American Sleep Disorders Association, 1997.

108. Chesson AL Jr, Wise M, Davila D, et al. Practice parameters for the treatment of restless legs syndrome and periodic limb movement disorder. An American Academy of Sleep Medicine Report. Standards of Practice Committee of the American Academy of Sleep Medicine. Sleep 1999;22(7):961–968.

109. Picchietti DL, Underwood DJ, Farris WA, et al. Further studies on periodic limb movement disorder and restless legs syndrome in children with attention-deficit hyperactivity disorder. Mov Disord 1999;14(6):1000–1007.

110. Hening W, Allen R, Earley C, Kushida C, Picchietti D, Silber M. The treatment of restless legs syndrome and periodic limb movement disorder. An American Academy of Sleep Medicine Review. Sleep 1999;22(7):970–999.

111. Picchietti DL, Walters AS. Moderate to severe periodic limb movement disorder in childhood and adolescence. Sleep 1999;22(3):297–300.

112. Picchetti D, Walters A, Underwood D, et al. Periodic limb movement disorder in attention-deficit hyperactivity disorder in children. Sleep Res 1997;26:469.

113. Picchietti DL, Underwood DJ, Farris WA, et al. Further studies on periodic limb movement disorder and restless legs syndrome in children with attention-deficit hyperactivity disorder. Mov Disord 1999;14:1000–1007.

114. Picchietti DL, England SJ, Walters AS, Willis K, Verrico T. Periodic limb movement disorder and restless legs syndrome in children with attention-deficit hyperactivity disorder. J Child Neurol 1998;13(12):588–594.

115. Chervin RD, Hedger KM. Clinical prediction of periodic leg movements during sleep in children. Sleep Med 2001;2:501–510.

116. Picchietti DL, Walters AS. Moderate to severe periodic limb movement disorder in childhood and adolescence. Sleep 1999;22:297–300.

117. Allen R, LaBuda M, Becker P, Earley C. Family history of RLS patients from two clinical populations. Sleep Res 1997;26:309

118. Allen RP, Barker PB, Wehrl F, Song HK, Earley CJ. MRI measurement of brain iron in patients with restless legs syndrome. Neurology 2001;56(2):263–265.

119. Connor JR, Wang XS, Patton SM, et al. Decreased transferrin receptor expression by neuromelanin cells in restless legs syndrome. Neurology 2004;62(9):1563–1567.

120. Comella CL. Restless legs syndrome: Treatment with dopaminergic agents. Neurology 2002;58(4 Suppl 1):S87–S92.

121. Littner MR, Kushida C, Anderson WM, et al. Practice parameters for the dopaminergic treatment of restless legs syndrome and periodic limb movement disorder. Sleep 2004;27(3):557–559.

122. Walters AS, Mandelbaum DE, Lewin DS, Kugler S, England SJ, Miller M. Dopaminergic therapy in children with restless legs/periodic limb movements in sleep and ADHD. Dopaminergic Therapy Study Group. Pediatr Neurol 2000;22(3):182–186.

123. Hardman JG, Limbird LE (Eds.) Goodman and Gilman's the Pharmacologic Basis of Therapeutics. 9th Ed. New York: Macmillan, 1996.

124. Earley CJ, Allen RP. Pergolide and carbidopa/levodopa treatment of the restless legs syndrome and periodic leg movements in sleep in a consecutive series of patients. Sleep 1996;19(10):801–810.

125. Allen RP, Earley CJ. Augmentation of the restless legs syndrome with carbidopa/levodopa. Sleep 1996;19(3):205–213.

126. Burg F, Ingelfinger J, Polin R, Gershon A. Gellis and Kagan's Current Pediatric Therapy. 17th Ed. Philadelphia: WB Saunders, 2002.

127. Walters AS, Hening W. Clinical presentation and neuropharmacology of restless legs syndrome. Clin Neuropharmacol 1987;10(3):225–237.

128. Guilleminault C, Cetel M, Philip P. Dopaminergic treatment of restless legs and rebound phenomenon. Neurology 1993;43(2):445.

129. Allen RP, Earley CJ. Restless legs syndrome: a review of clinical and pathophysiologic features. J Clin Neurophysiol 2001;18(2):128–147.

130. Earley CJ, Hyland K, Allen RP. CSF dopamine, serotonin, and biopterin metabolites in patients with restless legs syndrome. Mov Disord 2001;16(1):144–149.

131. Earley CJ, Connor JR, Beard JL, Malecki EA, Epstein DK, Allen RP. Abnormalities in CSF concentrations of ferritin and transferrin in restless legs syndrome. Neurology 2000;54(8):1698–1700.

132. Allen RP, Mignot E, Ripley B, Nishino S, Earley CJ. Increased CSF hypocretin-1 (orexin-A) in restless legs syndrome. Neurology 2002;59(4):639–641.

133. Simakajornboon N, Gozal D, Vlasic V, Mack C, Sharon D, McGinley BM. Periodic limb movements in sleep and iron status in children. Sleep 2003;26(6):735–738.

134. Stiasny K, Wetter TC, Winkelmann J, et al. Long-term effects of pergolide in the treatment of restless legs syndrome. Neurology 2001;56(10):1399–1402.

135. Montplaisir J, Nicolas A, Denesle R, Gomez-Mancilla B. Restless legs syndrome improved by pramipexole: a double-blind randomized trial. Neurology 1999;52(5):938–943.

136. Pelayo R, Chen W, Monzon S, Guilleminault C. Pediatric sleep pharmacology: you want to give my kid sleeping pills? Pediatr Clin North Am 2004;51(1):117–134.

137. Owens JA, Rosen CL, Mindell JA. Medication use in the treatment of pediatric insomnia: results of a survey of community-based pediatricians. Pediatrics 2003;111(5 Pt 1):e628–e635.

138. Ferber RA. Behavioral "insomnia" in the child. Psychiatr Clin North Am 1987;10(4):641–653.

139. Montgomery P, Stores G, Wiggs L. The relative efficacy of two brief treatments for sleep problems in young learning disabled (mentally retarded) children: a randomised controlled trial. Arch Dis Child 2004;89(2):125–130.

140. Ferber R. Childhood sleep disorders. Neurol Clin 1996;14(3):493–511.

141. Weissbluth M. Modification of sleep schedule with reduction of night waking: a case report. Sleep 1982;5(3):262–266.

142. Weissbluth M. Sleep learning: the first four months. Pediatr Ann 1991;20(5):228–234, 37–38.

143. Young A, Sears W, Levine B, Kodadek M, Davidson M. Key issues to address with bottle-feeding. Pediatr Nurs 2001;27(1):50–51.

144. Kahn A, Mozin MJ, Casimir G, Montauk L, Blum D. Insomnia and cow's milk allergy in infants. Pediatrics 1985;76(6):880–884.

145. Kahn A, Mozin MJ, Rebuffat E, Sottiaux M, Muller MF. Milk intolerance in children with persistent sleeplessness: a prospective double-blind crossover evaluation. Pediatrics 1989;84(4):595–603.

146. Carskadon MA. Sleep deprivation: health consequences and societal impact. Med Clin North Am 2004;88(3):767–776, x.

147. Fallone G, Seifer R, Acebo C, Carskadon MA. How well do school-aged children comply with imposed sleep schedules at home? Sleep 2002;25(7):739–745.

148. Carskadon MA, Harvey K, Duke P, Anders TF, Litt IF, Dement WC. Pubertal changes in daytime sleepiness. 1980. Sleep 2002;25(6):453–460.

149. Weitzman ED, Czeisler CA, Coleman RM, et al. Delayed sleep phase syndrome. A chronobiological disorder with sleep-onset insomnia. Arch Gen Psychiatry 1981;38(7):737–746.

150. Thorpy MJ, Korman E, Spielman AJ, Glovinsky PB. Delayed sleep phase syndrome in adolescents. J Adolesc Health Care 1988;9(1):22–27.

151. Regestein QR, Monk TH. Delayed sleep phase syndrome: a review of its clinical aspects. Am J Psychiatry 1995;152(4):602–608.

152. Shirayama M, Shirayama Y, Iida H, et al. The psychological aspects of patients with delayed sleep phase syndrome (DSPS). Sleep Med 2003;4(5):427–433.

153. Ancoli-Israel S, Schnierow B, Kelsoe J, Fink R. A pedigree of one family with delayed sleep phase syndrome. Chronobiol Int 2001;18(5):831–840.

154. Katzenberg D, Young T, Finn L, et al. A CLOCK polymorphism associated with human diurnal preference. Sleep 1998;21(6):569–576.

155. Hohjoh H, Takasu M, Shishikura K, Takahashi Y, Honda Y, Tokunaga K. Significant association of the arylalkylamine N-

acetyltransferase (AA-NAT) gene with delayed sleep phase syndrome. Neurogenetics 2003;4(3):151–153.

156. Archer SN, Robilliard DL, Skene DJ, et al. A length polymorphism in the circadian clock gene Per3 is linked to delayed sleep phase syndrome and extreme diurnal preference. Sleep 2003;26 (4):413–415.

157. Ebisawa T, Uchiyama M, Kajimura N, et al. Association of structural polymorphisms in the human period3 gene with delayed sleep phase syndrome. EMBO Rep 2001;2(4):342–346.

158. Katzenberg D, Young T, Lin L, Finn L, Mignot E. A human period gene (HPER1) polymorphism is not associated with diurnal preference in normal adults. Psychiatr Genet 1999;9(2):107–109.

159. Pedrazzoli M, Ling L, Finn L, et al. A polymorphism in the human timeless gene is not associated with diurnal preferences in normal adults. Sleep Res Online 2000;3(2):73–76.

160. Takahashi Y, Hohjoh H, Matsuura K. Predisposing factors in delayed sleep phase syndrome. Psychiatry Clin Neurosci 2000;54 (3):356–358.

161. Watanabe T, Kajimura N, Kato M, et al. Sleep and circadian rhythm disturbances in patients with delayed sleep phase syndrome. Sleep 2003;26(6):657–661.

162. Gottesmann C. Is the delayed sleep phase syndrome a physical or psychological disease? A case report of disappearance following a change of latitude. Psychiatry Clin Neurosci 2000;54(5):543–546.

163. Chesson AL, Jr., Littner M, Davila D, et al. Practice parameters for the use of light therapy in the treatment of sleep disorders. Standards of Practice Committee, American Academy of Sleep Medicine. Sleep 1999;22(5):641–660.

164. Hori T, Watanabe T, Kajimura N, Kato M, Sekimoto M, Takahashi K. Effects of phototherapy on the phase relationship between sleep and body temperature rhythm in a delayed sleep phase syndrome case. Psychiatry Clin Neurosci 2000;54(3):371–373.

165. Cole RJ, Smith JS, Alcala YC, Elliott JA, Kripke DF. Bright-light mask treatment of delayed sleep phase syndrome. J Biol Rhythms 2002;17(1):89–101.

166. Watanabe T, Kajimura N, Kato M, Sekimoto M, Takahashi K. Effects of phototherapy in patients with delayed sleep phase syndrome. Psychiatry Clin Neurosci 1999;53(2):231–233.

167. Nagtegaal JE, Laurant MW, Kerkhof GA, Smits MG, van der Meer YG, Coenen AM. Effects of melatonin on the quality of life in patients with delayed sleep phase syndrome. J Psychosom Res 2000;48(1):45–50.

168. Smits MG, van Stel HF, van der Heijden K, Meijer AM, Coenen AM, Kerkhof GA. Melatonin improves health status and sleep in children with idiopathic chronic sleep-onset insomnia: a randomized placebo-controlled trial. J Am Acad Child Adolesc Psychiatry 2003;42(11):1286–1293.

169. Paavonen EJ, Nieminen-von Wendt T, Vanhala R, Aronen ET, von Wendt L. Effectiveness of melatonin in the treatment of sleep disturbances in children with Asperger disorder. J Child Adolesc Psychopharmacol 2003;13(1):83–95.

170. Smits MG, Nagtegaal EE, van der Heijden J, Coenen AM, Kerkhof GA. Melatonin for chronic sleep onset insomnia in children: a randomized placebo-controlled trial. J Child Neurol 2001;16 (2):86–92.

171. Cartwright R. Sleep-related violence: does the polysomnogram help establish the diagnosis? 2000;1(4):331–335.

172. D'Alessandro R, Guarino M, Greco G, Bassein L. Risk of seizures while awake in pure sleep epilepsies: a prospective study. Neurology 2004;62(2):254–257.

173. Lahorgue Nunes M, Ferri R, Arzimanoglou A, Curzi L, Appel CC, Costa da Costa J. Sleep organization in children with partial refractory epilepsy. J Child Neurol 2003;18(11):763–766.

174. Kotagal P. The relationship between sleep and epilepsy. Semin Pediatr Neurol 2001;8(4):241–250.

175. Macleod S, Ferrie C, Zuberi SM. Symptoms of narcolepsy in children misinterpreted as epilepsy. Epileptic Disord. 2005; 7(1):13–17.

176. Montagna P. Nocturnal paroxysmal dystonia and nocturnal wandering. Neurology 1992;42(7 Suppl 6):61–67.

177. Hirsch E, Sellal F, Maton B, Rumbach L, Marescaux C. Nocturnal paroxysmal dystonia: a clinical form of focal epilepsy. Neurophysiol Clin 1994;24(3):207–217.

178. Provini F, Plazzi G, Lugaresi E. From nocturnal paroxysmal dystonia to nocturnal frontal lobe epilepsy. Clin Neurophysiol 2000;111(Suppl 2):S2–S8.

179. Sinclair DB, Wheatley M, Snyder T. Frontal lobe epilepsy in childhood. Pediatr Neurol 2004;30(3):169–176.

Ischemic Stroke in Childhood

19

Peter E. Anderson, PhD   *Gabrielle A. deVeber, MD, MSc*

A stroke is the result of a sudden occlusion or rupture of cerebral arteries or veins, with consequent focal cerebral damage and neurological deficits. A stroke can be either ischemic (i.e., secondary to an occlusion, termed a cerebral infarction) or hemorrhagic (i.e., intraparenchymal or resulting from subarachnoid bleeding). This chapter focuses on ischemic strokes.

There are two types of ischemic stroke: arterial ischemic stroke and sinovenous thrombosis. An arterial ischemic stroke occurs when there is an obstruction in the arterial system of the central nervous system. Sinovenous thrombosis, sometimes referred to as cerebrosinovenous thrombosis, occurs when there is an obstruction to the venous system of the brain. In both cases, blood flow to a specific brain area is interrupted, with resulting cerebral damage and neurological deficit(s). The ratio of arterial ischemic strokes to sinovenous thromboses is on the order of three to one (1).

Awareness of stroke in childhood continues to increase. The publication in the year 2000 of the special issues on cerebrovascular disorders by the *Journal of Child Neurology* and *Seminars in Pediatric Neurology* as well as the work of those involved in the clinical care and research of children with stroke have led to an increase in the reporting of child-

hood stroke and to a more complete understanding of the etiological factors and outcomes of childhood stroke. In addition, the development and availability of more effective forms of diagnostic technology has increased our understanding (2). Advances in other areas of medicine, which have made it possible for children who would not have survived earlier to survive, have also broadened the clinical spectrum of children who are at risk for stroke (e.g., premature births, severe cardiac disease, cardiac surgery, extracorporeal membrane oxygenation [ECMO], and trauma).

A note regarding the approach to this chapter—given the excellent review provided in the previous edition of this text, this chapter will emphasize the literature that has emerged since its publication (i.e., late 1990s).

EPIDEMIOLOGY

The first systematic epidemiological study of cerebrovascular disease in infants and children involved a review of the records of the Mayo Clinic (Rochester, Minnesota) from 1965 to 1974 (3). This population-based study produced an incidence rate of 2.52 cases per 100,000 children; that is, four cases of stroke over a 10-year period. The authors noted that neonatal strokes were not included and that the incidence of sickle cell anemia, a significant risk factor for stroke, was not seen in any of the hospitals in Rochester and that, therefore, the "true" incidence might be higher. Moreover, this study was completed before computerized tomography (CT) scans were developed so that this effective means of diagnosing stroke was not available. In a subsequent study by Broderick et al. involving infants and children residing in Greater Cincinnati, which took place in 1988–1989 (a period when CT/MRI was standard in the workup of a child

Acknowledgments:
This work was supported by Heart and Stroke Foundation of Ontario (NA4107, G.dV) and the Hospital for Sick Children Foundation (G.dV.). Dr deVeber is also supported with a Stroke Investigator award from the Heart and Stroke Foundation of Canada.
We thank Sarah Reiss and Maartje Salden for assistance with manuscript preparation, the members of the Children's Stroke Program at the Hospital for Sick Children, and our colleagues Drs. Michael Balthazor, Simone Kortstee, and Maureen Lovett for their support and critical review of the manuscript.

referred for stroke-like phenomena), the incidence rate was similar to that of the Rochester study, namely 2.7 strokes per 100,000. The study population was much larger than that of Rochester (295,577 children versus 15,834 children) (4). An incidence of 1.5 per 100,000 for intracerebral hemorrhage and subarachnoid hemorrhage and 1.2 per 100,000 for cerebral infarction was reported in this study.

A series of papers by Giroud and colleagues (5, 6) regarding the incidence of cerebrovascular disease in children in Dijon, France, reported far higher numbers of strokes in infants and children: 7.91 per 100,000 for ischemic stroke and 5.11 per 100,000 for hemorrhagic stroke. This series also reports a preponderance of ischemic stroke, differing with the findings of the Cincinnati study reported by Broderick. The authors noted that these differences might be explained by several factors. The data were gathered outside the main University Hospital, death certificates were reviewed for "unknown" causes of death, and "mild" stroke and strokes induced by trauma were included.

The Canadian Pediatric Ischemic Stroke Registry was conceived to obtain comprehensive and prospective epidemiological data on arterial ischemic stroke and cerebral sinovenous thrombosis in children. Given the participation of all 16 pediatric tertiary care centers in Canada, this is truly a national registry, encompassing a general population of approximately 31,000,000 citizens. The most recent figures from this registry report an incidence of 2.6 per 100,000 per year for arterial ischemic stroke (7) and 0.7 per 100,000 per year for sinovenous thrombosis (8), resulting in a total of 3.3 per 100,000 per year. A 60% male preponderance was also reported for ischemic stroke at all ages (7, 8).

ETIOLOGY

Stroke in infants and children can occur for a myriad of reasons. A thorough workup will typically result in identifying at least one etiologic factor, although in approximately 20% of cases, the cause will remain cryptogenic despite the most complete of investigations. It has often been reported that the most common cause of stroke in infants and children is cardiac disease, which is thought to account for approximately 15% of childhood stroke (9). For example, a series of 59 consecutive cases of childhood stroke reported a total of seven children with cardiac or transcardiac embolic strokes, a rate of 12% (10). Cardiac disease was listed as the primary risk factor for stroke in 19% of patients enrolled in the Canadian Pediatric Ischemic Stroke Registry, followed by coagulation disorders (14%), dehydration (11%), vasculitis (7%), infection (6%), dissection (5%), neoplasm (4%), metabolic disorder (3%), Moyamoya disease (2%), sickle cell anemia (2%), and perinatal complications (2%), with miscellaneous factors accounting for 4%. A risk factor could not be identified in 21% of participants in this registry (11, 12).

The search for a putative cause(s) of a stroke is of great importance and should extend beyond the obvious cause (e.g., an arterial dissection or congenital heart disease), as multiple risk factors are often found in ischemic strokes and the presence of multiple risk factors has been linked with both stroke recurrence and stroke outcome (12). There is frequently a preceding or concomitant condition, which by itself or in combination with its treatment results in cerebral insult, in addition to the stroke itself. It is sometimes difficult to separate out the primary and secondary causes of the cerebral insult. The adult literature, often used as a jumping off point for the treatment of children, is of limited use as the causes of stroke in adults can be quite different (e.g., although atherosclerosis and atrial fibrillation are common risk factors in adults, they are not listed as common in stroke in children).

CLINICAL PRESENTATION

Presentation of stroke varies with the age at which the lesion occurs, as well as the location and type of lesion. Infants with arterial ischemic strokes and sinovenous thrombosis often present with lethargy and seizures, while in older infants and toddlers symptoms may present with an abrupt onset and with focal neurological signs, such as facial droop or hemiparesis. If a stroke occurs in the prenatal or perinatal stroke period, motor signs may not emerge until several months later—between 4 to 8 months of age (13). A school-age or teenage child may describe more subtle symptoms, such as word finding difficulty or visual disturbance, headache, or a focal sensory deficit. There is some thought that transient ischemic attacks precede arterial ischemic strokes in up to one third of cases, although they are rarely diagnosed (7). In some cases, the symptoms of these transient ischemic attacks may be thought to be hysterical in nature, or a conversion disorder, given that the symptoms appear and then fade away, possibly to return again if there is another attack.

Seizures and lethargy are the most typical presentations of sinovenous thrombosis in the neonatal period (8). Older infants and children typically present with more varied symptomatology, related to increased intracranial pressure, with headache, visual disturbance papilledema, and, occasionally, sixth-cranial nerve palsy. Hemiparesis and seizures are common occurring in 35 to 45 and 48%, respectively (8).

As is the case with stroke in adult patients, there are a great number of etiologies for a stroke in the neonatal period or in childhood, which can be broken down into major categories) with several examples under each category, some of which will be described in the text (see Table 19.1).

SICKLE CELL DISEASE

Sickle cell disease is one of the numerous medical conditions that can precede a stroke. Cerebrovascular accidents are a frequent and major complication in patients with sickle cell disease. Sickle cell disease is the result of an abnormal

TABLE 19.1
RISK FACTORS FOR STROKE IN CHILDREN

Hematologic Disorders

Hemoglobinopathies (e.g., sickle cell anemia)
Immune thrombocytopenic purpura
Thrombotic thrombocytopenic purpura
Thrombocytosis
Polycythemia
Leukemia or other neoplasm
Disseminated intravascular coagulation

Vasculopathies

Postvaricella angiopathy
Ehlers-Danlos syndrome
Early atherosclerosis
Diabetes
Systemic hypertension
Hypernatremia
Superior vena cava syndrome
Homocystinuria
Pseudoxanthoma elasticum
Fabry disease
Arterial fibromuscular dysplasia
Moyamoya syndrome
Moyamoya disease
Postradiation vasculopathy
NADH-CoQ reductase deficiency
Williams syndrome

Vasculitis

Meningitis
Systemic lupus erythmatosus
Systemic infection
Polyateritis nodosa
Granulomatous angiitis
Takayasu's arteritis
Rheumatoid arthritis
Dermatomytosis
Inflammatory bowel disease
Drug abuse (cocaine, amphetamines)
Hemolytic-uremic syndrome

Vasospastic Disorders

Migraine
Ergot poisoning
Vasospasm with subarachnoid hemorrhage

Cardiac Disorders

Complex congenital heart defect
Ventricular/atrial septal defects
Patent ductus arteriosus
Patent foramen ovale
Aortic or mitral stenosis
Coarctation
Cardiac rhabdomymoma or myxoma
Rheumatic heart disease
Prosthetic heart valve
Bacterial endocarditis
Libman-Sacks endocarditis
Cardiomyopathy and myocarditis
Arrhythmias

Coagulation Disorders

Congenital coagulation defects
Prothrombotic medications (oral
   contraceptives, L-asparaginase)
Pregnancy/postpartum period
Lupus anticoagulant
Antithrombin III deficiency
Anticardiolipin antibodies
Lipoprotein abnormalities
Factor V Leiden
Protein S deficiency
Protein C deficiency
Liver dysfunction with coagulopathy
Vitamin K deficiency
Plasminogen deficiency
Hyperhomocystienemia
Hyperlipidemia

Trauma

Amniotic fluid/placental embolism
Child abuse
Fat or air embolism
Foreign body embolism
Cardiac catheterization
Carotid ligation (e.g., ECMO)
Vertebral trauma due to cervical rotation
Posttraumatic arterial dissection
Brain herniation and arterial compression
Intra-oral trauma
Arteriography
Carotid cavernous fistula

hemoglobin, which causes red blood cells to form a sickle shape. As the hemoglobin is deoxygenated, the stiff, inflexible sickle cells occlude small vessels and deprive the brain and other organs of oxygenated blood and result in infarction. Sickle cell anemia is the most common form of sickle cell disease in the United States, accounting for 60 to 70% of the cases, and the most likely to cause stroke is the HbSS genotype (14). This autosomal recessive disorder results from a mutation in the hemoglobin beta (HBB) gene. Other forms of sickle cell disease result from co-inheritance of Hb S with other abnormal globin beta chain variants. These include sickle-hemoglobin C disease (Hb SC) and two types of sickleβ-thalassemia (Hb Sβ^+-thalassemia and Hb Sβ°-thalassemia). Other globin beta chain variants such as D-Punjab and O-Arab also result in sickle cell disease when co-inherited with Hb S. In a Jamaican cohort of 310 patients of all genotypes ranging in age from 9 to 17 years, the overall estimate of incidence of stroke was 7.8%, a very high number (15).

Ohene-Frempong and colleagues (16) initiated the Cooperative Study of Sickle Cell Disease, a prospective longitudinal study that enrolled more than 4,000 patients between 1978 and 1988. Among all of these genotypes, the investigators found that the HbSS patients had the highest prevalence rate for stroke (4.01%) and an incidence rate for stroke of 0.61 per 100 patient years, although they emphasized that stroke occurred in all common genotypes. It should be noted that these findings included both ischemic and hemorrhagic stroke. In this study, a history of transient ischemic attack was a strong risk factor for a completed infarctive stroke, indicating that an aggressive stance toward the prevention of stroke should be adopted if evidence of a transient ischemic attack is present. A low steady-state hemoglobin concentration, elevated systolic blood pressure, and recent episode of acute chest syndrome or crisis were also considered as risk factors for an ischemic stroke. Finally, it was noted that sickle cell patients who had a stroke had a high risk of recurrent stroke, a risk that can be attenuated, but not eliminated, by chronic transfusion therapy (17).

MOYAMOYA DISEASE/SYNDROME

Another medical condition that predisposes one to stroke is Moyamoya disease. When Takeuchi and Shimizu first described Moyamoya disease in 1957, they used the technical term "hypoplasia of the bilateral internal carotid arteries" (18). In this report, they presented a case study of a 29-year-old man. Following the publication of this case study, many more reports followed, and in 1967, Suzuki and Takaku coined the phrase "Moyamoya disease" to describe the neuroradiological characteristics (19). Moyamoya, as the disease has been called since this time, is a Japanese expression meaning "something hazy, just like a puff of cigarette smoke drifting in the air" and refers to the cerebral angiogram of an individual with this rare disease.

Although the fine network of vessels at the base of the brain or the basal ganglia is the aspect of the disease that initially attracted the attention of neurosurgeons, the formation of these vessels is thought to be a secondary process of the disease induced by chronic ischemia (20). More specifically, the development of these Moyamoya disease vessels is seen as the brain's reaction to occlusion (blockage of a vessel or artery) or stenosis (narrowing of vessel or artery) as it tries to compensate for the decrease in cerebral blood flow to the areas distal to the sites of occlusion or stenosis by making collateral vessels (21). This specific response of the brain is unique to Moyamoya disease and is not seen in other cerebrovascular diseases (22).

The main feature of Moyamoya disease is the progressive occlusion or stenosis of one or more of the main arteries of the circle of Willis; namely, the terminal portion of the internal carotid artery, the proximal portion of the anterior, or the middle cerebral arteries, the result of which is chronic ischemia. Both stenosis or occlusion next to the Moyamoya vessels should be found bilaterally, according to the official diagnostic criteria (23). Of note to this review, the diagnostic criteria are based on the observable characteristics of the disease as measured by invasive and noninvasive devices. Alternatively, Moyamoya disease can be diagnosed by medical reports of associated diseases or the conditions of the patient at time of autopsy.

Moyamoya disease is rare, however, prevalence rates vary. In Asian countries such as Japan, China, and Korea, the incidence is higher than in European and American countries (24). For example, the estimated total number of Moyamoya disease patients in Japan in 1994 was 3,800, which represents an incidence of 1/1,000,000 each year (23). A questionnaire study provided an estimate of the incidence of Moyamoya disease across Europe as being one tenth of the Japanese incidence (25). A somewhat different picture is seen if one uses a pediatric stroke sample as the population of interest. A study of 59 pediatric stroke patients in France (10) found that four (7%) patients presented with Moyamoya symptomatology. The study also reported that the patients with Moyamoya disease had the highest risk of stroke recurrence (75%) relative to the other identified mechanisms causing stroke in childhood (10).

In a nationwide study of Moyamoya disease in Japan, four subtypes were identified: hemorrhagic (occurring in 33% of participants), infarctive (22%), transient ischemic attack (20%), and epileptic (12%) (26). The incidence of these subtypes varies depending on gender and age. The infarct subtype is more common among males as opposed to the hemorrhagic subtype, which is more common in females (26). Different studies show that hemorrhagic strokes are more common among adults than children (23, 27–29).

HUMAN IMMUNODEFICIENCY VIRUS

As the number of persons with human immunodeficiency virus (HIV) continues to grow, so the number of HIV-infected children grows. Approximately 20% of HIV-infected infants will develop acquired immunodeficiency syndrome (AIDS) in the first year of life, and approximately 90% will develop AIDS by 18 months of age. This progression to AIDS is important for pediatric stroke, as an estimated 1.3% of these children will go on to experience stroke (30), a combination of ischemic and hemorrhagic strokes. For example, in the case of a young lady with known AIDS who presented with new-onset seizures and a right hemiparesis, a combination of subacute hemorrhage and a complete occlusion of the left middle cerebral artery was diagnosed (31). These authors speculated that the cause of stroke in this case was a vasculopathy caused by the human immunodeficiency virus, an etiology similar to postvaricella vasculopathy (32). Interestingly, this patient returned after her hemiparetic symptoms worsened, at which time a new left frontal ischemic infarction was noted, with occlusion of both anterior cerebral arteries. The angiographic characteristics of this vasculopathy were described as "Moyamoya disease-like." Other authors stress that stroke and seizures can represent the presenting symptoms of pediatric HIV infection or AIDS, describing two such cases (33) and emphasizing that testing for HIV should be included in the investigation of stroke in a child who is at risk for HIV infection. A follow-up letter to this article proposed a cause for the vasculopathy and ischemic stroke, that being an "HIV-1-associated vasculitis-vasculopathy-hypoxia/ischemia sequence" (34). The supposition of these authors that cytotoxic T lymphocytes are responsible for the cascade of events culminating in ischemic stroke led to suggestions for therapeutic approaches in children with HIV infection, including those related to the HIV infection (e.g., antiretroviral medications, prophylactic immunomodulators) and to the cerebrovascular system (e.g., vasodilators, calcium-channel blockers).

PROTHROMBOTIC DISORDERS

Many genetic syndromes not only predispose a child to stroke (e.g., hyperhomocystienemia (35) but exert their own influence on the neuropsychological, behavioral, or psychiatric profile (e.g., Down syndrome (36)). Arterial ischemic strokes and sinovenous thrombosis can both be caused by thrombotic vascular occlusion. While vascular occlusive strokes in adults are typically the result of atherosclerosis, in children, they are often the result of another disease or risk factor, including prothrombotic disorders. Prothrombotic disorders are thought to be present in anywhere from 20 to 50% of childhood arterial ischemic strokes and from 33 to 99% in childhood sinovenous thrombosis. The fact that these disorders can be both a cause for the initial stroke but can also be a cause for recurrent strokes highlights the need for a thorough workup and evaluation when a child strokes. Relatively common prothrombotic disorders include deficiencies of antithrombin, protein C, protein S, plasminogen, the presence of Factor V Leiden, Prothrombin gene G20210A, dysfibrinogenemia, antiphospholipid antibodies, hyperhomocysteinemia, and elevated lipoprotein (37). Of note in this review is the approach provided by Chan and deVeber to suggested laboratory tests when faced with a child suspected of having or having a stroke (37).

DIFFERENTIAL DIAGNOSIS

When a child presents with a hemiparesis or seizure, there are, of course, many diagnostic options, one of which is stroke. Other causes for a hemiparesis could include the pressure exerted on brain structures by a brain tumor or an arteriovenous malformation, acute disseminated encephalomyelitis, or a progressive epileptic condition, such as Rasmussen's encephalitis, of which a progressive hemiparesis is a symptom. Todd's paralysis (a transient hemiparesis that can follow a seizure) should also be considered. Finally, a migraine may present with a hemiplegia, in addition to other symptoms (38).

The diagnosis of stroke is best confirmed by neuroimaging. Cranial ultrasound, which has unquestionable value in the diagnosis of periventricular and intraventricular hemorrhage in premature infants, has been shown to be too insensitive for the diagnosis of ischemic stroke in term newborns (39). Advances in other areas of neuroimaging, including magnetic resonance imaging (MRI) techniques such as diffusion weighted imaging and perfusion MRI, as well as magnetic resonance angiography, have enhanced the ability to identify and characterize ischemic strokes in children (2). Conventional angiography continues to be the gold standard for children with stroke; however, as magnetic resonance angiography images flow signal rather than vascular anatomy and has been shown to miss abnormalities that would be identified with conventional angiography (40).

When considering the consequences of stroke, there are many factors other than stroke to consider. For example, those children who develop a seizure disorder secondary to their stroke will most likely be prescribed an anticonvulsant medication(s), which are well known to have effects on cognitive functioning (41–44). Migraine headaches can precede stroke or result from a stroke, and, if severe, can have a debilitating effect on many aspects of functioning (45). The functioning of a child and family can also be significantly disrupted by the medical sequelae of a stroke (e.g., investigations for stroke etiology, such as phlebotomies, CT, or MRI scans), or the concern about stroke recurrence. Finally, it is not uncommon for children who are not walking or talking as other children do to be ostracized in their schools and neighborhoods secondary to the visible aftereffects of stroke. Keeping these additional factors in mind, the neurological, neuropsychological, behavioral, and psychiatric sequelae of stroke are considered.

NEUROLOGICAL SEQUALAE

In the adult population, 85% of patients with sinovenous thrombosis have been reported to have a good longterm (mean 6.5 years) outcome, based on the absence of neurologic signs and symptoms (46). However, in a study of 57 adults with sinovenous thrombosis, significant cognitive morbidity was reported at a mean 1.5-year follow-up (47).

Some information has been reported regarding the neurological outcome of sinovenous thrombosis in infants and children. In a literature review, neurologic sequelae were present in 27% of 124 survivors of childhood sinovenous thrombosis untreated with anticoagulant therapy (49). A prospective study utilizing a standardized neurological assessment found that 18% of 38 infants and children surviving sinovenous thrombosis had poor outcome, based on the presence of moderate or severe neurologic deficits (49). In the Canadian Registry, the neurologic outcomes in 61 neonates and 91 nonneonates at a mean interval from thrombosis of 1.6 years were as follows: 54% were normal, 38% had neurologic deficits, and 8% had died. The neurologic deficits (based on neurological examination only) included motor impairment in 80% of cases, cognitive impairment in 10%, developmental delay in 9%, speech impairment in 6%, visual impairment in 6%, and other impairments in 26% (8).

In children with ischemic arterial stroke, an altered level of consciousness, or seizures, and a completed or cortical completed middle cerebral artery stroke were significant risk factors for poor outcome, measured by both the presence of recurrent stroke and neurological impairment (50).

COGNITIVE/INTELLECTUAL/ NEUROPSYCHOLOGICAL SEQUALAE

Most investigations of intellectual outcome after childhood stroke focus on the effect of unilateral lesions. Coupled with this emphasis on unilateral lesions has been a focus on the perceived plasticity of the immature central nervous system, more specifically, a search for the age at which the traditional functional specialization of the left hemisphere for speech and language and the right hemisphere for visuospatial functioning emerges (51–54). Part and parcel of this approach has been the investigation of whether either hemisphere of the immature brain can take over for any cognitive functions if the lesion occurs early enough. For example, evidence has been presented suggesting that prenatally and perinatally acquired lesions in the left periventricular white matter shift the organization of speech to the right hemisphere, documented as right-hemisphere fMRI activation with left facial motor tract involvement (55).

Intellectual outcome after unilateral lesions that have taken place in infancy and childhood is typically reported as being within the average range, but below that of normal population means, and that of matched controls (54, 56–59). Hogan and colleagues (59) as well as Bates and colleagues (57) have summarized this body of research, examining the impact that a number of factors may have on poststroke outcome. For example, given the evidence to date, there does not appear to be a consistent significant effect for side of lesion, a result that is consistent across a number of studies (57, 60, 61). A lack of consistent results has also been found for variables including etiology of stroke and associated neurological disorders, in particular, seizures; lesion variables including extent of lesion, hemispheric lateralization of lesion, and location of lesion within the hemisphere; and variables related to the child, such as sex, age at onset, time since onset, and age at test; and socioeconomic status.

Children with focal stroke often appear to demonstrate a remarkable recovery from the insult (62). However, detailed studies of children with severe brain injuries do identify deficiencies in the area of discourse (connected language) (63–66). Chapman et al. found that the children with stroke performed more poorly than orthopedic controls when examined for language-structure (e.g., the length of utterance) as well as information-structure (the content and organization of the episodic structure, including being able to relay the core propositions, the gist propositions, and a macrolevel interpretation). This pattern of recovery in children, that is, the recovery of lexical and grammatical ability in the context of weakness in discourse macrolevel skills, is opposite to the pattern that typically found in adult stroke patients (67). These investigators also noted that there was a poorer outcome for discourse in those who had a stroke at an early age (up to 12 months of age) compared to those who had a stroke at 12 months of age or later. Moreover, the site- and size-of-lesion effects found in adult stroke populations were not observed. The implications of these findings for how these children will perform in an academic environment are clearly concerning and should be the focus of continuing investigation.

BEHAVIORAL SEQUALAE

As is the case with research into the cognitive or intellectual outcome of pediatric stroke, most of the research into the behavioral sequelae of pediatric stroke has focused on the discrepancy between lesions of the left or the right hemispheres. More specifically, left-sided lesions in adults tend to result in disturbances of language, calculations, and praxis, while right-sided lesions tend to result in the alteration of functions that are reliant on directed attention and visuospatial skills, modulation of affect, and the paralinguistic aspects of communication (68). Previous research into the "right hemisphere deficit syndrome" in children (68–72) generally supported these findings and suggested the presence of a fairly specific pattern of social and personality deficits, with difficulties being noted in social interaction/social withdrawal, attention, and arithmetic. The latter difficulty has also been described as a "nonverbal learning disability"(73).

In keeping with this line of research, children with early focal right-hemisphere lesions have been documented to have greater difficulties recognizing and identifying facial affect than both normal controls and children with early focal left-hemisphere lesions (74). Precursors of this social difficulty may also be seen in investigations of early temperament by Nass and Koch, who described babies with right-hemisphere lesions as consistently showing more negative temperament and mood than babies with left-hemisphere lesions (75).

While the number of investigations into the behavioral sequelae of strokes in infancy and childhood does not rival that of investigations into the intellectual outcome, some have been reported. Trauner and colleagues (76) found that children with early focal lesions differed from control children in the areas of general adjustment (i.e., cognitive and academic development), social skills, and social adjustment. These children were subdivided into those with left- and right-hemisphere lesions, with the resulting discrepancies failing to reach significance. The overall conclusion of these authors was that any early onset and focal brain lesion predisposes one to social and cognitive deficits. A subsequent study, reporting on the behavioral profile of children with prenatal or perinatal onset unilateral brain damage, found little difference between these children and controls (77). In fact, when the effect of IQ was removed from the analysis, there was no difference between the groups on any of the scales or subscales of the questionnaire used (78). These authors were careful, however, to avoid stating that such lesions do not have an impact on the behavioral profile of a child. They noted that their group of children with unilateral brain damage was mixed, with some lesions being left hemisphere, some right hemisphere, some frontal and some nonfrontal, and so on, and that the behavioral profiles of these subgroups may have "balanced out" across the other groups. They also stated that patients with bilateral or more extensive damage than that of the children in their study may be at a greater risk for behavioral dysfunction than their subjects were.

PSYCHIATRIC SEQUALAE

Changes in the psychiatric functioning of adults who have suffered a stroke have been widely reported, including personality changes, impaired social behaviors, decision-making deficiencies, and other executive functions following damage to the frontal lobes (79–81). The impact of side of lesion has also figured prominently in this literature, with left-hemisphere lesions commonly being associated with depression (82–85). Right-hemisphere lesions have been associated with difficulties comprehending or expressing emotion (79, 86, 87), as well as mania or hypomania (86, 88, 89). More recently, depression has been associated with stroke severity (i.e., a major hemispheral stroke syndrome, reflecting the severity of the neurological impairment), infarcts affecting the limbic system of the brain, presence of dementia, and female gender (90). Other investigators have also found that greater degrees of physical disability are related to depression and poor emotional outcome (91).

Adults who have suffered a stroke have been reported to have difficulty controlling their emotional responses, in some cases resulting in significant problems controlling anger and aggression (92, 93). Kim and colleagues have looked at the inability to control anger and aggression in adult stroke, comparing the ratings of close relatives or caretakers of adults poststroke to their estimates of the ability to control anger and aggression prior to the stroke

(92). They reported that 32% of those sampled were unable to control their anger or aggression, with some of these behaviors being spontaneous and some being environmentally triggered.

Poststroke changes in aggression and anger control, while observed clinically in pediatric populations, have not been formally reported in the pediatric stroke literature. We completed a pilot study, asking the parents of children with stroke to complete the aggression subscale of the Behavior Assessment System for Children Parent Rating Scales (BASC) (94) as well as a 5-point Likert scale to indicate whether there was a poststroke difference in their child's level of aggression or expression of anger, and whether this behavior interfered with family functioning (95). Of 26 completed questionnaires, 6 (23%) yielded a T-score equal to or greater than one standard deviation above the mean on the BASC aggression subscale, with two ratings exceeding a T-score of 65 (i.e., within the defined clinical range). More than one quarter of respondents reported that their child's current level of aggression or expression of anger disrupted the functioning of their family. These early data suggest that aggression and expression of anger is of clinical concern in a subset of children with stroke, to the point that families have stopped or changed their involvement in various activities as a result of concern about their child's ability to control his or her emotions.

In some case studies, lesions in specific areas have resulted in tic-like behaviors (96). Two boys who suffered subcortical strokes involving the right basal ganglia at the age of 8 years were described. In the case of one boy, the right caudate and putamen were affected, while in the other case, the head of the right caudate nucleus was lesioned. In both cases, the boys developed a left hemidystonia 2 weeks after the stroke, with the later emergence of tic-like behavior. Difficulties in the realm of focusing and attending were also noted.

A number of investigations have focused specifically on the psychiatric sequelae following a stroke in childhood. Max and colleagues have explored the prevalence of psychiatric morbidity in children with stroke relative to orthopedic controls (i.e., the subjects with stroke were matched individually to subjects with clubfoot or scoliosis). This group has also explored groups of children with stroke and similar controls for the presence of a psychiatric disorder that was not present prior to the child experiencing the stroke. When they considered general categories of psychiatric disorder, they found that 46% of their sample had poststroke ADHD, 31% had a poststroke anxiety disorder, 21% had a poststroke mood disorder, and 17% had a poststroke personality change (97). Strongly correlated with the development of a poststroke psychiatric disorder was an abnormal neurological exam (assessment of neurological severity was rated by seizure history, head circumference, degree of hemiplegia, and function of the unaffected side of the body), lower full-scale IQ (FSIQ) and verbal IQ (VIQ), socialization deficits (noted on the Socialization Domain of the Vineland Adaptive Behavior Scales), and increased family psychopathology (in first-degree relatives).

The children with attention deficit hyperactivity disorder (ADHD) were followed up in an accompanying study, designed to determine whether a commonality in lesion characteristics was present (98). Of 25 children with focal stroke lesions, 15 were noted to have ADHD or ADHD traits (that is, cases with symptoms that fell at a subsyndromal level or cases in which there was disagreement between raters). Lesion volume was not associated with the presence of ADHD traits. When the MRI scans of the 13 children with the largest lesions (greater than 10^3 cm were examined, it was found that ADHD traits were present in six of seven patients with lesions of the putamen compared to two of six patients with lesions that did not involve the putamen (Fisher exact test p = .1). These authors stress that the putamen is a part of dopamine-rich ventral or limbic striatum, and that this area of the brain has been related to ADHD in previous studies (99, 100), especially ADHD dominated by symptoms of inattention.

Max and colleagues have also reported that lifetime ADHD traits were significantly more common in children with stroke and no prior ADHD symptomatology than in orthopedic controls (46 versus 17%) (101). Inattention and apathy were identified as "core features" of the presence of ADHD traits in children with stroke, secondary to their performance across several neurocognitive measures.

REMEDIATION

As is apparent from the preceding review of the various types of outcome of stroke in infancy or childhood, it is clear that early views of the plasticity of the immature brain (i.e., that the earlier the insult to the brain, the more complete recovery) were overly optimistic (102–104). Indeed, it is clear that there are considerable and lasting changes and areas of deficit that these children and their families, as well as those working with them, will have to keep in mind. Effort must be directed toward the development of remediation and rehabilitation techniques to help these children if improvement in their functioning is to be seen. A major part of this effort to help these children is being able to provide an accurate assessment of their strengths and weaknesses in order (1) to document that they are in need of assistance and (2) to better guide and direct that assistance. We have found that providing them with a neuropsychological assessment is often ideal in determining the best way to approach helping these children.

The purpose of a neuropsychological assessment is to promote the development of independence, competence, and well-being for the child being assessed. In addition to careful consideration of the developmental and physical context that the child is in, it is important to assess a sufficient number of domains of functioning to be able to provide specific recommendations for the child and those

working with him or her. More specifically, determining the IQ of a child will not translate into specific recommendations for the development of language or visual-spatial functioning, for example. A typical neuropsychological assessment, therefore, includes the assessment of general cognitive/intellectual functioning, verbal or language functioning, visual-spatial functioning, attention/concentration, memory, sensory-perceptual, motor, academic achievement, executive functioning, and socioemotional functioning (see the following for cogent reviews of neuropsychological assessment (105–107)). Translating the assessment results into a form that is real to those involved, and that includes practical implications and treatment recommendations, is extremely important. For example, a 3-year-old with frontal infarcts would not be expected to differ much from another child that is 3 years old, as the functioning of the frontal lobes begins to become more important for the overall functioning of a child later in life, say when she or he is entering school. Therefore, from a practical perspective, the neuropsychologist may be able to point out subtle areas of current deficit and translate them as indicators of the difficulties yet to come (i.e., how attentional and organizational issues will play a greater role as the child ages) and provide recommendations about how to best work with the child to encourage the development of these skills and abilities.

Numerous resources are available for parents and those working with children with stroke that address specific areas of functioning, such as difficulties with academic subjects (e.g., reading or math) and difficulties with the development of executive functioning or social skills. For example, Stephen Nowicki and Marshall Duke have written an excellent series of books designed to promote the development of social skills (108–110).

CONCLUSION

It is important to realize that the pediatric stroke field is in its infancy, with the vast majority of the stroke literature coming from the adult/geriatric end of the age spectrum. However, definitive steps have been taken to move the field forward, including the aforementioned special issues (*Journal of Child Neurology*, Seminars in Pediatric Neurology), a text devoted to the field (111), conferences dedicated to pediatric stroke, such as the First International Conference on Cerebrovascular Disease in Children in 1998, and several multisite research initiatives, such as the Canadian Pediatric Ischemic Stroke Registry and a project directed toward the establishment of standards of practice and the initiation of further multicenter, multinational clinical trials for neonates and children with stroke, sponsored by the Child Neurology Society/Child Neurology Foundation.

It is also important to note that some steps have been taken in assessing outcome in some areas of functioning in children with stroke. For example, investigators are now exploring specific aspects of language functioning and finding areas of weakness, rather than relying on global measures of verbal functioning and concluding that performance based on this global measure was age appropriate. Early studies of behavioral or psychiatric outcome also often focused on generalities and found few or no differences between children with stroke and controls. More recent studies, such as those of Max and colleagues (97, 98, 101) have focused on specific areas of functioning (e.g., ADHD, anxiety disorders) and on more specific methods of assessment, again with the result of identifying areas of need that were previously masked by (imprecise) measures of global functioning. Continued developments along these lines will more clearly demarcate areas of need in children with stroke, which will, in turn, allow for the fine-tuning of efforts toward the development of specific methods of rehabilitation/remediation.

Over the coming years, it will be the goal of those working in the field of pediatric stroke to continue to inform the medical and lay world of the magnitude of childhood stroke and to emphasize the importance of early and accurate diagnosis, as well as early and effective intervention to improve the outcome for these children.

REFERENCES

1. DeVeber G, Roach S. Cerebrovascular disease. In: Maria BL, ed. *Current Management in Child Neurology*. Hamilton: BC Decker, 2001:356–360.
2. Hunter JV. Magnetic resonance imaging in pediatric stroke. Top Magn Reson Imaging 2002;13:23–38.
3. Schoenberg BS, Mellinger JF, Schoenberg DG. Cerebrovascular disease in infants and children: A study of incidence, clinical features, and survival. Neurology 1978;28:763–768.
4. Broderick J, Talbot GT, Prenger E, et al. Stroke in children within a major metropolitan area: The surprising importance of intracerebral hemorrhage. J Child Neurol 1993;8:250–255.
5. Giroud M, Lemesle M, Gouyon J-B, et al. Cerebrovascular disease in children under 16 years of age in the city of Dijon, France: A study of the incidence and clinical features from 1985 to 1993. J Clin Epidemiol 1995;48:1343–1348.
6. Giroud M, Lemesle M, Madinier G, et al. Stroke in children under 16 years of age: Clinical and etiological difference with adults. Acta Neurol Scand 1997;96:401–406.
7. deVeber G, Andrew M, and the Canadian Pediatric Ischemic Stroke Study Group. Canadian paediatric ischemic stroke registry: Analysis of children with arterial ischemic stroke [abstract]. Ann Neurol 2000;48:526.
8. deVeber G, Andrew M, Adams C et al. Cerebral sinovenous thrombosis in children. N Engl J Med 2001;345:417–423.
9. Ganesan V, Prengler M, McShane MA, et al. Investigation of risk factors in children with arterial ischemic stroke. Ann Neurol 2003;53:167–173.
10. Chabrier S, Husson B, Lasjaunias P, et al. Stroke in childhood: Outcome and recurrence risk by mechanism in 59 patients. J Child Neurol. 2000;15:290–294.
11. deVeber G, Adams M, Andrew M, and Canadian Pediatric Neurologists. Canadian Pediatric Ischemic Stroke Registry (Analysis III). Can J Neurol Sci 1995;22:S24.
12. Lanthier S, Carmant L, David M, et al. Stroke in children: The coexistence of multiple risk factors predicts poor outcome. Neurology 2000;54:371–378.
13. deVeber G. Stroke and the child's brain: An overview of epidemiology, syndromes and risk factors. Curr Opin Neurol 2002; 15:133–138.
14. Ohene-Frempong K. Stroke in sickle cell disease: Demographic, clinical and therapeutic considerations. Semin Hematol 1991; 28:213–219.
15. Balkaran B, Char G, Morris JS, et al. Stroke in a cohort of patients with homozygous sickle cell disease. J Pediatr 1992;120: 360–366.
16. Ohene-Frempong K, Weiner SJ, Sleeper LA, et al. Cerebrovascular accidents in sickle cell disease: Rates and risk factors. Blood 1998;91:288–294.
17. Pegelow CH, Adams RJ, McKie V, et al. Risk of recurrent stroke in patients with sickle cell disease treated with erythrocyte transfusions. J Pediatr 1995;126:896–899.
18. Takeuchi K, Shimizu K. Hypoplasia of the bilateral internal carotid arteries (in Japanese with English abstract). Brain Nerve 1957;9:37–43.
19. Suzuki J, Takaku A, Asahi M. Comments on "Moyamoya disease." In: Kudo T, ed. *A Disease With Abnormal Intracranial Vascular Networks*. Tokyo: Igakushoin, 1967:73–75.
20. Farrugia M, Howlett DC, Saks AM. Moyamoya disease. J Postgrad Med 1997;73:549–552.
21. Mugikura S, Takahashi S, Higano S, et al. The relationship between cerebral infarction and angiographic characteristics in childhood Moyamoya disease. Am J Neuroradiol 1999;20: 336–343.
22. Yoshimoto T, Houkin K, Takahashi A, et al. Angiogenic factors in Moyamoya disease. Stroke 1996;27:2160–2165.
23. Fukui M. Current state of study on Moyamoya disease in Japan. Surg Neurol 1997;47:138–143.
24. Goto F, Yonekawa Y. World-wide distribution of Moyamoya disease. Neurol Med Chir 1992;32:883–886.
25. Yonekawa Y, Ogata N, Kaku Y, et al. Moyamoya disease in Europe, past and present status. Clin Neurol Neurosur 1997;99: S58–S60.
26. Yamaguchi T, Tashito M, Sugi T, et al. Nation wide survey of obstruction of circle of Willis (in Japanese). In: Annual report of special working group of welfare ministry for Moyamoya disease in fiscal year 1979, 1980:9–16.
27. Choi JU, Kim DS, Kim EY, et al. Natural history of Moyamoya disease: Comparison of activity of daily living in surgery and non-surgery groups. Clin Neurol Neurosur 1997;99: S11–S18.
28. Han DH, Kwon O, Byun BJ, et al. A co-operative study: Clinical characteristics of 334 Korean patients with Moyamoya disease treated at neurosurgical institutes (1979–1994). Acta NeurochirurWien 2000;142:1263–1274.
29. Ikezaki K, Inamura T, Kawano T, et al. Clinical features of probable Moyamoya disease in Japan. Clin Neurol Neurosur 1997; 99:S173–S177.
30. Park YD, Belman AL, Kim T-S, et al. Stroke in pediatric acquired immunodeficiency syndrome. Ann Neurol 1990;28:303–311.
31. Narayan P, Samuels OB, Barrow DL. Stroke and pediatric human immunodeficiency virus infection: Case report and review of the literature. Pediatr Neurosurg 2003;37:158–163.
32. Askalan R, Laughlin S, Mayank S, et al. Chickenpox and stroke in childhood: A study of frequency and causation. Stroke 2001;32: 1257–1262.
33. Visudtibhan A, Visudhiphan P, Chiemchanya S. Stroke and seizures as the presenting signs of pediatric HIV infection. Pediatr Neurol 1999;20:53–56.
34. Legido A, Lischner HW, de Chadarevian J-P, et al. Correspondence: Stroke in pediatric HIV infection. Pediatr Neurol 1999; 21:588.
35. van Beynum IM, Smeitink JAM, den Heijer M, et al. Hyperhomocysteinemia: A risk factor for ischemic stroke in children. Circulation 1999;99:2070–2072.
36. Trauner D, Bellugi U, Chase C. Neurologic features of Williams and Down syndromes. Pediatr Neurol 1989;5:166–168.
37. Chan AKC, deVeber G. Prothrombotic disorders and ischemic stroke in children. Semin Pediatr Neurol 2000;7:301–308.
38. Kirkham FJ. Stroke and cerebrovascular disease in childhood. Current Paediatrics 2003;13:350–359.
39. Golumb MR, Dick PT, MacGregor DL, et al. Cranial ultrasonography has a low sensitivity for detecting arterial ischemic stroke in term neonates. J Child Neurol 2003;18:98–103.

40. Ganesan V, Savvy L, Chong WK, et al. Conventional cerebral angiography in children with ischemic stroke. Pediatr Neurol 1999;20:38–42.
41. Dooley JM, Camfield PR, Smith E, et al. Topiramate in intractable childhood onset epilepsy—a cautionary note. Can J Neurol Sci 1999;26:271–273.
42. Goldberg JF, Burdick KE. Cognitive side effects of anticonvulsants. J Clin Psychiatry 2001;62:27–33.
43. Hirsch E, Schmitz B, Carreno, M. Epilepsy, antiepileptic drugs (AEDs) and cognition. Acta Neurol Scand 2003;180: 23–32.
44. Sulzbacher S, Farwell JR, Temkin N, et al. Late cognitive effects of early treatment with phenobarbital. Clin Pediatr 1999;38: 387–94.
45. Ashkenazi A, Silberstein SD. The evolving management of migraine. Curr Opin Neurol 2003;16:341–345.
46. Preter M, Tzourio PM, Ameri A, et al. Long-term prognosis in cerebral venous thrombosis: Follow-up of 77 patients. Stroke 1996;27:243–246
47. de Bruijn SFTM, Budde M, Teunisse S, et al. Long-term outcome of cognition and functional health after cerebral venous sinus thrombosis. Neurology 2000;54:1687–1689.
48. deVeber G, Andrew M, Adams M, et al. Treatment of pediatric sinovenous thrombosis with low molecular weight heparin. Ann Neurol 1995;38:S32
49. deVeber GA, MacGregor D, Curtis R, et al. Neurologic outcome in survivors of childhood arterial ischemic stroke and Sinovenous thrombosis. J Child Neurol 2000;15:316–324.
50. Delsing BJP, Catsman-Berrevoets CE, Appel IM. Early prognostic indicators of outcome of ischemic childhood stroke. Pediatr Neurol 2001;24:283–289.
51. Anderson AL. The effect of laterality localization on focal brain lesions on the Wechsler-Bellevue subtests. J Clin Psychol 1951;7:149–153.
52. Bornstein RA, Matarazzo JD. Wechsler Verbal IQ versus Performance IQ differences in cerebral dysfunction: A literature review with emphasis on sex differences. J Clin Neuropsychol 1982;4: 319–334.
53. Warrington EK, James M, Maciejewski C. The WAIS as a lateralizing and localizing diagnostic instrument: A study of 656 patients with unilateral cerebral lesions. Neuropsychologia 1986; 24:223–239.
54. Vargha-Khadem F, Isaacs E, Muter V. A review of cognitive outcome after unilateral lesions sustained during childhood. J Child Neurol 1994;9:67–73.
55. Staudt M, Grodd W, Niemann G, et al. Early left periventricular brain lesions induce right hemispheric organization of speech. Neurology 2001;57:122–125.
56. Ballantyne AO, Scarvie KM, Trauner DA. Verbal and performance IQ patterns in children after perinatal stroke. Dev Neuropsychol 1994;10:39–50.
57. Bates E, Vicari S, Trauner D. Neural mediation of language development: Perspectives from lesion studies of infants and children. In: Tager-Flausberg H, ed. Neurodevelopmental Disorders. Cambridge, MA: The MIT Press, 1999:533–582.
58. Hetherington CR, Tuff L, Anderson PE, et al. (in press). Short-term intellectual outcome after arterial ischemic stroke and sinovenous thrombosis in childhood and infancy.
59. Hogan AM, Kirkham FJ, Isaacs EB. Intelligence after stroke in childhood: Review of the literature and suggestions for future research. J Child Neurol 2000;15:325–332.
60. Muter V, Taylor S, Vargha-Khadem F. A longitudinal study of early intellectual development in hemiplegic children. Neuropsychologia 1997;35:289–298.
61. Vargha-Khadem F, Isaacs E, Van der Werf S, et al. Development of intelligence and memory in children with hemiplegic cerebral palsy: The deleterious consequences of early seizures. Brain 1992;115:315–329.
62. Feldman H, Holland A, Kemp S, et al. Language development after unilateral brain injury. Brain Lang 1992;42:89–102.
63. Chapman SB, Max JE, Gamino JF, et al. Discourse plasticity in children after stroke: Age at injury and lesion effects. Pediatr Neurol 2003;29:34–41.
64. Brookshire B, Chapman SB, Song J, et al. Cognitive and linguistic correlates of children's discourse after closed head

injury: A three year follow-up. J Int Neuropsychol Soc 2000;6: 741–751.
65. Chapman SB, Culhane KA, Levin HS, et al. Narrative discourse after closed head injury in children and adolescents. Brain Lang 1992;43:42–65.
66. Chapman SB, Levin HS, Wanek A, et al. Discourse after closed head injury in young children. Brain Lang 1998;78:1–16.
67. Ulatowska HK, Allard L, Chapman SB. Narrative and procedural discourse in aphasia. In: Joanette Y, Brownell HH, eds. Discourse Ability and Brain Damage. New York, NY: Springer-Verlag, 1990: 180–198.
68. Weintraub S, Mesulam M-M: Developmental learning disabilities of the right hemisphere: Emotional, interpersonal, and cognitive components. Arch Neurol 1983;40:463–468.
69. Rourke BP, Fisk JL, Strang JD. Neuropsychological Assessment of Children: A Treatment-Oriented Approach. New York, NY: Guilford Press, 1986.
70. Tranel D, Hall LE, Olson S, et al. Evidence for a right-hemisphere developmental learning disability. Dev Neuropsychol 1987;3: 113–117.
71. Voeller KKS: Right-hemisphere deficit syndrome in children. Am J Psychiat 1986;143:1004–1009.
72. Voeller KKS: Clinical neurologic aspects of the right-hemisphere deficit syndrome. J Child Neurol 1995;10:S16–S22.
73. Johnson DJ, Myklebust HR. Learning Disabilities. New York, NY: Grune & Stratton, 1971.
74. Voeller KKS, Hanson JA, Wendt RN: Facial affect recognition in children: A comparison of the performance of children with right and left hemisphere lesions. Neurology 1988;38:1744–1748.
75. Nass R, Koch D: Temperament differences in toddlers with early unilateral right- and left-brain damage. Dev Neuropsychol 1987;3:93–99.
76. Trauner DA, Panyard-Davis JL, Ballantyne AO. Behavioral differences in school age children after perinatal stroke. Assessment 1996;3:265–276.
77. Trauner DA, Nass R, Ballantyne A. Behavioural profiles of children and adolescents after pre- or perinatal unilateral brain damage. Brain 2001;124:995–1002.
78. Achenbach TM. Manual for the child behavior checklist 4–18 years and 1991 profile. Burlington: Department of Psychiatry, University of Vermont, 1991.
79. Heilman KM, Bowers D, Valenstein E. Emotional disorders associated with neurological diseases. In: Heilman KM, Valenstein E, eds. Clinical Neuropsychology, 3rd Ed. New York, NY: Oxford University Press, 1993:461–497.
80. Mesulam MM. Frontal cortex and behavior. Ann Neurol 1986; 19:320–325.
81. Stuss DT, Benson DF. Neuropsychological studies of the frontal lobes. Psychol Bull 1984;95:3–28.
82. Nelson LD, Cicchetti D, Satz P, et al. Emotional sequelae of stroke: A longitudinal perspective. J Clin Exp Neuropsychol 1994;16:796–806.
83. Robinson RG, Kubos KL, Starr LB, et al. Mood disorders in stroke patients. Brain 1984;107:81–93.
84. Robinson RG, Lipsey JR, Rao K, et al. Two-year longitudinal study of post-stroke mood disorders: Comparison of acute-onset with delayed-onset depression. Am J Psychiatry 1986;146:1238–1244.
85. Ross ED, Rush AJ. Diagnosis and neuroanatomical correlates of depression in brain-damaged patients. Arch Gen Psychiatry 1981;38:1344–1354.
86. Borod J. Interhemispheric and intrahemispheric control of emotion: A focus on unilateral brain damage. J Consult Clin Psychol 1992;60:339–348.
87. Ross ED. Nonverbal aspects of language. Neurol Clin 1993;11: 9–23.
88. Gainotti G. Emotional behavior and hemispheric side of the lesion. Cortex 1972;8:41–55.
89. Robinson RG, Starkstein SE. Current research in affective disorders following stroke. J Neuropsychiatry Clin Neurosci 1990;2:1–14.
90. Desmond DW, Remien RH, Moroney JT, et al. Ischemic stroke and depression. J Int Neuropsychol Soc 2003;9:429–439.
91. Dennis M, O'Rourke S, Lewis S, et al. Emotional outcomes after stroke: Factors associated with poor outcome. J Neurol Neurosurg Psychiatry 2000;68:47–52.

92. Kim JS, Choi S, Kwan SU, et al. Inability to control anger or aggression after stroke. Neurology 2002;58:1106–1108.
93. Paradiso S, Robinson RG, Arndt S. Self-reported aggressive behavior in patients with stroke. J Nerv Ment Dis 1996;184: 746–753.
94. Reynolds CR, Kamphaus RW. *Behavioral Assessment System for Children*. Circle Pines, MN: American Guidance Service, 1992.
95. Anderson PE, Newton S, Fuijkschot E, et al. Parent reported change in aggression and expression of anger after childhood stroke: A pilot study. J Int Neuropsychol Soc 2003;9:140.
96. Kwak CH, Jankovic J. Tourettism and dystonia after subcortical stroke. Mov Disord 2002;4:821–825.
97. Max JE, Mathews K, Lansing AE, et al. Psychiatric disorders after childhood stroke. J Am Acad Child AdolescPsychiatry 2002;41: 555–562.
98. Max JE, Fox PT, Lancaster JL, et al. Putamen lesions and the development of attention-deficit/hyperactivity symptomatology. J Am Acad Child Adolesc Psychiatry 2002;41:563–571.
99. Teicher MH, Anderson CM, Polcari A, et al. Functional deficits in basal ganglia of children with attention-deficit/hyperactivity disorder shown with functional magnetic imaging relaxometry. Nat Med 2000;6:470–473.
100. Vaidya CJ, Austin G, Kirkorian G, et al. Selective effects of methylphenidate in attention deficit hyperactivity disorder: A functional magnetic resonance study. Proc Natl Acad Sci USA 1998;95:14494–14499.
101. Max JE, Mathews K, Manes FF, et al. Attention deficit hyperactivity disorder and neurocognitive correlates after childhood stroke. J Int Neuropsych Soc 2003;9:815–829.
102. Hebb DO. The effects of early experience on problem solving at maturity. Am Psychol. 1947;2:737–745.
Hebb DO. *The Organization of Behaviour*. New York, NY: McGraw-Hill, 1949.
103. Schnieder GE. Is it really better to have your brain lesion early? A revision of the "Kennard Principle." Neuropsychologia 1979;17: 557–583.
104. Baron IS, Fennell EB, Voeller KKS. *Pediatric Neuropsychology in the Medical Setting*. New York, NY: Oxford University Press, 1995.
105. Bernstein JH. Developmental neuropsychological assessment. In: Yeates KO, Ris MD, Taylor HG, eds. *Pediatric Neuropsychology: Research, Theory and Practice*. New York, NY: Guilford Press, 2000.
106. Rourke BP, Fisk JL, Strang JD. *Neuropsychological Assessment of Children: A Treatment-oriented Approach*. New York, NY: Guilford Press, 1986.
107. Nowicki S, Duke MP. *Helping the Child Who Doesn't Fit In*. Atlanta, GA: Peachtree, 1992.
108. Duke MP, Martin EA, Nowicki S. *Teaching Your Child the Language of Social Success*. Atlanta, GA: Peachtree, 1996.
109. Nowicki S. Duke MP, *Will I Ever Fit In? The Breakthrough Program for Conquering Adult Dyssemia*. New York: Free Press, 2002.
110. Roach ES, Riela AR. *Pediatric Cerebrovascular Disorders*, 2nd Ed. Armonk, NY: Futura, 1995.

Neuropsychiatric Aspects of Blindness and Severe Visual Impairment, and Deafness and Severe Hearing Loss in Children

20

Bryan H. King, MD   *Peter C. Hauser, PhD*   *Peter K. Isquith, PhD*

DEFINITION OF BLINDNESS/SEVERE VISUAL IMPAIRMENT

The population of children with blindness or severe visual impairment is a heterogeneous one. Visual impairment is measured on a continuum, and there is therefore no universally accepted criterion for defining "blindness." Consequently, in many parts of the world, definitions fall to those applied for legal purposes. In the United States, the first of these definitions was that of "economic blindness" (Schloss 1963; Jan, Freeman and Scott 1977). This definition has since been adopted by most of the Western cultures and defines blindness as the visual acuity in the best eye with correction of less than 20/200 or a defect in the visual field so that the widest visual diameter is less than 20 degrees. This legal definition of blindness was not developed for children but rather for determining the disability status of adults and thus there are distinct disadvantages in the assessment of youngsters. Moreover, until the age of 3 or 4 years, a child may satisfy criteria for legal blindness but nonetheless be quite able to function in society. Indeed even among children whose visual acuity satisfies criteria for legal blindness there remains extreme heterogeneity; congenitally blind children may be grouped together with those who retain some perception of light as well as children with some intact vision (Jan et al. 1977). Currently, the International Classification of Diseases (World Health Organization 1992) designates six categories to describe significant visual impairment with category 1 corresponding to the best possible corrected visual acuity being between 20/70 and 20/200; category 2 is between 20/200 and 20/400; category 3 is between 20/400 and 20/1200, which corresponds to finger counting at 1 meter; category 4, is between finger counting at 1 meter and mere light perception, and category 5, is "no light perception." A sixth category is reserved for "unspecified or undetermined degrees of visual impairment". Persons in categories 1 and 2 are also referred to as having "low-vision" and those in categories 3, 4, and 5 are referred to as having "blindness." Regarding visual field defects, if the field is no greater than 10 degrees but greater than 5 degrees around central fixation, individuals are placed in category 3. Persons with a field no greater than 5 degrees around central fixation are placed in category 4 even if their acuity is not impaired.

Incidence and Prevalence of Blindness in Children and Adolescents

In their landmark studies, Jan and colleagues (Jan, et al. 1977) surveyed the entire population of children born in British Columbia in the cohort 1944 through 1973 utilizing a questionnaire to record the etiology, sight, and type of lesion and associated handicaps. The legal definition of blindness was used and cortical blindness was excluded because of the commonly associated profound mental retardation in that context and the attendant difficulty in assessing visual function in those individuals. Four hundred fifty-four children were included in the study, the majority of whom, 382, had a congenital etiology for their blindness while the remaining 72 acquired their visual impairment in childhood. Of the total, one third were characterized as having no sight or light perception only and the remainder had some useful vision with the percentages being similar when the subgroups with congenital versus acquired blindness were compared. While the male–female ratio was essentially 1:1 in children with the congenital etiologies for their blindness, there was a relative preponderance of males among those with acquired visual impairment (60%). Among the children with visual impairment, the children with congenital etiologies were typically referred at less than 1 year of age and for those referred in the second year of age, the vast majority had suspected visual impairment at less than 1 year. Overall, looking at the annual incidence of congenital blindness in British Columbia during the 30-year study period, the investigators noted a figure of between one and eight per 10,000 population. The incidence rates increased during the late 1940s and early 1950s secondary to retrolental fibroplasia, prior to its identification as a side effect of exposure to high oxygen saturation in premature infants. The authors further observed that while the incidence generally stabilized over the latter part of their study to about two per 10,000 live births, the prevalence of blindness was clearly increasing, perhaps secondary to advances in pediatric care enabling more children with blindness to survive. More recent epidemiological studies have been reported from other groups of investigators.

Frick and Foster (2003) applied epidemiologic modeling to World Health Organization estimates for blindness and projected that there will be 2 million blind children (0 to 14-year olds) in 2010 and 2020. Causes of blindness in childhood, as for any disability, may be divided into genetic factors and those that operate in the neonatal, perinatal, or early childhood period. Molecular genetic aspects of blindness are reviewed in Black and Craig (1994); an example of a prenatal cause of blindness is an intrauterine infection like rubella. Retinopathy of prematurity would represent an early acquired cause, and vitamin A deficiency would contribute to blindness later in childhood. The differences in prevalence of blindness in children, which range from 0.3 per thousand population in developed countries, to 0.9 to 1.1 in developing countries, is largely accounted for by an increase in acquired (and preventable) causes of blindness including xerophthalmia, or vitamin A deficiency, in the context of protein malnutrition or malabsorption due to diarrhea. Together with xerophthalmia, trachoma, a chronic infection of the conjunctiva and cornea, and onchocerciasis, an infection due to a roundworm transmitted by black fly bites, are recognized as the main causes of blindness in developing countries (Vader 1992). Measles is the single leading cause of blindness among children in low-income countries and accounts for up to 60,000 cases per year (Semba and Bloem 2004). Frick and Foster (2003) estimate that the projected number of blind children in the world could be cut in half with implementation of the VISION 2020 initiative of the World Health Organization and the International Agency for the Prevention of Blindness, which specifically targets cataract, trachoma, onchocerciasis, vitamin A deficiency, and refractive errors. The application of traditional eye remedies with resultant corneal scarring and neonatal bacterial infections are also significant contributors to blindness in Africa and many parts of Asia (WHO 1992; Gilbert et al. 1995; Alemayehu et al. 1995).

Development of the Primate Visual System

The visual system in the primate is composed of the retina, optic nerves, optic chiasm, optic tracts, lateral geniculate nuclei, geniculostriate radiations, striate cortex (area 17), visual association cortex, and related interhemispheric connections (areas 18 to 21). All together, over one million axons comprise the optic nerve, an order of magnitude greater than comparable afferent neurons in the aural system (Glaser and Sadun 1990).

The first evidence of eye development in humans occurs at approximately the third week of gestation when the primordial optic bulbs extend from the prosencephalon. The "torus opticus" is the primitive optic chiasm and appears as a thickening between optic bulbs. Cup-shaped evaginations induce lens growth on contact with overlying surface ectoderm. By approximately 5 weeks, retinal development has begun, and cells in the retinal ganglion differentiate to send optic nerve fibers through the optic stalk into the chiasm, which is reached 2 weeks later. By seven weeks, a full complement of axons is contained in the optic nerve, and the optic disc and scleral openings are well defined (Glaser and Sadun 1990).

Neural connections in the visual system begin diffusely as the axons from the retinal ganglion cells terminate in the lateral geniculate nucleus (LGN) and form synapses throughout this structure. Through selective retraction and more directed growth, refinement of the network is achieved so that within the lateral geniculate nucleus, the retinotopic organization of the optic tract is maintained in vertical columns of cells called "projection lines," which have been described in all mammals studied to date. This refinement of connections is dependent upon signaling emanating from retinal ganglion cells, and recent studies reveal that synchronous bursts of action potentials from these cells can be detected long before photoreceptors have matured (Meister et al. 1991; Masland 1977; Galli and Maffei 1988).

Six distinct cellular laminae can be identified within the LGN. Ventrally, layers one and two receive contralateral and ipsilateral retinal projections, respectively, and are termed "magnocellular" because of their relatively larger neuron size. The remaining layers are termed "parvocellular." Functional studies of retinal ganglion cells which project to the magnocellular or parvocellular LGN ("M" or "P" pathways, respectively) reveal that the former are cells that detect motion, direction, speed, coarse stereopsis (depth perception), and pursuit (Tychsen 1994). The latter cells respond to color, shape, fine acuity, and fine stereopsis. Thus M-retinal ganglion cells transmit the "where" of visual stimuli, and P ganglion cells transmit the "what" (Tychsen 1994). From the LGN, magnocellular laminae project to area 4B of the striate cortex and then primarily to parietooccipital association cortex. Parvocellular laminae project to area 4A of the striate cortex, and then primarily to temporooccipital association cortex. These distinct occipitoparietal and occipitotemporal visual pathways are also described as the dorsal and ventral stream, respectively.

The maturation of M and P projections to the striate and extrastriate cortices occurs significantly after birth and this maturation is dependent upon visual stimulation. In their landmark studies, Hubel and Weisel (Wiesel and Hubel 1963, 1965) demonstrated that periods of critical sensitivity exist in the developing visual system during which the deprivation of adequate stimulation will prevent the progression toward normal adult characteristics. In their early work, kittens and adult cats were subjected to unilateral eye closure for varying durations. Susceptibility to the effects of eye closure, as determined by the number of cells in the striate cortex responding to visual stimulation from the previously closed eye, peaked over a period of 2 weeks. Eye closure for as little as 6 days during this interval effectively reduced the proportion of cells the eye could influence by over 90%. In the adult, eye closure for over 1 year produced no detectable effects (Hubel and Wiesel 1970). The finding of sensitive periods of development has been extended to the barn owl (Knudsen and Knudsen 1990), mouse (Gordon and Stryker 1996), rat (Stafford 1984), and nonhuman primates (Sloper 1993). In humans, stimulation in advance of a critical period does not hasten or enhance vision. In their comparative study of preterm infants and those delivered at term, van Hof-van Duin and colleagues (1992) found that visual experience before the expected term date had no measurable effect upon the development of visual acuity or in terms of accelerating the development of peripheral vision.

It has also become clear that multiple, partially overlapping sensitive periods exist for various functions of the primate visual system (Harwerth et al. 1986). The critical period for the rod system to respond to different light wavelengths differs from that for cone information processing, and different sensitive periods also exist for both spatial vision and for binocular vision (Harwerth et al.).

When sensory input from a given modality is disrupted during a critical period, significant changes in the distribution of the cortical map may occur. Rauschecker and colleagues (1993, 1994) have shown that auditory spatial discrimination is enhanced in cats deprived of visual stimulation associated with an enlargement of the cortical representation for auditory processing. Similar findings have been revealed in neuroimaging and electrophysiological studies in humans which demonstrate recruitment of occipital cortex for tactile manipulation and even tactile imagery, for example, imagining the "feel" of textures on the fingertips in early blind subjects, or even simply performing a Braille reading task (Theoret et al. 2004). Occipital recruitment has also been demonstrated for auditory tasks in subjects with congenital blindness.

Recently, Theoret and colleagues (2004) reviewed evidence to support the occurrence of neurophysiological changes that occur with blindness. Studies demonstrating better sound localization abilities for blind subjects in comparison to sighted controls not only demonstrate that vision is not critical to placing the origin of sounds in three-dimensional space, but also support the longstanding notion that compensatory enhancement of audition occurs in blindness. Moreover, the same compensatory advantage is evident in studies of tactile discrimination in blind and control subjects, and within the blind population, sensory thresholds are lower for the Braille-reading finger than for other fingers in a gratings orientation task (the ability to detect the direction of grooves cut into a metal surface).

Kauffman and colleagues (2002) conducted an elegant study in which sighted subjects were compared to blindfolded subjects with respect to the speed with which they learned to recognize Braille characters. Interestingly, blindfolding conferred a significant advantage (as measured by error rate of character recognition), after just 5 days. Thus, some plastic changes in the brain in response to sensory deprivation appear to occur quickly, and not to be exclusively confined to specific critical developmental windows. On the other hand, Sadato and colleagues (2002), have observed differences in activation of primary visual cortex with a tactile discrimination task in blind subjects as a function of the timing of their loss of sight (before or after 16 years of age). Consequently, they conclude that the first 16 years of life may be a critical period for cross-modal plasticity in primary visual cortex (e.g., from processing visual stimuli to processing tactile stimuli).

In human infants, the development of M-pathway visual functions precedes that for those mediated by the P-pathway. The former can be detected by motion-evoked visual evoked potential studies, as well as by examining optokinetic nystagmus pursuit and vergence eye movements and large disparity stereoscopic vision, all of which are evident at 3 to 5 months of age (Tychsen 1991). P-neurons in the lateral geniculate nucleus do not achieve adult-like dendritic morphology until 8 or 9 months (de Courten et al. 1982). The refinement of spatial contrast and color sensitivity which occur after 1 year of age are attributed to the ongoing development of P-neuron–mediated vision. Milestones in the development of vision are summarized in Table 20.1, where it can be seen that interrelationships between vision, motor development, and praxis become particularly apparent in later childhood.

The clinical principle that derives from the observations above is that early intervention is essential to the ultimate correction of visual disturbance. Surgery for congenital cataracts is now performed within days of diagnosis with optical correction and occlusion therapies instituted shortly thereafter, and outcomes from this aggressive approach have been characterized as "astounding" (Tyschen 1994). Studies with regard to the timing of intervention for strabismus or esotropia are also clear in suggesting that intervention after two years of age is significantly less successful in restoring binocularity in comparison to early treatment (6 to 18 months) (Sarniguet-Badoche 1984; Rethy and Rethy-Gal 1984; Ing 1984). Based upon these studies, one might also conclude that a role exists for early and frequent exposure to visual stimuli among children with severe visual impairment. Brodsky, Baker, and Hamed (1996) observe that visual stimulation as a therapeutic modality is somewhat controversial in terms of its usefulness owing to the largely anecdotal nature of reported outcomes. Such "visual stimulation therapy" follows from the premise that vision is in some respects a learned skill, and, either by recruiting neurons, increasing synaptic density or by some other means, such stimulation may help a child to maximize his or her rudimentary sight (Sonksen et al. 1991). Preliminary but certainly compelling results of tachistoscopic visual stimulation (presenting flashes of light repetitively for 1 to 2 hours daily for 6 months) in three adult patients with partial cortical blindness were reported by Pleger and colleagues (2003). Color and pattern recognition improved significantly and in a clinically meaningful way in two of the subjects, all of whom had sustained their occipital injuries fully two years prior to this therapeutic intervention; an interval that argues strongly against mere spontaneous recovery.

Circadian Rhythms

A number of studies have examined the effect of blindness on circadian rhythms, but few have involved children. Many groups have demonstrated that circadian rhythms including temperature, cortisol, melatonin, and sleep are free-running in blind individuals (Sack et al. 1992, Miles and Wilson 1977, Nakagawa et al. 1992). Since the free-running diurnal cycle approximates 25 hours, persons with sleep-wake cycle disorders will have periods in which they awaken during the night and sleep during daytime hours. Okawa and colleagues (1987) studied four congenitally blind children and observed free-running sleep-wake cycles in three and an irregular sleep-wake rhythm in the fourth child. Despite attempts to entrain the sleep-wake cycles in these patients to a 24-hour rhythm by the use of forced awakening, playing musical instruments, and tactile stimulation, only two of the children could maintain such a rhythm. The authors concluded that concurrent severe mental retardation in these children diluted the effectiveness of environmental manipulation to serve as a synchronizer. Nevertheless, exposure to bright light may have an effect on neuroendocrine function and mood even in the context of blindness. Czeisler and colleagues (1995) measured melatonin suppression by bright light in 11 blind patients without light perception in comparison to sighted controls. All of the subjects were blind in both eyes due to retinal pathology, congenital glaucoma, or acquired eye injury. In three of the 11 blind subjects, melatonin secretion was reduced by nearly 70% following light exposure just as for control subjects. Since these subjects were also unique in that they did not report periodic insomnia, the authors concluded that the visual subsystem by which melatonin secretion is suppressed may be functionally intact in some blind subjects despite the absence of conscious light perception. Effects of light exposure in blind subjects were also documented by Partonen and associates (1995), who observed that subjective sleepiness was reduced, and mood improved, in both controls and blind subjects after exposure to 3300 lux of bright light for 2 weeks. Differences did emerge, however, between sighted controls and blind subjects with respect to the body temperature response to light exposure.

There is a growing body of literature examining the effects of melatonin for sleep disturbance in persons with blindness. A recent double-masked, randomized trial of placebo, a physiological (0.14 mg) dose, and a pharmacological dose (2.2 mg) in a 7-year-old child with blindness associated with birth asphyxia and septo-optic dysplasia was noteworthy for significant improvement on the high dose of melatonin only (Cavallo et al. 2002).

Behavioral and Developmental Consequences of Blindness

The etiology and the timing of blindness or severe visual impairment is of tremendous importance in terms of predicting its developmental consequences, but few studies

TABLE 20.1
MILESTONES IN DEVELOPMENT OF SIGHT

Age	Visual Responses and Capabilities
30–34 wk gestation	Pupillary light reaction present, lid closure in response to bright light; vestibular eye rotations well developed.
0–1 mos	Attends to light and forms, limited fixation ability (visual acuity approx. 20/400), can discriminate color red from achromatic background; optokinetic nystagmus well developed, horizontal gaze.
	Beginning oculomotor coordination.
	Limited imitation of facial expression (tongue protrusion; open mouth).
1–2 mos	Can follow moving objects and light, attend to novelty and complex patterns, stare at faces.
	Beginning binocular coordination.
2–3 mos	Eyes can fixate, converge, and focus.
	Discriminate from among faces.
	Color discrimination includes blue, green, yellow, orange, red.
	Conjugate vertical gaze.
3–4 mos	Smoother eye movements and improved acuity.
	Can manipulate and examine objects.
	Blink response to visual threat.
4–5 mos	May shift focus from objects to body parts, attempt to reach for and approach objects. Explores the environment visually, tracks objects across entire field of vision.
	Development of binocularity (fusion and stereopsis).
	Accommodation well developed, differentiation of fovea completed.
5–6 mos	Can reach and grasp objects demonstrating eye-hand coordination.
6–7 mos	Visual attention can shift from object to object, can reach for and retrieve dropped objects.
	Eye movements become more fluid.
	Stereoacuity at near adult level; iris stromal pigment well developed.
7–8 mos	Can manipulate objects and look at results.
	Can follow movements.
9–10 mos	Excellent visual acuity, smooth accommodation.
	Can hunt for hidden objects around corners and play looking games.
11–18 mos	Ongoing refinement of optical skills and sharpening of acuity. Can put objects together.
	Cornea 95% of adult diameter.
1½–2 yrs	Can match objects, point to objects in a book, imitate strokes and actions with writing instrument.
2–2½ yrs	Can inspect objects at distance, imitate movements of others, match colors and like forms. Visual memory span is increased. Objects can be ordered by color.
	Snellen letter acuity at adult level.
2½–3 yrs	Can match geometric forms, draw crude circles, insert objects in proper holes and assemble two puzzle pieces.
	Eyeball 95% of adult diameter.
3–4 yrs	Can match identically shaped objects by size.
	Demonstrates good depth perception.
	Discriminates line lengths, can copy an X, discriminate most basic forms.
4–5 yrs	Eye-hand coordination is further refined.
	Can color, cut and paste, draw a square, and perceive detail in objects and pictures.
5–6 yrs	Can perceive relationships in pictures, abstract figures and symbols.
	Can copy symbols and match letters and words.
6–7 yrs	Can identify and reproduce abstract symbols.
	Perceive the constancy of letter and word styles.
	Associate words with pictures and read words on sight.

Sources: Brandt, 1994; Gonzales and Dweck, 1994; Adams et al., 1994; Birch and Petrig, 1996; Thorn et al., 1994; Bloch and Carchon, 1992; van Hof-van Duin et al., 1992; Robinson and Fielder, 1992; Meltzoff and Moore, 1983; Valenza et al., 1996; Serrano et al., 1992.

have looked specifically at developmental issues in children with a homogeneous etiology for their visual impairment.

Motor Development

In terms of its effect on behavior and early development, the absence of sight exerts profound influences on motor and adaptive function. In their early studies of preschool-

ers, Nesker and colleagues (Nesker Simmons, & Davidson 1985) were overwhelmed by the stark contrast of the motor activity of blind children in comparison to children with sight in a nursery setting. The nursery was described as extraordinarily quiet and sterile-looking, with everything remaining in its place even after the children had left. On balance, the blind children were characterized as less mobile, less verbal, and less socially aware than their 2- and

3-year-old sighted counterparts. Moreover, the investigators were also impressed with the degree of intervention required on the part of mothers or staff to encourage blind children to participate in activities other than stereotyped rocking, eye rubbing, or meaningless repetitive speech. These observations were interpreted to underscore the particularly important role that a blind child's care providers and the surrounding environment must play in facilitating developmental progress. Gross motor function appears to be uniformly delayed in blind children (Davidson 1983; Levtzion-Korach et al. 2000). The greatest delays are evident early, including precrawling, sitting, pulling to standing, and walking. Nearly all blind children reviewed by Davidson (1983) had substantial lags in the onset of walking that did not appear until a median age of 20 months. Levtzion-Korach and colleagues (2000) suggest that environmental enrichment may be helpful in hastening motor development, but caution that motor delays should be expected in children with blindness.

Social Development and Adaptive Function

In part, stereotyped and other self-stimulatory or maladaptive behaviors may be more frequently observed in visually impaired children because of the differences observed in how they bond to caregivers and form social attachments. For example, blind infants smiled at a caregiver's face only inconsistently, even at the age of 12 months and reacted to separation between 11 and 20 months of age. This represents a delay of approximately 6 months compared to their sighted peers (Davidson 1983). Warren (1994) notes that development of attachment is dependent not only upon the visually impaired child's construct of parents as distinguished from other persons, but also the parents' responsiveness to a child having a disability. In combination with other factors, such as extended hospitalization as a result of prematurity, effects upon the existing family structure, or financial strains, parents may be faced with numerous unanticipated difficulties in bonding with their disabled child. Compounding these stresses is the emotional readjustment associated with the "imperfection" of their infant. Observation of mother–infant interactions indicates that blind children receive less positive and more negative vocalization and affect from their mothers than sighted controls (Rogers and Puchalski 1984; Warren 1994).

Generally, the social maturity scores of children with visual impairments are lower than their age-matched sighted peers (Warren 1994). In a study comparing the social skills of visually impaired adolescents to sighted peers through the use of role plays, interviews, and rating scales, Van Hasselt, Hersen, and Kazdin (1985) found that, as a group, adolescents with visual impairment asked fewer open-ended questions, spoke for longer durations in social interactions, had greater speech disturbances, and experienced greater difficulty being assertive. Cole, Jenkins, and Shott

(1989) found that congenitally blind children were just as able to mask disappointment as their sighted peers. They had a greater tendency to make neutral comments or change the topic, and paid less attention to the quality of their facial expressions or awareness that others might "read" their expressions. Thus, some specific differences in social behavior are likely a product of the loss of visual information. Unfortunately, social development and adjustment have been inconsistently assessed in young blind children, despite evidence that problems presenting later are rooted during these formative years. Child and parent interviews, observations in naturalistic settings (home, school), and role play tests should all be considered for any visually impaired child who evidences deficits in social functioning.

Language Development

Preisler (1993) examined the development of communication in a cohort of blind children in comparison to children with deafness. She found that the development of communication was delayed in the blind infants and concluded that visual stimulation in infancy probably plays a more critical role in comparison to auditory stimulation in terms of its promotion of mother–infant interactions (Preisler 1995). Preisler further observed that in the period of early infancy (up to age 18 months) blind children did not use gestures like pointing or showing, gestures that would facilitate for caregivers the ability to understand preference and interest. The absence of these eye, finger, or hand-pointing gestures in blind infants challenges the ability for parents to elaborate on the expressed interests of their children by referring to mutually discernible external events. Although blind children may "point" with their head or upper torso in response to sounds, such gestures may frequently be lost or not understood by parents, resulting in the recommendation for specific education of caregivers with the use of video (Preisler and Palmer 1989; Preisler 1990). McConachie and Moore (1994) found delays in early language development in children with severe visual impairments. The ages at which children with severe visual impairment or blindness spoke their first word was at 15 and 18 months, respectively, with the first ten words being spoken at approximately 20 months of age for both groups. The latter compares to a 10-word vocabulary emerging at 15 months in a control group of sighted children. These authors also noted that the content of blind children's initial vocabulary differs subtly in quality in comparison to sighted children. There is reported to be a relative increase in the use of verbs, particularly to those referring to the children's own actions as well as an increased use of specific names instead of generalized labels for classes of objects or functions. In his review of the development of language in blind children, Hodapp (1998) elaborates on this point illustrating that "doggie," for example, may refer only to the blind child's pet, and not to dogs in general. While these observed differences in language could logically follow from the unique ways in which blind children must experience the world (Bigelow 1987), there may also be differences in cognitive abilities which may further influence the acquisition of language. Although it was once believed that blindness predisposed to the late acquisition of personal pronouns and other personal reference terms as well as frequent pronominal reversal, recent work has called this notion into question (Perez-Pereira 1999).

Cognitive Development

While blind children may progress through Piagetian stages of development in the same sequence as do sighted children, their development appears to be relatively slowed in comparison to sighted children particularly insofar as tasks involving classification and conservation are concerned (Hodapp 1998). Between 3 and 15% of the blind population are believed to function at or below the range of mild mental retardation, and intellectual disability is particularly common among children with blindness secondary to retinitis of prematurity and deaf-blindness due to rubella (Davidson 1983).

In terms of measuring intellectual functioning however, there are many problems that come with attempting to adapt intelligence quotient (IQ) tests to the population with severe visual impairment. Because of the inability to use subtests that rely on performance, many IQ instruments are simply inappropriate for persons with severe visual impairment. Some investigators have long cautioned against the widespread use of the Wechsler verbal scales to assess visually impaired children (Ammerman et al. 1986; Bauman and Kropf 1979; Margach and Kern 1969), and more recently Warren (1994) notes that use of verbal IQ tests, while common, is inappropriate for testing the intelligence of visually impaired children. In doing so, examiners ignore the existence of certain aspects of intelligence that cannot be captured by purely verbal means. The Perkins-Binet, a modification of the original Stanford-Binet, has items specifically selected for their appropriateness with children with visual impairment. Two versions have been developed: Form N for blind children and Form U for the partially sighted (Ammerman et al. 1986). The need for different versions is highlighted by Hull and Mason (1995), who found that congenitally blind children who had no better than light perception consistently did better on verbal memory tasks than did children with acquired blindness. Finally, some investigators have advocated using a "functional-ecological" or "behavior-analytic" approach as opposed to using test measures that have been insufficiently normed on visually impaired populations, particularly in the assessment of educational and social skills (Downing and Perino 1992, Van Hasselt 1985).

Beelman and Brambring (1998) described a home-based early intervention program for ten children (average age of 12 months) with congenital blindness and their parents that addressed blindness-specific issues like tactile and auditory object perception, and spatial orientation and mobility. Approaches were individualized based on assessment of the children's developmental level. Parents were also offered problem-oriented counseling as well as guidance and training on parent–child interactions like remaining in calling distance, verbal accompaniment of activities performed with the child, intensive body contact with the child, and guiding hands from behind when carrying out exercises or playing games. The intervention team visited families every 2 weeks for an average of 2 years. Results were quite mixed. Children who were born prematurely did not seem to benefit, but others showed significant acceleration of development, particularly with respect to orientation and mobility and cognitive and socioemotional development.

Neuroanatomy of Blindness and Behavior

It is possible to distinguish different behavioral presentations among children blind from damage to the retina, the anterior visual pathways, visual cortex, visual fields, and disorders of oculomotor control (Good and Hoyt 1989). Eye pressing is a behavior associated with retinal disease which is common in blindness (Williams 1969). Jan and colleagues (1983) examined a large cohort of blind children and found that eye pressing occurred exclusively in the context of retinal damage; specifically, Leber congenital amaurosis, retinitis of prematurity, retinal dysplasia, or retinal infections in utero. Children who engage in chronic eye pressing behavior may develop orbital fat atrophy or the orbits may in fact enlarge from the sustained pressure resulting in the appearance of sunken eyes. Jan and colleagues (1983, 1994) suggested that children engage in eye pressing behavior to stimulate visual cortex and took support for this assertion from the observation that children with defects in the visual pathways or with cortical atrophy do not engage in eye pressing. Additional support may be taken from the recent report of electrical stimulation of the retinal surface in patients blind from retinitis pigmentosa, which yielded light perception (a spot of light) localizing to the area stimulated (Humayun et al. 1996).

"Overlooking" behavior is the term given to describe the position a child with macular disease might adopt in lifting the chin up and appearing to look above the object of interest. This behavior occurs in the absence of nystagmus and has been interpreted by Taylor and colleagues (1983) as a compensatory response to the presence of some residual vision in the inferior fields. Some behaviors in blind children have also been linked to diseases of the anterior visual pathways and roving eye movements are one example. Typically these slow drifting movements are present from birth and indicate a lack of central fixation (Good and Hoyt 1989). The slow drifting nature of these movements makes them readily distinguishable from nystagmus, and roving movements and nystagmus do not coexist. Among children with visual impairment from cortical defects specific behaviors that may be observed are influenced in part by the frequently coexisting generalized brain damage and attendant neurologic abnormalities. Children with cortical impairment seem to prefer colors over shapes (Jan et al. 1987), and this preference is taken to derive from the bilateral representation of color vision, that is, color vision would be spared except when a very large cortical lesion is present. Children with visual impairment from cortical pathology also typically turn their heads away from an object when reaching to grab it, seeming to prefer peripheral vision over central. The anterior striate cortex is the cortical area that typically represents the peripheral visual field (Benton et al. 1980) and because it is often spared in cases of even severe cortical visual impairment, this may account for the head-turning by some children with cortical visual defects. "Blindsight" is the term given to explain the observation that cortically impaired children can sometimes ambulate and avoid objects even in the absence of detectable cortical vision (Campion et al. 1983). It is suggested that such blindsight might derive from the presence of an extrageniculostriate visual system, and while its specific function is debated, it has been suggested that such a system could mediate the unconscious awareness of motion in the peripheral field, spatial localization, and visuospatial orientation (Good et al. 1994; Brodsky, Baker, and Hamed, 1996).

Blindness, Stereotypy, and Autism

Stereotyped behavioral traits occur in the majority of children with blindness (Fazzi et al. 1999). Janson (1993) reviewed the link between retinal pathology and abnormal and stereotyped movements in children with blindness secondary to the retinitis of prematurity. Indeed, others have noted that children with congenital blindness are often at risk for behavioral and emotional disturbances including withdrawal, isolation, and even symptoms of autism. One survey of 24 congenitally blind children drawn from special schools found that nearly half of the sample of 3- to 9-year olds met criteria for autism (Brown et al. 1997). Some symptoms of autism in such populations occasionally are referred to as blindisms and include repetitive stereotyped behaviors and echolalia-like imitations as well as pronoun reversal, social withdrawal, and frequent self-stimulatory behaviors. As noted by Good and Hoyt (1989), and more recently by Fazzi and colleagues (1999), eye pressing and finger waving may actually heighten the sensitivity of retinal ganglion cells, appear to offer sensory input, and should not be viewed as inherently pathological. Janson (1993), too, suggests that such behaviors are normative in the blind population. Developmentally, eye rubbing, rocking, swaying, head turning and stereotyped hand gestures usually appear at the end of the first or during the second year of life. In comparison to children with autism, in blind children diagnosed with retinitis of prematurity, general development is frequently delayed and occasionally experienced as deviant. But while blind children may have difficulties in initiating interaction, they may

respond normally when contacted. The lack of functional communication in some children with autism and their stereotyped manipulation of certain objects is not characteristic of children with retinitis of prematurity or blindness from other causes (Sakuma 1975). That said, the incidence of autism in the context of blindness appears to be much greater than that in the general population (Hobson and Bishop 2003), and specific causes, such as retinitis of prematurity and Leber congenital amaurosis, may also be predisposing factors for autism (Rogers and Newhart-Larson, 1989).

The specific topography, rate of occurrence of stereotypy, and even the degree to which it interferes with attention and learning is generally not a good diagnostic indicator to determine whether a visually impaired child also has autism. That said, Hobson and Bishop (2003) studied the relationship between blindness and autism and suggested that the many sources of social impairment that come with blindness, both physical and environmental, may lead to impoverished interpersonal experiences that could predispose to autism. These investigators are nonetheless clear, however, that there are blind children who do not have autism, but who still have marked impairment in interpersonal engagement. Other factors, then, such as (1) echolalic and/or repetitive verbal behavior; (2) significant delays in social development, especially cooperative play and use of symbolism in toy play; (3) excessive need for sameness in activities, routine, or physical environment; (4) extreme tantrum behavior when attempts are made to change routine or redirect while engaged in ritualistic or stereotypic behavior; (5) excessive avoidance of physical contact and/or extreme clinginess with primary caregivers; and (6) unusual posturing or mannerisms are more significant determining criteria in the differential diagnosis of autism than the presence of stereotypic behaviors alone.

Blindness and Maladaptive Behaviors

In addition to stereotyped behaviors noted previously, maladaptive behaviors may occur in the context of blindness. Concurrent mental retardation increases the likelihood for self-injurious behavior, for example, which may be expressed as hand and arm biting; head-banging; hits to the head or body; dropping to the ground; skin picking, scratching, and excessive hand mouthing causing skin breakdown. Blind children are sometimes highly reactive to the sudden presence of others around them and may startle by headbutting or lashing out with their arms or hands (Van Hasselt 1987). Hitting, scratching, and pinching others has also been reported (Vollmer et al. 1992). Such behaviors place those around the child at risk for any number of injuries. Children with visual impairment may also reject objects presented to them by throwing the objects indiscriminately. Other impulsive behaviors may occur; for example, staff and parents working with visually impaired children have reported being struck in the face, nose, or chin as children jerk their heads quickly backward, striking the unprepared. In beginning orientation and mobility training with children and adolescents, especially individuals with concurrent language deficits who may not be able to perceive where others are in space, caregivers face the risk of being struck by a walking cane.

Psychopathology in Blindness

Blindness appears to be a risk factor for the development of behavioral and psychiatric disorders in children and adolescents but studies of psychopathology in blind children are few. Blacher and colleagues (1992), examining the factors that result in out-of-home placement for children with mental retardation, found that blindness alone was not highly contributory. Age (older children were more often placed), degree of retardation, reduced adaptive behavior, and increased maladaptive behaviors were much more significant factors resulting in placement. These data support Williams' (1969) inferences drawn from placements out of home and in hospital among children in England and Wales with severe visual defects, that upwards of 30% probably had some behavioral "maladjustment." Fine (1968, in Williams 1969) also observed similar percentages. Williams (1969) was clear in suggesting that there are no symptoms of psychiatric disorder unique to the child with blindness. Neurotic disorders, conduct disorders, autism, and hyperactivity could all be diagnosed in blind children. Reviewing the diagnoses associated with blind children between 7 and 13 years of age referred for psychiatric consultation (N = 17), Williams recounted nine cases of "free floating anxiety." aggressiveness (N = 8), irritability and distractibility (N = 8), and overactivity (N = 5). Although five of the children were said to exhibit autistic behavior, the diagnosis of autism was made in only one.

In their classic study, Jan and colleagues (1977) examined children and adolescents in British Columbia who met criteria for legal blindness. No exclusions were made in the presence of additional handicapping conditions and while these children were compared with a gender and age matched control group, they were not matched for IQ. The study also predated current diagnostic criteria for mental disorders, but global psychiatric assessments are listed in Table 21.2.

In addition to the previous distribution, 7% of the sample were judged to have abnormalities in thought process as judged by loose associations, another 7% were found to be pathologically preoccupied with certain topics, and 23% of the children were said to lack a sense of humor, being characterized as excessively serious. Nearly one third of the children examined had received some tranquilizing drug (unspecified), and one fifth of the sample continued to receive a psychoactive medication at the time of the study (excluding anticonvulsants) in comparison to 1% of controls. This study was also important in suggesting that the degree of visual impairment tended to impact on the likelihood of psychopathology, with the totally blind experiencing more

TABLE 20.2

PSYCHOPATHOLOGY IN CHILDREN WITH SEVERE VISUAL IMPAIRMENT (N = 86)

Diagnosis	n*	%
Normal	37	43
Mental retardation	16	18.6
Developmental disorder	13	15.1
Adjustment reaction	9	10.5
Personality disorder	7	8.1
Behavior disorder	6	7.0
Organic brain syndrome	5	5.8
Psychosis	3	3.5
Neurotic reaction	3	3.5
Special symptom reaction	2	2.3

Source: Adapted from Jan et al., 1977.
*15 children received two diagnoses.

dysfunction than their partially sighted peers. Ammerman and colleagues (1986) made the important point that some characteristics of blind children identified as pathologic, such as high scores on indices of anxiety, may in fact be appropriate responses to blindness when, for example, the fear in question includes a worry about running into things. Similarly, elevated measures of dependence may also be artifacts of the reality that finds children and young adults with blindness frequently dependent on supports from others in the environment to make their way in the world.

Indeed, because many parents may feel ill-equipped to adapt to the special needs of their visually impaired infants, they may unintentionally foster social dependence and inhibit haptic exploratory search in their children as they develop. Clinicians working with blind children should anticipate parents having difficulty leaving their child alone for the testing session, wanting to hold their child's hand during an interview, and having difficulty not answering for their child. While these protective behaviors are by no means universal, they underscore the importance of early intervention programs to teach parents how to permit their children to develop competence and independence.

Assessing the Need for Treatment

Treatment of the child with blindness should always follow from a comprehensive evaluation. In the context of developmental disabilities, and blindness in particular, a multidisciplinary approach is essential. Medical problems may present as behavioral difficulties, and the latter may occur as side effects of medical treatment. It does little good to bring a visually impaired, developmentally delayed child to a psychiatrist's or internist's office for medication evaluation, unless the purpose of the visit is to observe how the child reacts in novel, unfamiliar environments or to examine the child for particular medication side effects. A treating clinician will receive far more useful data by arranging for involved persons to collect observational data on selected target symptoms. To this end, teachers and parents, occupational therapists, nurses, social workers, psychologists, pediatricians, ophthalmologists, and child psychiatrists best function as a team in their approach to the child with blindness.

In determining whether children with visual impairments exhibit behavior that requires the attention and intervention of mental health professionals, it is necessary to determine how the observed symptoms interfere with the child's development or ability to achieve greater independence. Clinicians may wish to ask themselves the questions summarized in Table 21.3 regarding a presenting symptom.

If the behavior does appear to meet criteria for intervention, several factors must be considered initially: Is the behavior a symptom that may be treated medically? In children lacking effective language skills, self-injury may reflect their underlying physical discomfort, such as an ear infection. Clinicians should look for recent changes in the child's sleep, health, diet, or general level of functioning. Recent significant environmental or social changes (i.e., parents divorced, move to new home, arrival of new sibling, etc.) may also affect adaptive functioning. "Setting events" may also be an influencing factor. Such events refer to antecedent social or environmental conditions that alter the probability of behavior in the child's repertoire occurring (Durand 1990; Twardosz 1985). Increased problems may occur with students if their favorite staff happens to have the day off. Sometimes poor sleep is a problem, particularly in totally blind individuals. Insomnia may predispose them to irritability, poor attention span, and other behaviors, that may again increase the likelihood of maladaptive behaviors occurring.

Often children with both developmental delay and visual impairment develop fears associated with transitions between settings or activities. This difficulty can be compounded by the fact that different caregivers may be teaching the child at any given point in time and may not be sufficiently consistent in how they transition the child from one activity or place to another. In examining why transitions are difficult for students, it may be helpful to consider the following factors (Wright et al. 1994): (1) What is the child's tolerance for noise, physical crowding, changes in routine (Environment). (2) How do staff or peer interactions affect them? Does having different caregivers around make a difference? (Social). (3) What is the child's ability to communicate when frustrated? Are they ever with individuals who cannot understand how they communicate? (Communication). (4) What is their frustration tolerance level, how well do they control impulses, how do they respond when confronted with sudden changes? (Emotional). (5) How do they explore their environment, how long can they pay attention? What are the best ways to help them stay focused and motivated? (Cognitive). (6) How are transitions handled? What does waiting do to them? Do they understand where they are going and why? (Task-related).

Psychotherapeutic Interventions

There has been considerable growth and sophistication in the types and breadth of methods used in behavioral treatment. What began as consequence-driven, behavior reduction techniques involving punishment, aversive stimulation, or time-out has evolved into a multifaceted, highly positive, treatment approach. Behavioral treatment approaches should be a standard part of any treatment plan designed for the amelioration of stereotypic, self-injurious, and disruptive behaviors in children, and a growing literature attests to successful applications in treating children with visual impairment (Van Hasselt 1987). These treatments are derived from theories of social learning, classical and operant conditioning, and cognitive restructuring, and detailed reviews can be found elsewhere (Martin and Pear 1996; Thorpe and Olson 1990; Bellack and Hersen 1985). Contingent positive reinforcement is the most widely researched and effective tool available to caregivers working with visually impaired children. Review of treatment approaches for managing self-injury, stereotypic, and disruptive behaviors (Van Hasselt 1987) indicated over two thirds of the studies from 1970 on used positive reinforcement as part of the treatment of persons with visual impairment. For reinforcement to be effective, it must immediately follow the behavior to be increased. Having a child sign "eat" then taking him or her across the hall to receive food might be effective for a well-established behavior, but would be much less likely to teach the child to make the connection initially, resulting in an increase in spontaneous signing. To maximize the effectiveness of positive reinforcement, it is important to: (1) specify the exact behavior targeted for reward; (2) provide reward or signal the availability of reward immediately following emission of the target behavior; (3) vary the availability of reinforcing stimuli

TABLE 20.3

ASSESSMENT OF NEED FOR BEHAVIORAL INTERVENTIONS

Behavior	Example
Potentially of harm to the child?	Eye poking; darting into traffic; self-injurious behavior
Dangerous to others?	Startle-induced aggression; throwing objects; head-butting; scratching; pinching
Impairs acquisition of new skills or behaviors?	Stereotypies; noncompliance
Limits independence?	Difficulty with transitions; fear of separation
Distress to the individual?	Sleep disturbance; excessive fears
Disruptive to others?	Screaming; public masturbation
Socially inappropriate?	Taking others' food

and activities; (4) replace contrived rewards with naturally occurring rewards as the behavior becomes more frequent; (5) reduce the number of times the behavior is rewarded as it becomes more firmly established in the child's repertoire.

For children with sufficiently developed language skills, cognitive functioning, and the ability to form social attachments, supportive psychotherapy may be a useful addition to behavior therapy (Anders and Walton 1983). Often, it is necessary to work with families who may be reacting to the stress of having a handicapped child to help them cope more effectively with feelings that may prevent them from effectively participating in their child's behavioral treatment.

As with sighted individuals, exercise may be of benefit for visually impaired and blind individuals. Hanna (1986) reported that blind school children exhibit significant differences in lateral posture, biological functioning, and cardiovascular endurance relative to their sighted peers, and recommended recreational activities that make moderate demands on the cardiovascular system. Gleser and colleagues (1992) found that judo practice, in combination with group psychotherapy, occupational therapy, and physiotherapy, benefited school-aged mentally retarded blind children who exhibited improvement in developmental and motor skills as well as their social attitude. O'Cleirigh and colleagues (1994) also endorsed noncontingent exercise as an intervention warranting further attention.

Social Skills Training

Next to self-injurious and stereotypic behaviors, Van Hasselt (1987) found that the majority of studies in his review of behavioral treatments for blind children focused on disruptive behaviors. It is thus necessary to be sure that children and adolescents learn what is considered socially offensive behavior and learn how to suppress such behaviors in certain settings. Otherwise, others in the community will be less likely to interact with these individuals, increasing their sense of isolation and withdrawal. As reported by Van Hasselt (1987), maladaptive behaviors do not usually disappear on their own, but continue to interfere with interactions with others and with learning.

Treatment to improve social skills does not need to be burdensome or complicated. Providing increased opportunities for social interaction through prompting by teachers or parents is likely to result in the initiation of peer interaction and, once it begins, it is more likely to be sustained through continued positive feedback. Breaking certain activities down and providing assistance that is gradually reduced may also be helpful. Van Hasselt (1987) indicated that improvement in assertiveness skills could be accomplished with visually impaired female adolescents in less than a month. Sessions occurred five times weekly for 15 to 30 minutes and included modeling, direct instructions, behavioral rehearsal, performance feedback, and manual guidance. Targeted behaviors evidencing change included direction of gaze, posture, voice tone, and requests for behavior

change. A one-month follow-up evaluation showed a retreat toward baseline in some responses; however, once "booster" treatment sessions were implemented, further follow-up indicated these behaviors had returned to posttreatment levels. This experience highlights some of the primary considerations in improving prosocial behaviors: (1) Assessment is critical and specific behaviors to be changed must be targeted; (2) A single approach is less likely to be effective than a treatment package; (3) The techniques are not time-consuming or complex and may be implemented in a variety of situations; (4) Maintenance of treatment gains may require booster sessions; (5) Once social behaviors are established, naturally occurring consequences are likely to maintain such behaviors, but only if the child has sufficient opportunity to interact in a social environment.

Psychopharmacology

Little has been written about the use of psychotropic medications in children with blindness or severe visual impairment. It is well known, however, that there are ophthalmic effects of medications commonly used to treat mental disorders and, in particular, in the context of severe visual impairment, medications which impair accommodation have the potential of exerting significantly greater impact than would the same drugs administered to children with more in the way of visual reserve. Medications well known for such anticholinergic side effects include the tricyclic antidepressants, but the mood stabilizers, lithium carbonate and carbamazepine, as well as the neuroleptic drugs all have the potential to impair visual acuity through this mechanism. Sanabria-Bohorquez and colleagues (2001) have observed decreased cerebellar benzodiazepine receptor density in early blind subjects. There did not appear to be cortical differences in receptor density as assessed by flumazenil binding. The clinical implications of these observations are unclear, but may suggest a potential for differential sensitivity to therapeutic and motor or other side effects of benzodiazepines in persons who became blind early in life.

Geringer (1994) has reviewed psychiatric considerations in ophthalmology and noted a variety of potentially significant ophthalmic effects associated with commonly used psychotropic agents. While most of these effects have greater implications for adults with visual impairment, for example concerns about the use of agents with anticholinergic effects in the context of narrow angle glaucoma, it is worth noting that a variety of side effects with regard to the visual system have been described. These include for the antidepressants bilateral internuclear ophthalmoplegia (doxepin and amitriptyline), palinopsia (trazodone), impaired smooth pursuit eye movements, divergence paralysis and decrease in saccadic velocity associated with benzodiazepines in general, and glaucoma and allergic conjunctivitis associated with diazepam in particular (Donhowe 1984; Hughes and Lessel, 1990, Arai and Fujii 1990; Hyams and Keroub 1977).

Downbeat nystagmus, saccadic dysmetria, oculogyric crisis, opsoclonus, unilateral gaze palsy, papilledema and eye irritation all have been associated with lithium administration (Corbett et al. 1989; Deleu and Ebinger 1989; Sandyk 1984; Levine and Puchalski 1990). The use of carbamazepine has been associated with downbeat nystagmus, retinopathy and oculogyric crisis (Chrousos et al. 1987; Nielson and Syversen 1986). Among the neuroleptic drugs, oculogyric crises, corneal and lenticular deposits, pigmentary retinopathy and blinking blepharospasm, perhaps a tardive dyskinesia variant, have been reported (Hamilton 1985; Miller et al. 1982; Sachdev 1989).

In addition to particular issues with regard to the use of psychotropic medications in children with blindness, there are also considerations that need to be kept in mind with regard to the use of ophthalmic drugs and their possible psychiatric consequences. Among these drugs, the medications most likely to cause psychiatric symptoms include anticholinergic agents used for pupillary dilation, and beta-blockers, which may be used in the treatment of glaucoma. Among the anticholinergic eyedrops widely used are preparations of atropine, scopolamine, homatropine and cyclopentolate hydrochloride. The latter is most often associated with symptoms of irritability, restlessness, agitation, insomnia, and confusion, as well as occasionally more severe symptoms of depersonalization, delirium, paranoid thoughts, memory loss, and visual hallucinations (Geringer 1994). Among patients treated with beta-blockers, typically timolol for glaucoma, approximately 10% may report psychiatric symptoms, which include light-headedness, depression, fatigue, dissociative states, and loss of memory.

Conclusion

Research in the neurobiology of vision has contributed much to our understanding of basic brain function. Arguably, vision is the dominant sense in humans, and impairment of this modality can significantly alter cortical maps, sleep-wake cycles, and motor, language, and personality development. Blind children are at risk for psychiatric disorder. Advances in knowledge of the visual system have informed therapeutic approaches, but considerable work remains to advance our understanding of how best to prevent and remediate blindness and its attendant developmental consequences in children.

DEAF AND HARD-OF-HEARING CHILDREN AND ADOLESCENTS

Definition of Hearing Loss

Deafness can at once be simple and quite difficult to define, and choice of terminology can have important connotations for individuals with varying degrees of hearing loss. At the simplest level, "deaf" refers to the mechanical characteristics of hearing loss, with individuals exhibiting thresholds for sound detection sufficient to interfere with ability to detect and decipher speech (approximately 60 dB or greater), while "hard-of-hearing" individuals have lesser degrees of hearing loss such that they can still understand at least some speech, particularly with the benefit of hearing aids. Beyond level of hearing, however, hearing loss and associated terms such as deaf and hard of hearing can be defined by additional mechanical features including not only amount but also quality of residual hearing, timing of onset, etiology, whether or not the hearing loss occurs in isolation (nonsyndromic) or with other symptoms (syndromic), educational experience, linguistic choices, and cultural identification. In this discussion, hearing loss refers to the mechanical aspects of audition, "deaf" or "deafness" refers to hearing loss sufficient to prevent access to auditory inputs, "hard of hearing" refers to a more modest hearing loss that allows for auditory input, and "Deaf" refers to a cultural identification of oneself with the deaf community, a recognized cultural and linguistic minority. We avoid, however, the term "hearing impaired," as this has long been considered by many deaf and hard-of-hearing individuals to be an attempt by hearing professionals to concatenate two ends of the spectrum of hearing loss for simplicity and to medicalize a "disorder" or "disability"; a premise with which many such individuals disagree. The term can be considered offensive and clinicians are forewarned to remove "hearing impaired" from their lexicon.

Mechanical features of hearing loss include degree of loss measured in decibels (dB) and is described as normal when thresholds are between 0 and 26 dB, mild 27 to 40 dB, moderate 41 to 55 dB, moderately severe 56 to 70 dB, severe 71 to 90 dB, and profound for thresholds greater than 90 dB. The pattern of hearing loss across the frequency spectrum also plays an important role in the degree to which a child has access to spoken language via auditory channels. With primary speech frequencies ranging from 500 to 4,000 Hz, losses outside of that range have less impact on ability to detect and understand speech than losses within these speech frequencies. Hearing loss is also characterized as either conductive, sensorineural, or mixed. Conductive hearing loss stems from defects or disruption in the external or, more likely, middle ear components that conduct sound to the sensory organ (cochlea) within the inner ear. Sensorineural hearing loss stems from deficits in the inner ear or auditory (VIII) nerve. The majority of children with clinically significant hearing loss have sensorineural losses.

Stability of hearing thresholds over time has important implications for a child's access to, and development of, spoken language. Early intact hearing or only mild to moderate loss is more likely to provide the child with access to, and experience with, spoken language that can serve as a basis for spoken language development, even when the hearing loss progresses to a more severe degree once basic language abilities are developed. Quality of residual hearing also impacts ability to detect and discriminate sounds. It is possible to have a severe or profound hearing loss but with good discrimination such that the child benefits well from amplification, while it is also possible to have only a moderate to severe loss with poor discrimination such that amplification is unhelpful to the child in comprehending speech via aural channels. Hearing loss can be further defined by timing of onset, or as congenital, acquired prelingual, or postlingual. Congenital and acquired prelingual hearing loss is more likely to interfere with acquisition of spoken language, while postlingual, as the term implies, occurs after the child has developed spoken language. Postlingually, or adventitiously, deafened children have sufficient experience with their spoken language (e.g., English) to enable continued speech and knowledge of the language of their hearing peers.

Hearing loss can further be described as occurring in isolation (nonsyndromic) or with other symptoms (syndromic), and can be hereditary or acquired via a number of mechanisms, including intrauterine or neonatal infections such as cytomegalovirus or Rubella, later infections such as meningitis, or events such as anoxia. Certain hereditary forms of hearing loss, particularly those that are syndromic, are more often associated with other neurological deficits. Intrauterine and postnatal infectious causes of hearing loss are also often associated with neurological, behavioral or psychiatric deficits.

Epidemiology of Hearing Loss in Children and Adolescents

The epidemiology of hearing loss is based on fragmentary information (Nadol and Merchant 2001), but estimates suggest that both the incidence and prevalence of deafness are approximately 1 in 1,000. Although approximately 1 in 1,000 children are born with severe or profound deafness (Fraser 1964; Kitson and Fry 1990), as many as one in 300 children are born with at least some degree of hearing loss (Thiringer et al. 1984). Another 1 in 1,000 children become deaf before adulthood (Petit and Weil 2001).

Etiology of Hearing Loss

Hearing loss has many causes, including hereditary factors, anoxia, congenital and postnatal infections, and ototoxic drugs. Although etiologies have historically been difficult to determine and estimates vary widely across the few extant studies, substantial strides have been made in the past decade in the identification of genetic causes. This, in combination with interventions for prenatal infections such as rubella and alternatives for ototoxic drugs, has led to a marked increase in the incidence of known genetic causes of hearing loss in children. Etiology of hearing loss is an important historical factor in the clinical evaluation of deaf and hard-of-hearing children, as certain etiologies are likely

to carry additional neurological complications such as visual, motor, or cognitive deficits.

Hereditary Deafness

The number of genes involved in development and functioning of the hearing system are unknown, but is estimated to number in the hundreds or as many as 1,000 (Nance, 1980). Over 350 different genetic conditions associated with hearing loss are described in the literature (Martini, Mazzoli, and Kimberling 1997). These can be broken down further into syndromic, comprising some 30% of cases, and nonsyndromic, accounting for 70% of cases (Petit 1996). At least 50% of children born deaf have genetic bases for their hearing loss, and 70 to 80% of these are autosomal recessive, 15 to 20% are autosomal dominant, and 2 to 3% are X-linked or mitochondrial in origin (Morton 1991, Bussoli and Steel 1998). At least 30% of the causative genes have been identified.

Syndromic Hereditary Deafness

There are several hereditary syndromes that feature sensorineural hearing loss as a primary symptom, among them Waardenburg's and Usher's syndromes. Although there are a few recognizable syndromes involving hearing loss associated with in utero infection (e.g., rubella, cytomegalovirus), the majority of cases of syndromic deafness are genetically mediated.

Waardenburg's syndrome is an autosomal dominant genetic syndrome with four known subtypes (Nadol and Merchant 2001). Hearing loss in Waardenburg's syndrome varies, ranging from unilateral to bilateral and across the hearing spectrum, with a characteristic low frequency loss. Type I is associated with dystopia canthorum and heterochromia iridis along with sensorineural hearing loss and is attributed to a mutation of the PAX-3 gene at 2q35. Type II is similar in presentation but without dystopia canthorum and is attributed to mutation of the microphthalmia gene. Type III is referred to as Klein-Waardenburg and is similar to Type I with added abnormalities of upper limbs and is attributed to the PAX-3 gene at 2q35. Type IV, or Waardenburg-Shah, is akin to Type II but with Hirschsprung disease. The mechanism for Waardenburg's syndrome is thought to be genetically induced abnormal migration of melanocytes from the neural crest, leading to defective development of the stria vascularis and other cochlear structures (Merchant, McKenna, Baldwin, Milunsky, and Nadol, 2001).

Usher's syndrome is an autosomal recessive syndrome categorized into three subtypes, each with congenital hearing loss and onset of visual impairment later in life. Type I is characterized by congenital profound sensorineural hearing loss and onset of retinitis pigmentosa by age 10 years. Type II includes a sensorineural congenital hearing loss with a downsloping audiogram, no vestibular abnormalities and retinitis pigmentosa by age 10 to 20 years. Type III is characterized by progressive sensorineural hearing loss, some involvement of the vestibular system, and variable onset of retinitis pigmentosa. Nadol and Merchant (2001) describe several genetic mutations responsible for each type of Usher's syndrome.

There are many syndromic disorders attributed to inherited mitochondrial DNA mutations that involve hearing loss including MELAS syndrome (metabolic encephalopathy, lactic acidosis, and stroke-like episodes), MIDD syndrome (maternally inherited diabetes and deafness), MERRF syndrome (myoclonic epilepsy associated with ragged red fibers), and Kearns-Sayre syndrome.

Nonsyndromic Hereditary Deafness

Autosomal-recessive inheritance characterizes 80% of cases of nonsyndromic inherited deafness. Autosomal dominant inheritance occurs in nearly all of remaining cases, with X-linked and mitochondrial inheritance patterns comprising approximately 1% of cases (Petersen 2002). Some 53 loci for nonsyndromic recessive forms have been reported (Petit and Weil 2001), including a mutation in the GJB2 gene, which may account for hearing loss in as many as 50% of cases in some populations (McGuirt and Smith 1999). With respect to dominant patterns of transmission, 38 genes, consecutively numbered DFNA1-38 (autosomal dominant sensorineural deafness) have been mapped to 15 different chromosomes, whose functions relate to hair cell formation, potassium recycling into endolymph, several connexin (gap junction) proteins, and others (Petersen 2002). Autosomal recessive forms of deafness tend to be more severe, and sensorineural in etiology in comparison to the conductive loss that typifies most syndromic forms of deafness. Nonsyndromic causes of deafness are, almost by definition, less likely to be associated with other neurological, cognitive, behavioral, or psychiatric concerns.

Nonhereditary Causes

Although the incidence of non-hereditary forms of deafness continues to decrease, these are important etiologies as they are often associated with other, sometimes severe, neurological sequelae that affect behavioral, cognitive, and psychiatric functioning in children. Hearing loss can result from hyperbilirubinemia congenital infections such as cytomegalovirus and rubella, postnatal infections such as bacterial meningitis, prenatal, perinatal, or postnatal anoxia, ototoxic drugs such as aminoglycosides during pregnancy, or use of ototoxic drugs postnatally.

Congenital Infections

Select pathogens can infect the placenta and damage the developing fetal central nervous system resulting in neurological disorders including sensorineural hearing loss. Of the so-called TORCH infections (toxoplasmosis, others, rubella, cytomegalovirus and herpes; Nahmias 1974), cytomegalovirus (CMV) and rubella are the primary culprits.

Cytomegalovirus

CMV may be the most common cause of nonhereditary deafness. The incidence of acquired CMV infection in the population is 1 to 2% per year, with nearly 100% of adults infected at some point (Bale and Jordan 1989). The majority of healthy individuals with acquired CMV infections do not exhibit symptoms, and most infected neonates have no signs of infection at birth. Some 10% of neonates exhibit symptoms including jaundice, hepatomegaly, splenomegaly, rash, intrauterine growth retardation, and respiratory distress. Over 90% of these infants have neurological sequela, including microcephaly, chorioretinitis, seizures, hypo/hypertonia, cerebral palsy, mental retardation, and behavioral disorders (Boppana et al. 1992; Noyola et al. 2001; Pass et al. 1980). Sensorineural hearing loss occurs in approximately 40% of infants with congenital CMV infection (Istas, Demmler, Dobbins, and Stewart 1995). Imaging studies have shown periventricular calcifications in approximately 50% of infants with intrauterine infection and may also show periventricular leukomalacia, polymicrogyria, pachygyria, or lissencephaly (Bale 2002).

Rubella

Until the introduction of the rubella vaccine in 1969, rubella epidemics occurred at 6- to 9-year intervals and resulted in thousands of cases of congenital rubella syndrome (Bale 2002). This was the most common cause of hearing loss in children born in the early 1960s during a rubella pandemic. Since the vaccine, however, the incidence of congenital rubella syndrome has declined in the United States to less than 0.1 per 100,000 births (Schluter, Reer, Redd, and Dykewicz 1998). Unfortunately, rubella prevalence in central and eastern Europe, particularly in the former Soviet Union, has increased dramatically (Banatvala and Brown 2004). Moreover, recent concerns in the United Kingdom and United States regarding the safety of the measles-mumps-rubella vaccine have substantially reduced the uptake rate of the vaccine.

Infants born with congenital rubella syndrome exhibit a broad spectrum of symptoms including sensorineural hearing loss, cataracts, retinopathy, micro-ophthalmia, microcephaly, cardiac defects (myocarditis, patent ductus arteriosus, valvular stenosis, and septal defects). Neurological symptoms can include autistic features and mental retardation. Abnormalities are related to timing of infection during gestation (Ueda, Nishida, Oshmia, and Shepard 1979): cataracts and cardiac defects result from infection during the first 8 weeks and hearing loss results from infection during the first 16 weeks. Infections after the 16th week have few known sequelae, although hearing loss can occur. Although the incidence of congenital rubella syndrome in the United States has declined, it is more likely to occur in immigrants from countries without compulsory immunization (Schluter et al. 1998).

Herpes Simplex Virus

Neonatal herpes simplex infection occurs in 1 in 3,000 to 20,000 live births (American Academy of Pediatrics 2000) and is typically a result of viral exposure during birth. Sensorineural hearing loss results in most cases where the infection presents in disseminated fashion, in some 40% of children with encephalitis, and 25% of children with only localized infections (Whitley and Hutto 1985). Hearing loss in these cases is often accompanied by other neurological symptoms, including mental retardation, visual impairment, and seizures (Roizen 2003).

Other Etiologies

Bacterial Meningitis

Before vaccination programs, bacterial meningitis accounted for the majority of hearing loss in infants and children (Anderson and Taylor, 2000). While the incidence of specific forms of the illness has markedly decreased since introduction of vaccination for *Haemophilus influenzae* type b meningitis, there are as yet no vaccines for other forms of the disease, including pneumococcal meningitis, meningococcal meningitis, and group B streptococcal infections, the most common form of neonatal meningitis. While each form tends to affect children at different ages (e.g., group B streptococcal infections are often neonatal, while other forms occur between 1 month and 4 years), the majority of childhood infections occur during the critical language development period. For young children who contract meningitis, mortality rates are between 4 and 10% (Grimwood, Nolan, Bond, Anderson, Catroppa, and Keir 1996). Of the survivors, some 40% exhibit acute neurological complications (Grimwood et al. 1996, Taylor et al. 1990), although the majority have no residual effects (Taylor, Schatschneider, and Rich 1992). Hearing loss is the most common residual sequelae of bacterial meningitis. Baraff, Lee, and Schriger (1993) found that 16% of bacterial meningitis survivors had severe or profound hearing loss. This may be accompanied, however, by other neurological sequelae including mental retardation (6%), spasticity or paresis (4%), and seizure disorders (4%). Cognitive, language, behavioral and academic difficulties are seen in many children with histories of meningitis, with acute phase neurological symptoms and persistent hearing loss increasing risks for these difficulties. Longterm deficits have been documented in language, fine and gross motor function, perception, memory, executive function, and academic skills in postmeningitic children. Although language deficits may be associated with hearing loss itself, they are also seen in postmeningitic children without hearing loss, suggesting that language deficits may be a result of meningitis infection that are further compounded by hearing loss (Anderson and Taylor 2000). Anderson and Taylor also note that deficits may change over time, such that gross motor difficulties may be more apparent in the acute phase, but fine motor, language, perceptual and behavioral difficulties may emerge and persist in later years as environmental demands increase.

Prematurity

The incidence of sensorineural hearing loss as a result of perinatal/neonatal complications has increased substantially over the past 30 years, accounting for only some 2% of children with hearing loss in the 1960s but some 27% in the 1990s (Kile 1993). This is thought related in part to the increased survival of high-risk infants. In a study of etiological factors resulting in deafness in prematures less than 33 weeks gestational age, duration of intubation, ventilation, oxygen exposure, and acidosis contribute significantly to later hearing loss. Although bilirubin levels and aminoglycoside levels were not in themselves associated with later hearing loss, the risk of later hearing loss increased significantly when acidosis and/or aminoglycoside use occured during peak bilirubin levels (Marlow, Hunt, and Marlow 2000). (See also Chapter 23.)

Anatomy of the Hearing System

The human hearing system is composed of three distinct components: the external, middle, and inner ear. The external ear includes the auricle and external auditory canal, bringing sound from the external environment up to the tympanic membrane. The middle ear begins at the tympanic membrane, which transduces sound vibrations, or airwave pressure oscillations, into mechanical energy, transmitted from the membrane through the three ossicles (malleus, incus, and stapes) to the oval window. The oval window is the entry point of sound to the inner ear. At the oval window, the mechanical energy is again transduced to fluid vibrations in the endolymph, a potassium-rich fluid that fills the cochlea and the vestibule. The vestibule is responsible for balance and includes the saccule and utricle, which respond to linear acceleration, and three semicircular canals, which respond to rotational movements. The cochlea and vestibule contain sensory receptors termed hair cells or stereocilia. The hair cells are covered by acellular membranes: the tectorial membrane within the cochlea, otoconical membranes for the saccule and utricle, and cupulae for the semicircular canals. The hair cells and membranes move in response to endolymph vibrations within the cochlea and vestibule, resulting in depolarization and neurotransmitter release into synapses corresponding to the hair cells. This process generates signals that are transmitted along the auditory nerve (VIII). Sound intensity or amplitude and frequency or pitch are encoded via the hair cells in the cochlea, which are arranged *tonotopically* with hair cells near the base of the cochlea responding to high frequencies and those near the apex of the cochlea responding to low frequencies. This tonotopic organization is maintained throughout most of the auditory perceptual system.

Once signals enter the central auditory system via the auditory (VIII) nerve, they bifurcate at the cochlear nuclei and superior olivary complex, or brainstem auditory nuclei, into several separate monaural and binaural pathways. Monaural pathways capture spectral features (amplitude, frequency) of sound from one cochlea and arise from the cochlear nucleus, projecting via the acoustic stria to the contralateral inferior colliculus. Binaural pathways compare and contrast signals from both cochlea and are responsible for localization of sound and discrimination of sound in noise via two mechanisms: interaural timing and interaural level differences. Lower frequency sounds below 3,000 Hz are localized in space via timing differences from sound waves reaching the closer or more proximal ear in an earlier phase than the distal ear, while higher frequency sounds are loudest in the proximal ear and attenuated slightly by an auditory "shadow" created by the head. From a functional standpoint, binaural inputs are essential for sound localization and discrimination of foreground sounds from background noise. Thus, while frequency and volume of sound may be preserved in unilateral hearing loss, localization and discrimination is affected.

Binaural processing begins in the superior olivary complex, which receives ipsilateral excitatory input and contralateral inhibitory input from the cochlea. This information projects ipsilaterally to the lateral lemnisci where it is projected to both the ipsilateral inferior colliculus and to the contralateral lemnisci and on to the contralateral inferior colliculus. At the inferior colliculus, binaural and monaural pathways are combined and integrated and passed to the medial geniculate nucleus in the thalamus, which serves as a relay to the primary auditory cortex (Brodmann's area 41) in the posterior area of the superior temporal gyrus. Tonotopic organization is maintained within the auditory cortex, with low frequencies processed rostrally and high frequencies processed caudally.

The inferior colliculus also has several projections to the superior colliculus. This provides for integration of spatial sensory information from somatosensory, visual and auditory inputs. The auditory projections form an auditory map of space that parallels that of the visual map.

Descending auditory pathways provide control of auditory inputs and processing from the cortex down to the cochlear nuclei and directly to the hair cells within the cochlea. There are two primary pathways; one arising from the lateral division of the superior olivary complex whose function is not yet known, and one arising from the medial division of the superior olivary complex that is involved in modulating or attenuating sound from the cochlea.

Behavioral and Developmental Consequences of Deafness

Hearing loss, by itself, does not have any direct behavioral or developmental consequences. If a deaf or hard-of-hearing child is brought up in a visual sociolinguistic environment at home and school that compensates for their hearing loss, the child's development would be within normal limits. However, there are often indirect behavioral and developmental consequences of growing up with hearing loss in a world that relies heavily on audition such as environmental factors that hinder their language, academic, and psychosocial development. There are negative consequences when parents, teachers, and professionals have on these children when they do not know how to deal with a child or adolescent with hearing loss. These factors are discussed in depth in the following sections.

Motor Development

There is widespread agreement that deaf children's early gross and fine motor development is quantitatively and qualitatively similar to that of hearing children (Paul and Jackson 1993). In a study that focused on various aspects of motor skill development in 201 deaf (mean hearing loss = 96.94 dB) children and adolescents (ages 4 to 18), it was found that they had similar motor skills acquisition compared to hearing peers (Dummer, Haubenstricker, and Stewart 1996). Deaf children with sign language fluency have been found to perform better on tasks that require rapid manual speed compared to non-signers (Braden 1985, 1987). Deaf children of deaf parents are faster than deaf children of hearing parents, who in turn are faster than hearing children on these types of tasks (Braden 1988).

Language Development

Language access is perhaps the primary concern when dealing with hard-of-hearing or deaf children and adolescents. Some hard-of-hearing children are able to have full access to spoken language when fitted with hearing aids. Other hard-of-hearing individuals cannot understand speech from hearing alone but with hearing aids or cochlear implants they can lip read better; for example, the hearing aid or cochlear implant can help them identify the differences between the voiceless /s/ and voiced /z/ phonemes while lip reading. There remain to be some who receive no obvious benefits from hearing aids or cochlear implants. Those who do not attain normal hearing with hearing aids and those with cochlear implants often do not have the benefits of language acquisition in the periphery and they have only limited access to language when they are watching someone's lips.

Lip reading requires more attention and effort than passive listening and often requires guesswork. For example, one study demonstrated that deaf adolescents were able to guess pseudosyllables correctly with 30% accuracy through lip reading alone. The same subjects were able to correctly identify key words in sentences with low predictability with 25.5% accuracy and in highly predictable sentences with 49.2% accuracy (Nicholls and Ling 1982). Hearing aids and cochlear implants have been shown in a number of studies to improve the accuracy of lip reading in some children and adolescents (Geers and Brenner 1994). The intelligibility of deaf and hard-of-hearing individuals' speech varies widely depending on degree of hearing loss, age of onset of hearing loss, and how much the individual benefits from speech therapy (Ellis and Pakulski 2003; Monsen 1983).

Visual languages have emerged and visual codes have been developed because of the difficulties of providing adequate access to language through lip reading. American Sign Language (ASL) is the language of North American deaf communities (Padden and Humphries 1988). It evolved almost 200 years ago from its original pidgin form that included French Sign Language (*Langue des Signes Francaise*), a sign language that used to exist in Martha's Vineyard, Massachusetts, and Native American Indian sign languages (Lane 1984). Over the time, it creolized into a natural language that has a different grammatical structure than spoken English (Liddell 1980, 1995) and is different from sign languages in other countries, for example, British Sign Language.

The benefit of using ASL is that a child is able to learn a visual language as their primary language and later learn English as their second language (Hoffmeister 2000). When deaf and hard-of-hearing children are in a signing environment, they are able to passively acquire more language skills when watching others communicate with each other that they would otherwise miss in an auditory environment. Deaf and hard-of-hearing children who are born to deaf parents develop native fluency in ASL; however, less than 5% of deaf and hard-of-hearing individuals have at least one deaf parent (Mitchell and Karchmer 2002). They achieve the same language development milestones in ASL as children with no hearing loss (Caselli and Volterra 1994). Literature has shown that deaf children of deaf parents often develop better English literacy skills than those with hearing parents (Padden and Ramsey 2000) and it is believed that having fluency in one language (ASL) helps these children acquire a second language (English) at a faster rate compared to deaf children who attempt to acquire English as their first language.

There are visual codes that have been created to follow a similar word order as spoken English but involve different phonological and morphosyntactical structures such as Manually Coded English and Signing Exact English (Lucas and Valli 1989). They have been created to remove the need for bilingual education although English sign systems cannot achieve the exact same grammatical structure as English. There is also another coding system that minimizes the grammatical differences between its visual form and spoken English; that is, the cued English or cued Speech system (Cornett 1967, Fleetwood and Metzger 1998). The cued English system provides visual phonemes in the form of hand shapes, hand placements, and mouth shapes. While it is phonologically different from spoken English, it follows English's phonemic sequence and it shares the same morphological and syntactical structure. Deaf adolescents who use cued English have been shown to guess pseudosyllables and key words in low predictable and high predictable sentences with 83.5%, 96.2%, and 96.6% accuracy, respectively (Nicholls and Ling 1982). Similar results were found in a study with deaf children from Belgium who used cued French (Périer, Charlier, Hage, and Alergia 1990).

It is important for early detection of hearing loss and immediate accommodations in the home to provide language access and early educational intervention to treat their language delay. Deaf children who are born to a household that does not use a visual language almost always have a delay in their language development. The average age that hearing loss is detected is approximately 18 months (Mertens, Sass-Lehrer, and Scott-Olson 2000). The child's need for visual access to language usually is not addressed in the first 2 years of their lives. Often after diagnosis, professionals attempt to correct their hearing rather than focusing on providing visual access to language (with or without hearing aids or cochlear implants), which further hinders their language development.

The delay of deaf and hard-of-hearing children's English development includes their literacy development. The most recent national survey of 17- to 18-year-old deaf and hard-of-hearing students' reading achievement found the average reading level to be at the 4th grade equivalent (Holt, Traxler, and Allen 1997). If a psychiatric (i.e., lower intelligence) or neurological (i.e., cerebral palsy, epilepsy) disorder is also present, it can exacerbate the language delay. Often deaf and hard-of-hearing children are given a primary diagnosis of a learning disability and/or attentional disorder that is actually secondary to language delay. Deaf and hard-of-hearing children with limited access to language and a language delay often have difficulty paying attention or sitting still in class. Their academic development is often below their cognitive potential. Differential diagnosis is very difficult and many deaf and hard-of-hearing children are misdiagnosed with these types of disorders.

Cognitive Development

Myklebust (1964) proposed that the lack of auditory stimulation experienced by deaf individuals shifts the cognitive organization within the individual. Event-related potential (ERP), functional magnetic resonance imaging (fMRI), and cognitive behavioral studies have confirmed this hypothesis (e.g., Bavelier, Tomann, and Hutton 2000; Neville and Lawson 1987a, 1987b, 1987c; Proksch and Bavelier 2002). The cognitive reorganization of some functions does not seem to have an impact on intellectual functioning. Deaf and hard-of-hearing individuals' intellectual functioning has a similar distribution to that of hearing individuals (Braden 1994; Maller 1999).

The compensatory theory states that the loss of one sense may be met by a greater reliance upon, and therefore an enhancement of, the remaining senses (Grafman 2000; Neville 1990). Psychophysical studies within the visual domain in deaf individuals, compared to hearing individuals, have failed to validate this theory. Both groups have similar thresholds for brightness discrimination (Bross 1979), contrast sensitivity (Finney and Dobkins 2001), motion sensitivity (Bosworth and Dobkins 1999), and temporal discrimination (Bross and Sauerwein 1980; Poizner and

Tallal 1987). The cognitive differences found in deaf individuals are at the higher level perceptual processing rather than an enhancement of visual sensory thresholds.

Within the domain of executive functions, deaf children and adolescents demonstrate similar cognitive flexibility in nonverbal problem solving compared to age-matched hearing peers (Kelly 1995; Rosenstein 1960); however, a study of nonverbal problem solving involving multiple steps demonstrated that deaf and hard-of-hearing children and adolescents (ages 6 to 19) lagged behind their age-matched hearing peers (Luckner and McNeill 1994). Deaf and hard-of-hearing children have demonstrated similar executive abilities compared to age-matched peers in their ability to initiate behaviors and responses, plan, organize, self-monitor, and control their emotions (Rhine 2002). The area of executive functions that has been documented to be different between deaf and hearing individuals is within the area of impulse and attention control.

Earlier studies have claimed that deaf children are more impulsive than hearing children (Altshuler, Deming, Vollenweider, Rainer, and Tendler 1976; Chess and Fernandez 1980; Quellette 1988); however, these conclusions are not based on well-controlled experimental measures of impulse control; rather they are based on personality measures. Deaf children of deaf parents have impulsivity rates that are lower than those of deaf children of hearing parents (Harris 1978). Current psychological inventories on deaf and hard-of-hearing children's impulsivity, inattention, and ability to shift attention continue to illustrate higher incidences of impulsivity and difficulty shifting attention but not within clinical ranges (Rhine 2002). Similar results are found in continuous performance tasks that are often used by psychologists for ruling out attentional disorders (Parasnis, Samar, and Berent 2003).

The results of psychological assessment tests of attention contradict current cognitive neuroscience literature. Cognitive neuroscience literature has demonstrated that deaf individuals' attention and ability to inhibit distractors is better in some areas and different than that of hearing individuals. Deaf individuals have been shown to have an enhanced capacity to distribute attention over the whole visual field (Sireteanu and Rettenbach 2000) and are able to terminate their search faster when no target was present, without compromising their accuracy as compared with hearing subjects (Rettenbach, Diller, and Sireteanu 1999; Stivalet, Moreno, Richard, Barraud, and Raphel 1998). In studies that required deaf adults to attend to peripheral stimuli while ignoring centrally presented distractors, they did not demonstrate difficulty inhibiting these distractors. Instead, they demonstrated a superior ability, compared to hearing subjects, to selectively attend to the peripheral stimuli while ignoring the centrally presented distractors (Parasnis and Samar 1985; Reynolds 1993).

Other studies have demonstrated that deaf adults are faster and more accurate than hearing adults at detecting (Loke and Song 1991) and discriminating (Neville and Lawson 1987c) shapes presented in the periphery compared to the center of the visual field suggesting enhanced attention and increased vigilance in the periphery. Proksch and Bavelier (2002) report that deaf adults (native signers) allocate more attentional resources to the periphery compared to the center of the visual field. The allocation of attentional resources to the periphery seems to bring with it reduced resources at the center of the visual field. A similar allocation of attention was not found in hearing subjects who were native ASL signers, suggesting that sign language alone could not be responsible for this change. These results suggest that auditory deprivation from birth enhances the speed of orientating visual attention and attentional processing of the peripheral visual field. Deaf individuals' enhancement of visual attention in the periphery has been supported by ERP (Neville and Lawson 1987b) and fMRI studies (Bavelier et al. 2000).

Sign language experience has been shown to improve some cognitive functions. Deaf signers were found to have a longer spatial memory span than hearing nonsigners (Wilson, Bettger, Niculae, and Klima 1997), but deaf children with no exposure to sign language and hearing children were found to have a similar spatial memory span (Parasnis, Samar, Bettger, and Sathe 1996). Deaf signers are more accurate (McKee 1988) and faster (Emmorey, Kosslyn, and Bellugi 1993) in performing mental rotation skills than hearing nonsigners while deaf nonsigners performed similarly to hearing nonsigners (Chamberlain and Mayberry 1994). Deaf signers between the ages of 6 and 9 years old performed better at every age level than hearing children on a test that involves matching the frontal view of a target face with other views of the same person (Bellugi et al. 1990). Similar results were found in hearing adult signers (Bettger 1992) but not in deaf adult nonsigners (Parasnis et al. 1996). Deaf signers are more accurate than hearing nonsigners in discriminating between faces that were identical except for a change in a single facial feature (McCullough & Emmorey, 1999). Deaf and hearing signers are more accurate than hearing non-signers at remembering locations of faces in a matching pairs task but both groups did not differ in remembering locations of objects (Arnold and Murray 1998).

Psychological tests are designed to be used with hearing individuals and often when they are used with deaf individuals, they measure something other than what the test is intended to measure. This might be why the psychological literature that is based on psychological assessment instruments has shown deaf individuals to have attention and impulse control abilities lower than the norm. Well-controlled experiments have demonstrated that deaf individuals do not necessarily have attentional and impulse control difficulties but their upper level visual perceptual processing is different than that of hearing individuals. Auditory deprivation alone is responsible for some of these changes. As illustrated previously, sign language fluency can cause enhanced attentional, memory, and visual perceptual abilities.

Psychosocial Factors of Parent–Child Attachment

The diagnosis of a permanent medical condition often is difficult for any parents to accept without emotional distress. The diagnosis of hearing loss is no exception especially since communication difficulties are inherent in the diagnosis. Parents often go through a grieving process (Harvey 2003; Mertens et al. 2000; Schirmer 2001) and their attachment with their child is often different from the norm. There is substantial literature demonstrating that interactions between hearing mothers and their deaf or hard-of-hearing children are less than optimal. The mothers of deaf and hard-of-hearing children tend to be more involved in their childrearing than fathers. This usually includes learning how to communicate with the child. Azar (1995) demonstrated that there are marked differences in 20- to 40-month-old deaf children's relationships with their mothers compared to their fathers. It is crucial for fathers to realize the importance of their active participation in early intervention programs. Azar's study also demonstrated the more parents have a negative attitude toward deafness, the weaker the child's security of attachment.

Hearing mothers of deaf or hard-of-hearing children have been described as more rigid, intrusive, and negative; deaf or hard-of-hearing children of hearing mothers are less active, responsive, and involved compared to dyads in which both members are hearing (Meadow-Orleans 1990; Spencer and Gutfreund 1990). Hearing mother–hearing child dyads have shown more maternal structuring and hearing mother–hearing child nonhosility when compared to hearing mother and deaf or hard-of-hearing child dyads (Pipp-Siegel, Blair, Deas, Pressman, and Yoshinaga-Itano 1998).

Maternal sensitivity is related to gains in language competence in young deaf and hard-of-hearing children (Pressman, Pipp-Siegel, Yoshinaga-Itano, and Deas 1999) and to more broad indices of the affective climate between mothers and deaf and hard-of-hearing children (Greenstein, Greenstein, McConville, and Stellini 1975). Deaf and hard-of-hearing children who have mothers that are sensitive to their needs learn more vocabulary between the ages of 2 and 3 years compared to mothers who were less sensitive to their deaf or hard-of-hearing children's needs (Pressman, Pipp-Siegel, Yoshinaga-Itano, Kubicek, and Erode, 1998). Samuel (1996) found that maternal sign language skills and attitude toward deafness is positively correlated to deaf 15- to 18-year-old adolescents' positive sense of attachment to their mothers. Samuel's study also demonstrated that the deaf adolescents' attachment to parents and close peers predicted the adolescents' self-concept and social adjustment.

Deaf parents' relationship with their deaf or hard-of-hearing children is often dramatically different from that of hearing parents. Many deaf individuals consider being deaf as a part of their cultural identity rather than as a disability. Genetically deafened parents often go through a similar grieving process and have similar parent–child attachment issues when they have hearing children. In a study of 12- to 40-month-old deaf children of deaf parents, it was found that their ability to develop secure attachment and independence from their parents is the same as that of hearing children (Meadow, Greenberg, and Erting 1984).

Psychosocial Development

It has long been believed that deafness itself does not necessarily lead to lower self-esteem; it is the quality and quantity of communication the child receives that is positively correlated with self-esteem development (Schlesinger and Meadow 1972). Meadow (1980) claimed that the language delay of children with hearing loss who have hearing parents has a negative impact on their self-esteem and self-concept. Earlier studies have shown that if parents treated the child's hearing loss as a family issue it has a positive effect on the child's self-esteem (Bat-Chava 2002; Schlessinger 1978; Schlesinger and Meadow 1972). This means that the whole family plays an active role in communicating with the child rather than viewing the hearing loss as a deficient characteristic of the child.

In a meta-analytic review of 42 studies on self-esteem in deaf and hard-of-hearing individuals, it was found that deaf children with hearing parents who use sign language have better self-esteem than deaf children who have parents who do not sign (Bat-Chava 1993). A study conducted on adolescents from residential schools for the deaf found a significant positive correlation between the students' self-esteem and parents' signing skills. The students who had parents who did not sign had the lowest self-esteem whereas parents with some signing skills had children with higher self-esteem and those with the best signing skills had children with the highest self-esteem (Desselle 1994). A recent study with a sample of over 1,000 deaf students from Turkey found similar results (Polat 2003). Desselle (1994) found a significant positive relationship between deaf children's self-esteem and their reading achievement.

This meta-analysis (Bat-Chava) also found that deaf individuals have a response similar to that of other minority groups wherein the negative attitudes toward minorities is internalized and hinders development of self-esteem. Cocker and Major (1989) claimed that members of minority groups who identified with their minority group have higher self-esteem than those who do not. In Bat-Chava's (1993) meta-analysis, it was found that this was also true for deaf children; those who identified with deaf adults have higher self-esteem and deaf children born to deaf parents experience a similar upbringing to that of minority children with minority parents. Deaf children of deaf parents were found to have a higher self-esteem than deaf children of hearing parents (Bat-Chava 1993; Hilburn, Marini, and Slate 1997). However, the meta-analysis revealed that overall, deaf individuals have lower self-esteem compared to hearing individuals. Similar results have been found in studies of the self-esteem of deaf adults who have deaf parents compared to those who have hearing parents (Yachnik 1986).

Later onset of hearing loss has been associated with poor psychosocial adjustment and earlier onset has been associated with greater degree of satisfaction with self (Loeb and Sarigani 1986; Polat 2003). Some studies have found that higher degrees of hearing loss have been associated with higher degree of adjustment problems (Polat 2003), while others have found no differences (Frustenberg and Doyal 1994; Sinkkonen 1994). Literature has shown that the existence of additional disabilities has consistently been associated with more psychosocial and adjustment problems (Mertens 1993 et al; Polat 2003).

Psychopathology

In the past, many deaf people with poor written, spoken, or signed language skills were in psychiatric institutional care, often with no appropriate communication or formal diagnosis (Denmark 1985, 1994). Studies of adult deaf and hard-of-hearing psychiatric inpatients from the United States and other countries have shown a greater overall prevalence of mental illnesses than the hearing population and longer hospital stays (Vernon and Diagle-King 1999). Deaf children, particularly those from hearing families, may be exposed to an excess of the risk factors that can affect all children and lead to adjustment disorders in adolescence. These factors include academic failure, low self-esteem, inconsistent discipline, failure of age-appropriate development, and sexual and physical abuse. Most of these are secondary to negative attitudes to deafness and failure to develop age-appropriate language fluency (du Feu and Fergusson 2003).

Schlesinger and Meadow (1972) found that 31% of deaf children had mild to severe psychiatric disturbances while the hearing control group had an incidence rate of 9.7%. In a sample of 117 deaf children from ages 5 to 16 years old, Freeman, Malkin, and Hastings (1975) found a prevalence rate of 22% for moderate to severe psychiatric disturbances. They found that those who had psychiatric disturbances also had a higher prevalence of neurological disorders. Based on a study of 62 deaf children 11 to 16 years of age in the United Kingdom, the prevalence of psychiatric disorders was found to be as high as 50.3%. The prevalence was even higher in children in mainstream educational settings than in those attending schools for the deaf (Hindley, Hill, McGuigan, and Kitson 1994).

Fundudis, Kolvin, and Garside (1979) compared deaf, hard-of-hearing, and hearing children and found prevalence rates of psychiatric disturbances to be 54%, 28%, and 18%, respectively. However, Hindley (2000) stated that the degree of hearing loss generally does not appear to be a risk factor for psychiatric illnesses. Other studies have shown that the deaf and hard-of-hearing groups with higher prevalence of psychiatric disturbances come from dysfunctional families that involved substance abuse, physical abuse, verbal abuse, parent psychiatric difficulties, parent refusal to learn the child's language or communication (Goldberg, Lobb, and Kroll 1975; Powers, Elliott, Patterson, and Shaw 1995) and lower intelligence quotients (Schlesinger and Meadow 1972). Neurological problems associated with the cause of deafness can have disproportionately adverse effects for deaf children; for example, cerebral palsy can limit speech, signing and writing and epilepsy may reduce confidence and increase overprotectiveness from others (du Feu and Fergusson 2003).

Meadow (1980) claimed that behavioral disorders in deaf children occur at a rate three times higher than in hearing children. However, Bond (2000) has stressed that any problem behaviors are not a result of hearing loss per se; but the consequences of other factors such as the environment and the factors mentioned in the psychosocial development section of this chapter. Additionally, there is a higher prevalence of sexual and physical abuse perpetrated upon deaf and hard-of-hearing children and adolescents (Hindley 2000).

A recent large-scale survey of school administrators and teachers of deaf children estimated that approximately 8 to 11% of the deaf population is affected by learning disabilities (Schildroth and Hotto 1996). The actual incidence of learning disabilities might be lower since many deaf and hard-of-hearing children's learning difficulties are secondary to their hearing loss and language delay. It is difficult to differentiate a primary diagnosis of a learning disability from those that are secondary to hearing loss. Such evaluation needs to be conducted by a skilled psychologist who is familiar with and experienced in working with this population. Studies on the incidence of learning disabilities in this population have historically relied on teacher and parent reports rather than comprehensive psychological evaluations by qualified professionals.

There is no evidence for genetic aggregation of hearing loss and attention-deficit/hyperactivity disorder (ADHD), nor is there any evidence that auditory deprivation itself causes ADHD (Parasnis, Samar, and Berent 2003). However, some of the recognized causes of ADHD, such as anoxia and drug toxicity, are also causes of hearing loss (Mauk and Mauk 1992; Samar, Parasnis, and Berent 1998). The incidence of ADHD in hearing individuals has been estimated to be between 3 and 7% (Barkley 1997) and in deaf and hard-of-hearing individuals the incidence ranges from 3.5 to 38.7% with the highest rates of ADHD occurring in children with acquired hearing loss as opposed to hereditary hearing loss (Kelly, Forney, Parker-Fisher, and Jones 1993). The actual incidence of ADHD most likely is lower. It is difficult to survey the actual incidence because the frequent language delays found in this population can cause restlessness and difficulty following language dialogue in the classroom.

Psychological Assessment

There is an inherent ethical dilemma involved in the psychological evaluation of a deaf or hard-of-hearing patient (Maller 2003). Test instructions often need to be given in a visual mode (e.g., signing, cueing, or lip reading) or a combination of verbal and visual modalities, depending on which communication mode is most readily accessible to the patient. Almost every time a test is administered to this population, the standard administration procedures are modified and therefore violated (Braden 1994). The use of psychological tests with verbal content has been strongly discouraged when evaluating a patient from this population (Braden 1994; Maller 2003; Vernon and Brown 1964). Psychologists must realize that some non-verbal psychological tests continue to be a problem because they require verbal mediation strategies for correct or rapid responses and many require verbal instructions (Simeonsson, Wax, and White 2001).

Verbal items are often omitted from intelligence batteries and thus the only tests remaining are the non-verbal subtests (Blennerhassett 1990; Moores 1987). This poses a problem because subtests are not equally effective at measuring all aspects of intelligence, and cannot function alone as an appropriate representation of intelligence. The most widely used test with deaf children, the Wechsler Intelligence Scale for Children (WISC-III; Wechsler 1991, Braden and Hannah 1998; Gibbins 1989) has been reported to measure the construct of intelligence differently at the item and factor structure levels with deaf children (Maller 1999; Maller and Ferron 1997). Other intelligence batteries also have some validity issues (Maller 2003, Simeonsson, Wax, and White 2001). Deaf children are often misdiagnosed as mentally retarded or learning disabled when assessed by psychologists unfamiliar with the issues of intelligence testing in this population (Vernon and Andrews 1990).

There are not enough validated tests designed for the deaf and hard-of-hearing client that can be administered without modification. This ethical dilemma forces the psychologist to leave the safety of relying on each test's psychometric soundness and to rely more on clinical skills and judgment while taking into consideration the factors that might be affecting clients and their test scores. The psychological assessment of deaf and hard-of-hearing clients requires relatively more reliance on knowledge and qualitative data obtained through observations, to support clinical hypotheses, diagnoses, and recommendations. Psychiatrists who refer their patients for a psychological evaluation should seek psychologists who are familiar with the empirical literature and test modifications that are necessary to provide a valid evaluation of deaf and hard-of-hearing children and adolescents' psychological functioning.

Psychopharmacologic Interventions

There is surprisingly little literature reporting pharmacotherapy of mental disorders in children with deafness. Case reports exist for the use of various medications to treat maladaptive behaviors, for example, self-injury and aggression, in individuals with developmental disorders such as congenital rubella syndrome.

As is the case for children with blindness, concerns about medication side effects need to be firmly on the radar screen of the prescriber. Drugs that may affect visual acuity, for example, may be particularly disconcerting in persons who must rely on their vision for communication (Roberts and Hindley 1999). Similarly, medication-induced extrapyramidal symptoms carry obvious additional significance.

For those individuals whose deafness was the result of ototoxic drugs, the clinician may have to take extra care to explore a family's willingness to consider medication treatment given a likely bias against such intervention.

Psychotherapeutic Interventions

After the initial diagnosis of hearing loss, hearing parents of deaf and hard-of-hearing children often would benefit from psychotherapy to avoid psychopathological changes in the parent–child attachment. Family therapy is often beneficial because having a deaf or hard-of-hearing child frequently changes the family dynamics. In family therapy, it may be necessary to use an interpreter if the deaf or hard-of-hearing child or adolescent is most fluent in a signed language and the patient's family is not fluent in that language (ASL) or communication mode (cued or signed English) (Harvey 1984, 2003). The family therapist should also be knowledgeable about the family dynamics of having a deaf or hard-of-hearing child. In the case where a deaf or hard-of-hearing patient needs therapeutic intervention, it is necessary to seek a mental health professional who specializes in working with this unique population (Harvey 2003; Leigh, Corbett, Gutman, and Morere 1996; Sussman and Brauer 1999).

The use of mental health professionals who are not familiar with this population could lead to misdiagnosis and mistreatment. As previously mentioned, there are psychosocial, language, and cognitive factors that make this population different from hearing children and adolescents. It is also important for the patient to work with a mental health professional who can communicate directly with the patient. The use of sign language interpreters has a direct impact on the individual therapeutic process (Leigh et al. 1996). Therapists who have used interpreters acknowledge that it dilutes and distorts the patient–therapist relationship (Wohl 1995). There is an additional challenge of using interpreters with deaf or hard-of-hearing children because the patient would be looking at the interpreter, not the therapist (Sussman and Brauer 1999). There are additional problems when working with younger children who are not familiar with using interpreters.

The literature has shown that various psychotherapeutic approaches can be used to successfully treat deaf or hard-of-hearing children. These include psychoanalytic and insight-oriented therapies (Levin 1981; Rayson 1985) as well as humanistic oriented therapies, Adlerian therapy, cognitive therapy, and rational-emotive therapy (Anderson and Watson 1985; Gough 1990; Sussman 1988). The type of approach that would be best for any patient (hearing, hard-of-hearing, or deaf) would depend on their psychopathology, not their hearing status. Psychiatrists and parents usually do not have the flexibility to choose between a variety of approaches and professionals. Instead, they usually have to choose the mental health professional who specializes in working with this population. Sometimes, this means traveling long distances for such treatment.

If there are no professionals that specialize in this population, then it is necessary to accept the second best alternative which would be working with a mental health professional (with interpreting services if necessary) who does not have any experience working with this population. One common mistake made by therapists who are not familiar with treating deaf and hard-of-hearing children is that they often automatically assume that the core problem with the patient's psychopathology has something to do with their hearing loss. It is possible that a patient's hearing loss might be exacerbating their psychopathology but the patient's hearing loss often is not the primary problem.

It is important for professionals who work with deaf and hard-of-hearing individuals to realize that they are not only dealing with a disability group, but also a group that has a different lifestyle. There is a continuum within the deaf and hard-of-hearing community between those who identify with deaf culture and those who do not. Regardless of their cultural identification, there are similar psychosocial issues shared by members of this community. Literature on psychotherapy with cultural minorities is more relevant to this community than literature on disability groups. It is necessary for mental health professionals to provide culturally affirmative psychotherapy (Glickman 1996) when treating individuals from this community.

Conclusions

As with visual impairment, research in the neurobiology of hearing loss has contributed much to our understanding of basic brain function. Significant advances in molecular genetics have informed our understanding of the physiology of hearing. Neuropsychological studies will continue to look to individuals with deafness to better understand language and personality development. Deafness does not protect from psychiatric disorders, but recent work may place the prevalence closer to that for the general population than once believed. Considerable work remains with respect to characterizing specific psychiatric treatments in

this population, but individualized treatment approaches that are culturally sensitive are always indicated.

REFERENCES

Adams, R. J., Courage, M. L., Mercer, M. E. (1994). Systematic measurement of human neonatal color vision. *Vision Research, 34,* 1691–1701.

Alemayehu, W., Tekle-Haimanot, R., Forsgren, L., Erkstedt, J. (1995). Causes of visual impairment in central Ethiopia. *Ethiopian Medical Journal, 33,* 163–174.

Altshuler, K., Deming, W., Vollenweider, J., Rainer, J., & Tendler, R. (1976). Impulsivity and profound early deafness: A cross cultural inquiry. *American Annals of the Deaf, 121,* 331–345.

American Academy of Pediatrics. (2000). *2000 Red Book: Report of the Committee on Infectious Diseases,* 25th Ed. Elk Grove Village, IL: American Academy of Pediatrics.

Ammerman, R. T., Van Hasselt, V. B., & Hersen, M. (1986). Psychological adjustment of visually handicapped children and youth. *Clinical Psychology Review, 6,* 67–85.

Anders, T. F., & Walton, C. (1983). Psychotherapy with children. In M. D. Levine, W. B. Carey, A. C. Crocker, & R. T. Gross (Eds.). *Developmental Behavioral Pediatrics.* Philadelphia: WB Saunders.

Anderson, G. B., & Watson, D. (1985). *Counseling deaf people: Research and practice* (pp. 123–144). Little Rock, AR: Arkansas Rehabilitation Research and Training Center on Deafness and Hearing Impairment, University of Arkansas.

Anderson, V. A., & Taylor, H. G. (2000). Meningitis. In K. O. Yeates, M. D. Ris, & H. G. Taylor (Eds.), *Pediatric neuropsychology: Research, theory and practice* (pp 117–148). New York: The Guilford Press.

Arai, M., & Fujii, S. (1990). Divergence paralysis associated with the ingestion of diazepam. *Journal of Neurology 237,* 45.

Arnold, P., & Murray, C. (1998). Memory for faces and objects by deaf and hearing signers and hearing nonsigners. *Journal of Psycholinguistic Research, 27,* 481–497.

Azar, H. (1995). Attitudes toward deafness and security of attachment relationships among deaf children and their parents. *Early Education & Development, 2,* 181–191.

Bale Jr., J. F. (2002). Congenital infections. *Neurologic Clinics, 20,* 1039–1060.

Bale Jr., J. F., & Jordan, M. C. (1989). Cytomegalovirus. In P. J. Vinken, G. W. Bruyn, & H. L. Klawans (Eds.) *Handbook of clinical neurology* (pp. 263–279). Amsterdam: Elsevier.

Banatvala, J. E., Brown, D. W. G. (2004). Rubella. *Lancet, 363,* 1127–1137.

Baraff, L. J., Lee, S. I., & Schriger, D. L. (1993). Outcomes of bacterial meningitis in children: A meta-analysis. *Pediatric Infectious Disease Journal, 12,* 389–394.

Barkley, R. A. (1997). *ADHD and the nature of self-control.* New York: Guilford Press.

Bat-Chava, Y. (1993). Antecedents of self-esteem in deaf people: A meta-analytic review. *Rehabilitation Psychology, 38,* 221–234.

Bat-Chava, Y. (2002). Sibling relationships for deaf children: The impact of child and family characteristics. *Rehabilitation Psychology, 47,* 73–91.

Bauman, M. K., & Kropf, C. A. (1979). Psychological tests used with blind and visually handicapped persons. *School Psychology Review, 8,* 257–270.

Bavelier, D., Tomann, A., Hutton, C., Mitchell, T. V., Corina, D. P., Liu, G., & Neville, H. J. (2000). Visual attention to the periphery is enhanced in congenitally deaf individuals. *Journal of Neuroscience, 20,* 1–6.

Bellack, A. S., and Hersen, M. (Eds.). (1985). *Dictionary of behavior therapy techniques.* New York: Pergamon Press.

Bellugi, U., O'Grady, L., Lillo-Martin, D., O'Grady, M., van Hoek, K., & Corina, D. (1990). Enhancement of spatial cognition in deaf children. In V. Volterra & C. Erting (Eds.), *From gesture to language in hearing and deaf children* (pp. 278–298). New York: Springer-Verlag.

Bettger, J. (1992). *The effects of experience on spatial cognition: Deafness and knowledge of ASL.* Unpublished doctoral dissertation, University of Illinois, Urbana-Campaign.

Birch E, Petrig B. (1996). FPL and VEP measures of fusion, stereopsis and stereoacuity in normal infants. *Vision Research 36,* 1321–1327.

Blacher, J. B., Hanneman, R. A., and Rousey, A. B. (1992). Out-of-home placement of children with severe handicaps: a comparison of approaches. *American Journal on Mental Retardation, 96,* 607–616.

Blennerhassett, L. (1990). Intellectual assessment. In D. Moores & K. Meadow-Orlans (Eds.), *Educational and developmental aspects of deafness* (pp. 255–280). Washington, D. C.: Gallaudet University Press.

Bloch, H., Carchon, I. (1992). On the onset of eye-head coordination in infants. *Behavioural Brain Research 49,* 85–90.

Bond, D. E. (2000). Mental health in children who are deaf and have multiple disabilities. In P. Hindley & N. Kitson (Eds.)., *Mental health and deafness* (pp. 127–148). London: Whurr Publishers.

Boppana, S. B., Pass, R. F., Britt, W. J., et al. (1992). Symptomatic congenital cytomegalovirus infection: Neonatal morbidity and mortality. *Pediatric Infectious Disease Journal, 11,* 93–99.

Bosworth, R., & Dobkins, K. (1999). Left hemisphere dominance for motion processing in deaf signers. *Psychological Science, 10,* 256–262.

Braden, J. P. (1985). The relationship between choice reaction time and IQ in deaf and hearing children. *Dissertations Abstracts International, 46,* 2622A. (UMI No. DES85–24895).

Braden, J. P. (1987). An explanation of the superior performance IQs of deaf children of deaf parents. *American Annals of the Deaf, 132,* 263–266.

Braden, J. P. (1988). Understanding IQ differences between groups: Deaf children as a natural experiment in the nature-nurture debate. In D. H. Soklofske & S. B. Eysenck (Eds.), *Individual differences in children and adolescents: international research perspectives* (pp. 265–277).

Braden, J. P. (1994). *Deafness, Deprivation, and IQ.* New York: Plenum Press.

Braden, J. P., & Hannah, J. M. (1998). Assessment of hearing-impaired and deaf children with the WISC-III. In A. Prifitera & D. Saklofske (Eds.), *WISC-III Clinical Use and Interpretation* (pp. 175–201). San Diego: Academic Press.

Brodsky, M. C., Baker, R. S., Hamed, L. F. (1996). The apparently blind infant. In *Pediatric neuro-ophthalmology* (pp.1–41). New York: Springer.

Bross, M. (1979). Residual sensory capacities of the deaf: A signal detection analysis of a visual discrimination task. *Perceptual and Motor Skills, 48,* 187–194.

Bross, M., & Sauerwein, H. (1980). Signal detection analysis of visual flicker in deaf and hearing individuals. *Perceptual and Motor Skills, 51,* 839–843.

Brown, R., Hobson, R. P., Lee, A., Stevenson, J. (1997). Are there 'autistic-like' features in congenitally blind children? *Journal of Child Psychology and Psychiatry, and Allied Disciplines 38,* 693–703.

Browning Wright, D., Gurman, H. B., et al. (1994). *Positive intervention for serious behavior problems: Best practices in implementing the hughes bill (A. B. 2586) and the positive behavioral intervention regulations.* Sacramento, CA: Resources in Special Education.

Bussoli, T. J., & Steel, K. P., (1998). The molecular genetics of inhereited deafness- current and future applications. *Journal of Laryngology & Otology, 112,* 523–530.

Caselli, M. C., & Volterra, V. (1994) From communication to language in hearing and deaf children. In V. Volterra & C. J. Erting (Eds.), *From gesture to language in hearing and deaf children,* 2nd ed. (pp. 263–277). Washington, D. C.: Gallaudet University Press.

Chamberlain, C., & Mayberry, R. I. (1994). *Do the deaf "see" better? Effects of deafness on visuospatial skills.* Poster presented at TENNET V, Montreal, Quebec.

Chess, S., & Fernandez, P. (1980). Neurologic damage and behavior disorder in rubella children. *American Annals of the Deaf, 125,* 505–509.

Chrousos, G. A., Cowdry, R., Schuelein, M., et al. (1987). Two cases of downbeat nystagmus and oscillopsia associated with carbamazepine. *American Journal Ophthalmology 103,* 221.

Cole, P. M., Jenkins, P. A., and Shott C. T. (1989). Spontaneous expressive control in blind and sighted children. *Child Development, 60,* 683–688.

Corbett, J. J., Jacobsen, D. M., Thompson, H. S., et al. (1989). Down-beating nystagmus and other ocular motor defects caused by lithium toxicity. *Neurology 39,* 481.

Cornett, O. (1967). Cued speech. *American Annals of the Deaf, 112,* 3–13.

Czeisler, C. A., Shanahan, T. L., Klerman, E. B., Martens, H., Brotman, D. J., Emens, J. S., Klein, T., Rizzo, J. F. (1995). Suppression of melatonin secretion in some blind patients by exposure to bright light. *New England Journal of Medicine 332,* 6–11.

Davidson, P. W. (1983). Visual impairment and blindness. In M. D. Levine, W. B. Carey, A. C. Crocker, & R. T. Gross, R. T. (Eds.), *Developmental behavioral pediatrics* pp. 778–788. Philadelphia: WB Saunders.

de Courten C., Leuba G., Huttenlocher L.J., et al. (1982). Volumetric, neuronal and synaptic development of human primary visual cortex. *Neuroscience Letters (Supplement) 10,* S135.

Deleu, D., & Ebinger, G. (1989). Lithium-induced internuclear ophthalmoplegia. *Clinical Neuropharmacology 12,* 224.

Denmark, J. C. (1985). A study of 250 patients referred to a department of psychiatry for the deaf. *British Journal of Psychiatry, 146,* 282–286.

Denmark, J. C. (1994). *Deafness and mental health.* London: Jessica Kingsley Publishers.

Derby, K. M., Wacker, D. P., Sasso, G., Steege, M., Northup, J., Cigrand, K., & Asmus, J. (1992). Functional assessment techniques to evaluate aberrant behavior in an outpatient setting: a summary of 79 cases. *Journal of Applied Behavior Analysis, 3,* 713–721.

Desselle, D. D. (1994). Self-esteem, family climate and communication patterns in relation to deafness. *American Annals of the Deaf, 125,* 322–328.

Donhowe, S. P. (1984). Bilateral internuclear ophthalmoplegia from doxepin overdose. *Neurology 34,* 259.

Downing, J. E., & Perino, D. M. (1992). Functional versus standardized assessment procedures: Implications for educational programming. *Mental Retardation, 5,* 289–295.

du Feu, M., & Fergusson, K. (2003). Sensory impairment and mental health. *Advances in Psychiatric Treatment, 9,* 95–103.

Dummer, G. M., Haubenstricker, J. L., & Stewart, P. A. (1996). Motor skill performance of children who are deaf. *Adapted Physical Activity Quarterly, 13,* 400–414.

Durand, V. M. (1990). *Severe behavior problems: A functional communication training approach.* New York: Guilford Press.

Ellis, L. W., & Pakulski, L. (2003). Judgments of speech intelligibility and speech annoyance by mothers of children who are deaf or hard of hearing. *Perceptual & Motor Skills, 96,* 324–328.

Emmorey, K., Kosslyn, S. M., & Bellugi, U. (1993). Visual imagery and visual-spatial language: Enhanced imagery abilities in deaf and hearing ASL signers. *Cognition, 46,* 139–181.

Finney, E. M., & Dobkins, K. R. (2001). Visual contrast sensitivity in deaf versus hearing populations: Exploring the perceptual consequences of auditory deprivation and experience with a visual language. *Cognitive Brain Research, 11,* 171–183.

Fleetwood, E., & Metzger, M. (1998). *Cued language structure: An analysis of cued american english based on linguistic principles.* Silver Spring, MD: Calliope Press.

Fraser, G. R. (1964). Profound childhood deafness. *Journal of Medical Genetics, 1,* 118–161.

Freeman, R., Malkin, S., & Hastings, J. (1975). Psychosocial problems of deaf children and their families: A comparative study. *American Annals of the Deaf, 121,* 391–405.

Frick, K. D., & Foster, A. (2003). The magnitude and cost of global blindness: An increasing problem that can be alleviated. *American Journal of Ophthalmology 135,* 471–476.

Frustenberg, K., & Doyal, G. (1994). The relationship between emotional-behavioural functioning and personal characteristics on performance outcomes of hearing students. *American Annals of the Deaf, 139,* 410–414.

Fundudis, T., Kolvin, I., & Garside, R. (1979). *Speech retarded and deaf children: Their psychological development.* London: Academic Press.

Gardner, W. I., Graeber, J. L., & Cole, C. L. (1996). Behavior Therapies: A multimodal Diagnostic and Intervention Model. In J. W. Jacobson, & J. A. Mulick (Eds.). *Manual of diagnosis and professional practice in mental retardation* (pp., 355–370). Baltimore, MD: United Book Press.

Geers, A., & Brenner, C. (1994). Speech perception results: Audition and lipreading enhancement. *Volta Review, 95*, 97–108.

Gibbins, S. (1989). The provision of school psychological assessment services for the hearing impaired: A national survey. *The Volta Review, 91*, 95–103.

Gilbert, C., Rahi, J., Eckstein, M., Foster, A. (1995). Hereditary disease as a cause of childhood blindness: regional variation. *Ophthalmic Genetics 16*, 1–10.

Gilbert, C. E., Wood, M., Waddel, K., Foster, A. (1995). Causes of childhood blindness in East Africa: Results in 491 pupils attending 17 schools for the blind in Malawi, Kenya and Uganda. *Ophthalmic Epidemiology 2*, 77–84.

Gleser, J. M., Margulies, J. Y., Nyska, M., Porat, S., et al. (1992). Physical and psychosocial benefits of modified Judo practice for blind, mentally retarded children: A pilot study. *Perceptual & Motor Skills, 74*, 915–925.

Glickman, N. S. (1996). What is culturally affirmative psychotherapy? In N. S. Glickman, & M. A. Harvey (Eds.), *Culturally affirmative psychotherapy with deaf persons* (pp. 1–55). Mahwah, NJ: Lawrence Erlbaum Associates.

Goldberg, B., Lobb, H., & Kroll, H. (1975). Psychiatric problems of the deaf child. *Canadian Psychiatric Association Journal, 20*, 75–83.

Gonzales, L., & Dweck, H. S. (1994). Eye of the newborn: A neonatologist's perspective. In S. J. Isenberg, (Ed.), *The eye in infancy* (2nd ed., p. 2). St. Louis: Mosby.

Good, W. V., & Hoyt, C. S. (1989). Behavioral correlates of poor vision in children. *International Ophthalmology Clinics, 29*, 57–60.

Good, W. V., Jan, J. E., DeSa, L., Barkovich, A. J., Groenveld, M., & Hoyt, C. S. (1994). Cortical visual impairment in children. *Survey of Opthalmology 38*, 351–364.

Gordon, J. A., & Stryker, M. P. (1996). Experience-dependent plasticity of binocular responses in the primary visual cortex of the mouse. *Journal of Neuroscience, 16*, 3274–86.

Gough, D. L. (1990). Rational-emotive therapy: A cognitive-behavioral approach to working with hearing impaired clients. *Journal of Rehabilitation of the Deaf, 23*, 96–104.

Grafman, J. (2000). Conceptualizing functional neuroplasticity. *Journal of Communication Disorders, 33*, 345–356.

Greenstein, J., Greenstein, B., McConville, K., & Stellini, I. (1975). Maternal sensitivity and newborns' orientation responses as related to quality of attachment in North Germany. *Monographs of the Society of Child Development, 50* (1–2, serial no. 209).

Grimwood, K., Nolan, T., Bond, L., Anderson, V., Catroppa, C., & Keir, E. (1996). Risk factors for adverse outcomes of bacterial meningitis. *Journal of Pediatric Child Health, 32*, 457–462.

Hamilton, J. D. (1985). Thioridazine retinopathy within the upper dosage limit. *Psychosomatics, 26*, 823.

Hanna, R. S. (1986). Effect of exercise on blind persons. *Journal of Visual Impairment & Blindness, 80*, 722–725.

Harris, R. (1978). The relationship of impulse control to parent's hearing status, manual communication, and academic achievement in deaf children. *American Annals of the Deaf, 123*, 52–67.

Harvey, M. (1984). Family therapy with deaf persons: The systemic utilization of an interpreter. *Family Therapy, 23*, 205–213.

Harvey, M. (2003). *Psychotherapy and deaf and hard-of-hearing persons: A Systemic Model*, (2nd ed.). Mahwah, NJ: Lawrence Erlbaum Associates.

Harwerth, R. S., Smith III, E. L., Duncan, G. C., Crawford, J. L. J., & von Noorden, G. K. (1986). Multiple sensitive periods in the development of the primate visual system. *Science, 232*, 235–238.

Hilburn, S., Marini, I., & Slate, J. R. (1997). Self-esteem among deaf versus hearing children with deaf versus hearing parents. *Journal of American Deafness and Rehabilitation Association, 30*, 9–12.

Hindley, P, Hill, P. D., McGuigan, S., & Kitson, N. (1994). Psychiatric disorder in deaf and hearing impaired children and young people: A prevalence study. *Journal of Psychiatry and Psychology, 35*, 917–934.

Hindley, P. (2000). Child and adolescent psychiatry. In P. Hindley & N. Kitson (Eds.), *Mental health and deafness* (pp. 42–74). London: Whurr Publishers.

Hobson, R. P., & Bishop, M. (2003). The pathogenesis of autism: insights from congenital blindness. *Philosophical Transactions of the Royal Society of London. B Series, Biological sciences 358*, 335–344.

Hodapp, R. D. (1998) Blindness and visual impairments. In *Development and Disabilities*. New York: Cambridge University Press, in press.

Hoffmeister, R. J. (2000). A piece of the puzzle: ASL and reading comprehension in deaf children. In C. Chamberlain (Ed.), *Language acquisition by eye* (pp. 143–163). Mahwah, NJ: Lawrence Erlbaum Associates.

Holt, J. A., Traxler, C. B., & Allen, T. E. (1997). Interpreting the Scores: A User's Guide to the 9th Edition Stanford Achievement Test for Educators of Deaf and Hard-of-Hearing Students. *Gallaudet Research Institute Technical Report 97-1*. Washington, DC: Gallaudet University.

Hubel, D. H., & Wiesel, T. N. (1970). The period of susceptibility to the physiological effects of unilateral eye closure in kittens. *The Journal of Physiology 206*, 419–436.

Hughes, M. S., & Lessel, S. (1990). Trazadone-induced palinopsia. *Archives of Ophthalmology 108*, 399.

Hull, T., & Mason, H. (1995). Performance of blind children on digit-span tests. *Journal of Visual Impairment & Blindness, 89*, 166–169.

Humayun, M. S., de Juan, Jr., E., Dagnelie, G., Greenberg, R. J., Propst, R. H., & Phillips, D. H. (1996). Visual perception elicited by electrical stimulation of retina in blind humans. *Archives of Ophthalmology 114*, 40–46.

Hyams, S. W., & Keroub, C. (1977). Glaucoma due to diazepam. *American Journal of Psychiatry 134*, 447.

Ing, M. R. (1984). Early surgical alignment for congenital esotropia. In I. I. Strabismus, & R. D. Reinecke (eds.). (pp. 55–66). New York: Grune and Stratton.

Istas, A. S., Demmler, G. J., Dobbins, J. G., & Stewart, J. A. (1995). Surveillance for congenital cytomegalovirus disease: A Report from the National Congenital Cytomegalovirus Disease Registry. *Clinical Infectious Disease, 20*, 665–670.

Jan, J. E., Freeman, R. D., & Scott, E. P. (1977). *Visual impairment in children and adolescents* (pp. 29–47). New York: Grune and Stratton.

Jan, J. E., Good, W. V., Freeman, R. D., & Espezel, H. (1994). Eye-poking. *Developmental Medicine and Child Neurology 36*, 321–325.

Jones, T. W. (1984). Behavior modification studies with hearing-impaired students: A review. *American Annals of the Deaf, 129*, 451–458.

Kelly, D., Forney, J., Parker-Fisher, S., & Jones, M. (1993). The challenge of attention deficit disorder in children who are deaf or hard of hearing. *American Annals of the Deaf, 138*, 343–348.

Kelly, M. D. (1995). Neuropsychological assessment of children with hearing impairment on Trail Making, Tactual Performance, and Category Tests. *Assessment, 2*, 305–312.

Kile, J. E. (1993). Identification of hearing impairment in children: A 25-year review. *Infant Toddler Intervention, 3*, 155–160.

Kitson, N., & Fry, R. (1990). Prelingual deafness and psychiatry. *British Journal of Hospital Medicine, 44*, 353–356.

Knudsen, E. I., & Knudsen, P. F. (1990). Sensitive and critical periods for visual calibration of sound localization by barn owls. *Journal of Neuroscience 10*, 222–232.

Kujala, T., Alho, K., Kekoni, J., Hamalainen, H., Reinikainen, K., Salonen, O., Standertskjold-Nordenstam, C.-G., & Naatanen, R. (1995). Auditory and somatosensory event-related brain potentials in early blind humans. *Experimental Brain Research 104*, 519–526.

Lane, H. (1984). *When the mind hears: A history of the deaf*. New York: Vintage Books.

Leigh, R. J., Foley, J. M., Remler, B. F., et al. (1987). Oculogyric crisis: A syndrome of thought disorder and ocular deviation. *Annals of Neurology 22*, 13.

Leigh, I. W., Corbett, C. A., Gutman, V., & Morere, D. A. (1996). Providing psychological services to deaf individuals: A response to new perceptions of diversity. *Professional Psychology: Research and Practice, 27*, 364–371.

Levin, F. M. (1981). Insight-oriented psychotherapy with the deaf. In L. K. Stein, E. G. Mindel, & T. Jabaley (Eds.), *Deafness and mental health* (pp. 113–132). New York: Grune and Stratton.

Levine, S. H., & Puchalski, C. (1990). Pseudotumor cerebri associated with lithium therapy in two patients. *The Journal of Clinical Psychiatry 51*, 251.

Lewis, M. H., Gluck, J. P., Bodfish, J. W., Beauchamp, A. J., & Mailman, R. B. (1996). Neurobiological basis of stereotyped movement disorder. In R. L. Sprague, & K. M. Newell (Eds.), *Stereotyped movements: Brain and behavior relationships* (pp. 37–67). Washington, DC: American Psychological Association.

Liddell, S. K. (1980). *American Sign Language syntax*. The Haque: Mouton.

Liddell, S. K. (1995). Real, surrogate, and token space: Grammatical consequences in ASL. In K. Emmorey, & J. S. Reilly (Eds.), *Language, gesture, and space* (pp. 19–42). Hillsdale, NJ: Lawrence Erlbaum Associates.

Loke, W. H., & Song, S. (1991). Central and peripheral visual processing in hearing and nonhearing individuals. *Bulletin of the Psychonomic Society, 29*, 437–440.

Lucas, C., & Valli, C. (1989). Language contact in the American Deaf Community. In C. Lucas (Ed.), *The sociolinguistics of the deaf community* (pp. 11–40). New York: Academic Press.

Luckner, J. L., & McNeill, J. H. (1994). Performance of a group of deaf and hard-of-hearing students and a comparison group of hearing students on a series of problem solving tasks. *American Annals of the Deaf, 139*, 371–377.

Maller, S. J. (1999, April). *The validity of WISC-III subtest analysis for deaf children.* Paper presented at the annual meeting of the American Educational Research Association, Montreal.

Maller, S. J. (2003). Intellectual Assessment of Deaf People: A Critical Review of Core Concepts and Issues. In M. Marshark, & P. E. Spencer (Eds.), *Oxford handbook of deaf studies, language, and education* (pp. 451–463). New York: Oxford University Press.

Maller, S. J., & Ferron, J. (1997). WISC-III factor invariance across deaf and standardization samples. *Educational and Psychological Measurement, 7*, 987–994.

Margach, C., & Kern, K. C. (1969). Visual impairment, partial-sight and the school psychologist. *Journal of Learning Disabilities, 2*, 407–414.

Marlow, E. S., Hunt, L. P., & Marlow, N. (2000). Sensorineural hearing loss and prematurity. *Archives of Disease in Childhood Fetal & Neonatal Edition, 82*, 141–144.

Martin, G., & Pear, J. (1996). *Behavior modification: What it is and how to do it* (5th Ed.). Totowa, NJ: Prentice Hall.

Martini, A., Mazzoli, M., & Kimberling, W. (1997). An introduction to genetics of normal and defective hearing. *Annals of the New York Academy of Sciences, 830*, 361–374.

Mauk, G. W., & Mauk, P. P. (1992). Somewhere, out there: Preschool children with hearing impairment and learning disabilities. *Topics in Early Childhood Education: Hearing-Impaired Preschoolers, 12*, 174–195.

McCullough, S., & Emmorey, K. (1999). *Perception of emotional and linguistic facial expressions: A categorical perception study with deaf and hearing subjects.* Poster presented at the Psychonomic Society meeting, Los Angeles, CA.

McGuirt, W. T., & Smith, R. J. H. (1999). Connexin 26 as a cause of hereditary hearing loss. *American Journal of Audiology, 8*, 93–100.

McKee, D. E. (1988). An analysis of specialized cognitive functions in deaf and hearing signers. *Dissertation Abstracts International, 49*, 768.

Meadow, K. P. (1980). *Deafness and child development.* Berkeley, CA: University of California Press.

Meadow, K. P., Greenberg, M. T., & Erting, C. (1984). Attachment behavior of deaf children of deaf parents. *Journal of the American Academy of Child Psychiatry, 22*, 23–28.

Meadow-Orlans, K. P. (1990). Research on developmental aspects of deafness. In D. F. Moores & K. P. Meadow-Orlans (Eds.), *Education and developmental aspects of deafness* (pp. 283–298). Washington, DC: Gallaudet University Press.

Meister, M., Wong, R. O. L., Baylor, D. A., Shatz, C. J. (1991). Synchronous bursts of action potentials in ganglion cells of the developing mammalian retina. *Science, 252*, 939–943.

Meltzoff, A. N., & Moore, M. K. (1983). Newborn infants imitate adult facial gestures. *Child Development, 54*, 702–9.

Merchant, S. N., McKenna, M. J., Baldwin, C. T., Milunsky, A., & Nadol Jr., J. B. (2001). Otopathology in a case of type I Waardenburg's syndrome. *Annals of Otology, Rhinology & Laryngology, 110*, 875–882.

Mertens, D. M. (1993). A conceptual model for academic achievement. In D. F. Moores & K. P. Meadow-Orleans (Eds.), *Educational and developmental aspects of deafness* (pp. 25–72). Washington, DC: Gallaudet University Press.

Mertens, D. M., Sass-Lehrer, S., & Scott-Olson, K. (2000). Sensitivity in family-professional relationships: Potential experiences of families with young deaf and hard of hearing children. In P. Spencer, C. Erting & M. Marschark (Eds.). *The deaf child in the family and at school.* Mahwah, NJ: Erlbaum Associates.

Miller, F. S., Bunt-Miliam, A. H., & Kalina, R. E. (1982). Clinical-ultrastructural study of thioridazine retinopathy. *Ophthalmology, 89*, 1478.

Miller, L. R., Adrian, R. J., & de L'Auneand, W. R. (1982). Personality assessment of the early visually impaired utilizing the CPI and the MMPI. *International Journal of Rehabilitation Research, 5*, 66–69.

Mitchell, R. E., & Karchmer, M. A. (2002). Chasing the mythical ten percent: Parental hearing status of deaf and hard of hearing students in United States. *Sign Language Studies, 4*, 138–163.

Monsen, R. (1983). The oral speech intelligibility of hearing-impaired talkers. *Journal of Speech and Hearing Research, 48*, 286–296.

Moores, D. (1987). *Educating the deaf: Psychology, principles, and practices* (3rd ed.). Boston: Houghton Mifflin.

Morton, N. E. (1991). Genetic epidemiology of hearing loss. *Annals of the New York Academy of Sciences, 630*, 16–31.

Myklebust, H. R. (1964). *The psychology of deafness: Sensory deprivation, learning, and adjustment.* New York: Grune & Stratton.

Nadol, J. B., & Merchant, S. N. (2001). Histopathology and molecular genetics of hearing loss in the human. *International Journal of Pediatric Otorhinolaryngology, 61*, 1–15.

Nahmias, A. J. (1974). The TORCH complex. *Hospital Practice, May*, 65–72.

Nance, W. E. (1980). The genetic analysis of profound prelingual deafness. *Birth Defects, 16*, 263–269.

Nesker Simmons, J., Davidson, I. F. (1985). Perspectives on intervention with young blind children. *Child: Care, Health and Development, 11*, 183–193.

Neville, H. J., & Lawson, D. S. (1987a). Attention to central and peripheral visual space in a movement detection task: An event-related potential and behavioral study: I. Normal hearing adults. *Brain Research, 405*, 253–267.

Neville, H. J., & Lawson, D. S. (1987b). Attention to central and peripheral visual space in a movement detection task: An event related potential and behavioral study: II. Congenitally deaf adults. *Brain Research, 405*, 268–283.

Neville, H. J., & Lawson, D. S. (1987c). Attention to central and peripheral visual space in a movement decision task: III. Separate effects of auditory deprivation and acquisition of a visual language. *Brain Research, 405*, 284–294.

Nicholls, G. H., & Ling, D. (1982). Cued speech and the reception of spoken language. *Journal of Speech and Hearing Research, 25*, 262–269.

Nielson, N. V., & Syversen, K. (1986). Possible retinotoxic effect of carbamazepine. *American Journal of Ophthalmology 103*, 221.

Noyola, D. E., Demmler, G. J., Nelson, C. T. et al. (2001). Early predictors of neurodevelopmental outcome in symptomatic congenital cytomegalovirus infection. *Journal of Pediatrics, 138*, 325–331.

O'Cleirigh, C. M., McAdam, D. B., & Cuvo, A. J. (1994). Behavioral interventions to reduce stereotypic behaviors of persons with visual impairments: a methodological review and critical analysis. *Progress in Behavior Modification, 29*, 27–52.

Okawa, M., Nanami, T., Wada, S., Shimizu, T., Hishikawa, Y., Sasaki, H., Nagamine, H., & Takahashi, K. (1987). Four congenitally blind children with circadian sleep-wake rhythm disorder. *Sleep 10*, 101–110.

Pace, G. M., Ivancic, M. T., Edwards, G. L., Iwata, B. A., & Page, T. J. (1985). Assessment of stimulus preference and reinforcer value with profoundly retarded individuals. *Journal of Applied Behavior Analysis, 18*, 249–255.

Padden, C. A., & Humphries, T. (1988). *Deaf in america: Voices from a culture.* Cambridge, MA: Harvard University Press.

Padden, C. A., & Ramsey, C. (2000). American Sign Language and reading ability in deaf children. In C. Chamberlain (Ed.), *Language acquisition by eye* (pp. 165–189). Mahwah, NJ: Lawrence Erlbaum Associates.

Parasnis, I., & Samar, V. J. (1985). Parafoveal attention in congenitally deaf and hearing young adults. *Brain and Cognition, 4*, 313–327.

Parasnis, I., Samar, V. J., & Berent, G. P. (2003). Deaf adults without attention deficit hyperactivity disorder display reduced perceptual sensitivity and elevated impulsivity on the Test of Variables of Attention (T.O.V.A.). *Journal of Speech, Language, and Hearing Research, 46*, 1166–1183.

Parasnis, I., Samar, V. J., Bettger, J. G., & Sathe, K. (1996). Does deafness lead to enhancement of visual spatial cognition in children? Negative evidence from deaf nonsigners. *Journal of Deaf Studies & Deaf Education, 1*, 145–152.

Partonen, T, Vakkuri, O., Lamberg-Allardt, C. (1995). Effects of exposure to morning bright light in the blind and sighted controls. *Clinical Physiology 15*, 637–646.

Pass, R. F., Stagno, S., Meyers, G. J., et al. (1980). Outcome of symptomatic congenital cytomegalovirus infection: results of long-term, longitudinal follow-up. *Pediatrics, 66*, 758–762.

Paul, P. V., & Jackson, D. W. (1993). *Toward a psychology of deafness: theoretical and empirical perspectives.* Boston: Allyn and Bacon.

Perez-Pereira, M. (1999). Deixis, personal reference and the use of pronouns by blind children. *Journal of Child Language 26*, 655–680.

Périer, O., Charlier, B., Hage, C., & Alegria, J. (1990). Evaluation of the effects of prolonged cued speech practice upon the reception of spoken language. *Cued Speech Journal, 4*, 39–46.

Peterson, M. B. (2002). Non-syndromic autosomal-dominant deafness. *Clinical Genetics, 62*, 1–13.

Petit, C. (1996). Genes responsible for human hereditary deafness: symphony of a thousand. *Nature Genetics, 14*, 385–391.

Petit, C., & Weil, D. (2001). Deafness. *Encyclopedia of Life Sciences.* Nature Publishing Group. Available at: www.els.net.

Pipp-Siegel, S. (1998). Assessing the quality of relationships between parents and children: The Emotional Availability Scales. *The Volta Review, 100*, 237–249.

Pipp-Siegel, S., Blair, N. L., Deas, A. M., Pressman, L., & Yoshinaga-Itano, C. (1998). Touch and emotional availability in hearing and deaf or hard of hearing toddlers and their hearing mothers. *The Volta Review, 100*, 279–298.

Poizner, H., & Tallal, P. (1987). Temporal processing in Deaf signers. *Brain and Language, 30*, 52–62.

Polat, F. (2003). Factors affecting psychosocial adjustment of deaf students. *Journal of Deaf Studies and Deaf Education, 8*, 325–339.

Powers, A. R., Elliott, R. N., Patterson, D., & Shaw, S. (1995). Family environment and deaf and hard-of-hearing students with mild additional disabilities. *Journal of Childhood Communication Disorders, 17*, 15–19.

Preisler, G. M. (1993). A descriptive study of blind children in nurseries with sighted children. *Child: Care, Health and Development, 19*, 295–315.

Pressman, L., Pipp-Siegel, S., Yoshinaga-Itano, C., Deas, A. M. (1999). Maternal sensitivity predicts language gain in preschool children who are deaf and hard of hearing. *Journal of Deaf Studies and Deaf Education, 4*, 294–304.

Pressman, L., Pipp-Siegel, S., Yoshinaga-Itano, C., Kubicek, L., & Erode, R.N. (1998). A comparison of the links between emotional availability and language gain in young children with and without hearing loss. *The Volta Review, 100*, 251–277.

Proksch, J., & Bavelier, D. (2002). Changes in the spatial distribution of visual attention after early deafness. *Journal of Cognitive Neuroscience, 14*, 687–701.

Quellette, S. (1988). The use of projective drawing techniques in the personality assessment of prelingually deafened young adults: A pilot study. *American Annals of the Deaf, 133*, 212–218.

Rauschecker, J. P., & Korte, M. (1993). Auditory compensation for early blindness in cat cerebral cortex. *Journal of Neuroscience 13*, 4538–4548.

Rauschecker, J. P., & Kniepert, U. (1994). Auditory localization behavior in visually deprived cats. *The European Journal of Neuroscience 6*, 149–160.

Rayson, B. C. (1985). Psychodynamic psychotherapy with deaf clients. In G. B. Anderson, & D. Watson (Eds.), *Counseling deaf people: Research and practice* (pp. 123–144). Little Rock, AR: Arkansas Rehabilitation Research and Training Center on Deafness and Hearing Impairment, University of Arkansas.

Rethy, S., & Rethy-Gal, S. (1984). Decreasing behavioral flexibility (of adjustment to strabismus) as the cause of resistance against treatment during the first year of life. In I. I. Strabismus, R. D. Reinecke (Eds.), (pp. 91–101). New York: Grune and Stratton.

Rettenbach, R., Diller, G., & Sireteanu, R. (1999). Do deaf people see better? Texture segmentation and visual search compensate in adults but not in juvenile subjects. *Journal of Cognitive Neuroscience, 11*, 560–583.

Reynolds, H. N. (1993). Effects of foveal stimulation on peripheral visual processing and laterality in deaf and hearing subjects. *American Journal of Psychology, 106*, 523–540.

Rhine, S. (2002). *Assessment of Executive Function.* Unpublished master's thesis, Gallaudet University, Washington, D.C.

Rincover, A. (1978). Sensory extinction: a procedure for eliminating self-stimulatory behavior in developmentally disabled children. *Journal of Abnormal Psychology, 6*, 299–310.

Roberts, C. R., & Hindley, P. (1999). Practitioner review: The assessment and treatment of deaf children with psychiatric disorders. *Journal of Child Psychology and Psychiatry 40*, 151–167.

Robinson, J., & Fielder, A. R. (1992). Light and the neonatal eye. *Behavioural Brain Research 49*, 51–55.

Rogers, S. J., & Newhart-Larson, S. (1989). Characteristics of infantile autism in five children with Leber's congenital amaurosis. *Developmental Medicine and Child Neurology 31*, 598–608.

Rogers, S. J., & Puchalski, C. B. (1984). Social characteristics of visually impaired infants' play. *Topics in Early Childhood Special Education, 3*, 52–56.

Roizen, N. J. (2003). Nongenetic causes of hearing loss. *Mental Retardation and Developmental Disabilities Research Reviews, 9*, 120–127.

Rosenstein, J. (1960). Cognitive abilities of deaf children. *Journal of Speech and Hearing Research, 3*, 108–119.

Sachdev, P. S. (1989). Blinking-blepharospasm after long-term neuroleptic treatment. *The Medical Journal of Australia 150*, :341.

Sadato, N., Okada, T., Honda, M., & Yonekura, Y. (2002). Critical period for cross-modal plasticity in blind humans: A functional MRI study. *NeuroImage 16*, 389–400.

Sakuma, M. (1975). A comparative study by the behavioral observation for sterotypy in the exceptional children. *Folia Psychiatrica et Neurologica Japonica, 29*, 371–91.

Samar, V. J., Parasnis, I., & Berent, G. P. (1998). Learning disabilities, attention deficit disorders, and deafness. In M. Marschark, & D. Clark (Eds.), *Psychological perspectives on deafness* (Vol. 2, pp. 199–242). Mahwah, NJ: Erlbaum Lawrence Associates.

Samuel, K. A. (1996). The relationship between attachment in deaf adolescents, parental sign communication and attitudes, and psychosocial adjustment. *Dissertation Abstracts International, 57*, 2182B. (UMI No. 9623718).

Sandyk, R (1984). Oculogyric crisis induced by lithium carbonate. *European Neurology 23*, 92.

Sarniguet-Badoche, J. M. (1984). Early medical treatment of strabismus before the age of 18 months. In I. I. Strabismus, & Reinecke, R. D. (Eds.), (pp. 83–89). New York: Grune and Stratton.

Schildroth, A. N., & Hotto, S. A. (1996). Annual survey of deaf and hard-of-hearing children and youth: Changes in student characteristics, 1984–85 and 1994–95. *American Annals of the Deaf, 141*, 68–71.

Schirmer, B. R. (2001). *Psychological, social, and educational dimensions of deafness.* Needham, MA: Allyn & Bacon.

Schlesinger, H. S., & Meadow, K. P. (1972). *Sound and sign: Childhood deafness and mental health.* Berkeley, CA: University of California Press.

Schloss, I. P. (1963). Implications of altering the definition of blindness. Research Bulletin No 3 (pp. 111–116). New York: American Foundation for the Blind.

Schluter, W. W., Reer, S. E., Redd, S. C., Dykewicz, C. A. (1998). Changing epidemiology of congenital rubella syndrome in the United States. *Journal of Infectious Disease, 178*, 636–641.

Semba, R. D., & Bloem, M. W. (2004). Measles blindness. *Survey of Ophthalmology 49*, 243–255.

Serrano, J. M., Iglesias, J., & Loeches, A. (1992). Visual discrimination and recognition of facial expressions of anger, fear, and surprise in 4- to 6-month-old infants. *Developmental Psychobiology, 25*, 411–25.

Simeonsson, R. J., Wax, T.M., & White, K. (2001). Assessment of children who are deaf or hard of hearing. In R. J. Simeonsson & S. L. Rosenthal (Eds.), *Psychological and developmental assessment: Children with disabilities and chronic conditions* (pp. 248–266). New York: Guilford Press.

Sinkkonen, J. (1994). *Hearing Impairment, Communication And Personality Development.* Helsinki: Department of Child Psychiatry, University of Helsinki.

Sireteanu, R., & Rettenbach, R. (2000). Perceptual learning in visual search generalizes over tasks, locations, and eyes. *Vision Research, 40*, 2925–2949.

Sloper, J. J. (1993). Edridge-Green Lecture. Competition and cooperation in visual development. *Eye, 7*, 319–31.

Sonksen, P. M., Petrie, A., Drew, K. J. (1991). Promotion of visual development in severely visually impaired babies. Evaluation of a developmentally based programme. *Developmental Medicine and Child Neurology 33*, 320–335.

Spencer, P. E., & Gutfreund, M. K. (1990). Directiveness in mother-infant interactions. In D. F. Moores & K. P. Meadow-Orlans (Eds.), *Educational and developmental aspects of deafness* (pp. 350–364). Washington, DC: Gallaudet University Press.

Spencer, P. T., Erting, C. J., & Marschark, M. (Eds.) (2000). *The deaf child in the family at school*. Mahwah, NJ: Lawrence Erlbaum Associates.

Stafford, C. A. (1984). Critical period plasticity for visual function: definition in monocularly deprived rats using visually evoked potentials. *Ophthalmic and Physiological Optics, 4*, 95–100.

Stivalet, P., Moreno, Y., & Richard, J., Barraud, P. A., & Raphel, C. (1998). Differences in visual search tasks between congenitally deaf and normally hearing adults. *Cognitive Brain Research, 6*, 227–232.

Sussman, A. E. (1988). Approaches in counseling and psychotherapy revisited. In D. Watson, G. Long, M. Taff-Watson, & M. Harvey (Eds.), *Two decades of excellence 1967–1987: A Foundation for the future* (pp. 2–15). Little Rock, AR: American Deafness and Rehabilitation Association.

Sussman, A. E., & Brauer, B. A. (1999). On being a psychotherapist with deaf clients. In I. W. Leigh (Ed.), *Psychotherapy with deaf clients from diverse groups* (pp. 3–22). Washington, DC: Gallaudet University Press.

Taylor, H. G., Mills, E. L., Ciampi, A., du Berger, R., Watters, G. V., Gold, R., MacDonald, N., & Michaels, R. H. (1990). The sequelae of Haemophilus influenzae meningitis in school age children. *New England Journal of Medicine, 323*, 1657–1663.

Taylor, H. G., Schatschneider, C., Rich, D. (1992). Sequelae of Haemophilus influenzae meningitis: Implications for the study of brain disease and development. In M. Tramontana & S. Hooper (Eds.), *Advances in child neuropsychology*, (Vol. 1, pp. 50—108). New York: Springer-Verlag.

Thiringer, K., Kankhunen, A., Liden, G., & Niklasson, A. (1984). Perinatal risk factors in the etiology of hearing loss in preschool children. *Developmental Medicine and Child Neurology, 26*, 799–807.

Thorn, F., Gwiazda, J., Cruz, A. A. V., Bauer, J. A., & Held, R (1994). The development of eye alignment, convergence, and sensory binocularity in young infants. *Investigative Ophthalmology & Visual Science, 35*, 544–553.

Thorpe, G. L., & Olson, S. L. (1990). *Behavior therapy: Concepts, procedures and applications*. Needham Heights, MA: Ayllon and Bacon.

Twardosz, S. (1985). Setting Events. In A. S., Bellack, and M., Hersen, (Eds.), *Dictionary of behavior therapy techniques*. New York: Pergamon Press.

Tychsen, L. (1994). Development of vision. In S. J., Isenberg, (Ed.), *The eye in infancy*, (2nd ed., pp. 121–130). St. Louis: Mosby.

Ueda, K., Nishida, Y., Oshmia, K., & Shepard, T. H. (1979). Congenital rubella syndrome: Correlation of gestational age at time of maternal rubella with type of defect. *Journal of Pediatrics, 94*, 763–765.

Ungerleider, L. G., & Haxby, J. V. (1994). "What" and "where" in the human brain. *Current Opinion in Neurobiology 4*, 157–165.

Vader, L. A. (1992). Vision and vision loss. *Nursing Clinics of North America, 27*, 705–714.

Valenza, E., Simion, F., Cassia, V. M., & Umilta, C. (1996). Face preference at birth. *Journal of Experimental Psychology: Human Perception and Performance, 22*, 892–903.

Van Hasselt, V. B. (1987). Behavior therapy for visually handicapped persons. *Progress in Behavior Modification, 21*, 13–44.

Van Hasselt, V. B., Hersen, M., & Kazdin, A. E. (1985). Assessment of social skills in visually-handicapped adolescents. *Behaviour Research & Therapy, 23*, 53–63.

Van Hasselt, V. B., Kazdin, A. E., Hersen, M., Simon, J., & Mastantuono, A. K. (1985). A behavioral-analytic model for assessing social skills in blind adolescents. *Behaviour Research & Therapy, 23*, 395–405.

van Hof-van Duin, J., Heersema, D. J., Groenendaal, F., Baerts, W., & Fetter, W. P. F. (1992). Visual field and grating acuity development in low-risk preterm infants during the first 2 1/2 years after term. *Behavioural Brain Researach 49*, 115–122.

Vernon, M., & Andrews, J. F. (1990). *The psychology of deafness: Understanding deaf and hard of hearing people*. New York: Longmans.

Vernon, M., & Brown, D. W. (1964). A guide to psychological tests and testing procedures in the evaluation of deaf and hard-of-hearing children. *Journal of Speech and Hearing Disorders, 29*, 414–423.

Vernon, M., & Diagle-King, B. (1999). Historical overview of inpatient care of mental patients who are deaf. *American Annals of the Deaf, 144*, 51–61.

Vollmer, T. R, Iwata, B. A., Smith, R. G., Rodgers, T. A. (1992). Reduction of multiple aberrant behaviors and concurrent development of self-care skills with differential reinforcement. *Research in Developmental Disabilities, 3*, 287–299.

Vollmer, T. R, Marcus, B. A., & LeBlanc, L. (1994). Treatment of self-injury and hand mouthing following inconclusive functional analysis. *Journal of Applied Behavior Analysis, 2*, 331–344.

Wechsler, D. (1991). WISC-III: *Manual for Wechsler Intelligence Scale for Children* (3rd ed.). San Antonio, TX: Psychological Corporation.

Whitley, R. J., & Hutto, C. (1985). Neonatal herpes simplex virus infections. *Pediatrics Review, 7*, 119–126.

Wiesel, T.N., & Hubel, D.H. (1965). Extent of recovery from the effects of visual deprivation in kittens. *Journal of Neurophysiology 28*, 1060–1072.

Wilson, M., Bettger, J., Niculae, I., & Klima, E. (1997). Modality of language shapes working memory: Evidence form digit span and spatial span in ASL signers. *Journal of Deaf Studies and Deaf Education, 2*, 150–160.

Wohl, J. (1995). Traditional individual psychotherapy with ethnic minorities. In J. F. Aponte, R. Y. Rivers, & J. Wohl (Eds.), *Psychological interventions and cultural diversity* (pp. 74–91).

World Health Organization. (1992). *Prevention of Childhood Blindness* (pp. 2–25). Geneva: World Health Organization.

Movement Disorders

21

Ergun Y. Uc, MD   Robert L. Rodnitzky, MD

BASAL GANGLIA

The basal ganglia are a group of gray matter structures symmetrically placed in a deep paracentral location within the brain. The chief nuclei of the basal ganglia are the striatum and the pallidum (1, 2). The terms "striatum" and "neostriatum" refer to the caudate and putamen. The term "dorsal striatum" refers to most of the caudate and putamen, while the term "ventral striatum" refers to the ventral parts of the caudate and putamen, the nucleus accumbens septi, and the striatal part of the olfactory tubercle. The terms "pallidum" and "paleostriatum" refer to globus pallidus (composed of the globus pallidus interna and globus pallidus externa). The term "corpus striatum" refers to the caudate, putamen, and globus pallidus. The putamen and globus pallidus together compose the "lentiform nucleus." The term "extrapyramidal system" refers to the basal ganglia and an array of subcortical structures and brainstem nuclei (red nucleus, subthalamic nucleus, substantia nigra pars compacta, and substantia nigra pars reticulata, reticular formation, and portions of the ventral tier thalamic nuclei) to which they are connected (Fig. 21.1).

Neurotransmitters in the Basal Ganglia

Dopamine is widely distributed throughout the brain, but over 80% of this neurotransmitter located in the brain is concentrated in the striatum (3). Besides the nigrostriatal pathway, other dopamine-containing pathways include the mesolimbic (from the medial portion of the substantia nigra pars compacta and ventral tegmental area to the ventral striatum, rostral caudate nucleus, the olfactory tubercle, and the amygdaloid nucleus), the mesocortical (from the medial portion of the substantia nigra pars compacta and ventral tegmental area to the prefrontal and the cingulate cortex), the tuberoinfundibular, and the hypothalamospinal pathways.

Five distinct receptors for dopamine (D1 to D5) have been cloned (3). The D1 family is composed of D1 and D5 receptors, and the D2 family of D2, D3, and D4 receptors. The various dopamine receptor subtypes are distributed in different parts of the brain and subserve distinct functions (Table 21.1). The D1 and D2 receptors are found mainly in the striatum and mediate dopamine signals involved in motor control. Presynaptic dopamine receptors, known as autoreceptors, are of the D2 subtype and provide feedback inhibition of dopamine synthesis and dopaminergic neuron firing when stimulated by the release of the neurotransmitter from the presynaptic nerve terminal. The D3 receptors are abundant in limbic connections. The D4 receptors are also found in the frontal cortex and seem to play a role in behavior. The atypical antipsychotic clozapine blocks D4 receptors but has low affinity for D2 receptors, accounting for its very low potential to cause parkinsonism. D5 receptors are located throughout the cortex, thalamus, and striatum.

Glutamate is the predominant excitatory neurotransmitter of the basal ganglia. The main output pathways of the basal ganglia involve gamma-aminobutyric acid (GABA). Acetylcholine is present in the striatal interneurons. There are also noradrenergic inputs from the locus coeruleus and serotonergic inputs from the raphe nucleus to the basal ganglia. Many more neuropeptides and neuromodulators, whose functions are largely unknown, are found in the basal ganglia (3).

Functional Anatomy

Frontal-subcortical circuits mediate motor activity, eye movements, cognition, behavior, and limbic function (4). Their interconnections represent parallel reentrant circuits that convey information from different regions of the cortex, through the basal ganglia and then via the thalamus back to the cortex. These circuits have been named according to their

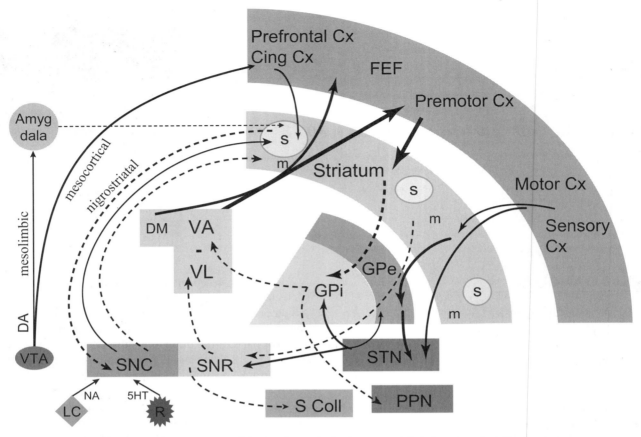

Figure 21.1 The interaction of the basal ganglia, brainstem nuclei, thalamus, and cerebral cortex. DA, dopamine; SNC(R), substantia nigra pars compacta (reticulata); GPE(I), globus pallidus externa (interna); STN, subthalamic nucleus; CM, centromedian; PF, parafascicular; VL(A), ventral lateral (anterior) nuclei of thalamus, SC, superior colliculus; s, striosome; m, matrix; DA, dopamine; 5HT, serotonine; NA, noradrenaline; LC, locus ceruleus; RN, Raphe nucleus; VTA, ventral tegmental area; Cing, cingulate; cx, cortex. Dash arrows represent inhibitory (GABAergic) pathways, solid arrows excitatory (glutamatergic) pathways.

function or cortical site of origin: the motor circuit, the oculomotor circuit originating in the frontal eye fields, the dorsolateral prefrontal and lateral orbitofrontal (cognition and behavior), and anterior cingulate (limbic) circuits (Fig. 21.2). Within these circuits, information flows through two parallel (direct and indirect) pathways whose balance of activity is critical for normal function. The putamen is the predominant striatal structure for the motor circuit; caudate for the oculomotor, dorsolateral prefrontal, and lateral orbitofrontal circuits; and the ventral striatum for the limbic circuit. The striatum can be further subdivided into neurochemically distinct compartments known as striosomes and

TABLE 21.1
DOPAMINE RECEPTORS

	D1 Family		D2 Family		
	D1	**D5**	**D2**	**D3**	**D4**
Effector pathways	↑ cAMP	↑ cAMP	↓ cAMP	↓ cAMP	↓ cAMP
Channel			↑ K$^+$, ↓ Ca^{2+}	↑ K$^+$	
mRNA distribution	Caudate, putamen, nuc. accumbens, olfactory tubercle	Hypothalamus, hypocampus	Caudate, putamen, nuc, accumbens, olfactory tubercle	Hypothalamus, nuc. accumbens, olfactory tubercle	Frontal cordex, medulla, midbrain
Chromosome	5	4	11	3	11

Source: Modified from Kuhar et al., *Basic Neurochemistry*, 6th ed. Philadelphia, PA: Lippincott Williams & Wilkins, 1999.

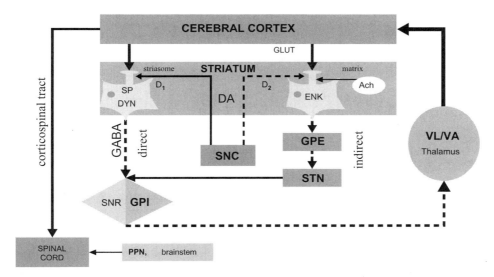

Figure 21.2 The motor frontal-subcortical circuit. SNC(R), substantia nigra pars compacta (reticulata); GPE(I), globus pallidus externa (interna); STN, subthalamic nucleus; VL(A), ventral lateral (anterior) nuclei of thalamus; DA, dopamine; D₁ (D₂), dopamine receptor type; GLU, glutamate; GABA, gamma-aminobutyric acid; Ach, acetylcholine; DYN, dynorphin; SP, substance P; ENK, enkephalin. Dash arrows represent inhibitory (GABAergic) pathways, solid arrows excitatory (glutamatergic) pathways.

matrix (1, 2). Striosomes form branched three-dimensional labyrinths that constitute only 10 to 20% of the striatum and are mainly present in the head of the caudate. They stain for acetylcholinesterase and have higher levels of mu opiod receptors, D1 dopamine receptors, and the neuropeptides Substance P and dynorphin. Striosomal neurons communicate with substantia nigra pars compacta and the limbic regions. The matrix, on the other hand, gives rise to the direct and indirect striatal output pathways and receives corticostriatal inputs from sensory cortices, motor and premotor areas, and association cortex as well as thalamic input.

The frontal-subcortical motor circuit (Fig. 21.3) originates in primary motor, supplementary motor, and primary sensory cortices. The excitatory glutamatergic corticostriatal pathway mainly terminates on the heads of the dendritic spines of the medium spiny neurons, whereas the dense dopaminergic input from the substantia nigra pars compacta terminates principally on the shafts of the spines, thus modulating the effect of cortical inputs. The medium spiny neurons constitute about 95% of the striatal neurons and send GABAergic projections to globus pallidus externa and globus pallidus interna/substantia nigra pars reticulata. The remaining striatal neurons (interneurons) are restricted to the striatum and include large aspiny cholinergic cells, among others. The cholinergic interneurons in the striatum synapse on the soma and the shafts of the dendrites of the medium spiny neurons and exert an opposite effect to dopamine in terms of modulation of the glutamatergic corticostriatal input, which probably constitutes the basis of anticholinergic treatment in Parkinson's disease. The neurons projecting to the globus pallidus interna/substantia nigra pars reticulata (*direct*

pathway) express Substance P and dynorphin and predominantly have D1 receptors, which activate the synthesis of cyclic adenosine monophosphate when stimulated by dopamine. Thus, stimulation of D1 receptors is "excitatory" and increases the inhibitory output to the globus pallidus interna/substantia nigra pars reticulata. The *indirect* pathway originates from the medium spiny neurons that express the neuropeptide enkephalin and have a preponderance of D2 receptors, which are "inhibitory." This pathway is completed by an inhibitory GABAergic projection from the globus pallidus externa to the subthalamic nucleus, and an excitatory, glutamatergic projection from the subthalamic nucleus to the globus pallidus interna/substantia nigra pars reticulata. Thus, dopamine stimulation of the indirect pathway leads to a reduction in the excitatory drive from the subthalamic nucleus to the globus pallidus interna/substantia nigra pars reticulata through double inhibition. Dopaminergic stimulation provides a positive feedback for cortically initiated movements via the direct pathway and a negative feedback for undesired movement. The relative balance of activity in the direct and indirect pathways regulates the inhibitory output from globus pallidus interna/substantia nigra pars reticulata to the ventral thalamus. Thus, one important mechanism by which the basal ganglia exert motor control is by determining the level of excitatory activity of the thalamus on the motor cortex at the origin of the pyramidal (corticospinal) system.

Despite its highly simplified nature and its serious shortcomings, this model of basal ganglia function (5) has fostered the formulation of hypotheses for the study of movement disorders and provided an important rationale

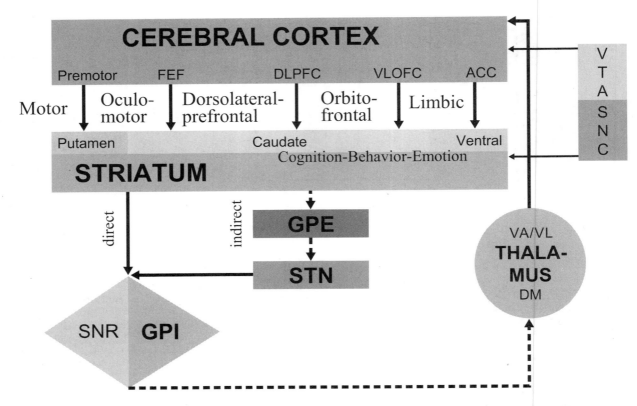

FRONTAL-SUBCORTICAL CIRCUITS (BASAL GANGLIA LOOPS)

Figure 21.3 Basal ganglia loops. DA, dopamine; SNC(R), substantia nigra pars compacta (reticulata); GPE(I), globus pallidus externa (interna); STN, subthalamic nucleus; CM, centromedian; PF, parafascicular; VL(A), ventral lateral (anterior) nuclei of thalamus; SC, superior colliculus; s, striosome; m, matrix; DA, dopamine; 5HT, serotonine; NA, noradrenaline; LC, locus ceruleus; RN, Raphe nucleus; VTA, ventral tegmental area; Cing, cingulate; cx, cortex. Dash arrows represent inhibitory (GABAergic) pathways, solid arrows excitatory (glutamatergic) pathways.

for the successful revival of surgical treatment for Parkinson's disease. In Parkinson's disease, loss of dopaminergic innervation of the striatum decreases the activity of the direct pathway, reducing the inhibition of the globus pallidus pars interna and substantia nigra pars reticulata. At the same time, activity in the indirect pathway is augmented, leading to increased excitatory input to the globus pallidus pars interna/substantia nigra pars reticulata from subthalamic nucleus. Together, these effects produce strong inhibition of the ventral thalamus and reduced excitation of motor cortex. As predicted by this model, surgical procedures that impair the function of globus pallidus pars interna and subthalamic nucleus improve parkinsonian symptoms such as bradykinesia and rigidity. Pathologic lesions of the subthalamic nucleus such as an infarction markedly increase motor activity, leading to ballismus, while surgical intervention in this structure utilizing deep brain stimulation seldom results in this abnormal movement. In adult-onset Huntington's disease, the enkephalinergic striatal projection neurons are more vulnerable to degeneration, causing severe impairment of the indirect pathway, with relative preservation of the direct pathway. This leads to unopposed inhibition of globus pallidus pars

interna/substantia nigra pars reticulata and increased motor output, a possible basis for chorea.

With regard to psychiatric disorders, such as Tourette's syndrome, obsessive-compulsive disorder (OCD), schizophrenia, and attention deficit hyperactivity disorder (ADHD) (6), dysfunction of the basal ganglia leads to a disruption of cognitive control and impaired inhibition of competing inappropriate thoughts and behaviors. OCD is thought to be associated with abnormal activation of striosomes, the compartment that is preferentially connected with the orbitofrontal and anterior cingulate cortex (7).

HYPOKINETIC MOVEMENT DISORDERS

Juvenile Parkinsonism

Juvenile parkinsonism, a heterogeneous entity, is clinically and pathologically distinct from young-onset Parkinson's disease (8). In addition to cardinal features of parkinsonism (rest tremor, bradykinesia, rigidity), many patients with juvenile parkinsonism have one or more atypical features including opthalmoparesis, seizures, and dementia leading to a diagnosis of one of the childhood encephalopathies. Some have identifiable causes such as drug toxicity, encephalitis, or tumors leading to the diagnosis of secondary parkinsonism. The secondary and hereditary/metabolic causes of juvenile parkinsonism show great overlap with childhood dystonias (Table 21.2).

Mutations of the parkin gene on chromosome 6q25–27, which codes for a ubiquitin ligase, are the most common cause of autosomal recessive juvenile parkinsonism across many different ethnic groups (9). In autosomal recessive juvenile parkinsonism related to the parkin mutations, classic parkinsonism is usually accompanied by foot dystonia, hyperreflexia, a good response to levodopa, and the early appearance of levodopa-induced dyskinesias (9). Lewy bodies are generally absent in this disorder. In chil-

dren and adolescents, autosomal recessive juvenile parkinsonism associated with the parkin mutation, self-mutilation, anorexia nervosa, depression, and suicidality has been described (13).

A mutation on the DJ-1 gene has been identified as another cause of autosomal recessive parkinsonism, albeit with a slightly older age of onset (10). Anxiety disorder is commonly associated with this form of parkinsonism (11).

The treatment of juvenile parkinsonism, similar to that used for idiopathic Parkinson's disease, is predominantly centered on preparations of levodopa combined with a peripheral DOPA decarboxylase inhibitor such as carbidopa or benzeraside to increase bioavailability and decrease peripheral side effects. Adjunctive therapies include catecholamine-O-methyl transferase (COMT) inhibitors

TABLE 21.2
ETIOLOGIC CLASSIFICATION OF DYSTONIA

1. Primary (Idiopathic)

a. *DYT1 dystonia:* Oppenheim's dystonia, dystonia musculorum deformans
b. *Other DYT dystonias*
c. *Sporadic:* Usually adult-onset and focal

2. Dystonia Plus

a. Dystonia with parkinsonism
  i. Dopa-responsive dystonia (DYT5)
  ii. Dopamine agonist-responsive dystonia
  iii. Rapid-onset dystonia-parkinsonism (DYT12)
b. Myoclonus-dystonia syndrome (DYT11)

3. Secondary Dystonia

a. *Drug-induced:* Neuroleptic induced (acute, tardive), anticonvulsants, levodopa
b. *Toxic:* Manganese, carbon monoxide, carbon disulfide, cyanide, methanol, 3-nitroproprionic acid
c. *Infectious:* Viral encephalitis, postinfectious, Reye's syndrome, subacute sclerosing leukoencephalopathy, wasp sting encephalopathy, HIV
d. *Focal central nervous system lesions:* Trauma, stroke, arteriovenous malformation, tumor affecting the basal ganglia, thalamus, cortex, brainstem or spinal cord
e. *Physical causes:* Hypoxia, perinatal cerebral injury, electric shock, peripheral injury
f. *Autoimmune:* Multiple sclerosis, antiphospholipid syndrome, Sjogren syndrome
g. *Metabolic:* Hypoparathyroidism
h. *Psychogenic*

4. Heredodegenerative Disorders

a. *Autosomal dominant:* Juvenile Parkinson's disease, Huntington's disease (Westfahl variant), Machado-Joseph disease (SCA3), Dentatorubro-pallidoluysian atrophy, other spinocerebellar degenerations
b. *Autosomal recessive:* Wilson's disease, Niemann-Pick type C, juvenile neuronal ceroid-lipofuscinosis (Batten's disease), GM1 and GM2 gangliosidosis, metachromatic leukodystrophy, Lesch-Nyhan syndrome, homocystinuria, glutaric acidemia, Hartnup's disease, ataxia telangiectasia, aeurodegeneration with iron accumulation (formerly Hallervorden-Spatz syndrome), neuroacanthocytosis
c. *X-linked recessive:* Lubag (dystonia-parkinsonism), deafness-dystonia syndrome (Mohr-Tranebjaerg syndrome)
d. *X-linked dominant:* Rett's syndrome
e. *Mitochondrial:* Leigh's disease, Leber's disease, deafness-dystonia-retardation-blindness syndrome

such as entacapone to prolong the effect of levodopa, dopamine agonists such as pramipexole, ropinirole, pergolide, or bromocriptine, anticholinergics (benztropine mesylate or trihexyphenydil) MAO-B inhibitors such as selegiline, and amantadine, an adenosine 2B type glutamate receptor inhibitor. In many instances, initial therapy with an agonist rather than levodopa is used in this patient group to forestall the development of dyskinesias and offer the putative benefit of neuroprotection (12). Some patients with parkin-related juvenile parkinsonism are remarkably responsive to anticholinergic drugs (13).

HYPERKINETIC MOVEMENT DISORDERS

Tremor

Tremor is a rhythmic, alternating movement of a body part. It can be described by its frequency and amplitude, as well as by the circumstances under which it occurs. Resting tremor (e.g., Parkinson's disease) occurs in a body part in complete repose, postural tremor when the involved body part is being maintained in position against gravity (e.g., essential tremor, enhanced physiologic tremor), and kinetic tremor when the affected limb or body part is in motion (e.g., essential tremor, cerebellar tremor). When a single position or a specific activity causes tremor, the terms "position-specific" and "task-specific" tremor are used.

Physiologic Tremor

Physiologic tremor is present in all individuals at all ages but under normal circumstances it is not apparent and is not associated with disability. Circumstances such as anxiety, fatigue, hypoglycemia, hyperthyroidism, alcohol withdrawal, or drug effects (e.g., adrenergic agents, stimulants) can result in enhanced physiologic tremor, which is clearly visible and potentially disabling.

Essential Tremor

Essential tremor, an autosomal dominant trait, is the most common movement disorder seen in clinical practice. No structural or cellular abnormalities responsible for essential tremor have been identified, but functional imaging studies suggest increased reverberations in the olivocerebellar circuits that can be enhanced or suppressed by reflex pathways. Approximately 5% of all new essential tremor cases arise during the first two decades of life, as early as age 2 years. Most cases emerge during late childhood and adolescence with a male predominance (14). It virtually always presents with a gradual onset, postural, distal upper extremity 4 to 12 Hz tremor and may occasionally affect the head or the voice.

Essential tremor should be treated when it results in functional disability or social embarrassment. In most cases of childhood essential tremor, no pharmacologic

therapy is recommended (14), in part because of the side effect profile of antitremor medications and their modest efficacy in most cases. Primidone and propranolol are the two first-line drugs in the treatment of essential tremor. Benzodiazepines and gabapentin offer a modest benefit, and topiramate has shown some promise for this condition (15). Drug-resistant essential tremor in adults can be treated with surgical interventions including thalamotomy and thalamic deep brain stimulation of the ventral intermediate nucleus of the thalamus. Thalamic deep brain stimulation has been successfully performed in children for indications such as severe chorea or dystonia, but to our knowledge it has not been performed in the pediatric age group for essential tremor.

Dystonia

Dystonia is a sustained abnormal movement that is much slower than chorea and often has a twisting appearance due to abnormal cocontraction of agonist and antagonist muscles. When severe or chronic, dystonia may lead to a relatively fixed position of the involved body parts, resulting in a characteristic posture. When patients voluntarily attempt to move the involved part in the direction opposite to a dystonic movement, a rhythmic or arrhythmic oscillation may develop during this "tug of war" resulting in a dystonic tremor. Dystonia that is worsened during attempted voluntary movement is referred to as action dystonia. Dystonia can be described by the body parts or regions that are involved. Focal dystonia refers to the involvement of an isolated body part such as a hand, while segmental dystonia implies that adjacent body parts such as the neck and arm are affected, and generalized dystonia indicates involvement of limbs bilaterally or one limb and a nonadjacent body part.

Dystonic movements increase with fatigue and stress and improve with relaxation, hypnosis, and sleep. Most patients discover that they can reduce dystonic muscle contractions by using tactile or proprioceptive stimuli such as touching the involved or an adjacent body part. These maneuvers are known as "sensory tricks."

Some children and adolescents may experience a sudden marked increase in the severity of dystonia, which can lead to rhabdomyolysis and myoglobinuria. These episodes are known as a dystonic storm or status dystonicus and require treatment in an intensive care unit due to the risk of renal failure and death (16).

A detailed etiological classication of dystonia is presented in Table 21.2. In primary (idiopathic) dystonia, there are no other systemic and neurologic abnormalities except for tremor, and there is no identifiable exogenous cause or other inherited/degenerative disease. In dystonia-plus, other neurologic signs such as parkinsonism or myoclonus may occur; however, these disorders are of neurochemical nature and unassociated with apparent neurodegeneration. Secondary dystonia is due to acquired/exogenous causes. Heredodegenerative disorders are caused by a genetic abnormality and are typically associated with morphological brain changes.

Primary dystonia results from a functional disturbance of the basal ganglia, particularly in the striatal control of the globus pallidus (and substantia nigra pars reticulata), causing altered thalamic control of cortical motor planning and executive function, as well as abnormal regulation of brainstem and spinal cord inhibitory interneuronal mechanisms (17).

In a child with typical primary dystonia, diagnostic evaluation can be started with DYT1 DNA testing after genetic counseling is obtained, followed by a levodopa trial if DYT1 is ruled out. If the patient does not respond to levodopa, serum ceruloplasmin and slit-lamp examination for Keyser-Fleischer ring should be obtained to rule out Wilson's disease. If history and examination suggest a structural lesion, neuroimaging with brain magnetic resonance imaging (MRI) should be obtained. If history and examination suggest other metabolic or inherited disorders, genetic testing, lactate/pyruvate, serum and urinary amino acids in, urine organic acids, cerebrospinal fluid analysis, electromyography/nerve conduction velocities, electroencephalogram, red blood cell smear for acanthocytes, antiphospholipid antibody, lysosomal analysis, alpha-fetoprotein, biopsies of skin, muscle, nerve, or bone marrow should be considered as guided by the clinical clues.

DYT1 Dystonia

DYT1 dystonia (primary torsion dystonia, dystonia musculorum deformans, Oppenheim's dystonia) is an autosomal dominant disease with a penetrance rate of 30 to 40%. A guanine-adenine-guanine (GAG) deletion in the gene coding for Torsin A, a protein of unknown function, on chromosome 9q34, accounts for ~90% of childhood-onset limb dystonia in those of Ashkenazi Jewish descent and approximately 40 to 60% of early-onset limb dystonia in the non-Jewish population (18).

DYT1 dystonia starts at a relatively young age, with an average age of onset around 12 years. In the great majority of cases, the disorder affects a limb first, but craniocervical or axial onset may also be the initial sign. Cases with lower extremity onset usually present at a younger age and, over time, tend to generalize (16). Psychiatric disorders have been reported to be associated with DYT1, particularly major depressive disorder. Heiman et al. reported on a large sample of individuals with the DYT1 mutation, contrasting manifesting carriers, symptomatic carriers, and noncarriers. In comparison to noncarriers (who shared many of the same environmental and psychosocial factors) the risk for recurrent major depression was three times as high in carriers, regardless of whether they had motor signs or not. The increased risk was quite specific for recurrent major depressive disorder, and did not include other affective disorders such as bipolar disorder, single episode major depressive disorder, or any combination of mood disorders (16a). Carriers of the DYT1 gene also have subtle deficits in learn-

ing sequences, although they do not differ from controls in terms of motor accuracy or timing. Positron emission tomograpy (PET) study revealed increased activation in the left premotor cortex and right supplementary motor area, with reduction in the posterior medial cerebellum(16b).

Dystonia-Plus Syndromes

Dopa-Responsive Dystonia (DYT5)

Dopa-responsive dystonia presents in mid-childhood with dystonia affecting the gait, hyperreflexia, and parkinsonism signs (19) that show a dramatic and sustained response to low-dosage levodopa without emergence of motor fluctuations (16). Patients progressively worsen throughout the day, becoming more dystonic and parkinsonian by evening, but improve the next morning after overnight sleep. Dopa-responsive dystonia is an autosomal disorder with marked phenotypic heterogeneity (20), affecting females more than males with gender-related incomplete penetrance.

Mutations in the guanosine triphosphate (GTP) cyclohydrolase I gene on chromosome 14q22.1–q22.2 that codes for a cofactor of tyrosine hydroxylase account for many cases of dopa-responsive dystonia (21). These mutations are heterogeneous and may also affect other genes involved in dopamine synthesis (22). Approximately 40 to 50% of patients with Dopa-responsive dystonia have no known mutations (23).

Aromatic L-amino acid decarboxylase deficiency, also known as dopamine agonist-responsive dystonia, is characterized by reduced metabolism of 3,4-dihydroxyphenylalanine (DOPA) to dopamine and 5-hydroxytryptophan to serotonin (24). This autosomal recessive disorder begins in infancy with dystonia-parkinsonism, hypotonia, hyperhidrosis, miosis, and ptosis, as well as episodes of oculogyria and paroxysmal movements. Diurnal fluctuations with sleep benefit is present in 50% of cases.

Myoclonus-Dystonia Syndrome (DYT11)

Autosomal dominant myoclonus-dystonia syndrome, perhaps the same disorder as essential myoclonus (25), is caused by mutations in the ε-sarcoglycan gene on chromosome 7q21 (26). It may start at any age and primarily affects the upper body with alcohol-responsive myoclonus. It progresses slowly and then tends to plateau (25). There is also a sporadic form of this condition that is not associated with mutations in the ε-sarcoglycan gene (27).

Rapid-Onset Dystonia-Parkinsonism (DYT12)

Rapid-onset dystonia-parkinsonism is an autosomal dominant disorder mapped to chromosome 19q13 (28) and characterized by sudden onset of dystonia and parkinsonism during adolescence or early adulthood. The symptoms evolve over hours or days and generally stabilize within a few weeks, with slow or no subsequent progression. There is little or no response to levodopa. The concentration of homovanillic acid in the cerebrospinal fluid is low in patients with rapid-onset dystonia-parkinsonism and in some carriers (29), but PET studies indicate no loss of presynaptic dopaminergic nerve terminals (30).

Heredodegenerative Dystonia

Niemann-Pick Type C

Niemann-Pick type C (juvenile dystonic lipidosis) is a rare neurovisceral disorder that is clinically and genetically heterogeneous (31). The disorder typically presents in late childhood and culminates in death in the second decade, but some cases start in the neonatal period and some with adult-onset have been reported. Characteristic clinical signs are hepatosplenomegaly and vertical supranuclear gaze palsy, usually accompanied by neonatal jaundice, dystonia, ataxia, or seizures. Foam cells in the bone marrow are characteristic but not pathognomonic. A decreased rate of cholesterol esterification in skin fibroblasts and abundant staining of free, lysosomal cholesterol by filipin are diagnostic (32). The translocation of low-density lipoprotein-derived cholesterol from lysosomes to the endoplasmic reticulum and the Golgi apparatus is impaired due to mutations in the Niemann-Pick type C1 gene on chromosome 18q11–12, which codes for a transmembrane pump (33) in the vast majority of cases. Mutations in the Niemann-Pick type C2 gene encoding for a lysosomal protein (HE2) with cholesterol-binding properties (34) account for the rest. Niemann-Pick type C1 and Niemann-Pick type C2 cannot be differentiated clinically or histochemically.

Mitochondrial Disorders

Leigh syndrome is caused by defects in mitochondrial respiratory chain enzymes such as cytochrome C oxidase (COX), pyruvate dehydrogenase complex, Complex I, Complex II, and biotinidase (35, 36). It presents during childhood or early adolescence and causes widespread neurological dysfunction, including ataxia, spasticity, optic atrophy, developmental delay, psychomotor retardation, and psychiatric manifestations. Dystonia, although rarely a presenting sign, is the most common (86%) movement disorder, followed by parkinsonism, tremor, chorea, athetosis, myoclonus, and tics (37, 38). The diagnosis is supported by serum lactic acidosis and necrotic lesions in the basal ganglia on neuroimaging studies (38). Ragged red fibers on muscle biopsy, mutations on mitochondrial DNA analysis, defective oxidative phosphorylation on phosphorus magnetic resonance spectroscopy of muscle, and elevated cerebrospinal fluid lactate are useful ancillary tests. There is no specific treatment.

Amino Acid Disorders

Glutaric acidemia, type I (39), is an autosomal recessive condition caused by deficiency of glutaryl-CoA dehydrogenase (GCDH). The gene, glutaryl-CoA dehydrogenase has been mapped to 19p13.2 (39a).

It usually presents at some point between age 6 and 18 months with hypotonia and associated loss of head control, followed by progressive dystonia (opisthotonic posturing, facial grimacing, tongue thrusting, and limb dys-

tonia) with relative preservation of intellect. Macrocephaly is a common finding. Metabolic stress such as fever and viral illness may lead to a dystonic storm that may be accompanied by encephalopathy and ketosis. The encephalopathy results in striatal necrosis primarily affecting medium spiny neurons (39b). Glutaric acid concentration is increased in the blood, urine, and CSF. The presence of 3-hydroxyglutaric acid in urine is a unique finding. Deficient glutaryl-CoA dehydrogenase activity in cultured skin fibroblasts confirms the diagnosis. Dietary restriction of glutarigenic amino acids (lysine, tryptophan, and hydroxylysine), L-carnitine, and riboflavin is recommended as a therapeutic measure. Propionic acidemia (40) and methylmalonic acidemia may also cause similar basal ganglia dysfunction and dystonia or chorea (41).

Secondary Dystonia

Acute Dystonic Reactions

Acute dystonic reactions typically involve the muscles of the mouth, face, eyes, and neck with resultant combinations of retrocollis, trismus, tongue protrusion, and upward or lateral deviation of the eyes. They occur after exposure to dopamine receptor blocking agents including neuroleptic agents such as haloperidol and antiemetic agents such as prochlorperazine. Acute dystonic reactions occur in over 50% of cases within the first day after exposure to dopamine receptor blocking agents and approximately 90% within 5 days (42). The atypical neuroleptic agents are generally associated with a lower incidence of acute dystonic reactions. Risk factors include young age, male gender, a primary psychotic disorder, and prior dystonic reactions. The risk of acute dystonic reactions may be greater after administration of very potent dopamine receptor blocking agents such as haloperidol or discontinuance of a concurrently administered anticholinergic drug.

The treatment of acute dystonic reactions is parenteral intravenous diphenhydramine or benztropine. A second-line, but usually effective therapy is intravenous diazepam. The impressive immediate response to these therapies helps confirm the diagnosis as well. After acute resolution of symptoms, it is wise to continue oral anticholinergic agents for 2 weeks, especially if a long-acting dopamine receptor blocking agent was used or if dopamine receptor blocking agent therapy will need to be continued.

Posttraumatic Dystonia

Dystonia can occur after significant craniocerebral trauma resulting in thalamic or basal ganglia lesions (16, 43). Dystonia can appear after head trauma within a few days of the insult, but is more commonly delayed, sometimes as long as several years. Once established, the dystonic movements may progress over a period of years. Injury at a young age is associated with a longer latency to onset of subsequent movement disorder, a greater tendency to development of generalized dystonia, and a greater probability of altered handedness, perhaps due to age-related neuroplasticity

(43). The delayed appearance of dystonia can be due to resolution of hemiparesis or aberrant neural connections. Focal dystonia and hemidystonia are the most common clinical patterns seen in these patients.

Treatment of Dystonia

The symptomatic treatment of dystonia is often difficult and characterized by incomplete responses. Dystonia may be greatly improved by the treatment of specific underlying causes such as the dramatic response of dopamine responsive dystonia to low doses of levodopa. In this regard, a trial of levodopa is recommended for all children with primary dystonia. The anticholinergic medication trihexyphenidyl has been used with good success in some patients with dystonia, but high doses (30 to 60 mg/day or more) are often required to obtain maximum benefit (44). The most common side effects are dry mouth, constipation, decreased concentration, and blurred vision. If there is inadequate benefit from levodopa or trihexyphenidyl, baclofen alone or in combination with trihexyphenidyl may be beneficial (45). The most common side effect of baclofen is sedation. Benzodiazepines may also be beneficial, but often the benefit is limited by side effects or tolerance. Botulinum toxin injections may be highly effective, especially if impairment or disability is attributable to a few muscle groups. An intrathecal baclofen pump can be tried for severe primary or secondary dystonia that is refractory to medications. However, success is not universal, there are potentially serious side effects, and maintenance can be difficult (46). Stereotaxic surgery (pallidotomy or pallidal deep brain stimulation) has been used with increasing success for a select group of patients, especially those with primary dystonia (47–49), but it should still be considered investigational (50). Some patients with secondary dystonia may be more responsive to thalamic stimulation (51).

Chorea

Chorea is characterized by arrhythmic, nonstereotypic, rapid and distally predominant flinging movements that randomly flow from one body part to another. In pure chorea, there is no sustained quality to any of these rapid movements, as is usually the case in Sydenham's chorea. In other forms of chorea, such as that often seen in Huntington's disease or levodopa-induced dyskinesia, there is a slower, slightly sustained component to the movement, described as choreoathetosis. When this slowing results in still more prominent sustained postures superimposed on chorea, the term "choreodystonia" is used. Ballism is considered by most authorities to be a severe form of chorea in which larger amplitude movements are seen with a predilection for proximal portions of the limbs. When chorea or ballism involve only one side of the body, the terms "hemichorea" and "hemiballism" are used. Chorea can be caused by disorders of the basal ganglia that are inherited, autoimmune, infectious, metabolic, toxic, traumatic, or neoplastic.

Huntington's Disease

Huntington's disease is an autosomal dominant condition caused by a cytosine-adenine-guanine (CAG) trinucleotide expansion mutation on chromosome 4 in the gene coding for huntington, a protein of unknown function. The Huntington's disease phenotype is not always penetrant for repeat sizes of 36 to 39, but is fully penetrant for alleles with repeats of 40 or more (52). Although Huntington's disease can begin in adolescence or even earlier in childhood, or as late as age 70, most affected individuals begin to manifest clinical signs of the illness during the third or fourth decade of life. Longer repeat lengths appear to correlate with earlier onset and more rapid disease progression (53). The phenomenon of progressively earlier onset in successive generations of affected individuals, known as anticipation, is felt to be due to a further increase in CAG repeat length during meiosis, especially when the gene has been paternally inherited (54), as seen in up to 80% of juvenile-onset Huntington's disease (55).

In addition to chorea, motor impersistence (inability to sustain tongue protrusion or apply a continuous grip to the examiner's fingers) and a dancing-type gait with poor balance are common. With progression of the illness, chorea may become less prominent and be replaced by rigidity and dystonia. Abnormalities of ocular motility including slowed saccades, jerky pursuit, and impaired ability to initiate rapid refixation saccades may also be among the early findings.

Cognitive, behavioral, and psychiatric symptoms including executive dysfunction, irritability, depression, impulsiveness, mania, and psychosis typically appear after the development of motor abnormalities, but on occasion can be the presenting signs (56). CT or MRI scans of the brain typically reveal prominent atrophy of the head of the caudate. The duration of the illness from clinical onset to death is usually between 15 and 20 years.

The earliest cognitive manifestations of Huntington's disease in asymptomatic carriers occurs in deficits in attention, working memory, verbal learning, verbal longterm memory and learning of random associations (56a).

Juvenile Huntington's disease is characterized by the onset of clinical symptoms prior to the age of 20 years. Affected individuals in this age group differ from the adult phenotype in that they more commonly present with an akinetic-rigid syndrome (Westphal variant), have an increased risk of seizures, suffer from learning disabilities, and have rapid progression of disease (57). A child who presented with major depression at age 10 years, which then evolved into severe motor dysfunction at age 14, has been described (57a).

The identification of presymptomatic Huntington's disease carriers by genetic testing is a complex issue with many ethical ramifications. Pre- and posttest psychological and genetic counseling is required for asymptomatic individuals (58). Predictive testing in children under the age of 18 years is almost never recommended.

There is not yet any curative therapy for Huntington's disease. Both the irritability and depression associated with

Huntington's disease are responsive to treatment with selective serotonin reuptake inhibitors. Benzodiazepines may also be useful for irritability. Symptoms of psychosis can be improved with standard neuroleptic agents, but the chronic use of these agents can result in development of tardive dyskinesia or parkinsonism. Atypical neuroleptic drugs with a lower potential for extrapyramidal side effects such as olanzapine (59) or clozapine (60) can also be used. Clozapine must be used with great caution because of its potentially serious complication of agranulocytosis. Mild chorea does not require therapy, but more severe chorea that interferes with motor skills or socialization should be treated using neuroleptics or dopamine-depleting agents. Levodopa or dopamine agonists are useful in treating akinesia and rigidity, but they may exacerbate or uncover chorea. Supportive treatment using physical and speech therapy may help with the management of dysphagia, speech, and gait disorders (61).

Fetal striatal transplantation has not provided clear benefit despite survival of transplanted cells and has been associated with a high incidence of serious complications (62). Coenzyme Q10 demonstrated a trend toward slowing the functional decline in Huntington's disease (63). Caspase inhibitors to prevent the development of the neuronal toxicity associated with the mutant protein are being evaluated (64).

Sydenham's Chorea

Sydenham's chorea typically occurs within 4 to 8 weeks after an episode of Group A beta-hemolytic streptococcal infection. Some have drawn an analogy between this condition and the childhood neurobehavioral disorders collectively termed PANDAS (pediatric autoimmune neuropsychiatric disorders associated with streptococcal infection) (65). Although an autoimmune etiology has not been unequivocally proven, the presence of serum antineuronal antibodies in Sydenham's chorea (66) and the reported success of immunomodulating therapies such as plasma exchange support this notion (67). With the advent of effective antibiotic therapy for streptococcal infections, the incidence of Sydenham's chorea in the United States has declined markedly. Sydenham's chorea typically develops in early childhood with a mean age at onset of 9 years. Carditis is present in a large majority of patients (68), its detection is enhanced by echocardiography (69). The chorea itself is usually bilateral, although asymmetric, and in up to 20% of cases it appears as hemichorea. Other neurologic signs and symptoms include dysarthria, hypotonia, and hypometric saccades. Behavioral abnormalities such as obsessive compulsive symptoms, emotional lability, and personality changes are common and often appear weeks before and occasionally after the onset of chorea. One survey found that 82% of children with Sydenham's chorea met diagnostic criteria for OCD (70). The behavioral and motoric symptoms usually resolve within 9 months, sometimes leaving behind subtle signs of chorea. Up to 50% of patients experience recurrent episodes of chorea, sometimes precipitated by subsequent streptococcal infections, therapy with oral contraceptives, or pregnancy. The reappearance or persistence of the original chorea suggests that an acute attack of Sydenham's chorea can result in irreversible changes in the basal ganglia in some patients (71).

Diagnostic studies are of limited use in evaluating Sydenham's chorea. Evidence of Group A beta-hemolytic streptococcal infection, such as a positive throat culture or an elevated antistreptolysin titer, is not consistently present by the time chorea appears, often several months after the acute infection. Although 10% of patients gave a history of sore throat, group A streptococci were isolated in only 1.4% of patients at the time of chorea onset (72). Anti-DNAse B titers remain elevated for as long as a year and are therefore more likely to be abnormal at the onset of chorea. MRI scans of the brain in Sydenham's chorea demonstrate increased size of the caudate, putamen, and globus pallidus (73) and occasionally show increased signal in the basal ganglia (74). The specificity of antineuronal antibodies for Sydenham's chorea is not proven (75).

No specific therapy is required for mild chorea in this self-limited condition. Valproic acid (76) or carbamazepine (77) may help moderately severe or persistent chorea. For still more severe or refractory chorea, neuroleptic therapy may be required. Pimozide may be the agent of choice because of its more favorable side effect profile in children. When other therapies fail, oral or intravenous corticosteroids, or rarely other immunomodulating therapies such as plasma exchange and Intravenous immunoglobulin, have been used (67). Penicillin remains the most appropriate primary and secondary prophylaxis for recurrent streptococcal infection (78).

Tardive Dyskinesia

Tardive dyskinesia consists of a variety of involuntary movements appearing in a patient currently or recently exposed (usually greater than 3 months) to chronic neuroleptic therapy or another dopamine receptor blocking agent. In addition to classic tardive dyskinesia, children are prone to develop withdrawal dyskinesias when dopamine receptor blocking agent therapy is discontinued. In one of the largest recent series, 5.9% of children receiving antipsychotic therapy with neuroleptics had tardive dyskinesia, and 14.5% of those whose treatment was stopped developed withdrawal dyskinesias (79). Risk factors for developing tardive dyskinesia or withdrawal dyskinesias in children, other than exposure to typical neuroleptics (80), include a high drug dosage, underlying CNS dysfunction, history of extrapyramidal side effects, concurrent anticholinergic use, and rapid antipsychotic dose taper, as well as presence of autism or a history of perinatal complications (81). Withdrawal dyskinesias can appear within a few days to 2 months after dopamine receptor blocking agent withdrawal but most commonly is seen after about 2 weeks. The value of slow dopamine receptor blocking agent taper in avoiding withdrawal dyskinesias is not well established (80, 81). Tardive dyskinesia seems to be rare in patients receiving antipsychotic agents for Tourette's syndrome (82).

The vast majority of children with tardive dyskinesia have involuntary, choreiform movements of the face, lips, tongue, and jaw, often resulting in a typical masticatory pattern, while the extremities or the trunk are involved in less than half of the cases (79, 81). The differential diagnosis of the classical choreic tardive syndrome in children includes Wilson's disease, Sydenham's chorea and chorea gravidarum, systemic lupus, Huntington's disease, hyperthyroidism, and lesion of the subthalamic nucleus or its efferent or afferent connections.

Dopamine receptor hypersensitivity or a shift in the balance of dopamine receptor subtype function (83, 84), as well as a complementary mechanism involving GABA insufficiency in the basal ganglia (85) has been postulated to explain the pathophysiologic basis of tardive dyskinesia.

Early discontinuance of the neuroleptic or reduction to the lowest required dosage is thought to improve the chances for permanent remission and diminished clinical disability (86), but the benefit of this approach has not been proven in controlled trials (87). The chances for improvement after discontinuance of the dopamine receptor blocking agent may be higher in younger patients and in those with a shorter duration of therapy. Total withdrawal of neuroleptics must be balanced against the risk of reemergence of the underlying psychiatric disorder. One option is to change therapy to an atypical neuroleptic such as clozapine or olanzapine that is less likely to induce tardive dyskinesia. These agents can be used either to replace the more typical antipsychotic agent that is required for continued therapy or, in a patient who no longer requires neuroleptic therapy, can be used to simply suppress the dyskinetic movements. In adult patients, suppressive medical therapy with dopamine-depleting agents such as reserpine (88) and tetrabenazine (89) has been tried with some success. Preliminary clinical studies have suggested that thiamine (90), gabapentin (91), branched chain amino acids (92), or vitamin E (93, 94) may be helpful. Although various benzodiazepines have been proposed as therapy for tardive dyskinesia, an extensive literature review indicated that benzodiazepines were not better than placebo (95). Tardive dystonia may respond to anticholinergic therapy; when the cervical muscles are involved, botulinum toxin injections are very effective (96).

Neuroacanthocytosis

Neuroacanthocytosis, previously referred to as choreoacanthocytosis, presents during childhood or any time during adult life, most commonly in the fourth decade, and has an average survival of 10 years after disease onset (97). The gene (VPS13A) has been mapped to chromosome 9q21 (98) and encodes chorein, an evolutionarily conserved protein that is involved in protein sorting. In addition to chorea, dystonia, tics, and parkinsonism can be seen. A characteristic orofaciolingual movement, "feeding dystonia," can sometimes be so profound as to lead to mutilation of the lips and tongue. Other neurologic abnormalities include seizures and a variety of neuropsychiatric symptoms including personality change, impulsivity, executive dysfunction (99), and peripheral neuropathy (100). Peripheral smear reveals spiculated erythrocytes known as acanthocytes, sometimes only seen by scanning electron microscopy (101). Creatine kinase levels are typically elevated and correlate with the generalized muscle atrophy seen in this condition. MRI shows caudate and cortical atrophy, as well as striatal hyperintensity on T2-weighted sequences (102).

Other Genetic Causes of Chorea

Benign hereditary chorea presents in the first decade of life is an isolated, nonprogressive autosomal dominant chorea that is mapped to chromosome 14q (103). Chorea can occasionally be seen in patients with trinucleotide repeat expansion disorders other than Huntington's disease. A subtype of dentatorubropallidoluysian atrophy, an autosomal dominant condition common in Japan but only infrequently observed in the Western Hemisphere, may mimic Huntington's disease (104). Chorea seen in autosomal dominant spinocerebellar ataxia types 1 (105) and 2 (106) is not the predominant neurologic finding. Several conditions, clinically similar to Huntington's disease but genetically distinct, have been identified, consistent with the observation that approximately 1 to 7% of patients with phenotypically classical Huntington's disease do not have expanded CAG repeats in the IT15 gene on chromosome 4p (107).

Chorea Associated With Systematic Illness

Chorea can occur in patients with systematic lupus erythematous or the antiphospholipid syndrome (108). Although chorea associated with antiphospholipid syndrome can occur at any time in life, it is somewhat more likely to appear in childhood. Once thought to be due entirely to vasculitis and ischemia, the finding of striatal hypermetabolism in patients with antiphospholipid syndrome–related chorea and the response of the symptoms to immunosuppressive therapy suggest that this syndrome may be the result of an immune-mediated striatal excitatory effect instead (109).

Hyperthyroidism occasionally causes chorea (110), or even less commonly paroxysmal chorea (111). AIDS can be associated with chorea or hemichorea through a variety of mechanisms, including basal ganglia abscess, HIV encephalopathy, and progressive multifocal leukoencephalopathy (112). Children undergoing cardiac surgery with deep hypothermia and extracorporeal circulation are at risk for developing postoperative chorea that may resolve within a few weeks or persist indefinitely (113).

Ballism

The large amplitude, proximally predominant flinging movements that are characteristic of ballism are felt to exist on a clinical continuum with the smaller amplitude, more distally predominant movements of chorea. The fact that these two different types of abnormal involuntary movements are pathophysiologically related is strengthened by the observation that both may exist in the same individual at the same time, and ballism, as it improves, may evolve into chorea. Structural causes of hemiballism include stroke, multiple sclerosis, abscess, neoplasm, Moyamoya disease, or arteriovenous malformation that affect subthalamic nucleus, or less commonly striatum, thalamus, and cerebral cortex. A host of other pathologies including encephalitis, systemic lupus erythematosus, basal ganglia calcification, nonketotic hyperglycemia, or minor systemic infection in children with static encephalopathy can also result in hemiballism (114, 115). Hemiballism should be treated aggressively using dopamine blocking or depleting drugs, valproic acid, or even thalamic deep brain stimulation (116) to prevent physical injury, extreme exhaustion, or cardiac symptoms.

Myoclonus

Myoclonus is a lightning-like movement produced by a sudden and brief muscle contraction (positive myoclonus) or a muscle inhibition (negative myoclonus) (117). Asterixis is an example of negative myoclonus. Myoclonus can be classified according to its distribution (focal, multifocal, segmental, or generalized), activation characteristics (spontaneous, reflex, or action), temporal profile (continuous or intermittent, rhythmic or arrhythmic), site of origin (cortical, subcortical [brainstem, reticular], spinal, or peripheral), and etiology (physiologic, essential, epileptic, or symptomatic).

Posthypoxic myoclonus, reflex myoclonus seen in neurodegenerative diseases such as neuronal ceroid lipofuscinosis, and epilepsia partialis continua are examples of cortical myoclonus. Subcortical myoclonus is usually generalized and may be associated with an exaggerated startle response (hyperekplexia). Examples of subcortical myoclonus include reticular reflex myoclonus, essential myoclonus, palatal myoclonus, and uremic myoclonus (118). Symptomatic palatal myoclonus usually persists during sleep, whereas essential palatal myoclonus disappears with sleep (119). Essential palatal myoclonus frequently is associated with an ear-clicking sound. Symptomatic palatal myoclonus is often associated with hypertrophy of the inferior olive that develops subsequent to a lesion involving the dentate-olivary pathway in the Guillain-Mollaret triangle (118) with accompanying impairment of cerebellar or brainstem function (119). The differential diagnosis of startle syndromes also includes reticular reflex myoclonus, startle epilepsy, exaggerated startle in Tourette's syndrome, and hereditary hyperekplexia. This latter syndrome is an autosomal dominant disorder of childhood, caused by disinhibition of motor neurons resulting from mutations on chromosome 5 in the gene for the glycine receptor (120), leading to impaired glycine- and GABA (A)-receptor transmission. Clonazepam is the treatment of choice (121). In essential myoclonus, there are no other significant neurological signs or symptoms.

Generalized myoclonus is believed to reflect discharges arising from the brainstem reticular formation. Segmental myoclonus consists of spontaneous and rhythmic (1 to 3 Hz) contractions of several contiguous muscle groups due to discharges from the brainstem or the spinal cord (122). Segmental myoclonus, usually, is symptomatic due to a tumor, demyelinating process, spondylosis, infection, or a degenerative condition (122). An irritative lesion affecting a nerve root or a peripheral nerve may give rise to peripheral myoclonus (123). Hemifacial spasm, an example of this condition, is most frequently attributed to compression of the facial nerve at the root exit zone by an ectatic blood vessel, possibly resulting in ephaptic transmission. It is characterized by involuntary, irregular, clonic, or tonic movements of muscles innervated by the seventh cranial nerve on one side of the face (124).

Physiologic myoclonus (sleep myoclonus, anxiety or exercise-induced muscle jerks, hiccups, and benign infantile myoclonus) is a normal phenomenon that is not associated with disability (125).

The most common causes of epilepsia partialis continua include cortical stroke and Rasmussen's encephalitis, a disorder of childhood or adolescence caused by focal cortical lesion or inflammation, possibly from viral infection (126). Other epileptic myoclonias include childhood myoclonic epilepsies such as juvenile myoclonic epilepsy of Janz, benign familial myoclonic epilepsy, and progressive myoclonic epilepsy (117). The progressive forms of epileptic myoclonus, seizures, and myoclonus may ultimately be accompanied by encephalopathy after time (117).

Symptomatic myoclonus is frequently associated with an identifiable static or progressive encephalopathy, often one of the dementing syndromes (127). The underlying causes include storage diseases, spinocerebellar degeneration, basal ganglia degeneration, degenerative dementias, spongiform encephalopathy, malabsorption syndromes, focal central nervous system lesions, and encephalopathies due to mitochondrial, viral, metabolic, endocrinologic, toxic, traumatic, hypoxic, or paraneoplastic causes (128). The progressive myoclonus epilepsies belong to the category of symptomatic myoclonus. They are clinically characterized by stimulus sensitive myoclonus, epilepsy, and progressive neurologic deterioration in cognitive, motor, and psychiatric domains depending on the etiology (129). Dentatorubropallidoluysian atrophy is a trinucleotide repeat—a CAG repeat expansion in 12p13.31. Mitochondrial encephalomyopathy with ragged red fibers (MERRF) arises from a RNA Lys mutation in mitochondrial DNA. With the exception of these two disorders, the progressive myoclonus epilepsies are mostly autosomal recessive disorders (129). Specific mutations have been identified in Lafora disease (gene for laforin or dual specificity phosphatase on 6q), Unverricht-Lundborg disease (cystatin B in 21q), Jansky-Bielschowsky ceroid lipofuscinoses (CLN2 gene for tripeptidyl peptidase 1 in 11q15), Finnish variant of late infantile ceroid lipofuscinoses (CLN5 gene in 13q), juvenile ceroid lipofuscinoses or Batten disease (CLN3 gene in 16p), a subtype of Batten disease, and infantile ceroid lipofuscinoses of the Haltia-Santavuori type (both caused by mutations in palmitoyl-protein thiosterase gene at 1p) (129). Ramsay Hunt syndrome (dyssynergia cerebellaris myoclonica, progressive myoclonic ataxia) is characterized by combination of ataxia and myoclonus with infrequent seizures and absence of dementia. Its differential diagnosis overlaps with that of progressive myoclonus epilepsies (130). A variety of drugs and toxins can cause myoclonus (131, 132). The most common of these are listed in Table 21.3.

Valproic acid and clonazepam probably improve myoclonus largely via their GABAergic activity (133). Levetiracetam, an agent that increases adenosine metabolism and modulates acetylcholine levels, has shown promising efficacy in the treatment of cortical myoclonus (134) and progressive myoclonus epilepsies (135), possibly by reducing corticospinal excitability at the motor cortex level (136). Posthypoxic myoclonus may respond dramatically to 5-hydroxytryptophan, a direct precursor of serotonin, supporting the serotonin deficiency hypothesis for its etiology (137). Primidone, phenobarbital, diazepam, carbamazepine, baclofen, and phenytoin have also been used for various types of myoclonus (131).

Tics and Tourette's Syndrome

Tourette'syndrome, first characterized in 1885 by George Gilles de la Tourette, is a relatively common, but complex hereditary neurobehavioral disorder of unknown cause. It is characterized by motor and vocal tics starting in childhood that often are accompanied by behavioral problems such as OCD, ADHD, and lack of impulse control (138, 139). The clinical expression is often different in various members of the family (140). Tourette's syndrome is the most common cause of tics and affects males approximately three times as frequently as females. Prevalence estimates range from 0.7 to 4.2% (138).

TABLE 21.3
ETIOLOGICAL CLASSIFICATION OF MYOCLONUS

1. Physiological Myoclonus

Sleep jerks, exercise-induced, hiccough, benign infantile myoclonus

2. Essential Myoclonus

Hereditary (may include myoclonus dystonia syndrome), sporadic

3. Epileptic Myoclonus

  a. **Component of epilepsy:** Isolated epileptic myoclonic jerks, epilepsia partialis continua, photosensitive myoclonus, myoclonic absence
  b. **Myoclonic epilepsies of childhood and adolescense:** Infantile spasms, Lennox-Gastaut syndrome (myoclonic astatic epilepsy), Aicardi's infantile myoclonus epilepsy, Janz's juvenile myoclonus epilepsy, benign familial myoclonic epilepsy
  c. **Progressive myoclonus epilepsy**

4. Symptomatic Myoclonus

  a. **Hereditary:** Progressive myoclonus epilepsy (Lafora body disease, Unverricht-Lundborg disease, neuronal ceroid lipofuscinosis, dentadorubropallidoluysian atrophy), Friedreich's ataxia, ataxia telangiectasia, Wilson's disease, Hallervorden-Spatz disease, Huntington's disease, mitochondrial encephalopathies such as MERRF sialidosis, lipidoses (GM2 gangliosidosis, Tay-Sachs, Krabbe's)
  b. **Neurodegenerative:** Parkinson's disease, Alzheimer's disease, corticobasal ganglionic degeneration, multiple system atrophy, progressive supranuclear palsy, pallidal degenerations
  c. **Acquired:**
    i. *Drugs:* Selective serotonin reuptake inhibitors, tricyclic antidepressants, lithium, levodopa, valproic acid, carbamazepine, phenytoin, morphine
    ii. *Metabolic:* Hepatic failure, renal failure, hypoglycemia, hyponatremia, dialysis syndrome, nonketotic hyperglycemia
    iii. *Toxins:* Bismuth, heavy metals, methyl bromide, DDT
    iv. *Physical encephalopathies:* Posthypoxic (Lance-Adams), posttraumatic, heat stroke, electric shock, decompression injury
    v. *Focal CNS lesions:* Stroke, tumor, trauma, multiple sclerosis affecting the cortex, thalamus, brainstem (palatal myoclonus), or spinal cord (segmental or spinal myoclonus)
    vi. *Infectious:* Viral encephalitis (arbovirus, herpes simplex), subacute sclerosing panencephalitis, Creutzfeldt-Jakob disease, postinfectious
    vii. *Psychogenic*

DDT, dichlorodiphenyltrichloroethane; MERRF, myoclonic epilepsy and ragged red fibers.

Other tic disorders include transient tic disorder, chronic tic disorder, and secondary tics due to an identifiable cause. Both transient tic disorder and chronic tic disorder are idiopathic and typically start before age 18 years (141). Patients with transient tic disorder have single or multiple motor or vocal tics that occur for at least 4 weeks, but for no longer than 12 consecutive months. Patients with chronic tic disorder have single or multiple motor or vocal tics, but not both, that have been present for more than 1 year, during which time there was never a tic-free period of more than 3 consecutive months.

Clinical Features

Tics and Motor Symptoms

Tics, the clinical hallmark of Tourette's syndrome, are sudden, brief, intermittent, involuntary or semivoluntary movements (motor tics) or sounds (phonic or vocal tics) (138). They typically consist of simple or coordinated, repetitive or sequential movements, gestures, and utterances that mimic fragments of normal behavior. Simple motor tics involve a limited number of muscles and can further be classified as clonic (brief, jerking movements such as blinking, nose twitching, or jerking of the head and limbs), dystonic (slow, briefly sustained abnormal postures such as blepharospasm, oculogyric movements, bruxism, torticollis, and shoulder rotation), or tonic (isometric contractions such as tensing of abdominal or limb muscles). Complex motor tics, a sequence of intense and coordinated movements, may resemble normal, purposeful motor acts or gestures that are incorporated into the flow of movement, but with inappropriate timing. Specific examples of complex motor tics include obscene gestures (copropraxia) or imitation of movements of others (echopraxia). Examples of typical simple vocal tics are sniffing, throat clearing, grunting, screaming, coughing, and blowing. Complex vocal tics may include seemingly meaningful but inappropriate utterances and verbalizations. Specific examples include shouting of obscenities (coprolalia), repetition of someone else's words or phrases (echolalia), and repetition of one's own utterances (palilalia).

Tics are often preceded by premonitory sensations or psychological symptoms that are temporarily relieved after the execution of the tic. These sensations may consist of localizable paresthesias, or discomfort such as a burning feeling in the eye before an eye blink, tension, or sore throat before throat clearing. Premonitory psychologic symptoms include urges, as well as anxiety or a fear of a catastrophic event if tics are not promptly or properly executed. Patients may need to repeat a particular tic until this uncomfortable feeling is relieved, suggesting a compulsive component.

Tourette's syndrome patients can temporarily suppress the frequency and severity of their tics volitionally or by concentrating on mental or physical tasks. Upon relaxation after a period of tic suppression (e.g., coming home from school), the tics may rebound. Suggestibility and exacerbation with stress, excitement, boredom, or fatigue are other distinguishing features (138). Tics can be socially disabling by causing embarrassment and interference in interactions with others or physically disabling by causing pain or discomfort (138).

The definitive criteria for the diagnosis of Tourette's syndrome (142) are (1) onset before the age 21 years; (2) presence of both multiple motor tics and one or more phonic tics at some time during the illness, although not necessarily concurrently; (3) occurrence of tics many times a day, nearly every day, or intermittently throughout a period of more than 1 year; (4) change of the anatomical location, number, frequency, type, complexity, or severity of tics over time; (5) exclusion of other medical conditions that can cause tics; and (6) confirmation of the tics by a reliable examiner at some point during the illness by direct examination or watching an audiovisual recording.

Tourette's syndrome typically begins between ages 3 and 8 years and is manifested by age 11 years in the large majority of cases (143). Tics usually become most severe around 10 years of age and then start declining thereafter. By age 18 years, half of Tourette's syndrome patients are free of tics (144), especially by their own assessment, but careful examination suggests that 50% of them continue to have subtle tics (145). Males demonstrate substantially more variability in improvement but overall tend to improve more than females (146). In females, there has been no consistent correlation between hormonal levels and fluctuations in tics or OCD symptoms (147). In children with developmental stuttering, one should look for clues for Tourette's syndrome, since careful study has suggested that such signs may be present but undiagnosed in almost 50% of cases (148). Except for tics, the neurologic examination in Tourette's syndrome is normal. Tics are evident in all stages of sleep, and sleep abnormalities are observed in Tourette's syndrome (149). Table 21.4 displays the clinical classification and etiology of tic disorders.

Behavioral-Cognitive Symptoms

Although intellectual ability is generally normal in Tourette's syndrome, specific cognitive deficits such as visuomotor integration problems, impaired fine motor skill, and executive dysfunction may be present (150). The presence of comorbid conditions, notably ADHD and OCD, appear to significantly increase the likelihood of learning problems or cognitive impairment. Behavioral disorders such as ADHD, OCD, or both, are apparent at some time during the course of Tourette's syndrome in the majority (60 to 80%) of patients (151, 152). Anxiety and mood disorders may also be observed (153). They usually interfere with personal, academic, and professional life more than the tics and may lead to social and emotional maladjustment if untreated. Impaired attention in Tourette's syndrome can result from a number of different factors: comorbid ADHD, the intrusive thoughts associated with OCD, the mental effort required to suppress tics and premonitory urges, and as a result of sedation caused by the drugs used to treat tics.

TABLE 21.4
ETIOLOGICAL CLASSIFICATION OF TICS

Primary

- Tourette's syndrome
- Chronic (>1 year) tic disorder: Similar to Tourette's except that patients have only either motor or vocal tics, but not both
- Transient (<1 year) tic disorder: Similar to chronic tic disorder except total duration of the illness
- Adult-onset tic

Secondary Tics

- *Drugs:* Stimulants (amphetamines, methylphenydate, cocaine), levodopa, dopamine blockers (tardive tourettism), carbamazepine, phenytoin, phenobarbital, lamotrigine
- *Infectious/immunologic:* Encephalitis, Sydenham's chorea, neurosyphilis, Creutzfeldt-Jakob disease
- *Hereditary:* Huntington's disease, neuroacanthocytosis, Hallervorden-Spatz disease, Wilson's disease, tuberous sclerosis, primary dystonia, and chromosomal anomalies such as Down syndrome, Klinefelter syndrome, and fragile X syndrome
- *Others:* Developmental disorders with mental retardation and behavioral problems, head trauma, carbon monoxide poisoning, stroke, schizophrenia, neurodegenerative diseases

Related Disorders

- Stereotypies, habits, and mannerisms
- Akathisia
- Hyperekplexia
- Jumping Frenchmen of Maine, latah, myriachit
- Obsessive-compulsive disorder

Additional cognitive, behavioral and neurological abnormalities are seen in patients with Tourette's syndrome who have comorbid ADHD (152). Associated poor impulse and anger control may lead to temper outbursts, rage, inappropriate sexual aggressiveness, and antisocial or oppositional behavior. Episodic rage can cause significant morbidity (154). Self-injurious behavior (139) and migraine headaches (155) are also associated with Tourette's syndrome. A less well appreciated but not unexpected fact is that parents of children with Tourette's syndrome have a markedly increased caregiver burden and are themselves at risk for psychiatric morbidity (156).

Pathogenesis

Although postmortem neuropathological examinations of Tourette's syndrome brains (157) and standard anatomical neuroimaging studies have not revealed any specific abnormalities, various biochemical, functional imaging, neurophysiological, and genetic studies suggest that it is an inherited, developmental disorder of synaptic neurotransmission resulting in the disinhibition of cortico-striatal-thalamic-cortical circuitry (138, 158, 159). The caudate nucleus and the inferior prefrontal cortex have been implicated in the pathogenesis of Tourette's syndrome, as well as in that of OCD and ADHD (138, 159, 160).
Volumetric MRI studies in Tourette's syndrome show loss of the normal asymmetry of the basal ganglia, which are

usually larger on the right, suggesting a developmental abnormality (160). Functional MRI studies reveal decreased neuronal activity during periods of suppression in the ventral globus pallidus, putamen, and thalamus and increased activity in prefrontal, parietal, temporal, and cingulate cortical areas; areas normally involved in the inhibition of unwanted impulses (160). PET studies show a nonspecific pattern of increased motor cortical activity, as in other hyperkinetic disorders, as well as a specific brain network characterized by a reduction in the activity of limbic basal ganglia (especially caudate) thalamocortical projection systems (161). There is temporally-related aberrant activity in the interrelated sensorimotor, language, executive, and paralimbic circuits during tics that may account for the initiation and execution of diverse motor and vocal behaviors, as well as for the urges that often accompany them (162).

Using back-averaging electroencephalographic techniques, the involuntary nature of tics has been demonstrated in many Tourette's syndrome patients by the absence of the premovement potential (Bereitschafts potential) before the execution of motor tics. Its presence, however, in other patients, suggests evidence of a voluntary component to some tics (163). The shortened cortical silent period and defective intracortical inhibition demonstrated by transcranial magnetic stimulation may explain the decreased motor inhibition and intrusive phenomena seen in Tourette's syndrome and OCD (164, 165). The inability to inactivate secondary motor areas when no movement is performed possibly explains Tourette's syndrome patients' involuntary urges to move, resulting in interference with accurate planning of voluntary behavior (166).

An alteration of neurotransmitters in Tourette's syndrome has been suggested based on the relatively consistent clinical responses to pharmacologic modulation of the dopaminergic system in patients with the disorder. Increased binding of 3H-mazindol to presynaptic dopamine-uptake-carrier sites indicates dopaminergic hyperinnervation of the ventral striatum and the associated limbic system (167). High [18F] Fluorodopa accumulation in the caudate nucleus and the substantia nigra and ventral tegmental area provides evidence of high presynaptic dopaminergic activity (168). However, the response of some Tourette's syndrome patients to dopamine agonist therapy (169) calls into question the role of dopamine overactivity. In addition to dopamine, other neurotransmitters have been implicated in the pathophysiology of Tourette's syndrome. Low levels of serotonin in the brainstem, low levels of glutamate in the globus pallidus, and low levels of cyclic adenosine monophosphate in the cortex have been demonstrated in the few brains available for postmortem study (157, 167).

Studies of twin have found a ~90% concordance for tics and Tourette's syndrome, providing strong evidence of a genetic etiology (170). Bilineal transmission is present in 25 to 41% of families with Tourette's syndrome (171, 172). Ethnic differences in the nature and frequency of vulnerable alleles for Tourette's syndrome and related disorders are suggested by the finding that the rates of Tourette's syndrome and related disorders in Japan are much lower than those in studies on twin and family studies in the United States and Western Europe (173). Genetic studies suggest a rather complex inheritance pattern with elements of gender-specific penetrance (males are more affected than females) and the possibility of multiple susceptibility genes (174–177). Nongenetic prenatal factors also affect the phenotype since low birth weight (170), maternal life stress, and nausea and vomiting during the first trimester of pregnancy (178) correlate with tic severity.

Some Tourette's syndrome patients have been shown to have elevated titers of antibodies to group A beta-hemolytic streptococcus (179), possess the B-lymphocyte antigen D8/17 (180), or display increased levels of antineuronal antibodies against putamen (181), suggesting an immunologic pathogenesis. The most recent attempts to passively transfer antineuronal antibodies from the serum of Tourette's syndrome patients to animals have been unsuccessful (182). Classification of Tourette's syndrome under the controversial category of pediatric autoimmune neuropsychiatric disorders associated with streptococcus infections (PANDAS) has been proposed (65). However, well-designed and adequately controlled studies will be needed to determine whether there is a true etiologic relation between streptococcal infection and the onset or exacerbation of childhood neuropsychiatric disorders such as Tourette's syndrome and whether the use of immune-modifying therapies for these conditions is rational (183).

Treatment

Behavioral therapy, a beneficial ancillary modality (184), and adjustments in the home, school, and classroom environments through education play an important part in the management of patients with Tourette's syndrome and are helpful in improving self-esteem and increasing motivation (185). Pharmaceutical treatment should only be started when symptoms begin to interfere with peer relationships, social interactions, academic or job performance, or activities of daily living and should be tailored to the individual needs of the patient by targeting the most troublesome symptom first (138). Each medication and dosage regimen should be given an adequate trial to avoid unnecessary changes that might be made in response to normal variations in symptoms during the natural course of the disease.

Treatment of Tics

Neuroleptics are the most effective agents for treating tics. However, given that their side effects include tardive dyskinesia, parkinsonism, sedation, depression, weight gain, school phobia, and hepatotoxicity, they should be used judiciously. The goal should be to relieve tic-related discomfort or embarrassment and to achieve a degree of control of tics that allows the patient to function as normally as possible, rather than elimination of all the tics. Haloperidol and pimozide are the only neuroleptic drugs currently approved by the Food and Drug Administration for the treatment of Tourette's syndrome. Pimozide has been found to be superior to haloperidol for controlling tics at equivalent doses, while causing fewer side effects (186). However, pimozide may prolong the QT interval and requires periodical monitoring with electrocardiography.

Risperidone (187–189) and ziprasidone (190) have been found to be beneficial in placebo-controlled, double-blind studies. Other neuroleptics such as quetiapine (191), fluphenazine, thioridazine, trifluoperazine, molindone, thiothixene, or tiapride are also used. Tetrabenazine, a drug that depletes monoamine and blocks the dopamine receptors, is a powerful antic drug that, unlike the conventional neuroleptics, has not been demonstrated to cause tardive dyskinesia (192). However, worsening of hyperkinetic movement disorders while on tetrabenazine has been observed in a small subset of patients (193).

Baclofen (194) and pergolide (169) have also been demonstrated to be modestly useful in Tourette's syndrome by placebo-controlled, double-blind studies. Other drugs found to be useful in the treatment of tics include clonazepam, quetiapine, olanzapine, cannabinoids, nicotine gum, and transdermal nicotine patches, but none of these drugs have been studied in well-designed, placebo-controlled trials (195). Focal motor and vocal tics have also been treated successfully with injections of botulinum toxin in the affected muscles (196–198). Such local chemical denervation not only ameliorates involuntary movements but may also eliminate the premonitory sensory component. However, tic reduction may not necessarily translate into global subjective improvement (196). Although stereotactic surgery has not generally been found to be useful in the treatment of tics (199), preliminary reports of successful thalamatomy (200) and high-frequency deep-brain stimulation of the thalamus (201) in severe, refractory Tourette's syndrome are encouraging.

Treatment of Coexisting Behavioral Symptoms

Central nervous system stimulants, such as methylphenidate, controlled-release methylphenidate, dextroamphetamine, a mixture of amphetamine salts, and pemoline, are very effective in the treatment of ADHD (202). Potential side effects include nervousness, irritability, insomnia, anorexia, abdominal pain, headaches, and rare hepatotoxicity (pemoline) (203). Previous concerns over the safety of stimulants used to treat Tourette's syndrome have largely been erased (204). The initial increase of severity and intensity of tics with stimulant use is usually not sustained (205, 206), but if necessary, dopaminergic blockers can be added for exacerbation of tics.

If central nervous system stimulants are not well tolerated or are contraindicated, presynaptic alpha$_2$-adrenergic agonists can be considered. Clonidine, also available as a transdermal patch, and guanfacine (longer acting, less sedative, and better tolerated) reduce the symptoms of ADHD and impulse-control problems and may also ameliorate tics (207–209). The most frequently encountered side effects of clonidine and guanfacine include sedation, dry mouth, itchy eyes, dizziness, headaches, fatigability, and postural hypotension. A randomized, double-blind clinical trial found that methylphenidate and clonidine (particularly in combination) are effective for ADHD in children with comorbid tics (210). Other drugs occasionally used in the treatment of mild cases of ADHD disorder include selegiline (211) and tricyclic antidepressants, such as imipramine, nortriptyline, and desipramine.

The selective serotonin-reuptake inhibitors (SSRIs) are the most effective drugs for OCD (212) and can also help with associated anxiety and social phobias (213). In some refractory cases they may need to be combined with buspirone, clonazepam, lithium, or neuroleptics (214). With such combinations, one should be vigilant to monitor for serotonin syndrome (confusion, hypomania, agitation, myoclonus, hyperreflexia, sweating, tremor, diarrhea, and fever), withdrawal phenomena, and possible extrapyramidal side effects (215). Limbic leucotomy or cingulotomy may be considered as a last resort in extremely severe and refractory OCD (216).

Paroxysmal Dyskinesias

Paroxysmal dyskinesias manifest as episodic chorea, dystonia, ballism, or a mixture of these abnormal involuntary movements (217). The patient is generally normal in between the episodes. Although some paroxysmal dyskinesias respond well to therapy, they often go untreated because they are commonly misdiagnosed as being psychogenic. Paroxysmal dyskinesias are classified as "paroxysmal kinesigenic dyskinesia," referring to disorders induced by sudden movement, or "paroxysmal nonkinesigenic dyskinesia," indicating those in which it is not (217). Those cases in which exercise is the precipitating cause are described as paroxysmal exercise-induced dyskinesia. The term "paroxysmal hypnogenic dyskinesia" is used when dyskinesias occur only during sleep. The majority of paroxysmal dyskinesias are idiopathic (primary, familial), while approximately 20% are classified as symptomatic (secondary) due to trauma, vascular lesions, multiple sclerosis, kernicterus, and encephalitis (218).

Paroxysmal kinesigenic dyskinesia starts in childhood and is characterized by a distinct predominance of males (219). Family history is present in about a quarter of cases and usually follows an autosomal dominant pattern of inheritance (219). Typical paroxysmal kinesigenic dyskinesia (220) and the syndrome of benign familial infantile convulsions and paroxysmal choreoathetosis (221) have been linked to the pericentromic region of chromosome 16 (16p12–q12) and are also referred to as dystonia 10 (DYT10). Rolandic epilepsy with paroxysmal exercise-induced dystonia and writer's cramp has also been mapped to this area (221a).

Attacks in paroxysmal kinesigenic dyskinesia usually consist of episodes of dystonia or choreodystonia precipitated by a sudden change in position such as moving from a sitting to standing position. Startle, hyperventilation, vigorous exercise, or a sudden change in the speed of an ongoing movement can also induce an attack (219). A premonitory phase consisting of tingling or other sensory phenomena that is generalized or felt in the body part that subsequently becomes dyskinetic occurs in most cases (219). Attacks commonly involve the hemibody and rarely generalize. Speech can be affected but there is no change in consciousness. Typically, paroxysmal kinesigenic dyskinesia attacks last from seconds to 1 to 2 minutes and occur up to dozens of times per day with a subsequent refractory period. Some patients can abort or prevent an attack by stopping moving or starting their movement slowly. The large majority of patients with paroxysmal kinesigenic dyskinesia respond dramatically to low doses of anticonvulsants, especially to carbamazepine or phenytoin (219). The attack frequency of paroxysmal kinesigenic dyskinesia diminishes over time with potential remission in adulthood (222).

Paroxysmal nonkinesigenic dyskinesia presents in childhood with intermittent episodes of involuntary movements that are a mixture of dystonia and chorea (222). These episodes are much more infrequent then those in paroxysmal kinesigenic dyskinesia but usually last for a few hours. The attacks can be spontaneous, but more often there are one or more precipitants such as stress, fatigue, alcohol, or caffeine. It may be possible to abort an attack by going to sleep (223). Similar to paroxysmal kinesigenic dyskinesia, there is a male predominance and a tendency for improvement with age. The pattern of inheritance is autosomal dominant with linkage to chromosome 2q, classified as DYT8 (224). In sporadic cases, adulthood onset and female predominance has been noted (225). Another paroxysmal condition—referred to as choreoathetosis/spasticity, episodic movement disorder, or DYT9—is linked to chromosome 1p. These patients have accompanying perioral paresthesias, diplopia, headache, generalized myoclonus with seizures, and spastic paraparesis (226). Paroxysmal nonkinesigenic dyskinesia is more difficult to treat than paroxysmal kinesigenic dyskinesia (217). Clonazepam is useful in some patients (225). Patients usually do not benefit from anticonvulsants, but occasionally individuals respond to levodopa suggestive of an abnormality of dopamine metabolism in this disorder (227).

Paroxysmal exercise-induced dyskinesia is provoked by ongoing exertion such as walking for at least 10 to 15 minutes. The dyskinetic episode usually lasts 5 to 30 minutes (228). The attacks are usually dystonic and appear in the body part involved in the exercise, such as leg dystonia after prolonged walking or jaw dystonia after chewing gum, and then wane in 10 to 15 minutes after stopping the offending exercise (229). Exposure to cold (230), or passive movements and vibration (231) may also precipitate attacks. Both sporadic and autosomal dominant cases have been described, the latter being more common (228). Anticonvulsants, levodopa, acetazolamide, and trihexiphenidyl have been used with limited success (228).

Paroxysmal hypnogenic dyskinesia is sporadic or familial (232–235). Affected individuals awaken often with a shout or cry and then exhibit dystonic and ballistic movements lasting up to 45 seconds, usually with no detectable concurrent EEG abnormalities. Several attacks can occur each night (232). Most cases, especially the familial ones, have autosomal nocturnal frontal lobe epilepsy, which has been linked to chromosomes 15q24 (236) and 20q13.2 (237), genes coding for the acetylcholine receptor (234, 235). Discharges arise from the mesial frontal lobe explaining the difficulty in detecting EEG abnormalities on surface recordings (235). Carbamazepine is an effective therapy for most cases of paroxysmal hypnogenic dyskinesia (235).

Stereotypies

A stereotypy is a voluntary repetitive movement. Like tics, the movement may be simple or complex. Typical stereotypies include hand ringing, repetitive lip pursing, and body rocking. This form of excessive movement is common in individuals with moderate or severe mental retardation, autism, or Rett syndrome and can also be seen as a part of the symptom complex of tardive dyskinesia. Such repetitive behaviors can be also induced environmentally in confined settings.

Confinement in adulthood results in a functional disorder that rapidly dissipates when normal conditions are restored, but confinement in infancy may have a more lasting effect (238).

Rett Syndrome

Rett syndrome is one of the leading causes of mental retardation and developmental regression in girls. The majority of cases of sporadic Rett syndrome are caused by mutations in the gene encoding methyl-CpG-binding protein 2 (*MeCP2*) (239) that likely regulates gene expression and chromatin structure. The type of the specific mutation coupled with possible variation in X-chromosome inactivation appears to determine phenotype–genotype correlations (240). After the first 6 months of life, there is developmental slowing and loss of social interest accompanied by decelerating brain growth. This is followed by a severe dementia and loss of hand skills, development of stereotypies such as frequent hand wringing, apraxia and ataxia, autistic features, irregular breathing with hyperventilation, and seizures. Patients stabilize somewhat during the preschool to school years, associated with more emotional contact but also abnormalities of the autonomic and skeletal systems. After the age of 15 to 20 years, a late motor deterioration occurs with dystonia and spasticity, but seizures become milder (241).

OTHER MOVEMENT DISORDERS

Wilson's Disease

Wilson's disease is an autosomal recessive disorder due to mutations in the ATP7B gene on chromosome 13q, which encodes for a copper-transporting P-type adenosinetriphosphatase (ATPase) (242). More than 200 mutations of the Wilson's disease gene have been detected, and most patients are compound heterozygotes who carry at least two mutations (243). Correlations between genotype and phenotype are weak. The disease occurs in every ethnic and geographic population, with a worldwide prevalence of ~1 in 30,000 and a heterozygous carrier frequency of ~1 in 90 (243).

The abnormality in copper-transporting P-type ATPase leads to a marked reduction in biliary copper excretion. Initially, copper accumulates in the liver, causing progressive damage, but ultimately it overflows, producing toxic effects in the brain and other sites, including the eye, kidney, bones, and bone marrow. Symptoms usually start between the ages of 11 and 25 years but can occur as early as 4 years of age and rarely as late as in the sixth decade. The clinical features are age dependent (244). In about half of patients, usually children, the clinical onset may be heralded by hepatic disturbances. The initial manifestations of the illness are neurological in about 40% of patients (usually after the age of 12 years) and psychiatric in about 15% (245). Both modes of presentation are almost always accompanied by Kayser-Fleischer rings, golden brown copper depositions in the cornea. The diagnosis of Wilson's disease may occasionally be made when Kayser-Fleischer rings are observed during routine ophthalmologic examination by slit-lamp (246). Kayser-Fleischer rings may be absent in patients presenting only with hepatic symptoms. In about 5% of patients, the clinical onset reflects neither a hepatic nor a central nervous system disturbance (247) but rather atypical features such as primary or secondary amenorrhea. In about half of Wilson's disease patients, the initial symptoms are misinterpreted resulting in an average delay of the diagnosis by 2 years.

In children, the initial neurologic symptoms usually consist of progressive dystonia, rigidity, and dysarthria. Tremor that typically involves the proximal upper extremity ("wing-beating tremor") is the most common presenting neurological feature in adults. Many patients with neurological signs of Wilson's disease develop prominent disorders of speech, swallowing and facial expression. Dysarthria can be a manifestation of lingual and facial dystonia, parkinsonism with hypophonia, or a result of cerebellar involvement with features of scanning speech. Facial dystonia often results in a peculiar grinning appearance. An akinetic-rigid state resembling Parkinson's disease can be seen, but chorea is uncommon. Rarely, seizures are part of the syndrome.

Psychiatric or behavioral abnormalities occur in the majority of patients with Wilson's disease. Although psychiatric symptoms are the presenting sign in a relatively small percentage, they emerge somewhat later in the course of the disease in the majority of patients. Symptoms range from relatively mild behavioral manifestations in about 45.9%, which include personality change, irritability and emotional lability or aggression. Depression may occur in 27%. Other less frequent psychiatric symptoms include anxiety, psychosis, and catatonia (247a). In one study, depressive symptomatology was shown to be negatively correlated with presynaptic serotonin transporter availability (247b). Dementia and psychosis may also occur. The dopamine blocking drugs used to treat psychiatric symptoms of Wilson's disease may incorrectly be considered the etiology of later-developing extrapyramidal symptoms.

Diagnosis

Wilson's disease should be considered in any young patient with an unexplained liver disease or a movement disorder, cognitive dysfunction, or psychiatric abnormalities. The most useful laboratory screening test for Wilson's disease is plasma ceruloplasmin, which usually is less than 20 mg/dl. Normal ceruloplasmin levels, however, can be present in up to 5% of Wilson's disease patients (248), and low ceruloplasmin levels can be seen in patients with other forms of severe liver disease. The serum copper level is usually less than 100 µg/dl in Wilson's disease, and 24-hour urine excretion of copper is usually above 100 µg/24 hours (normal less than 50) (243). Since serum and urine copper levels are influenced by dietary intake of copper, these tests are not entirely reliable in the diagnosis of Wilson's disease. The diagnosis is confirmed by the demonstration of either

a serum ceruloplasmin level <20 mg/dL *and* Kayser-Fleischer rings, or a serum ceruloplasmin level <20 mg/dL *and* copper concentration in a liver biopsy sample >250 µg/g dry weight (243, 247). Other abnormalities in Wilson's disease include hemolytic anemia, hematuria, abnormalities in liver and renal function, increased excretion of amino acids in the urine, and elevated CSF levels of copper. MRI scans of the brain are usually abnormal (249) and may show decreased signal intensity on T1-weighted scans, and on T2-weighted scans hyperintensity in the striatum and superior colliculi. A characteristic, but rare MRI finding is increased signal intensity in the midbrain tegmentum (except for the red nucleus) and in the lateral substantial nigra pars reticulata, giving the appearance of "face of the giant panda" on T2-weighted images (250). Due to the high number of possible mutations over the entire length of the gene, commercial genetic testing is not feasible. However, genetic testing of full siblings of Wilson's disease patients can be useful in identifying presymptomatic individuals and starting prophylactic treatment (251).

Postmortem examination of the brain shows Alzheimer type II astrocytes in the striatum, and Opalski cells in the gray matter (252, 253) with 10- to 15-fold increased concentration of copper in all brain regions.

Treatment

Pharmacological treatment is aimed at preventing or reversing the copper deposition. The strategies include a low copper diet, removing copper by the use of chelating agents (D-penicillamine, trientine hydrochloride, British Antilewisite-BAL, and tetrathiomolybdate), and maintenance therapy with zinc salts that compete for intestinal copper absorption and stimulate the production of the copper-sequestering protein metallothionein in the liver (243). Penicillamine therapy can result in initial worsening due to mobilization of copper stores. Symptomatic therapies for the movement disorders associated with Wilson's disease include levodopa for parkinsonism and anticholinergics or botulinum toxin for dystonia.

Liver transplantation is indicated in cases of fulminant hepatitis and Coombs-negative hemolytic anemia or if progressive hepatic insufficiency occurs despite adequate treatment with penicillamine or trientine (254). Although an improvement of the neurologic picture has been seen in almost 80% of cases, the decision to perform liver transplantation in patients with Wilson's disease solely on the basis of neurological impairment must be considered experimental (255).

Wilson's disease treatment must be continued for life. Inadequate treatment or interruption of therapy can be fatal or cause an irreversible relapse.

Hallervorden-Spatz Syndrome

Hallervorden-Spatz syndrome, now referred to as neurodegeneration with brain iron accumulation (256), is an autosomal recessive disorder that usually presents in childhood and is characterized by dystonia, parkinsonism, and iron accumulation in the brain (257). Additional features may include spasticity, progressive intellectual impairment, retinitis pigmentosa or optic atrophy (258), tourettism, or hemiballism (259). Many patients with this disease have mutations in the gene encoding pantothenate kinase 2 (*PANK2*); these patients are said to have pantothenate kinase-associated neurodegeneration (257). Hypoprebetalipoproteinemia, acanthocytosis, retinitis pigmentosa, and pallidal degeneration (HARP syndrome) are part of the pantothenate kinase-associated neurodegeneration disease spectrum (260).

There is considerable clinical variation from patient to patient and even within the same family (261). The disease is progressive. Patients who become symptomatic in early childhood have the most rapid progression. Adults progress more slowly, with the mean survival being 11 years (262). Those who present in late childhood progress at an intermediate rate. In a large series of patients with neurodegeneration with brain iron accumulation, all patients with the classical syndrome (characterized by early onset with rapid progression) and approximately one third of those with atypical disease (later onset with slow progression) had *PANK2* mutations (257). Patients with atypical disease who had *PANK2* mutations were more likely to have prominent speech-related and psychiatric symptoms than patients with classic disease or mutation-negative patients with atypical disease. Predicted levels of *PANK2* protein correlated with the severity of disease (257). On T2-weighted MRI of the brain, all patients with neurodegeneration with brain iron accumulation, whether classic or atypical, have hyperintensity within the hypointense medial globus pallidus ("eye of the tiger" pattern (263)), a pattern not seen in any patients without *PANK2* mutations (257).

The pathology of neurodegeneration with brain iron accumulation/pantothenate kinase-associated neurodegeneration includes iron accumulation, demyelination, and gliosis especially in the globus pallidus and pars reticulata of the substantia nigra. Swollen axons, also known as axonal spheroids, and Lewy-type bodies are present (264, 265). Both the Lewy-like bodies and the axonal spheroids seen in this disorder have been found to contain α-synuclein, linking this disease to the class of degenerative conditions collectively termed the synucleinopathies, which also includes Parkinson's disease (266).

There is no curative therapy for neurodegeneration with brain iron accumulation or pantothenate kinase-associated neurodegeneration. Iron chelation therapy has not been successful in this condition. Symptomatically, dystonia responds to levodopa, dopamine agonists, or anticholinergic agents in some patients (258). Sterotactic pallidotomy has been reported to be a benefit for relieving painful dystonia and improving limb function in a single case (267). Levodopa may also be useful to treat parkinsonism in late-onset patients (268). Antioxidant therapies have been proposed to treat this disorder, based on histologic evidence of oxidative stress and lipid peroxidation that has been found in autopsy studies (269).

Psychogenic Movement Disorders

Psychogenic movement disorders are defined as abnormal movements for which no organic cause can be found or is likely. In this respect, they are ultimately considered to be due to a somatoform disorder or a result of overt malingering. The diagnosis is often suggested by abnormal movements that conform to a pattern of onset, intermittency, inconstancy, medication responsiveness, or anatomic distribution that is not seen in any of the recognized organic movement disorder syndromes. In addition to these atypical clinical features, a variety of behavioral or historical risk factors have been associated with the development of psychogenic movement disorders (270), such as a history of psychiatric treatment, suicide attempt, self-injurious behavior, drug or alcohol use, physical or sexual abuse, previous somatization, exposure to a person with an organic movement disorder, or medicolegal conflict over the current or a past illness. Added to these risk factors are accompanying clinical findings such as false weakness or anatomically unlikely sensory loss. Yet the clinician must be aware that 100% accuracy cannot be achieved even when the maximal numbers of predictors are present. Confounding issues include patients with bonafide movement disorders who also manifest concurrent psychogenic movements or bizarre exaggerations of a true underlying abnormal movement, which then dominates the clinical syndrome (271).

Tremor is the most commonly encountered psychogenic movement disorder followed by dystonia (272). Psychogenic tremor often changes frequency or direction within the span of a few minutes and often displays an intermittency that cannot be associated with any apparent precipitating factors such as a specific position or motor activity. A common feature of psychogenic dystonia is abrupt onset, rapid progression, and immediate progression to a fixed dystonic posture.

The treatment of a psychogenic movement disorder involves informing the patient, family members, and caregivers of the diagnosis and the relatively high degree of certainty of its correctness. A confrontational approach must be avoided and commentary on the validity of other physician's opinions should not be central to the discussion, as opposed to the current diagnostic process and conclusions. Referral to a mental health professional with an interest and expertise in these disorders should be suggested as an option. Despite this approach, experience has suggested that these disorders are often relatively refractory to therapy. Poor outcome with respect to resolution of these movements appears to be associated with long duration of symptoms, insidious onset of movements, and psychiatric comorbidity (273).

REFERENCES

1. Afifi AK. Basal ganglia: functional anatomy and physiology. Part 1. Journal of Child Neurology 1994; 9(3):249–260.
2. Afifi AK. Basal ganglia: functional anatomy and physiology. Part 2. Journal of Child Neurology 1994; 9(4):352–361.
3. Sian J, Youdim MB, Riederer P, Gerlach M. Neurotransmitters and disorders of basal ganglia. In: Siegel GJ, Agranof BW, Albers RW, Fisher SK, Uhler MD, eds. Basic Neurochemistry: Molecular, Cellular and Medical Aspects. Philadelphia: Lippincott Williams & Wilkins, 1999: 917–948.
4. Alexander GE, DeLong MR, Strick PL. Parallel organization of functionally segregated circuits linking basal ganglia and cortex. Annual Review of Neuroscience 1986; 9:357–381.
5. Albin RL, Young AB, Penney JB. The functional anatomy of disorders of the basal ganglia. Trends in Neurosciences 1995; 18(2): 63–64.
6. Casey BJ, Tottenham N, Fossella J. Clinical, imaging, lesion, and genetic approaches toward a model of cognitive control. Developmental Psychobiology 2002; 40(3):237–254.
7. Graybiel AM, Rauch SL. Toward a neurobiology of obsessive-compulsive disorder. Neuron 2000; 28(2):343–347.
8. Uc EY, Rodnitzky RL. Juvenile parkinsonism. Seminars in Pediatric Neurology 2003; 10(1):62–67.
9. Lucking CB, Durr A, Bonifati V, Vaughan J, De Michele G, Gasser T, et al. Association between early-onset Parkinson's disease and mutations in the parkin gene. French Parkinson's Disease Genetics Study Group. New England Journal of Medicine 2000; 342 (21):1560–1567.
10. Bonifati V, Rizzu P, van Baren MJ, Schaap O, Breedveld GJ, Krieger E, et al. Mutations in the DJ-1 gene associated with autosomal recessive early-onset parkinsonism. Science 2003; 299 (5604):256–259.
11. Abou-Sleiman PM, Healy DG, Quinn N, Lees AJ, Wood NW. The role of pathogenic DJ-1 mutations in Parkinson's disease. Annuals of Neurology 2003; 54(3):283–286.
12. Whone AL, Moore RY, Piccini PP, Brooks DJ. Plasticity of the nigropallidal pathway in Parkinson's disease. Annuals of Neurology 2003; 53 (2):206–213.
13. Khan NL, Graham E, Critchley P, Schrag AE, Wood NW, Lees AJ, et al. Parkin disease: a phenotypic study of a large case series. Brain 2003; 126(Part 6):1279–1292.
14. Louis ED, Dure LS, Pullman S. Essential tremor in childhood: a series of nineteen cases. Movement Disorders 2001; 16(5): 921–923.
15. Gatto EM, Roca MC, Raina G, Micheli F. Low doses of topiramate are effective in essential tremor: a report of three cases. Clinical Neuropharmacology 2003; 26(6):294–296.
16. Uc EY, Rodnitzky RL. Childhood dystonia. Seminars in Pediatric Neurology 2003; 10(1):52–61
16a. Heiman, GA, OttmanR, Saunders-Pullman RJ, Ozelius LJ, Risch NJ, Bressman SB. Increased risk for recurrent major depression in DYT1 dystonia mutation carriers. Neurology 2004; 63:631–637
16b. Ghilardi MF, Carbon M, Silvestri G, Dhawan V, Tagliati M, Bressman S, Ghez C, Eidelberg D. Impaired sequence learning in carriers of DYT1 dystonia mutation. Annuals Neurology 2003; 54: 102–109.
17. Berardelli A, Rothwell JC, Hallett M, Thompson PD, Manfredi M, Marsden CD. The pathophysiology of primary dystonia. Brain 1998; 121(Part 7):1195–1212.
18. Ozelius LJ, Hewett JW, Page CE, Bressman SB, Kramer PL, Shalish C, et al. The early-onset torsion dystonia gene (DYT1) encodes an ATP-binding protein. Nature Genetics 1997; 17(1):40–48.
19. Nygaard TG, Marsden CD, Fahn S. Dopa-responsive dystonia: long-term treatment response and prognosis. Neurology 1991; 41(2 (Part 1):174–181.
20. Grotzsch H, Schnorf H, Morris MA, Moix I, Horvath J, Prilipko O, et al. Phenotypic heterogeneity of dopa-responsive dystonia in monozygotic twins. Neurology 2004; 62(4):637–639.
21. Ichinose H, Ohye T, Takahashi E, Seki N, Hori T, Segawa M, et al. Hereditary progressive dystonia with marked diurnal fluctuation caused by mutations in the GTP cyclohydrolase I gene. Nature Genetics 1994; 8(3):236–242.
22. Furukawa Y. Update on dopa-responsive dystonia: locus heterogeneity and biochemical features. Advances in Neurology 2004; 94:127– 138.
23. Furukawa Y, Kish SJ. Dopa-responsive dystonia: recent advances and remaining issues to be addressed. Movement Disorders 1999; 14(5):709–715.
24. Pons R, Ford B, Chiriboga CA, Clayton PT, Hinton V, Hyland K, et al. Aromatic L-amino acid decarboxylase deficiency: clinical features, treatment, and prognosis. Neurology 2004; 62(7): 1058–1065.
25. Gasser T. Inherited myoclonus-dystonia syndrome. Advances in Neurology 1998; 78:325–334.
26. Zimprich A, Grabowski M, Asmus F, Naumann M, Berg D, Bertram M, et al. Mutations in the gene encoding epsilon-sarcoglycan cause myoclonus-dystonia syndrome. Nature Genetics 2001; 29(1):66–69.
27. Valente EM, Misbahuddin A, Brancati F, Placzek MR, Garavaglia B, Salvi S, et al. Analysis of the epsilon-sarcoglycan gene in familial and sporadic myoclonus-dystonia: evidence for genetic heterogeneity. Movement Disorders 2003; 18(9):1047–1051.
28. Kramer PL, Mineta M, Klein C, Schilling K, de Leon D, Farlow MR, et al. Rapid-onset dystonia-parkinsonism: linkage to chromosome 19q13. Annals of Neurology 1999; 46(2):176–182.
29. Brashear A, Butler IJ, Hyland K, Farlow MR, Dobyns WB. Cerebrospinal fluid homovanillic acid levels in rapid-onset dystonia-parkinsonism. Annals of Neurology 1998; 43(4):521–526.
30. Brashear A, Mulholland GK, Zheng QH, Farlow MR, Siemers ER, Hutchins GD. PET imaging of the pre-synaptic dopamine uptake sites in rapid-onset dystonia-parkinsonism (RDP). Movement Disorders 1999; 14(1):132–137.
31. Uc EY, Wenger DA, Jankovic J. Niemann-Pick disease type C: two cases and an update. Movement Disorders 2000; 15(6):1199–1203.
32. Patterson MC, Vanier MT, Suzuki K, Morris JA, Carstea ED, Neufeld EB, et al. Niemann-Pick disease type C: a lipid trafficking disorder. In: Scriver CR, Beaudet AL, Sly WS, Vale J, eds. The Metabolic and Molecular Bases of Inherited Disease. New York: McGraw Hill, 2001: 3611–3633.
33. Davies JP, Chen FW, Ioannou YA. Transmembrane molecular pump activity of Niemann-Pick C1 protein. Science 2000; 290 (5500):2295–2298.
34. Naureckiene S, Sleat DE, Lackland H, Fensom A, Vanier MT, Wattiaux R, et al. Identification of HE1 as the second gene of Niemann-Pick C disease. Science 2000; 290(5500):2298–2301.
35. Pequignot MO, Desguerre I, Dey R, Tartari M, Zeviani M, Agostino A, et al. New splicing-site mutations in the SURF1 gene in Leigh syndrome patients. Journal of Biological Chemistry 2001; 276(18):15326–15329.
36. Tatuch Y, Christodoulou J, Feigenbaum A, Clarke JT, Wherret J, Smith C, et al. Heteroplasmic mtDNA mutation (T--G) at 8993 can cause Leigh disease when the percentage of abnormal mtDNA is high. American Journal of Human Genetics 1992; 50 (4):852–858.
37. Lera G, Bhatia K, Marsden CD. Dystonia as the major manifestation of Leigh's syndrome. Movement Disorders 1994; 9(6): 642–649.
38. Macaya A, Munell F, Burke RE, De Vivo DC. Disorders of movement in Leigh syndrome. Neuropediatrics 1993; 24(2):60–67.
39. Baric I, Zschocke J, Christensen E, Duran M, Goodman SI, Leonard JV, et al. Diagnosis and management of glutaric aciduria type I. Journal of Inherited Metabolic Disease 1998; 21(4):326–340.
39a. Biery BJ, Goodman SI. Mutation in glutaryl-CoA dehdrogenase (GCDH) in glutaric academia type I. (Abstract) American Journal of Human Genetics 1992;51 (Suppl.): A165.
39b. Funk CB, Prasad AN, Frosk P, Sauer S, Kolker S, Greenberg CR, Del Bigio MR. Neuropathological, biochemical and molecular findings in a glutaric academia type 1 cohort. Brain 2005; 711–722.
40. Nyhan WL, Bay C, Beyer EW, Mazi M. Neurologic nonmetabolic presentation of propionic acidemia. Archives of Neurology 1999; 56(9):1143–1147.
41. Heidenreich R, Natowicz M, Hainline BE, Berman P, Kelley RI, Hillman RE, et al. Acute extrapyramidal syndrome in methylmalonic acidemia: "metabolic stroke" involving the globus pallidus. Journal of Pediatrics 1988; 113(6):1022–1027.

42. Rodnitzky RL. Drug-induced movement disorders. Clinical Neuropharmacology 2002; 25(3):142–152.

43. Scott BL, Jankovic J. Delayed-onset progressive movement disorders after static brain lesions. Neurology 1996; 46(1):68–74.

44. Burke RE, Fahn S, Marsden CD. Torsion dystonia: a double-blind, prospective trial of high-dosage trihexyphenidyl. Neurology 1986; 36(2):160–164.

45. Greene P. Baclofen in the treatment of dystonia. Clinical Neuropharmacology 1992; 15(4):276–288.

46. Walker RH, Danisi FO, Swope DM, Goodman RR, Germano IM, Brin MF. Intrathecal baclofen for dystonia: benefits and complications during six years of experience. Movement Disorders 2000; 15(6):1242–1247.

47. Lozano AM, Kumar R, Gross RE, Giladi N, Hutchison WD, Dostrovsky JO, et al. Globus pallidus internus pallidotomy for generalized dystonia. Movement Disorders 1997; 12(6):865–870.

48. Vitek JL, Zhang J, Evatt M, Mewes K, DeLong MR, Hashimoto T, et al. GPi pallidotomy for dystonia: clinical outcome and neuronal activity. Advances in Neurology 1998; 78:211–219.

49. Kumar R, Lozano AM, Montgomery E, Lang AE. Pallidotomy and deep brain stimulation of the pallidum and subthalamic nucleus in advanced Parkinson's disease. Movement Disorders 1998; 13(Suppl 1):73–82.

50. Volkmann J, Benecke R. Deep brain stimulation for dystonia: patient selection and evaluation. Movement Disorders 2002; 17(Suppl 3):S112–S115.

51. Krauss JK, Yianni J, Loher TJ, Aziz TZ. Deep brain stimulation for dystonia. Journal of Clinical Neurophysiology 2004; 21(1):18–30.

52. Anonymous. ACMG/ASHG statement; Laboratory guidelines for Huntington's disease genetic testing. American Journal of Human Genetics 2002; G2:1243–1247.

53. Brandt J, Bylsma FW, Gross R, Stine OC, Ranen N, Ross CA. Trinucleotide repeat length and clinical progression in Huntington's disease. Neurology 1996; 46(2):527–531.

54. Ranen NG, Stine OC, Abbott MH, Sherr M, Codori AM, Franz ML, et al. Anticipation and instability of IT-15 (CAG)n repeats in parent-offspring pairs with Huntington disease. American Journal of Human Genetics 1995; 57(3):593–602.

55. Nance MA, Myers RH. Juvenile onset Huntington's disease—clinical and research perspectives. Mental Retardation & Developmental Disabilities Research Reviews 2001; 7(3):153–157.

56. Rosenblatt A, Leroi I. Neuropsychiatry of Huntington's disease and other basal ganglia disorders. Psychosomatics 2000; 41(1):24–30.

56a. Lemiere J, Decruyenaere M, Evers-Kiebooms G, Vandenbussche E, Dom R. Cognitive changes in patients with Huntington's disease (HD) and asymptomatic carriers of the HD mutation–a longitudinal follow-up study. Journal of Neurology 2004: 935–942.

57. Foroud T, Gray J, Ivashina J, Conneally PM. Differences in duration of Huntington's disease based on age at onset. Journal of Neurology, Neurosurgery & Psychiatry 1999; 66(1):52–56.

57a. Duesterhus P, Schimmelmann BG, Wittkugel O, Schulte-Markwort M, Huntington disease: a case study of early onset presenting as depression. Journal of American Academy Child and Adolescent Psychiatry. 2004;43: 1293–1297.

58. Anonymous. Guidelines for the molecular genetics predictive test in Huntington's disease. International Huntington Association (IHA) and the World Federation of Neurology (WFN) Research Group on Huntington's Chorea. Neurology 1994; 44:1533–1536.

59. Bonelli RM, Niederwieser G, Tribl GG, Koltringer P. High-dose olanzapine in Huntington's disease. International Clinical Psycho Pharmacology 2002; 17:91–93.

60. van Vugt JP, Siesling S, Vergeer M, van der Velde EA, Roos RA. Clozapine versus placebo in Huntington's disease: a double blind randomised comparative study. Journal of Neurology, Neurosurgery & Psychiatry 1997; 63(1):35–39.

61. Moskowitz CB, Marder K. Palliative care for people with late-stage Huntington's disease. Neurologic Clinics 2001; 19(4):849–865.

62. Hauser RA, Furtado S, Cimino CR, Delgado H, Eichler S, Schwartz S, et al. Bilateral human fetal striatal transplantation in Huntington's disease. Neurology 2002; 58(5):687–695.

63. The Huntington Study Group. A randomized, placebo-controlled trial of coenzyme Q10 and remacemide in Huntington's disease. Neurology 2001; 57(3):397–404.

64. O'Brien T, Lee D. Prospects for caspase inhibitors. Mini Reviews in Medicinal Chemistry 2004; 4(2):153–165.

65. Swedo SE, Leonard HL, Garvey M, Mittleman B, Allen AJ, Perlmutter S, et al. Pediatric autoimmune neuropsychiatric disorders associated with streptococcal infections: clinical description of the first 50 cases. American Journal of Psychiatry 1998; 155(2):264–271.

66. Church AJ, Dale RC, Cardoso F, Candler PM, Chapman MD, Allen ML, et al. CSF and serum immune parameters in Sydenham's chorea: evidence of an autoimmune syndrome? Journal of Neuroimmunology 2003; 136(1–2):149–153.

67. Loiselle CR, Singer HS. Genetics of childhood disorders: XXXI. Autoimmune disorders, part 4: is Sydenham chorea an autoimmune disorder? Journal of the American Academy of Child & Adolescent Psychiatry 2001; 40(10):1234–1236.

68. Cardoso F, Eduardo C, Silva AP, Mota CC. Chorea in fifty consecutive patients with rheumatic fever. Movement Disorders 1997; 12(5):701–703.

69. Elevli M, Celebi A, Tombul T, Gokalp AS. Cardiac involvement in Sydenham's chorea: clinical and Doppler echocardiographic findings. Acta Paediatrica 1999; 88(10):1074–1077.

70. Swedo SE, Leonard HL, Schapiro MB, Casey BJ, Mannheim GB, Lenane MC, et al. Sydenham's chorea: physical and psychological symptoms of St Vitus dance. Pediatrics 1993; 91(4):706–713.

71. Church AJ, Cardoso F, Dale RC, Lees AJ, Thompson EJ, Giovannoni G. Anti-basal ganglia antibodies in acute and persistent Sydenham's chorea. Neurology 2002; 59(2):227–231.

72. Carapetis JR, Currie BJ. Rheumatic chorea in northern Australia: a clinical and epidemiological study. Archives of Disease in Childhood 1999; 80(4):353–358.

73. Giedd JN, Rapoport JL, Kruesi MJ, Parker C, Schapiro MB, Allen AJ, et al. Sydenham's chorea: magnetic resonance imaging of the basal ganglia. Neurology 1995; 45(12):2199–2202.

74. Ikuta N, Hirata M, Sasabe F, Negoro K, Morimatsu M. High-signal basal ganglia on T1-weighted images in a patient with Sydenham's chorea. Neuroradiology 1998; 40(10):659–661.

75. Morshed SA, Parveen S, Leckman JF, Mercadante MT, Bittencourt Kiss MH, Miguel EC, et al. Antibodies against neural, nuclear, cytoskeletal, and streptococcal epitopes in children and adults with Tourette's syndrome, Sydenham's chorea, and autoimmune disorders. Biological Psychiatry 2001; 50(8):566–577.

76. Genel F, Arslanoglu S, Uran N, Saylan B. Sydenham's chorea: clinical findings and comparison of the efficacies of sodium valproate and carbamazepine regimens. Brain Development 2002; 24:73–76.

77. Harel L, Zecharia A, Straussberg R, Volovitz B, Amir J. Successful treatment of rheumatic chorea with carbamazepine. Pediatric Neurology 2000; 23(2):147–151.

78. Rullan E, Sigal LH. Rheumatic fever. Current Rheumatology Reports 2001; 3(5):445–452.

79. Connor DF, Fletcher KE, Wood JS. Neuroleptic-related dyskinesias in children and adolescents. Journal of Clinical Psychiatry 2001; 62(12):967–974.

80. Kumra S, Jacobsen LK, Lenane M, Smith A, Lee P, Malanga CJ, et al. Case series: spectrum of neuroleptic-induced movement disorders and extrapyramidal side effects in childhood-onset schizophrenia. Journal of the American Academy of Child & Adolescent Psychiatry 1998; 37(2):221–227.

81. Campbell M, Armenteros JL, Malone RP, Adams PB, Eisenberg ZW, Overall JE. Neuroleptic-related dyskinesias in autistic children: a prospective, longitudinal study. Journal of the American Academy of Child & Adolescent Psychiatry 1997; 36(6):835–843.

82. McMahon WM, Filloux FM, Ashworth JC, Jensen J. Movement disorders in children and adolescents. Neurology Clinics 2002; 20(4): viii, 1101.

83. Van Kampen JM, Stoessl AJ. Dopamine D(1A) receptor function in a rodent model of tardive dyskinesia. Neuroscience 2000; 101(3):629–635.

84. Silvestri S, Seeman MV, Negrete JC, Houle S, Shammi CM, Remington GJ, et al. Increased dopamine D2 receptor binding after

long-term treatment with antipsychotics in humans: a clinical PET study. Psychopharmacology 2000; 152(2):174–180.

85. Delfs JM, Ellison GD, Mercugliano M, Chesselet MF. Expression of glutamic acid decarboxylase mRNA in striatum and pallidum in an animal model of tardive dyskinesia. Experimental Neurology 1995; 133(2):175–188.

86. Jeste DV, Krull AJ, Kilbourn K. Tardive dyskinesia: managing a common neuroleptic side effect. Geriatrics 1990; 45(12):49–54.

87. McGrath JJ, Soares KV. Neuroleptic reduction and/or cessation and neuroleptics as specific treatment for tardive dyskinesia. Cochrane Database Systematic Review 2000; 2. CD000208

88. Duvoisin RC. Reserpine for tardive dyskinesia. New England Journal of Medicine 1972; 286(11):611.

89. Ondo WG, Hanna PA, Jankovic J. Tetrabenazine treatment for tardive dyskinesia: assessment by randomized videotape protocol. American Journal of Psychiatry 1999; 156:1279–1281.

90. Lerner V, Miodownik C, Kaptsan A, Cohen H, Matar M, Loewenthal U, et al. Vitamin B(6) in the treatment of tardive dyskinesia: a double-blind, placebo-controlled, crossover study. American Journal of Psychiatry 2001; 158(9):1511–1514.

91. Hardoy MC, Hardoy MJ, Carta MG, Cabras PL. Gabapentin as a promising treatment for antipsychotic-induced movement disorders in schizoaffective and bipolar patients. Journal of Affective Disorders 1999; 54(3):315–317.

92. Richardson MA, Small AM, Read LL, Chao HM, Clelland JD. Branched chain amino acid treatment of tardive dyskinesia in children and adolescents. Journal of Clinical Psychiatry 2004; 65 (1):92–96.

93. Barak Y, Swartz M, Shamir E, Stein D, Weizman A. Vitamin E (alpha-tocopherol) in the treatment of tardive dyskinesia: a statistical meta-analysis. Annals of Clinical Psychiatry 1998; 10(3):101–105.

94. Soares KV, McGrath JJ. Vitamin E for neuroleptic-induced tardive dyskinesia. Cochrane Database Systematic Review 2001;(4): CD000209.

95. McGrath JJ, Soares KV. Benzodiazepines for neuroleptic-induced tardive dyskinesia. Cochrane Database Systematic Review 2000; (2):CD000205.

96. Brashear A, Ambrosius WT, Eckert GJ, Siemers ER. Comparison of treatment of tardive dystonia and idiopathic cervical dystonia with botulinum toxin type A. Movement Disorders 1998; 13(1): 158–161.

97. Hardie RJ, Pullon HW, Harding AE, Owen JS, Pires M, Daniels GL, et al. Neuroacanthocytosis. A clinical, haematological and pathological study of 19 cases. Brain 1991; 114(Part 1A):13–49.

98. Ueno S, Maruki Y, Nakamura M, Tomemori Y, Kamae K, Tanabe H, et al. The gene encoding a newly discovered protein, chorein, is mutated in chorea-acanthocytosis. Nature Genetics 2001; 28 (2):121–122.

99. Kartsounis LD, Hardie RJ. The pattern of cognitive impairments in neuroacanthocytosis: a frontosubcortical dementia. Archives of Neurology 1996; 53(1):77–80.

100. Ohnishi A, Sato Y, Nagara H, Sakai T, Iwashita H, Kuroiwa Y, et al. Neurogenic muscular atrophy and low density of large myelinated fibres of sural nerve in chorea-acanthocytosis. Journal of Neurology, Neurosurgery & Psychiatry 1981; 44(7):645–648.

101. O'Brien C, Sung JH, McGeachie RE, Lee MC. Striatonigral degeneration: clinical, MRI, and pathologic correlation. Neurology 1990; 40(4):710–711.

102. Okamoto K, Ito J, Furusawa T, Sakai K, Tokiguchi S, Homma A, et al. CT and MR findings of neuroacanthocytosis. Journal of Computer Assisted Tomography 1997; 21(2):221–222.

103. Breedveld GJ, Percy AK, MacDonald ME, de Vries BB, Yapijakis C, Dure LS, et al. Clinical and genetic heterogeneity in benign hereditary chorea. Neurology 2002; 59(4):579–584.

104. Warner TT, Williams LD, Walker RW, Flinter F, Robb SA, Bundey SE, et al. A clinical and molecular genetic study of dentatorubropallidoluysian atrophy in four European families. Annals of Neurology 1995; 37(4):452–459.

105. Namekawa M, Takiyama Y, Ando Y, Sakoe K, Muramatsu SI, Fujimoto KI, et al. Choreiform movements in spinocerebellar ataxia type 1. Journal of the Neurological Sciences 2001; 187 (1–2):103–106.

106. Geschwind DH, Perlman S, Figueroa CP, Treiman LJ, Pulst SM. The prevalence and wide clinical spectrum of the spinocerebellar ataxia type 2 trinucleotide repeat in patients with autosomal dominant cerebellar ataxia. American Journal of Human Genetics 1997; 60(4):842–850.

107. Stevanin G, Camuzat A, Holmes SE, Julien C, Sahloul R, Dode C, et al. CAG/CTG repeat expansions at the Huntington's disease-like 2 locus are rare in Huntington's disease patients. Neurology 2002; 58(6):965–967.

108. Brey RL, Holliday SL, Saklad AR, Navarrete MG, Hermosillo-Romo D, Stallworth CL, et al. Neuropsychiatric syndromes in lupus: prevalence using standardized definitions. Neurology 2002; 58(8):1214–1220.

109. Paus S, Potzsch B, Risse JH, Klockgether T, Wullner U. Chorea and antiphospholipid antibodies: treatment with methotrexate. Neurology 2001; 56(1):137–138.

110. Pozzan GB, Battistella PA, Rigon F, Zancan L, Casara GL, Pellegrino PA, et al. Hyperthyroid-induced chorea in an adolescent girl. Brain & Development 1992; 14(2):126–127.

111. Yen DJ, Shan DE, Lu SR. Hyperthyroidism presenting as recurrent short paroxysmal kinesigenic dyskinesia. Movement Disorders 1998; 13(2):361–363.

112. Piccolo I, Causarano R, Sterzi R, Sberna M, Oreste PL, Moioli C, et al. Chorea in patients with AIDS. Acta Neurologica Scandinavica 1999; 100(5):332–336.

113. Gherpelli JL, Azeka E, Riso A, Atik E, Ebaid M, Barbero-Marcial M. Choreoathetosis after cardiac surgery with hypothermia and extracorporeal circulation. Pediatric Neurology 1998; 19(2): 113–118.

114. Vidakovic A, Dragasevic N, Kostic VS. Hemiballism: report of 25 cases. Journal of Neurology, Neurosurgery & Psychiatry 1994; 57 (8):945–949.

115. Beran-Koehn MA, Zupanc ML, Patterson MC, Olk DG, Ahlskog JE. Violent recurrent ballism associated with infections in two children with static encephalopathy. Movement Disorders 2000; 15(3):570–574.

116. Tsubokawa T, Katayama Y, Yamamoto T. Control of persistent hemiballismus by chronic thalamic stimulation. Report of two cases. Journal of Neurosurgery 1995; 82(3):501–505.

117. Fahn S, Marsden CD, Van Woert MH. Definition and classification of myoclonus. Advances in Neurology 1986; 43:1–5.

118. Shibasaki H. Electrophysiological studies of myoclonus. Muscle & Nerve 2000; 23(3):321–335.

119. Deuschl G, Toro C, Valls-Sole J, Zeffiro T, Zee DS, Hallett M. Symptomatic and essential palatal tremor. 1. Clinical, physiological and MRI analysis. Brain 1994; 117(Part 4):775–788.

120. Becker L, von Wegerer J, Schenkel J, Zeilhofer HU, Swandulla D, Weiher H. Disease-specific human glycine receptor alpha1 subunit causes hyperekplexia phenotype and impaired glycine- and GABA(A)-receptor transmission in transgenic mice. Journal of Neuroscience 2002; 22(7):2505–2512.

121. Ryan SG, Sherman SL, Terry JC, Sparkes RS, Torres MC, Mackey RW. Startle disease, or hyperekplexia: response to clonazepam and assignment of the gene (STHE) to chromosome 5q by linkage analysis. Annals of Neurology 1992; 31(6):663–668.

122. Jankovic J, Pardo R. Segmental myoclonus. Clinical and pharmacologic study. Archives of Neurology 1986; 43(10): 1025–1031.

123. Seidel G, Vieregge P, Wessel K, Kompf D. Peripheral myoclonus due to spinal root lesion. Muscle & Nerve 1997; 20(12): 1602–1603.

124. Wang A, Jankovic J. Hemifacial spasm: clinical findings and treatment. Muscle & Nerve 1998; 21(12):1740–1747.

125. Caviness JN. Myoclonus. Mayo Clinic Proceedings 1996; 71(7): 679–688.

126. Antel JP, Rasmussen T. Rasmussen's encephalitis and the new hat. Neurology 1996; 46(1):9–11.

127. Caviness JN, Alving LI, Maraganore DM, Black RA, McDonnell SK, Rocca WA. The incidence and prevalence of myoclonus in Olmsted County, Minnesota. Mayo Clinic Proceedings 1999; 74 (6):565–569.

128. Caviness JN. Primary care guide to myoclonus and chorea. Characteristics, causes, and clinical options. Postgraduate Medicine 2000; 108(5):163–166.

129. Delgado-Escueta AV, Ganesh S, Yamakawa K. Advances in the genetics of progressive myoclonus epilepsy. American Journal of Medical Genetics 2001; 106(2):129–138.

130. Marsden CD, Harding AE, Obeso JA, Lu CS. Progressive myoclonic ataxia (the Ramsay Hunt syndrome). Archives of Neurology 1990; 47(10):1121–1125.

131. Blindauer K. Myoclonus and its disorders. Neurologic Clinics 2001; 19(3):723–734.

132. Jimenez-Jimenez FJ, Garcia-Ruiz PJ, Molina JA. Drug-induced movement disorders. Drug Safety 1997; 16(3):180–204.

133. Frucht S, Fahn S. The clinical spectrum of posthypoxic myoclonus. Movement Disorders 2000; 15 (Suppl 1):2–7.

134. Agarwal P, Frucht SJ. Myoclonus. Current Opininions in Neurology 2003; 16(4): 515–521.

135. Crest C, Dupont S, Leguern E, Adam C, Baulac M. Levetiracetam in progressive myoclonic epilepsy: An exploratory study in 9 patients. Neurology 2004; 62(4):640–643.

136. Sohn YH, Kaelin-Lang A, Jung HY, Hallett M. Effect of levetiracetam on human corticospinal excitability. Neurology 2001; 57 (5):858–863.

137. Hallett M. Physiology of human posthypoxic myoclonus. Movement Disorders 2000; 15 (Suppl 1):8–13.

138. Jankovic J. Tourette's syndrome. New England Journal of Medicine 2001; 345(16):1184–1192.

139. Robertson MM. Tourette syndrome, associated conditions and the complexities of treatment. Brain 2000; 123 (Part 3):425–462.

140. Kurlan R. Hypothesis II: Tourette's syndrome is part of a clinical spectrum that includes normal brain development. Archives of Neurology 1994; 51(11):1145–1150.

141. American Psychiatric Association. Tourette's disorder. Diagnostic and Statistical Manual of Mental Disorders, 4th ed., Text Revision (DSM-IV-TR). Washington, DC: American Psychiatric Association, 2000: 111–114.

142. The Tourette Syndrome Classification Study Group. Definitions and classification of tic disorders. Archives of Neurology 1993; 50(10):1013–1016.

143. Robertson MM. The Gilles de la Tourette syndrome: the current status. British Journal of Psychiatry 1989; 154:147–169.

144. Leckman JF, Zhang H, Vitale A, Lahnin F, Lynch K, Bondi C, et al. Course of tic severity in Tourette syndrome: the first two decades. Pediatrics 1998; 102(1 Part 1):14–19.

145. Pappert EJ, Goetz CG, Louis ED, Blasucci L, Leurgans S. Objective assessments of longitudinal outcome in Gilles de la Tourette's syndrome. Neurology 2003; 61(7):936–940.

146. Burd L, Kerbeshian PJ, Barth A, Klug MG, Avery PK, Benz B. Long-term follow-up of an epidemiologically defined cohort of patients with Tourette syndrome. Journal of Child Neurology 2001; 16(6):431–437.

147. Kompoliti K, Goetz CG, Leurgans S, Raman R, Comella CL. Estrogen, progesterone, and tic severity in women with Gilles de la Tourette syndrome. Neurology 2001; 57(8):1519.

148. Abwender DA, Trinidad KS, Jones KR, Como PG, Hymes E, Kurlan R. Features resembling Tourette's syndrome in developmental stutterers. Brain & Language 1998; 62(3):455–464.

149. Cohrs S, Rasch T, Altmeyer S, Kinkelbur J, Kostanecka T, Rothenberger A, et al. Decreased sleep quality and increased sleep related movements in patients with Tourette's syndrome. Journal of Neurology, Neurosurgery & Psychiatry 2001; 70(2):192–197.

150. Como PG. Neuropsychological function in Tourette syndrome. Advances in Neurology 2001; 85:103–111.

151. Coffey BJ, Park KS. Behavioral and emotional aspects of Tourette syndrome. Neurologic Clinics 1997; 15(2):277–289.

152. Shin MS, Chung SJ, Hong KE. Comparative study of the behavioral and neuropsychologic characteristics of tic disorder with or without attention-deficit hyperactivity disorder (ADHD). Journal of Child Neurology 2001; 16(10):719–726.

153. Kurlan R, Como PG, Miller B, Palumbo D, Deeley C, Andresen EM, et al. The behavioral spectrum of tic disorders: a community-based study. Neurology 2002; 59(3):414–420.

154. Budman CL, Rockmore L, Stokes J, Sossin M. Clinical phenomenology of episodic rage in children with Tourette syndrome. Journal of Psychosomatic Research 2003; 55(1):59–65.

155. Barabas G, Matthews WS, Ferrari M. Tourette's syndrome and migraine. Archives of Neurology 1984; 41(8):871–872.

156. Cooper C, Robertson MM, Livingston G. Psychological morbidity and caregiver burden in parents of children with Tourette's disorder and psychiatric comorbidity. Journal of the American Academy of Child & Adolescent Psychiatry 2003; 42(11): 1370–1375.

157. Swerdlow NR, Young AB. Neuropathology in Tourette syndrome: an update. Advances in Neurology 2001; 85:151–161.

158. Leckman JF, Cohen DJ, Goetz CG, Jankovic J. Tourette syndrome: pieces of the puzzle. Advances in Neurology 2001; 85:369–390.

159. Peterson BS, Staib L, Scahill L, Zhang H, Anderson C, Leckman JF, et al. Regional brain and ventricular volumes in Tourette syndrome. Archives of General Psychiatry 2001; 58(5):427–440.

160. Peterson BS. Neuroimaging studies of Tourette syndrome: a decade of progress. Advances in Neurology 2001; 85:179–196.

161. Eidelberg D, Moeller JR, Antonini A, Kazumata K, Dhawan V, Budman C, et al. The metabolic anatomy of Tourette's syndrome. Neurology 1997; 48(4):927–934.

162. Stern E, Silbersweig DA, Chee KY, Holmes A, Robertson MM, Trimble M, et al. A functional neuroanatomy of tics in Tourette syndrome. Archives of General Psychiatry 2000; 57(8): 741–748.

163. Hallett M. Neurophysiology of tics. Advances in Neurology 2001; 85:237–244.

164. Ziemann U, Paulus W, Rothenberger A. Decreased motor inhibition in Tourette's disorder: evidence from transcranial magnetic stimulation. American Journal of Psychiatry 1997; 154(9): 1277–1284.

165. Greenberg BD, Ziemann U, Cora-Locatelli G, Harmon A, Murphy DL, Keel JC, et al. Altered cortical excitability in obsessive-compulsive disorder. Neurology 2000; 54(1):142–147.

166. Serrien DJ, Nirkko AC, Loher TJ, Lovblad KO, Burgunder JM, Wiesendanger M. Movement control of manipulative tasks in patients with Gilles de la Tourette syndrome. Brain 2002; 125(Part 2):290–300.

167. Singer HS. Current issues in Tourette syndrome. Movement Disorders 2000; 15(6):1051–1063.

168. Ernst M, Zametkin AJ, Jons PH, Matochik JA, Pascualvaca D, Cohen RM. High presynaptic dopaminergic activity in children with Tourette's disorder. Journal of the American Academy of Child & Adolescent Psychiatry 1999; 38(1):86–94.

169. Gilbert DL, Sethuraman G, Sine L, Peters S, Sallee FR. Tourette's syndrome improvement with pergolide in a randomized, double-blind, crossover trial. Neurology 2000; 54(6):1310–1315.

170. Hyde TM, Aaronson BA, Randolph C, Rickler KC, Weinberger DR. Relationship of birth weight to the phenotypic expression of Gilles de la Tourette's syndrome in monozygotic twins. Neurology 1992; 42(3 Part 1):652–658.

171. Hanna PA, Janjua FN, Contant CF, Jankovic J. Bilineal transmission in Tourette syndrome. Neurology 1999; 53(4):813–818.

172. Lichter DG, Dmochowski J, Jackson LA, Trinidad KS. Influence of family history on clinical expression of Tourette's syndrome. Neurology 1999; 52(2):308–316.

173. Kano Y, Ohta M, Nagai Y, Pauls DL, Leckman JF. A family study of Tourette syndrome in Japan. American Journal of Medical Genetics 2001; 105(5):414–421.

174. Simonic I, Nyholt DR, Gericke GS, Gordon D, Matsumoto N, Ledbetter DH, et al. Further evidence for linkage of Gilles de la Tourette syndrome (GTS) susceptibility loci on chromosomes 2p11, 8q22 and 11q23–24 in South African Afrikaners. American Journal of Medical Genetics 2001; 105(2):163–167.

175. The Tourette Syndrome Association International Consortium for Genetics. A complete genome screen in sib pairs affected by Gilles de la Tourette syndrome. American Journal of Human Genetics 1999; 65(5):1428–1436.

176. Zhang H, Leckman JF, Pauls DL, Tsai CP, Kidd KK, Campos MR, et al. Genomewide scan of hoarding in sib pairs in which both sibs have Gilles de la Tourette syndrome. American Journal of Human Genetics 2002; 70(4):896–904.

177. Petek E, Windpassinger C, Vincent JB, Cheung J, Boright AP, Scherer SW, et al. Disruption of a novel gene (IMMP2L) by a breakpoint in 7q31 associated with Tourette syndrome. American Journal of Human Genetics 2001; 68(4):848–858.

178. Leckman JF, Dolansky ES, Hardin MT, Clubb M, Walkup JT, Stevenson J, et al. Perinatal factors in the expression of Tourette's syndrome: an exploratory study. Journal of the American Academy of Child & Adolescent Psychiatry 1990; 29(2):220–226.

179. Swedo SE, Leonard HL, Mittleman BB, Allen AJ, Rapoport JL, Dow SP, et al. Identification of children with pediatric autoimmune neuropsychiatric disorders associated with streptococcal infections by a marker associated with rheumatic fever. American Journal of Psychiatry 1997; 154(1):110–112.

180. Murphy TK, Goodman WK, Fudge MW, Williams RC, Jr., Ayoub EM, Dalal M, et al. B lymphocyte antigen D8/17: a peripheral marker for childhood-onset obsessive-compulsive disorder and Tourette's syndrome? American Journal of Psychiatry 1997;154 (3):402–407.

181. Singer HS, Giuliano JD, Hansen BH, Hallett JJ, Laurino JP, Benson M, et al. Antibodies against human putamen in children with Tourette syndrome. Neurology 1998; 50(6):1618–1624.

182. Loiselle CR, Lee O, Moran TH, Singer HS. Striatal microinfusion of Tourette syndrome and PANDAS sera: failure to induce behavioral changes. Movement Disorders 2004; 19(4):390–396.

183. Kurlan R, Kaplan EL. The pediatric autoimmune neuropsychiatric disorders associated with streptococcal infection (PANDAS) etiology for tics and obsessive-compulsive symptoms: hypothesis or entity? Practical considerations for the clinician. Pediatrics 2004; 113(4):883–886.

184. Piacentini J, Chang S. Behavioral treatments for Tourette syndrome and tic disorders: state of the art. Advances in Neurology 2001; 85:319–331.

185. Peterson BS, Cohen DJ. The treatment of Tourette's syndrome: multimodal, developmental intervention. Journal of Clinical Psychiatry 1998; 59 (Suppl 1):62–72.

186. Sallee FR, Nesbitt L, Jackson C, Sine L, Sethuraman G. Relative efficacy of haloperidol and pimozide in children and adolescents with Tourette's disorder. American Journal of Psychiatry 1997; 154(8):1057–1062.

187. Dion Y, Annable L, Sandor P, Chouinard G. Risperidone in the treatment of Tourette syndrome: a double-blind, placebo-controlled trial. Journal of Clinical Psychopharmacology 2002; 22(1):31–39.

188. Gaffney GR, Perry PJ, Lund BC, Bever-Stille KA, Arndt S, Kuperman S. Risperidone versus clonidine in the treatment of children and adolescents with Tourette's syndrome. Journal of the American Academy of Child & Adolescent Psychiatry 2002; 41(3):330–336.

189. Bruggeman R, van der LC, Buitelaar JK, Gericke GS, Hawkridge SM, Temlett JA. Risperidone versus pimozide in Tourette's disorder: a comparative double-blind parallel-group study. Journal of Clinical Psychiatry 2001; 62(1):50–56.

190. Sallee FR, Kurlan R, Goetz CG, Singer H, Scahill L, Law G, et al. Ziprasidone treatment of children and adolescents with Tourette's syndrome: a pilot study. Journal of the American Academy of Child & Adolescent Psychiatry 2000; 39(3):292–299.

191. Mukaddes NM, Abali O. Quetiapine treatment of children and adolescents with Tourette's disorder. Journal of Child & Adolescent Psychopharmacology 2003; 13(3):295–299.

192. Jankovic J, Beach J. Long-term effects of tetrabenazine in hyperkinetic movement disorders. Neurology 1997; 48(2):358–362.

193. Jankovic J, Orman J. Tetrabenazine therapy of dystonia, chorea, tics, and other dyskinesias. Neurology 1988; 38(3):391–394.

194. Singer HS, Wendlandt J, Krieger M, Giuliano J. Baclofen treatment in Tourette syndrome: a double-blind, placebo-controlled, crossover trial. Neurology 2001; 56(5):599–604.

195. Lang AE. Update on the treatment of tics. Advances in Neurology 2001; 85:355–362.

196. Marras C, Andrews D, Sime E, Lang AE. Botulinum toxin for simple motor tics: a randomized, double-blind, controlled clinical trial. Neurology 2001; 56(5):605–610.

197. Kwak CH, Hanna PA, Jankovic J. Botulinum toxin in the treatment of tics. Archives of Neurology 2000; 57(8):1190–1193.

198. Scott BL, Jankovic J, Donovan DT. Botulinum toxin injection into vocal cord in the treatment of malignant coprolalia associated with Tourette's syndrome. Movement Disorders 1996; 11 (4):431–433.

199. Rauch SL, Baer L, Cosgrove GR, Jenike MA. Neurosurgical treatment of Tourette's syndrome: a critical review. Comprehensive Psychiatry 1995; 36(2):141–156.

200. Babel TB, Warnke PC, Ostertag CB. Immediate and long term outcome after infrathalamic and thalamic lesioning for intractable Tourette's syndrome. Journal of Neurology, Neurosurgery & Psychiatry 2001; 70(5):666–671.

201. Vandewalle V, van der LC, Groenewegen HJ, Caemaert J. Stereotactic treatment of Gilles de la Tourette syndrome by high frequency stimulation of thalamus. Lancet 1999; 353 (9154):724.

202. Manos MJ, Short EJ, Findling RL. Differential effectiveness of methylphenidate and Adderall in school-age youths with attention-deficit/hyperactivity disorder. Journal of the American Academy of Child & Adolescent Psychiatry 1999; 38(7): 813–819.

203. Efron D, Jarman F, Barker M. Side effects of methylphenidate and dexamphetamine in children with attention deficit hyperactivity disorder: a double-blind, crossover trial. Pediatrics 1997; 100(4):662–666.

204. Kurlan R. Tourette's syndrome: are stimulants safe? Current Neurology and Neuroscience Reports 2003; 3(4):285–288.

205. Law SF, Schachar RJ. Do typical clinical doses of methylphenidate cause tics in children treated for attention-deficit hyperactivity disorder? Journal of the American Academy of Child & Adolescent Psychiatry 1999; 38(8):944–951.

206. Gadow KD, Sverd J, Sprafkin J, Nolan EE, Grossman S. Long-term methylphenidate therapy in children with comorbid attention-deficit hyperactivity disorder and chronic multiple tic disorder. Archives of General Psychiatry 1999; 56(4):330–336.

207. Scahill L, Chappell PB, Kim YS, Schultz RT, Katsovich L, Shepherd E, et al. A placebo-controlled study of guanfacine in the treatment of children with tic disorders and attention deficit hyperactivity disorder. American Journal of Psychiatry 2001;158 (7):1067–1074.

208. Taylor FB, Russo J. Comparing guanfacine and dextroamphetamine for the treatment of adult attention-deficit/hyperactivity disorder. Journal of Clinical Psychopharmacology 2001; 21(2):223–228.

209. Hunt RD, Arnsten AF, Asbell MD. An open trial of guanfacine in the treatment of attention-deficit hyperactivity disorder. Journal of the American Academy of Child & Adolescent Psychiatry 1995; 34(1):50–54.

210. The Tourette's Syndrome Study Group. Treatment of ADHD in children with tics: a randomized controlled trial. Neurology 2002; 58(4):527–536.

211. Feigin A, Kurlan R, McDermott MP, Beach J, Dimitsopulos T, Brower CA, et al. A controlled trial of deprenyl in children with Tourette's syndrome and attention deficit hyperactivity disorder. Neurology 1996; 46(4):965–968.

212. Hollander E. Treatment of obsessive-compulsive spectrum disorders with SSRIs. British Journal of Psychiatry, Suppl 1998;(35): 7–12.

213. Fluvoxamine for the treatment of anxiety disorders in children and adolescents. The Research Unit on Pediatric Psychopharmacology Anxiety Study Group. New England Journal of Medicine 2001; 344(17):1279–1285.

214. Goodman WK, Ward HE, Murphy TK. Biologic approaches to treatment-refractory obsessive-compulsive disorder. Psychiatric Annals 1998; 28:641–649.

215. Kurlan R. Acute parkinsonism induced by the combination of a serotonin reuptake inhibitor and a neuroleptic in adults with Tourette's syndrome. Movement Disorders 1998; 13(1): 178–179.

216. Baer L, Rauch SL, Ballantine HT, Jr., Martuza R, Cosgrove R, Cassem E, et al. Cingulotomy for intractable obsessive-compulsive disorder. Prospective long-term follow-up of 18 patients. Archives of General Psychiatry 1995; 52(5):384–392.

217. Demirkiran M, Jankovic J. Paroxysmal dyskinesias: clinical features and classification. Annals of Neurology 1995; 38(4): 571–579.

218. Blakeley J, Jankovic J. Secondary paroxysmal dyskinesias. Mov Disord 2002; 17(4):726–734.

219. Houser MK, Soland VL, Bhatia KP, Quinn NP, Marsden CD. Paroxysmal kinesigenic choreoathetosis: a report of 26 patients. Journal of Neurology 1999; 246(2):120–126.

220. Bennett LB, Roach ES, Bowcock AM. A locus for paroxysmal kinesigenic dyskinesia maps to human chromosome 16. Neurology 2000; 54(1):125–130.

221. Szepetowski P, Rochette J, Berquin P, Piussan C, Lathrop GM, Monaco AP. Familial infantile convulsions and paroxysmal choreoathetosis: a new neurological syndrome linked to the pericentromeric region of human chromosome 16. American Journal of Human Genetics 1997; 61(4):889–898.

221a. Guerrini R, Bonanni P, Nardocci N, Parmeggiani L, Piccirilli M, De Fusco M, et al. Autosomal recessive rolandic epilepsy with paroxysmal exercise-induced dystonia and writer's cramp: delineation of the syndrome and gene mapping to chromosome 16p12–11.2. Annuals of Neurology 1995;45:344–l353.

222. Bhatia KP. Familial (idiopathic) paroxysmal dyskinesias: an update. Seminars in Neurology 2001; 21(1):69–74.

223. Byrne E, White O, Cook M. Familial dystonic choreoathetosis with myokymia: a sleep responsive disorder. Journal of Neurology, Neurosurgery & Psychiatry 1991; 54(12):1090–1092.

224. Fouad GT, Servidei S, Durcan S, Bertini E, Ptacek LJ. A gene for familial paroxysmal dyskinesia (FPD1) maps to chromosome 2q. American Journal of Human Genetics 1996; 59(1):135–139.

225. Bressman SB, Fahn S, Burke RE. Paroxysmal non-kinesigenic dystonia. Advances in Neurology 1988;'50:403–413.

226. Auburger G, Ratzlaff T, Lunkes A, Nelles HW, Leube B, Binkofski F, et al. A gene for autosomal dominant paroxysmal choreoathetosis/spasticity (CSE) maps to the vicinity of a potassium channel gene cluster on chromosome 1p, probably within 2 cM between D1S443 and D1S197. Genomics 1996; 31(1):90–94.

227. Fink JK, Hedera P, Mathay JG, Albin RL. Paroxysmal dystonic choreoathetosis linked to chromosome 2q: clinical analysis and proposed pathophysiology. Neurology 1997; 49(1):177–183.

228. Bhatia KP, Soland VL, Bhatt MH, Quinn NP, Marsden CD. Paroxysmal exercise-induced dystonia: eight new sporadic cases and a review of the literature. Movement Disorders 1997; 12(6): 1007–1012.

229. Munchau A, Valente EM, Shahidi GA, Eunson LH, Hanna MG, Quinn NP, et al. A new family with paroxysmal exercise induced dystonia and migraine: a clinical and genetic study. Journal of Neurology, Neurosurgery & Psychiatry 2000; 68(5):609–614.

230. Wali GM. Paroxysmal hemidystonia induced by prolonged exercise and cold. Journal of Neurology, Neurosurgery & Psychiatry 1992; 55(3):236–237.

231. Plant GT, Williams AC, Earl CJ, Marsden CD. Familial paroxysmal dystonia induced by exercise. Journal of Neurology, Neurosurgery & Psychiatry 1984; 47(3):275–279.

232. Lugaresi E, Cirignotta F. Hypnogenic paroxysmal dystonia: epileptic seizure or a new syndrome? Sleep 1981; 4(2):129–138.

233. Lee BI, Lesser RP, Pippenger CE, Morris HH, Luders H, Dinner DS, et al. Familial paroxysmal hypnogenic dystonia. Neurology 1985; 35(9):1357–1360.

234. Tinuper P, Cerullo A, Cirignotta F, Cortelli P, Lugaresi E, Montagna P. Nocturnal paroxysmal dystonia with short-lasting attacks: three cases with evidence for an epileptic frontal lobe origin of seizures. Epilepsia 1990; 31(5):549–556.

235. Scheffer IE, Bhatia KP, Lopes-Cendes I, Fish DR, Marsden CD, Andermann E, et al. Autosomal dominant nocturnal frontal lobe epilepsy. A distinctive clinical disorder. Brain 1995; 118(Part 1): 61–73.

236. Phillips HA, Scheffer IE, Crossland KM, Bhatia KP, Fish DR, Marsden CD, et al. Autosomal dominant nocturnal frontal-lobe epilepsy: genetic heterogeneity and evidence for a second locus at 15q24. American Journal of Human Genetics 1998;63(4): 1108–1116.

237. Phillips HA, Scheffer IE, Berkovic SF, Hollway GE, Sutherland GR, Mulley JC. Localization of a gene for autosomal dominant nocturnal frontal lobe epilepsy to chromosome 20q13.2. Nature Genetics 1995; 10(1):117–118.

238. Ridley RM. The psychology of perserverative and stereotyped behaviour. Progress in Neurobiology 1994; 44(2):221–231.

239. Neul JL, Zoghbi HY. Rett syndrome: a prototypical neurodevelopmental disorder. Neuroscientist 2004; 10(2):118–128.

240. Schanen C, Houwink EJ, Dorrani N, Lane J, Everett R, Feng A, et al. Phenotypic manifestations of MECP2 mutations in classical and atypical Rett syndrome. American Journal of Medical Genetics 2004; 126A(2):129–140.

241. Dunn HG, Macleod PM. Rett syndrome: review of biological abnormalities. Canadian Journal of Neurological Science 2001; 28(1):16–29.

242. Thomas GR, Forbes JR, Roberts EA, Walshe JM, Cox DW. The Wilson disease gene: spectrum of mutations and their consequences. Nature Genetics 1995; 9(2):210–217.

243. Schilsky ML. Diagnosis and treatment of Wilson's disease. Pediatric Transplantation 2002; 6(1):15–19.

244. Stremmel W, Meyerrose KW, Niederau C, Hefter H, Kreuzpaintner G, Strohmeyer G. Wilson disease: clinical presentation, treatment, and survival. Annals of Internal Medicine 1991; 115(9):720–726.

245. Brewer GJ. Recognition, diagnosis, and management of Wilson's disease. Proceedings of the Society for Experimental Biology & Medicine 2000; 223(1):39–46.

246. Liu M, Cohen EJ, Brewer GJ, Laibson PR. Kayser-Fleischer ring as the presenting sign of Wilson disease. American Journal of Ophthalmology 2002; 133(6):832–834.

247. Scheinberg IH. Wilson's disease. In: Braunwald E, Fauci AS, Isselbacher KJ, Kasper DL, Hauser SL, Longo DL, et al., eds. Harrison's Online. New York: McGraw-Hill, 2001: DOI 10.1036/1096–7133, ch 348.

247a. Akil M, Schwartz JA, Dutchak D, Yuzbasiyan-Gurkan V, Brewer. The psychiatric presentations of Wilson's disease. The Journal of Neuropsychiatry and Clinical Neurosciences 1991:3:377–382.

247b. Dening TR, Berrios GE. Wilson's Disease. Psychiatric Symptoms in 195 cases Archives of General Psychiatry. 1989;46:1126–1134.

247c. Hesse S, Barthel H,l Hermann W, Murai T, Kluge R, Wagner A, Sabri O, Eggers B. Regional serotonin transporter availability and depression are correlated in Wilson's disease. Journal of Neural Transmission 2003;110:923–933.

248. Cox DW. Genes of the copper pathway. American Journal of Human Genetics 1995; 56(4):828–834.

249. Giagheddu M, Tamburini G, Piga M, Tacconi P, Giagheddu A, Serra A, et al. Comparison of MRI, EEG, EPs and ECD-SPECT in Wilson's disease. Acta Neurologica Scandinavica 2001; 103(2): 71–81.

250. Hitoshi S, Iwata M, Yoshikawa K. Mid-brain pathology of Wilson's disease: MRI analysis of three cases. Journal of Neurology, Neurosurgery & Psychiatry 1991; 54(7):624–626.

251. Wu ZY, Lin MT, Murong SX, Wang N. Molecular diagnosis and prophylactic therapy for presymptomatic Chinese patients with Wilson disease. Archives of Neurology 2003; 60(5):737–741.

252. Bertrand E, Lewandowska E, Szpak GM, Hoogenraad T, Blaauwgers HG, Czlonkowska A, et al. Neuropathological analysis of pathological forms of astroglia in Wilson's disease. Folia Neuropathologica 2001; 39(2):73–79.

253. Bertrand E, Lechowicz W, Szpak GM, Lewandowska E, Czlonkowska A, Dymecki J. Quantitative study of pathological forms of astroglia in Wilson's disease. Folia Neuropathologica 1997; 35(4):227–232.

254. Bellary S, Hassanein T, Van Thiel DH. Liver transplantation for Wilson's disease. Journal of Hepatology 1995; 23(4):373–381.

255. Stracciari A, Tempestini A, Borghi A, Guarino M. Effect of liver transplantation on neurological manifestations in Wilson disease. Archives of Neurology 2000; 57(3):384–386.

256. Hayflick SJ. Unraveling the Hallervorden-Spatz syndrome: pantothenate kinase-associated neurodegeneration is the name. Current Opinion in Pediatrics 2003; 15(6):572–577.

257. Hayflick SJ, Westaway SK, Levinson B, Zhou B, Johnson MA, Ching KH, et al. Genetic, clinical, and radiographic delineation of Hallervorden-Spatz syndrome. New England Journal of Medicine 2003; 348(1):33–40.

258. Swaiman KF. Hallervorden-Spatz syndrome. Pediatric Neurology 2001; 25(2):102–108.

259. Carod-Artal FJ, Vargas AP, Marinho PB, Fernandes-Silva TV, Portugal D. Tourettism, hemiballism and juvenile Parkinsonism: expanding the clinical spectrum of the neurodegeneration associated to pantothenate kinase deficiency (Hallervorden Spatz syndrome). Review of Neurology 2004; 38(4):327–331.

260. Ching KHL, Westaway SK, Gitschier J, Higgins JJ, Hayflick SJ. HARP syndrome is allelic with pantothenate kinase-associated neurodegeneration. Neurology 2002; 58:1673–1674.

261. Gouider-Khouja N, Miladi N, Belal S, Hentati F. Intrafamilial phenotypic variability of Hallervorden-Spatz syndrome in a Tunisian family. Parkinsonism and Related Disorders 2000; 6: 175–179.

262. Dooling EC, Schoene WC, Richardson EP, Jr. Hallervorden-Spatz syndrome. Archives of Neurology 1974; 30:70–83.

263. Hayflick SJ, Westaway SK, Levinson B, Zhou B, et al. Genetic, clinical, and radiographic delineation of Hallervorden Spatz syndrome. New England Journal of Medicine 2003; 348(1):33–40.

264. Koeppen AH, Dickson AC. Iron in the Hallervorden-Spatz syndrome. Pediatric Neurology 2001; 25(2):148–155.

265. Tripathi RC, Tripathi BJ, Bauserman SC, Park JK. Clinicopathologic correlation and pathogenesis of ocular and central nervous system manifestations in Hallervorden-Spatz syndrome. Acta Neuropathologica 1992; 83(2):113–119.

266. Galvin JE, Giasson B, Hurtig HI, Lee VM, Trojanowski JQ. Neurodegeneration with brain iron accumulation, type 1 is characterized by alpha-, beta-, and gamma-synuclein neuropathology. American Journal of Pathology 2000; 157(2):361–368.

267. Justesen CR, Penn RD, Kroin JS, Egel RT. Stereotactic pallidotomy in a child with Hallervorden-Spatz disease. Case report. Journal of Neurosurgery 1999; 90(3):551–554.

268. Tuite PJ, Provias JP, Lang AE. Atypical dopa responsive parkinsonism in a patient with megalencephaly, midbrain Lewy body disease, and some pathological features of Hallervorden-Spatz disease. Journal of Neurology, Neurosurgery & Psychiatry 1996; 61(5):523–527.

269. Chiueh CC. Iron overload, oxidative stress, and axonal dystrophy in brain disorders. Pediatric Neurology 2001; 25(2): 138–147.

270. Gosser DS, Stern MB. The psychogenic movement disorders: theoretical and clinical considerations. In: Adler CH, Ahlskog JE, eds. Parkinson's Disease and Movement Disorders. Totowa, NJ: Humana Press, 2000: 435–451.

271. Ranawaya R, Riley D, Lang A. Psychogenic dyskinesias in patients with organic movement disorders. Movement Disorders 1990; 5(2):127–133.

272. Factor SA, Podskalny GD, Molho ES. Psychogenic movement disorders: frequency, clinical profile, and characteristics. Journal of Neurology, Neurosurgery & Psychiatry 1995; 59(4):406–412.

273. Feinstein A, Stergiopoulos V, Fine J, Lang AE. Psychiatric outcome in patients with a psychogenic movement disorder: a prospective study. Neuropsychiatry, Neuropsychology, & Behavioral Neurology 2001; 14(3):169–176.

Epilepsy Syndromes in Childhood

22

Rochelle Caplan, MD   *Erin Lanphier, PhD*

INTRODUCTION

Epilepsy occurs in 4 per 1,000 children (Hauser and Hesdorffer, 1990) with a lifetime incidence of 4 to 9 /1,000 in 10-year-old children (Murphy et al., 1995). Since epilepsy is a recurrent chronic disorder that involves the brain, child clinicians need to be aware of the neurological and behavioral aspects of this disorder to understand the impact of this illness on the child and his or her family.

The Commission on Classification and Terminology of the International League Against Epilepsy (1989) divided the epileptic syndromes by seizure types (i.e., partial, focal, or localized versus generalized) and by etiology into idiopathic (primary) or symptomatic (secondary) (Table 22.1). Using the Commission classification, this chapter describes the clinical and behavioral aspects of the most common epileptic syndromes in childhood and adolescence. It then reviews the clinical manifestations, associated disorders, diagnosis, and treatment of pseudoseizures in childhood and adolescence. The chapter concludes with a brief discussion on how epilepsy affects school achievement, cognition, and language in children.

LOCALIZATION-RELATED EPILEPSIES AND SYNDROMES

Symptomatic

Temporal Lobe Epilepsy (TLE)

Seizures originating from the temporal lobe can be simple partial, complex partial, secondarily generalized, or a combination of the above (Commission, 1989). As described for adolescents and adults, the etiology of temporal lobe

epilepsy in childhood includes mesial temporal sclerosis, tumors, and cortical dysplasia (Aso et al., 1994; Porter et al., 2003; Wyllie et al., 1993). However, dual pathology involving both mesial temporal sclerosis (hippocampal pathology) and cortical dysplasia is more common in children with temporal lobe epilepsy (Bocti et al., 2003; Mohamed et al., 2001).

Nonetheless, the younger the cohort of children, the more infrequent is mesial temporal (hippocampal) sclerosis. Magnetic resonance imaging (MRI) studies show that only 46% of children and 44% of adolescents with temporal lobe epilepsy have focal atrophy of the hippocampal head or body; whereas the remaining patients in these age groups have asymmetry of total hippocampal volumes (Mohamed et al., 2001). As described for adults, the presence of mesial temporal sclerosis in childhood is associated with a history of febrile convulsions and status epilepticus (Aso et al., 1994; Harvey et al., 1993; Scott et al., 2001; Wyllie et al., 1993).

In terms of ictal semiology, simple partial seizures of temporal origin present with sensory (e.g., rising unpleasant epigastric sensation, olfactory or auditory hallucinations or illusions), autonomic (e.g., nausea, vomiting), or psychic symptoms (e.g., forced thinking, déja vue, déja entendu) (Commission, 1989). Complex partial seizures last less than 1 minute and present with loss of consciousness, a motor arrest, oroalimentary automatisms followed by other automatisms, and postictal confusion or amnesia (Commission, 1989).

In contrast to adults, the clinical manifestations of temporal lobe epilepsy in children are not homogenous and motor phenomena, such as tonic, clonic, hypermotor movements as well as epileptic spasms, occur (see the review in Fogarasi et al., 2002). Other ictal manifestations of temporal lobe seizures in children include shouting, tonic

TABLE 22.1
CLASSIFICATION OF EPILEPSY AND EPILEPTIC SYNDROMES

1. Localization-Related Epilepsies

   a. **Partial (Focal)**
     Temporal lobe epilepsy
     Frontal lobe epilepsy
     Parietal lobe epilepsy
     Occipital lobe epilepsy
   b. **Idiopathic**
     Benign rolandic with centro-temporal spike
     Childhood epilepsy with occipital paroxysms
     Primary reading epilepsy
   c. **Symptomatic**
     Chronic progressive epilepsia partialis continua of childhood (Kojewnikow's syndrome)

2. Generalized Epilepsies and Syndromes

   a. **Idiopathic**
     Benign neonatal familial convulsions
     Benign neonatal convulsions
     Benign myoclonic epilepsy in infancy
     Childhood absence epilepsy
     Juvenile absence epilepsy
     Juvenile myoclonic epilepsy
     Epilepsy with grand mal seizures on awakening
     Other generalized epilepsies not defined previously
   b. **Cryptogenic or symptomatic**
     West syndrome (infantile spasms)
     Lennox-Gastaut syndrome
     Epilepsy with myoclonic-astatic seizures
     Epilepsy with myoclonic absences
   c. **Symptomatic**
     Epilepsies and syndromes undetermined whether focal or generalized
     Neonatal seizures
     Severe myoclonic epilepsy in infancy
     Epilepsy with continuous spike-waves during slow wave sleep
     Acquired epileptic aphasia (Landau-Kleffner syndrome)

3. Special Syndromes

     Febrile convulsions
     Isolated seizures or isolated status epilepticus
     Seizures with acute metabolic or toxic event

Source: Adapted from Commission on Classification and Terminology of the International League Against Epilepsy, 1989.

posturing, versive seizures, vomiting, eye deviation, and laughing, but these are more infrequent in children (Aso et al., 1994; Olbrich et al., 2002).

In terms of auras, like adults, children with temporal lobe epilepsy due to mesial temporal sclerosis have abdominal or gustatory auras (Wyllie et al., 1993) or rising epigastric sensation (Aso et al., 1994); whereas those without mesial temporal sclerosis have more complex auras with somatosensory and visual phenomena, dizziness, or headache (Aso et al., 1994; Wyllie et al., 1993). The automatisms of complex partial seizures are, however, more infrequent and simpler in children compared to adults and are limited to lip smacking and fumbling hand gestures

(Mohammed et al., 2001; Wyllie et al., 1993). Secondary generalization occurs infrequently in 2 to 24% of the seizures of children with temporal lobe epilepsy (Aso et al., 1994; Wyllie et al., 1993).

Whereas the EEG of adolescents with temporal lobe epilepsy present with unilateral anterior temporal interictal spikes, the anterior temporal spikes of children with temporal lobe epilepsy are associated with mid/posterior temporal, bilateral temporal, extratemporal, or generalized spikes in 60% of the cases (Mohammed et al., 2001).

Studies on the course and outcome of pediatric temporal lobe epilepsy indicate that these are difficult-to-control seizures and usually do not remit spontaneously (Aso et al.,

1994). A retrospective chart study of 120 children, ages 1 to 18 years revealed that failure of the first antiepileptic drug (AED) trial accurately predicts refractory pediatric TLE at the 2-year follow-up (Dlugos et al., 2001). Bilateral temporal interictal sharp waves and bilateral hippocampal sclerosis on MRI are associated with a tendency for lower seizure-free outcome at the 2.6 year follow-up (Mohamed et al., 2001).

In terms of long-term outcome, in a prospective study Lindsay et al. (1979a) reported that one third of 100 children with temporal lobe epilepsy were seizure free as adults. However, they might have included cases of benign focal epilepsy of childhood (discussed later), an entity unknown at that time, in their sample (Kotagal et al., 1987). Aso et al. (1994) described a similar course in children with mesial temporal sclerosis and in those with other underlying etiologies. This finding led Aso et al. (1994) to conclude that, irrespective of the underlying pathology, pediatric complex partial seizures originating from the temporal lobe have a bad prognosis.

Behavioral Aspects of Temporal Lobe Epilepsy

Several older studies suggest that children with temporal lobe epilepsy have characteristic behavioral disturbances (Hoare, 1991; Lindsay et al., 1979a, 1979b, 1984; Rutter et al., 1970; Stores, 1978a; Stores et al., Taylor, 1975), particularly if they have left-sided foci (Lindsay et al., 1979b, 1984; Stores, 1978a). These include hyperactivity, antisocial behavior, and aggression (Hoare, 1991; Rutter et al., 1970; Stores, 1978), and a schizophrenia-like psychosis (Caplan et al., 1991; Lindsay et al., 1979a and b).

Antisocial behavior was related to male sex, poor seizure control, low IQ, and childhood rages (Lindsay et al., 1979a, 179b; Stores, 1978a, 1978b). Lindsay et al. (1979a) reported that 10% of children with temporal lobe epilepsy developed psychosis by adulthood, in particular, if they had experienced cataclysmic rage attacks and hyperkinetic reactions in childhood. The schizophrenia-like psychosis appeared to be associated with hallucinations, delusions, and illogical thinking but not with loose associations or negative signs of schizophrenia (Caplan et al., 1991, 1992a). Unlike adults with temporal lobe epilepsy and schizophrenia-like psychosis (Dongier, 1959; Kristensen and Sindrup, 1978; Landolt, 1958; Pakalnis et al., 1987; Slater et al., 1963), middle childhood onset of interictal psychosis was not associated with a long latency period, seizure control, or normalization of EEG (Caplan et al., 1991). Despite these behavioral difficulties, a prospective study by Lindsay et al. (1979a, 1979b) demonstrated a significant reduction of behavioral disturbances in adulthood compared to adolescence, particularly if seizures were controlled prior to age 12 years.

In contrast to these findings, Kaminer et al. (1988) were unable to demonstrate increased psychopathology in adolescents with temporal lobe epilepsy compared to adolescents with asthma. Other researchers were unable to identify differences in measures of psychopathology in children with temporal lobe and generalized epilepsy (Hermann et al., 1988; Whitman et al., 1982). Camfield et al. (1979) found that dysfunction on neuropsychological tests rather than lateralization of the temporal lobe focus was related to differences in the psychopathology profile of children with epilepsy.

Studies indicate high rates of psychopathology in children with complex partial seizures, many of whom have temporal lobe epilepsy. Sixty percent of the children have an axis I diagnosis compared to age- and gender-matched normal control subjects (Caplan et al., 2004). Subtle verbal difficulties, not seizure variables, are a robust predictor of these behavioral problems (Caplan et al., 2004). Of note, this high rate of behavioral problems is not specific for children with TLE and is also found in childhood absence epilepsy (Caplan et al., 1998; Ott et al., 2001, 2003).

Shortterm follow-up 3 months after surgery of 21 surgically treated children with intractable epilepsy, 13 of whom had anterior temporal lobectomy, showed significant improvement in parent-based internalizing, externalizing, attention, and thought problems of the Child Behavior Checklist (Achenbach, 1991) compared to presurgical measures and to a control group of medically treated children with comparable psychopathology scores (Lendt et al., 2000). A good seizure outcome predicted these behavioral changes similar to the findings of earlier studies indicating reduced aggression in surgically treated TLE children with seizure control (Green, 1977; Hopkins and Klug, 1991; Lindsay et al., 1984). However, none of these earlier studies used standardized psychiatric instruments to follow the postoperative behavioral changes of a representative sample of children undergoing temporal lobectomy.

In contrast, seizure variables were unrelated to the findings of a follow-up study of 30 children who had anterior temporal lobectomy compared to 21 medically controlled children with intractable TLE. There were no psychosocial differences between the groups 1 year after surgery other than a trend toward promotion of independence and less satisfaction with the family of the surgical patients (Smith et al., 2004).

Lower IQ scores and impaired performance on neuropsychological tests are also found in both new onset (Hermann et al., 2005) and chronic childhood temporal lobe epilepsy (Caplan et al., 2004; Schoenfeld et al., 1999). These neuropsychological deficits have been associated with reduction in total white matter volume in the chronic patients (Hermann et al., 2002) but not in the new onset patients (Hermann et al., 2005). Parent reports support attentional difficulties, particularly in children with left-sided lesions (Duval et al., 2002).

In children who had temporal lobe epilepsy surgery, earlier reports indicated unchanged cognition and memory (Miranda and Smith, 2001; Williams et al., 1998), decline in memory and language (Szabo et al., 1998), or improved attention and memory (Lendt et al., 1999; Mabbott and Smith, 2003). Smith et al. (2004) found no difference at the 1-year follow-up in cognition and behavior in children who had undergone epilepsy surgery compared to medical control subjects. Compared to children with other epilepsy syndromes (e.g., frontal lobe epilepsy, childhood absence epilepsy), children with temporal lobe epilepsy have significantly worse memory function and reduced performance on most verbal and visual tasks (Nolan et al., 2004).

In addition, these children have significantly impaired linguistic skills when compared to either normal (Caplan et al., 2004) or sibling-control subjects (Schoenfeld et al., 1999). In formulating and organizing their thoughts, they also perform poorly compared to age- and gender-matched normal subjects (Caplan et al., 2002a). Additionally, they monitor and correct communication breakdowns more infrequently than do the normal children (Caplan et al., 2001).

Diagnosis

A child who presents with abdominal, gustatory, somatosensory, or psychic aura automatisms, such as lip smacking or hand gestures, decreased level of awareness, and postictal amnesia, might have temporal lobe epilepsy. An EEG finding of focal interictal spikes or sharp waves in the temporal area using scalp or depth electrodes will confirm the diagnosis.

The differential diagnosis should include other seizure disorders, such as childhood absence epilepsy if the child presents with absences; frontal lobe epilepsy if the child presents with aura, motor seizures, or tonic versive seizures; benign focal epilepsy if the seizures are nocturnal and involve the orofacial area; and benign occipital epilepsy if the child presents with visual aura. Psychic symptoms, like hallucinations, illusions, and forced thinking, that occur during temporal lobe epilepsy auras need to be differentiated from those that occur in psychoses, such as schizophrenia, manic depressive disorder, psychosis not otherwise specified, or dissociative psychosis associated with posttraumatic stress disorder.

Ictal psychic symptoms are stereotyped and consistent across ictal episodes. In contrast, the form and content of the hallucinations, illusions, and abnormal thoughts of psychotic children vary over time. Furthermore, children with ictal auditory hallucination usually do not recall the content of their hallucinations. Psychotic children describe the content, albeit bizarre, of their auditory hallucinations. Ictal psychic phenomena cause marked subjective distress to children who perceive them as an unreal experience. In the acute phase of psychosis, children might respond with subjective distress and insight as to the unreal nature of the experience. The child with chronic psychosis, however, does not become upset and has poor reality testing when he or she experiences hallucinations, illusions, or forced thinking.

Finally, forced thinking should be differentiated from the obsessions of obsessive-compulsive disorder. Forced thinking and obsessions can both cause subjective distress in the child. Unlike the epileptic child with stereotyped forced thinking, the child with obsessive-compulsive disorder usually has more than one obsession, and these obsessions change over time.

Treatment

The drugs commonly used in children with temporal lobe epilepsy include carbamazepine and valproic acid, and more recently lamotrigine, topiramate, oxcarbazepine, and gabapentin (French et al., 2004). Children who fail to respond to the first AED have a high rate of treatment failure (89%) to a subsequent AED trial (Dlugos et al., 2001). Anterior temporal lobectomy (Clusmann et al., 2004; Sinclair et al., 2004) and vagal nerve stimulation have variable success rates. Normal intelligence at baseline and tumor as etiology are associated with better outcome in pediatric epilepsy surgery that also includes anterior temporal lobectomy (Gashlan et al., 1999; Sherman et al., 2003).

Frontal Lobe Epilepsy

A good understanding of the clinical and behavioral aspects of this epileptic syndrome is important because they often involve bizarre behaviors (Chauvel et al., 1995; Delgado-Escueta et al., 1994) that are labeled as hysteria (Saygi et al., 1992; Stores et al., 1991) or other psychiatric syndromes (Boone et al., 1988; Sinclair et al., 2004). In addition to bizarre behaviors, this syndrome poses diagnostic difficulties because the ictal and interictal scalp EEG is often normal, particularly in patients with mesial or orbital frontal lobe epilepsy (Shigematsu et al., 1992; Van Ness, 1993; Williamson et al., 1985).

Typically, frontal lobe seizures are characterized by auras, bilateral coarse and upper extremity movements, rare oroalimentary automatisms, short duration of less than 1 minute, minimal postictal confusion, and frequent seizures (Kotagal et al., 2003; Laskowitz et al., 1995; Quesney et al., 1992; Salanova et al., 1995; Wieser et al., 1992; Williamson, 1992, 1995). The clinical presentation of frontal lobe seizures depends on the anatomical location of the focus and ipsilateral or bilateral seizure spread.

There are different opinions on the anatomical classification of frontal lobe seizures (Quesney et al., 1992), and in some cases the epileptic zone might be a continuum rather than a discrete focus (Quesney et al., 1990). Penfield and Jasper (1954) originally classified them into focal motor seizures, supplementary motor seizures, and psychomotor seizures, and this classification is supported by Wieser et al.'s (1983) cluster analysis of psychomotor seizures and by more recent studies (Chauvel et al., 1995; Salanova et al., 1995).

Focal motor seizures involve unilateral clonic movements of the face followed by the arm, speech arrest, blinking, version of the head and eyes, but no loss of consciousness (Salanova et al., 1995). Seizures originating in the supplementary motor area occur in clusters at night (Bancaud and Talairach, 1992; Wieser et al., 1992) and present with somatosensory auras, unilateral or bilateral posturing and tonic movements that spread to the whole body, vocalizations from simple groaning to shouted obscenities, laughing, crying, and version of the head and eyes (Laskowitz et al., 1995; Salanova et al., 1995; Williamson et al., 1985). Patients with supplementary motor seizures maintain consciousness prior to generalization of the seizure and spread to the other side (Bancaud and Talairach, 1992; Morris et al., 1988; Wieser et al., 1992).

Complex partial seizures occur if the seizure focus is in the frontal opercular convexity or the anterofrontal region (Quesney et al., 1992). Complex partial seizures of frontal origin have a sensory aura with a feeling of pins and needles, tingling, or sensation of heaviness or light headedness on the contralateral side (Quesney et al., 1992). The patient can also experience whole body dizziness, fear, or visual phenomena. During a seizure, the patient stares ahead with partial or complete unresponsiveness, vocalizes, has bilateral tonic arm movements, laughs, cries, makes pedaling bicycle movements, or turns the head and eyes contralateral to the seizure focus (Salanova et al., 1995).

Seizures from the mesial frontal cortex produce emotional and autonomic manifestations, such as aura with panic or fear and changes in sympathetic tone. Seizures of orbitofrontal origin are silent until they spread to the adjacent cingulate or insular regions and then produce autonomic signs (i.e., facial reddening, tachycardia), olfactory hallucinations, or oroalimentary automatisms (Laskowitz et al., 1995). The presence of sexual automatisms reflects involvement of the anterior cingulate gyrus (Stoeffels et al., 1980). Finally, frontal lobe seizures from the frontal pole present with a motionless stare, loss of postural tone, and secondary generalization (Laskowitz et al., 1995).

Preschool children with frontal lobe epilepsy have frequent short seizures that occur at night or during sleep with motor manifestations and automatisms, such as moaning, groaning, and crying, but rare secondary generalization and laughing or pedal movements (Fogarasi et al., 2002). In older children asymmetric tonic posturing, contralateral head/eye deviation, and unilateral clonic jerking were associated with reduced blood flow in dorsolateral, front central, and medial frontal regions while vocalization, hyperventilation, truncal flexion, and complex gestural automatisms were found in children with reduced blood flow in orbital and polar frontal regions (Harvey et al., 1993). Seizures occur mainly in sleep and are associated with bilateral ictal and interictal epileptiform EEG findings (Lawson et al., 2002).

Behavioral Aspects of Frontal Lobe Epilepsy
There have been no studies on the psychiatric aspects of frontal lobe seizures in children to date. Children with complex partial seizures with EEG evidence for frontal involvement have more severe formal thought disorder (Caplan et al., 1992) and discourse deficits (Caplan et al., 1994) than those with temporal involvement. Two case re-

ports (Boone et al., 1988; Stores et al., 1991) describe sexual disinhibition, pressured and tangential speech, screaming, aggression, disorganized behavior, and nightmares in children with frontal lobe epilepsy. Children with frontal lobe epilepsy appear to have more deficits in planning and executive function (Culhane-Shelburne et al., 2002), but no difference in language scores (Blanchette and Smith, 2002) compared to those with temporal lobe epilepsy.

Diagnosis
This is a difficult disorder to diagnose (Bass et al., 1995; Riggio and Harner, 1992). One should entertain a diagnosis of frontal lobe epilepsy in a child if he or she presents with brief sudden unresponsiveness without loss of consciousness and continued understanding of spoken language during the episode with either clonic or tonic motor phenomena that involve the face and arms and become bilateral. The presence of vocalizations, laughing, crying, or rarely pedaling movements could be suggestive of this diagnosis. A normal EEG with scalp electrodes does not rule out the diagnosis of frontal lobe epilepsy.

The two main disorders to consider in the differential diagnosis are complex partial seizures of temporal origin and pseudoseizures. The aura, stare, and automatisms of frontal lobe epilepsy might resemble the complex partial seizures of temporal lobe origin. Unlike complex partial seizures of temporal lobe origin, the amnesia of complex partial seizures of frontal origin is more pronounced than the degree of loss of consciousness (Chauvel et al., 1995). Furthermore, frontal complex partial seizures have associated unilateral or bilateral tonic posturing and bicycling movements, partial rather than complete loss of consciousness, and contralateral head and eye deviation. In contrast, patients with complex partial seizures of temporal lobe origin have more oroalimentary and repetitive hand automatisms and looking around (Salanova et al., 1995).

Among the similarities of pseudoseizures and frontal lobe seizures, children with both disorders present with unresponsiveness or partial loss of consciousness and no EEG correlates during continuous video-EEG monitoring of these episodes. In addition, the vocalizations of children with frontal lobe seizures can be interpreted as emotional lability or dissociative phenomena in children with pseudoseizures. Among the differences between these two disorders, pseudoseizures have a prolonged onset and duration and usually do not occur during sleep, whereas frontal lobe seizures start suddenly, last less than 1 minute, and are nocturnal. The motor phenomena of pseudoseizures involve thrusting or rolling rather than the rhythmic flexion and extension of clonic movements in frontal lobe epilepsy. Children with pseudoseizures, in contrast to frontal lobe epilepsy, have a primary conflict that involves difficulty expressing negative affect and a secondary gain that reinforces their pseudoseizures. In some cases, however, it is difficult to differentiate between these disorders, particularly when a child has both disorders. Continued video-EEG monitoring with depth electrodes is helpful in providing a definitive diagnosis of frontal lobe epilepsy in these children (Bass et al., 1995).

Finally, the presence of sensory, gustatory, or olfactory hallucinations underscore the importance of ruling out psychotic disorders, such as schizophrenia, psychosis not otherwise specified, manic psychosis, or another organic psychosis as previously described in the section on temporal lobe epilepsy.

Treatment
Typically this is a difficult disorder to treat medically or surgically (Fish et al., 1993: Kral et al., 2001).

Benign Rolandic Epilepsy
Benign rolandic epilepsy begins in childhood between ages 3 and 10 years and remits by age 16 years (Blom and Heijbel, 1992; Lerman and Kivity, 1975; Loiseau et al., 1988; Kramer and Lerman, 2001). This form of epilepsy is frequent in childhood and accounts for 15 to 25% of all epileptic syndromes in children under age 12 years (Astradsson et al., 1998; Cavazutti, 1980). Benign rolandic epilepsy occurs more frequently in children with a history of febrile seizures (Degen and Degen, 1990; Gregory and Wong, 1984; Kajitani et al., 1992; Lerman and Kivity, 1975), a family history of febrile seizures (Kajitani et al., 1992), or benign rolandic epilepsy (Heijbel et al., 1975). It is also frequent in children with fragile X syndrome (Berry-Kravis, 2002). MRI studies might reveal hippocampal asymmetries and white matter abnormalities (Lundberg et al., 1999).

Benign rolandic seizures usually occur nocturnally during sleep (Drury and Beydoun, 1991). The children have brief and mild tonic–clonic seizures of the face, lips, tongue, pharyngeal and laryngeal muscles, speech arrest, saliva pooling and drooling, and no loss of consciousness (de Weerd and Arts, 1993; Iannetti et al., 1994; Lerman and Kivity, 1991). Although partial, these seizures tend to generalize (de Weerd and Arts, 1993; Iannetti et al., 1994; Kajitani et al., 1992). Daytime seizures that are simple/partial, involving the face and tongue, occur in one third of the children (Camfield and Camfield, 2002).

The EEG findings include normal background, as well as interictal spikes or blunted monomorphic sharp waves (Drury and Bedoun, 1991; Lüders et al., 1989). Similar EEG findings occurring in 1.3 to 2.4% of normal children (Cavazutti, 1980) are thought to reflect central nervous system immaturity in terms of brain excitability and inhibition (Ferri et al., 2000). The cortical generators for rolandic discharges are localized in the sulcal or gyral cortices on either side of the central sulcus of the precentral motor cortex, closer to hand secondary somatosensory cortex than to primary cortex (Jung et al., 2003; Lin et al., 2003). Spike propagation involves spreading across the central sulcus (Jung et al., 2003). Spikes in the high central region are associated with hand involvement, whereas those in the low central region are associated with oromotor phenomena and drooling (Legarda et al., 1994). Studies demonstrate rare or no association between this syndrome and childhood absence epilepsy (Dimova and Daskalova, 2002; Gelisse et al., 1999).

Most children with benign rolandic epilepsy have few seizures, 15% have one seizure, 56% have two to six seizures, and 29% have more than six seizures (Ambrosetto et al., 1987). The children who present with a generalized convulsive seizure and with a long interval between the first and second seizure have the best prognosis (Ambrosetto et al., 1987). The course is benign in 95 to 100% of the children.

Behavioral Aspects of Benign Rolandic Epilepsy
Although these children were thought to have normal psychomotor development and functioning, parents recognize difficulties with concentration, temperament, and impulsiveness (Croona et al., 1999). In addition, neuropyschological testing reveal significantly lower scores on immediate and delayed recall of auditory-verbal and visual material, verbal fluency, problem-solving ability, visuospatial constructional ability, and Raven's Coloured-Progressive Matrices compared to age- and gender-matched normal control subjects (Croona et al., 1999; Deonna et al., 2000). The findings of some investigators, however, imply preferential impairment of executive function in these children (Chevalier et al., 2000), cognitive impairment and attentional difficulties in children with EEG evidence of a prolonged slow focus, and strong activation of spike and wave discharges at night (Saint-Martin et al., 2001). Given the small sample size of these studies, the possible role of carbamazepine on these findings needs to be considered (Seidel and Mitchell, 1999).

Diagnosis
A diagnosis of benign rolandic epilepsy should be considered when a child presents with a history of hemifacial nocturnal seizures with normal EEG background activity and midtemporal spikes. From the clinical perspective, these seizures differ from complex partial seizures of temporal origin because they are partial motor seizures and do not involve loss of consciousness. Like benign rolandic epilepsy, frontal lobe epilepsy that involves the supplementary motor area also occurs during sleep. However, children with benign rolandic seizures do not have posturing and tonic movement, vocalizations, laughing, crying, and version of the head and eyes. The possibility of facial and eye movements during REM sleep should also be ruled out.

Regarding midtemporal spikes, these are not pathognomonic for benign rolandic epilepsy (van der Meij et al., 1992) and, as previously mentioned, occur in children who have no clinical epileptic manifestations (de Weerd and Arts, 1993; Ferri et al., 2000). Midtemporal spikes are also found in children with neurological disorders, such as cerebral palsy, epilepsy, developmental delays, and attention deficit hyperactivity disorder (van der Meij et al., 1992).

Finally, parental anxiety and misinterpretation of children's myoclonic movements during sleep can be easily differentiated from benign rolandic epilepsy. Myoclonic jerks involve large groups of muscles other than the face and do not present with a consistent pattern.

Treatment
Although carbamazepine, valproic acid, and levetiracetam have been successfully used in these children, randomized trials have been conducted only with gabapentin (Bourgeois et al., 1998) and sulthiame (Rating et al., 2000).

Benign Occipital Epilepsy
This form of epilepsy presents with visual, motor, and migrainous symptoms with unilateral or bilateral spike-wave complexes in the occipital regions that are inhibited by eye-opening (Lerman and Kivity, 1991). In 25% of cases the seizures are precipitated by going from light to dark or vice versa (Gastaut, 1985). Benign occipital epilepsy has greater morbidity than benign rolandic epilepsy. Antiepileptic drugs control about 60% of the cases of benign occipital seizures, and seizures stop between ages 13 and 19 years (Lerman and Kivity, 1991; Oguni et al., 2001).

The benign form of the disease, most frequent in 4- to 8-year-old boys (Beaumanoir and Nahory, 1983; Lerman and Kivity, 1989), involves nocturnal motor seizures with tonic deviation of the head and eyes, clonic (i.e., nystagmoid) eye movements, and loss of consciousness, which can be prolonged (Lerman and Kivity, 1991). In Panayiotopulous syndrome, autonomic symptoms (e.g., ictal vomiting), lateral eye deviation, and impairment of consciousness, followed by hemi- or generalized seizures occur more frequently in girls (Lada et al., 2003).

Children older than 8 years have the Gastaut type with a more protracted course of illness with diurnal seizures, visual symptoms, migrainous symptoms, and preserved or impaired consciousness (Lerman and Kivity, 1991; Martinovic, 2001; Tsai et al., 2001). The visual symptoms include partial or complete loss of vision, elementary or complex visual hallucinations, and visual illusions (i.e., micropsia, macropsia, metamorphosia) (Gastaut, 1982; Gastaut and Zifkin, 1984; Lerman and Kivity, 1991; Panayiotopoulos, 1989). The symptoms of migraine can be ictal or postictal and include a diffuse nonpulsatile headache and vomiting (Gastaut, 1985; Lerman and Kivity, 1991).

The EEG findings typically entail unilateral or bilateral spikes or sharp waves in posterior head regions. Non-REM sleep, closed eyes, or lack of visual fixation activate, and REM sleep and eye opening inhibit the epileptic discharges (Lerman and Kivity, 1991). Among children with early onset occipital seizures (e.g., Panayiotopoulous syndrome), occipital spike focus is seen in younger children, ages 2 to 5 years; whereas independent frontopolar, occipital, and centroparietotemporal spike foci appear between ages 6 to 10 years (Ohtsu et al., 2003). These EEG patterns are unrelated to the prognosis.

Behavioral Aspects of Benign Occipital Epilepsy
To date, the single study that examined neuorpsycholgoical functioning in 21 children with this disorder found lower attention, memory, and intellectual functioning compared to 21 children without epilepsy with whom they were matched by age, gender, and socioeconomic status (Gulgonen et al., 2000).

Diagnosis
A diagnosis of benign occipital epilepsy should be considered in children who have nocturnal adversive seizures with loss of consciousness, diurnal seizures with visual, autonomic, and migrainous symptoms, but preserved or somewhat impaired consciousness, and EEG evidence of posterior epileptic discharges that disappear with eye opening. Based on the clinical symptoms, this syndrome should be differentiated from supplementary motor epilepsy, temporal lobe epilepsy with autonomic manifestations (e.g., abdominal epilepsy), migraine, occipital lobe tumor, and psychotic disorders.

Unlike occipital epilepsy, the nocturnal tonic deviation of the head and eyes in supplementary motor epilepsy is associated with somatosensory auras, posturing and tonic movement, vocalizations, laughing, and crying. Children with temporal lobe epilepsy with autonomic symptoms do not have tonic deviation of the eyes. Compared to migraine, children with benign occipital epilepsy have visual hallucinations and illusions, not scotomata. Their headache is diffuse, not pulsatile.

If unilateral, the EEG findings of benign occipital epilepsy could mimic those of a cortical lesion in the occipital lobe. During an attack of migraine, there might be slowing rather than posterior sharp waves or spikes on the EEG. Activation of the epileptic discharges on EEG by closed eyes and nonREM sleep do not occur in other conditions.

Finally, the visual hallucinations of psychotic disorders are complex, variable, and associated with auditory hallucinations, not with symptoms of migraine.

Treatment
Most patients respond well to classic AEDs (Oguni et al., 2001).

Chronic Progressive Epilepsia Partialis Continua of Childhood (Rasmussen's Syndrome)
Rasmussen encephalitis, a progressive disorder of unproven viral or autoimmune etiology (Park and Vinters, 2003; Pardo et al., 2004; Watson et al., 2004), presents with increasingly intractable unilateral seizures, emerging hemiparesis that sometimes progresses to hemiplegia, and a downhill cognitive course (Granata et al., 2003a; Honavar et al., 1992; Oguni et al., 1991; Rasmussen and Andermann, 1989; Vining et al., 1993). The onset occurs in childhood, adolescence, or adulthood (Honavar et al., 1992; McLachlan et al., 1993; Rasmussen and Andermann), but in 85% of cases the illness begins before age 10 years (Rasmussen and Andermann).

There is a characteristic progression observed in both the MRI scan and EEG. By 4 months after the onset of symptoms, the MRI reveals focal contralateral white matter hyperintensity with cortical atrophy that always involves the insula and in most cases, the head of the caudate (Granata et al., 2003a). As the disorder progresses, there is increasing MRI signal intensity. Subsequently, signal intensity decreases, with or without progressive unilateral cortical atrophy (Kim et al., 2002). Initially the EEG reveals focal slowing and ictal and interictal multifocal spikes. Over the next few months there is progressive slowing and voltage attentuation, with unilateral multifocal independent spikes. Contralateral asynchronous slow waves were often noted.

Behavioral Aspects of Rasmussen Syndrome

Despite earlier normal development, children with Rasmussen's syndrome have impaired cognitive (Honavar et al., 1992; Vining et al., 1993) and linguistic function (Caplan et al., 1999; Vargha-Khadem et al., 1991).

Diagnosis

Diagnosis is based on the evolving clinical picture of intractable unilateral motor seizures with epilepsia partialis continua, contralateral increased signal intensity with or without cortical atrophy on MRI, and brain biopsy. The histological hallmarks of Rasmussen encephalitis include chronic inflammation, microglial nodules, and focal patchy gliosis.

Treatment

AEDs usually do not control the seizures. Treatment with hemispherectomy (Jonas et al., 2004; Rasmussen and Andermann, 1989) and immunomodulatory treatments (Granata et al., 2003b) appear to stop progression of the disorder (Honavar et al., 1992). Postsurgical improvement in the communication deficits of children with Rasmussen encephalitis is associated with later age of onset and shorter duration of illness prior to surgery (Caplan et al., 1999).

Generalized Epilepsies and Syndromes Idiopathic (With Age-Related Onset) Childhood Absence Epilepsy

An absence is a brief change in the state of consciousness during which the child suddenly stops ongoing activity and stares vacantly (Lockman, 1989). Typical absence seizures (also known as petit mal) occur frequently and are associated with automatisms of the eyes (i.e., eyelid fluttering) and face (i.e., twitching of the perioral muscles), unchanged tone, and generalized spike and wave discharges at a rate of three per second on a normal EEG background (Holmes et al., 1987; Lockman). Atypical absence seizures last longer, are associated with a decrease in postural tone or tonic activity, greater than three per second spike and wave ictal recordings, abnormal interictal EEGs, and multiple seizure types (Holmes et al., 1987). Hyperventilation can induce typical absence seizures, but not atypical absence seizures. Both typical and atypical absence seizures start and stop suddenly without postictal symptoms (Erba and Browne, 1983; Holmes et al., 1987). During a typical or atypical absence, the child maintains receptive and expressive speech (Holmes et al., 1987). In petit mal status, however, the child might experience cognitive clouding and difficulties with comprehension and expression of language.

Typical absence seizures are found in school-age children, more frequently in girls than boys (Camfield et al., 1996) They remit in 64 to 90% of the cases if therapy is adequate and given for at least 2 years (Bouma et al., 1996; Camfield and Camfield, 2002; Siren et al., 2002; Wirrell et al., 1996, 2001). Predictors of good remission include the absence of generalized tonic clonic seizures, absence status, cognitive problems, myoclonic seizures, abnormal background, and a family history of generalized tonic clonic seizures

Behavioral Aspects of Absence Seizures

Children with absence seizures have high rates of psychopathology including disruptive disorders (i.e., attention-deficit hyperactivity disorder, oppositional defiant disorder, conduct disorder), anxiety/affective disorders, and comorbid disruptive and anxiety/affective disorders (Caplan et al., 1998). They have difficulties using language to organize and formulate their thinking (Caplan et al., 2001, 2002a), as well as problems with general cognition (Mandelbaum and Burack, 1997; Pavone et al., 2001), attention (Levav et al., 2002), memory, particularly nonverbal memory (Nolan et al., 2004; Pavone et al.), and performance IQ (Caplan et al., 2004). As previously mentioned, children with atypical absence seizures usually have mental retardation or developmental delay (Holmes et al., 1987).

Diagnosis

A child who presents with brief staring spells during middle childhood, eyelid fluttering or twitching of the perioral muscles, no loss of tone, generalized three per second spike and wave on EEG, and induction of episodes by hyperventilation has typical absence seizures. From the neurological perspective, typical absence seizures should be differentiated from the absences of complex partial seizures. In contrast to children with typical absence seizures, hyperventilation will not induce the absence episodes of children with complex partial seizures. In addition, children with complex partial absences also have lip smacking and hand fumbling automatisms, postictal amnesia or tiredness, and focal interictal spikes rather than generalized 3 Hz spike and wave complexes. EEG findings of 3 Hz spike and wave together with eye opening and eyelid flutter differentiate typical absence seizures from hyperventilation-induced high-amplitude rhythmic slowing also associated with loss of awareness but with automatisms, such as yawning, smiling, and fidgeting (Lum et al., 2002).

From a behavioral perspective, children with typical absence seizures might first be noticed by the teacher who will complain that the child is inattentive or has lost ground in his or her studies. Unlike the child with attention-deficit hyperactivity disorder (ADHD), children with typical absence seizures do not have a history of hyperactivity, impulsiveness, and distractibility since the toddler period, and they are unaware of their attentional difficulties. Children with a learning disorder will report specific learning difficulties; whereas the child with typical absence seizures will be unaware of why he or she is having learning difficulties.

Finally, the stares of autistic children that precede or occur together with their stereotyped behaviors, such as hand flapping, could be misinterpreted as absences. Children with typical absences do not have stereotyped behaviors other than the stare, eyelid fluttering, or twitching of lip muscles. Unlike autistic children, they do not have impaired communication skills and poor social relationships. Children with atypical absence seizures might have developmental delays like autistic children; however, unlike the brief staring associated with the stereotypies of autistic children, the staring spells of children with atypical absence seizures are long and associated with some loss of tone.

Treatment

Monotherapy ethosuximide, valproic acid, and lamotrigine control typical absences in 70%, 75%, and 50 to 60% of the cases, respectively (see the review in Panayiotopoulos, 2001; Coppola et al., 2004; Henriksen and Johannessen, 1982; Wirrell et al., 2001) with no cognitive or behavioral adverse effects (Mandelbaum and Burack, 1997). In contrast, atypical absence seizures are more difficult to control, particularly in children with early onset or with late onset and lower intelligence, necessitating antiepileptic drug polytherapy.

Juvenile Myoclonic Epilepsy

Juvenile myoclonic epilepsy affects 7% of adolescents with epilepsy; 3 to 8% of whom had childhood absence epilepsy (see the review in Renganathan and Delanty, 2003). The clinical seizures and/or the EEG abnormalities may be observed in relatives (Delgado-Escueta et al., 1994; Obeid, 1994). Juvenile myoclonic epilepsy is an inherited disorder that is genetically heterogenous, and is associated with mutations in a number of genes, including the short arm of chromosome 6 (Greenberg et al., 2000; Sander et al., 1997). Relatively few cases can be linked to single genes and most cases appear to be the result of the interaction of complex genetic and environmental factors (Zifkin, Andermann, Andermann, 2005).

All cases have myoclonic jerks that occur shortly after awakening in the neck and upper extremities without loss of consciousness. In addition to sudden awakening, sleep deprivation, photic stimulation, alcohol consumption, menses, and stress precipitate the jerks (Dreifuss, 1989). Usually these jerks are undiagnosed because adolescents interpret them as clumsiness or nervousness (Gordon, 1994). The jerks are usually bilateral but can be unilateral, arrhythmic, and repetitive. A massive myoclonic jerk can make the patient fall to the ground with brief loss of consciousness and no postictal phenomena (Lockman, 1989).

The disorder becomes progressive with onset of clonic seizures and generalized tonic-clonic seizures in 90 to 95% of the cases. The symmetric and violent generalized tonic-clonic seizures have a long tonic component (see the review in Renganathan and Delanty, 2003). Absences occur in 40% of the cases.

Ictal EEGs reveal bilateral diffuse spikes at a rate of 16 to 24 Hz (Delgado-Escueta et al., 1994) that can be preceded by asymptomatic spike and wave complexes and followed by 1 to 3Hz spike and slow wave complexes. The interictal EEG is also abnormal with 4 to 6 Hz multiple spike and slow wave complexes. Photic stimulation leads to a generalized paroxysmal EEG discharge in about 30 to 40% of the cases. Some of these patients also have absence seizures, which often are undiagnosed because they are unaccompanied by behavioral phenomena (Voeller, 1995).

The prognosis is excellent with AED treatment (Gordon, 1994) in 80 to 90% of the cases. Intractability occurs in patients who have all three seizure types and behavior problems (see the review in Renganathan and Delanty, 2003).

Behavioral Aspects of Juvenile Myoclonic Epilepsy

Other than clumsiness, nervousness, or ill-defined attentional difficulties prior to the onset of generalized tonic clonic convulsions, there have been no studies to date on the behavioral aspects in adolescents with juvenile myoclonic epilepsy.

Diagnosis

Several studies emphasize the long lag time between onset of the syndrome and correct diagnosis (Asconape and Penry, 1984; Gordon, 1994; Obeid, 1994). When presented with an adolescent with poorly defined complaints about clumsiness, nervousness, and difficulties concentrating, one should ascertain if the clumsiness is precipitated by sleep deprivation, photic stimulation, or alcohol consumption. A positive family history and characteristic ictal and interictal EEG findings will help confirm the diagnosis of juvenile myoclonic epilepsy.

Among the neurological disorders, one needs to rule out nonepileptic myoclonus and movement disorders. Unlike myoclonic seizures, myoclonus is not precipitated by sensory stimuli, continues during sleep, has no EEG correlates, and does not remit in response to AEDs. The jerks of movement disorders, such as Tourette's disorder, dystonia, or chorea, involve repetitive involuntary movements of parts of the body rather than isolated movements of large muscle groups. In addition, tics, dystonia, and chorea usually disappear during sleep. Finally, complaints of poor self-esteem (associated with clumsiness and poor concentration) can present in adolescents with psychiatric disorders, such as depression, schizophrenia, or adjustment disorder. The early stages of juvenile myoclonic epilepsy might suggest the prodrome of one of these psychiatric disorders.

Treatment

The treatment response to valproic acid is excellent (Gordon, 1994; Dreifuss, 1989; Obeid, 1994). Topiramate and vagal nerve stimulation have been used in intractable patients with success (see the review in Renganathan and Delanty, 2003).

Cryptogenic or Symptomatic Infantile Spasms (West Syndrome)

Infantile spasm is a generalized seizure disorder with clusters of flexion, extension, or brief tonic seizures often associated with hypsarrhythmia, high voltage slowing, and multifocal spikes on EEG (Commission, 1989). This syndrome usually begins by age 4 to 8 months (Glaze et al., 1988; Jeavons and Bower, 1964; Riikonen, 1982) and is cryptogenic (e.g., normal prior development, no known causative factors, normal neuroimaging) in 20% and symptomatic in 80% of the cases associated with a variety of etiological causes (see Hrachovy and Frost, 2003 for a review).

Although regarded as a generalized seizure disorder (Commission, 1989), focal cortical abnormalities due to cortical dysplasia (Alvarez et al., 1987; Cusmai et al., 1988), tumors (Branch and Dyken, 1979; Mimaki et al., 1983), or other etiologies underlie the symptomatic form of infantile spasms. The origin of the pathology, whether interaction of focal cortical and brainstem pathology, brainstem, or basal ganglia pathology (Avazini et al., 2002; Chugani, 2002; Hrachovy and Frost, 1989), increased proconvulsant activity in both cortical and brainstem regions (Lado and Moshe, 2002), or abnormal release of corticotrophin release hormone (Brunson et al., 2002) continue to be debated.

The rate of spontaneous remission is 25% and occurs from 1 to12 months after the onset of infantile spasms (Hrachovy et al., 1991). Although 51% of the children continue to have seizures (see the review in Frost and Hrachovy, 2003), infantile spasms and hypsarrhythmia are age-specific phenomena (Yamatogi and Ohtahara, 1981). If treatment does not control infantile spasms, the children develop other seizures and the EEG no longer shows the hypsarrhthymia characteristic of infantile spasms (Yamatogi and Ohtahara, 1981). Ultimately, 25% of children with infantile spasm develop Lennox-Gastaut syndrome (see the review in Frost and Hrachovy, 2003).

Behavioral Aspects of Infantile Spasms

In the absence of early seizure control (Kivity et al., 2004), the developmental outcome for these children is poor (Dulac et al., 1986, 1993; Favatta et al., 1987; Fois et al., 1984; Glaze et al., 1988; Guzzetta et al., 1993; Jeavons and Bower, 1964; Hrachovy et al., 1991; Jonas et al., 2004; Kurokawa et al., 1980; Lacy and Penry, 1976; Matsumoto et al., 1981; Riikonen, 1982; Vigevano et al., 1993). Children who respond to medical treatment with seizure control (Koo et al., 1993; Riikonen, 1982; Schlumberger and Dulac, 1994) have a better developmental outcome than those who do not respond. In addition to seizure control, there is evidence that developmental regression at the onset of the illness (Dulac et al., 1993; Guzetta et al.,), delayed development prior to

the onset of infantile spasms (Guzetta et al., 1993; Koo et al.; Ohtahara et al., 1993; Riikonen, 1982; Schlumberger and Dulac, 1994), and impaired visually mediated social interaction following ACTH treatment (Dulac et al., 1993) are associated with a poor cognitive outcome.

About 6% of children with infantile autism had hypsarrhythmia in the first year of life (Olsson et al., 1988). Follow-up of children with infantile spasms also reveals varying degrees of impaired social relationships (Caplan et al., 2002b; Dulac et al., 1993; Jambaque et al., 1993) and autism (Askalan et al., 2003; Riikonen, 2001). Riikonen (1982) reported that about 10% of the infantile subjects they followed met criteria for infantile autism, particularly those with EEG and CT evidence for temporal lobe abnormalities. About two thirds of children with infantile spasms who have autism also meet criteria for hyperkinetic disorder (Riikonen and Amnell, 1981), and about 15% of children with infantile spasms have severe "nonautistic" overactivity (Caplan and Gillberg, 1998).

Diagnosis

A 4- to 8-month-old infant with onset of clusters of unilateral or bilateral jerks, after normal or abnormal development, with and without developmental arrest, should have an EEG to rule out infantile spasms as soon as possible. Table 22.2 lists the neurological disorders to be included in the differential diagnosis of infantile spasms.

TABLE 22.2

DIFFERENTIAL DIAGNOSIS OF INFANTILE SPASMS IN INFANCY

1. Other Seizure Disorders

    a. Febrile seizures
    b. Nonfebrile seizures
        (i)   Generalized tonic–clonic seizures
        (ii) Partial seizures
        (iii) Benign myoclonus
        (iv) Myoclonic epilepsy
             Benign
             Severe

2. Neurocutaneous Disorders Causing Seizures in Infancy

    a. Neurofibromatosis
    b. Sturge-Weber syndrome
    c. Tuberous sclerosis
    d. Incontinentia pigmenti
    e. Linear nevus sebaceous syndrome

3. Dystonia

    a. Glutaric aciduria
    b. Transient paroxysmal dystonia of infancy

4. Breatholding spells

    a. Cyanotic
    b. Pallid

Treatment

The classical and most successful shortterm treatment of infantile spasms is with ACTH, but vigabatrin is also possibly effective (see the review in Mackay et al., 2004). Prednisone, valproic acid, other AEDs (felbamate, nitrazapam, topiramate), and their combinations have been variably successful (Mackay et al.). The longterm developmental outcome is related to early rather than late control of infantile spasms, the absence of underlying pathology as in symptomatic infantile spasms, and no early developmental regression (Mackay et al.)

Lennox-Gastaut Syndrome

This epileptic syndrome is characterized by early onset of intractable seizures (tonic, generalized tonic–clonic, atypical absence, atonic and myoclonic), bilateral slow spike and wave complexes (1.5 to 2Hz) while awake, and paroxysmal fast activity (8–26Hz) during nonREM sleep on EEG (see the review in Markland, 2003). About 25% of children with infantile spasms go on to develop Lennox-Gastaut syndrome. Follow-up of children with Lennox-Gastaut syndrome reveals continued seizures in about 60% (Goldsmith et al., 2000) and mental retardation in about half, particularly in children with minor motor seizures and multifocal independent spikes (Ohtsuka et al., 1990).

Behavioral Aspects of Lennox-Gastaut Syndrome

Children with Lennox-Gastaut syndrome usually have marked language delays. As in other cases of mental retardation, the children are sometimes irritable and hyperactive. These behavioral symptoms might decrease with seizure control and exacerbate with increased seizure frequency or when the children are on high doses of AED polytherapy.

Diagnosis

A diagnosis of Lennox-Gastaut syndrome is based on the EEG finding of interictal slow spike and wave discharges in a child with early onset of poorly controlled mixed seizures and developmental delay.

Treatment

Until the development of new AEDs and vagal nerve stimulation, the treatment response of children with this syndrome was poor. Benzodiazepines such as nitrazapam and clonazapam were somewhat successful in decreasing the seizure frequency of these children. Although felbamate improved control of drop attacks and tonic seizures (Felbamate Study Group, 1993), its use in children has been limited by the need for frequent blood studies due to possible aplastic anemia. Among the new AEDs, lamotrigine and topiramate improve seizure control in these patients (see the review in French et al., 2004). Vagal nerve stimulation led to a median reduction of seizure frequency in 50 children by 42% (Frost et al., 2001) and to a significant 4.5-month increase in the mental age of children with more than a 50% reduction in their seizures (Majoie et al., 2001).

Epilepsies and Syndromes Undetermined Whether Focal or Generalized

Landau-Kleffner Syndrome (Acquired Epileptic Aphasia)

All children with this syndrome have aphasia and epileptiform abnormalities on EEG (Landau and Kleffner, 1957; see the review in Galanopoulou et al., 2000). About two thirds of the children develop clinical seizures (Beaumanoir, 1985; Bishop, 1985) that are focal motor or generalized tonic clonic seizures (Hirsch et al., 1990), easy to control (Gascon et al., 1973; Landau and Kleffner), and resolve by age 15 years (Beaumanoir, 1985). Due to the benign course of the clinical seizures, this syndrome is classified as one of the benign epilepsy syndromes. The course of the aphasia, however, is fluctuating with remissions and exacerbations (Billard et al., 1991; Deonna et al., 1977; Paquier et al., 1992). A few children make some speech and language gains, but most children continue to be aphasic. Children with a later onset of Landau-Kleffner syndrome have a better prognosis (Bishop, 1985).

The syndrome occurs in males more than in females and begins between ages 5 to 7 years (Nevšímalová et al., 1992). In most cases the aphasia appears after normal language development and presents with word deafness or auditory agnosia (Aicardi, 1986; Bishop, 1985; Deonna et al., 1977; Dlouhă and Nevšímalová, 1990; Gascon et al., 1973; Landau and Kleffner, 1957). These children appear not to hear what is being said to them by their parents, who then increase the volume of their speech. The child's responsivity to verbal language decreases gradually and he or she becomes unresponsive. In addition to expressive difficulties, 90% of these children have receptive difficulties (Deonna et al., 1989). Older children who acquired reading and writing skills before the onset of their aphasia lose these skills (Rapin et al., 1977). Most children with Landau-Kleffner syndrome do not learn to write or to sign (Deonna et al., 1989). Some children use gestures and other forms of nonverbal communication to get their needs met.

The EEG abnormalities typically involve bilateral independent temporal or temporoparietal spike and wave discharges, bilateral 1 to 3 Hz spike wave activity maximal over the temporal areas, generalized sharp waves or spike wave discharges, and multifocal or unilateral spikes (Bishop, 1985; Deonna et al., 1977; Nakano et al., 1989; Paquier et al., 1992). These EEG abnormalities are continuous or nearly continuous during sleep, and in some cases they meet the criteria for electrical status epilepticus.

It is unclear if there is a causal relationship between the three components of this syndrome: aphasia, epileptiform abnormalities involving the temporal lobe, and seizures. Among the theories on the etiology of this syndrome, some suggest that continuous convulsive discharge (Deonna, 1991; Dulac et al., 1983; Gordon, 1990; Landau and Kleffner, 1957; Pateau et al., 1999), focal subacute encephalitis (Gascon et al., 1973; Perniola et al., 1993; Ravnik, tis (Gascon et al., 1973; Perniola et al., 1993; Ravnik, 1985), cerebral arteritis (Pascual-Castroviejo, 1990), deficits in high level auditory processing (Bishop, 1985), or an encephalopathic process (Holmes et al., 1981; Perniola et al., 1993) cause the aphasia.

Behavioral Aspects of Landau-Kleffner Syndrome

Children with this syndrome develop mild to pronounced behavioral disturbances (Humphrey et al., 1975) including hyperactivity, aggression, depression (Sawhney et al., 1988; White and Sreenivasan, 1987), and psychosis (Dugas et al., 1982; Gordon, 1990; Humphrey et al., 1975; Zivi et al., 1990).

Diagnosis

This diagnosis should be considered when faced with a child who presents with gradual loss of expressive language skills after a period of normal development, in the context of seizures and epileptiform EEG abnormalities. Among the behavioral disorders, children with developmental dysphasia have a history of impaired language development and an increased rate of EEG abnormalities while awake (Nasr et al., 2001) and during sleep (Echenne et al., 1992). Unlike autistic children, children with Landau-Kleffner syndrome are socially relating and responsive and use nonverbal communication to make their needs known. Like children with Landau-Kleffner syndrome, some autistic children develop seizures and epileptiform abnormalities (Tuchman and Rapin, 1997; Caplan and Gillberg, 1998).

Among the neurological disorders, children with onset of Rasmussen encephalitis during the toddler period lose language, like children with Landau-Kleffner syndrome. However, they present with difficult-to-control sensorimotor seizures, which may be almost continuous. Language loss occurs after the onset of seizures in these young cases of Rasmussen encephalitis. In contrast, the seizures of Landau-Kleffner syndrome can begin before, during, or after the onset of aphasia (Deonna et al., 1977; Gascon et al., 1973; Landau and Kleffner, 1957).

A tumor that involves the speech areas might cause loss of language skills and seizures (Nass et al., 1993). Imaging findings of a space-occupying lesion would help make the definitive diagnosis. There are no typical magnetic resonance imaging (MRI) (Sankar et al., 1990), single-photon emission computed tomography (Guerreirro et al., 1996; Tauma et al., 1995), or positron emission tomography findings (Rintahaka et al., 1995; Sankar et al., 1990) in children with Landau-Kleffner syndrome.

Children with the syndrome of continuous spike and wave sleep, to be discussed next, have marked behavioral changes other than language loss, and their EEG abnormalities occupy 85% of slow wave sleep and disappear during REM sleep. In contrast, the epileptiform discharges of children with Landau-Kleffner syndrome are activated at sleep onset and during REM (Genton and Guerrini, 1993).

Treatment

Valproate, ethosuximide, and some benzodiazepines alleviate the seizures not the aphasia of children this syndrome. Treatment with steroids (Lerman et al., 1991; Marescaux et al., 1990), ACTH (Perniola et al., 1993), nifedipine (Pascual-Castroviejo, 1990), sulthiame (Wakai et al., 1997), and subpial resection (Sawheny et al., 1995) has been associated with improved language skills in these children.

Continuous Spike and Wave During Slow-Wave Sleep

Continuous spike and wave during slow sleep syndrome occurs in 0.5% of children (Morikawa et al., 1985) and involves behavioral changes, intellectual deterioration, seizures, and continuous spike and wave during at least 85% of slow-wave sleep (Bureau et al., 1990; Perez et al., 1993; Tassinari et al., 1982). Due to the long duration of the epileptic discharges during slow-wave sleep, this syndrome has also been called electrical status epilepticus during slow-wave sleep (Tassinari et al., 1982).

This syndrome begins in children, ages 4 to 6 years, after normal or abnormal development and presents with subtle behavioral or intellectual changes followed by marked deterioration of behavior and intellect (Perez et al., 1993; Tassinari et al., 1982). Children with continuous spike and wave sleep have motor seizures, nocturnal partial motor seizures or generalized convulsive seizures, and subsequent development of absences or atypical absences, which are well controlled with AEDs and remit by age 15 years (Boel and Caesar, 1989; see the review in Galanopoulou et al., 2000; Perez et al., 1993).

Sleep EEGs reveal continuous generalized spike and wave during 85% of slow-wave sleep. Awake EEGs, however, may be normal (Perez et al., 1993; Tassinari et al., 1982), or reveal sporadic generalized spike and wave (Boel and Caesar, 1989), or focal paroxysmal discharges (see the review in Galanopoulou et al., 2000).

Behavioral Aspects of Continuous Spike and Wave Sleep

In 25% of the children, the behavioral changes are the first sign and include inattention, hyperactivity, impulsiveness, loss of sense of danger, aggressiveness, mood changes, disinhibition, mouthing of objects, reduced play, and perseveration (Perez et al., 1993). In others, subtle cognitive changes first occur (Boel and Caesar, 1989; Perez et al., 1993; Roulet et al., 1991) with subsequent downhill cognitive deterioration (see the review in Galanopoulou et al., 2000). Several studies have described language disturbances in 40 to 60% of the cases with an expressive aphasia (see the review in Galanopoulou et al., 2000).

Diagnosis

This syndrome should be considered in children who present with gradual onset of inattention, hyperactivity, impulsiveness, behavioral regression, intellectual deterioration, and seizures after prior normal or abnormal development. A sleep EEG will provide a definitive diagnosis. The differential diagnosis should include neurological disorders that cause dementia in children (Table 22.3), benign seizure syndromes, such as Landau-Kleffner syndrome, and psychiatric disorders, such as disintegrative psychosis, pervasive developmental disorder, and schizophrenia.

Among the neurological disorders, the onset of Landau-Kleffner involves gradual appearance of auditory agnosia and later onset of aggressive and hyperactive behavior (Landau and Kleffner, 1957). In contrast, children with continuous spike and wave sleep present with behavioral disturbances or cognitive deficits, as well as expressive aphasia (see the review in Galanopoulou et al., 2000). Their communicative deficits involve the form and content of their speech, as well as their expressive skills (Boel and Caesar, 1989; Genton and Guerrini, 1993; Paquier et al., 1992; Perez et al., 1993; Tassinari et al., 1982). The characteristic EEG findings of continuous spike and wave sleep are generalized and occur only in slow-wave sleep compared to the focal temporo-parietal epileptic discharges in Landau-Kleffner syndrome that are found in the sleep and awake states (Genton and Guerrini, 1993).

Among the psychiatric disorders, children with disintegrative psychosis, also known as Heller's syndrome or de-

mentia infantilis, have marked regression in multiple areas of their functioning following at least 2 years of normal development (American Psychiatric Association, 1994, p. 74). The children have associated mental retardation, EEG abnormalities, and seizure disorder. In some cases, one of the disorders listed in Table 22.3 might cause this syndrome. In most cases, however, extensive investigation does not reveal an underlying cause.

Most of the cases of pervasive developmental disorder begin in infancy or during the toddler period and involve impaired development of communication and social reciprocal interaction skills, as well as stereotyped, behavior, interests, and activities (American Psychiatric Association, 1994, pp. 70–71). In contrast, they clearly demonstrate a gradual and progressive regression in behavioral and cognitive functioning from the previous normal or abnormal baseline. Finally, they might present with disorganized behavior and what might appear to be formal thought disorder (Perez et al., 1993). However, they do not have hallucinations or delusions, and their cognitive deficits are apparent.

Treatment

Although clinical seizures respond well to AEDs, control of the electrical status is more difficult and has been achieved with high doses of ACTH and prednisone, ethosuximide, benzodiazepines, and combinations of AEDs (see the review in Galanopoulou et al., 2000). Reports differ on the efficacy of treatment of the electrical status on the children's behavior and cognition. Some researchers describe reversibility of the behavioral and cognitive changes with control of the electrical status (Bureau et al., 1990; Tassinari et al., 1982). Others (Perez et al., 1993; Boel and Caesar, 1989) have found behavioral and cognitive improvements but noticeable residual deficits in these areas of functioning.

PSEUDOSEIZURES

Definition and Incidence

Pseudoseizures, epileptic-like phenomena due to psychological causes, have also been called hysterical seizures, psychogenic seizures, and more recently nonepileptic events. The term "pseudoseizure," unlike the terms "hysterical" and "psychogenic," refers to the clinical phenomenology rather than to the psychological cause of these episodes. Pediatric pseudoseizures can be due to an underlying conversion disorder, a factitious disorder, misinterpretation of seizures by the adults who care for the child, or a Munchausen-syndrome by proxy. In children under age 5 years, the majority of cases of nonepileptic seizures involve daydreaming, physiological events, such as inattention/daydreaming, stereotyped movements, hypnic jerks, and parasomnias that are misinterpreted by parents as epileptic seizures (Kotagal et al., 2003).

Despite the morbidity and marked cost to health care services, only few studies and case reports describe

---

> **TABLE 22.3**
> ### NEUROLOGICAL DISORDERS ASSOCIATED WITH CHILDHOOD DEMENTIA

1. Infectious Diseases

   a. Subacute sclerosing panencephalitis (SSPE)

2. Disorders of Gray Matter

   a. Ceroid lipifuscinosis
   b. Heller syndrome
   c. Huntington disease
   d. Mitochondrial disorders
   e. Xeroderma pigmentosum

3. Disorders of White Matter

   a. Adrenoleuokodystrophy
   b. Alexander disease
   c. Cerebrotendinous xanthomatosis

4. Lysosomal Enzyme Disorders

   a. Mucopolysaccharidoses
     (i) Hunter syndrome
     (ii) Sly disease
   b. Sphingolipidoses
     (i) Gaucher disease
     (ii) Juvenile Tay-Sachs
     (iii) Late-onset Krabbe's disease
     (iv) Late-onset sulfatide lipidoses
     (v) Sphingomyelin lipidosis
   c. Glycoprotein Degradation Disorders
     (i) Aspartylglycosaminuria
     (ii) Mannosidosis

pseudoseizures in children and adolescents (see the review in Papavasiliou et al., 2004). About 12.5% of children referred to a pediatric neurology inpatient service (Schneider and Rice, 1979) and 15.2% referred to a pediatric epilepsy monitoring service (Kotagal et al., 2002) are given a diagnosis of pseudoseizures.

The disorder is more common in children with confirmed epileptic seizures (19–46%) (Kotagal et al., 2002) and in nonepileptic children who are exposed to this disorder through a family member, a neighbor, or a friend (Goodyer, 1985). There are both age- and sex-related differences in the incidence of pseudoseizures. Pseudoseizures occur more frequently in adolescents than in younger children (Finalyson and Lucas, 1979; Gross and Huerta, 1980; Mohr and Bond, 1982). In adolescence, but not in middle childhood, pseudoseizures occur more commonly in girls (Finalyson and Lucas, 1979; Gross and Huerta, 1980; Kotagal et al., 2002; Mohr and Bond, 1982) who also tend to have a more chronic course than boys (Schneider and Rice, 1979). In middle childhood, a high rate of prior head trauma was noted in boys with pseudoseizures (Pakalnis and Paolicchi, 2003b),

Clinical Manifestations

Although pseudoseizures mimic all seizure types, earlier studies suggested that in middle childhood they most commonly present with atypical movements and behaviors (Sas-

sower and Duchowny, 1992), whereas in early adolescence pseudoseizures begin to mimic generalized tonic–clonic convulsions and complex partial seizures (Sassower and Duchowny). One study found no significant difference across ages in the presentation of motor pseudoseizures compared to unresponsive events (Kotagal et al., 2002).

Table 22.4 compares the clinical manifestations of epileptic and pseudoseizures. Despite differences in the clinical manifestations of epileptic and pseudoseizures, these are not always clear-cut and one cannot base the diagnosis of pseudoseizures solely on the clinical picture (see Diagnosis).

In terms of onset, epileptic seizures start suddenly or after a brief aura that is stereotyped and consistent across epileptic events. In contrast, pseudoseizures begin gradually with a buildup of anxiety or some other emotion, a "weird" poorly defined feeling, or hyperventilation. Typically, pseudoseizures do not occur when the child is alone. Epileptic seizures, however, occur when the child is alone or with others.

Generalized tonic–clonic seizures often begin with a cry followed by a sudden fall to the ground, which injures the patient. Pseudoseizure patients might cry out after slumping to the ground without sustaining any bodily injuries. During a motor seizure, the clonic-like movements of the child with pseudoseizures look more like thrusting, jerking, or side-to-side rolling movements that are unsynchronized

TABLE 22.4
CLINICAL MANIFESTATIONS IN EPILEPTIC AND PSEUDOSEIZURES

Clinical Manifestations	Epileptic Seizures	Pseudoseizures
Onset		
Premonition	Brief stereotyped aura	Ill-defined "weird" feeling
Evolution	Sudden	Gradual
Environment	Anywhere, with or without people present	Only in presence of others
Description of Seizure		
Generalized tonic–clonic	Cry, sudden fall, injury	Slumps, cry, no injury
Motor component	Synchronized clonic movements	Unsynchronized, thrusting, jerking, side-to-side rolling
Complex partial	Automatic, quasipurposive	Varied
	Motionless stare	Wavering stare
Level of consciousness		
Ictal	Marked change, unresponsive	Inconsistent response
Postictal	Tiredness, confusion, irritability	Resumption of activities
Repeated seizures	Clouding of consciousness	Clearheaded
Continence		
Urinary	Frequent	Rare
Fecal	Infrequent	Infrequent
End of seizure	Abrupt	Waxes and wanes
Duration	Brief	Brief to hours

compared to the synchronized and brisk movements of the clonic phase. The distribution of these movements does not follow known anatomical patterns. Other motor behaviors described in pseudoseizures include episodic staring, blinking, grimacing, laughing, crying, hand and head movements, and unresponsiveness (Wyllie et al., 1990).

The automatic and quasipurposive behaviors of complex partial seizures are sometimes difficult to differentiate from the complex behaviors that occur in children with pseudoseizures. Pseudoseizures that resemble complex partial seizures involve a wavering rather than a motionless stare with a preoccupied look. There are marked changes in the level of consciousness in children with generalized or complex partial seizures, and they do not respond to environmental stimuli. Children with pseudoseizures appear unresponsive, but might respond inconsistently to their environment.

In addition to differences in onset and clinical manifestations, urinary or fecal incontinence occur during epileptic seizures, not pseudoseizures. Epileptic seizures are brief events that last seconds to minutes and end abruptly. The duration of pseudoseizures varies and can last as long as hours with waxing and waning of symptoms.

The postictal period also differentiates between these two conditions. The child with pseudoseizures resumes previous activities without confusion or tiredness. In contrast, epileptic seizures are often accompanied by postictal sleeping, confusion, or irritability. If the child with pseudoseizures has repeated events, he or she is clearheaded between events, whereas the child with repeated epileptic seizures becomes more obtunded and confused.

Associated Psychopathology

A wide range of psychopathology is associated with pseudoseizures including conversion, affective, and anxiety disorders (Kotagal et al., 2002; Wyllie et al., 1999). Learning disorders or poor school achievement, as well as environmental stressors in the family or social milieu, are consistent findings in children with pseudoseizures. Sexual or physical abuse is also described (Gudmundsson et al., 2001; Pakalnis and Paolicchi, 2003a, 2003b; Wyllie et al., 1999).

Pseudoseizures Due to Conversion Disorder

In a conversion disorder (American Psychiatric Association, 1994, p. 457), the child's seizures or convulsions suggest that he or she has epilepsy and suffers significant distress or impairment from these attacks. Appropriate investigations do not confirm the epileptic basis for these episodes. Psychological factors in the form of conflicts or stressors, however, initiate or exacerbate these attacks. The child with a conversion disorder does not intentionally produce or feign the seizures.

The underlying primary conflict in pseudoseizures usually involves the child's difficulty expressing negative feelings, such as anger. Social difficulties, strife with parents, learning difficulties (Silver, 1982), or sexual abuse (Alper et al., 1993) can give rise to the negative feelings associated with the primary conflict. Expression of the primary conflict through seizures usually leads to significant attention from caregivers, friends, teachers, and others. This secondary gain reinforces the conversive symptoms and prevents the child from dealing with his or her problems in an adaptive manner.

The children's affective response can often be described as "la belle indifference." They usually minimize or deny any concern about the problems and difficulties in their lives even when these are significant. These children, however, respond with concern only about their attacks.

In terms of outcome, given the maladaptive nature of the symptoms of this disorder, a definitive diagnosis is needed as soon as possible. Wyllie et al. (1990) reported a good outcome in 14 of 18 children and adolescents diagnosed with nonepileptic seizures who had their symptoms for a mean duration of 7 months. Rather than duration of illness, Gudmundsson et al. (2001) found that among psychiatrically hospitalized children with pseudoseizures, more types of seizures, younger age at presentation, and female gender were associated with a better outcome.

Misinterpretation of Children's Behavior

Misinterpretation of the child's behaviors as epileptic seizures can reflect parental anxiety (Meadow, 1989). Several investigators have shown that the primary reason for nonepileptic events in children, particularly those with impaired intellectual function, was misinterpretation of behavior by parents and caretakers (Duchowny et al., 1988; Holmes et al., 1983; Neil and Alvarez, 1986). These behaviors included staring episodes, abnormal reactions to environmental stimuli, and repetitive movements, such as rocking, shaking, or arm waving. Unusual movements based on abnormal muscle tone were also often misinterpreted as seizures (Holmes et al., 1983; Neil and Alvarez, 1986). Unlike Munchausen syndrome by proxy (discussed later), these cases usually present with only one episode of factitious complaints. In addition, the parent's main concern is that their child recover rather than that the child be put through repeated medical examinations and procedures to determine that he or she is ill, as in the Munchausen syndrome by proxy.

Factitious Disorders

Factitious disorders (American Psychiatric Association, 1994, p. 474) involve intentional production or feigning of seizure symptoms specifically to assume the sick role. Unlike malingering, there are no external incentives for these behaviors, such as avoiding a legal responsibility like going to school. More commonly, the parent rather than the child has the factitious disorder and imposes a diagnosis of epilepsy on the child, as in Munchausen syndrome by proxy. To date, many of the cases of Munchausen syndrome by proxy present with seizures (see the review in Barber and Davis, 2002). In Meadow's original series

(1984) of 76 cases, 32 children had a primary diagnosis of epilepsy. In 21 cases the mothers fabricated the symptoms of the illness. In 11 cases the mothers caused seizures by suffocation, carotid sinus pressure, or use of drugs. Sixteen of the children in Meadow's sample had medical symptoms other than seizures. In Rosenberg's (1987) series, 42% of the 117 cases presented with seizures. It is important to note that Munchausen syndrome by proxy can also occur in a child with genuine epilepsy.

Unlike other disorders, clinicians do not usually observe the seizures of children with epilepsy and need to rely on parental report for a description of the clinical manifestations of the child's seizure (Meadow, 1984). Since it is difficult to confirm parental reports, it is relatively easy for a parent to fabricate a history of seizures and a lack of response to AEDs in the child (Meadow, 1984).

These cases present with a history of uncontrolled seizures, an inconsistent description of the child's seizures, repeated normal EEG recordings, repeated consultation with different physicians, particularly if the physician determines that there is no evidence that the child has epilepsy. Only the parent, not medical or school personnel have observed the child's seizures. The mothers of these children (McGuire and Feldman, 1989), sometimes employed in the health care field, are often very knowledgeable about epilepsy, EEG findings, and the use of AEDs. They are concerned and devoted to the child and appear at ease in the hospital and even form close relationships with hospital staff. The fathers usually are absent or play no role in the process so that they appear to be in "passive collusion" (Meadow, 1991) with the mother. In some cases of Munchausen syndrome by proxy, the father has been described as the perpetrator (Makar and Squier, 1990).

Diagnosis

The possibility of pseudoseizures should be entertained in cases of unexpectedly poor seizure control despite adequate AED levels, inconsistent seizure pattern, marked change in clinical presentation of seizures, and normal EEG recordings. A definitive diagnosis of the disorders underlying pseudoseizures is based on the lack of correlation between "seizure" behaviors and epileptic activity on video/EEG. Some researchers claim that provocative testing with suggestion can be a good and inexpensive tool to diagnose pseudoseizures in adults (Bazil et al., 1994) and in children (Sassower and Duchowny, 1992). Studies in adults attest to the reduced sensitivity of prolactin in differentiating epileptic from nonepileptic seizures (Shukla et al., 2004; Willert et al., 2004). However, although an increase in prolactin occurring 10 minutes after a seizure is a somewhat sensitive (64%) indicator of epileptic seizures (generalized tonic–clonic, complex partial), a negative serum prolactin within the first 100 minutes is highly predictive (98%) that a child did not have an epileptic seizure or had a pseudoseizure (Banjeree et al., 2004).

From the psychiatric perspective, to make a diagnosis of conversion, one must demonstrate both a primary conflict and secondary gain. The absence of a correlation between clinical seizures and epileptic activity on video-EEG alone is not indicative of pseudoseizures due to conversion if there is no evidence for both primary and secondary conflicts.

A diagnosis of misinterpretation of a child's behaviors as seizures is also best diagnosed by video-EEG. Psychiatric evaluation of the parent(s) and child can help rule out conversion and factitious disorder. It will also help determine underlying parental anxiety or difficulty coping with the child's epilepsy or behavior.

The diagnosis of Munchausen syndrome by proxy involves careful demonstration that the parent, usually the mother, has fabricated or is causing the child's symptoms. To do this, one has to methodically document all information obtained from the mother and check it for consistency in terms of dates, times, and descriptions of seizures. In addition, one needs to obtain information on previous and current AED blood levels to determine if the mother is overmedicating or undermedicating the child (Meadow, 1991). Furthermore, one should contact physicians who have previously cared for the child and find out if the mother left these physicians after they concluded that there was no evidence of a seizure disorder. Video-EEG recordings of the child's "seizures" and parent child interactions can provide important information on the factitious nature of the disorder and the mother's inability to parent (Epstein et al., 1987). A detailed psychiatric evaluation of the mother and child are also needed to make a definitive diagnosis of Munchausen syndrome by proxy.

Differential Diagnosis

When presented with a child who might have pseudoseizures, it is important to rule out neurological, sleep, and systemic disorders that might mimic seizures. For more detailed reviews of these disorders, see Sassower and Duchowny (1992), Mahowald and Rosen (1990), and Oppenheimer and Rosman (1983). Table 22.5 lists the diagnoses that should be considered in the differential diagnosis of pseudoseizures.

Neurological Disorders

Among the neurological disorders, movement disorders could mimic seizures, particularly if they are associated with sudden movements or tonic posturing. Unlike epileptic and pseudoseizures, none of these disorders are associated with change in state of consciousness even when they present with bilateral symptoms. Moreover, the symptoms of movement disorders occur when the child is alone or with others and change over time. Like pseudoseizures, however, the symptoms might last from seconds to hours. A family history of a movement disorder might support this diagnosis.

Migraine in middle childhood is not always associated with a headache and can present with confusion or disorientation (Gascon and Barlow, 1970), a transient hemi-

TABLE 22.5
DIFFERENTIAL DIAGNOSIS OF PSEUDOSEIZURES

1. Neurological Disorders

   a. Epilepsy and status epilepticus
   b. Migraine
      (i) Confusional
      (ii) Abdominal
   c. Movement disorders
      (i) Familial paroxysmal choreoathetosis
      (ii) Tic disorder

2. Systemic Disorders

   (i) Breath-holding spells
   (ii) Cardiogenic syncope
   (iii) Cardiac arrhythmias

3. Sleep Disorders

   (i) Night terrors
   (ii) Somnambulism
   (iii) Narcolepsy
   (iv) Cataplexy
   (v) Hypnogogic hallucinations and sleep paralysis
   (vi) Nocturnal myoclonus

paresis that might mimic a Todd's paralysis, and visual aura (Bodensteiner, 1990), symptoms that occur in children with pseudoseizures. It is important to note that migraine and epilepsy frequently coexist in the same child (Septien et al., 1991). Although migraine and epilepsy can cause a headache, a migrainous headache occurs at the beginning and an epileptic headache at the end of the episode. Migraine headache in the child is usually associated with a family history of migraine.

Children with vertigo appear pale and complain of nausea, vomiting, dizziness, and ataxia (Basse, 1964). Unlike children with pseudoseizures, these children look sick, are frightened, and cling to their parents (Dunn and Snyder, 1976).

Sleep Disorders

Night terrors present as crying or screaming, a state of panic, semipurposeful, and automatic behaviors that occur while the child is in deep sleep and unable to be roused. They might mimic a pseudoseizure, but the child with night terrors returns to sleep with no recollection for the night's events. Children with pseudoseizures remember their episodes and they occur in front of other people. The child with sleep walking gets out of bed with a glassy look in the eyes, walks around the house, and can be easily led back to bed. Sleep studies provide a definitive diagnosis by demonstrating that night terrors occur in stage 3 or 4 of nonREM sleep and sleep walking in REM sleep.

Children with narcolepsy fall asleep suddenly and might also have drop attacks due to sudden loss of muscle tone

(cataplexy), hypnagogic hallucinations, and sleep paralysis. Unlike pseudoseizures, rapid eye movements herald the onset of the narcolepsy, and sudden fright or excitement usually induce the cataplectic attacks.

Systemic Disorders

There are cardiopulmonary, autonomic, gastrointestinal, and metabolic disorders that can mimic seizures. Of these, syncope or fainting occurs most commonly in school-aged children. Syncope is often precipitated by an intense emotional stimulus, a systemic illness, or a mechanical cause, such as prolonged standing. Like pseudoseizures, the loss of consciousness of syncope occurs gradually, and the child becomes limp and usually falls backward without rigidity, clonus, incontinence, or physical injury. Children who present with these symptoms should have a cardiac evaluation to determine if they have cardiogenic or simple syncope. Some children might need Holter monitoring to rule out arrhythmias.

Breath-holding spells or infantile syncope should be considered in the differential diagnosis of pseudoseizures in young children. They begin between the ages of 6 and 18 months and subside by age 6 years in most cases (Lombroso and Lerman, 1967). In the cyanotic type, the child usually starts to cry vigorously because of some frustration or a sudden fright, then becomes apneic and cyanotic, loses consciousness, and the limbs become rigidly extended. The child regains consciousness in less than 1 minute. About 20% of children with breath-holding spells develop syncope later in life (Lombroso and Lerman, 1967). The child with pallid infantile syncope responds to a fright without crying but with pallor, loss of consciousness, and associated clonic jerks.

Treatment

Wyllie et al. (1990) suggest that psychiatric intervention should not begin until a definitive diagnosis of pseudoseizures is made. A psychiatric evaluation can begin as soon as the epileptologist thinks that the child might have pseudoseizures. Typically, this occurs after the first few days of telemetry. Once the psychiatric and neurological diagnostic procedures confirm a diagnosis of pseudoseizures, the child and family should be given diagnostic feedback. In giving the feedback, the pediatric neurologist should first inform the child and family of the nonictal nature of the child's seizures. The psychiatrist then explains the possible psychogenic basis for the child's attacks. The pseudoseizures are no longer called seizures, but "attacks," "episodes," or "the problem" (Aylward, 1984). It is important to ensure that the child and parents do not perceive the feedback as suggesting that the child has been faking the attacks (Aylward). In addition, the feedback should provide the child with an easy out without losing face (Aylward). Many parents have difficulty accepting a psychiatric diagnosis of pseudoseizures and need to be helped to accept this diagnosis.

The aims of psychiatric treatment are to stop the child's episodes and to teach the child adaptive coping strategies for dealing with his or her difficulties expressing negative affect or anger. Decreasing in the amount of attention and secondary gain the child receives during his or her episodes will usually reduce the frequency of attacks. To achieve this goal, one has to work with both the parents and siblings. If the child is having episodes at school, the psychiatrist also needs to work with the teachers and school nurse. A behavioral approach is often helpful in decreasing the secondary gain. In parallel with the psychiatric intervention, the child's AEDs should be gradually decreased or maintained at a lower dose if the child also has epilepsy.

In cases where the frequency of pseudoseizures is so high that it impairs the functioning of the child and family, psychiatric hospitalization needs to be considered. Once the frequency of episodes has decreased sufficiently so the child can function, one needs to work psychotherapeutically with the child and family. The length of treatment is dependent on the severity of the child's underlying emotional difficulties and those of his immediate family.

In Munchausen syndrome by proxy cases, once the diagnosis has been confirmed, the responsible physician needs to report the case to the local child protection authorities and then confront the mother with this diagnosis in the presence of the child protective services. Child protective services need to remove the child from the parents' care to ensure the child's safety and the child's AEDs are gradually withdrawn. The length and indications for treatment of the child and parent(s) vary in different cases.

PEDIATRIC EPILEPSY: SCHOOL ACHIEVEMENT, COGNITION, LANGUAGE, AND BEHAVIOR

The previous sections of this chapter characterized the phenomenology, clinical, and behavioral manifestations of different epilepsy syndromes in childhood and adolescence. This section reviews the impact of epilepsy on children's academic, cognitive, linguistic, and psychosocial functioning. Using a developmental and integrative perspective, it also examines how children's developmental level and neurocognitive functioning interact with their academic and psychosocial functioning.

Academic Achievement and School Factors

School, with its focus on academic achievement, acquisition of knowledge, and socialization, represents one of the primary developmental contexts and tasks for children and adolescents, including those with epilepsy. The sequelae associated with management of a chronic illness like epilepsy can substantially affect children's school experience in the areas of academic underachievement, increased remedial

placement, grade retention, and negative student attitudes toward school and learning (Olson et al., 2004).

Academic underachievement is prevalent in pediatric epilepsy (Fastenau et al., 2004). Epilepsy patients have a higher risk of learning disorders (Motamedi and Meador, 2003) and score significantly below both their healthy peers and those with other chronic illness across academic content areas. For example, Austin et al. (1999) found, in a 4-year longitudinal study, that children with epilepsy performed significantly worse than children with asthma on measures of reading, mathematics, language, and vocabulary. Subjects with the highest seizure severity performed most poorly on the measures of academic achievement. Antonello (1999) found that, after adjusting for IQ, 9- to 13-year-old children with epilepsy read more slowly than healthy children, and those with left-side complex partial seizures, as compared to either right-side complex partial seizures or primary generalized epilepsy, showed the most impairment in math and reading skills. Williams et al. (1996a) demonstrated that children with poorly-controlled complex partial seizures performed more poorly on measures of reading and attention than did children with better controlled seizures. In contrast to the preceding findings, Mitchell et al. (1991) found no relation between either seizure severity or duration of illness on academic achievement.

The academic underachievement of children with epilepsy places them at increased risk for grade retention and special education services. Bailet and Turk (2000) found that children with idiopathic epilepsy had higher rates of grade retention and placement in special education classes than did their healthy siblings. Likewise, Oostrom et al. (2002) found, both before diagnosis and over a period of 1 year after diagnosis, significantly more children with epilepsy, 51 versus 27% of their healthy classmates, required special education services. School difficulties, such as poor grades, remediation, or retention, can decrease a child's self-esteem and affect his or her learning style (Aldenkamp, 1983). Sturniolo and Galletti (1994) showed that emotional maladjustment in children with idiopathic epilepsy was associated with poor school performance. Similarly, Oostrom et al. (2003) found that children with epilepsy had poor motivation and attitude toward school and felt less socially accepted at school than did their healthy classmates.

The academic and school-related difficulties experienced by children with epilepsy reflect the interrelations among psychosocial and neuropsychological factors. For example, Fastenau et al. (2004) found both a direct association of neuropsychological functioning with achievement (e.g., verbal, memory, and executive function factors strong relation to reading, math, and writing) as well as a moderating role of family functioning on academic achievement in pediatric epilepsy patients ages 8 to 15 years. Specifically, a supportive and organized home environment moderated the impact of neuropsychological deficits on children's academic achievement (Fastenau al.), conceivably by requiring consistent homework completion, regular sleep, and medication schedules. Williams et al. (2001) noted that the academic underachievement of children with epilepsy may be related to lower self-esteem, inattention, or memory inefficiency. Controlling for intelligence in a sample of 65 children with well-controlled epilepsy, Williams et al. (2001) found that attention was the only variable associated with achievement scores. The lower academic achievement and school problems may be related to both cognitive and psychosocial factors.

Cognition

Because epilepsy disrupts brain maturation, it has been thought to produce nonspecific cognitive consequences (Lassonde et al., 2000). Past and current research has documented a link between epilepsy and cognitive impairment in children (e.g., see the review in Nolan et al., 2003). To understand how pediatric epilepsy disrupts cognitive functioning and subsequently children's academic performance and behavioral adjustment, we briefly review the complex relation between epilepsy and cognition, focusing first on general cognitive function. However, because cognitive impairment may affect a variety of neurocognitive skills (e.g., attention, perception, concept formation, reading, thought process, learning, memory, and problem solving) (Motamedi and Meador, 2003), the specific neurocognitive skills of attention, memory, and executive functions, as well as how seizure variables modify children's cognitive abilities, are also reviewed.

While generally within the normal range, the IQ scores of children with epilepsy are distributed more toward the lower end of functioning (Black and Hynd, 1995; Motamedi and Meador, 2003). Caplan et al. (2004) found that 5- to 16-year-old children with complex partial seizures earned significantly lower standardized IQ and language scores than healthy subjects while controlling for demographic and perinatal factors. Using a test-retest design, Bjornaes et al. (2001) assessed the long-term consequences of refractory seizures on intellectual functioning and found that mean IQ scores decreased in children with epilepsy. One possible explanation for the cognitive impairment noted in children with epilepsy is not that they are experiencing cognitive decline, but rather acquiring skill at a slower rate or have a decreased capacity to learn compared to healthy peers (Cornaggia and Gobbi, 2002).

Assessment of seizure variables (e.g., seizure type, frequency, severity, localization of seizure activity, age at onset, duration, and number of AEDs) is somewhat challenging as seizure variables are themselves interrelated (e.g., number of AEDs may reflect seizure severity). In addition, seizure variables, such as the severity of the child's seizure disorder, might differentially affect child adjustment, and, in turn, cognitive functioning. Nonetheless, this research has yielded additional understanding of the link

between pediatric epilepsy and cognition. For example, generally, there appears to be a positive association between severity of epilepsy and cognitive impairment. Several clinical studies have indicated that high seizure frequency (e.g., Caplan et al., 2004; Hermann, 1982; Rodin et al., 1986; Seidenberg, 1989), early onset (Schoenfeld et al., 1999; Smith et al., 2002), or a history of status epilepticus (Singhi et al., 1992) are associated with poor academic performance and lower IQ in children with epilepsy. Cornaggia and Gobbi (2002) and Schoenfeld et al. (1999) noted that cognitive impairment was more pronounced in children with a higher lifetime total number of seizures, particularly if they had multiple seizure types (Cornaggia and Gobbi).

Finally, use of multiple AEDs in children with epilepsy is a marker for intractable seizures, severity of epileptic disorder, multiple seizure types, and often early onset of epilepsy. While treatment with AEDs may improve learning by reducing the number of seizures, negative side effects of AEDs such as sleepiness, slowed reaction time, and attentional difficulties may also impair learning and cognitive performance (Cornaggia and Gobbi, 2002). Although beyond the scope of this chapter, it is important to note that, because some AEDs produce global changes in excitatory neurotransmitters, such as glutamate (Ortinski and Meador, 2004), and others in inhibitory neurotransmitters, such as gabba amino butyric acid (Keller et al., 2002), they might cause or exacerbate both cognitive and behavioral difficulties in children with epilepsy.

Executive Function
As with seizure severity, seizure variables, such as type of seizure disorder and localization of epileptic focus may differentially affect the nature of the cognitive impairment experienced by children with epilepsy. Executive functions are one neurocognitive skill in which this has been examined. Research has documented executive function like deficits (e.g., impairment of planning, working memory, impulse control, attention, and set shifting) in children with epilepsy, similar to the deficits seen in children diagnosed with ADHD and adults with frontal lobe lesions (Hernandez et al., 2002; Lassonde et al., 2000). Not surprisingly, this has most often been noted in children with frontal lobe epilepsy, a rare form of pediatric epilepsy. For example, Culhane-Shelburne et al. (2002) found that children with this seizure disorder showed deficits in planning and executive functions but not in verbal and nonverbal memory, while the opposite pattern was true for children with TLE. Similarly, Hernandez and colleagues (2002, 2003) found that children with frontal lobe epilepsy, as compared to temporal lobe or generalized epilepsy, had more deficits in the executive function tasks of planning and impulse control, performance speed, motor coordination rigidity, and more intrusion and interference errors on a task of verbal recall. Finally, Riva et al. (2002) noted that children with frontal lobe epilepsy with a left, in compari-

son to a right-sided EEG foci showed more deficits in categorization, verbal long-term memory, and detailed visuol-spatial analysis. More studies are needed to replicate these findings given that the sample sizes for the previously cited studies have all been relatively small, ranging from 8 in the Riva et al.'s (2002) study to 32 in the Hernandez et al. (2002, 2003) research.

Attention

Attention, an important aspect of general cognition and component of executive functions, encompasses sustained, selective, or divided attention. Attention problems are frequently seen in children with both new onset and chronic epilepsy (Caplan et al., 2004; Dunn et al., 2003; Oostrom et al., 2003). In his early studies on children with epilepsy, Stores (1973, 1978b) described parent and teacher reports of inattention and hyperactivity, but no evidence for impaired vigilance, impulsivity, or distractibility based on laboratory measures. Semrud-Clikeman and Wical (1999) found that children with comorbid complex partial seizure disorder and ADHD had increased reaction time and made significantly more errors of omission and commission than did healthy children, but were similar in performance on these attentional tasks to children diagnosed with only epilepsy or ADHD. Similarly, medically and surgically treated children with epilepsy evidenced slow reaction time, increased errors of omission, and variability in response, but no increase in errors of commission (Aldenkamp et al., 2000; Billingsley et al., 2000; Mitchell et al., 1993; Oostrom et al., 2003; Semrud-Clikeman and Wical 1999; Lendt et al., 2002).

The attentional problems of children with epilepsy and ADHD are related to lower IQ scores (Kinney et al., 1989; Williams et al., 1996b), impaired memory (Billingsley et al., 2000), and poor school performance (Oostrom et al., 2003; Williams et al., 2001). From an integrative perspective, Oostrom et al. (2003) found that children with prior school or behavioral difficulties and those whose parents responded maladaptively to the new epilepsy diagnosis performed more poorly on a reaction time task than did patients without these additional risk factors. According to Motamedi and Meador (2003), the attentional difficulties of children with epilepsy may affect their encoding of new information leading to memory problems. Finally, from a practical perspective, Kadis et al. (2004) suggested that attentional problems may also underlie everyday memory problems found in children with intractable epilepsy.

Memory

Memory, a specific neurocognitive ability, represents the complex skills of information storage and retrieval. General conceptualizations of memory include its division into short- and longterm memory, with the latter further subdivided into implicit and explicit (semantic and episodic) memory. Decreased memory skills have been reported in children with epilepsy (e.g., Nolan et al., 2004). For example, Pavone et al. (2001) found nonverbal and delayed memory disturbances in 16 children with absence epilepsy compared to matched control subjects. Williams et al. (2001b) assessed the verbal memory of 8- to 13-year-old children with well controlled seizures: 44 children with complex partial seizures and 21 with generalized seizures. They found that children with both seizure types performed better on short-term memory tasks than long-term delayed recall tasks, although no differences in memory performance were noted based on seizure type. In contrast, Nolan et al. (2004) found that syndrome type differentially affected memory functioning in children with epilepsy. Specifically, of the 70 subjects, ages 6 to 18, with absence, frontal lobe, or temporal lobe epilepsy, those with TLE evidenced significantly worse verbal memory functioning than the other two groups. Moreover, Nolan et al. (2004) found that longer duration of intractable epilepsy was associated with reduced memory ability. Finally, Lespinet et al. (2002) found that children with epilepsy onset at age 5 or before showed substantial verbal and nonverbal memory deficits, whereas subjects with onset at age 10 or older evidenced minor deficits consistent with lateralization (i.e., verbal deficits with left TLE and nonverbal deficits with right TLE).

Other researchers have assessed the link between pediatric epilepsy and memory in subjects undergoing epilepsy surgery using a presurgical and postsurgical test–retest design. Using this paradigm, Mabbott and Smith (2003) assessed the verbal and visual memory of 44 children and adolescents with focal epilepsy who underwent either right, left, or extratemporal excisions and found that all surgical groups improved on the visual memory task of facial recognition after surgery. In contrast, Kuehn et al. (2002), also using a presurgical and postsurgical test–retest design, found no significant improvement in the memory functioning of 20 subjects with temporal and 6 with extratemporal resections. Unlike what has been found in adults, they did not find that children with surgically treated left TLE had more verbal and those with right TLE had more visual memory deficits.

Cognition and Psychopathology

As noted earlier, both general and more specific epilepsy-related cognitive impairments are detrimental to children's academic achievement. Likewise, cognitive impairments, ranging from minimal to more severe, also affect the psychosocial and behavioral functioning of children with epilepsy. In children with average IQ scores who had complex partial seizures, Caplan et al. (2004) found that mild verbal IQ deficits, but not seizure variables, predicted psychopathology. Buelow et al. (2003) found pediatric epilepsy patients with an IQ of 85 or lower had more behavior and mental health problems than children with higher IQ scores. In the most severe form, the presence of epilepsy and mental retardation increases the severity of psychopathology in children (see the review in Caplan and Austin, 2000).

Language

Language, communication, and speech delays are a pervasive type of developmental difficulty, which may result from specific language impairment, cognitive impairment, hearing impairment, or chronic illness (Watkins, 1994) such as epilepsy. Language delays may include difficulties in the areas of expressive, receptive or pragmatic skills, phonological and grammatical rules, word learning, semantics, recognizing and using speech regularities, vocabulary, using clarification responses, repairing conversational breakdowns, and modifying speech to fit the social situation (Rice, 1991). These same types of language difficulties are seen in children with epilepsy.

Farwell et al. (1985) found that 6- to 16-year-old children with epilepsy made more mistakes on language-related tasks than on other cognitive tasks. Regarding children with complex partial seizures, Antonello (1999) found they had both expressive and receptive language delays, while Schoenfeld et al. (1999) found they performed significantly worse than their siblings on linguistic tasks of word knowledge, category fluency, and response to commands of increasing length and complexity, even after controlling for IQ. In addition, Caplan et al. (2001, 2002a, 2004) reported that children with epilepsy had both basic and higher-level linguistic deficits. Despite average IQ scores, they had significantly lower language age scores than normal children (Caplan et al., 2004), as well as more illogical thinking, discourse deficits, and poor monitoring and correction of communication breakdowns (Caplan et al., 2001, 2002a). Evidence for significantly more language deficits in younger compared to older children with epilepsy led Caplan et al. (2001) to conclude that epilepsy syndromes, particularly complex partial seizures and primary generalized epilepsy, impact the ongoing development of children's communicative skills. Moreover, Saltzman et al. (2002) found that a higher proportion of children with seizure onset prior to age 5 showed speech deficits as compared to children with seizure onset after age 5.

From an integrative perspective, linguistic impairments exert comprehensive deficits on the cognitive and psychosocial functioning of children with epilepsy. Wheless et al. (2002) noted that language development may be disrupted in children with epilepsy given the disorder's negative effect on intellectual functioning. Impairment in specific linguistic skills may also, in turn, impact children's memory and learning. Likewise, impaired linguistic functioning has lasting negative consequences on the academic and social adjustment of children with epilepsy (Wheless et al., 2002). For example, Caplan et al. (2004) noted that verbal deficits were predictive of behavioral difficulties in children with complex partial seizures. More specifically, the presence of illogical thinking and discourse deficits, as noted in the Caplan et al. studies (2001, 2002a), might increase the social difficulties of these children because their peers have difficulty following what they are talking about.

Developmental and Integrative Summary

From an integrative perspective, epilepsy has a profound impact on children's adjustment across the developmental domains of academic achievement, cognition, language, and psychosocial functioning. Moreover, the way in which epilepsy influences these domains of functioning varies depending on the interrelations among these factors and the child's developmental level. For example, throughout childhood, seizures have important implications for brain development in that they may interfere with neural maturation and subsequently with brain structure, which may then have both immediate and lifelong cognitive implications (e.g., Hermann and Seidenberg, 2002). In middle childhood, seizures may negatively impact children's ongoing acquisition of higher level cognitive and linguistic skills, as well as their success in achievement and socialization tasks, which are tantamount to maturational success during this developmental period. Finally, evidence for continued maturation of brain regions involved in higher level integrative functions, such as language and cognition during adolescence (Gogtay et al., 2004; Sowell et al., 2003), points to the potential negative cognitive impact of epilepsy on older youth. In addition, the adolescent maturational challenge of developing a self-identity and autonomy may also be compromised in youth with epilepsy given their increased dependence on parents and necessary adherence to seizure-reducing medication and schedule routines.

Although a review of the social and family factors relevant to pediatric epilepsy is beyond the scope of this chapter, it is important to briefly note that peer and family influences may differentially affect the interaction of epilepsy with neurocognitive and psychosocial factors across children's developmental level. For example, the unpredictability and possible severe consequences of seizures causes anxiety and fear for parents of children with epilepsy (e.g., Austin et al., 1993; Ziegler, 1985). Thus, parents must negotiate the difficult task of providing adequate supervision without being overanxious or overprotective, thereby limiting children's participation in typical socialization experiences and development of age-appropriate autonomy. In contrast, a supportive and stable family environment may serve a protective function and promote positive adjustment for children with epilepsy (Fastenau et al., 2004).

REFERENCES

Achenbach T: Manual for the Child Behavior Checklist and Revised Child Behavior Profile. Burlington, Vermont: Department of Psychiatry, University of Vermont, 1991.

Asconape J, Penry JK: Some clinical and EEG aspects of benign juvenile myoclonic epilepsy. Epilepsia 25:108–114, 1984.

Aicardi J: Epilepsy in Children. New York: Raven Press, 1986, p 124.

Aldenkamp A, van Bronswijk K, Braken M, et al: A clinical comparative study evaluating the effect of epilepsy versus ADHD on timed cognitive tasks in children. Neuropsychol Dev Cogn Sect C Child Neuropsychol 6:209–217, 2000.

Aldenkamp AP: Epilepsy and learning behavior. In Advances in Epileptology: XIVth Epilepsy International Symposium. Edited by Parsonage M, Grant RHE, Craig, AG, Ward AA, Jr. New York: Raven Press, 1983, pp. 221–229.

Alper K, Devinsky O, Perrine K, et al: Nonepileptic seizures and childhood sexual and physical abuse. Neurology 43:1950–1953, 1993.

Alvarez LA, Shinnar S, Moshe SL: Infantile spasms due to unilateral cerebral infarcts. Pediatrics 6:1024–1026, 1987.

Ambrosetto G, Rossi PG, Tassinari CA: Predictive factors of seizure frequency and duration of antiepileptic treatment in rolandic epilepsy: a retrospective study. Brain Dev 9:300–304, 1987.

American Psychiatric Association: Diagnostic and Statistical Manual of Mental Disorders, 4th ed. Washington, DC, American Psychiatric Association Press, 1994.

Antonello JL: Epilepsy and reading in children. Dissertation Abstracts International 60: (3, a) 1999, p. 644.

Askalan R, Mackay M, Brian L, et al: Prospective preliminary analysis of the development of autism and epilepsy in children with infantile spasms. J Child Neurol 18:165–170, 2003.

Aso K, Watanabe K, Maeda N, et al: Temporal lobe epilepsy of childhood onset. Jpn J Psychiatry Neurol 48:217–220, 1994.

Astradsson A, Olafsson E, Ludvigssion P, et al: Icelandic epilepsy: an incidence study in Iceland. Epilepsia 39:884–886, 1998.

Austin JK, Huberty JT, Huster GA, et al: Does academic achievement in children with epilepsy change over time? Dev Med Child Neurol 41:473–479, 1999.

Austin JK, Dunn DW, Levstek DA: First seizures: concerns and needs of parents and children. Epilepsia 34 (6):24, 1993.

Avanzini G, Panzica F, Franceschetti S: Brain maturational aspects relevant to pathophysiology of infantile spasms. Int Rev Neurobiol 49:353–365, 2002.

Aylward GP: Description of a therapeutic approach to pseudoseizures in adolescents. Community Ment Health J 20:155–158, 1984.

Bailet LL, Turk WR: The impact of childhood epilepsy on neurocognitive and behavioral performance: a prospective longitudinal study. Epilepsia 41:426–431, 2000.

Bancaud J, Talairach J: Clinical semiology of frontal lobe seizures. Adv Neurol 57:3–58, 1992.

Banerjee S, Paul P, Talib VJ: Serum prolactin in seizure disorders. Indian Pediatr 41:827–831, 2004.

Barber MA, Davis PM: Fits, faints, or fatal fantasy? Fabricated seizures and child abuse. Arch Dis Child 86 :230–233, 2002.

Bass N, Wyllie E, Comair Y, et al: Supplementary sensorimotor area seizures in children and adolescents. J Pediatrics 126:537–544, 1995.

Basse LS: Benign paroxysmal vertigo of childhood. Brain 87:141–152, 1964.

Bazil CW, Kothari M, Luciano D, et al: Provocation of nonepileptic seizures by suggestion in a general seizure population. Epilepsia 35: 768–770, 1994.

Beaumanoir A: The Landau-Kleffner syndrome in Epileptic Syndromes, in Infancy, Childhood, and Adolescence. Edited by Roger J, Dravet C, Bureau M, Dreifuss FE, Wolf P. London-Paris, John Libbey Eurotext, 1985, pp. 181–191.

Beaumanoir A, Nahory A: Les epilepsies benignes partielles: 41 cas d'epilepsie partielle frontal a evolution favorable. Revue EEG Neurophysiologique 13:207–211, 1983.

Berry-Kravis E: Epilepsy in fragile X syndrome. Dev Med Child Neurol 44:724–728, 2002.

Beydoun A, Garofalo EA, Drury I: Generalized spike-waves, multiple loci and clinical course in children with EEG features of benign epilepsy of childhood with centrotemporal spikes. Epilepsia 33: 1091–1096, 1992.

Billard C, Loisel ML, Gillet P, et al: Relationship between acquired neuropsychological deficits and nocturnal EEG abnormalities in a case of Landau-Kleffner syndrome. ANAE 3:39–43, 1991.

Billingsley R L, Smith M L, McAndrews MP: Material-specific and non-specific attention deficits in children and adolescents following temporal-lobe surgery. Neuropsychologia 38:292–303, 2000.

Bishop DVM: Age of onset and outcome of "acquired aphasia with convulsive disorder" (Landau-Kleffner syndrome). Dev Med Child Neurol 27:705–712, 1985.

Bjornaes H, Stabell K, Henriksen O, et al: The effects of refractory epilepsy on intellectual functioning in children and adults: a longitudinal study. Seizure 10:250–259, 2001.

Black KC, Hynd GW: Epilepsy and the school aged child: cognitive-behavioral characteristics and effects on academic performance. School Psychology Quarterly 10:345–358, 1995.

Blanchette N, Smith ML: Language after temporal or frontal lobe surgery in children with epilepsy. Brain Cogn 48:280–284, 2002.

Blom S, Heijbel J: Benign epilepsy of children with centro-temporal EEG foci: A follow-up study in adulthood of patients initially diagnosed as children. Epilepsia 23:629–631, 1992.

Blomquist HK, Zetterlund B: Evaluation of treatment in typical absence seizures. The roles of long-term EEG monitoring and ethosuximide. Acta Peda Scand 74:409–415, 1985.

Bocti C, Robitaille Y, Diadori P, Lortie A, Mercier C, Bouthillier A, Carmant L: The pathological basis of temporal lobe epilepsy in childhood. Neurology 60:191–195, 2003.

Bodensteiner JB: Visual symptoms in childhood migraine. J Child Neurol 5:190, 1990.

Boel M, Caesar P: Continuous spikes and waves during slow sleep: A 30 months follow-up study of neuropsychological recovery and EEG findings. Neuropediatrics 20:176–180, 1989.

Boone KB, Miller BL, Rosenberg L, et al: Neuropsychological and behavioral abnormalities in an adolescent with frontal lobe seizures. Neurology 38:583–586, 1988.

Bourgeois B, Brown LW, Pellock JM, et al: Gabapentin (Neurontin) monotherapy in children with benign childhood epilepsy with centrotemporal spikes (BECTS): a 36-week, double-blind, placebo-controlled study. Epilepsia 39(suppl 6):163, 1998.

Bouma PA, Westendorp RG, van Dijk JG, Peters AC, Brouwer OF: The outcome of absence epilepsy: a meta-analysis. Neurology 47:802–808, 1996.

Braathen G, Theorell K, Persson A, et al: Valproate in the treatment of absence epilepsy in children: A study of dose-response relationships. Epilepsia 29:548–552, 1988.

Branch CE, Dyken PR: Choroid plexus papilloma and infantile spasms. Ann Neurol 5:302–304, 1979.

Brunson KL, Avishai-Eliner S, Baram TL: ACTH treatment of infantile spasms: mechanisms of its effects in modulation of neuronal excitability. Int Rev Neurobiol 49:185–197, 2002.

Buelow JM, Austin JK, Perkins SM, et al: Behavior and mental health problems in children with epilepsy and low IQ. Dev Med Child Neurol 45:683–692, 2003.

Camfield P, Camfield C. Epileptic syndromes in childhood: clinical features, outcomes, and treatment. Epilepsia 43:27–32, 2002.

Camfield CS, Chaplin S, Doyle AB, et al: Side effects of phenobarbital in toddlers: behavior and cognitive aspects. J Pediatrics 95: 361–365, 1979.

Caplan R, Siddarth P, Gurbani S, et al: Psychopathology and pediatric complex partial seizures: seizure-related, cognitive, and linguistic variables. Epilepsia 45:1273–1281, 2004.

Caplan R, Guthrie D, Komo S, et al: Social communication in pediatric epilepsy. J Child Psychol Psychiatry 43:245–253, 2002a.

Caplan R, Siddarth P, Mathern G, et al: Developmental outcome with and without successful intervention. Int Rev Neurobiol 49:269–284, 2002b.

Caplan R, Guthrie D, Komo S et al: Conversational repair in pediatric complex partial seizure disorder. Brain Lang 78:82–93, 2001.

Caplan R, Austin JK: Behavioral aspects of epilepsy in children with mental retardation. Ment Retard Dev Disabil Res Rev 6:293–299, 2000.

Caplan R, Curtiss S, Chugani HC et al: Pediatric Rasmussen encephalitis: Social communication, language, PET, and pathology before and after hemispherectomy. Brain Cogn 39:116–132, 1999.

Caplan R, Gillberg C: Child psychiatric disorders. In Epilepsy: A Comprehensive Textbook. Edited by Engel J Jr., Pedley T. New York: Raven Press, vol. 2, pp. 2125–2139, 1998.

Caplan R, Guthrie D, Shields WD, et al: Formal thought disorder in pediatric complex partial seizure disorder. J Child Psychitry Psychol 33:1399–1412, 1992a.

Caplan R, Shields WD, Mori L, et al: Middle childhood onset of interictal psychoses: Case studies. J Am Acad Child Adolesc Psychiatry 30:6:893–896, 1991.

Cavazutti GB: Epidemiology of different types of epilepsy in school age of Modena, Italy. Epilepsia 2:57–62, 1980.

Chauvel P, Vignal JP, Chodkiewicz JP, et al: The clinical signs and symptoms of frontal lobe seizures. Phenomenology and Classification. In Epilepsy and the functional Anatomy of the Frontal Lobe. Edited by Jasper HH, Riggio S, Godman-Rakic PS. New York: Raven Press, 1995, pp. 115–125.

Chevalier H, Metz-Lutz MN, Segalowitz SJ: Impulsivity and control of inhibition in benign focal childhood epilepsy (BFCE). Brain Cogn 43:86–90, 2000.

Chugani HT: Pathophysiology of infantile spasms. Adv Exp Med Biol 497:111–121, 2002.

Clusmann H, Kral T, Gleissner U, et al: Analysis of different types of resection for pediatric patients with temporal lobe epilepsy. Neurosurgery 54:847–859, 2004.

Commission on Classification and Terminology of the International League Against Epilepsy: Proposal for revised clinical and electroencephalographic classification of epileptic seizures. Epilepsia 30:389–399, 1989.

Coppola G, Licciardi F, Sciscio N, Russo F, Carotenuto M, Pascotto A: Lamotrigine as first-line drug in childhood absence epilepsy: a clinical and neurophysiological study. Brain Dev 26:26–29, 2004.

Cornaggia CM, Gobbi G: Epilepsy and learning disorders. In the Neuropsychiatry of Epilepsy. Edited by Trimble M, Schmitz B. New York: Cambridge University Press, 2002, pp. 62–69.

Croona C, Kihlgren M, Lundberg S, et al: Neuropsychological findings in children with benign childhood epilepsy with centrotemporal spikes. Dev Med Child Neurol 41:813–818, 1999.

Culhane-Shelburne K, Chapieski L, Hiscock M et al: Executive functions in children with frontal and temporal lobe epilepsy. J Int Neuropsychol Soc 8:623–632, 2002.

Cusmai R, Dulac O, Diebler C: Lesions focales dans les spasmes infantiles. Neurophysiology Clinique 18:235–241, 1988.

da Silva EA, Chugani DC, Muzik O, et al: Landau-Kleffnersyndrome: metabolic abnormalities in temporal lobe are a common feature. J Child Neurol 12:489–495, 1997.

Degen R, Degen HE: Some genetic aspects of rolandic epilepsy: waking and sleep. Epilepsia 31:795–801, 1990.

Delgado-Escueta AV, Serratosa JM, Liu A, et al: Progress in mapping human epilepsy genes. Epilepsia 35:S29–40, 1994.

Deonna T, Zesiger P, Davidoff V, et al: Benign partial epilepsy of childhood: a longitudinal neuropsychological and EEG study of cognitive function. Dev Med Child Neurol 42:595–603, 2000.

Deonna TW: Acquired epileptiform aphasia in children (Landau-Kleffner syndrome). J Clin Neurophysiol 7:288–298, 1991.

Deonna TW, Peter C, Ziegler AL: Adult follow-up of the acquired aphgasia-epilepsy syndrome in childhood. Report of 7 cases. Neuropediatrics 20:132–138, 1989.

Deonna T, Beaumanoir A, Gaillard F, Assal G: Acquired aphasia in childhood with seizure disorder: A heterogenous syndrome. Neuropediatrics 8:263–273, 1977.

de Weerd AW, Arts WFM: Significance of centro-temporal spikes on the EEG. Acta Neurological Scandinavia 87:429–433, 1993.

Dimova PS, Daskalov DS: Coincidence of rolandic and absence features: rare, but not impossible. J Child Neurol 17:838–846, 2002.

Dlouhá O, Nevšimalová S: Speech disorder and hearing in Landau-Kleffner syndrome. Česk Otolaryngol 39:114–120, 1990.

Dlugos DJ, Sammel MD, Strom BL, Farrar JT: Response to first drug trial predicts outcome in childhood temporal lobe epilepsy. Neurology 26;57:2259–2264, 2001.

Dongier S: Statistical study of clinical and electroencephalographic manifestations of 536 psychotic episodes occurring in 516 epileptics between clinical seizures. Epilepsia 1:117–142, 1959.

Dreifuss FE: Juvenile myoclonic epilepsy: characteristics of a primary generalized epilepsy. Epilepsia 30:S1–S7, 1989.

Drury I, Beydoun A: Benign epilepsy of childhood with monomorphic sharp waves in centrotemporal and other locations. Epilepsia 32:662–667, 1991.

Duchowny MS, Resnic TJ, Deray M, et al: Video EEG diagnosis of repetitive behavior in childhood and its relationship to seizures. Ped Neurology 2:162–164, 1988.

Dugas M, Masson M, Le Heuzey MF, et al: Aphasi 'acquise' de l'enfant avec épilepsie (syndrome de Landau et Kleffner): douze observations personelles. Revue Neurologique (Paris) 138:755–780, 1982.

Dulac O, Plouin P, Jambaque I: Predicting favorable outcome in idiopathic West syndrome. Epilepsia 34:747–756, 1993.

Dulac O, Chiron C, Luna D, et al: Vigabatrin in childhood epilepsy. J Child Neurol 6 (Suppl):2S30–2S37, 1991.

Dulac O, Plouin P, Jambaque I, et al: Spasmes infantiles epileptique benins. Rev EEG Neurophysiol Clin 16:371–382, 1986.

Dulac O, Billard C, Arthuis M: Aspects électro-cliniques et évolutifs de l'épilepsie dans le syndromes aphasie-épilepsi. Archives Francais Pediatrie 40:229–308, 1983.

Dunn DW, Austin JK, Harezlak J, et al: ADHD and epilepsy in childhood. Dev Med Child Neurol 45:50–4, 2003.

Dunn DW, Snyder CH: Benign paroxysmal vertigo of childhood. Am J Diseases Child 130:1099, 1976.

Duval J, Braun CM, Daigneault S, Montour-Proulx I: Does the child behavior checklist reveal psychopathological profiles of children with focal unilateral cortical lesions? Appl Neuropsychol 9:74– 83, 2002.

Echenne B, Cheminal R, Rivier F, et al: Epileptic electroencephalographic abnormalities and developmental dysphasias: a study of 32 patients. Brain Dev 14:216–225, 1992.

Epstein M, Markowitz R, Gallo D, et al: Munchausen syndrome by proxy: considerations in diagnosis and confirmation by video surveillance. Pediatrics 80:220–224, 1987.

Erba G, Browne TR: Atypical absence, myoclonic, atonic, and tonic seizures and the Lennox-Gastaut syndrome. In Epilepsy: Diagnosis and Management. Edited by Browne TR, Feldman RG. Boston, Little, Brown, 1983, pp. 75–94.

Farwell JR, Dodrill CB, Batzel LW: Neuropsychological abilities of children with epilepsy. Epilepsia 26:395–400, 1985.

Fastenau PS, Shen J, Dunn DW, et al: Neuropsychological predictors of academic underachievement in pediatric epilepsy: moderating roles of demographic, seizure, and psychosocial variables. Epilepsia 45:1261–1272, 2004.

Favatta I, Leuzzi V, Curatolo P: Mental outcome in West syndrome: Prognostic value of some clinical factors. J Mental Def Res 31:9–15, 1987.

Felbamate Study Group in the Lennox-Gastaut Syndrome: Efficacy of felbamate in childhood epileptic encephalopathy (Lennox-Gastaut syndrome). N Engl J Med 328:29–33, 1993.

Ferri R, Del Gracco S, Elia M, Musumeci SA: Age-related changes of cortical excitability in subjects with sleep-enhanced centrotemporal spikes: a somatosensory evoked potential study. Clin Neurophysiol 111:591–599, 2000.

Finalyson GW, Lucas A: Pseudoepileptic seizures in children and adolescents. Mayo Clinic Proc 54:83–87, 1979.

Fish DR, Smith SJ, Quesney LF, et al: Surgical treatment of children with medically intractable frontal or temporal lobe epilepsy: results and highlights of 40 years experience. Epilepsia 34:244–247, 1993.

Fogarasi A, Jokeit H, Faveret E, et al: The effect of age on seizure semiology in childhood temporal lobe epilepsy. Epilepsia 43:638–643, 2002.

Fois A, Malandrini F, Balestri P, et al: Infantile spasms—long term results of ACTH treatment. Eur J Pediatr 142:1–55, 1984.

French JA, Kanner AM, Bautista J, et al: Efficacy and tolerability of the new antiepileptic drugs II: treatment of refractory epilepsy: report of the Therapeutics and Technology Assessment Subcommittee and Quality Standards Subcommittee of the American Academy of Neurology and the American Epilepsy Society. Neurology 62: 1261–1273, 2004.

Frost JD Jr, Hrachovy RA: Infantile spasms. Boston: Kluwer Academic, 2003.

Frost M, Gates J, Helmers SL, et al: Vagus nerve stimulation in children with refractory seizures associated with Lennox-Gastaut syndrome. Epilepsia 42:1148–1152, 2001.

Funakoshi A, Morikawa T, Maramatsu R, et al: A prospective WISC-R study in children with epilepsy. Jap J Psychiat Neurol 42:562–564, 1988.

Galanopoulou AS, Bojko A, Lado F, Moshe, SL: The spectrum of neuropsychiatric abnormalities associated with electrical status epilepticus in sleep. Brain Dev 22:279–295, 2000.

Gascon G, Victor D, Lombroso C, et al: Language disorder, convulsive disorders, and electroencephalographic abnormalities. Arch Neurol 28:56–162, 1973.

Gascon G, Barlow C: Juvenile migraine, presenting as acute confusional state. Pediatrics 45:628–635, 1970.

Gashlan M, Loy-English I, Ventureyra EC, Keene D: Predictors of seizure outcome following cortical resection in pediatric and adolescent patients with medically refractory epilepsy. Childs Nerv Syst 15:45–50, 1999.

Gastaut H: Benign epilepsy of childhood with occipital parozysms. In Epileptic syndromes in Infancy, Childhood, and Adolescence. Edited by Roger J, Dravet C, Bureau M, Dreifuss FE, Wolf P. London: John Libbey Eurotext, 1985, pp. 159–170.

Gastaut H, Zifkin BG: Ictal visual hallucinations of numerals. Neurology 34:950–953, 1984.

Gastaut H: A new type of epilepsy: benign parital epilepsy of childhood with occipital spike-waves. Clinical Electroencephalography 12:13–22, 1982.

Gelisse P, Genton P, Bureau M, et al: Are there generalised spike waves and typical absences in benign rolandic epilepsy? Brain Dev 21:390–396, 1999.

Genton P, Guerrini R: What differentiates Landau-Kleffner syndrome from the syndrome of continuous spikes and waves during slow sleep. Arch Neurol 50:1008–1009 (letter), 1993.

Glaze DG, Hrachovy RA, Frost JD: Prospective study of outcome of infants with infantile spasms treated during controlled studies of ACTH and prednisone. J Pediatr 112:389–396, 1988.

Gogtay N, Giedd JN, Lusk L, et al: Dynamic mapping of human cortical development during childhood through early adulthood. Proc Natl Acad Sci USA 101:8174–8179, 2004.

Goldsmith IL, Zupac ML, Buchhalter JR: Long-term seizure outcome in 74 patients with Lennox-Gastaut syndrome: effects of incorporating MRI head imaging in defining the cryptogenic subgroup. Epilepsia 41:395–399, 2000.

Goodyer IM: Epileptic and pseudoepileptic seizures in childhood and adolescence. J Amer Acad Child Psychiatry 24:3–9, 1985.

Gordon N: Review: juvenile myoclonic epilepsy. Child Care Health Dev 20:71–76, 1994.

Gordon N: Acquired aphasia in childhood: the Landau-Kleffner syndrome. Dev Med Child Neurol 32:270–274, 1990.

Granata T, Gobbi G, Spreafico R, et al: Rasmussen's encephalitis: early characteristics allow diagnosis. Neurology 60:422–425, 2003a.

Granata T, Fusco L, Gobbi G, et al: Experience with immunomodulatory treatments in Rasmussen's encephalitis. Neurology 61:1807–1810, 2003b.

Green JR: Surgical treatment of epilepsy during childhood and adolescence. Surg Neurol 8:71–80, 1977.

Greenberg, DA, Durner M, Keddache M, et al: Reproducibility and complications in gene searches: linkage on chromosome 6, heterogeneity, association, and maternal inheritance in juvenile myoclonic epilepsy. Am J Hum Genet 66:508–516, 2000.

Gregory DL, Wong PK: Topographical analysis of the centro-temporal discharges in benign rolandic epilepsy of childhood. Epilepsia 25:705–711, 1984.

Gross M, Huerta E: Functional convulsions masked as epileptic disorder. J Pediat Psychol 511:71–79, 1980.

Gudmundsson O, Prendergast M, Foreman D, Cowley S: Outcome of pseudoseizures in children and adolescents: a 6-year symptom survival analysis. Dev Med Child Neurol 43:547–551, 2001.

Guerreiro MM, Camargo EE, Kato M, et al: Brain single photon emission computed tomography imaging in Landau-Kleffner syndrome. Epilepsia 37:60–67, 1996.

Gulgonen S, Demirbilek V, Korkmaz B, Dervent A, Townes BD: Neuropsychological functions in idiopathic occipital lobe epilepsy. Epilepsia 41:405–411, 2000.

Guzzetta F, Crisafulli A, Isaya Crino M: Cognitive assessment of infants with West syndrome: how useful is it for diagnosis and prognosis? Dev Med Child Neurol 35:379–387, 1993.

Harvey AS, Hopkins LJ, Bowe JM, et al: Frontal lobe epilepsy: Clinical seizure characteristics and localization with ictal ^{9m}Tc-HMPAO SPECT. Neurology 43: 1966–1980, 1993.

Hauser WA, Hesdorffer DC: Epilepsy, Frequency, Causes, and Consequences. New York: Demos Publications, 1990, pp. 2–51.

Heijbel J, Blom S, Rasmuson M: Benign epilepsy of childhood with centrotemporal EEG foci: A genetic study. Epilepsia 16:285–293, 1975.

Helmstaedter C: Neuropsychological aspects of epilepsy surgery. Epilepsy & Behavior 5:45–55, 2004.

Henriksen O, Johannessen SI: Clinical and pharmacokinetic observations on sodium valproate. A 5-year follow-up study in 100 children with epilepsy. Acta Neurol Scand 65:504–523, 1982.

Hermann BP: Neuropsychological functioning and psychopathology in children with epilepsy. Epilepsia 23:545–554, 1982.

Hermann BP, Whitman S, Hughes JR, et al: Multietiological determinants of psychopathology and social competence in children with epilepsy. Epil Res 2:51–60, 1998.

Hermann B, Seidenberg M: Neuropsychology and temporal lobe epilepsy. CNS Spectr 7:343–348, 2002.

Herman BP, Seidenberg M, Jones JE, Sheth R, Koehn M, Hansen R, et al: Neuropsychological Status of Children With New Onset Epilepsy. Annual meeting of International Neuroscience Society, 2005.

Hernandez MT, Sauerwein HC, Jambaque I, et al: Deficits in executive functions and motor coordination in children with frontal lobe epilepsy. Neuropsychologia 40:384–400, 2002.

Hernandez MT, Sauerwein HC, Jambaque I, et al: Attention, memory, and behavioral adjustment in children with frontal lobe epilepsy. Epilepsy Behav 4:522–536, 2003.

Hirsch E, Marescaux C, Maquet P, et al: Landau-Kleffner syndrome : A clinical and EEG study of five cases. Epilepsia 31:756–767, 1990.

Hoare P, Kerley S: Psychosocial adjustment of children with chronic epilepsy and their families. Dev Med Child Neurol 33:201–215, 1991.

Holmes GL, McKeever M, Adamson M: Absence seizures in children: clinical and electrographic features. Ann Neurol 21:268–273, 1987.

Holmes GL, McKeever M, Russman BS: Abnormal behavior or epilepsy? Use of longterm EEG and video monitoring with severely to profoundly mentally retarded patients with seizures. Am J Ment Retard 87:456–458, 1983.

Holmes GL, McKeever M, Saunders Z: Epileptiform activity in aphasia of childhood: An epiphenomenon. Epilepsia 22:631–639, 1981.

Honavar M, Janota I, Polkey CE: Rasmussen's encephalitis in surgery for epilepsy. Dev Med Child Neurol 34:3–14, 1992.

Hopkins IJ, Klug GL: Temporal lobectomy for the treatment of intractable complex partial seizures of temporal lobe origin in early childhood. Dev Med Child Neurol 33:26–31, 1991.

Hrachovy RA, Frost JD Jr: Infantile epileptic encephalopathy with hypsarrhythmia (infantile spasms/West syndrome). J Clin Neurophysiol 20:408–425, 2003.

Hrachovy RA, Glaze DG, Frost JD: A retrospective study of spontaneous remission and long-term outcome in patients with infantile spasms. Epilepsia 32:212–214, 1991.

Hrachovy RA, Frost JD Jr: Infantile spasms: a disorder of the developing nervous system. In: Kellaway P, Noebels JL, eds. Problems and concepts in developmental neurophysiology. Baltimore, MD: Johns Hopkins University Press, 1989:131–147.

Humphrey EL, Knopstein R, Bumpass ER: Gradually developing aphasia in children. J Am Acad Child Psychiatry 14:652–665, 1975.

Hurst DL, Rolan RD: The use of felbamate to treat infantile spasms. J Child Neurol 10:134–136, 1995.

Iannetti P, Raucci U, Bastile LA, et al: Benign epilepsy of childhood with centrotemporal spikes and unilateral developmental opercular dysplasia. Childs Nerv Sys 10:264–269, 1994.

Jambaque I, Chiron C, Dulac O, et al: Visual inattention in West syndrome: A neuropsychological and neurofunctional imaging study. Epilepsia 34:692–700, 1993.

Jeavons PM, Bower BD: Infantile Spasms: A Review of the Literature and a Study of 112 Cases. London: Heineman, 1964.

Jonas R, Nguyen S, Hu Bet, et al: Cerebral hemispherectomy: hospital course, seizure, developmental, language, and motor outcomes. Neurology 62:1712–1721, 2004.

Jung KY, Kim JM, Kim DW: Patterns of interictal spike propagation across the central sulcus in benign rolandic epilepsy. Clin Electroencephalogr 34:153–157, 2003.

Kadis DS, Stollstorff M, Elliott I, et al: cognitive and psychological predictors of everyday memory in children with intractable epilepsy. Epilepsy Behav 5:37–43, 2004.

Kajitani T, Takafumi K, Sumita M, et al: Relationship between epilepsy of children with centro-temporal EEG foci and febrile convulsions. Brain Dev 14:230–234, 1992.

Kaminer Y, Apter A, Lerman P, et al: Psychopathology and temporal epilepsy in adolescents. Acta Psychiat Scand 77:640–644, 1988.

Keller SS, Wieshmann UC, Mackay CE, et al: voxel based morphometry of grey matter abnormalities in patients with medically intractable temporal lobe epilepsy: effects of side of seizure onset and epilepsy duration. J Neurol Neurosurg Psychiatry 73:648–655, 2002.

Kim SJ, Park YD, Pillai JJ, et al: Longitudinal MRI study in children with Rasmussen syndrome. Pediatr Neurol 27:282–288, 2002.

Kinney RO, Shaywitz BA, Shaywitz SE, et al: Epilepsy in children with attention deficit disorder: cognitive, behavioral, and neuroanatomic indices. Pediatr Neurol 6:31–37, 1990.

Kivity S, Lerman P, Ariel R, et al: Long-term cognitive outcomes of a cohort of children with cryptogenic infantile spasms treated with high-dose adrenocorticotropic hormone. Epilepsia 45:255–262, 2004.

Koo B, Hwang PA, Logan WJ: Infantile spasms: outcome and prognostic factors of cryptogenic and symptomatic groups. Neurology 43: 2322–2327, 1993.

Kotagal P, Arunkumar G, Hammel J, et al: Complex partial seizures of frontal lobe onset statistical analysis of ictal semiology. Seizure 12: 268–281, 2003.

Kotagal P, Costa M, Wyllie E, et al: Paroxysmal nonepileptic events in children and adolescents. Pediatrics 110:e46, 2002.

Kotagal P, Rothner D, Erenberg G, et al: Complex partial seizures of childhood onset. A five-year follow-up study. Arch Neurol 44: 1177–1180, 1987.

Kral T, Kuczaty S, Blumcke I, et al: Postsurgical outcome of children and adolescents with medically refractory frontal lobe epilepsies. Childs Nerv Syst 17:595–601, 2001.

Kramer U, Lerman P: Benign childhood epilepsy with centro-temporal spikes. Harefuah 140:776–779, 805, 2001.

Kristensen O, Sindrup EH: Psychomotor epilepsy and psychosis I. Physical aspects. Acta Neurolog Scand 57:361–377, 1978.

Kuehn SM, Keene DL, Richards PM, et al: Are there changes in intelligence and memory functioning following surgery for the treatment of refractory epilepsy in childhood? Childs Nerv Syst 18:306–310, 2002.

Kurokawa T, Goya N, Fukuyama Y, et al: West syndrome and Lennox-Gastaut syndrome: a survey of natural history. Pediatrics 65:81–88, 1980.

Lacy JR, Penry JK: Infantile Spasms. New York: Raven Press, 1976.

Lada C, Skiadas K, Theodorou V, Loli N, Covanis A. A study of 43 patients with panayiotopoulos syndrome, a common and benign childhood seizure susceptibility. Epilepsia 44:81–8, 2003.

Lado FA, Moshe SL: Role of subcortical structures in the pathogenesis of infantile spasms: what are possible subcortical mediators? Int Rev Neurobiol 49:115–140, 2002.

Landau WM, Kleffner FR: Syndrome of acquired aphasia with convulsive disorder. Neurology 7:523–530, 1957.

Landolt H: Serial electroencephalographic investigations during psychotic episodes in epileptic patients and during schizophrenic attacks. In Lectures on Epilepsy. Edited by De Haas L. New York: Elsevier Science, 1958, pp. 91–133.

Laskowitz DT, Sperling MR, French JA, et al: The syndrome of frontal lobe epilepsy: Characteristics and surgical management. Neurology 45:780–787, 1995.

Lassonde M, Sauerwein HC, Jambaque I, et al: Neuropsychology of childhood epilepsy: pre-and postsurgical assessment. Epileptic Disord 2:3–13, 2000.

Lawson JA, Cook MJ, Vogrin S, et al: Clinical, EEG, and quantitative MRI differences in pediatric frontal and temporal lobe epilepsy. Neurology 58:723–729, 2002.

Legarda S, Jayakar P, Duchowny M, et al: Benign rolandic epilepsy: high central and low central subgroups. Epilepsia 25:1125–1129, 1994.

Lendt M, Gleissner U, Helmstaedter C, et al: Neuropsychological outcome in children after frontal lobe epilepsy surgery. Epilepsy Behav 3:51–59, 2002.

Lendt M, Helmstaedter C, Kuczaty S, et al: Behavioural disorders in children with epilepsy: early improvement after surgery. J Neurol Neurosurg Psychiatry 69:739–744, 2000.

Lendt M, Helmstaedter C, Elger CE. Pre-and postoperative neuropsychological profiles in children and adolescents with temporal lobe epilepsy. Epilepsia 40:1543–1550, 1999.

Lerman P, Kivity S: The benign parital nonrolandic epilepsies. J Clin Neurophysiol 8:272–287, 1991.

Lerman P, Kivity S: Benign focal epilepsy of childhood. Archives of Neurology 32:261–264, 1975.

Lerman P, Lerman-Sagie T, Kivity S: Effect of early cortico-steroid therapy for Landau-Kleffner syndrome. Dev Med Child Neurol 33:257–266, 1991.

Lespinet V, Bresson C, N'Kaoua B, et al: Effect of age of onset of temporal lobe epilepsy on the severity and the nature of preoperative memory deficits. Neuropsychologia 40:1591–600, 2002.

Levav M, Mirsky AF, Herault J, et al: Familial association of neuropsychological traits in patients with generalized and partial seizure disorders. J Clin Exp Neuropsychol 24:311–326, 2002.

Lin YY, Chang KP, Hsieh JC, et al: Magnetoencephalographic analysis of bilaterally synchronous discharges in benign rolandic epilepsy of childhood. Seizure 12:448–455, 2003.

Lindsay JJ, Glaser G, Richards P, et al: Developmental aspects of focal epilepsies of childhood treated by neurosurgery. Dev Med Child Neurol 26:574–587, 1984.

Lindsay JJ, Ounsted C, Richards P: Long-term outcome in children with temporal lobe seizures. III. Psychiatric aspects in childhood and adult life. Dev Med Child Neurol 21:630–636, 1979a.

Lindsay JJ, Ounsted C, Richards P: Long-term outcome in children with temporal lobe seizures I: Social outcome and childhood factors. Dev Med Child Neurol 21:285–298, 1979b.

Lockman LA: Absence, myoclonic, and atonic seizures. Pediatr Clin North Am 36:331–341, 1989.

Loiseau P, Duche B, Cordova S, et al: Prognosis of benign childhood epilepsy with centro-temporal spikes: A follow-up study of 168 patients. Epilepsia 29:229–235, 1988.

Lombroso CT, Lerman P: Breatholding spells (cyanotic and pallid infantile syncope). Pediatrics 39:563, 1967.

Lüders H, Lesser RP, Dinner D, et al: Benign rolandic epilepsy of childhood. In Epilepsy electroclinical syndromes. Edited by Lüders H. Berlin, Springer-Verlag, 1989, pp. 303–346.

Lum LM, Connolly MB, Farrell K, Wong PK: Hyperventilation-induced high-amplitude rhythmic slowing with altered awareness: a video-EEG comparison with absence seizures. Epilepsia 43:1372–1378, 2002.

Lundberg S, Eeg-Olofsson O, Raininko R, et al: Hippocampal asymmetries and white matter abnormalities on MRI in benign childhood epilepsy with centrotemporal spikes. Epilepsia 40: 1808–1815, 1999.

Mabbott DM, Smith ML: Material-specific memory in children with temporal and extratemporal lobectomies. Neuropsychologia 41: 995–1007, 2003.

Mackay MT, Weiss SK, Adams-Webber T, et al: Practice parameter: medical treatment of infantile spasms: report of the American Academy of Neurology and the Child Neurology Society. Neurology 62:1668–1681, 2004.

Maezawa M, Seki T, Yamawaki H, et al: Long-term prognosis of absence seizures. A follow-up study of more than five years. Brain Dev (Tokyo) 7:179,1985.

Mahowald MW, Rosen GM: Parasomnias in children. Pediatrician 17: 21–31, 1990.

Majoie HJ, Berfelo MW, Aldenkamp AP, et al: Vagus nerve stimulation in children with therapy-resistant epilepsy diagnosed as Lennox-Gastaut syndrome: clinical results, neuropsychological effects, and cost-effectiveness. J Clin Neurophysiol 18:419–428, 2001.

Makar AF, Squier PJ: Munchausen syndrome by proxy: father as a perpetrator. Pediatrics 85:370–373, 1990.

Mandelbaum D, Burack G: The effect of seizure type and medication on cognitive and behavioral functioning in children with idiopathic epilepsy. Dev Med Child Neurol 39:731–735, 1997.

Marescaux C, Hirsch E, Finck S, et al: Landau-Kleffner syndrome: a pharmacological study for five cases. Epilepsia 31:768–777, 1990.

Markand ON: Lennox-Gastaut syndrome (childhood epileptic encephalopathy). J Clin Neurophysiol 20:426–441, 2003.

Martinovic Z: Clinical correlations of electroencephalographic occipital epileptiform paroxysms in children. Seizure 10(5):379–381, 2001.

Matsumoto A, Watanabe K, Negoro T, et al: Longterm prognosis after infantile spasms: a statistical study of prognostic factors in 200 cases. Dev Med Child Neurol 23:51–65, 1981.

McGuire TL, Feldman KW: Psychological morbidity of children subjected to Munchausen syndrome by proxy. Pediatrics 83:289–292, 1989.

McLachlan RS, Girvin JP, Blume WT, et al: Rasmussen's chronic encephalitis in adults. Arch Neurol 50:269–274, 1993.

Meadow R: Neurological and developmental variants of Munchausen syndrome by proxy. Dev Med Child Neurol 33:267–272, 1991.

Meadow R: Munchausen syndrome by proxy. Brit Med J 299:248–250, 1989.

Meadow R: Fictitious epilepsy. Lancet 2:25–28, 1984.

Mimaki T, Ono J, Yabauchi H: Temporal lobe astrocytoma with infantile spasms. Ann Neurol 14:695–695, 1983.

Miranda C, Smith ML: Predictors of intelligence after temporal lobectomy in children with epilepsy. Epilepsy Behav 2:13–19, 2001.

Mitchell WG, Zhou Y, Chavez JM, et al: Effects of antiepileptic drugs on reaction time, attention, and impulsivity in children. Pediatrics 91:101–105, 1993.

Mitchell WG, Chavez JM, Lee H, et al: Academic underachievement in children with epilepsy. J Child Neurol 6:65–72, 1991.

Mohamed A, Wyllie E, Ruggieri P, et al: Temporal lobe epilepsy due to hippocampal sclerosis in pediatric candidates for epilepsy surgery. Neurology 56:1643–1649, 2001.

Mohr P, Bond MH: A chronic epidemic of hysterical blackouts in a comprehensive school. Brit Med J 284:961–996, 1982.

Morikawa T, Seino M, Osawa T, et al: Five children with continuous spike-waves during sleep. In Epileptic Syndromes in Infancy, Childhood, and Adolescence. Edited by Roger J, Dravet C, Bureau M, Dreifuss FE, Wolf P. London: John Libbey Eurotext, 1985, pp. 205–212.

Morris H, Dinner D, Lüders H, Wyllie E, Kramer R: Supplementary motor seizures: clinical and elcetrogphic findings. Neurology 38: 1075–1088, 1988.

Motamedi G, Meador K: Epilepsy and cognition. Epilepsy Behav 4:25–38, 2003.

Murphy CC, Trevathan E, Yeargin-Allsopp MY: Prevalence of epilepsy and epileptic seizures in 10-year-old children: results from the Metropolitan Atlanta Developmental Disabilities Study. Epilepsia 36:866–872, 1995.

Nakano S, Okuno T, Mikawa H: Landau-Kleffner syndrome. EEG topographic studies. Brain Dev (Tokyo) 11:43–50, 1989.

Nasr JT, Gabis L, Savatic M, Andriola MR: The electroencephalogram in children with developmental dysphasia. Epilepsy Behav 2:115–118, 2001.

Nass R, Heier L, Walker R: Landau-Kleffner syndrome: temporal lobe tumor resection results in good outcome. Pediatr Neurol 9:303–305, 1993.

Neil JC, Alvarez N: Differential diagnosis of epileptic versus pseudoepileptic seizures in disabled persons. Appl Res Ment Retard 7: 285–298, 1986.

Nevšímalová S, Tauberová A, Doutlík S, et al: A role of autoimmunity in the etiopathogenesis of Landau-Kleffner syndrome? Brain Dev 14:342–345, 1992.

Nolan MA, Redoblado MA, Lah S, et al: Intelligence in childhood epilepsy syndromes. Epilepsy Res 53:139–150, 2003.

Nolan M, Redoblado M, Lah S, Sabaz M, et al: Memory function in childhood epilepsy syndromes. J Paediatr Child Health 40:20–27, 2004.

Obeid T: Clinical and genetic aspects of juvenile absence epilepsy. J Neurol 241 487–491, 1994.

Oguni H, Andermann F, Rasmussen T: The natural history of the syndrome of chronic encephalitis and epilepsy: A study of the MNI series of forty-eight cases. In Chronic Encephalitis and Epilepsy: Rasmussen's Syndrome. Edited by Andermann F. Stoneham, MA: Butterworth, 1991, pp. 7–35.

Oguni H, Hayashi K, Funatsuka M, Osawa M: Study on early-onset benign occipital seizure susceptibility syndrome. Pediatr Neurol 25: 312–318, 2001.

Ohtahara S, Ohtsuka Y, Yamatogi Y, et al: Prenatal etiologies of West syndrome. Epilepsia 34:716–722, 1993.

Ohtahara S, Ohtsuka Y, Yoshinaga H, et al: Lennox-Gastaut Syndrome: etiological considerations. In The Lennox-Gastaut Syndrome. Edited by Niedermeyer E, Degen R. New York: AR Liss, 1988, pp. 47–63.

Ohtsu M, Oguni H, Hayashi K, Funatsuka M, Imai K, Osawa M. Epilepsia: EEG in children with early-onset benign occipital seizure susceptibility syndrome: Panayiotopoulos syndrome. Epilepsia 44: 435–442, 2003.

Ohtsuka Y, Amano R, Mizukawa M, et al: Long-term prognosis of the Lennox-Gastaut Syndrome. Jap J Psychiat Neurol 44:257–264, 1990.

Olbrich A, Urak L, Groppel G, et al: Semiology of temporal lobe epilepsy in children and adolescents. Value in lateralizing the seizure onset zone. Epilepsy Res 48:103–110, 2002.

Olson AL, Seidler AB, Goodman D: School professionals' perceptions about the impact of chronic illness in the classroom. Arch Pediatr Adolesc Med 158:53–58, 2004.

Oostrom KJ, Smeets-Schouten A, Kruitwagen CL, et al: Not only a matter of epilepsy: early problems of cognition and behavior in children with "epilepsy only"—a prospective, longitudinal, controlled study starting at diagnosis. Pediatrics 112:1338–1344, 2003.

Oostrom KJ, Schouten A, Kruitwagen CL, et al: Attention deficits are not characteristic of schoolchildren wit newly diagnosed idiopathic or cryptogenic epilepsy. Epilepsia 43:301–310, 2002.

Oppenheimer EY, Rosman NP: Seizures and seizure-Like states in the child: An approach to emergency management. Emergency Med Clin North Am 1:125–140, 1983.

Ortinski P, Meador KJ: Cognitive side effects of antiepileptic drugs. Epilepsy & Behavior 5:60–65, 2004.

Ott D, Caplan R, Guthrie D, et al: Measures of psychopathology in children with complex partial seizures and primary generalized epilepsy with absence. J Amer Acad Child Adolesc Psychiatry 40:907–914, 2001.

Pakalnis A, Paolicchi J: Frequency of secondary conversion symptoms in children with psychogenic nonepileptic seizures. Epilepsy Behav 4:753–756, 2003a.

Pakalnis A, Paolicchi J: Psychogenic seizures after head injury in children. J Child Neurol 15:78–80, 2003b.

Pakalnis A, Drake ME, Kuruvilla J, et al: Forced normalization: Acute psychosis after seizure control in seven patients. Arch Neurol 44: 289–292, 1987.

Panayiotopoulos CP: Treatment of typical absence seizures and related epileptic syndromes. Paediatr Drugs 3:379–340, 2001.

Panayiotopoulos CP: Benign nocturnal childhood occipital epilepsy: A new syndrome with nocturnal seizures, tonic deviation of the eyes and vomiting. J Child Neurol 4:43–48, 1989.

Papavasiliou A, Vassilaki N, Paraskevoulakos E, et al: Psychogenic status epilepticus in children. Epilepsy Behav 5:539–546, 2004.

Paquier PF, van Dongen HR, Loonen CB: The Landau-Kleffner syndrome or "acquired aphasia with convulsive disorder." Long-term follow-up of six children and a review of the recent literature. Arch Neurol 49:354–359, 1992.

Pardo CA, Vining EP, Guo L, et al: The pathology of Rasmussen syndrome: stages of cortical involvement and neuropathological studies in 45 hemispherectomies. Epilepsia 45:516–526, 2004.

Park SH, Vinters HV: Ultrastructural study of Rasmussen encephalitis. Ultrastruct Pathol 26:287–292, 2003.

Pascual-Castroviejo I: Nocardipine in the treatment of acquired aphasia and epilepsy. Dev Med Child Neurol 32:930, 1990.

Pateau M, Granstrom G, Blomstedt V, et al: Magnetoencephalography in presurgical evaluation of children with the Landau-Kleffner syndrome. Epilepsia 40:326–335, 1999.

Pavone P, Bianchini R, Trifiletti RR, Incorpora G, Pavone A, Parano E: Neuropsychological assessment in children with absence epilepsy. Neurology 56:1047–1051, 2001.

Penfield W, Jasper H: Epilepsy and the Functional Anatomy of the Human Brain, 1st ed. Boston, Little and Brown, 1954.

Perez ER, Davidoff V, Desplan PA, et al: Mental and behavioral deterioration of children with epilepsy and CSWS: Acquired epileptic frontal syndrome. Dev Med Child Neurol 35:661–674, 1993.

Perniola I, Margari L, Buttiglione M, et al: A case of Landau-Kleffner syndrome secondary to inflammatory demyelinating disease. Epilepsia 39:551–556, 1993.

Porter BE, Judkins AR, Clancy RR, et al: Dysplasia: a common finding in intractable pediatric temporal lobe epilepsy. Neurology 61:365–368, 2003.

Quesney LF, Constain M, Rasmussen T: Seizures from dorsolateral frontal lobe. Adv Neurol 57:233–243, 1992.

Quesney LF, Constain M, Fish DR, et al: Frontal lobe epilepsy—a field of recent emphasis. Am J EEG Technology 30:177–193, 1990.

Rapin I, Mattis S, Rowan AJ, et al: Verbal auditory agnosia in children. Dev Med Child Neurol 19:192–207, 1977.

Rasmussen T, Andermann F: Update on the syndrome of "chronic encephalitis" and epilepsy. Cleve Clin J Med 56 (Suppl Part 2):S181–S184, 1989.

Rating D, Wolf C, Bast T: Sulthiame as monotherapy in children with benign childhood epilepsy with centrotemporal spikes: a 6-month, double-blind, placebo-controlled study: Sulthiame Study Group. Epilepsia 41:1284–1288, 2000.

Ravnik I: A case of Landau-Kleffner syndrome: Effect of intravenous diazepam. In Epileptic Syndromes in Infancy, Childhood, and

Adolescence. Edited by Roger J, Dravet C, Bureau M, Dreifuss FE, Wolf P. London: John Libbey Eurotext, 1985, pp. 192–193.

Renganathan R, Delanty N: Juvenile myoclonic epilepsy: under-appreciated and under-diagnosed. Postgrad Med J 79:78–80, 2003.

Rice ML: Children with specific language impairment: Toward a model of teachability. In A Krasnegor, DM Rumbaugh, RL Schiefelbusch & M Studdert-Kennedy (Eds.). Biological and behavioral determinants of language development. Hillsdale, NJ: Lawrence Erlbaum Associates, 1991, pp. 447–480.

Riggio S, Harner RN: Frontal Lobe Epilepsy. Neuropsychiatry, Neuropsychol Behavioral Neurol 5:283–293, 1992.

Riikonen R: A long-term follow-up study of 214 children with the syndrome of infantile spasms. Neuropediatrics 13:14–23, 1982.

Riikonen R, Amnell G: Psychiatric disorders in children with earlier infantile spasms. Dev Med Child Neurol 23:747–760, 1981.

Rintahaka PJ, Chugani HT, Sankar R: Landau-Kleffner syndrome with continuous spikes and waves during slow-wave sleep. J Child Neurol 10:127–133, 1995.

Riva D, Saletti V, Nichelli F, et al: Neuropsychologic effects of frontal lobe epilepsy in children. J Child Neurol 17:661–667, 2002.

Rodin EA, Schmaltz S, Twitty G: Intellectual functions of patients with childhood-onset epilepsy. Dev Med Child Neurol 26:25–33, 1986.

Rosenberg D: Web of deceit: a literature review of Munchausen by proxy. Child Abuse Negl 11:547–563, 1987.

Roulet E, Deonna T, Gaillard F, et al: Acquired aphasia, dementia, and behavior disorder with epilepsy and continuous spike and waves during sleep in a child. Epilepsia 32:495–503, 1991.

Rutter M, Graham P, Yule W: A neuropsychiatric study in childhood. London: S.I.M.P./William Heinemann Medical Books, 1970.

Saint-Martin AD, Seegmuller C, Carcangiu R, et al: Cognitive consequences of Rolandic Epilepsy Epileptic Disord 3 Spec No 2:SI59–65, 2003.

Salanova V, Morris HH, Van Ness P, et al: Frontal lobe seizures: Electroclinical syndromes. Epilepsia 36:16–24, 1995.

Salanova V, Andermann F, Olivier A, et al: Occipital lobe epilepsy: Electrocortical manifestations, electrocorticography, cortical stimulation and outcome in 42 patients treated between 1930 and 1991. Brain 115:1655–1680, 1992.

Saltzman J, Smith ML, Scott K: The impact of age at seizure onset n the likelihood of atypical language representation in children with intractable epilepsy. Brain Cogn 48:517–520, 2002.

Sander T, Bockenkamp B, Hildmann T, et al: Refined mapping of the epilepsy susceptibility locus EJM1 on chromosome 6. Neurology 49:842–847, 1997.

Sankar R, Chugani H, Lubens P, et al: Heterogeneity in the patterns of cerebral glucose utulization in children with Landau-Kleffner syndrome. Neurology 40:257, 1990.

Sassower K, Duchowny M: Psychogenic seizures and nonepileptic phenomena in childhood. Epilepsy and Behavior. New York: Wiley-Liss, 1992, pp. 223–235.

Sawhney IM, Robertson IJ, Polkey CE, et al: Multiple subpial transection: a review of 21 cases. J Neurol Neurosurg Psychiatry 58:344–349, 1995.

Sawhney IM, Suresh N, Dhand UK, et al: Acquired aphasia with epilepsy: Landau-Kleffner syndrome. Epilepsia 29:283–287, 1988.

Saygi S, Katz A, Marks DA, et al: Frontal lobe partial seizures and psychogenic seizures: Comparison of clinical and ictal characteristics. Neurology 42:1274–1277, 1992.

Schlumberger E, Dulac O: A simple, effective and well-tolerated treatment regime for West syndrome. Dev Med Child Neurol 36:863–872, 1994.

Schneider S, Rice DR: Neurologic manifestations of childhood hysteria. The J Pediatrics 94:153–156, 1979.

Schoenfeld J, Seidenberg M, Woodard A, et al: Neuropsychological and behavioral status of children with complex partial seizures. Dev Med Child Neurol 41:724–731, 1999.

Scott RC, Gadian DG, Cross JH, et al: Quantitative magnetic resonance characterization of mesial temporal sclerosis in childhood. Neurology 56:1659–1665, 2001.

Seidel WT, Mitchell WG: Cognitive and behavioral effects of carbamazepine in children: data from benign rolandic epilepsy. J Child Neurol 4:716–723, 1999.

Seidenberg M: Childhood epilepsies: neuropsychological, psychosocial, and intervention aspects. "Academic achievement and school performance of children with epilepsy." In Herman BP, Seidenberg M, eds. New York: John Wiley & Sons, 1989.

Semrud-Clikeman M, Wical B: Components of attention in children with complex partial seizures with and without ADHD. Epilepsia 40:211–215, 1999.

Septien L, Pelletier JL, Brunotte F, et al: Migraine in patients with a history of centro- temporal epilepsy in childhood: a Hm-PAO SPECT study. Cephalalgia 11:281–284, 1991.

Sherman E, Slick DJ, Connolly MB, Steinbok P, Martin R, Strauss E, Chelune GJ, Farrell K: Reexamining the effects of epilepsy surgery on IQ in children: use of regression-based change scores. J Int Neuropsychol Soc 9:879–886, 2003.

Shigematsu H, Nakmura H, Yagi K, et al: Neuroimaging study of frontal lobe epilepsies. Jpn J Psychiatry Neurol 46:462–466, 1992.

Shukla G, Bhatia M, Vivekanandhan S, et al: Serum prolactin levels for differentiation of nonepileptic versus true seizures: limited utility. Epilepsy Behav 5:517–521, 2004.

Silver LB: Conversion disorder with pseudoseizures in adolescence: A stress reaction to unrecognized and untreated learning disabilities. J Am Acad Child Psychiatry 21:508–512, 1982.

Sinclair DB, Wheatley M, Snyder T: Frontal lobe epilepsy in childhood. Pediatr Neurol 30:169–176, 2004.

Sinclair DB, Aronyk KE, Snyder TJ, et al: Pediatric epilepsy surgery at the University of Alberta: 1988–2000. Pediatr Neurol 29:302–311, 2003.

Singhi PD, Bansal U, Singhi S, et al: Determinants of IQ profile in children with idiopathic generalized epilepsy. Epilepsia 33:1106–1114, 1992.

Siren A, Eriksson K, Jalava H, Kilpinen-Loisa P, Koivikko M: Idiopathic generalised epilepsies with 3 Hz and faster spike wave discharges: a population-based study with evaluation and long-term follow-up in 71 patients. Epileptic Disord 4:209–216, 2002.

Slater E, Beard AW: The schizophrenia-like psychoses of epilepsy. Brit J Psychiatry 109:95–150, 1963.

Smith ML, Elliott IM, Lach L: Cognitive, psychosocial, and family function one year after pediatric epilepsy surgery. Epilepsia 45:650–660, 2004.

Smith ML, Elliott IM, Lach L: Cognitive skills in children with intractable epilepsy: comparison of surgical and nonsurgical candidates. Epilepsia 43:631–637, 2002.

Sowell ER, Peterson BS, Thompson PM, et al: Mapping cortical change across the human life span. Nat Neurosci 6:309–315, 2003.

Stoeffels C, Munari C, Bonis A, et al: Manifestations génitales et "sexualles" lors des crises épileptiques partielles chex l'homme. Revue EEG Neurophysiologique 10:386–392, 1980.

Stores G, Zaiwalla Z, Bergel N: Frontal lobe complex partial seizures in children: A form of epilepsy at particular risk of misdiagnosis. Dev Med Child Neurol 33:998–1009, 1991.

Stores G: School-children with epilepsy at risk for learning and behavioral problems. Dev Med Child Neurol 20:502–508, 1978a.

Stores G, Hart J, Piran N: Inattentiveness in schoolchildren with epilepsy. Epilepsia 19:169–175, 1978b.

Stores, G: Studies of attention and seizure disorders Dev Med Child Neurol 15:376–382, 1973.

Sturniolo MG, Galletti F: Idiopathic epilepsy and school achievement. Arch Dis Child 70:424–428, 1994.

Szabo CA, Wyllie E, Stanford LD, et al: Neuropsychological effect of temporal lobe resection in preadolescent children with epilepsy. Epilepsia 39: 814–819, 1998.

Takeoka M, Riviello JJ Jr, Duffy FH, et al: Bilateral volume reduction of the superior temporal areas in Landau-Kleffnersyndrome. Neurology 263:1289–1292, 2004.

Tassinari CA, Bureau M, Dravet C, et al: Electrical status epilepticus during sleep in children (ESES). In Sleep and Epilepsy. Edited by Sterman MB, Shouse MN, Passouant P. New York: Academic Press, 1982, pp. 465–479.

Taylor DC: Aggression and epilepsy. J Psychosom Res 13:229–236, 1975.

Tsai ML, Lo HY, Chaou WT: Clinical and electroencephalographic findings in early and late onset benign childhood epilepsy with occipital paroxysms. Brain Dev 23:401–405, 2001.

Tuchman RF, Rapin I: Regression in pervasive developmental disorders: seizures and epileptiform electroencephalogram correlates. Pediatrics 99:560–566, 1997.

Tuchman RF, Rapin I, Shinnar S. Autistic and dysphasic children. II. Epilepsy. Pediatrics 88:1219–1225, 1991. Pediatrics 88: 1219–1225, 1991 van der Meij W, van Huffelen AC, Willemse J, et al: Rolandic spikes in the interictal EEG of children: Contribution to diagnosis, classification and prognosis of epilepsy. Dev Med Child Neurol 34:893–903, 1992.

Van Ness PC: Frontal and parietal lobe epilepsy. In The Treatment of Epilepsy: Principles and Practice. Edited by Wyllie E. Philadelphia, Lea and Febiger, 1993, pp. 525–532.

Vargha-Khadem F, Isaacs EB, Papaleloudi H, et al: Development of language in six hemispherectomized patients. Brain 11:473–495, 1991.

Vigevano F, Fusco L, Cusmai R, et al: The idiopathic form of West syndrome. Epilepsia 34:743–746, 1993.

Vining EPG, Freeman JM, Brandt J, et al: Progressive unilateral encephalopathy of childhood (Rasmussen's syndrome): A reappraisal. Epilepsia 34:639–650, 1993.

Voeller KKS: Epilepsy. In Pediatric Neuropsychology in the Medical Setting. Edited by Baron IS, Fennell EB, Voeller KKS. New York: Oxford University Press, 1995, pp. 241–291.

Wakai S, Ito N, Ueda D, et al: Landau-Kleffner syndrome and sulthiame. Neuropediatrics 28:135–136 1997.

Watkins RV: Specific language impairments in children: an introduction. In R V Watkins and ML Rice (Eds.), Specific language impairments in children (pp. 1–15) Baltimore, MD US: Paul H. Brookes, 1994.

Watson R, Jiang Y, Bermudez I, et al: Absence of antibodies to glutamate receptor type 3 (GluR3) in Rasmussen encephalitis. Neurology 63:43–50, 2004.

Wheless JW, Simos PG, Butler IJ: Language dysfunction in epileptic conditions. Semin Pediatr Neurol 9:218–228, 2002.

White J, Sreenivasan V: Epilepsy-aphasia syndrome in children: an unusual presentation to psychiatry. Can J Psychiatry 32:599–601, 1987.

Whitman S, Hermann BP, Black RB, et al: Psychopathology and seizure type in children with epilepsy. Psychol Med 12:843–853, 1982.

Wieser HG, Swartz BE, Delgado-Escueta AV, et al: Differentiating frontal lobe seizures from temporal lobe seizures. In Advances in Neurology, Vol. 57: Frontal Lobe Epilepsy. Edited by Chauvel P, Delgado-Escueta AV. New York: Raven Press, 1992, pp. 267–285.

Wieser HG: Electroclinical Features of the Psychomotor Seizure. Stuttgart. New York: G. Fischer, 1983.

Willert C, Spitzer C, Kusserow S, et al: Serum neuron-specific enolase, prolactin, and creatine kinase after epileptic and psychogenic nonepileptic seizures. Acta Neurol Scand 109:318–323, 2004.

Williams J, Phillips T, Griebel ML, et al: Factors associated with academic achievement in children with controlled epilepsy. Epilepsy Behav 2:217–223, 2001a.

Williams J, Phillips T, Griebel ML, et al: Patterns of memory performance in children with controlled epilepsy on the CVLT-C. Neuropsychol Dev Cogn Sect C Child Neuropsychol 1:15–20, 2001.

Williams J, Griebel ML, Sharp GB, et al: Cognition and behavior after temporal lobectomy in pediatric patients with intractable epilepsy. Pediatr Neurol 19:89–94, 1998.

Williams J, Sharp G, Bates S, et al: Academic achievement and behavioral ratings in children with absence and complex partial epilepsy. Edu Treat Child 19:143–152, 1996a.

Williams J, Sharp G, Lange B, et al: The effects of seizure type, level of seizure control, and antiepileptic drugs on memory and attention skills in children with epilepsy. Developmental Neuropsychology 12:241–253, 1996b.

Williamson PD: Frontal lobe epilepsy: some clinical characteristics. Adv Neurol 66:127–150, 1995.

Williamson PD: Frontal lobe seizures: Problems of diagnosis and classification. Adv Neurol 57:289–309, 1992.

Williamson PD, Spencer DD, Spencer SS, et al: Complex partial seizures of frontal origin. Ann Neurol 18:497–504, 1985.

Wirrell EC: Natural history of absence epilepsy in children. Can J Neurol Sci 30:184–188, 2003.

Wirrell EC, Camfield CS, Camfield PR, et al: Long-term psychosocial outcome in typical absence epilepsy. Sometimes a wolf in sheeps' clothing. Arch Pediatr Adolesc Med 151:152–158, 1997.

Wirrell EC, Camfield CS, Camfield PR, Gordon KE, Dooley JM: Long-term prognosis of typical childhood absence epilepsy: remission or progression to juvenile myoclonic epilepsy. Neurology 47:912–918, 1996.

Wyllie E, Glazer JP, Benbadis S, et al: Psychiatric features of children and adolescents with pseudoseizures. Arch Pediatr Adolesc Med 153:244–248, 1999.

Wyllie E, Chee M, Granström ML, et al: Temporal lobe epilepsy in early childhood. Epilepsia 34:859–868, 1993.

Wyllie E, Friedman D, Rothner AD, et al: Psychogenic seizures in children and adolescents: Outcome after diagnosis by ictal video and electroencephalographic recording. Pediatrics 85:480–484, 1990.

Yamatogi Y, Ohtahara S: Age-dependent epileptic encephalopathy: a longitudinal study. Folia Psychiatr Neurol Jpn 35:321–332, 1981.

Ziegler RG: Risk factors in childhood epilepsy. Psychother Psychosom 44:185–190, 1985.

Zifkin B, Andermann E, Andermann F: Mechanisms, genetics, and pathogenesis of juvenile myoclonic epilepsy. Surr Opin Neurol 2005:147–153.

Zivi A, Broussaud G, Daymas S, et al: Syndrome aphasie acquise-épilepsie avec psychose: Á propos d'une observation. Annals Pediatrie (Paris) 37:391–394, 1990.

Prematurity and Cerebral Palsy

23

Agnes H. Whitaker, MD   *Judith F. Feldman, PhD*   *John M. Lorenz, MD*
Naomi Breslau, PhD   *Nigel Paneth, MD*

Prematurity and cerebral palsy are related but distinct topics in pediatric neuropsychiatry. While prematurity is a risk factor for cerebral palsy, at least half of all persons with cerebral palsy are born at term (Nelson & Grether, 1999). Therefore, a separate section is devoted to each condition. Side by side, the two topics offer a clinically relevant framework for reviewing the relation between abnormalities in early brain development and neurobehavioral outcomes.

PREMATURITY

Prematurity, that is birth at less than 37 weeks of gestation, is an essential topic in pediatric neuropsychiatry for several reasons. First, preterm birth is a common event, affecting about 1 in every 10 families in the United States (Mattison Damus, Fiore, Petrini, & Alter, 2001). Second, preterm birth provides a window into the genetics and epigenetics of human brain development, injury, plasticity, and recovery (Luciana, 2003). Third, preterm birth is the second leading cause of neonatal death, the first leading cause of morbidity in infancy and early childhood, and a risk factor for morbidity at least into young adulthood (Msall & Tremont, 2002b).

Definitions

Gestational age (GA) has traditionally been defined as the number of gestational weeks (GW) since the first day of the last menstrual period as recalled by the mother. Fetal size, as assessed with early ultrasound, is also now used to esti-

mate GA. Premature refers to birth at <37 GW, and very premature to birth at <32 weeks (Green et al. 2005). The lower limit of viability is now considered to be 22 to 23 GW. Because GA is a major determinant of birthweight (BW) and because the latter is more accurately and easily measured, researchers often use BW rather than GA to define high risk samples.

GA and BW, although related characteristics of an infant, are not synonymous. GA is essentially an index of organ maturity, while BW is an index of overall growth. A baby is born at low birth weight (LBW; < 2,500 g) either because it was delivered preterm or because it grew slowly in utero or some combination of the two. Infants with BW in the lowest 10th percentile of birthweight for GA or BW or two standard deviations or more below the mean for GA are termed small for gestational age (SGA). One disadvantage of using a LBW sample for studying predictors and sequelae of preterm birth is that nearly half of heavier LBW infants (1,500 to 2,500 grams) are full-term but SGA. By contrast, at least 96.8% of infants born at 1,500 g, or below, were born preterm. Therefore studies of prematurity usually use samples that are very low birthweight (VLBW) (<1,500 grams; 3lbs 5oz) or extremely low birthweight (ELBW) (< 1,000 grams or 2lbs 3 oz) or even smaller. In the literature, VLBW and ELBW are often used interchangeably with "preterm."

The age of a preterm neonate is often expressed as postmenstrual age in weeks, GA + postnatal age. When comparing preterms in the first year of life to normative data or to full-term infants, clinicians and researchers commonly use corrected age rather than chronological age. Corrected age is defined as postnatal age minus the number of weeks by which delivery was premature. Beyond age one, the value of correcting for prematurity is a matter of some debate (den Ouden, Rijken, Brand, Verloove-Vanhorick, & Ruys, 1991).

Trends in Incidence, Prevalence, Mortality, and Morbidity

Between 1980 and 2000, the prevalence of preterm births in this country rose 17% (from 10.0 to 11.8%), while infant mortality declined 45% (from 12.6 to 6.9%), most markedly among the extremely preterm (Mathews, Menacker, & MacDorman, 2002). At the same time, the rates of major disabilities such as cerebral palsy, mental retardation, blindness, and deafness among children born preterm remained steady at around 10%. As a result, the actual numbers of children with major disabilities related to prematurity has increased (Hack & Fanaroff, 2000).

The major disabilities associated with preterm birth are usually detected by age 2 years. The risk of major disability increases markedly with decreasing BW/GA (see Table 23.1). Many less severe but still impairing outcomes, including learning, attention, and behavior problems, are not apparent until school age or beyond, and also show a BW/GA gradient (Msall & Tremont, 2002b). These high prevalence/low severity problems are all too common (Allen, 2002).

Preterm Delivery

About 25% of preterm deliveries (PTD) are therapeutic, that is due to medical intervention for maternal or fetal problems. The the remaining 75% are due to premature rupture of membranes (25%) or spontaneous preterm delivery (Moutquin, 2003).

TABLE 23.1

SEVERE DISABILITY IN LOW BIRTH WEIGHT SHOWS A BIRTH WEIGHT GRADIENT

BW Category	Adjusted Odds Ratio	95% Confidence Interval
450–749	97.50	(70.37, 135.11)
750–999	40.01	(31.59, 50.68)
1,000–1,499	15.84	(13.66, 18.36)
1,500–2,499	3.29	(3.04, 3.56)
2,500–2,999	1.39	(1.30, 1.48)
3,000–4,749	1.00	(Reference Category)
4,750–6,000	1.52	(1.11, 2.08)

Source: Florida 1998 Birth Cohort. (Adapted with permission from Thompson, J. R., Carter, R. L., Edwards, A. R., Roth, J., Ariet, M., Ross, N. L., et al. (2003). A population-based study of the effects of birth weight on early developmental delay or disability in children. Am J Perinatol 20: 321–332.)

TABLE 23.2

EPIDEMIOLOGICAL RISK FACTORS FOR AND ASSOCIATIONS WITH PRETERM BIRTH

Risk Factors

h/o previous preterm birth (the earlier the birth, the higher the risk)
multiple gestation
maternal in utero exposure to diethylstilbestrol

Associations

maternal social disadvantage
maternal infection (genital urinary tract, periodontitis)
African-American ethnicity
single marital status
cigarette smoking
second trimester bleeding
low pre-pregnancy BMI (esp., among white women)
maternal age <20 y and >35 y
artificial reproductive technology
mother doing physically demanding work

Risk factors for Preterm Delivery

Table 23.2 lists risk factors for preterm delivery (Berkowitz & Papiernik, 1993). The largest single risk factor is previous preterm delivery. Women with a history of prior preterm delivery are at risk for spontaneous delivery of another preterm baby in 15 to 80% of subsequent pregnancies depending on the population studied (Carr-Hill & Hall, 1985; Cunningham, et al., 1997; Ekwo, Gosselink, & Moawad, 1992). Mothers who were themselves preterm are more likely to have a preterm infant, and the risk increases as the mother's own birth GA decreases. It is likely that in most cases preterm delivery reflects a gene-gene interaction or gene-environment interaction (Ward, 2003).

In the United States, for poorly understood reasons, African American mothers have a rate of preterm birth (17.0%) that is nearly twice that of other ethnic/racial groups. Puerto Rican mothers have the next highest rate (13.5%); Cuban American, Mexican American, Central and South American mothers have rates similar to non-Hispanic whites (10.4%). Among both African American and nonHispanic white women, the risk of preterm delivery is inversely related to education, income, and occupation (Mathews et al., 2002). The mechanisms by which social disadvantage increases risk for preterm delivery are poorly understood.

Large scale prevention programs in the 1980s and 1990s based on detection and remediation of social and medical risk factors in Table 23.2 did not reduce the rates of preterm delivery. Research is now focusing on gene–environment interactions and pathological pathways more proximate to the the event of preterm delivery (Lockwood & Kuczynksi, 2001; Rondo, et al., 2003).

Management of Preterm Delivery

Tocolysis is presently the cornerstone of management for threatened spontaneous PTD. Tocolytic agents either inhibit uterine muscle stimulators or stimulate the inhibitors. At best, they can prolong pregnancy for up to 72 hours. While this may improve survival at the lower extremes of GA, the safety and effectiveness of tocolytics remain controversial (Gyetvai, Hannah, Hodnett, & Ohlsson, 1999).

Complications of Premature Birth

Environmental Stress in the Neonatal Intensive Care Unit

The intensive care required to salvage more immature neonates is associated with stress. Examples include equipment that limit positive interactions with caregivers, high noise levels, constant bright light, and pain (Perlman, 2001). The hospital course often is prolonged; the average hospital stay for VLBW infants less than 28 weeks GA is approximately 100 days (Stevenson, et al., 1998). Evidence from animal studies suggests that even in the absence of medical complications or focal brain injury, sustained environmental stress may have adverse effects on brain development and behavior (Anand & Scalzo, 2000; Grunau, 2002).

Medical Complications

Largely as a result of organ immaturity, the preterm neonate is at high risk for developing medical complications that may adversely affect neurobehavioral outcomes either directly or indirectly through brain injury. These include low Apgar score, pulmonary complications, prolonged bradycardia and hypotension, hypothyroxinemia of prematurity,

hyperbilirubinemia, retinopathy of prematurity, necrotizing enterocolitis, and malnutrition (Perlman, 2001).

Neonatal Seizures

About 4% of preterm neonates have seizures, a higher rate than in older preterm or full-term neonates (Sheth, 1998). Compared to seizures in term neonates, seizures in preterm neonates are more likely to be accompanied by autonomic signs (changes in blood pressure, pulse, and respiration). While between 20 to 40% of term neonates who suffer seizures develop disability, almost 90% of preterm neonates with clearly defined seizures do so (Scher et al., 1993). Animal studies suggest that recurrent neonatal seizures are associated with longterm changes in cerebral excitability and mossy fiber sprouting in the hippocampus in the absence of evident cell loss (de Rogalski, Minokoshi, Silveira, Cha, & Holmes, 2001).

Prematurity and Brain Development

Growing evidence suggests that *prenatal* brain injury may precede and even be a contributory trigger for preterm delivery. The evidence for this is strongest for inflammatory insults due to intrauterine infections. Intrauterine infection has been implicated in the white matter damage associated with cerebral palsy (Leviton, et al., 1999).

At this time far more is known about the risks that preterm birth carries for *postnatal* brain development. As shown in Figure 23.1, the brain of a preterm infant born at 25 GW has only just begun the major events of brain organization and myelination, which start at around 20 and 24

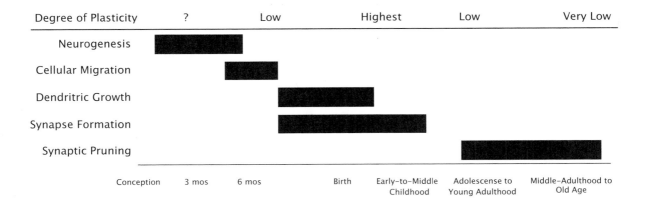

Figure 23.1 Plasticity in relation to stages of neurodevelopment. In the human, brain development proceeds in a sequence, as described in the text. This sequence begins with neurogenesis and ends with synaptic pruning. Following early brain damage, plasticity varies according to when the injury took place in the sequence. Animal studies suggest that plasticity will be low during the period of cell migration, corresponding to the second and third trimesters of pregnancy (second panel) and during adulthood (last panel) when synaptic networks have stabilized. Plasticity will be highest prior to synaptic stabilization during early and middle childhood (third panel). From Luciana, M (2003) Cognitive development in children born preterm: Implications for theories of brain plasticity following early injury. *Development and Psychopathology*, 15:1017-1047; (Reprinted with the permission of Cambridge University Press)

weeks, respectively, and continue postnatally for several years after birth and into adulthood. At 25 weeks, the human brain has only a thin layer of cortex, with barely visible gyri and immature Sylvian fissures; myelination is incomplete. Thrust into a physical environment for which it is not yet prepared, the preterm infant born at 25 weeks must accomplish ex utero the entire third trimester of brain development; a daunting challenge for an immature organism.

The preterm brain has certain site-specific vulnerabilities due to the timing of birth in relation to the stages of brain development (Perlman, 2003; Volpe, 2001). These vulnerabilities affect at least seven anatomic structures or regions. The first two, the germinal matrix and the cortical subplate, are transient brain structures that set the stage for both brain organization and myelination; the third, the subcortical white matter, is important both for connectivity and for cortical organization; the remaining four, the basal ganglia, the hippocampus, the cerebellum, and the cerebral cortex, are important gray matter structures.

Patterns of Neuropathological, Qualitative Brain Imaging, and Clinical Findings

Progress in understanding the relation between brain injury and later disabilities and impairments in preterm infants requires iterative cross-walks between two types of studies: those that examine the relation between brain imaging abnormalities and postmortem findings and those that examine the relation between brain imaging abnormalities and outcomes in survivors. Although quantitative brain imaging methods (discussed later) are emerging as important research tools, qualitative brain imaging methods such as ultrasonography (US) and magnetic resonance imaging (MRI) remain the clinical standards and have been the most extensively studied in relation to postmortem findings and clinical outcomes.

Based on postmortem exam, brain lesions in the preterm infant can be classified into four general categories: (1) hemorrhages in nonparenchymal areas of the brain, (2) white matter damage, (3) ventricular enlargement, and (4) lesions in other brain locations—cerebellum, basal ganglia, hippocampus, brain stem, and cortex.

Hemorrhages in Nonparenchymal Areas of the Brain

This category groups together the two most usual sites of origin of hemorrhage in the preterm brain, the germinal matrix and (less often) the choroid plexus with two common loci for their extension, the intraventricular and subarachnoid spaces. Cranial US through the anterior fontanelle typically visualizes germinal matrix hemorrhage (GMH) and intraventricular hemorrhage (IVH), while the other two are commonly encountered at autopsy.

Postmortem study of infants who were scanned before death confirmed that US echodensities in the periventricular region and in the ventricles were related to GMH/IVH

(Figure 23.2). In the early 1980s, GMH/IVH was present in up to 40% of VLBW infants, but its prevalence has fallen to around 25%. The balance of evidence suggests that premature infants with US evidence of GMH/IVH and no other brain lesions, experience relatively small elevations in risk of neurodevelopmental disorder in some studies (Pinto-Martin, et al., 1995; Whitaker, et al., 1996) and no elevation in risk at all in other studies (Kitchen, et al., 1985; Papile, Musick-Bruno, & Schafer A, 1983). This absence of adverse impact may reflect recovery due to reversion of astrocytes to radial glia and reactivation of radial glia in the germinal layers (Ganat, Soni, Chacon, Schwartz, & Vaccarino, 2002; Vaccarino & Ment, 2004).

White Matter Damage

White matter damage (WMD) encompasses a variety of neuropathologic entities, hemorrhagic and nonhemorrhagic, held together by one common feature: they tend to target developing white matter. One important neuropathologic form of white matter damage is periventricular leukomalacia (PVL). PVL is focal coagulation necrosis in the periventricular regions. More recent neuropathologic studies also refer to a more diffuse form of white matter damage whose characteristic histopathology is marked astrocytosis and activated microglial cells (Okoshi, et al., 2001). The mechanisms implicated in diffuse white matter damage (e.g., excitotoxicity, oxidative stress, inflammation) are similar to those for focal white matter damage.

Focal White Matter Damage

On neonatal US, PVL appears as echodensities and echolucencies in the periventricular region of the brain parenchyma, (Figure 23.2) frequently accompanied by ventricular enlargement. Recent advances in neonatal intensive care may have resulted in a decrease in the prevalence of focal abnormalities on US and MRI (Heuchan, Evans, Henderson Smart, & Simpson, 2002; Volpe, 2003).

In a regional LBW cohort born 1984 to 1987 and screened with serial cranial US, focal white matter damage occurred in around 8% of the survivors. Focal white matter damage was associated with markedly increased risk of disabling cerebral palsy by age 2 (Pinto-Martin, Riolo, Cnann, Holzman, & Paneth, 1993) and mental retardation by age 6 (Whitaker, et al., 1996). In LBW infants without disabling cerebral palsy or mental retardation, focal white matter damage was associated at age 6 with visual perceptual impairments and with attention deficit hyperactivity disorder (Whitaker, et al., 1996; Whitaker, et al., 1997), and, at ages 6 and 9, with minor motor problems but not general intelligence (Pinto-Martin, Whitaker, Feldman, Van Rossem, & Paneth, 1999).

Stewart et al. (1983) observed similar findings in a hospital-based cohort screened with serial cranial US and prospectively examined at 1, 4, 8, and 14 to 15 years in London. MRI findings at the adolescent follow-up indicate that,

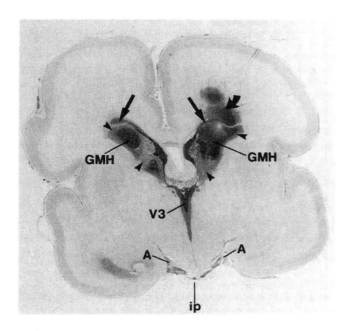

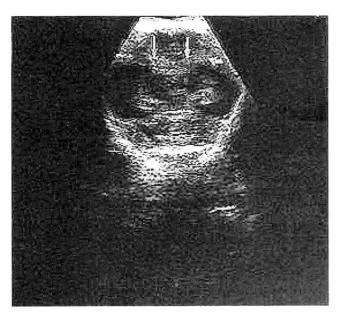

Figure 23.2 Germinal matrix and intraventricular hemorrhages and parenchymal hemorrhagic infarction: pathologic section (a) and in vivo sonogram (b). There are bilateral germinal matrix hemorrhages (GMH) extrinsically compressing and narrowing the frontal horns of the lateral ventricles, which contain ventricular hemorrhage (a—large arrows). The sonogram suggests bilateral intraventricular hemorrhages within the frontal horns (b—vertical arrows), but the adjacent germinal matrix hemorrhages cannot be delineated because the spared normal germinal matrix (a—arrowheads), which separates them from the intraventricular hemorrhage, cannot be visualized separately on sonography. The left frontal parenchymal hemorrhagic infarction (a—curved arrow) appears as a focus of increased echogenicity on sonography (b—curve arrow) contiguous to the echogenic lateral ventricle. Intraventricular hemorrhage is visible within the third ventricle (V3), and subarachnoid hemorrhage can be seen within the interpeduncular (ip) and ambient (A) cisterns on the pathologic section but not on sonography. (From Nigel Paneth et al. (2004). *Brain Damage in the Preterm Infant. Clinics in Developmental Medicine* (No. 131). Figure 7.7 p. 131. Reprinted with permission from Lippincott Williams & Wilkins.)

while neonatal US accurately identified serious permanent brain lesions, it missed a large proportion of abnormalities. When compared to full-term controls, preterms without major disabilities were far more likely to have abnormalities on MRI; indeed 55% of the preterms had unequivocally abnormal scans and 15 had equivocal scans as read by neuroradiologists blind to US findings or control status (Stewart et al., 1999). Thinning or atrophy of the corpus callosum, one of the commonest abnormalities, was seen in 42% of the preterms but in only 14% of age and sex matched controls who had been born at term (Stewart et al., 1999). Of great interest, qualitative MRI abnormalities at adolescence were related to behavioral problems and premorbid adjustment, but not to neurological outcomes or to neuropsychological test performance (with the single exception of word production) (Rushe, et al., 2001). Another hospital-based study, found a comparable rate of qualitative abnormalities on MRI (42.5%) in a sample of preterm adolescents, but no relation of these abnormalities to ADHD, low IQ, or dyspraxia (Cooke & Abernethy, 1999).

Many preterm infants imaged with MRI at term age have diffuse excessive high signal intensity (DEHSI) in the white matter (Counsell, Rutherford, Cowan, & Edwards, 2003). Counsell, Allsop, et al. (2003) have argued that DEHSI in preterm infants represents diffuse white matter abnormality. Reviewing a series of studies of diffuse white matter damage in preterm infants, Volpe (2003) has argued that diffuse white matter damage, similar to focal white matter damage, represents injury to preoligodendrocytes by infection or ischemia or an interaction between the two (Counsell, Rutherford, et al., 2003). Death of these cells accounts for the subsequent failure of white matter development as identified by diffusion weighted MRI imaging and of myelination, as identified on conventional MRI.

The diffuse white matter damage may explain some of the milder impairments seen by school age in preterm survivors. A recent study found that school-age children who were born preterm and escaped major disability had diffuse abnormality of cerebral white matter on MRI that was closely correlated with minor motor impairment but not with full scale IQ (Abernethy, et al. 2003).

Ventricular Enlargement (VE)

VE is the third general category of brain abnormality found on postmortem in preterm infants. Traditionally VE and hydrocephalus have been interpreted as sequelae of IVH. But there is increasing evidence that VE often, perhaps even always, reflects some degree of diffuse white matter damage that leads to a paucity of myelin producing oligodendrocytes and finally late VE (hydrocephalus *ex vacuo*). Evidence that VE is usefully viewed as a form of white matter damage is provided by Leviton and Gilles (1997).

Ment et al. (1999) demonstrated a strong association of US evidence of VE with adverse neurodevelopmental outcome at age 4.5 years. In their study, 56% of infants with VE demonstrated IQ scores below 70 as compared with 13%

of those without VE. Stewart and Kirkbride (1996) found that 14-year-old adolescents born preterm had both a high incidence of VE and poor school performance.

Lesions in Other Brain Locations
The fourth neuropathological category includes the forms of brain abnormalities about which we know the least. Peneth et al. (1994) found that 28% of 74 neonatal deaths in a regional cohort of infants weighing less than 2 kg had cerebellar hemorrhages at autopsy, 17% had basal ganglia necrosis and 16% had lesions of the brain stem.

Linear echogenicity within the basal ganglia and thalamus of preterm infants occurs in approximately 5% of preterm infants. (Chamnanvanakij, Rogers, Luppino, Broyles, Hickman, & Perlman, 2000). At 18 months adjusted age, preterm infants with Linear echogenicity as compared to a control group matched for BW and GA, had significantly lower scores on the mental and motor scores of the Bayley scales and on a rating of motor quality.

In one consecutive series, cerebellar hemorrhage occurred in 28% on LBW infants (Paneth et al., 2004, p. 183). Follow-up to age 4 has found that cerebellar hemorrhage was associated with cognitive rather than motor deficits (Merrill, Piecuch, Fell, Barkovich, & Goldstein, 1998). A retrospective study of MRI abnormalities in a preterm birth cohort, found cerebellar infarction and atrophy as evidenced on MRI in about 8% and 5% of the infants, respectively (Mercuri, et al., 1997), almost always accompanied by MRI abnormalities elsewhere in the brain, the most common being IVH.

Because lesions of the brain stem are not generally imaged in life, their contribution to development cannot as yet be assessed.

The cortex, which is only millimeters wide in infants born at the junction of the second and third trimester, has rarely been described as a site of gross structural lesions on postmortem in premature infants. However, histopathological postmortem work in human infants suggests that focal white matter damage may lead to reorganization of both local and distant neocortical gray matter (Marin-Padilla, 1997). This may explain the relation between US evidence of focal white matter damage and both general and specific cognitive deficits.

Magnetic Resonance Imaging: Diffusion Tensor Imaging, Volumetric, and Functional Studies

Neonatal Studies
Using diffusion tensor imaging, Huppi et al. (1998a) and Huppi, et al. (2001) found rapid changes in the microstructural organization of white matter between 28GW and term as well as both local and distal effects of focal white matter damage on the development of white matter fiber tracts.

Using quantitative volumetric MRI, Huppi et al. (1998) found that the preterm brain undergoes the developmen-

tal changes between 28GW and term that would normally occur during the third trimester. These changes include an increase in the volume, surface area, and sulcation of the cerebral cortex and an increase in the volume of the cerebral white matter. They also found, however, that both the volume of the myelinated white matter and the volume of cerebral cortical gray matter were reduced at term in preterm infants who previously had sustained focal WMD (termed PVL by the investigators); these findings are consistent with neuropathological studies (Marin-Padilla, 1997)

One study suggests that, even in the absence of focal white matter damage, cortical surface area and complexity is impeded in preterm infants (Ajayi-Obe, Saeed, Cowan, Rutherford, & Edwards, 2000). In a sample of 14 extremely preterm infants in which none of the infants had focal WMD and but seven had isolated GMH/IVH, they found that the cerebral cortex of the preterm infants at 38 to 42 weeks postmenstrual age, had less surface area and was less complex in terms of folding than that of term infants. At age 2, 40% of the preterms had global developmental delay, but none had major neuromotor deficits

School Age
In a study that compared 25 preterm 8-year-olds to 39 term controls using volumetric analyses, one investigator (Peterson, et al., 2002) found that several cortical regions, most prominently the sensorimotor regions and also premotor, midtemporal, parietooccipital, and subgenual cortices, were significantly smaller in the preterm group compared with term controls. Other structures also found to have smaller volumes in preterms were the cerebellum, basal ganglia, amygdalae, hippocampus, and corpus callosum. Structures having larger volumes in preterms were the occipital and temporal horns of the ventricles. The findings in the preterm group were associated with lower GA at birth. Sensorimotor and midtemporal cortical volumes correlated significantly with full scale, verbal and performance IQ. The authors suggest that the volume reduction is due to more subtle problems in blood or oxygen delivery than acute hemorrhage or severe asphyxia.

The same investigators (Peterson, et al., 2002), using functional MRI, found that the brain activation patterns of 8–year-old preterms during semantic processing resembled those of term controls during phonemic processing. These findings were interpreted as indicating that preterm children may process meaningful language as though it were meaningless sounds. However, the possibility that the unusual activation patterns in the preterms might reflect a more general cognitive dysfunction or lag was not ruled out, given that the preterms also had somewhat lower IQs than the term children.

Adolescents
A quantitative MRI study of very preterm adolescents found a 6.0% decrease in whole brain volume, an 11.8% decrease

in cortical gray matter volume, and decreases in right (15.6%) and left (12.1%) hippocampal volumes compared to full-term controls (Nosarti, et al., 2002). This study did not examine the relation between brain volumes and cognition. Another study of the same sample found that preterm subjects had significantly reduced cerebellar volume compared to term-born controls (Allin, et al., 2001). While there was no relation between cerebellar volume and motor neurological signs, cerebellar volume was significantly related to several cognitive test scores, including full scale IQ.

Adults

A study using computational morphometry found that lateral ventricular volume was significantly greater (by 41%) in VLBW adults compared to sibling controls (Allin, et al., 2004). The ratio of gray to white matter was significantly greater (by 10%) in those with VLBW, suggesting an abnormality in the organization of the cerebral cortex. Within the VLBW group there was a strong relation of greater lateral ventricular volume with less gray matter in subcortical nuclei and limbic cortical structures and less periventricular white matter. They conclude that the brains of VLBW adults have an abnormal distribution of gray matter and abnormal interregional and intraregional connectivity, and that these abnormalities result from the way normal brain development interacts with early brain lesions (Marin-Padilla, 1997; 1999). The relation between volumetric MRI abnormalities in adulthood and cognitive or motor test performance has not yet been reported.

Noting that thinning or atrophy of the corpus callosum, particularly the posterior portion, is one of the most common brain abnormalities found in very preterm survivors. Santhouse et al. (2002) examined the functional significance of perinatal corpus callosum damage in preterm adults. They compared seven very preterm males with callosal damage as previously identified by qualitative MRI scan at adolescence to nine very preterm males without evidence of callosal damage and to seven full-term controls with respect to activation patterns on auditory and visual tasks requiring callosal transfer. The very preterm males with callosal damage had significantly different activation patterns compared with the two comparison groups. On the visual task, the group with callosal damage manifested additional activity in the right dorsolateral prefrontal cortex, which the investigators interpret as consistent with the recruitment of working memory to compensate for impaired callosal function. On the auditory task, the group with callosal damage manifested a deficit of activity in the right temporal lobe, which the investigators interpret as consistent with left hemisphere or bilateral representation of timbre discrimination rather than the right hemisphere specialization found in normals. Overall, the investigators suggest that their findings point to neural compensation that is specific to the sensory modality involved and suggest the plasticity of the brain in the face of early brain damage.

Plasticity of the Preterm Brain

One of the more striking impressions that one carries away from the literature on brain imaging and outcomes in preterm survivors is the subtlety of the cognitive and motor impairments relative to the dramatic regional reductions in white and grey matter as measured on MRI. This suggests a remarkable plasticity of the preterm brain. Principles of plasticity following early brain injury in term infants have been reviewed recently by Stiles et al. (2005). For a comprehensive review of evidence for brain plasticity in preterm survivors, the reader is referred to Luciana (2003).

Neurobehavioral Sequelae of Preterm Birth

Survivors from the start of the modern era of neonatal care are now entering young adulthood. Outcome studies discussed next are mainly limited to these and later cohorts; that is, from the 1980s and beyond. Where evidence is available, outcomes are related to early biological and social risk factors. Excellent reviews of the methodological issues in preterm outcome research are available (Aylward, 2002; Kiely & Paneth, 1981; Saigal, 2000).

Need for Special Educational Services and Placements

School-related difficulties are among the most common problems confronting children born prematurely and at VLBW. More than half of VLBW and 60 to 70% of ELBW children require special educational assistance at some point in their school career (Aylward, 2002); by adolescence, ELBW children will have exceeded their peers in use of remedial or special educational services by eightfold to 10-fold. Similar figures for disabilities and special educational needs, and their inverse relation to birthweight, have been reported from numerous regional and population-based studies (Bowen, Gibson, & Hand, 2002; Buck, Msall, Schisterman, Lyon, & Rogers, 2000; Corman & Chaikind, 1998; Horwood, Mogridge, & Darlow, 1998; Klebanov, Brooks-Gunn, & McCormick, 1994; Pinto-Martin, et al., 2004; Saigal, et al., 2003).

Performance on Achievement Tests

By the middle school years ELBW children are about three to five times more likely than their age mates to have a problem with reading, writing, or spelling. Even among those scoring in the normal range of intelligence, children born prematurely are likely to have lower scores on tests of academic achievement (Taylor, Hack, Klein, & Schatschneider, 1995). In regional samples of ELBW children followed to school age in four different countries, below-normal scores on standardized tests ranged from 19 to 54% for reading, from 24 to 69% for arithmetic, and from 35 to 61% for spelling (Saigal, et al., 2003). Achievement deficits present in the early or middle-school years have been found to persist through high school (Breslau, Paneth, & Lucia, 2004; Saigal, et al., 2003).

Achievement is often especially low in arithmetic (Breslau, Johnson, & Lucia, 2001; Elgen & Sommerfelt, 2002; Rickards, Kelly, Doyle, & Callanan, 2001). In a preliminary attempt to locate the neurological substrate of this specific mathematical deficit, one study used MRI morphometry to compare two groups of preterm adolescents, matched on gender, age, and relevant perinatal variables; one with mathematical ability scores below expectation, based on intelligence testing, and another with math scores at expected levels. There was less grey matter in a specific area of the left parietal lobe in the preterms with below-expectation math scores (Isaacs, Edmonds, Lucas, & Gadian, 2001).

General Cognitive Abilities

In a regional birth cohort of LBW infants (Whitaker, et al., 1997), the prevalence of mental retardation (MR) was 5%; twice the amount expected based on population norms. In that cohort, focal white matter damage was the most powerful predictor of severe to moderate MR, followed by germinal matrix/intraventricular hemorrhage and by mechanical ventilation. Social disadvantage was not a predictor of severe to moderate MR.

When children with major disabilities are excluded from consideration, preterm children as a group, generally have mean scores falling in the average (or low average) range on a variety of tests of general cognitive ability; however, they also show a fairly consistent deficit (varying from 5 to 15 points) relative to their term-born peers (Aylward, 2002). A recent meta-analysis of 15 follow-up studies found the weighted mean difference between groups to be about 10 points (2/3 of a SD) (Bhutta, Cleves, Casey, Cradock, & Anand, 2002). A 10-point downward shift of the mean for the distribution of IQ implies an increment of about 21% in the proportion of preterms scoring below normal (i.e., having an IQ < 85).

Language

Between infancy and preschool, preterm children are more likely than full-term peers to have phonological and articulation problems (Briscoe, Gathercole, & Marlow, 1998). However, findings from older preterm children generally have been mixed. For example, at early school age, two population-based studies found normal language development in preterm samples (Scottish Low Birthweight Study Group, 1992; Whitaker, et al., 1996). Other studies have found delays in language ability and sentence repetition in early and middle childhood (Allin, et al., 2001; Breslau, Chilcoat, DelDotto, Andreski, & Brown, 1996; Largo, Molinari, Pinto, Weber, & Duc, 1986; Le Normand & Cohen, 1999; Wolke & Meyer, 1999).

Some studies report comparatively poor performance for preterm children in only selected aspects of language. According to a recent review (Aylward, 2002), preterms more consistently show deficits relative to term controls on tests of expressive language and on tests of complex grammar and syntax, than they do on tests of receptive language.

Motor Problems

In the neonatal period, a choreiform movement disorder has been discribed in a subgroup of premature infants with chronic lung disease. Although the abnormal movements improve with time, survivors exhibit cognitive problems (Perlman & Volpe, 1989).

By age 2, most cases of disabling cerebral palsy (DCP) are evident. DCP is the most serious of the motor impairments for which those born extremely preterm are at excess risk, occurring in about 10% of this population. Disabling CP is strongly related to focal white matter damage on neonatal cranial US. Nondisabling CP, principally mild spastic diplegia, is only modestly related to focal white matter damage (Pinto-Martin et al., 1996).

By middle and late childhood, milder motor impairments, such as those which contribute to the hidden disability associated with prematurity are evident (Bracewell & Marlow, 2002). Many of these less severe types of disability are often grouped together as Developmental Coordination Disorder (DCD). There is not yet a consensus on how to operationalize DCD; because of differing criteria and tests used in different studies, prevalence figures are uncertain. A recent report from a geographically-defined cohort in the U.K. (Foulder-Hughes & Cooke, 2003) found motor impairment to be diagnosed in up to 42.7% of 7 to 8 year olds born at < 32 GW.

In another regional cohort study of LBW children (Pinto-Martin, et al., 1999), assessments at 6 and 9 years of age with a motor problems inventory showed that the mean problem scores of nondisabled children in all birthweight groups were at or above the cutpoint identifying the top 10% of the standardization sample at both ages, and showed a significant birthweight gradient, with the highest problem scores in the lowest birthweight groups. In this same study, motor problems at both ages were significantly associated with neonatal US findings of focal white matter damage independently of other prenatal, perinatal, and neonatal risk factors (see also Levene, et al., 1992; Marlow, Roberts, & Cooke, 1989; Sullivan & McGrath, 2003).

Opthalmological Problems and Visual Impairment

Strabismus and refractive disorders (especially myopia) affect, respectively, nearly 15% and 20% of preterm children. Those with retinopathy of prematurity are at highest risk. More severe impairments include amblyopia, retinal detachment, optic nerve injury, and cortical injury. Together with strabismus and myopia, these impairments affect up to one third of nondisabled VLBW adolescents (Powls, Botting, Cooke, Stephenson, & Marlow, 1997). An additional 30% have impaired visual function on tests of contrast sensitivity and stereopsis. Overall, 64% of VLBW children had abnormalities on at least one measure as compared to 36% of NBW children. Poor contrast sensitivity and strabismus were related to poor motor skills, while poor contrast sensitivity and poor visual acuity were related to lower IQ. Reduced contrast sensitivity was the most sensitive predictor of impaired motor and cognitive function. White matter damage on US and MRI was related to strabismus, but not to reduced contrast sensitivity,

Visual–Perceptual and Visual–Motor Impairment

Preterms perform poorly on a broad range of visual–perceptual and visual–motor tests (Hård, Niklasson, Svensson, & Hellström, 2000; Luoama, Herrgard, & Martikainen, 1992). Poor performance on both a test of visual–motor skill and a motor-free test of visual–perceptual skills was associated with neonatal US evidence of focal white matter damage in nondisabled LBW 6-year-olds (Whitaker, et al., 1996).

Hearing

The prevalence of sensorineural hearing loss (SNHL) in very premature infants ranges from 0 to 9% and increases with decreasing GA (Msall and Tremont, 2002). SNHL is associated with severe respiratory illness and prolonged hospitalization; it has been suggested that this association might be a consequence of auditory nerve damage caused by noise levels in the NICU. Neonatal hyponatremia is also associated with SNHL.

Attention

In infancy, preterms have consistently been found to have less mature attention, as reflected in their longer looks and fewer shifts of gaze compared to controls matched on socio-economic status and age post-conception (Rose, Feldman, & Jankowski, 2004); these less mature patterns were found to be associated with aspects of medical risk in the preterm group, including days on oxygen and with mechanical ventilation. Preterm infants with respiratory distress syndrome, compared to preterms without RDS and to full-term infants, have also been found to have smaller heart rate responses, indicative of less intense attention, during periods of orienting to and sustained looking at a stimulus (Richards, 1994).

Findings for laboratory measures of attention in childhood, findings have been somewhat inconsistent. One study (Herrgard, Luoma, Tuppurainen, Karjalainen, & Martikainen, 1993) found no difference between preterms (< 32 weeks) and full-term controls on several attention tests. Another (Breslau, Brown, et al., 1996) found no difference between LBW and normal birthweight (NBW) groups on tests of sustained attention. Other studies have found performance on attention measures to be related to neonatal medical morbidity in preterms and to be poorer in LBW or VLBW children compared to NBW controls (Taylor, et al., 1995), though some of these findings, with the exception of accuracy on a vigilance test, disappeared when IQ was controlled (Taylor, Klein, Schatschneider, & Hack, 1998). In another study (Breslau, Chilcoat, et al., 1996) the poorer performance of preterms compared to controls withstood control for IQ on a test of focused attention, but not vigilance.

Processing Speed

Speed of information processing has been considered to be a fundamental component of individual differences in cognition generally. It is sometimes thought to be the basis for *g*, the factor representing the shared variance (correlation) among all cognitive tests and is important to the correlation between intelligence and achievement. As assessed with an encoding speed task, perceptual speed tasks, reaction time tasks, and decision time tasks, preterms have been found to be slower than full-terms at school-age (Rose & Feldman, 1996). Interestingly, when assessed with a choice reaction time task at age 11, preterm children were actually faster than full-terms when there was but one response choice, but became increasingly slower as the choices multiplied.

Memory

Memory is not a unitary construct; some types of memory have been found to be more affected in those born prematurely than others. Forms of memory that are particularly affected by prematurity are those dependent on structures in the medial temporal lobe (the hippocampus, dentate gyrus, subicular complex, and the adjacent perirhinal, entorhinal, and parahippocampal cortices). Collectively, these forms of memory are known as declarative (or explicit) memory and are characterized by recollection of facts (semantic memory) and events (episodic memory) and, in principle, are capable of entering consciousness. By contrast, forms of memory that do not depend on the medial temporal lobe, collectively known as nondeclarative (or implicit) memory, are nonconscious, and have not been found to be affected by premature birth. Nondeclarative memory is a catch-all category that includes procedural memory (skills and habits), classical conditioning, and nonassociative learning, among other things.

One of the most widely studied types of declarative memory is recognition, the capacity to distinguish things previously encountered from new ones. This type of memory has been shown to be particularly affected by prematurity even in its earliest-appearing form, in infancy (Nelson, 1995; Rose, et al., 2004). Several other forms of declarative memory have also been found deficient in preterm relative to full-term groups, including list learning, recall, memory span, working memory, and so on (Curtis, Lindeke, Georgieff, & Nelson, 2002; Luciana, Lindeke, Georgieff, Mills, Nelson, 1999; Taylor, Klein, Minich, & Hack, 2000). Everyday memory (a form of episodic memory), has been found to be impaired, compared to full-term controls, in preterm adolescents who were also found to have reduced bilateral hippocampal volumes on MRI, despite equivalent head size and an otherwise neurologically normal presentation (Isaacs, et al., 2000).

Executive Function

Executive function (or executive control) tasks require inhibition, planning, and/or application of strategies; good performance is thought to depend on mature functioning of frontal lobe structures. The few studies thus far which have examined executive function in preterm children found their performance poor compared to controls (Frisk & Whyte, 1994; Luciana, et al., 1999). A more precipitous decline in the performance of VLBW children compared to controls has been found with increasingly difficult memory tasks (Rose & Feldman, 1996). This exaggerated decline in response to cognitive challenge may be one of the factors behind the delayed emergence of some academic problems in children with VLBW.

Behavior and Psychopathology

Regulatory Problems in the NICU

Neurobehaviorally, there are several respects in which preterm/very low birthweight newborns, as a group, have been found to perform more poorly than full-term/normal birthweight peers, even when both groups are examined at equivalent postmenstrual ages. For example, when assessed at 40 weeks postmenstrual age with MRI and a modification of the Neonatal Behaviorial Assessment Scale (NBAS) (Als, Duffy, McAnulty, 1988), healthy preterm infants were found to have not only less grey and white matter differentiation and myelination, but also significantly poorer functioning, in four neurobehavioral areas: autonomic regulation, motor responsiveness, state organization, and attention compared to full-term controls. Yet, these same preterms had actually improved in both respects over earlier assessments done at birth. However, the NBAS and similar tests have little or no test–retest reliability and no predictive validity for later development. Thus it is unclear what they imply, if anything, about any long-term impact of prematurity.

Behavior Problems

Parents and teachers have often reported elevated levels of behavior problems in preterm children (for reviews see Buka, Lipsitt, & Tsuang, 1992; Chapieski & Evankovich, 1997. Though they can be detected earlier (Rose, Feldman, Rose, Wallace, & McCarton, 1992), behavior problems in preterms become more noticeable and impairing during the school years, when high levels of such problems interfere with normal activities and learning.

One of the most widely used behavior problem scales, the Child Behavior Checklist (Achenbach, 1991), assesses eight problem dimensions which are grouped into broader areas of behavioral difficulty. When preterm children are found to have more problems overall than controls, they most often show elevated scores on the Social and Attention Problem scales. The degree to which these problems may be characteristic of preterms was underscored in a recent paper which compared behavior problems obtained by parent report among school-aged children born at < 1,000g from four different countries: the U.S., Canada, the Netherlands, and Germany (Hille, et al., 2001). Despite somewhat different approaches to early socialization and education of children in these four countries and the administration of the same instrument in different languages, the behavioral profiles of the ELBW cohorts were strikingly similar, suggesting that social and attention problems, in particular, are common sequelae of prematurity across cultures. Another study, however, suggested that the elevation in preterms on the attention problems scale of the CBCL may be found mostly among children in the lower end of the socioeconomic spectrum (Breslau & Chilcoat, 2000).

Psychopathology

A number of studies have used structured psychiatric diagnostic interviews to assess a range of psychiatric disorders in preterm/LBW survivors. A consistent finding has been an excess of Attention Deficit Hyperactivity Disorder (ADHD) in preterm/LBW survivors relative to term/normal birthweight controls (Botting, Powls, Cooke, & Marlow, 1997; Breslau, 1995; Szatmari, Saigal, Rosenbaum, & Campbell, 1993; Szatmari, Saigal, Rosenbaum, Campbell, & King, 1990). Breslau, et al. (1996a) found that urban, but not suburban LBW survivors had an excess of ADHD relative to normal birthweight controls at age 6. In a large regional LBW birth cohort, independent predictors of ADHD at age 6 included neonatal cranial US consistent with white matter damage as well as male sex, a proximal measure of social disadvantage and both maternal smoking and mild alcohol consumption during pregnancy (Whitaker, et al., 1997).

The relation of prematurity and LBW to substance use is inconsistent. One community-based study (Chilcoat & Breslau, 2002) found a significantly higher incidence of drug use among 11-year-old boys (but not girls) with LBW compared to NBW controls (OR = 2.0), while a regional cohort followed to adulthood (Cooke, 2004) found less self-reported alcohol and drug use in preterms compared to controls, but equivalent rates of smoking. Another study (Hack, et al., 2002) found that adults born at VLBW were less likely than normal birthweight controls to report alcohol and drug use. It is not clear, however, whether the apparently encouraging findings regarding alcohol and drug use might reflect ongoing dependence of VLBW survivors on their families due to residual cognitive and social problems (Harrison, 2002).

A metanalysis has suggested that LBW is a modest but definite risk factor for schizophrenia (Kunugi, 2001). However, other studies have found that prematurity, but not LBW, is associated with risk for schizophrenia. One study found that, in patients with schizophrenia, prematurity (but not poor fetal growth), was associated with premorbid social withdrawal and an early age at illness onset, whereas poor fetal growth (but not prematurity) was associated with low educational achievement (Smith, et al., 2001).

Quality of Life in Adolescence and Adulthood

Despite their objectively greater functional impairment, preterm groups do not necessarily report more negative perceptions of quality of life (QOL) than full-term controls. For example, in a Canadian cohort of ELBW adolescents and NBW controls, although the mean score on a health-related quality of life scale was higher in controls, the vast majority of the ELBW group viewed their QOL as satisfactory (Saigal, et al., 1996), and the ELBW teenagers did not differ from their controls in self-esteem (Saigal, Lambert, Russ, & Hoult, 2002). Similarly, preterms and full-terms followed to adulthood in the U.K. reported no difference in six of eight QOL domains (physical functioning and general health being the two exceptions). One study of preterms even reported the counter-intuitive relation of better self-perceived QOL to more severe neonatal cranial US findings, based on birth record search (Feingold, Sheir-Neiss, Melnychuk, Bachrach, & Paul, 2002). And, even when preterm adolescents did rate their QOL as poorer than full-term peers, they were not unduly worried about their future (Walther, den Ouden, & Verloove-Vanhorick, 2000). Saigal et al. (1996) suggested that disabled preterm children may adjust their expectations downward so that they perceive their quality of life to be better than an outsider might see it.

Special Topics

Small for Gestational Age (SGA)

As noted earlier, SGA refers to an infant having weight at birth in the lowest portion (generally, the lowest 10%) of a weight-for-gestational-age reference standard. A more stringent standard, namely, the lowest 2% of a weight-for-gestational-age distribution, has been proposed on the grounds that higher percentages may include infants who are merely genetically small. Intrauterine growth restriction (IUGR) refers to an SGA infant for whom there is also evidence of a pathologic restriction of fetal growth due to adverse genetic or environmental influences. (Henrickson & Clausen, 2002).

A disproportionate number of adults who were born with IUGR seem predisposed to hypertension, heart disease, obesity, and type II diabetes (McClellan & Novak, 2001). According to the fetal origins hypothesis (a.k.a., the Barker Hypothesis or fetal programming), these adult disease states are thought to result from fetal adaptations to poor nutritional status that are harmful under conditions of good nutrition later on (Barker, 1995). However, this literature is controversial (Paneth, Ahmed, & Stein, 1996; Paneth & Susser, 1995).

Evidence regarding cognitive compromise in children born with IUGR is inconsistent, and may have to do with quality of postbirth nutrition; for a review, see Grantham-McGregor (1998). Evidence regarding behavioral and emotional problems also is mixed. In a study from Western Australia (Zubrick, et al., 2000), severe IUGR children had significantly elevated risk for mental disorder (OR 2.9; 95% CI: 1.18, 7.12). Meanwhile, the British Cohort Study, which used the 5th percentile of weight-for-gestational-age as the cutpoint for defining SGA, found no longterm social or emotional consequences (Strauss, 2000). This was also the case for a large multicenter Scandinavian cohort (Sommerfelt, et al., 2001). In this latter cohort, SGA versus AGA status explained only 1% of variance in a summary score of child behavior problems

Male Vulnerability

National birth registry data indicate an excess of males among preterm births (Ingemarsson, 2003). A recent meta-analysis of results from such studies found an overall OR (95%CI) of 1.12 (1.09, 1.15) for the association of maleness with prematurity (Zeitlin, et al., 2002). Males are also more likely to develop complications associated with preterm birth, in particular pulmonary morbidities and intracranial hemorrhage and, in consequence, their rates of neonatal mortality are higher than for females (Vatten & Skjaerven, 2004).

In studies examining longterm outcomes of prematurity, males have been found to have higher rates of neurosensory disability (Whitfield et al., 1977), poorer general cognitive ability (Hindmarsh, O'Callaghan, Mohay, & Rogers, 2000), and academic performance (Johnson & Breslau, 2000; O'-Callaghan, et al., 1996) than their female counterparts. Preterm males with sonographically identified perinatal brain injury have been found to have IQ scores at age 4 to 5 years about half a standard deviation lower than girls with the same degree of perinatal injury (Raz, et al., 1995).

Catch Up

With respect to physical growth, recent population-based studies have found that, despite some catch-up, growth parameters continue to be below normal into adolescence for a higher proportion of ELBW survivors than their term controls (Ford, Doyle, Davis, & Callanan, 2000).

With respect to cognitive growth, findings are mixed. For the most severely affected preterm children (e.g., those with ELBW and those with PL/VE), cognitive abilities generally either decline or remain stable at their initially low levels relative to peers. Meanwhile, for those without major complications and those born at heavier birth weights, subsequent interventions and socioeconomic circumstances play a major role in determining whether performance relative to peers improves, declines, or remains the same as they grow older. Most studies find that, while rates of severe disabilities tend to remain stable over age, there is an overall trend for increasing rates of more subtle problems through early, middle, and high-school ages (Saigal, 2000). This trend is exemplified in a full-population cohort of children born at < 1,500g or < 32 GW followed to age 14 (Walther, et al., 2000). In that cohort, problems in basic functions (e.g., speech, mobility) decreased from age 5 to 10 years of age while psychological problems (negative mood, poor concentration) increased (Theunissen, et al., 2000).

Summary of Prematurity

Preterm birth now affects 1 in 10 families in the United States and is a major risk factor for major disability and impairment, especially at the lower extremes of gestational age. The largest single risk factor for preterm delivery is a previous preterm delivery, pointing to a genetic contribution. Thus far, however, the causes of preterm delivery remain a mystery, frustrating efforts at prevention. In preterm infants, white matter damage, both focal and diffuse, is a risk factor for motor disability and impairment; white matter damage also may affect the organization of important grey matter structures, such as the cortex. Even in the absence of known brain injury, the brains of healthy preterms differ from those of term infants and these differences are apparent in different age groups, including adults. The functional significance of these differences requires further study. It is important to note, that at least half of preterm survivors are doing remarkably well and most are satisfied with their quality of life.

CEREBRAL PALSY

Cerebral palsy, the most common physical disability of childhood in developed countries, affects one in 500 school-age children (Stanley, Blair, & Alberman, 2000). The disabling forms of cerebral palsy exact an enormous toll from individuals, their families, and society (Honeycutt, Dunlap, Chen, & Homsi, 2004), while milder forms of motor impairment place an individual at risk for social isolation during school-age years (Skinner & Piek, 2001).

Background

Definitions

The term cerebral palsy describes a group of disorders of the development of movement and posture, causing activity limitation, that are attributed to non-progressive disturbances that occurred in the developing fetal or infant brain. The motor disorders of cerebral palsy are often accompanied by disturbances of sensation, cognition, communication, perception, and/or behavior, and/or by a seizure disorder (Bax M, et al., 2005). Postneonatal events such as meningoencephalitis, trauma, or occlusion of a cerebral artery account for only 12 to 21% of cases of CP in developed countries, but are more common in the developing world (Emond, Golding, & Peckham, 1989).

The manifestation of motor impairment due to brain injury or anomalies may change over time. Abnormalities of motor tone or movement in the first several weeks or months after birth may gradually improve during the first year. Conversely, relatively nonspecific motor signs, such as

hypotonia, that are seen in this early period may evolve over the 2 years into spasticity and extrapyramidal abnormalities.

Based on the predominant type of motor impairment, CP is classified as spastic, dyskinetic, ataxic, or mixed (see Table 23.3). For infants born in the Western world since 1980, spastic CP is the most frequent type and accounts for approximately 85% of cases, with estimates ranging from 76 to 93% (Colver & Sethumadhavan, 2003; Mutch, et al., 1992; Paneth & Kiely, 1984). Spasticity is defined as a velocity-dependent resistance of muscle to stretch, or excessive inappropriate involuntary muscle activity, associated with upper motor neuron paralysis or syndrome. Spasticity develops when injury to the corticospinal tracts decreases cortical excitatory input to reticulospinal and corticospinal tracts. This in turn decreases the number of effective motor units, producing aberrant muscle control and weakness. At the same time, the loss of descending inhibitory output through the reticulospinal tract and other systems increases the excitability of gamma and alpha neurons, producing spasticity (see Sanger, 2003).

Spastic CP is classified further, according to its topography, into quadriplegia (involvement of all four limbs), diplegia (significant leg involvement with less prominent effect on the arms), and hemiplegia (involvement of an ipsilateral arm and leg). The term double hemiplegia implies bilateral involvement characterized by greater involvement of the arms than the legs. Movement disorders (such as dystonia) can coexist with the predominant motor impairment. Because at present there is no reliable objective measure of muscle tone, the topographic classification of spasticity is somewhat unreliable between clinicians.

The inclusion of a measure of functional motor capacity in the diagnostic process improves the rate of diagnostic agreement between clinicians; the rate of agreement is greater for disabling than nondisabling forms of CP. For this reason, it has been argued that only disabling CP should be included in case registers for epidemiological studies of CP (Palisano, et al., 1997b). A simple five-level system for rating activity restriction that correlates highly with the International Classification of Impairments, Disabilities, and Handicap (WHO, 1980). Levels I and II correspond to nondisabling or mildly disabling CP, while Levels III to V correspond to moderately to severely disabling CP (Palisano, et al., 1997b). Children with spastic hemiplegia typically are mildly disabled (activity restricted), children with spastic diplegia, choreoathetoid CP, and mild ataxia are moderately disabled, while children with spastic quadriplegia are severely disabled (Palisano, et al., 1997a).

Trends in Incidence and Prevalence

The prevalence of CP in the Western world is about 2 to 3 per 1,000 live births (Stanley, et al., 2000). Information about the prevalence and time trends of CP has been most completely described for patients in the United Kingdom,

TABLE 23.3
CEREBRAL PALSY: CLASSIFICATION, ASSOCIATED FEATURES, AND RISK FACTORS

Type/Frequency/* Age at Dx	Motor Features/ Functional Level	Epilepsy	Other Features	Risk Factors
Spastic CP—80% of all cases	• Pyramidal signs, with distal weakness, hypertonicity, and hyperreflexia (*damage to cortico-spinal tracts*)			
Spastic Quadriplegia (0.2 /1,000 live births) First year of life	• All 4 extremities involved (though legs may be slightly worse than arms) • Usually nonambulatory	50–95%	• Dysphagia	• Intrauterine infection • Preterm birth • Hypoxic ischemic encephalopathy
Spastic Diplegia (0.7 / 1,000 live births)	• Legs extremities more involved than arms • 10% nonambulatory	16–27%	• Hydrocephalus Strabismus	• Preterm birth
Spastic Hemiplegia (0.6 / 1,000 live births) First 2 years of life	• One side of body involved (arm may be worse than leg) • Usually will walk independently	30–50%	• Small hand and foot on affected side with sensory loss Homonymous hemiopsia	• Coagulation disorders
Dyskinetic CP—15% of cases (0.3 / 1,000 live births)	• Extrapyramidal signs; insupressible, stereotyped involuntary movements (*basal ganglia damage*)			• Hypoxic-ischemic encephalopathy
Hyperkinetic / Choreoathetoid Age 3–5 years	• Purposeless massive involuntary movements with motor overflow • Usually ambulatory	rare	• Increased by stress Absent during sleep	• Kernicterus • Hypoxic-ischemic encephalopathy
Dystonic Age 5–10 years	• Abnormal and distorted postures; fluctuating muscle tone • Usually ambulatory	rare	• Increased by voluntary movement • Diminished by distraction and sleep	
Ataxic CP— 5 % of cases (0.1 / 1,000 live births)	• Axial hypotonia, truncal oscillations, intention tremor ± scanning speech (*cerebellar signs*)			
Simple Ataxia	• Ambulatory with broad-based gait	rare		• IUGR
Disequilibrium Syndrome	• Dysmetria and difficulty in posture, equilibrium	rare		• Genetic
Mixed CP	• Spastic /dystonic is common • Ataxic / diplegic			

*School age prevalence per thousand live births.

Sweden, and Australia. For the period from 1967 to the early and mid-1980s, data from these countries showed an increase in the live birth prevalence of CP in children with low birthweight with a leveling off thereafter (Hagberg, Hagberg, Beckung, & Uvebrant, 2001; Stanley & Watson, 1992). The only population-based study of CP in the United States has found a modest increase in the prevalence of CP, but only in normal birthweight one year survivors (Winter, Autry, Boyle, & Yeargin-Allsopp, 2002).

CP occurs more commonly in children who are born very preterm than in mildly premature children. A recent study in Sweden found that of 241 children with CP, 36% were born at less than 28 GW, 25% at 28 to 32 GW, and 2.5% at 32 to 38 GW and 37% at term. Of these 241 children, 33% were hemiplegic, 44% diplegic, and 6% quadriplegic (Hagberg, et al., 2001).

In developed countries, the natural history of CP has improved over the past 50 years. If appropriate health care is available, affected children without significant comorbidities have life spans approaching that of the general population However, life span is shorter in persons with quadriplegia, hydrocephalus, lack of basic functional skills, refractory seizures, and profound mental retardation (Hutton & Pharoah, 2002).

Clinical Patterns, Pathological Findings, and Imaging Studies

Full-Term Infants

Spastic hemiplegia is most typical of full-term infants. Cerebral injury in the distribution of the middle cerebral artery is the most common finding on postmortem and in patients evaluated with CT and MRI (Scher, Belfar, Martin, & Painter, 1991; van Bogaert, Baleriaux, Christophe, & Szliwowski, 1992; Wiklund & Uvebrant, 1991). These studies find necrosis and atrophy with or without gliosis, but it is not known when the ischemic or hemorrhagic disturbance began. For reasons not understood, right-sided hemiplegia occurs as twice as frequently as left-sided hemiplegia (Ment, Duncan, & Ehrenkranz, 1984).

Periventricular atrophy suggesting white matter abnormality is present in some children with hemiplegic CP and gross malformations of cerebral development are found in about one sixth. The CT or MRI is normal in another one quarter to one third of children with presumed congenital hemiplegia. The lack of areas of injury or abnormality on brain imaging supports the idea that some CP is related to abnormalities of brain development at the microscopic level. Consistent with this possibility, no abnormalities of any kind were found in the obstetrical history of a majority of infants with hemiplegia in two separate studies (Cohen & Duffner, 1981; Levy, Abroms, Marshall, & Rosquette, 1985).

In patients with quadriplegic CP, MRI findings include multiple cystic lesions in the white matter, diffuse cortical atrophy, cavities that communicate with the lateral ventricles, and hydrocephalus (Truwit, Barkovich, Koch, & Ferriero, 1992). Choreoathetoid forms of CP, which often include spasticity, tend to occur in term infants. Dystonia of the extremities often also co-occurs with spasticity but is often missed. On postmortem the histopathological appearance of the basal ganglia often resembles marble (status marmoratus). Persistently hypotonic or atonic CP suggests the involvement of the cerebellar pathways. Long tract signs such as brisk tendon reflexes and extensor plantar responses frequently accompany the hypotonia.

Preterm Infants

Until recently, the predominant view was that spastic quadriplegia was typically (although not invariably) associated with term delivery, while spastic diplegia was typically (although not invariably) associated with preterm delivery. This view accorded with what was known, based on neuropathological studies and early brain imaging, about the differing typical distribution of white matter injury in term and preterm infants. Parasaggital white matter injury in term infants and periventricular white matter injury in preterm infants have been attributed to gestational age-related differences in regional vulnerability of white matter to injury. However, recent epidemiological and brain imaging studies cast some doubt on this picture. Epidemiological studies of cohorts born since 1980 and found that spastic cases with predominantly lower limb involvement (about 33%) were equally distributed among preterm and term infants (Colver & Sethumadhavan, 2003). Moreover, in recent MRI studies of children with spastic CP, there has been no clear association between periventricular white matter injury and spastic diplegia or between parasaggital white matter injury and quadriplegia (Krageloh-Mann, 2000). Figure 23.3 shows examples of neuroimaging and neuropathology of the cerebral palsies with brief clinical descriptions.

Risk Factors and Pathogenesis

The view that intrapartum asphyxia was the predominant cause of CP was entrenched in the lay and professional mind until fairly recently (Gibbs, Rosenberg, Warren, Galen, & Rumack, 2004). This misconception gradually yielded to a series of important neuroepidemiological studies, beginning in the late 1970s with the Collaborative Perinatal Project (Nelson & Ellenberg, 1978) and including, in the United States, the Neonatal Brain Hemorrhage Study (Pinto-Martin, et al., 1993), the California Cerebral Palsy Project (Cummins, Nelson, Grether, & Velie, 2003; Grether, Nelson, Walsh, Willoughby, & Redline, 2003) and the Developmental Epidemiology Network (Leviton et al., 1999). In an attempt to evaluate the relative contribution of different risk factors, epidemiologists have used analytic models that evaluate later events (for example those occurring during delivery) in the light of earlier events (e.g., maternal characteristics before pregnancy, first trimester events) (Nelson & Ellenberg, 1986). As a result of these studies, we now know that the brain insults causing CP can occur prenatally, perinatally, postnatally or in some combination of these. (Kuban & Leviton, 1994) Table 23.4 summarizes epidemiologic risk factors for CP classified according to whether they occur before pregnancy, during pregnancy, or during the perinatal period.

At this time most cases of CP cannot be prevented. In a contemporary case series representing 217 cases of systematically assessed CP over a 10-year period, a plausible risk factor was identified in 82.0% of cases (Shevell, Majnemer, & Morin, 2003). The five most common factors were periventricular leukomalacia (white matter damage) 24.9%, intrapartum asphyxia 21.7%, cerebral dysgenesis 17.1%, intracranial hemorrhage 12.9%, and vascular, 9.7%. A single factor was found for 66.4% of the cases and multiple factors in 15.6% of cases. The risk factor profile varied according to the topography of the CP, gestational age, and source of the patients. Features associated with the

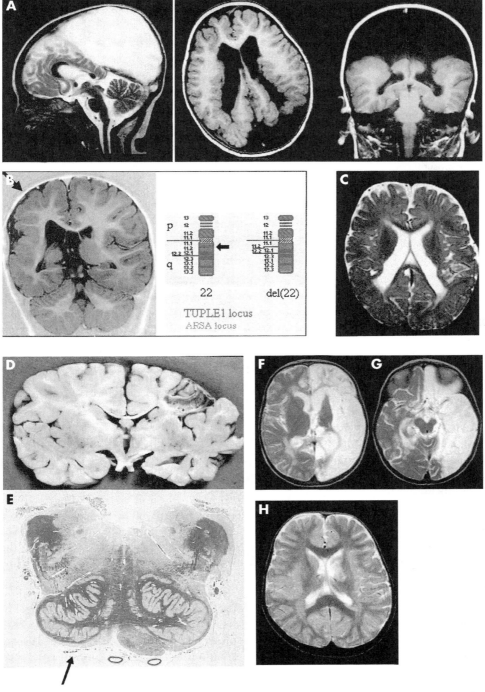

Figure 23.3 Neuroimaging and neuropathology of the "cerebral palsies." Note the heterogeneity of brain disorders. (A) Bilateral schizencephaly with grey matter lining the ventricles. This boy had visual function but it is not clear where the "visual cortex" is located. Note the effects on the corpus calosum. He had some head and trunk control but no mobility. His main clinical problem was intractable seizures and feeding difficulties. (B) Right hemisphere polymicrogyria (arrow) secondary to 22q deletion presenting as a classical left hemiplegia in the second six months of life. This girl has no fits, no feeding difficulty and no speech problems. She is not prone to infection. She walked at a typical age for hemiplegia (18–22 months). The left hemisphere is normal. This is yet another example of the importance of scanning children with CP. (C) Periventricular leucomalacia (PVL). Scan taken at 10 months age. Born prematurely at 27 weeks gestation. Note how the posterior horns of the lateral ventricles abut on the cerebral cortex along with an extremely thin corpus calosum. There is high signal change in what remains of the white matter. In contrast with hydrocephalus, the ventricles have sharp outlines indicating they are not under pressure. (D) Coronal section through hemisphere of 8-month-old infant showing old left cortical-subcortical infarct with thin internal capsule. (E) Transverse section through the medulla of the same infant as in panel D. Note the virtual absence of the pyramid on the right (arrow, E) due to a loss of descending corticospinal tracts. (F) Devastating destruction of the left hemisphere from herpes simplex encephalitis at 18 months of age. This girl lost the power of speech, feeding, sitting, and walking in the acute phase but regained all these over the following year. She is prone to seizures which are controlled with anticonvulsants. Despite her tremendous recovery, she has a dense right homonymous hemianopia and hemiplegia (without neglect) with learning difficulties. Note the smaller left cerebral peduncle in panel G. (H) Left postvaricella "capsular infarct" in a male toddler. The lesion involves the internal capsule, lentiform nucleus, and thalamus. All of these pathologies may be said to contribute to the "cerebral palsies". (From Jean-Pierre Lin. The cerebral palsies: a physiological approach. from the J. Neurol Neurosurg Psychiatry 2003;74: i23–i29. With permission from the BMJ Publishing Group)

TABLE 23.4

EPIDEMIOLOGIC RISK FACTORS FOR CEREBRAL PALSY

Maternal history of long intervals between menses
Short or unusually long interpregnancy interval
Pregnancy bleeding
Maternal history of fetal loss
Prenatal methylmercury exposure
Prenatal or perinatal stroke
Congenital rubella
Congenital toxoplasmosis
Fetal growth retardation
Chorioamnionitis
Premature separation of the placenta
Preterm birth
Multiple birth
Low Apgar Score
Transient Hypothyroxinemia of the Preterm
Hyperbilirubinemia
Newborn encephalopathy
Hypocapnia from mechanical ventilation

child's CP such as microcephaly, neonatal complications, and prior or concurrent epilepsy, were observed to be predictive of etiologic yield (Shevell, et al., 2003). At the level of the individual patient, the identification of risk factors provides answers to questions about recurrence risks, may reduce unnecessary investigations and empowers the family and child by providing knowledge.

Neonatal Markers for CP

On neonatal neurological exam, qualitative abnormalities of spontaneous motor activity in newborns and young infants are thought by some authorities to be early predictive markers for later spastic CP; in particular, infants who later develop spastic CP have an absence of fidgety movements, a spontaneous movement pattern that is normally present from 3 to 5 months (Ferrari, et al., 2002).

With respect to brain imaging in the neonatal period, current practice parameters recommend routine screening with cranial US on all preterm infants of < 30 GW (Ment, et al., 2002). Screening should be done once between 7 and 17 days of age and repeated between 36 and 40 weeks postmenstrual age so as to detect intraventricular hemorrhage, focal white matter damage (sometimes referred to as periventricular leukomalacia), and low pressure ventriculomegaly, which provide prognostic information on long-term developmental outcome. In term infants with clinical signs of encephalopathy, a history of birth trauma, low hematocrit, or coagulopathy, MRI should be done between days 2 and 8 to asses the location and extent of injury. In particular, basal ganglia and thalamic lesions identified by conventional MRI are associated with poor developmental outcomes (Ment, et al., 2002).

The Initial Diagnosis of CP

Practice parameters for the evaluation of cerebral palsy have recently been published by the American Academy of Neurology (Ashwal, et al., 2004). (See Figure 23.4.)

History and Physical Exam

The chief complaint typically is a concern that the child is not attaining motor milestones at the expected time in the first 2 to 3 years of life. At the outset of the diagnostic process, a careful history must ascertain that the child is not losing motor function given that a number of symptoms and signs are common to both CP and neurodegenerative/metabolic disorders (Gupta & Appleton 2001). A review of family history, maternal history, and pregnancy experience is necessary

The physical exam localizes the motor abnormalities to the brain as opposed to the motor unit (anterior horn cell, peripheral nerve, nerve–muscle junction, muscle). The observations on which the diagnosis of CP is based include motor function (e.g., ability to sit independently, ability to walk) and muscle tone and reflexes (e.g., deep tendon, primitive and protective reflexes). Dynamic deformities and movement disorders can be accentuated during ambulation or other activities.

CP usually is not difficult to diagnose in the patient who has not attained motor milestones, who is not losing function, and whose muscle tone is generally high. However, one commonly encounters patients who have not met milestones and whose muscle tone is normal or low. In these cases, important findings on exam that would be consistent with CP include persistence of the primitive reflexes past the time that they should have vanished or the failure to develop protective reflexes at the expected time. For example, the Moro reflex and tonic neck reflex should not be obtainable after 6 months of age; side protective reflexes should be elicitable after 5 months of age and the parachute reflex after 10 months. If the primitive reflexes have disappeared at the appropriate time and if the protective reflexes have emerged as expected, then one should think of a motor unit disease, such as spinal muscular atrophy or congenital myopathy rather than CP (Russman, 1992).

The diagnosis of CP in the hypotonic child can be especially difficult, and may require repeated examinations and more than one opinion. An important sign in the physical exam is that of hand preference. A child should not cross the midline when reaching for an object until after 1 year of age and should not show hand preference until 18 to 24 months of age. Evidence of handedness prior to this time suggests a hemiplegia (Russman, 1992).

The physical exam should establish whether signs of CP are present and if so permit classification of the type of CP (quadriplegia, hemiplegia, diplegia, ataxic, etc.). The normal examination in the first 6 months of life does not exclude the possibility of mild or moderately severe

EVALUATION OF THE CHILD WITH CEREBRAL PALSY

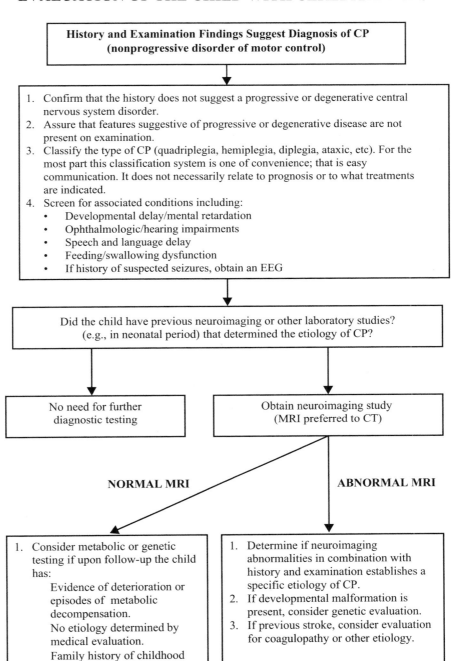

Figure 23.4 Algorithm for the evaluation of the child with cerebral palsy (CP). Screening for associated conditions (mental retardation, vision/hearing impairments, speech and language delays, oral motor dysfunction, and epilepsy) is recommended. Neuroimaging (MRI preferred to CT) is recommended for further evaluation if the etiology of the child's CP has not been previously determined. In some children, additional metabolic or genetic testing may be indicated. From: Ashwal S, Russman BS, Blasco PA, Miller G, Sandler A, Shevell M, et al. Practice parameter: diagnostic assessment of the child with cerebral palsy: report of the quality standards subcommittee of the American Academy of Neurology and the Practice Committee of the Child Neurology Society. *Neurology*, 62:851-863. (Reprinted with the permission of the American Academy of Neurology)

The new emergence of neurological abnormality after the first 6 months of life can be attributed to progressive myelination, which is reflected in changes in the neurological exam. While most severe cases of CP are identified by 24 months of age, some cases, particularly of dystonic CP, do not become manifest until adolescence; in these cases the static lesion or anomaly was present early in development but clinically silent until uncovered by brain maturation.

Screening for conditions that commonly co-occur with CP such as mental retardation, ophthalmologic abnormalities, hearing impairments, speech and language disorders, and disorders of oral-motor functioning should be part of the initial assessment.

Laboratory Tests

Current practice parameters (Ashwal, et al., 2004) recommend brain imaging as a first step in order to determine whether a brain abnormality exists that may, in turn, suggest and etiology and prognosis. MRI is preferred to CT because of the higher yield in suggesting an etiology and timing of insult leading to CP (see Brain Imaging, below). MRI has been found to identify major brain malformations in up to 12% of cases. Because these malformations (e.g., lissencephaly, schizencephaly, or pachygyria) are increasingly associated with specific genetic disorders, their presence in children with CP indicates the need for further genetic testing. Cerebral malformations are also found in certain neurometabolic disorders (e.g., peroxisomal disorders); these disorders can present within the first years of life with motor impairment that may appear to be nonprogressive. Metabolic disorders that may be misdiagnosed as CP are reviewed by Gupta and Appleton (2001).

Even in the absence of cerebral malformation, metabolic and genetic testing should be considered in the following situations: (a) absence of a definite preceding prenatal, perinatal, or postnatal insult, (b) presence of a positive family history of CP, (c) occurrence of developmental regression (loss of abilities), (d) presence of oculomotor abnormalities, involuntary movements, ataxia, muscle atrophy, or sensory loss. Because the incidence of cerebral infarction is high in children with hemiplegic CP, testing for coagulation disorders may be considered. Currently EEG is not recommended except when there is clinical suspicion of seizures (Ashwal, et al., 2004).

Disclosure

Research evidence indicates that, when interviewed, around half of parents of children with physical disability report dissatisfaction with the manner in which the disclosure was handled (Sloper & Turner, 1993). Evidence-based clinical guidelines for the sensitive disclosure of a diagnosis of CP have been advanced by Baird, McConachie, and Scrutton (2000), and the reader is urged to consult them.

Prognosis for Motor Function

When the diagnosis of CP is disclosed to parents, their first question is often "Will my child walk?" As reviewed by Sala and Grant (1995), three major factors (primitive reflexes and postural reactions, gross motor skills, and topography of CP) contribute to the inability to ambulate independently. Specifically, the persistence of primitive reflexes and absence of postural reactions by age of 2 is associated with poor prognosis for independent ambulation. Sitting without support by the age of 2 years is associated with attainment of ambulation. Children with spastic hemiplegia will walk independently, those with spastic diplegia will walk independently 85% of the time, and those with spastic quadriplegia are the least likely to walk independently. It must be noted, however, that there is wide variation in estimates of the likelihood of ambulation in children with spastic quadriplegia, ranging from 0 to 72% (Bottos & Gericke, 2003). In addition to these clinical criteria, a reliable and valid prognostic system that uses the GMFM is now available at www.canchild.org (Rosenbaum, et al., 2002).

Once achieved, independent walking is not necessarily maintained though adolescence and adulthood. Those who reach independent walking by the age of 3 years have a higher chance of maintaining the ability to walk than those who did not achieve it by that age. Important factors that influence the maintenance of ambulatory capacity are joint deterioration, physiological, or psychological burnout and surgery (Bottos, Feliciangeli, Scuito, Gericke, & Vianello, 2001).

On the other hand, CP diagnosed in the first 2 years of life may resolve during early childhood, especially if the functional impairment is mild (Ford, Kitchen, Doyle, Rickards, & Kelly, 1990). In the Collaborative Perinatal Project, 118 out of 229 children who had signs of CP at 1 year of age were found to be free from motor handicap when reexamined at age 7. Mild CP resolved in 72% of cases, but only 3% of severe cases resolved. However, mental retardation and nonfebrile seizures were almost 10 times more likely in children with resolved CP than in children with no history of CP (Nelson & Ellenberg, 1982). Thus it appears that even the child who improves is at risk for associated conditions.

Implications of Early Motor Status for Intervention and Management

By the age of 3 years, children generally fall into one of three groups: (1) those who are not sitting independently, but do exhibit locomotion patterns that require at least some trunk control such as crawling and bottom shuffling, (2) those who are sitting independently, but who have yet to develop independent walking and, (3) those who have already achieved independent walking (Bottos & Gericke, 2003).

For children in the first group, some authorities feel that the clinician and family should not wait to see whether the child will eventually become an independent walker due to maturation and therapy. These children need assistive devices to promote motor independence (typically this means a powered wheelchair). Without such assistance, their development will be hampered by ineffective mobility, fatigue, and reliance upon others. For children in the second group, physiotherapy may be indicated, together with the use appropriate orthoses and orthopedic surgery. After the age of 7 years, physiotherapy aimed at promoting walking should be limited, because independent walking is unlikely to be achieved after that age, particularly when spasticity is present. Even when walking is attained, assistive mobility devices should be used to widen the child's motor autonomy and avoid early physiological burnout. This is particularly true for those with mild and moderate motor impairment who may be more likely to struggle to keep up with peers. Children in the third group need close monitoring and need to have periodic session of physiotherapy well into adulthood in order to prevent deformities (Bottos & Gericke, 2003).

When gross motor impairment is minimal and orthopedic care is not indicated, it may be preferable to not make a formal diagnosis of CP because the diagnosis may carry the stigma of associated problems that may not be present, such as mental retardation (Russman, 1992). However, parents may need to be advised that other professionals they encounter may use the term CP, so the reasons for not making a formal diagnosis should be openly explained to the parents.

Cognitive Implications of CP

In most patients a prognosis about intellectual development must be deferred pending the development of language. Testing language is based on testing earling intelligence and early tests depend inordinately on visuomotor skills. Therefore in questionable situations a prognosis cannot and should not be rendered until after age 5 years. In the athetoid patient who might have a severe dysarthria, a prognosis about intelligence should be postponed until school age. An examiner experienced with the severely disabled dyskinetic population should perform the evaluation because the motor disability could lead to misleading scores. While severe cognitive impairment is rare among those with hemiparesis (about half of whom generally score in the normal range), it predominates among those with quadriparesis (Fennell & Dikel, 2001). Cognitive impairment is most severe among those with seizure activity (Vargha-Khadem, Isaacs, van der Werf, Robb, & Wilson, 1992).

In general, children with CP tend to have lower performance than verbal IQ scores (Fedrizzi, et al., 1996; Goodman & Yude, 1996; Ito, et al., 1996; Muter, Taylor, & Vargha-Khadem, 1997); the difference is unrelated to side of lesion (Muter, et al., 1997). However, it is the performance portion of the IQ tests used in these studies that most depends on motor skills. Tests with a yes/no or multiple-choice format, where answers can be indicated with minimal motor input and with no penalty for slow response times, allow clear separation of motor and cognitive abilities. Two recent studies using such techniques demonstrated greater visual–perceptual than language impairment in children with CP (Sabbadini, Bonanni, Carlesimo, & Caltagirone, 2001; Stiers, et al., 2002). In one of these studies patients indicated answers using prosthetic pointing devices (Sabbadini, et al., 2001). In this study, eight individuals with severe neuromotor and verbal disabilities performed comparably to 19 controls matched for mental age on all tests of language except for comprehension of syntactically complex sentences.

Psychosocial Issues in CP

Children with chronic functional limitations have considerably more difficulties in the social and behavioral aspects of their lives than typical children. Intellectual and behavioral problems in children with hemiplegic CP reported by teachers in mainstream schools indicate that such children are at a high risk for rejection by peers, for lack of friends, and for victimization (Yude & Goodman, 1999).

Brain damage is a risk factor for childhood psychiatric disorder. In the Isle of Wight study, children with CP were three times more likely to have a psychiatric disorder than peers in the general population. This finding was not accounted for by differences in IQ or physical handicap (Rutter, 1989), suggesting that brain injury accounted for the behavioral difficulties. A more recent population-based study found that parent-reported behavior problems were five times more likely in children with CP than in children with no health problems; behavior problems were even more common in children with both CP and mental retardation. The most frequent problems were dependency and headstrong and hyperactive behavior (McDermott, et al., 1996). The pharmacologic treatment of ADHD symptomatology in children with CP has received little attention. A single controlled study found that methylphenidate resulted in animprovement in ADHD symptoms, as assessed by both parent and teacher ratings (Gross-Tsur, Shalev, Badihi, & Manor, 2002.

Medical Management of CP

Assisting persons with CP requires a team approach in which the family and patient are leaders whenever possible.

Motor Function, Mobility, and Posture

The elimination of spasticity allows many patients with CP to use what selective motor control they possess more functionally. Spasticity associated with CP can lead to musculoskeletal complications such as contracture, pain, and subluxation.

Management of spasticity in the patient with CP involves multiple approaches, including environmental interventions such as minimizing sleep deprivation, alleviating pain, therapeutic use of heat, and/or deep tissue massage and reducing prolonged periods of immobility. Multiple oral medications are used to treat spasticity but have limited efficacy in most patients due to unacceptable side effects. Injectable neuromuscular blocking agents balance muscle power across joints by effecting selective denervation of muscles and nerves; botulinum toxin A is now the most widely used blocking agent (Bottos, Benedetti, Salucci, Gasparroni, & Giannini, 2003; Edgar, 2001). Neurosurgical interventions include the baclofen pump and selective dorsal rhizotomy. Placement of a pump to allow the delivery of baclofen directly to the spinal cord is more effective at reducing spasticity and dystonia without the cognitive side effects that are frequently seen with oral administration of the drugs. Selective dorsal rhizotomy involves the selective ablation of dorsal nerve rootlets and results in reduced tone in the lower extremities. Surgical tendon release is also used widely to help ambulation in CP (Koman, Smith, & Shilt, 2004). However, little careful evaluation has been done of the comparative efficacy of these modalities. Specialty organizations such United Cerebral Palsy Association and the American Academy for Cerebral Palsy and Developmental medicine have Web sites (www.ucpa.org and www. aacpdm.org, respectively) that can be informative and helpful to parents.

Epilepsy

Children with CP are at excess risk for epilepsy. In the general pediatric population, the prevalence of epilepsy is 3 to 6 per 1,000. By contrast, in a population-based study of children with CP, the prevalence of epilepsy was observed to be 38%. All children with quadriplegic CP and about one third of children with other types of CP developed epilepsy. Children with mental retardation have a higher frequency of epilepsy than those without mental retardation (Carlsson, Hagberg, & Olsson, 2003).

General Treatment Principles

The WHO model of health and disease focuses on the promotion of function and participation as the broad goals of medicine. It provides an important framework to guide modern thinking about treatment for children with CP (World Health Organization, 2001).

First, communication skills must be promoted. Without this ability, even with a normal intellect, the patient is isolated. Treatment of children with CP in the past has often focused on improving motor function, and communication has been relatively neglected (Russman, 1992).

Second, the achievement of functional abilities that facilitate autonomy must be emphasized. The liberal use of adaptive equipment may support early development of capacities with the important effect of improving overall development. The common concern that making things too easy for children will inhibit normal function is without basis. Robust evidence exists that the provision of powered mobility to children with disability as young as 36 months can have positive impact on social, language and play skills and promote independent movements (Butler, 1991).

Third, modern services for persons with CP need to be offered within a family-centered model in which parents and providers work together as partners. Parents' satisfaction with services is inversely related to their stress in their dealing with their child's treatment; their satisfaction is greater and their stress less with family centered as compared to other treatment models (King, Rosenbaum, & King, 1996). There is also an association between family-centered service and parents' mental health (King, King, Rosenbaum, & Goffin, 1999).

Finally, goal setting should be a collaborative effort between parents (and older children) and health care providers. CP is a chronic condition that requires intensive planning for full participation in the community. "This challenge is one that must be addressed by the whole community, and should involve the imagination and political will of professionals and families from all areas of society. To do less would be marginalize young people with CP and to squander the developmental and functional gains they have made in their developing years" (Rosenbaum, 2003, p. 973).

REFERENCES

Abernethy, L. J., Klafkowshi, G., Foulder-Hughes, L., Cooker, R. W. (2003). Magnetic resonance imaging and T2 relaxometry of cerebral white matter and hippocampus in children born preterm. *Pediatric Research*, 54: 868–874.

Achenbach, T. M. (1991). *Manual for the child behavior checklist/4-18 and 1991 profile.* Burlington, VT: University of Vermont, Department of Psychiatry.

Ajayi-Obe, M., Saeed, N., Cowan, F. M., Rutherford, M. A., & Edwards, A. D. (2000). Reduced development of cerebral cortex in extremely preterm infants. *Lancet*, 356: 1162–1163.

Allen, M. C. (2002a). Overview: Prematurity. *Mental Retardation & Developmental Disabilities Research Reviews*, 8: 213–214.

Allin, M., Henderson, M., Suckling, J., Nosarti, C., Rushe, T., Fearon, P., Bullmore, E. T., et al. (2004). Effects of very low birthweight on brain structure in adulthood. *Developmental Medicine & Child Neurology*, 46:46–53.

Allin, M., Matsumoto, H., Santhouse, A. M., Nosarti, C., Al Asady, M. H., Stewart, A. L., et al. (2001). Cognitive and motor function and the size of the cerebellum in adolescents born very pre-term. *Brain*, 124: 60–66.

Als, H., Duffy, F. H., & McAnulty, G. B. (1988). The APIB, an assessment of functional competence in preterm and fullterm newborns regardless of gestational age at birth. II. *Infant Behavior and Development*, 11: 319–331.

Anand, K. J., & Scalzo, F. M. (2000). Can adverse neonatal experiences alter brain development and subsequent behavior? *Biology of the Neonate*, 77: 69–82.

Ashwal, S., Russman, B. S., Blasco, P. A., Miller, G., Sandler, A., Shevell, M., et al. (2004). Practice parameter: diagnostic assessment of the child with cerebral palsy: report of the quality standards subcommittee of the American Academy of Neurology and the Practice Committee of the Child Neurology Society. *Neurology*, 62: 851–863.

Aylward, G. P. (2002). Cognitive and neuropsychological outcomes: More than IQ scores. *Mental Retardation and Developmental Disabilities Research Reviews*, 8: 234–240.

Baird, G., McConachie, H., & Scrutton, D. (2000). Parents' perceptions of disclosure of the diagnosis of cerebral palsy. *Archives of Disease in Childhood*, 83: 475–480.

Barker, D. J. (1995). Fetal origins of coronary heart disease. *British Medical Journal*, 311: 171–174.

Berkowitz, G. S. and Papiernik, E. (1993) Epidemiology of preterm birth. Epidemiologic Reviews. 15:414-443

Bhutta, A. T., Cleves, M. A., Casey, P. H., Cradock, M. M., & Anand, K. J. S. (2002). Cognitive and behavioral outcomes of school-aged children who were born preterm—A meta-analysis. *J—Journal of the American Medical Association*, 288: 728–737.

Botting, N., Powls, A., Cooke, R. W. I., & Marlow, N. (1997). Attention deficit hyperactivity disorders and other psychiatric outcomes in very low birthweight children at 12 years. *Journal of Child Psychology and Psychiatry*, 38: 931–941.

Bottos, M., & Gericke, C. (2003). Ambulatory capacity in cerebral palsy: prognostic criteria and consequences for intervention. *Developmental Medicine & Child Neurology*, 45: 786–790.

Bottos, M., Benedetti, M. G., Salucci, P., Gasparroni, V., & Giannini, S. (2003). Botulinum toxin with and without casting in ambulant children with spastic diplegia: a clinical and functional assessment. *Developmental Medicine & Child Neurology*, 45: 758–762.

Bottos, M., Feliciangeli, A., Sciuto, L. Gericke, C., & Vianello, A. (2001). Functional status of adults with cerebral palsy and implications for treatment of children. *Developmental Medicine & Child Neurology*, 43: 516–528.

Bowen, J. R., Gibson, F. L., & Hand, P. J. (2002). Educational outcome at 8 years for children who were born extremely prematurely: A controlled study. *Journal of Paediatrics and Child Health*, 38: 438– 444.

Bracewell, M., & Marlow, N. (2002). Patterns of motor disability in very preterm children. *Mental Retardation & Developmental Disabilities Research Reviews*, 8: 241–248.

Breslau, N. (1995). Psychiatric sequelae of Low Birth Weight. *Epidemiologic Review*, 17:96–106.

Breslau, N., Brown, G. G., DelDotto, J. E., Kumar, S., Ezthuthachan, S., Andreski, P., et al. (1996). Psychiatric Sequelae of Low Birth Weight at Six Years of Age. *Journal of Abnormal Child Psychology*, 24: 385–400.

Breslau, N., & Chilcoat, H. D. (2000). Psychiatric sequelae of low birth weight at 11 years of age. *Biological Psychiatry*, 47: 1005–1011.

Breslau, N., Chilcoat, H., DelDotto, J. E., Andreski, P., & Brown, G. G. (1996). Low Birth Weight and Neurocognitive Status at Six Years of Age. *Biological Psychiatry*, 40: 389–397.

Breslau, N., Johnson, E. O., & Lucia, V. C. (2001). Academic achievement of low birthweight children at age 11: The role of cognitive abilities at school entry. *Journal of Abnormal Child Psychology*, 29: 273–297.

Breslau, N., Paneth, N., & Lucia, V. C. (2004). The lingering academic deficits of low birthweight children. *Pediatrics*, 114: 1035–1040.

Briscoe, J., Gathercole, S. E., & Marlow, N. (1998). Short-term memory and language outcomes after extreme prematurity at birth. *Journal of Speech, Language, & Hearing Research*, 41: 654–666.

Buck, G. M., Msall, M. E., Schisterman, E. F., Lyon, N. R., & Rogers, B. T. (2000). Extreme prematurity and school outcomes. *Paediatric and Perinatal Epidemiology*, 14: 324–331.

Buka, S. L., Lipsitt, L. P., & Tsuang, M. T. (1992). Emotional and behavioral development of low-birthweight infants. In S.L.Friedman & M. D. Sigman (Eds.), *The Psychological Development of Low Birthweight Children* (pp. 187–214). Norwood, NJ: Ablex.

Butler, C. (1991). Walking: at what cost? In K.Jaffe (Ed.), *Pediatric Rehabilitation*. Physical Medicine and Rehab Clinics of North America (No 4. ed.) Philadelphia: WB Saunders.

Carlsson, M., Hagberg, G., & Olsson, I. (2003). Clinical and aetiological aspects of epilepsy in children with cerebral palsy. *Developmental Medicine & Child Neurology*, 45: 371–376.

Carr-Hill, R. A., & Hall, M. H. (1985). The repetition of spontaneous preterm labour. British *Journal of Obstetrics & Gynaecology*, 92: 921–928.

Chamnanvanakij, S., Rogers, C. G., Luppino, C. L., Broyles, S. R., Hickman, J. and Perlman J. M. (2000). Linear hyperechogenicity within the basal ganglia and thalamus of preterm infants. *Pediatric Neurology*, 23:129-133.

Chapieski, M. L., & Evankovich, K. D. (1997). Behavioral effects of prematurity. *Seminars in Perinatology*, 21: 221–239.

Chilcoat, H. D., & Breslau, N. (2002). Low birth weight as a vulnerability marker for early drug use. *Experimental and Clinical Psychopharmacology*, 10: 104–112.

Cohen, M. E., & Duffner, P. K. (1981). Prognostic indicators in hemiparetic cerebral palsy. *Annals of Neurology*, 9: 353–357.

Colver, A. F., & Sethumadhavan, T. (2003). The term diplegia should be abandoned. *Archives of Disease in Childhood*, 88: 286–290.

Cooke, R. W., & Abernethy, L. J. (1999). Cranial magnetic resonance imaging and school performance in very low birth weight infants in adolescence. *Archives of Disease in Childhood Fetal & Neonatal Edition*, 81: F116–F121.

Cooke, R. W. I. (2004). Health, lifestyle, and quality of life for young adults born very preterm. *Archives of Disease in Childhood*, 89: 201–206.

Corman, H., & Chaikind, S. (1998). The effect of low birthweight on the school performance and behavior of school-aged children. *Economics of Education Review*, 17: 307–316.

Counsell, S. J., Allsop, J. M., Harrison, M. C., Larkman, D. J., Kennea, N. L., Kapellou, O., et al. (2003). Diffusion-weighted imaging of the brain in preterm infants with focal and diffuse white matter abnormality. *Pediatrics*, 112: 1–7.

Counsell, S. J., Rutherford, M. A., Cowan, F. M., & Edwards, A. D. (2003). Magnetic resonance imaging of preterm brain injury. *Archives of Disease in Childhood—Fetal and Neonatal Edition*, 88: F269–F274.

Cummins, S. K., Nelson, K. B., Grether, J. K., & Velie, E.M. (1993). Cerebral palsy in four northern California counties, births 1983 through 1985. *Journal of Pediatrics*, 123: 230–237.

Cunningham, F. G., MacDonald, P. C., Gant, N. F., Leveno, K. J., Gilstrap, L. C., & Hawkins, G. D. V. (1997). Parturition. In *Williams Obstetrics* (20th ed., pp. 261–317). Stamford, CT: Appleton & Lange.

Curtis, W. J., Lindeke, L. L., Georgieff, M. K., & Nelson, C.A. (2002). Neurobehavioural functioning in neonatal intensive care unit graduates in late childhood and early adolescence. *Brain*, 125: 1646–1659.

de Rogalski, L.I., Minokoshi, M., Silveira, D. C., Cha, B. H., & Holmes, G. L. (2001). Recurrent neonatal seizures: relationship of pathology to the electroencephalogram and cognition. *Brain Research Developmental Brain Research*, 129: 27–38.

den Ouden, L., Rijken, M., Brand, R., Verloove-Vanhorick, S. P., & Ruys, J. H. (1991). Is it correct to correct? Developmental milestones in 555 "normal" preterm infants compared with term infants. *Journal of Pediatrics*, 118: 399–404.

Edgar, T. S. (2001). Clinical utility of botulinum toxin in the treatment of cerebral palsy: comprehensive review. *Journal of Child Neurology*, 16: 37–46.

Ekwo, E. E., Gosselink, C. A., & Moawad, A. (1992). Unfavorable outcome in penultimate pregnancy and premature rupture of membranes in successive pregnancy. *Obstetrics & Gynecology*, 80: 166–172.

Elgen, I., & Sommerfelt, K. (2002). Low birthweight children: coping in school? *Acta Paediatrica*, 91: 939–945.

Emond, A., Golding, J., & Peckham, C. (1989). Cerebral palsy in two national cohort studies. *Archives of Disease in Childhood*, 64: 848– 852.

Fedrizzi, E., Inverno, M., Grazia Bruzzone, M., Botteon, G., Saletti, V., & Farinotti, M. (1996). MRI features of cerebral lesions and cognitive functions in preterm spastic diplegic children. *Pediatric Neurology*, 15: 207–212.

Feingold, E., Sheir-Neiss, G., Melnychuk, J., Bachrach, S., & Paul, D. (2002). HRQL and severity of brain ultrasound findings in a cohort of adolescents who were born preterm. *Journal of Adolescent Health*, 31: 234–239.

Fennell, E. B., & Dikel, T. N. (2001). Cognitive and neuropsychological functioning in children with cerebral palsy. *Journal of Child Neurology*, 16: 58–63.

Ferrari, F., Cioni, G., Einspieler, C., Roversi, M. F., Bos, A. F., Paolicelli, P. B., et al. (2002). Cramped synchronized general movements in preterm infants as an early marker for cerebral palsy. [see comment]. *Archives of Pediatrics & Adolescent Medicine*, 156: 460–467.

Ford, G. W., Doyle, L. W., Davis, N. M., & Callanan, C. (2000). Very low birth weight and growth into adolescence. *Archives of Pediatrics Adolescent Medicine*, 154: 778–784.

Ford, G. W., Kitchen, W. H., Doyle, L. W., Rickards, A. L., & Kelly, E. (1990). Changing diagnosis of cerebral palsy in very low birthweight children. *American Journal of Perinatology*, 7: 178–181.

Foulder-Hughes, L. A., & Cooke, R. W. I. (2003). Motor, cognitive, and behavioural disorders in children born very preterm. *Developmental Medicine and Child Neurology*, 45: 97–103.

Frisk, V., & Whyte, H. (1994). The long-term consequences of periventricular brain damage on language and verbal memory. *Developmental Neuropsychology*, 10: 313–333.

Ganat, Y., Soni, S., Chacon, M., Schwartz, M. L., & Vaccarino, F. M. (2002). Chronic hypoxia up-regulates fibroblast growth factor ligands in the perinatal brain and induces fibroblast growth factor-responsive radial glial cells in the sub-ependymal zone. *Neuroscience*, 112: 977–991.

Gibbs, R. S., Rosenberg, A. R., Warren, C. J., Galan, H. L., & Rumack, C. M. (2004). Suggestions for practice to accompany neonatal encephalopathy and cerebral palsy. *Obstetrics & Gynecology*, 103: 778–779.

Goodman, R., & Yude, C. (1996). IQ and its predictors in childhood hemiplegia. *Developmental Medicine & Child Neurology*, 38: 881–890.

Grantham-McGregor, S. M. (1998). Small for gestational age, term babies, in the first six years of life. *European Journal of Clinical Nutrition*, 52 Sup 1: S59–S64.

Green, N. S., Damus, K., Simpson, J. L., et al. and the March of Dimes Scientific Advisory Committee on Prematurity (2005) American Journal of Obstetrics and Gynecology 193:626-635.

Grether, J. K., Nelson, K. B., Walsh, E., Willoughby, R. E., & Redline, R. W. (2003). Intrauterine exposure to infection and risk of cerebral palsy in very preterm infants. *Archives of Pediatrics & Adolescent Medicine*, 157: 26-32.

Gross-Tsur, V., Shalev, R. S., Badihi, N., & Manor, O. (2002). Efficacy of methylphenidate in patients with cerebral palsy and attention-deficit hyperactivity disorder (ADHD). *Journal of Child Neurology*, 17: 863-866.

Grunau, R. (2002). Early pain in preterm infants. A model of long-term effects. *Clinics in Perinatology*, 29: 373-394.

Gupta, R., & Appleton, R. E. (2001). Cerebral palsy: not always what it seems. *Archives of Disease in Childhood*, 85: 356-360.

Gyetvai, K., Hannah, M. E., Hodnett, E. D., & Ohlsson, A. (1999). Tocolytics for preterm labor: a systematic review. *Obstetrics & Gynecology*, 94: 869-877.

Hack, M., & Fanaroff, A. A. (2000). Outcomes of children of extremely low birthweight and gestational age in the 1990s. *Seminars in Neonatology*, 5: 89-106.

Hack, M., Flannery, D. J., Schluchter, M., Cartar, L., Borawski, E., & Klein, N. (2002). Outcomes in Young Adulthood for Very-Low-Birth-Weight Infants. *New England Journal of Medicine*, 346: 149-157.

Hagberg, B., Hagberg, G., Beckung, E., & Uvebrant, P. (2001). Changing panorama of cerebral palsy in Sweden. VIII. Prevalence and origin in the birth year period 1991-94. *Acta Paediatrica*, 90: 271-277.

Harrison, H. (2002). Letter to the editor re "Outcomes in young adulthood for very-low-birth-weight infants." *New England Journal of Medicine*, 347: 141.

Hård, A. L., Niklasson, A., Svensson, E., & Hellström, A. (2000). Visual function in school-aged children born before 29 weeks of gestation: a population-based study. *Developmental Medicine & Child Neurology*, 42: 100-105.

Henriksen, T., & Clausen, T. (2002). The fetal origins hypothesis: placental insufficiency and inheritance versus maternal malnutrition in well-nourished populations. *Acta Obstetricia et Gynecologica Scandinavica*, 81: 112-114.

Herrgard, E., Luoma, L., Tuppurainen, K., Karjalainen, S., & Martikainen, A. (1993). Neurodevelopmental profile at five years of children born at <=32 weeks gestation. *Developmental Medicine and Child Neurology*, 35: 1083-1096.

Heuchan, A. M., Evans, N., Henderson Smart, D. J., & Simpson, J. M. (2002). Perinatal risk factors for major intraventricular haemorrhage in the Australian and New Zealand Neonatal Network, 1995-97. *Archives of Disease in Childhood Fetal & Neonatal Edition*, 86: F86-F90.

Hille, E. T., Den Ouden, A. L., Saigal, S., Wolke, D., Lambert, M., Whitaker, A., et al. (2001). Behavioural problems in children who weigh 1000 g or less at birth in four countries. *Lancet*, 357: 1641-1643.

Hindmarsh, G. J., O'Callaghan, M. J., Mohay, H. A., & Rogers, Y. M. (2000). Gender differences in cognitive abilities at 2 years in ELBW infants. *Early Human Development*, 60: 115-122.

Honeycutt, A., Dunlap, L., Chen, H., & Homsi, G. (2004). Economic costs associated with mental retardation, cerebral palsy, hearing loss, and vision impairment—United States, 2003. *Morbidity and Mortality Weekly Report*, 53: 57-59.

Horwood, L. J., Mogridge, N., & Darlow, B. A. (1998). Cognitive, educational, and behavioural outcomes at 7 to 8 years in a national very low birthweight cohort. *Archives of Disease in Childhood—Fetal and Neonatal Edition*, 79: F12-F20.

Huppi, P. S., Maier, S. E., Peled, S., Zientara, G. P., Barnes, P. D., Jolesz, F. A., et al. (1998a). Microstructural development of human newborn cerebral white matter assessed in vivo by diffusion tensor magnetic resonance imaging. *Pediatric Research*, 44: 584-590.

Huppi, P. S., Murphy, B., Maier, S. E., Zientara, G. P., Inder, T. E., Barnes, P. D., et al. (2001). Microstructural brain development after perinatal cerebral white matter injury assessed by diffusion tensor magnetic resonance imaging. *Pediatrics*, 107: 455-460.

Huppi, P. S., Warfield, S., Kikinis, R., Barnes, P. D., Zientara, G. P., Jolesz, F. A., et al. (1998b). Quantitative magnetic resonance imaging of brain development in premature and mature newborns. *Annals of Neurology*, 43: 224-235.

Hutton, J. L., & Pharoah, P. O. (2002). Effects of cognitive, motor, and sensory disabilities on survival in cerebral palsy. *Archives of Disease in Childhood*, 86: 84-89.

Ingemarsson, I. (2003). Gender aspects of preterm birth. *BJOG: an International Journal of Obstetrics and Gynaecology*, 110 Suppl 20:34-38.

Isaacs, E. B., Edmonds, C. J., Lucas, A., & Gadian, D. G. (2001). Calculation difficulties in children of very low birthweight: A neural correlate. *Brain*, 124: 1701-1707.

Isaacs, E. B., Lucas, A., Chong, W. K., Wood, S. J., Johnson, C. L., Marshall, C., et al. (2000). Hippocampal volume and everyday memory in children of very low birth weight. *Pediatric Research*, 47: 713-720.

Ito, J., Saijo, H., Araki, A., Tanaka, H., Tasaki, T., Cho, K., et al. (1996). Assessment of visuoperceptual disturbance in children with spastic diplegia using measurements of the lateral ventricles on cerebral MRI. *Developmental Medicine & Child Neurology*, 38: 496-502.

Johnson, E. O. & Breslau, N. (2000). Increased risk of learning disabilities in low birthweight boys at age 11 years. *Biological Psychiatry*, 47: 490-500.

Kiely, J. L., & Paneth, N. (1981). Follow-up studies of low-birthweight infants: Suggestions for design, analysis and reporting. *Developmental Medicine & Child Neurology*, 23: 96-101.

King, G., King, S., Rosenbaum, P., & Goffin, R. (1999). Family-centered caregiving and well-being of parents of children with disabilities: Linking process with outcome. *Journal of Pediatric Psychology*, 24: Feb-53.

King, S. M., Rosenbaum, P. L., & King, G. A. (1996). Parents' perceptions of caregiving: development and validation of a measure of processes. *Developmental Medicine & Child Neurology*, 38: 757-772.

Kitchen, W. H., Ford, G. W., Murton, L. J., Rickards, A., Ryan, M. M., Lissenden, J. V., et al. (1985). Mortality and two year outcome of infants of birthweight 500-1500 g: Relationships with neonatal cerebral ultrasound data. *Australian Paediatric Journal*, 21: 253-259.

Klebanov, P. K., Brooks-Gunn, J., & McCormick, M. C. (1994). School achievement and failure in very low birth weight children. *Developmental and Behavioral Pediatrics*, 15: 248-256.

Koman, L. A., Smith, B. P., & Shilt, J. S. (2004). Cerebral Palsy. *Lancet*, 363: 1619-1631.

Kunugi, H. N. (2001). Obstetric complications and schizophrenia: prenatal underdevelopment and subsequent neurodevelopmental impairment. *British Journal of Psychiatry*, 178: S25-S29.

Largo, R. H., Molinari, L., Pinto, L. C., Weber, M., & Duc, G. (1986). Language development of term and preterm children during the first five years of life. *Developmental Medicine and Child Neurology*, 28: 333-350.

Le Normand, M. T., & Cohen, H. (1999). The delayed emergence of lexical morphology in preterm children: the case of verbs. *Journal of Neurolinguistics*, 12: 235-246.

Levene, M., Dowling, S., Graham, M., Fogelman, K., Galton, M., & Phillips, M. (1992). Impaired motor function (clumsiness) in 5 year old children: Correlation with neonatal ultrasound scans. *Archives of Disease in Childhood*, 67: 687-690.

Leviton, A., & Gilles, F. (1997).Ventriculomegaly, delayed myelination, white matter hypoplasia and "periventricular" leukomalacia: How are they related? *Pediatric Neurology*, 15: 127-135.

Leviton, A., Paneth,N., Reuss, M. L., Susser, M., Allred, E. N., Dammann, O., et al. (1999). Maternal infection, fetal inflammatory response, and brain damage in very low birth weight infants. Developmental Epidemiology Network Investigators. *Pediatric Research*, 46: 566-575.

Levy, S. R., Abroms, I. F., Marshall, P. C., & Rosquete, E. E. (1985). Seizures and cerebral infarction in the full-term newborn. *Annals of Neurology*, 17: 366-370.

Lockwood, C. J., & Kuczynski, E. (2001). Risk stratification and pathological mechanisms in preterm delivery. *Paediatric and Perinatal Epidemiology*, 15: 78-89.

Luciana, M. (2003). Cognitive development in children born preterm: Implications for theories of brain plasticity following early injury. *Development and Psychopathology*, 15: 1017-1047.

Luciana, M., Lindeke, L., Georgieff, M., Mills, M., & Nelson, C. (1999), Neurobehavioral evidence for working-memory deficits in school-aged children with histories of prematurity. *Developmental Medicine & Child Neurology*, 41: 521-533.

Luoma, L., Herrgard, E., & Martikainen, A. (1998). Neuropsychological analysis of the visuomotor problems in children born preterm at , or iqual to 32 weeks of gestation: a 5-year prospective follow-up. *Developmental Medicine and Child Neurology*, 40: 21–30.

Marin-Padilla, M. (1997). Developmental neuropathology and impact of perinatal brain damage. II: white matter lesions of the neocortex. *Journal of Neuropathology & Experimental Neurology*, 56: 219–235.

Marin-Padilla, M. (1999). Developmental neuropathology and impact of perinatal brain damage. III: gray matter lesions of the neocortex. *Journal of Neuropathology & Experimental Neurology*, 58: 407–429.

Marlow, N., Roberts, B. L., & Cooke, R. W. I. (1989). Motor skills in extremely low birthweight children at the age of 6 years. *Archives of Disease in Childhood*, 64: 839–847.

Mathews, T. J., Menacker, F., & MacDorman, M. F. (2002). Infant mortality statistics from the 2000 period linked birth/infant death data set. *National Vital Statistics Reports*, 50: 1–28.

Mattison, D. R., Damus, K., Fiore, E., Petrini, J., & Alter, C. (2001). Preterm delivery: a public health perspective. *Pediatric and Perinatal Epidemiology*, 15: 7–16.

McClellan, R., & Novak, D. (2001). Fetal nutrition: how we become what we are. *Journal of Pediatric Gastroenterology & Nutrition*, 33: 233–244.

McDermott, S., Coker, A. L., Mani, S., Krishnaswami, S., Nagle, R. J., Barnett-Queen, L. L., et al. (1996). A population-based analysis of behavior problems in children with cerebral palsy. *Journal of Pediatric Psychology*, 21: 447–463.

Ment, L. R., Bada, H. S., Barnes, P., Grant, P. E., Hirtz, D., Papile, L. A., et al. (2002). Practice parameter: neuroimaging of the neonate: report of the Quality Standards Subcommittee of the American Academy of Neurology and the Practice Committee of the Child Neurology Society. *Neurology*, 58: 1726–1738.

Ment, L. R., Duncan, C. C., & Ehrenkranz, R. A. (1984). Perinatal cerebral infarction. *Annals of Neurology*, 16: 559–568.

Ment, L. R., Vohr, B., Allan, W., Westerveld, M., Katz, K. H., Schneider, K. C., et al. (1999). The etiology and outcome of cerebral ventriculomegaly at term in very low birth weight preterm infants. *Pediatrics*, 104: 243–248.

Mercuri, E., He, J., Curati, W. L., Dubowitz, L. M., Cowan, F. M., & Bydder, G. M. (1997). Cerebellar infarction and atrophy in infants and children with a history of premature birth. *Pediatric Radiology*, 27: 139–143.

Merrill, J. D., Piecuch, R. E., Fell, S. C., Barkovich, A. J., & Goldstein, R. B. (1998). A new pattern of cerebellar hemorrhages in preterm infants. *Pediatrics*, 102: E62.

Moutquin, J-M. (2003). Classification and heterogeneity of preterm birth. *BJOG: an International Journal of Obstetrics & Gynaecology*, 110: 30–33.

Msall, M. E., & Tremont, M. R. (2002a). Measuring functional outcomes after prematurity: Developmental impact of very low birth weight and extremely low birth weight status on childhood disability. *Mental Retardation and Developmental Disabilities Research Reviews*, 8: 258–272.

Msall, M. E., & Tremont, M. R. (2002b). Measuring functional outcomes after prematurity: developmental impact of very low birth weight and extremely low birth weight status on childhood disability. *Mental Retardation & Developmental Disabilities Research Reviews*, 8: 258–272.

Mutch, L., Alberman, E., Hagberg, B., Kodama, K., & Perat, M. V. (1992). Cerebral palsy epidemiology: where are we now and where are we going? *Developmental Medicine & Child Neurology*, 34: 54– 551.

Muter, V., Taylor, S., & Vargha-Khadem, F. (1997). A longitudinal study of early intellectual development in hemiplegic children. *Neuropsychologia*, 35: 289–298.

Nelson, C. A. (1995). The ontogeny of human memory - a cognitive neuroscience perspective. *Developmental Psychology*, 31: 723–738.

Nelson, K. B., & Ellenberg, J. H. (1978). Epidemiology of cerebral palsy. In B. S. Schoenberg (Ed.), *Advances in Neurology* (pp. 421–435). New York: Raven Press.

Nelson, K. B., & Ellenberg, J. H. (1982). Children who 'outgrew' cerebral palsy. *Pediatrics*, 69: 529–536.

Nelson, K. B., & Ellenberg, J. H. (1986). Antecedents of cerebral palsy. Multivariate analysis of risk. *New England Journal of Medicine*, 315: 81–86.

Nelson, K. B., & Grether, J. K. (1999). Causes of cerebral palsy. *Current Opinion in Pediatrics*, 11: 487–491.

Nosarti, C., Al Asady, M. H., Frangou, S., Stewart, A. L., Rifkin, L., & Murray, R. M. (2002). Adolescents who were born very preterm have decreased brain volumes. *Brain*, 125: 1616–1623.

O'Callaghan, M. J., Burns, Y. R., Gray, P. H., Harvey, J. M., Mohay H., Rogers, Y. M., et al. (1996). School performance of ELBW children: a controlled study. *Developmental Medicine and Child Neurology*, 38: 917–926.

Okoshi, Y., Itoh, M., Takashima, S. (2001) Characteristic neuropathology and plasticity in periventricular leukomalacia. *Pediatric Neurology*, 256: 221-226.

Palisano, R. J., Rosenbaum, P. L., Walter, S. D., Russell, D. J., Wood, E. P., & Galuppi, B. E. (1997a). Development and reliability of a system to classify gross motor function in children with cerebral palsy. *Developmental Medicine & Child Neurology*, 39: 214–223.

Palisano, R. J., Rosenbaum, P. L., Walter, S. D., Russell, D. J., Wood, E. P., & Galuppi, B. E. (1997b). Development and reliability of a system to classify gross motor function in children with cerebral palsy. *Developmental Medicine & Child Neurology*, 39: 214–223.

Paneth, N. & Kiely, J. (1984). The frequency of cerebral palsy: a review of population studies in industrialised nations since 1950. In F. Stanley & E. Alberman (Eds.), *The epidemiology of the cerebral palsies* (pp. 46–56). London, England: Spastics International.

Paneth, N., & Susser, M. (1995). Early origin of coronary heart disease (the "Barker hypothesis"). *British Medical Journal*, 310: 411–412,.

Paneth, N., Ahmed, F., & Stein, A. D. (1996). Early nutritional origins of hypertension: a hypothesis still lacking support. *Journal of Hypertension—Supplement* 14: S121–S129.

Paneth, N., Rudelli, R., Monte, W., et al. White matter necrosis in very low birthweight infants: Neuropathologic and ultrasonographic findings in infants surviving six days or more. J Pediatrics 1990; 116:975-984.

Paneth, N., Bishai, S., Qui, H., et al. (2003) Reliability of cerebral palsy diagnosis across international cohorts of low birth weight infants. Developmental Medicine and Child Neurology 45:628-633.

Papile, L. A., Musick-Bruno, G., & Schafer, A. (1983). Relationship of cerebral interventricular hemorrhage and early childhood neurologic handicaps. *Journal of Pediatrics*, 103: 273–277.

Perlman, J. M. (2001). Neurobehavioral Deficits in Premature Graduates of Intensive Care—Potential Medical and Neonatal Environmental Risk Factors. *Pediatrics*, 108:1339–1348.

Perlman, J. M. (2003). The genesis of cognitive and behavioral deficits in premature graduates of intensive care. *Minerva Pediatrica*, 55: 89–101.

Perlman, J. M., & Volpe, J. J. (1989). Movement disorder of premature infants with severe bronchopulmonary dysplasia: A new syndrome. *Pediatrics*, 84: 215–218.

Peterson, B. S., Vohr, B., Kane, M. J., Whalen, D. H., Schneider, K. C., Katz, K. H., et al. (2002). A functional magnetic resonance imaging study of language processing and its cognitive correlates in prematurely born children. *Pediatrics*, 110: 1153–1162.

Pinto-Martin, J.A., Riolo, S., Cnaan, A., Holzman, C., Susser, M.W., and Paneth, N. (1995). Cranial ultrasound prediction of disabling and non-disabling cerebral palsy at age two in a low birthweight population. Pediatrics, 95:249-254.

Pinto-Martin, J., Whitaker, A., Feldman, J., Cnaan, A., Zhao, H., Rosen-Bloch, J., et al. (2004). Special education services and school performance in a regional cohort of low-birthweight infants at age nine. *Paediatric and Perinatal Epidemiology*, 18: 120–129.

Pinto-Martin, J. A., Riolo, S., Cnaan, A., Holzman, C., Susser, M. W., & Paneth, N. (1995). Cranial ultrasound prediction of disabling and non-disabling cerebral palsy at age two in a low birthweight population. *Pediatrics*, 95: 249–254.

Pinto-Martin, J. A., Whitaker, A. H., Feldman, J. F., Van Rossem, R., & Paneth, N. (1999). Relation of cranial ultrasound abnormalities in low-birthweight infants to motor or cognitive performance at ages 2, 6, and 9 years. *Developmental Medicine & Child Neurology*, 41: 826–833.

Powls, A., Botting, N., Cooke, R. W., Stephenson, G., & Marlow, N. (1997). Visual impairment in very low birthweight children. *Archives of Disease in Childhood—Fetal & Neonatal Edition*, 76: F82–F87.

Raz, S., Lauterbach, M. D., Hopkins, T. L., Porter, C. L., Riggs, W. W., & Sander, C. J. (1995). Severity of perinatal cerebral injury and developmental outcome: A dose-response relationship. *Neuropsychology*, 9: 91–101.

Richards, J. E. (1994). Baseline respiratory sinus arrhythmia and heart rate responses during sustained visual attention in preterm infants from 3 to 6 months of age. *Psychophysiology*, 31: 235–243.

Rickards, A. L., Kelly, E. A., Doyle, L. W., & Callanan, C. (2001). Cognition, academic progress, behavior, and self-concept at 14 years of very low birth weight children. *Developmental and Behavioral Pediatrics*, 22: 11–18.

Rondo, P. H., Ferreira, R. F., Nogueira, F., Ribeiro, M. C., Lobert, H., & Artes, R. (2003). Maternal psychological stress and distress as predictors of low birth weight, prematurity and intrauterine growth retardation. *European Journal of Clinical Nutrition*, 57: 266–272.

Rose, S. A., & Feldman, J. F. (1996). Memory and processing speed in preterm children at eleven years: A comparison with full-terms. *Developmental Psychology*, 67: 2001–2005.

Rose, S. A., Feldman, J. F., & Jankowski, J. J. (2004). Infant visual recognition memory. *Developmental Review*, 24: 74–100.

Rose, S. A., Feldman, J. F., Rose, S. L., Wallace, I. F., & McCarton, C. (1992). Behavior problems at 3 and 6 years: Prevalence and continuity in full-terms and preterms. *Development and Psychopathology*, 4: 361–374.

Rosenbaum, P. (2003). Cerebral palsy: what parents and doctors want to know. *British Medical Journal*, 326: 970–974.

Rosenbaum, P. L., Walter, S. D., Hanna, S. E., Palisano, R. J., Russell, D. J., Raina, P., et al. (2002). Prognosis for Gross Motor Function in Cerebral Palsy: Creation of Motor Development Curves. *J: The Journal of the American Medical Association*, 288: 1357–1363.

Rudelli, R., Bingham, P., Paneth, N., & Kairam, R. (1987). The intracerebellar hemorrhage—germinal matrix/choroid plexus hemorrhage association in very low birthweight neonates. *Journal of Neuropathology and Experimental Neurology*, 46: 344.

Rushe, T. M., Rifkin, L., Stewart, A. L., Townsend, J. P., Roth, S. C., Wyatt, J. S., et al. (2001). Neuropsychological outcome at adolescence of very preterm birth and its relation to brain structure. *Developmental Medicine and Child Neurology*, 43: 226–233.

Russman, B. S. (1992). Disorders of motor execution I: Cerebral Palsy. In R. B. David (Ed.), *Pediatric Neurology for the Clinician* (pp. 469–480). Norwalk, CN.: Appleton & Lange.

Rutter, M. (1989). Isle of Wight revisited: Twenty-five years of child psychiatric epidemiology. *Journal of the American Academy of Child and Adolescent Psychiatry*, 28: 633–653.

Sabbadini, M., Bonanni, R., Carlesimo, G. A., & Caltagirone, C. (2001). Neuropsychological assessment of patients with severe neuromotor and verbal disabilities. *Journal of Intellectual Disability Research*, 45: 169–179.

Saigal, S. (2000). Follow-up of very low birthweight babies to adolescence. *Seminars in Neonatology*, 5: 107–118.

Saigal, S., den Ouden, L., Wolke, D., Hoult, L., Paneth, N., Streiner, D. L., et al. (2003a). School-age outcomes in children who were extremely low birth weight from four international population-based cohorts. *Pediatrics*, 112: 943–950.

Saigal, S., Feeny, D., Rosenbaum, P., Furlong, W., Burrows, E., & Stoskopf, B. (1996). Self-perceived health status and health related quality of life of extremely low-birth-weight infants at adolescence. *Journal of the American Medical Association*, 276: 453–459.

Saigal, S., Lambert, M., Russ, C., & Hoult, L. (2002). Self-esteem of adolescents who were born prematurely. *Pediatrics*, 109: 429–433.

Sala, D.A. & Grant, A.D. (1995). Prognosis for ambulation in cerebral palsy. *Developmental Medicine and Child Neurology*, 37:1020–1026.

Sanger, T. D. (2003). Pathophysiology of pediatric movement disorders. *Journal of Child Neurology*, 18: S9–S24.

Santhouse, A. M., Ffytche, D. H., Howard, R. J., Williams, S. C., Stewart, A. L., Rooney, M., et al. (2002). The functional significance of perinatal corpus callosum damage: an fMRI study in young adults. *Brain*, 125: 1782–1792.

Scher, M. S., Aso, K., Beggarly, M. E., Hamid, M. Y., Steppe, D. A., & Painter, M. J. (1993). Electrographic seizures in preterm and full-term neonates: clinical correlates, associated brain lesions, and risk for neurologic sequelae. *Pediatrics*, 91: 128–134.

Scher, M. S., Belfar, H., Martin, J., & Painter, M. J. (1991). Destructive brain lesions of presumed fetal onset: antepartum causes of cerebral palsy. *Pediatrics*, 88: 898–906.

Scottish Low Birthweight Study Group. (1992). The Scottish Low Birthweight Study: II. Language attainment, cognitive status, and behavioural problems. *Archives of Disease in Childhood*, 67: 682–686.

Sheth, R. D. (1998). Frequency of neurologic disorders in the neonatal intensive care unit. *Journal of Child Neurology*, 13: 424–428.

Shevell, M. I., Majnemer, A., & Morin, I. (2003). Etiologic yield of cerebral palsy: a contemporary case series. *Pediatric Neurology*, 28: 352–359.

Skinner, R. A., & Piek, J. P. (2001). Psychosocial implications of poor motor coordination in children and adolescents. *Human Movement Science*, 20: 73–94.

Sloper P & Turner S. (1993) Determinants of parental satisfaction with disclosure of disability. *Developmental Medicine & Child Neurology*, 35: 816–825.

Smith, G. N., Flynn, S. W., McCarthy, N., Meistrich, B., Ehmann, T. S., MacEwan, G. W., et al. (2001). Low birthweight in schizophrenia: prematurity or poor fetal growth? *Schizophrenia Research*, 47: 177–184.

Sommerfelt, K., Andersson, H. W., Sonnander, K., Ahlsten, G., Ellertsen, B., Markestad, T., et al. (2001). Behavior in term, small for gestational age preschoolers. *Early Human Development*, 65: 107–121.

Stanley, F. J., Blair, E., & Alberman, E. (2000). *Cerebral palsies: epidemiology and causal pathways. (Vols. 151)* London, England: MacKeith Press.

Stanley, F. J., & Watson, L. (1992). Trends in perinatal mortality and cerebral palsy in Western Australia, 1967 to 1985. *British Medical Journal*, 304: 1658–1663.

Stevenson, D. K., Wright, L. L., Lemons, J. A., Oh, W., Korones, S. B., Papile, L. A., et al. (1998). Very low birth weight outcomes of the National Institute of Child Health and Human Development Neonatal Research Network, January 1993 through December 1994. *American Journal of Obstetrics & Gynecology*, 179: 1632–1639.

Stewart, A. L., Rifkin, L., Amess, P. N., Kirkbride, V., Townsend, J. P., Miller, D. H., et al. (1999). Brain structure and neurocognitive and behavioural function in adolescents who were born very preterm. *Lancet*, 353: 1653–1657.

Stewart, A. L., Thorburn, R. J., Hope, P. L., Goldsmith, M., Lipscomb, A. P., & Reynolds, E. O. (1983). Ultrasound appearance of the brain in very preterm infants and neurodevelopmental outcome at 18 months of age. *Archives of Disease in Childhood*, 58: 598–604.

Stiers, P., Vanderkelen, R., Vanneste, G., Coene, S., De Rammelaere, M., & Vandenbussche, E. (2002). Visual-perceptual impairment in a random sample of children with cerebral palsy. *Developmental Medicine & Child Neurology*, 44: 370–382.

Stiles, J., Reilly, J., Paul, B., & Moses, P. (2005) Cognitive development following early brain injury: evidence for neural adaptation. *Trends in Cognitive Sciences*, 9:136-143.

Strauss, R. S. (2000). Adult functional outcome of those born small for gestational age - Twenty-six-year follow-up of the 1970 British Birth Cohort. *Journal of the American Medical Association*, 283: 625–632.

Sullivan, M. C., & McGrath, M. M. (2003). Perinatal morbidity, mild motor delay, and later school outcomes. *Developmental Medicine and Child Neurology*, 45: 104–112.

Szatmari, P., Saigal, S., Rosenbaum, P., & Campbell, D. (1993). Psychopathology and adaptive functioning among extremely low birthweight children at eight years of age. *Development and Psychopathology*, 5: 345–357.

Szatmari, P., Saigal, S., Rosenbaum, P., Campbell, D., & King, S. (1990). Psychiatric disorders at five years among children with birthweights < 1000g: A regional perspective. *Developmental Medicine and Child Neurology*, 32: 954–962.

Taylor, H. G., Hack, M., Klein, N., & Schatschneider, C. (1995). Achievement in children with birth weights less than 750 grams with normal cognitive abilities: evidence for specific learning disabilities. *Journal of Pediatric Psychology*, 20: 703–719.

Taylor, H. G., Klein, N., Minich, N. M., & Hack, M. (2000). Verbal memory deficits in children with less than 750 g birth weight. *Child Neuropsychology*, 6: 49–63.

Taylor, H. G., Klein, N., Schatschneider, C., & Hack, M. (1998). Predictors of early school age outcomes in very low birth weight children. *Developmental and Behavioral Pediatrics*, 19: 238–243.

Theunissen, N. C. M., den Ouden, A. L., Meulman, J. J., Koopman, H. M., Verloove-Vanhorick, S. P., & Wit, J. M. (2000). Health status development in a cohort of preterm children. *The Journal of Pediatrics,* 137: 534–539.

Truwit, C. L., Barkovich, A. J., Koch, T. K., & Ferriero, D. M. (1992). Cerebral palsy: MR findings in 40 patients. *American Journal of Neuroradiology,* 13: 67–78.

Vaccarino, F. M., & Ment, L. R. (2004). Injury and repair in developing brain. *Archives of Disease in Childhood—Fetal & Neonatal Edition,* 89: F190–F192.

van Bogaert, P., Baleriaux, D., Christophe, C., & Szliwowski, H. B. (1992). MRI of patients with cerebral palsy and normal CT scan. *Neuroradiology,* 34: 52–56.

Vargha-Khadem, F., Isaacs, E., van der Werf, S., Robb, S., & Wilson, J. (1992). Development of intelligence and memory in children with hemiplegic cerebral palsy. The deleterious consequences of early seizures. *Brain,* 115: 315–329.

Vatten, L. J., & Skjærven, R. (2004). Offspring sex and pregnancy outcome by length of gestation. *Early Human Development,* 76: 47–54.

Volpe, J. J. (2001). *Neurology of the Newborn.* (4th ed.) Philadelphia, W.B. Saunders Company.

Volpe, J. J. (2003). Cerebral white matter injury of the premature infant—More common than you think. *Pediatrics,* 112: 176–180.

Walther, F. J., Den Ouden, A. L., & Verloove-Vanhorick, S. P. (2000). Looking back in time: Outcome of a national cohort of very preterm infants born in The Netherlands in 1983. *Early Human Development,* 59: 175–191.

Ward, K. (2003). Genetic factors in preterm birth. *BJOG: an International Journal of Obstetrics & Gynaecology,* 110: 117.

Whitaker, A., Van Rossem, R., Feldman, J., Schonfeld, I. S., Pinto-Martin, J., Torre, C., et al. (1997). Psychiatric outcomes in low birthweight children at age six: Relation to neonatal cranial ultrasound abnormalities. *Archives of General Psychiatry,* 54: 847– 856.

Whitaker, A. H., Feldman, J. F., Van Rossem, R., Schonfeld, I. S., Pinto-Martin, J. A., et al. (1996). Neonatal cranial ultrasound abnormalities in LBW infants: Relation to cognitive outcomes at age six. *Pediatrics,* 98: 719–729.

Whitfield, M. F., Grunau, R. V. E., and Holsti, L. (1997) Extremely premature (<800 g) schoolchildren; multiple areas of hidden disability. *Arch Dis Child,* 7: F85-F90.

Wiklund, L. M., & Uvebrant, P. (1991). Hemiplegic cerebral palsy: correlation between CT morphology and clinical findings. *Developmental Medicine & Child Neurology,* 33: 512–523.

Winter, S., Autry, A., Boyle, C., & Yeargin-Allsopp, M. (2002). Trends in the prevalence of cerebral palsy in a population-based study. *Pediatrics,* 110: 1220–1225.

Wolke, D., & Meyer, R. (1999). Cognitive status, language attainment, and prereading skills of 6-year-old very preterm children and their peers: the Bavarian Longitudinal Study. *Developmental Medicine and Child Neurology,* 41: 94–109.

World Health Organization. (2001). International classification of impairment, activity, and participation. Geneva, Switzerland: WHO.

Yude, C., & Goodman, R. (1999). Peer problems of 9- to 11-year-old children with hemiplegia in mainstream schools. Can these be predicted? *Developmental Medicine & Child Neurology,* 41:4–8.

Zeitlin, J., Saurel-Cubizolles, M. J., de Mouzon, J., Rivera, L., Ancel, P. Y., Blondel, B., et al. (2002). Fetal sex and preterm birth: are males at greater risk? *Human Reproduction,* 17: 2762–2768.

Zubrick, S.R., Kurinczuk, J. J., McDermott, B. M. C., McKelvey, R. S., Silburn, S. R., & Davies, L. C. (2000). Fetal growth and subsequent mental health problems in children aged 4 to 13 years. *Developmental Medicine & Child Neurology,* 42:14–20.

Traumatic Brain Injury

24

Sharon Arffa, PhD, MPPM

Traumatic brain injury in children and adolescents reflects a complex interplay of neurobiological and psychosocial factors; it is not a unitary entity. The child's age at the time of injury plays a significant role in the etiology and severity of the trauma, as well as in associated medical complications and outcome. Subsequent development, as well as psychosocial factors, also has an impact on recovery. There are also substantial methodological issues related to the measurement of the severity of the injury and the outcome.

In this chapter, the multiple mechanisms of injury and the unique features of the immature brain are reviewed. In addition, outcome studies are critically evaluated. This information provides a framework for a rational approach to the choice of treatments. To provide a broad conceptual framework, this chapter deals with studies of adults with traumatic brain injury as well. The response of the child's nervous system to other forms of brain injury (e.g., strokes) is reviewed. The neurocognitive and neurobehavioral outcomes are considered separately and cover issues such as severity of injury, age at injury, lesion location, and the influence of psychosocial factors. Finally, guidelines for the diagnosis and management of neurobehavioral disorders secondary to traumatic brain injury are discussed.

TERMINOLOGY

The terms *head injury* and *brain injury* are frequently used synonymously with traumatic brain injury but are less precise. Head injury also includes lacerations or external trauma to the face and head, as well as intracranial events; brain injury, a less specific term, is applicable to nontraumatic insults, such as cerebrovascular events or tumors. *Traumatic brain injury*, a far more precise term, is defined as physical damage or impairment in function of the brain secondary to the exchange of acute mechanical energy. This definition typically excludes brain injury resulting from

birth trauma; poisoning and asphyxia; soft tissue injuries to the face and scalp; or nondepressed skull fracture (Fife et al. 1986). *Concussion* is an elusive term with a history that dates to the middle ages. It has come to mean different things over the years but in 1966, the Congress of Neurologic Surgeons developed a consensual definition recognizing a concussion as an immediate and transient disruption of neural function. This is essentially synonymous with mild traumatic brain injury, and both terms are used in this chapter.

Traumatic brain injury is further classified as either "open" or "closed." These two types of traumatic brain injury differ substantially in both the pattern of brain injury and the associated neurobehavioral outcome. *Open* traumatic head injury occurs when the skull has been penetrated, such as with missile wounds or depressed fractures. In missile wounds, the extent of the neuroanatomic disruption is dependent on the path and velocity of the object or bullet, the scatter of bone chips, and the contusion and cerebral edema resulting from the entry wound (Bigler 1991). In contrast, *closed* traumatic brain injury typically results from rapid acceleration and deceleration injuries of the brain within the cranium as a result of high-speed accidents with sudden impact. In this situation, damage to the brain results from cerebral edema, hemorrhage, and ischemia (Jennett and Teasdale 1981).

CLASSIFICATION AND MEASUREMENT IN TRAUMATIC BRAIN INJURY

Level of consciousness, overall somatic injury, extent and duration of posttraumatic amnesia, other cognitive and neurobehavioral disturbances, and degree of neurocognitive dysfunction in the early posttraumatic period, and severity of injury are extremely important factors in determining outcome. A number of scales for measuring such factors have been developed.

Level of Consciousness

There is a spectrum of altered levels of consciousness, ranging from the fully conscious state to a confusional state, to stupor and coma (Plum and Posner 1980). Coma is a state in which patients lie with eyes closed and show a lack of awareness and responsiveness to external and internal stimuli. Comatose patients do not react to noxious stimuli with defensive, localized movements and do not speak (Salcman 1990).

Level of consciousness is extremely difficult to assess in very young infants. For example, stupor can be difficult to distinguish from normal sleepiness. Moreover, the motor examination is easily misinterpreted. Even in the presence of massive brain damage or increased intracranial pressure, babies may appear normal; they open their eyes and move spontaneously. Bicycling movements; rhythmic movements of the lower extremities; may be misinterpreted as normal activity but may actually be a manifestation of seizure activity in young infants. Limb withdrawal to pain; a primitive reflex; may be misinterpreted as well. The neurological examination in the infant should assess visual fixation and sucking responses, and cry (unconscious infants do not cry). A vigorous cry and facial grimace to trapezium pinch appears to be the most reliable measure of level of consciousness in young infants (Bruce and Zimmerman 1989; Ewing-Cobbs et al. 1995).

The Glasgow Coma Scale (Teasdale and Jennett 1974) continues to be the standard index to assess initial level of consciousness. Severity of injury in traumatic brain injury frequently has been defined by initial Glasgow Coma Scale score, either alone or in conjunction with other indices. This scale is also used to track recovery from coma in patients with traumatic brain injury. The Glasgow Coma Scale assesses function in three domains: eye opening, verbal response, and motor response. It yields a range of scores, from 3 to 15. Coma is defined as a score of 8 or less (Eisenberg and Werner 1987).

For the very young and preverbal child, the Glasgow Coma Scale is inappropriate. It is a less reliable and less successful predictor of outcome in children than in adults, in part because the same score in adults and children may not represent the same degree of primary irreversible brain damage (Bruce 1983). For example, an infant would not score more than a 4 on the motor examination (flexor withdrawal) and more than a 2 on the verbal examination (incomprehensible sounds). However, modifications of the Glasgow Coma Scale have been developed for infants and toddlers (Raimondi and Hirschauer 1984; Yager et al. 1990). These include recording ocular responses and reinterpreting "verbal response" to encompass vocalizations, crying, fixation, and following in response to speech and to exclude meaningful communications.

The Children's Coma Scale (Table 24.1) contains these modifications and eliminates from the motor examination segment the requirement of following commands. Although matching of anatomic level to coma severity level is inexact, there are significant differences between the Glasgow and Children's Coma Scales. Higher integrative cortical functions are not assessed by the Children's Coma Scale, and brain-stem functions are emphasized. The Glasgow Coma Scale (and the Children's Coma Scale) becomes more reliable when patients are measured at the same time postinjury, preferably on arrival at the emergency room (Kraus and Sorenson 1994).

Overall Somatic Injury

Because traumatic brain injury is often associated with injuries to other areas of the body, measures have been devised to obtain an index of overall injury severity, which facilitates triage and helps in the assessment of longterm outcome potential. The Abbreviated Injury Severity Scale (Joint Committee on Injury Scaling 1980) measures cumulative damage across six body regions, including the head. Severity ratings on this scale include loss of consciousness, length of coma, and neuroradiological findings (Tables 24.2 and 24.3). A revision, the Injury Severity Score (Table 24.4), is the most commonly used multiple injury assessment technique. The Injury Severity Score is calculated by summing the squares from the three most severely injured body regions. A high Injury Severity Score is correlated with both disability and mortality (Baker et al. 1974a).

Posttraumatic Amnesia

Posttraumatic amnesia refers to the period following recovery from coma in which continuous memories are not stored (Russell and Smith 1961). In this sense, posttraumatic amnesia is synonymous with anterograde amnesia, although Russell and colleagues included both length of coma and anterograde amnesia in their measurement of posttraumatic amnesia.

The duration of posttraumatic amnesia has become an important benchmark for prediction of outcome (Williams 1992). The period of posttraumatic amnesia is, on average, four times longer than the coma stage (Guthkelch 1979). In the dense stage of posttraumatic amnesia, patients who are able to speak repeatedly ask the same questions and do not remember having had meals or visits from close family members. In the second stage, information may be retained for short periods but is not permanently stored. Later, a few important events, such as the visit of a close friend or a medical procedure, may be recalled.

The recovery of islands of memory can be mistakenly identified as the end of posttraumatic amnesia. For example, a patient may remember arriving in the ambulance or being prepared for surgery, but nothing else until the next day (Gronwall 1989). Since it is difficult to verify subjective memories without the presence of an eyewitness, it is also difficult to distinguish confabulation from true recall. Weinstein and Lyerly (1968) reported that confabulation

TABLE 24.1
COMPARISON OF GLASGOW COMA SCALE (GCS) AND CHILDREN'S COMA SCALE (CCS)

A. GCS	CCS	B. GCS	CCS
Eye opening	Ocular pursuit	15	
4 Spontaneous	4 Pursuit	14	
3 Speech	3 Extraocular muscles intact, pupils reactive	13	
		12	11
		11	
2 Pain	2 Fixed pupils or extraocular muscles impaired	10	
		9	
1 None	1 Fixed pupils and extraocular muscles paralyzed	8	10
		7	9
Verbal response	Verbal response	6	8
5 Oriented	3 Cries		5
4 Confused	2 Spontaneous respirations	4	7
3 Inappropriate	1 Apneic		6
2 Incomprehensible			5
1 None			4
Motor response	Motor response	3	3
6 Obeys commands	4 Flexes and extends		
5 Localizes pain	3 Withdraws from pain		
4 Flexor withdrawal	2 Hypertonic		
3 Extension	1 Flaccid		

C. Testable functions

	Higher integrative	Cortical	Subcortical	Brain stem
GCS	12–15	9–11	5–8	3–4
CCS	None	11	8–10	3–7

Note: **A.** Number allocations to neurological observations. Ocular pursuit, rather than eye opening, is measured in the CCS. Verbal responses measured in the CCS include crying and respiration; speech is not required. Following commands or localizing pain is not measured in the CCS Motor Response section.
B. The GCS ranges from 3 to 15; the CCS ranges from 3 to 11.
C. Comparison of integrative, cortical, subcortical, and brainstem functions as expressed by coma scores on the respective scales. Higher integrative cortical functions are indicated by GCS of 12 to 15, whereas those functions are not assessed by the CCS. Increased emphasis on brain-stem function is also noted in the Children's Coma Scale.
Source: Reprinted from Raimondi AJ, Hirschauer J. Head injury in the infant and toddler: Coma Outcome Scale. *Child's Brain* 11:12–35, 1984. Used with permission.

occurred in 60% of a sample of patients with severe head injury. Therefore, the conservative approach is to consider the possibility of confabulation in all patients with significant head injuries.

To avoid some of the problems of assessing subjective memories, posttraumatic amnesia can be defined as disorientation to person, place, and time. However, disorientation is not the same as posttraumatic amnesia, and the two can be dissociated. For example, a patient may correctly answer questions about person, place, and time but have no recollection of having been asked. For adults, the point at which they can accurately report what has happened to them and the circumstances of their hospitalization and accurately state the month, year, day of month, and day of week has been taken as the resolution of posttraumatic amnesia (Gronwall 1989).

The Children's Orientation and Amnesia Test (Ewing-Cobbs et al. 1989) (Fig. 24.1) is designed to evaluate posttraumatic amnesia in children ages 3 through 15 years. It is a short, 16-item measure that assesses general orientation, temporal orientation, and immediate and remote memories. It has been normed for ages 3 through 15 years and can be repeated daily to assess recovery. The end of posttraumatic amnesia is defined by a criterion score. Before the development of the Children's Orientation and Amnesia Test, posttraumatic amnesia measurement in children was estimated through parent and child interviews. The duration of posttraumatic amnesia, as measured by the Children's Orientation and Amnesia Test, was found to be related to neurological indicators of severity as well as to memory functioning 1 year after injury (Ewing-Cobbs et al. 1989).

Other Cognitive and Neurobehavioral Factors

The term *posttraumatic amnesia* has been criticized because it addresses only memory disturbance; while arousal, attention, mood, and behavior may be altered during this stage as well (Trzepacz 1994). A patient who is emerging

TABLE 24.2

ABBREVIATED INJURY SEVERITY SCALE (AISS)

Abbreviated injury score:	1 Minor	2 Moderate	3 Severe, not life-threatening	4 Severe, life-threatening	5 Critical, survival uncertain
External					
Abrasion/ contusion	**Minor abrasion/ contusion** — Superficial or unspecified, ≤25 cm² on face or 50 cm² on body	**Major abrasion/ contusion** — >25 cm² on face or >50 cm² on body			
Laceration	**Superficial or unspecified laceration** — Not into subcutaneous tissue regardless of length, or — Into subcutaneous tissue but <5 cm on face or ≤10 cm on body	**Deep laceration** — Into subcutaneous tissue and >10 cm on body or >5 cm on face			
Burns	1° burn up to 100%; 2° or 3° burn <6% total body	2° or 3° burn to 6–15% total body	2° or 3° burn to 16–34% total body	2° or 3° burn to 26–35% total body	2° or 3° burn to 36–90% total body
Head					
Level of consciousness on admission or initial observation	**Awake, with** — No prior unconsciousness, but may have headache/ dizziness due to head trauma	**Awake, with** — Prior unconsciousness, but length of time unspecified, or — Amnesia (no recollection of crash), or — Unconsciousness <15 minutes OR **Lethargic, stuporous, or obtunded, but can be aroused by verbal stimuli, and** — No prior unconsciousness, or — Unconsciousness <15 minutes OR **When level of unconsciousness is unknown, and** — Unconsciousness <15 minutes **Medical diagnosis is listed as concussion with no other description**	**Awake, with** — Prior unconsciousness, but length unspecified/amnesia, or — Unconsciousness 15 minutes with neurological deficit, or — Unconsciousness 15–59 minutes OR **Lethargic, stuporous, obtunded, but can be aroused by verbal stimuli, and** — No prior unconsciousness, or — Unconsciousness <15 minutes with neurological deficit, or — Unconsciousness 15–59 minutes, or — Prior unconsciousness/loss of consciousness unspecified OR	**Awake, with** — Unconsciousness 15–59 minutes with neurological deficit OR **Lethargic, stuporous, obtunded, but can be aroused by verbal stimuli, and** — Unconsciousness 15–59 minutes, or — Prior unconsciousness for unspecified length of time, or — Unspecified loss of consciousness involving neurological deficit OR **Unconscious on admission or initial observation (unresponsive to verbal commands)** — 1–24 hours (includes one calendar day when hours cannot be estimated)	**Unconscious and unresponsive to verbal stimuli** — Inappropriate movements (decerebrate, decorticate, flaccid, no response to pain no matter the length of unconsciousness) — 1–24 hours (includes one calendar day when hours cannot be estimated)/ appropriate movements, but only to painful stimuli (no matter the length of unconsciousness with neurological deficit)

Head injuries

Ear canal injury
Eyes (F)
— Conjunctiva abrasion/ contusion/laceration
— Corneal abrasion/contusion
— Lid abrasion/ contusion/ laceration
— Vitreous/retina/canaliculus (tear duct) laceration
— Choroid rupture
— Uvea injury
Gingiva (F)
— (Gum) contusion/laceration
Lip (F)
— Contusion/laceration/ no matter how extensive
Mandible (F)
— Fracture unspecified
— Ramus fracture
Nose (F)
— Fracture
Teeth (F)
— Avulsion/ dislocation/fracture
Superficial tongue (F)
— Laceration

Fracture of vault (frontal, occipital, parietal sphenoid, temporal, or unspecified)
— Closed, undisplaced, diastatic, linear, simple, unspecified
Ear
— Inner/middle ear injury
— Ossicular bone dislocation
— Tympanic membrane rupture
— Avulsion of pinna
Eye (F)
— Cornea laceration
— Sclera laceration/rupture
Alveolar ridge (bone) (F)
— Fracture with or without tooth injury
Avulsion gingiva/lid/lip (F)
Mandibular fracture (F)
— Ramus if open displaced/ comminuted
— Body with or without Ramus involvement
— Subcondylar
Maxilla fracture (F)
— Closed/ unspecified/Le Fort I/zygomatic fracture
Tongue (F)
— Deep and/or extensive laceration

Fracture of base (basilar ethmoid, orbital roof, sphenoid, temporal) without cerebrospinal fluid leak
— Comminuted compound, depressed or displaced fracture of vault
Cerebellum or cerebrum
— Confusion
— Injury involving any of the following, but no further anatomic description: subarachnoid hemorrhage, edema, brain swelling, subpial hemorrhage, hygroma, ischemia, infarction
Zygomatic fracture (F)
— Open/displaced/ comminuted
Eye (F)
— Avulsion
— Optic nerve avulsion/ laceration
— Tear
Mandibular fracture (F)
— Ramus involvement/mandible fracture
— Subcondylar/body with or without ramus involvement for anyone displaced/ comminuted

Unconsciousness, unresponsive to verbal commands, and
— Length of unconsciousness unspecified, or
— Unconsciousness <1 hour
When level of consciousness is unknown, and
— Unconsciousness 15–59 minutes, or
— Unconsciousness <15 minutes with neurological deficit

— Appropriate movements, but only on painful stimuli (no matter the length of unconsciousness), or
— Length of unconsciousness unspecified/unconsciousness < 1 hour with neurological deficit
When level of consciousness on admission or initial observation is unknown, but unconscious for
— 1–24 hours (includes one calendar day when hours cannot be estimated)
— 15–59 minutes with neurological deficit

Fracture of base (basilar ethmoid, orbital roof, sphenoid, temporal) with cerebrospinal leak or pneumocephalus
Fracture of vault (frontal occipital, parietal, sphenoid, temporal, unspecified)
— open/dura torn/ cerebrospinal fluid leak/pneumocephalus or brain exposed
Cerebellum or cerebrum
— Laceration
— Hematoma, epidural/ subdural ≤100 cc, or unspecified
— Hematoma, intracerebral, intracerebellar (including petechial and subcortical hematoma)
Le Fort III (F)

When initial level of unconsciousness is unknown, but unconscious for
— 1–24 hours (includes one calendar day when hours cannot be estimated) with neurological deficit
— >24 hours

Brain stem
— Compression/ contusion/injury involving hemorrhage
Cerebellum or cerebrum
— Hematoma, epidural/ subdural > 100 cc
— Diffuse brain injury (white matter shearing injury)

(continued)

TABLE 24.2
(continued)

Abbreviated injury score:	1 Minor	2 Moderate	3 Severe, not life-threatening	4 Severe, life-threatening	5 Critical, survival uncertain
Neck	**Pharynx** — Contusion/ laceration/ puncture/rupture **Throat** (inner soft tissue) — Abrasion/ contusion/ laceration (not involving major artery) **Trachea** — Contusion	**Pharynx** — Contusion with hematoma/ laceration with hemorrhage — Contusion/esophagus/larynx/ thyroid gland	**Trachea** crush **Thyroid gland** — Laceration	**Laceration** of trachea/carotid artery/subclavian artery **Larynx** — Crush/fracture/ laceration	**Esophagus/larynx/ trachea** — Avulsion/rupture
			Orbit fracture open/displaced, comminuted (F) Le Fort II (F)		
		Nose (F) — Fracture open/displaced/ comminuted			
Thorax	**Rib** — Contusion/fracture	**Rib** — Fracture open/displaced/ >two adjacent ribs up to flail chest **Sternum** — Fracture	**Lung/pericardium** — Contusion with or without unilateral hemothorax **Lung** — Laceration superficial or unspecified **Unilateral hemothorax/ pneumothorax** with rib cage or thoracic cavity injury **Sternum** —Fracture open/displaced/ comminuted	**Chest wall (soft tissue)** Perforation/ puncture Lung — Contusion with hemomediastinum/ pneumomediastinum/ bilateral hemothorax or pneumothorax **Myocardium** — Contusion **Pericardium** — Contusion with hemomediastinum/ pneumomediastinum or tamponade/perforation/ puncture/rupture/ laceration/bilateral hemothorax or pneumothorax **Bilateral hemothorax or pneumothorax** **Hemomediastinum/ pneuomediastinum** Flail chest ("sucking chest" wound)	**Laceration** —Aorta/bronchus/ coronary artery/lung (deep and/or extensive)/myocardium (including multiple chambers)/pulmonary artery or vein/superior or inferior vena cava/ pericardium if involving hemodiastinum/ pneumomediastinum or tamponade **Puncture/rupture** —Aorta/intracardia valve or septum/ myocardium involving multiple chambers/superior or inferior vena cava/ pericardium if involving hemodiastinum/ pneumomediastinum or tamponade

Region					
					Lung — Laceration superficial or unspecified with hemothorax/pneumothorax —**Inhalation burn**	**Perforation** — Aorta/bronchus/myocardium/pericardium if involving hemodiastinum/pneumo-mediastinum or tamponade **Rupture bronchus** **Inhalation burn** requiring mechanical respiratory support **Myocardium contusion** —If severe or involving hemodiastinum/pneumomediastinum
Abdomen/pelvic contents	**Superficial or unspecified laceration/perforation of abdominal wall** (no organ involvement) **Abrasion/contusion**/superficial or unspecified **Laceration or perforation** of scrotum/vagina/vulva/perineum **Contusion** of penis **Rupture** of scrotum	**Abdominal wall avulsion** **Deep and/or extensive laceration or perforation** of abdominal wall (no organ involvement)/scrotum **Contusion** of stomach **Contusion/superficial or unspecified laceration** of ureter	**Abdominal wall musculature rupture** **Contusion** of "biliary tract" (gall-bladder, hepatic, cystic, and common bile ducts)/colon/ duodenum/jejunum/ileum/kidney (with or without hematuria)/liver/bladder/mesentery/pancreas/peritoneum/ rectum/spleen/ urethra/uterus **Superficial or unspecified laceration/perforation** of bladder/ureter/penis/ diaphragm **Deep and/or extensive laceration/perforation** of perineum/ureter/vagina/vulva **Avulsion** of scrotum/ureter **Retroperitoneum injury** involving hemorrhage or hematoma	**Superficial or unspecified laceration/perforation of** "biliary tract"/colon/ duodenum/jejunum/ileum/kidney/liver/pancreas/peritoneum/rectum (superficial over entire rectal wall, extraperitoneal) **Deep and/or extensive laceration/perforation of** bladder/mesentery/penis/ stomach/urethra/uterus **Avulsion** of bladder/mesentery/penis/spleen/stomach/testes/urethra/uterus (not pregnant, or in 1st trimester)/ ovary **Rupture** of spleen/stomach/ urethra/uterus (not pregnant, or in 1st trimester)/bladder (intraperitoneal) **Rupture/tear** ovarian/fallopian tube **Laceration** of spleen	**Avulsion/deep and/or extensive laceration/ perforation/rupture** of "biliary tract"/colon/ duodenum/jejunum/ ileum/kidney/liver/ pancreas (with or without duodenum involvement) **Deep and/or extensive laceration/rupture** of peritoneum/rectum **Laceration** of intraabdominal or intrapelvic major vessel **Avulsion/rupture** of uterus (in 2nd or 3rd trimester)	
Spine	**Acute strain with no fracture or dislocation** cervical/thoracic/lumbar spine		**Dislocation (subluxation) + fracture** spinous or transverse process (or unspecified) of cervical/thoracic/lumbar spine **Minor compression fracture** T1–12/L1–L5 (<20% loss in height of anterior vertebral body/unspecified)	**Cervical cord** contusion with transient neurological signs (muscle weakness, paralysis, loss of sensation) **Disc herniation (rupture) with nerve root damage** of cervical/thoracic/lumbar spine	**Cervical cord lesion** incomplete with preservation of significant sensation and/or motor function	**Cervical cord** crush/ laceration or total transection with or without fracture and/or dislocation C4 or below **Complete cervical cord lesion** (quadriplegia or paraplegia)

(continued)

TABLE 24.2 (continued)

Abbreviated injury score:	1 Minor	2 Moderate	3 Severe, not life-threatening	4 Severe, life-threatening	5 Critical, survival uncertain
			Dislocation (subluxation) and/or fracture of lamina/body/facet/pedicle/odontoid of cervical/thoracic/lumbar spine Nerve root/trunk brachial plexus/lumbar plexus/sacral plexus avulsion/laceration/rupture, injury with unknown lesions Compression fracture of more than one vertebrae and/or >20% loss of height of anterior body T1–12, L1–5		Cord/cauda equina crush/laceration/total transection (paraplegia)
Extremities and bony pelvis	Contusion/sprain of acromioclavicular joint/elbow/shoulder (glenohumeral joint)/sternoclavicular joint/wrist (carpus)/ankle Contusion fibula/knee Sprain finger/foot/hip/toe Fracture/dislocation finger/toe	Dislocation/laceration into joint of acromioclavicular joint/elbow (dislocation of radial head)/hand (laceration involving flexor or extensor tendons)/sternoclavicular joint/wrist/heel (dislocation subtalar; laceration involving Achilles tendon)/patella (laceration or rupture) Fracture of clavicle/acromion/hand (carpal or metacarpal)/humerus/radius (including Colles)/scapula/ulna/fibula (head, neck, shaft, or lateral malleolus)/ foot (metatarsal talar, tarsal, or unspecified)/heel (calcaneus) patella/ pelvis closed or unspecified) with or without dislocation of any of the combination of the ilium, ischium, coccyx, sacrum, pubic, ramus/tibia (shaft, malleolus, plateau, condyles)	Crush of acromioclavicular joint/arm forearm/elbow/hand/shoulder/sternoclavicular joint/wrist/ankle/foot/heel/knee/below knee Amputation upper extremity above or below elbow/hand/foot forearm/lower extremity below knee Dislocation of shoulder/wrist (radiocarpal, intercarpal, pericarpal)/ankle/knee/elbow (if involving olecranon)/hip (with or without fracture of acetabulum, femoral head, neck, or intertrochanteric) Fracture of humerus/radius (including Colles)/ulna (with any one combination of open, displaced, comminuted, or involving radial nerves)/femur (condyle, head, neck, shaft with or without sciatic nerve involvement)	Crush of pelvis Crush/amputation above knee (traumatic partial or complete)	

Laceration into joint of shoulder/ankle/knee

Muscle rupture of biceps

Amputation/crush of finger/toe

Acromioclavicular separation

Contusion of fibula with peroneal nerve injury ("footdrop")

Rupture of collateral or cruciate ligaments of the knee

Fracture of tibia, fibula, or pelvis

Fracture and/or dislocation of sacroiliac

Separation (fracture) of symphysis pubis

Rupture of knee collateral or cruciate ligaments

Rupture of ankle collateral ligaments and/or Achilles tendon

Laceration of axillary/brachial femoral/popliteal artery

Nerve laceration of upper (median, radial, ulnar) or lower (femoral, tibial, sciatic peroneal) extremity involving two or more nerves in same extremities

Muscle avulsion or laceration of multiple major muscle tendons in upper and lower (except patella or Achilles) extremities

Laceration or rupture of complete patellar tendon

Note: This table is a simplified chart incorporating Abbreviated Injury Scale criteria for grading the severity of an injury in seven body regions.

aInjuries scored as facial injuries in the Injury Severity Score are noted with an **(F).**

Source: Greenspan L, McLellan BA, Greig H. Abbreviated injury scale and injury severity score: a scoring chart. J Trauma 25:60–64, 1985. Used with permission.

TABLE 24.3
ABBREVIATED INJURY SEVERITY SCALE–MAXIMUM INJURY

External	Secondary or tertiary burns including incineration >91% of total body
Head	Crush or ring fracture, crush/laceration brain stem (hypothalamus, medulla, midbrain, pons)
Neck	Decapitation
Thorax	Total severance aorta, chest massively crushed
Abdomen/Pelvis	Spinal cord crush/laceration or total transection
Spine	Spinal cord crush/laceration or total transection with or without fracture C3 or above

Note: This chart depicts maximum injury (i.e., injury severity score of 75 automatically assigned) for the six body regions of the injury Severity Scale: (1) external injuries refer to burns, contusion, lacerations, and abrasions; (2) head and neck injuries include injuries to the cervical spine, spinal cord, skull, brain, and ears; (3) face injuries include injuries to the mouth, eye, nose, and facial bones; (4) chest injuries include injuries to internal chest cavity organs, diaphragm, thoracic spine, or rib cage; (5) abdominal or pelvic content injuries include injuries to the internal abdominal cavity organs and lumbar spine; (6) injuries to extremities and pelvic girdle include sprains, fractures, amputations, and dislocations except those to skull, spinal cord, or rib cage. Note that the regions for the Abbreviated Injury Scale do not always coincide with the Injury Severity Scale regions.
Source: Greenspan L, McLellan BA, Greig H. Abbreviated injury scale and injury severity score: a scoring chart. J Trauma 25:60–64, 1985. Used with permission.

from coma displays inability to focus attention, disorientation, memory disturbance, higher-order cognitive deficits (such as concreteness), agitation or lethargy, and emotional lability (Goethe and Levin 1984; Trzepacz 1994). A disturbance in sleep/wake cycle and a fluctuating course of cognitive and neurobehavioral problems may be found as well. Hallucinations; defined as sensory perceptions without external stimulation of visual, auditory, olfactory, gustatory, or tactile organs that are perceived as real by the patient; are not commonly experienced by patients with traumatic brain injury but have been documented (Goethe and Levin 1984). Delirium, as defined in DSM-IV (American Psychiatric Association 1994), refers to an abnormal state of consciousness preceding stupor and coma, marked by restlessness, affective instability, cognitive deficits, disorientation, and disturbances of the sleep/wake cycle. Although delirium occurs in the course of recovery from trau-

matic brain injury, this term is used only infrequently in this context.

Several different instruments have been developed to evaluate these neurobehavioral factors during recovery from traumatic brain injury. The Neurobehavioral Rating Scale (Levin et al. 1987b) (Fig. 24.2), which is used to monitor broader psychiatric symptoms during recovery, contains 27 clinician-rated items addressing cognitive disturbance, mood alteration, and perceptual disturbance. The Ranchos Los Amigos Scale of Cognitive Functioning (Hagen et al. 1972) (Table 24.5) is commonly used in cases of traumatic brain injury, particularly at rehabilitation centers. It provides a tool for assessing behaviors typical of the eight stages of recovery, from deep coma to purposeful, appropriate behavior. Although clinically useful, it is not sufficiently quantifiable to be appropriate for research (Lehr 1990).

Degree of Neurocognitive Dysfunction in the Early Posttraumatic Period

The resolution of posttraumatic amnesia is followed by the early posttraumatic period (Gronwall 1989). Although generally oriented in time and able to remember events from the previous day, the patient may show slowing in reaction time and mental processes, susceptibility to distraction, and poor concentration. Because rapid improvement can occur during this early stage and attention span is still limited, lengthy neurocognitive evaluations are impractical. However, a brief battery of neuropsychological tests can be useful in documenting the degree of neurocognitive dysfunction and in determining disposition. One such battery (reviewed in Arffa 1995) includes brief attentional tasks such as the Wechsler Intelligence Scale for Children–III or IV (WISC-III; Wechsler 1991; WISC-IV, Wech-

TABLE 24.4
SCORING GRID FOR DETERMINING INJURY SEVERITY SCORE (ISS)

Body region	Abbreviated Injury Score	Squared
Head/Neck		
Face		
Chest		
Abdomen/pelvic contents		
Extremities/pelvic girdle		
External		
Total ISS*		

*Based on sum of squares of three most severely injured body regions.
Source: Greenspan L, McLellan BA, Greig H. Abbreviated injury scale and injury severity score: a scoring chart. J Trauma 25:60–64, 1985. Used with permission.

Children's Orientation and Amnesia Test

INSTRUCTIONS:

Begin by introducing yourself by name (e.g., Dr._____) and ask the child to be sure to remember your name. Points for correct responses (shown in parentheses after each question) are scored and entered in the columns on the extreme right side of the test form. Enter the total points accrued for the items in the lower right corn of the test form. Children ages 3–7 years are administered only the General Orientation and Memory sections of the te The entire test is administered to children ages 8–15 years.

GENERAL ORIENTATION: **POINT**

1. What is your name? First (2)_____ Last (3)_____   _____

2. How old are you? (3)_____ When is your birthday? Month (1)____ Day (1)____   _____

3. Where do you live? City (3)_____ State (2)_____   _____

4. What is your father's name? (5)_____ What is your mother's name? (5)_____   _____

5. What school do you go to? (3)_____What grade are you in? (2)_____   _____

6. Where are you now? (5)_____(may rephrase question: Are you at home now?
    Are you in the hospital? If rephrased, the child must correctly answer both questions.)   _____

7. Is it daytime or nighttime? (5)_____   _____

TEMPORAL ORIENTATION:

8. What time is it now? (5)_____(correct = 5; <hour off = 4; 1 hour off = 3; >1 hour off = 2;
    2 hours off = 1)   _____

9. What day of the week is it? (5)_____(correct = 5; 1 off = 4; 2 off = 3; 3 off = 2; 4 off = 1)   _____

10. What day of the month is it? (5)_____(correct = 5; 1 off = 4; 2 off = 3; 3 off = 2; 4 off = 1)   _____

11. What is the month? (10)_____(correct = 10; 1 off = 7; 2 off = 4; 3 off = 1)   _____

12. What is the year? (15)_____(correct = 15; 1 off = 10; 2 off = 5; 3 off = 1)   _____

MEMORY:

13. Say these numbers after me in the same order. (Discontinue when the child fails both series of
    digits at any length. Score 2 points if both digit series are correctly repeated; score 1 point if
    only one is correct.) 3 5____; 58 42____; 643 926____; 7,216 3,279____; 35,296 81,493____;
    539,418 724,856____; 8,129,365 4,739,128 (14)   _____

14. How many fingers am I holding up? Two fingers (2)____Three fingers (3)____10 fingers (5)____   _____

15. Who is on *Sesame Street*?(10)_____(can substitute other major television show)   _____

16. What is my name? (10)_____   _____

Figure 24.1 Children's orientation and amnesia test. Reprinted from Ewing-Cobbs L, Levin HS, Fletcher JM, et al. The Children's Orientation and Amnesia Test: relationship to severity of acute head injury and to recovery of memory. Neurosurgery 27:683–691, 1990. Used with permission.

Neurobehavioral Rating Scale

DIRECTIONS: Place an X in the appropriate column to represent level of severity of each symptom.

	Not present	Very mild	Mild	Moderate	Moderately severe	Severe	Extremely severe

1. **Inattention/reduced alertness:**
   Fails to sustain attention, easily distracted, fails to notice aspects of environment, difficulty directing attention, and decreased alertness

2. **Somatic concern:**
   Volunteers, complains, or elaborates about somatic symptoms (headache, dizziness, blurred vision) and about physical health in general

3. **Disorientation:**
   Confusion or lack of proper association for person, place, or time

4. **Anxiety:**
   Worry, fear, and overconcern for present or future

5. **Expressive deficit:**
   Word-finding disturbance, anomia, pauses in speech, effortful and agrammatic speech, and circumlocution

6. **Emotional withdrawal:**
   Lack of spontaneous interaction, isolation, and deficiency in relating to others

7. **Conceptual disorganization:**
   Thought processes confused, disconnected, disrupted, tangential social communication, and perseverative

8. **Disinhibition:**
   Socially inappropriate comments and/or actions, including aggressive/sexual content, or inappropriate to the situation, and outbursts of temper

9. **Guilt feelings:**
   Self-blame, shame, and remorse for past behavior

10. **Memory deficit:**
    Difficulty learning new information, rapidly forgets recent events, although immediate recall (forward digit span) may be intact

11. **Agitation:**
    Motor manifestations of overactivation (kicking, arm flailing, picking, roaming, restlessness, and talkativeness)

Figure 24.2 Neurobehavioral rating scale. Reprinted from Levin HS, High WM, Goethe KE, et al. The neurobehavioral rating scale: assessment of the behavioral sequelae of closed head injury by the clinician. J Neurol Neurosurg Psychiatry 50:183–193, 1987. Used with permission.

	Not present	Very mild	Mild	Moderate	Moderately severe	Severe	Extremely severe
12. Inaccurate insight and self-appraisal: Poor insight, exaggerated self-opinion, and overrates level of ability and underrates personality change in comparison with evaluation by clinicians and family							
13. Depressive mood: Sorrow, sadness, despondency, and pessimism							
14. Hostility/uncooperativeness: Animosity, irritability, belligerence, disdain for others, and defiance of authority							
15. Decreased initiative/motivation: Lacks normal initiative in work or leisure; fails to persist in tasks, and is reluctant to accept new challenges							
16. Suspiciousness: Mistrust, belief that others harbor malicious or discriminatory intent							
17. Fatigability: Rapidly fatigues on challenging cognitive tasks or complex activities; lethargic							
18. Hallucinatory behavior: Perceptions without normal external stimulus correspondence							
19. Motor retardation: Slowed movements or speech (excluding primary weakness)							
20. Unusual thought content: Unusual, odd, strange, and bizarre thought content							
21. Blunted affect: Reduced emotional tone, reduction in normal intensity of feelings, and flatness							
22. Excitement: Heightened emotional tone, increased reactivity							
23. Poor planning: Unrealistic goals, poorly formulated plans for the future, disregards prerequisites (e.g., training), and fails to take disability into account							
24. Lability of mood: Sudden change in mood that is disproportionate to the situation							
25. Tension: Postural and facial expression of heightened tension, without the necessity of excessive activity involving the limbs or trunk							
26. Comprehension deficit: Difficulty in understanding oral instructions on single or multistage commands							
27. Speech articulation deficit: Misarticulation, slurring, or substitution							

Figure 24.2 *(continued)*

sler 2003), Digit Span and Arithmetic subtests, the Verbal and Visual Memory subtests from the Wide Range Assessment of Memory and Learning (Sheslow and Adams 1990), and executive function tests such as the Wisconsin Card Sorting Test (Heaton et al. 1993) and the Controlled Oral Word Fluency Test (see Lezak 1994).

Level of Severity

Assessment of severity is probably the most important measurement in traumatic brain injury. Incidence and outcome researchers typically rely on categories of "mild," "moderate," and "severe" when studying differences in rates of traumatic brain injury, sequelae, and recovery. The severity of the injury is defined in terms of its consequences and not the characteristics of the injury itself (e.g., velocity or angle of the blow).

There is no uniformly accepted classification of severity, and this is one of the major sources of variability in outcome research (Levin et al. 1995). Traditionally, severity has been assessed on the basis of initial level of consciousness, duration of coma, and extent of posttraumatic amnesia (Goethe and Levin 1984). However, other definitions have taken into account necessity for brain surgery, length of hospitalization, abnormalities on neuroradiological examination, and even quantitative analysis of computed tomography (CT) (see, e.g., Marshall et al. 1991).

"Mild" traumatic brain injury is frequently defined as a transient loss or altered state of consciousness and amnesia, but specific criteria have varied widely. Kraus and Sorenson (1994) found that in 35% of research studies from 1984 to 1994, mild traumatic brain injury was defined as no loss of consciousness, whereas in 36% of studies a loss of consciousness of 15 to 60 minutes was required. The Glasgow Coma Scale score used as the criterion for mild traumatic brain injury has also varied. In 59% of the research reports reviewed by Kraus and Sorenson (1994), a Glasgow Coma Scale score of 13, 14, or 15 was used as the criterion for mild traumatic brain injury, whereas in 24% a Glasgow Coma Scale score of 8 or 9 to 15 was used. The duration of posttraumatic amnesia is also quite variable in definitions of mild traumatic brain injury. Chadwick and colleagues (1980), for example, specified a posttraumatic amnesia duration of more than 1 hour to less than 1 week as indication of mild injury, whereas Asarnow and colleagues (1991) used a criterion of less than 4 hours.

"Moderate" traumatic brain injury is generally defined as a loss of consciousness lasting more than 30 minutes and less than 24 hours (Annegars et al. 1980). Kraus and colleagues (1984) also required a hospital stay of 4 to 8 hours and neurosurgery or abnormal CT. Most commonly, a Glasgow Coma Scale score of 9 to 12 is used to define moderate traumatic brain injury.

TABLE 24.5
RANCHOS LOS AMIGOS SCALE OF COGNITIVE FUNCTIONING

EARLY STAGES OF RECOVERY
Level I—no response
The patient appears to be in deep sleep, with no eye opening or response to external stimulation.
Level II—generalized response
The patient reacts nonpurposefully and inconsistently to stimulation.
Level III—localized response
The patient reacts purposefully to stimulation but is inconsistent. He or she may turn his or her head toward sound.

MIDDLE STAGES OF RECOVERY
Level IV—confused/agitated
The patient shows heightened activity level. Aggression or excessive irritation disproportionate to stimulation may occur. Patient is confused and is severely limited in ability to process information. No self-care functions.
Level V—confused/inappropriate/not agitated
The patient is alert and able to respond to simple commands in a fairly consistent manner. He or she is highly distractible and cannot sustain and focus attention. Memory is severely compromised, and new information is not learned. When aphasia is not present, the patient makes inappropriate verbalizations. The patient may be able to assist with self-care functions.
Level VI—confused/appropriate
Goal-directed behaviors may be observed, but these involve overlearned or automatized skills such as feeding or brushing teeth. Attention and memory are improving but are still impaired. The patient may be inconsistently oriented and recognizes caretakers.

LATE STAGES OF RECOVERY
Level VII—automatic/appropriate
The patient may be able to follow a routine when prompted and may be independent or semi-independent, with self-care. The patient, however, lacks insight into his or her condition and shows poor judgment and problem-solving skills.
Level VIII—purposeful/appropriate
The patient is completely oriented, is independent, and is capable of self-care. Memory has improved; the patient can recall past events and shows capacity for new learning. Some continued compromise in reasoning and judgment may be present.

Source: Adapted with permission from the Adult Brain Injury Service of the Ranchos Los Amigos Medical Center, Downey, CA.

TABLE 24.6

SUGGESTED CRITERIA FOR SEVERITY RATINGS IN TRAUMATIC BRAIN INJURY

Severity of TBI	Length of Coma	Initial GCS Score	Duration of PTA	CT Criteria
Minimal	No LOC		1–5 min; confusion with or without amnesia	
Very mild	No LOC		5–60 mins	
Mild	30 mins	13–15	1–24 hrs	Negative
Moderate	30 mins–24 hrs	9–12	>24 hrs, but <7 days	Negative/positive
Severe	>24 hrs	3–8	8–28 days	Positive
Very severe	>24 hrs	3–8	>28 days	Positive

Note: Three gradations of mild injury are suggested; in minimal and very mild severity levels, medical attention may or may not be sought. TBI = traumatic brain injury; GCS = Glasgow Coma Scale (see Table 24.1); PTA = posttraumatic amnesia; CT = computed tomography; LOC = loss of consciousness.

"Severe" traumatic brain injury has been defined as loss of consciousness lasting longer than 24 hours (Annegars et al. 1980, Whitman et al. 1984) and depressed level of consciousness initially (i.e., Glasgow Coma Scale score ≤ 8) (Kraus et al. 1984, Rimel et al. 1981). Very severe traumatic brain injury has been defined as loss of consciousness or posttraumatic amnesia lasting longer than 7 days (Qennett 1983).

More recently, the utility of more gradations in the measurement of traumatic brain injury severity has been noted, particularly in the area of sports related concussion (Cantu 1998, Kelly 1995, Johnston et al. 2001). Suggested criteria of severity levels are presented in Table 24.6.

Advances in neurodiagnostic imaging may help in refining severity ratings. For example, with the expanding use of magnetic resonance imaging (MRI), which can identify surface contusions, many mild injuries may be reclassified as moderate.

EPIDEMIOLOGY

Our understanding of traumatic brain injury in children has been advanced through descriptive epidemiology. Knowledge of the incidence, developmental trends, and risk factors of pediatric brain injury is useful in a number of ways. Awareness of medical sequelae common to certain types of injury in population subsets can facilitate medical decision making. Furthermore, the premorbid characteristics of the child and family can help the neuropsychiatrist identify risk factors for neuropsychological or psychiatric sequelae and aid in planning for the care and treatment of the child. Perhaps most important, public awareness of the magnitude of the problem can be advanced, and effective prevention programs can be developed.

Despite the methodological problems associated with the definition of traumatic brain injury and case ascertainment, estimates of incidence rates have been more similar than dissimilar. In six reports on the epidemiology of head trauma in the general population, the incidence ranged from 180 to 295 per 100,000. In each study, males outnumbered females, the peak age was most frequently cited as 15 to 19 years, and motor vehicle accident was the most frequent cause of injury (Frankowski et al. 1985). The incidence of traumatic brain injury in pediatric populations is similar to that reported for adults. A mortality rate of 10 per 100,000 children (Annegars 1983) places head trauma as the major cause of death in children. However, children and adolescents are consistently reported to have a lower mortality rate than adults (Goldstein and Levin 1987) and a much lower rate than the elderly (Annegars et al. 1980; Jennett et al. 1980). The death rate in males was estimated to be four times that in females (Frankowski 1985).

Mortality statistics show only one part of the picture. Approximately 100,000 to 170,000 children are hospitalized each year with traumatic brain injury, and six times that number visit the emergency room (Eiben et al. 1984; Kraus et al. 1986). These figures indicate that traumatic brain injury is a major public health problem and represents a significant health-related financial burden (Gottschall 1993). Kraus and associates (1990) reported that the costs of hospital care alone for pediatric traumatic brain injury exceed 1 billion per year. All the direct costs (other medical costs, nursing costs, and pharmaceuticals) add an additional 1,810 million in the 0- to 4-year-old range, 4,026 million in the 5- to 14-year range, and 8,934 million in the 15- to 24-year ranges (Rice and MacKenzie 1989).[1]

The rate, severity, and mechanisms of traumatic brain injury vary with the child's age. A steadily increasing rate of injury was recognized up through age 14 years, with a dramatic peak occurring beginning at age 15 (Kraus et al. 1986; Rivera and Mueller 1986) (Fig. 24.3). Ninety-three percent of all head trauma in children (Kraus et al. 1986), compared with 80% in adults (Kraus and Sorenson 1994),

---

[1] Indirect costs fill such categories as loss of output and productivity in the workforce, caretaker opportunity costs, costs incurred from mental/social sequelae such as homelessness, incarceration, increases in other health expenditures, and costs from tranfer payments such as welfare and disability.

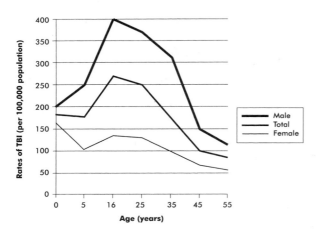

Figure 24.3 Incidence rates of traumatic brain injury (TBI) by age and sex. Adapted from Kraus JF, Black MA, Hessol N, et al. The incidence of acute brain injury and serious impairment in a defined population. Am J Epidemiol 119:186–201, 1984. Used with permission.

has been classified as mild. Mild injury is most common in 10- to 14-year-old children, but nearly the same proportion of mild injuries occurs in children ages 5 to 9 years. The peak incidence of severe and moderate injury occurs at age 15 years, but a relatively high proportion of such injuries also occurs in infants younger than 1 year of age (Fig. 24.4). Males are known to have a much higher rate of traumatic brain injury than females, but ratios vary, from as high as 4:1 to 1:1, as a function of age and mechanism of injury. In infancy, males are injured as frequently as females, but beginning at age 5 years, there are significantly more head injuries in boys than in girls (Fife et al. 1986).

Falls and transport-related accidents account for up to 83% of all traumatic brain injuries in children, although the proportion attributed to falls and transport injuries

varies widely from study to study (Kraus 1995). Injuries sustained during sports and recreation, assault, child abuse, and some types of birth injury account for the remainder of traumatic brain injuries in children.

The risk of traumatic brain injury associated with a specific mechanism varies as a function of age. In infancy, traumatic brain injury from child abuse accounts for most cases; in the preschool age group, falls are the predominant mechanism; and in the early elementary school age group, pedestrian accidents are the most common source of traumatic brain injury. In 10- to 14-year-old children, there is a dramatic increase in injuries from sports and bicycle accidents. Beginning at age 15 years, motor vehicle accidents in which the victim is an occupant become the most frequent cause of traumatic brain injury (Kraus et al. 1986; Rivera and Mueller 1986). The mechanisms of all forms of traumatic brain injury, and for severe traumatic brain injury only, in 1,544 children admitted to Allegheny General Hospital, a large western Pennsylvania trauma center, from 1987 to 1994 are outlined in Figures 24.5 and 24.6 (Arffa 1995).

Demographic risk factors for all childhood injury include poverty, single-parent households, and congested living conditions. A parental history of psychiatric disorder, drug and alcohol abuse, or physical illness is another risk factor. Unsupervised play is also reported frequently among children with traumatic brain injury and can be a direct cause of the injury (Chadwick et al. 1981; Klonoff and Paris 1974). Children with cognitive problems are at greater risk for a history of traumatic brain injury than are peers with normal cognition. Children with traumatic brain injury are more likely to have a history of behavior disorder (Bijur and Haslum 1995; Brown et al. 1981; Chadwick et al. 1981; Klonoff 1971; Klonoff and Paris 1974; Arffa & Goldstrum 2003a,b), although Pelco and colleagues (1992) and Donders (1992) did not find this relationship. Arffa (1995) found that in a series of 100

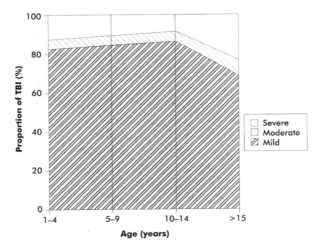

Figure 24.4 Traumatic brain injuries (TBI) by age and severity. Reprinted from Kraus JF, Fife D, Cox P, et al. Incidence, severity, and external causes of pediatric brain injury. Am J Dis Child 140:687–693, 1986. Copyright 1986, American Medical Association. Used with permission.

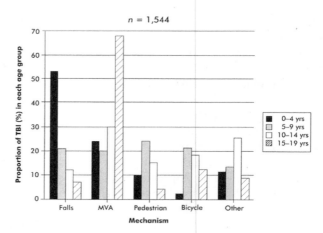

Figure 24.5 Mechanism of traumatic brain injuries (TBI) by age, for 1,544 patients hospitalized at a northeastern trauma center from 1987 to 1994. MVA = motor vehicle accidents. Cases of child abuse were not recorded; bicycle-related injuries include accidents involving bicycles and motor vehicles.

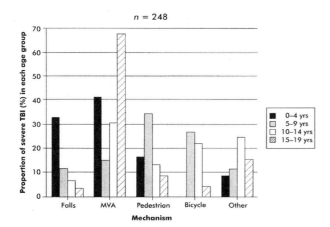

Figure 24.6 Mechanism of *severe* traumatic brain injuries (TBI) (GCS = 3–8) by age, for 248 patients hospitalized at a northeastern trauma center from 1987 to 1994. MVA = motor vehicle accidents. Cases of child abuse were not recorded; bicycle-related injuries include accidents involving bicycles and motor vehicles.

pediatric patients with traumatic brain injury from 1993 to 1995, 55 had a history of either school learning difficulties or behavior or emotional disturbance. Arffa and Goldstrum (2003a) found injured preschoolers had higher rates of developmental and behavioral problems than controls, but head injured preschoolers actually had significantly greater history of developmental delay before their injuries.

Child behavioral characteristics associated with high traumatic brain injury rates include impulsivity, aggression, and attention-seeking behavior. In contrast, in the toddler age group, behavioral factors are related to the home environment (Matheny 1987). A history of previous traumatic brain injury is also associated with an increased risk of further traumatic brain injury (Annegars 1983). The occurrence of multiple episodes of traumatic brain injury is strongly related to socioeconomic factors and the behavioral characteristics of the child, such as hyperactivity and aggression (Bijur and Haslum 1995).

Falls

Falls account for 4% of deaths in children (Table 24.7). Psychosocial factors are prominent in falls (Sieban et al. 1971; Spiegel and Lindaman 1977). The rate of death is higher in urban areas, where falls may occur from greater heights (Kottmeier 1995; Reynolds et al. 1971). Children survive falls from comparable heights more often than do adults (Barlow et al. 1983), although some of the highest fatality rates occur among very young children (Reynolds et al. 1971). Overall mortality rates from falls in 1.6% (Wang et al. 2001), and intracranial injury is most always the cause of death. Falls account for a significant proportion of nonfatal cases of pediatric traumatic brain injury as well (Annegars et al. 1980; Rivera and Mueller 1986). Children under the age of 4 years, particularly males, are

susceptible (Kottmeier 1995). Most falls occur during the summer, and they occur more often during the afternoon (Barlow et al. 1983). The incidence of walker injuries is especially high during infancy (Rieder et al. 1986). Falls from windows are more common in toddlers, and falls from fire escapes or roofs are more common in older children (Barlow et al.).

The physical characteristics of the young child in a free fall are thought to contribute to the higher number of central nervous system (CNS) injuries and skull fractures in this age group. The proportionately larger and heavier head of the child leads to a head-first orientation in the fall and head-first impact. Injury from head-first impact is likely to be more severe than that from a transverse fall, in which the force is distributed over a larger body surface (Kottmeier 1995).

Motor Vehicle Accidents

Motor vehicle accidents are a major source of fatal injuries (Annegars 1983). Thirty percent of deaths in children under the age of 18 years are due to motor vehicle accidents (Pautle et al. 1995). The percentage of injuries related to motor vehicle accidents increases progressively with age (Frankowski 1985). From ages 15 to 19 years, males outnumber females in motor vehicle accidents by 2.1:1 (Fife et al. 1986), and the rate of fatalities is higher among males.

To understand the biomechanics of motor vehicle accidents, it is useful to separate the accident into three or four separate "collisions" (Pautle et al. 1995). The first impact to the vehicle is followed closely by the occupant's impacting a portion of the vehicle. A third collision occurs internally as the brain strikes the interior of the cranium.

Frontal impact of the vehicle carries the greatest risk to occupants. Further insult can occur as unrestrained objects in the vehicle are propelled forward into the occupant. An unrestrained occupant is thrown forward until, in frontal collisions, the head meets the windshield. The rear seat is commonly thought to be safer because there are no steering wheels, dashboards, or windshields, but fatality rates for backseat occupants are approximately equal to those for front-seat occupants (Still et al. 1992). Injuries also occur from noncrash events. Excluding frontal collisions, the risk of fatality is actually greater in noncrash events than in collisions (Peterson and Royer 1991). Children are frequently fatally injured by ejection, or falls from the vehicle (Howard et al., 2003). Sudden stops or swerves can also lead to impact within the vehicle (Pautle et al. 1995).

The younger child's relatively large head, higher center of gravity, and weak neck and shoulder muscles can make him or her more susceptible to acceleration and deceleration injuries (Ward 1995a). When unrestrained, the child can become a projectile, moving head first until stopped by a stationary object (Pautle et al. 1995).

TABLE 24.7

CHARACTERISTICS OF THE COMMON MECHANISMS OF TRAUMATIC BRAIN INJURY IN CHILDREN AND ADOLESCENTS

Mechanism	Mortality	Morbidity	Biomechanics	Pathophysiology/Complications
Falls	Account for 4% of deaths in children; higher (13–20%) mortality in urban areas because of tall buildings; mortality highest among young children, but older children survive better than adults[1–3]	13–69% of all traumatic brain injuries in children[4]; 1.7:1 male:female ratio; major cause of head injury in children 4 years and younger; common in summer months[5,6]; Psychosocial factors prominent (i.e., low-socioeconomic, urban housing, single-family household)[7,8]	Larger and heavier head of preschooler leads to head-first orientation, resulting in greater central nervous system injury and skull fracture[2]	Fracture most common, followed by central nervous system injury[2] Deceleration injuries with falls from heights[2] Intracranial mass lesions common in older children[9]
Motor vehicle accidents	Account for 30% of all deaths in children; highest mortality in children 15–19 years of age and in males[10,11]	Account for 25%–77% of all traumatic brain injuries in children, depending on the study[4] Morbidity increases with age: highest (70%) in males 15–19 years of age[12,13]	"3 or 4 impacts": 1) to vehicle, 2) to occupant, 3) to brain hitting interior of cranium, and 4) from flying objects[11] Injuries greatest in frontal impact and unrestrained occupants; rear seat ≤ front seat fatalities, and morbidity is increased in ejection from vehicle[11,14,15] Child becomes projectile when unrestrained[11]	Deceleration injuries potentiated in young children because of large, heavy head and weak shoulder muscles[16]
Pedestrian accidents	Dominant mechanism of traumatic brain injury death in children ages 1–9 years[12,18]	Children ages 5–9 years (pedestrian mechanism accounts for 39% of all head injury in this age range) and males most at risk[12,17] Driver negligence and careless crossing by child implicated[19–21]	Older children are thrown onto hood, often sustaining multiple impact injuries; small children roll under vehicle[22]	Multifocal injuries may be present in cases of multiple impact
Bicycle/sports accidents	Greater mortality in bicycle–motor vehicle accident[10,23,24] Equestrian sports have 2.5% mortality rate[41]	11% of all and 3% of severe traumatic brain injuries are recreationally related,[10,23–26] more severe in adolescents 70% of bicycle injuries are in children younger than 10 years of age; sports injuries occur more frequently and are more severe in adolescence[10,23–26, 38]; common in males, in summer months, and between 3:00 and 9:00 PM[25]; All-terrain vehicles: more severe injury in younger child[27] Football most hazardous, up to 200,000 concussions[39]; high schoolers fare worse than collegiates 40 injuries reduced with better coaching standards[28,29]	Most bicycle-motor vehicle accident victims make contact with front end of vehicle; children younger than 12 years of age often hit from left side[25] Second impact syndrome controversial[42]	More severe injuries occur in unhelmeted cyclist[25,27]

(continued)

TABLE 24.7

(continued)

Mechanism	Mortality	Morbidity	Biomechanics	Pathophysiology/ Complications
Child abuse	1,000 to 2,500 cases per year[30] Most common in young children[31–34]	64% of all and 95% of severe traumatic brain injuries in children 2 years of age and younger[31–34] Males and females at equal risk[35]	Shaken baby syndrome includes violent shaking and impact[36–38]	

[1]Barlow et al. 1983; [2]Kottmeier 1995; [3]Reynolds et al. 1971; [4]Kraus 1995; [5]Annegars et al. 1980; [6]Rivera and Mueller 1986; [7]Sieban et al. 1971; [8]Spiegel and Lindaman 1977; [9]Teasdale and Jennett 1974; [10]Annegars 1983; [11]Pautle et al. 1995; [12]Frankowski 1985; [13]Fife et al. 1986; [14]Peterson et al. 1995; [15]Still et al. 1992; [16]Ward 1995a; [17]Rivera and Barber 1985; [18]Tanz and Christoffel 1985; [19]Stevenson et al. 1992; [20]Baker et al. 1974; [21]Wolfe and O'Day 1982; [22]MacKay 1992; [23]Friede et al. 1985; [24]Kraus et al. 1987; [25]Spaite et al. 1991; [26]Fife et al. 1983; [27]Wesson et al. 1995; [28]Mueller and Blythe 1987; [29]Albright et al. 1985; [30]Cohn 1983; [31]Billmire and Myers 1985; [32]Duhaime et al. 1992; [33]Hahn et al. 1983; [34]Kraus et al. 1990; [35]U. S. Department of Health and Human Services 1989; [36]Caffey 1972; [37]Duhaime et al. 1992; [38]Sato et al. 1989; [38]Conn et al 2003; [39]Mueller and Blythe 1987; [40]Collins et al 2002; [41]Ghosh et al. 2000; [42] McCrory 2001.

Pedestrian Accidents

Injuries resulting from pedestrian accidents are most common in older preschoolers and young school-age children (Frankowski 1985). In this age range, fatalities occur more frequently from pedestrian accident injuries than from passenger motor vehicle accident injuries (Rivera and Barber 1985; Tanz and Christoffel 1985). Among those sustaining injury in pedestrian accidents, boys outnumber girls by 1.7:1 (Rivera and Barber). Most often, the child is struck by the front of the automobile and is thrown forward onto the hood. The child may continue rolling and sliding, potentially incurring additional impact injuries. Small children may roll under the vehicle (MacKay 1992). Injuries occur most frequently when children dart out into the street rather than cross at intersections (Rivera and Barber; Stevenson et al. 1992). Driver negligence and alcohol use by drivers contribute to these accidents and the resultant injuries (Baker et al. 1974b; Wolfe and O'-Day 1982).

Sports-Related Injuries

As many as 11% of pediatric head injuries and 3% of severe head injuries are recreationally related (Annegars 1983; Waller 1985). Compared with motor vehicle accidents and falls, sports injuries account for a much lower percentage of traumatic brain injury in children under age 12 years (Bruce et al. 1982), but the percentage increases greatly in adolescence (Conn et al, 2003; Poirier and Wadsworth, 2000). Adolescents also suffer more severe sports-related injuries, and among those sustaining such injuries, males significantly outnumber females. Although contact sports have the highest risk of concussion, there are reports of substantial concussion in winter sports, sports with risk of falls such as gymnastics, and nonorganized sports like rollerblading (Kushner 2001). Of all injuries incurred in the sport, mild traumatic brain injury accounts for 7.3% of injuries in football, 4.4% in wrestling, 3.9% in boys soccer, 4.3% in girls soccer, 3.6% in girls basketball, and 2.5% in field hockey (Powell and Barber-Foss 1999).

Football is the most hazardous organized sporting activity, with two thirds of football-related deaths resulting from traumatic brain injury (Mueller and Blythe 1987). High school football players alone have 200,000 concussions per year. High school football players were more cognitively impaired after concussion than their college cohorts, suggesting a more protracted recovery pattern in this age group, yet few are required to stop playing, and many have multiple concussions (Collins et al 2002; Field et al 2003; Langburt et al 2001; Genuardi and King 1995; Gerberich et al. 1983; Thurman et al. 1998). Better standards for football helmets and rules regarding blocking and tackling have helped to reduce the head and spinal cord injuries associated with football (e.g., Albright et al. 1985).

Hockey contributes about five concussions per 1,000 player/game hours (Goodman et al 2001). Heading is a factor in soccer related injuries, and although subjective complaints are high (Tysvaer and Storli 1981), cognitive function does not appear significantly disrupted (Janda et al. 2002). Golf injuries are caused by impact with the ball or club and 37 traumatic brain injuries in children 3 to 13 were reported in a single emergency room in a 7-month period in the United Kingdom (MacGregor 2002). New sporting fads are novel sources of traumatic brain injury. The "scooter phenomenon" lead to 19 concussions in children and adolescents in a single year in one Swiss town (Mankovsky et al. 2002). More snowboarding injuries are concussive injuries, while skiers injure other body parts more often (Skokan et al. 2003). Sledding may be one of the largest contributors of concussion in children (Hackam et al. 1999). Of inline skating injuries, head and neck injury occurred only in 16% of cases in a Canadian town (Nguyen and Letts 2001). An average of 31 pediatric equestrian injuries per year in a Boston hospital, and head injuries are second to orthopedic injuries in frequency, and carry a 2.5% mortality rate (Ghosh et al. 2000). Use of motorbikes and all-terrain vehicles is more likely to result in traumatic brain injury when the vehicles are driven on roadways and when the driver is unhelmeted, inexperienced, and young (Wesson et al. 1995).

Incidence rates of bicycle injury are considerably higher when injuries due to collision with a motor vehicle are included. Nearly 70% of all bicycle-related head injuries occur in children under age 15 years (Friede et al. 1985, Kraus et al. 1987; Spaite et al. 1991). Preschoolers make up only 5% of bicycle-related injuries and are less likely to be injured in the street, although they sustain traumatic brain injury at the same frequency and the same level of severity as older children (Powell et al. 1997). Among those sustaining bicycle-related injuries, boys outnumber girls by 3:1 (Kraus et al. 1987; Spaite et al. 1991). Most victims make contact with the front end of the vehicle, but they also are often hit from the left side when darting out into the street; this is true particularly among children younger than 12 years of age. Injury most often occurs in spring and summer months and between 3:00 and 9:00 PM. (Annegars 1983; Fife et al. 1983). Unhelmeted children are more likely to sustain more severe injuries (Sosin et al, 1996; Spaite et al. 1991).

Gunshot injuries are often listed under sports-related injuries even though a majority occur not in the context of recreation, but with accidental discharge or as an act of violence. Thirty-two head and neck gunshot wounds in children 3 to 17 were identified over 3 years in Houston, Texas, and carried a very high mortality rate even with low velocity missiles (Kountakis et al. 1996).

Child Abuse

Twelve- to 14-year-old children are more likely than children of other ages to be the target of physical abuse, but severe and fatal injuries occur most often in infants and young children. As many as 64% of all, and 95% of serious, traumatic brain injuries in the first and second years of life are thought to result from nonaccidental injury (Billmire and Myers 1985; Duhaime et al. 1992; Hahn et al. 1983; Keenan et al. 2003; Kraus et al. 1990). Nonaccidental injury causes 2,000 to 5,000 deaths per year (Cohn 1983). Males and females are equally affected, although females may suffer more abusive incidents. Abuse is more common in

families with psychosocial adversity, such as poverty and poor living conditions (U.S. Department of Health and Human Services 1989).

Behavioral indicators of abused preschoolers include social withdrawal, dependence, overcompliance, lack of curiosity, and flattened affect. Alternatively, modeling of aggressive behavior, hyperactivity, and agitation have been reported. Abusive parents often know little about normal child development. The more the child is perceived as different, the more likely he or she is to be abused. Therefore, children who were born prematurely and/or have congenital defects, mental retardation, developmental delay, or frequent physical illnesses are at greater risk for abuse (Cohn 1983; Helfer and Kempe 1987).

PATHOPHYSIOLOGY

It has become the convention to separate primary causes of traumatic brain injury from their sequelae, even though secondary complications may occur within minutes of the initial insult, and the brain tissue damage from the primary impact develops over hours and even days after the injury (Honig and Albers 1994; Jennett and Teasdale 1981; Pang 1985; Teasdale and Mendelow 1984).

Primary Brain Damage

Primary injuries result from events that take place within the first few milliseconds of an injury. Skull fractures and brain contusions or lacerations can occur on impact. The term *contusion* is used to describe a wide range of blunt injuries, from a small bruise on the crests of the gyri to a large coalescing clot, better termed an *intracerebral hemorrhage* (Jennett and Teasdale 1981; Teasdale and Mendelow 1984). The condition of the cranium does not correlate well with the severity of brain damage. Although localized contusions and lacerations often occur beneath depressed or compound skull fractures, the extent of injury can be limited, and clouding of the sensorium or loss of consciousness can be absent (Harwood-Nash et al. 1971; Jennett and Teasdale 1981; Miller and Jennett 1968).

Also, extensive contusions, lacerations, and hemorrhage can occur without skull fracture. Lacerations of the brain and rupture of the blood vessels can result from pulling and stretching during movement after an injury, and contusions often result from impact of the brain against the inner surface of the skull. Contusions commonly affect the undersurface of the frontal lobes and the tips of the temporal lobes, most likely because the brain impacts against the bony protuberances of the anterior cranial fossa and sphenoid region (Miller and Becker 1982). Even with a blow to the back of the head, frontal and temporal contusions will occur much more frequently than occipital lesions.

Contrecoup injuries are thought to occur from the brain and skull recoiling from impact (Pang 1985). In infants younger than age 5 months, surface contusions and contre-coup are uncommon (Ward 1995a).

Diffuse axonal injury is currently thought to be one of the primary mechanisms of damage in closed traumatic brain injury. This has been studied primarily through animal models and histological exam after death as non-invasive procedures are not available (Smith et al. 2003). Acceleration and sudden deceleration of the brain, and, even more important, rotation of the brain around its axis, cause stretching and tearing of the long white matter tracts (Adams et al. 1989; Povlishock 1992, 1993; Teasdale and Mendelow 1984). Damaged axons, even those not mechanically ruptured at the time of impact, undergo a cascade of well-known cellular changes leading to cell death (Jennett and Teasdale 1981; Povlishock 1992). Ommaya (1982) thought that the surface of the brain was affected in milder injuries and that more central areas were affected in more severe concussions. The role of axonal damage is supported by studies which found that the duration of unconsciousness is related to degree of axonal injury, with widespread severe damage leading to deep or persistent coma (Teasdale and Mendelow 1984). Although definitive research on the elastic properties of the neuron has yet to be conducted, young children may be more vulnerable to diffuse axonal injuries because unmyelinated fibers may be more vulnerable to shearing (Ward 1995b).

Mild Traumatic Brain Injury

Mild traumatic brain injury has been associated with well-known neurocognitive and neuropsychiatric symptom patterns, yet its pathophysiology remained an enigma until recently. Both animal and human research studies have revealed cellular and subcellular changes, vascular changes, and neurochemical reactions that can account for the morbidity in concussion. The exact mechanism remains elusive, and there may indeed be several varieties of mild traumatic brain injury. Mechanical impact stretches the axon, affects the axonal cytoskeleton, causing sudden neuronal depolarization, which disrupts axonal transport (Shetter and Demakis 1979). A cascade of neurochemical, ionic, and metabolic changes ensue (Hovda et al. 1995). Neuroexcitatory amino acids, such as glutamate and aspartate, are released, increasing glycolysis, resulting in metabolic depression (Christman et al. 1994; Povlishock 1992, 1993; Povlishock and Coburn 1989). Reuptake is inhibited causing increased receptor cell firing, and oxygen free radicals; nitric oxide can be particularly damaging when released in excess. Vascular changes have also been reported. Blood-brain barrier breakdown results in ischemic degeneration in the hippocampus in animal models of severe brain injury (Ward 1964), which may account for memory disruption. Hippocampal micro-hemorrhaging was found on autopsy of an adult male with symptomatic, prolonged mild traumatic brain injury, who died from an unrelated condition (Bigler 2003). Cerebral blood flow abnormalities appear

responsible for some ongoing postconcussive symptoms, as evidenced by reduced cerebral circulation time (Taylor 1966) and vasoconstriction (Gilbert 1968). Intracranial pressure alterations are not prominent in mild traumatic brain injury (Denny-Brown and Russell 1941), nor is it associated with diffuse axonal injury (Adams et al. 1982).

In mild traumatic brain injury, damaged axons are scattered throughout the white matter and are surrounded by healthy brain tissue. This unique situation, in which damaged neurons are contained in an intact environment, may precipitate a regenerative process observed as reactive sprouting and growth cone formation. The progress of this regenerative response appears to correlate with functional recovery. However, the neurophysiological factors responsible for neuronal recovery are complex and numerous, and beyond the scope of this chapter (see Bach Y Rita for an excellent review, 2003).

Secondary Brain Damage

Secondary brain damage occurs as a result of later-developing lesions or physiological processes stemming from the primary injury. Intracranial factors include hematomas, brain swelling, infection, subarachnoid hemorrhage, hydrocephalus, and seizures. Extracranial factors include respiratory failure and cardiovascular compromise with hypoxia. With a given Glasgow Coma Scale score, outcome will be poorer and will involve injuries to other organ systems when secondary brain damage is sustained, but the complex relationship between multiple organ or bodily system compromise and brain injury is not well defined (Bruce 1995).

Epidural hematomas often result from a tear of the meningeal artery. These hemorrhages can expand very rapidly and require prompt surgical evacuation. Epidural hematomas are somewhat more common in children and adolescents and are associated with an 18% mortality rate (Ward 1995a). Subdural hematomas are rare in childhood and are associated with greater overall severity of traumatic brain injury than in adults. The exception is subdural hemorrhages in infants, which are frequent sequelae of child abuse (Caffey 1972, Ward 1995a).

Brain swelling results from two mechanisms. Increased cerebral blood volume leads to failure of vascular autoregulation in the brain. There is also true cerebral edema, which can be vasogenic or cytotoxic. Both brain swelling and mass lesions increase brain volume and can lead to increased intracranial pressure. The brain attempts to accommodate the added volume and increasing intracranial pressure by making adjustments to blood flow and cerebrospinal fluid. When brain volume exceeds the capacity of this autoregulation, intracranial pressure rises rapidly (Fig. 24.7). Subsequent compromise in cerebral perfusion pressure and cerebral blood flow can lead to ischemic damage. Such ischemia is associated with poorer outcome and is characterized on CT scan by a low-density

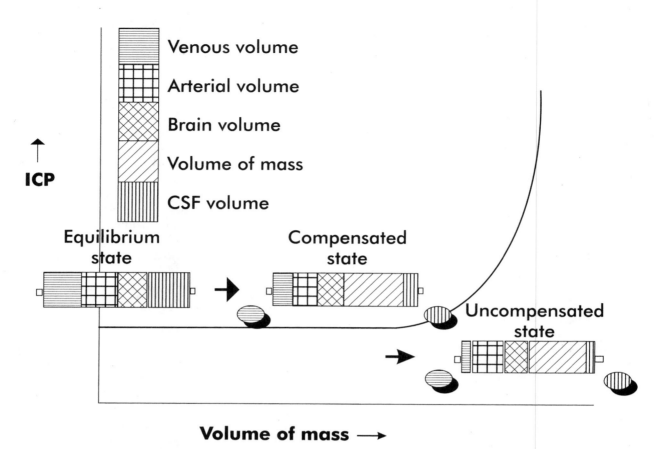

Figure 24.7 Intracranial pressure-volume of mass curve indicating change to uncompensated state. When mass increases, some compartments decrease to compensate. Intracranial pressure (ICP) increases rapidly when brain mass exceeds the capacity of the systems to compensate. CSF = cerebrospinal fluid. Reprinted from Ward JD. Craniocerebral injuries, in *Management of Pediatric Trauma.* Edited by Buntain WL. Philadelphia: WB Saunders, 1995, pp. 178–188. Used with permission.

brain ratio and an indistinct separation of white and gray matter (Bruce 1995).

Ischemic injury can also result from increased intracranial pressure; brain shift that compresses or damages arteries; arterial spasm; and complications from extracranial events, such as respiratory compromise or frank apnea. Ventricular enlargement is commonly seen months to years after severe brain injury and results from atrophy of the white matter. Progressive hydrocephalus is rare but can be caused by scarring. Abscess formation within the brain is a complication of penetrating traumatic brain injury and is usually prevented by debridement of the brain and closure of the dura and skin (Reitan and Wolfson 1986; Teasdale and Mendelow 1984).

After traumatic brain injury, early seizures occur in 6% of mild and 35% of severe traumatic brain injuries in children (Bruce 1993). Seizures associated with mild traumatic brain injury are unique to childhood (Jennett and Teasdale 1981). Early seizures are more common in children under age 5 years; they generally occur within the first 24 hours and do not predict outcome (Hauser 1983). One third of patients have only a single seizure.

Early seizures should be distinguished from later-onset epilepsy, which develops in 5% of patients with traumatic brain injury. Partial seizures are more common than generalized seizures. Localized scar tissue within the brain is one source proposed for this complication. However, vascular lesions, gliosis, disruption of glial–neuronal relationships, and disruption of inhibiting systems are also thought to be causes of posttraumatic epilepsy. Epilepsy occurs more commonly following penetrating head injury and is more likely to occur as the level of severity increases. Individuals with intracerebral hematoma and prolonged loss of consciousness also are more likely to develop epilepsy. Injuries to the posterior frontal and parietal regions are more likely to result in later-onset epilepsy (Hauser 1983; Jennett and Teasdale 1981). It is common for adults with a history of early seizures to develop later-onset epilepsy, but this is not the case for pediatric patients.

Child Abuse

Shaken baby syndrome is characterized by acute subdural hematoma and retinal hemorrhages. Shaking a young infant causes deceleration and rotational force injuries and is believed to involve an impact injury as well (Caffey 1972; Duhaime et al. 1992; Sato et al. 1989). Apnea and hypoxia are common consequences of inflicted brain damage. Immediate medical attention is often not sought following abuse, and this can set the stage for a cascade of secondary damage to ensue. The unconscious child is put to bed and breathing is further compromised, leading to further increased intracranial pressure and ischemia. Medical attention may not be sought until the situation has progressed to deep coma. At presentation, the infant may be in coma or cardiac arrest, with bulging fontanelles and retinal hemorrhage, but often no external evidence of head injury (Bruce 1995). CT scan may show subdural hemorrhage and low-density brain swelling, and MRI often shows multifocal hemorrhage (Bruce and Zimmerman 1989). Infants who present with reduced consciousness have a poor outcome (Reece and Sege 2000): one third will die, one third will have severe disability, and one third will have a moderate to good recovery (Bruce 1995).

Several physical signs are considered pathognomonic for abuse. Subdural hematoma is a case in point. In infancy, subdural hematoma is an infrequent result of falls, even from heights. Metaphyseal fractures and failure to thrive are signs that raise the possibility of abuse in a given child (Figs. 24.8 and 24.9). Fractures and wounds at different stages of healing, and external marks that conform to the shape of a hand, teeth, or object, are also suggestive of abuse. In addition, parents often give vague or contradictory accounts of the "accident" (Billmire and Myers 1985; Hettler & Greenes, 2003).

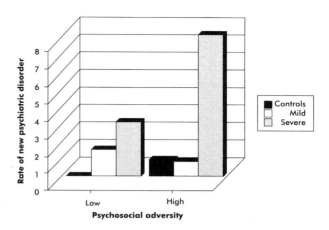

Figure 24.9 Cranial computed tomography (CT) image from 2-month-old infant who was born at 36 weeks' gestation with inflicted traumatic brain injury. Patient was brought to the emergency department in status epilepticus, and CT showed bilateral subdural hematomas. Skeletal survey showed healing fractures in the tibia and femur. Courtesy of I. Jarjour, M.D., Allegheny General Hospital, Pittsburgh, Pennsylvania.

Sports-Related Injuries

When the athlete's head is at rest and struck by another object (as in a "left hook"), maximal damage is usually sustained beneath the site of cranial impact. When the athlete is in motion and strikes his or her head with a moving object, maximal injury is sustained opposite the site of impact or *countra-coup*. Shearing from rotational forces can be significant in high velocity impacts. The

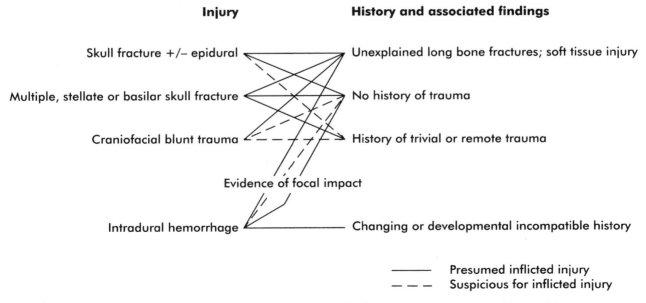

Figure 24.8 An algorithm for determining presence of inflicted injury in very young children. *Solid lines* indicate a "presumed" inflicted injury, and *dashed lines* indicate less conclusive or "suspicious" findings. Reprinted from Duhaime AC, Alario AJ, Lewander WJ, et al. Head injury in very young children: mechanisms. injury types, and ophthalmologic findings in 100 hospitalized patients younger than 2 years of age. *Pediatrics* 90:179–185, 1992, p. 180. Reproduced by permission of *Pediatrics*.

athlete who sees the blow coming will tense his neck muscles, and thereby suffer less of these rotational-related injuries (Cantu 1986).

The previous section on the pathophysiology of mild traumatic brain injury explains much of what occurs in sports-related injury. However, the concepts of second-impact syndrome is unique to the sports literature. "Vascular congestion syndrome" was initially reported by Kelly (1991) after a high school football player died from uncontrollable increases in intracranial pressure after sustaining two concussions in a game. There are 25 to 30 putative cases of second impact syndrome (Cantu and Voy 1995; Mueller et al. 1996), but McCrory (2001) recently critically reviewed these data. McCrory studied the case reports of athletes who had severe, unexplained cerebral swelling after concussion, and found many did not have conclusive evidence of a concussion in temporal proximity to the offending insult. He also recognizes that the syndrome is, curiously, seen only in the United States, while other countries may report significantly higher rates of concussive injuries during sporting. All the published cases of second impact syndrome occurred in adolescents, and this age group may have a higher rate of cerebral swelling and disturbed autoregulation after mild traumatic brain injury regardless of whether there was a second impact.

Another concept unique to sports-related traumatic brain injury is *dementia pugilistica*, identified initially from the sport of boxing, and due to repeated blows to the head, is characterized by chronic headache, imbalance, fatigue, dysarthria, and neurocognitive and functional deficits. Distinct neuroanatomical abnormalities have been found throughout the brain (Stiller and Weinberger 1985) in adults. The sport is uncommon in pediatric circles.

On a final note, many studies suggest that regular helmet use and design specific to the sport can ameliorate the occurrence and severity of sports-related concussion.

OUTCOME

Recovery is related to the severity of initial brain damage, primarily diffuse axonal injury. A secondary mass lesion that initially depresses consciousness may cause only reversible brain injury if treated promptly. Whereas children may be less vulnerable to mass lesions, they may be more susceptible to bilateral diffuse brain swelling and to subsequent ischemic injuries (Bruce et al. 1978, 1979). Ischemia is probably the most pernicious of the secondary complications. Recent human trauma research efforts in neuropharmacology have been aimed at introducing agents, such as free radical inhibitors, early in medical treatment to attempt to attenuate some of the secondary damage that ensues in the immediate surround of ischemic lesions (Honig and Albers 1994). There have been some limited, favorable outcome data, but studies with children are extremely rare (Ward 1995b).

The Glasgow Coma Scale is a useful method of grading severity and predicting outcome in adults (Levin et al. 1990; Taylor 1992), although in the 13 to 15 range, GCS is unrelated to later neuropsychiatric sequelae (McCullagh et al. 2001). However, this scale is less reliable in pediatric cases, especially those involving infants and preschoolers (Bruce 1983), and it is not entirely clear that the scale predicts cognitive outcome in this population. Length of posttraumatic amnesia may serve as a better predictor of neurocognitive outcome than length of coma in adults (Shores 1989), and it predicts later memory function in children (Ewing-Cobbs et al. 1990). Neurological indices of pupillary and brainstem reflexes are good predictors of independence, whereas hemiparesis and early seizures are not (Eisenberg 1985; Hauser 1983; Levin et al. 1990). Elevated intracranial pressure portends a poor outcome.

Overall Outcome

The Glasgow Outcome Scale (Jennett and Bond 1975) has become the standard instrument to measure outcome after traumatic brain injury in adults. Outcome is divided into five categories: (1) death, (2) persistent vegetative state, (3) severe disability, (4) moderate disability, and (5) good recovery. A lower rate of severe injuries during childhood (Kraus et al. 1986) and multiple medical problems in the elderly may contribute to this trend in overall mortality rates (Goldstein and Levin 1987). Although considerable discrepancy exists among research reports, most evidence suggests that mortality rates may be lower in children compared with in adults, when rates are equated for severity of injury (Alberico et al. 1987; Bruce et al. 1979; Kraus et al. 1986; Luerssen et al. 1988). Nevertheless, infancy does appear to be a vulnerable period, with a high rate of mortality from severe injury (see, e.g., Luerssen et al. 1988).

Infants and children are generally recognized to have a greater potential for neurological recovery than adults, especially with anoxic and ischemic insults (Ashwal et al. 1992). The persistent vegetative state following traumatic brain injury is rare in childhood (occurring in fewer than 1% of children admitted to hospitals for traumatic brain injury), and 90% of pediatric traumatic brain injury survivors will recover to a moderately disabled state or better after 3 years (Bruce et al. 1978, 1979). Because children, compared with adults, are less likely to die and because they recover well physically and are less likely to be left with permanent neurological sequelae such as aphasia, it has been commonly assumed that traumatic brain injury is less pernicious in childhood. This is not the case, however, when one looks at academic, neuropsychological, or psychiatric criteria (Fletcher et al. 1995). Neuropsychological studies suggest that cognitive deficits in childhood may linger, and to a greater degree than in adulthood (Brink et al. 1970; Fletcher et al. 1987). The Glasgow Outcome Scale apparently is not sensitive to unique factors in childhood such as the effect that brain injury has on disrupting later development of function (Fletcher et al. 1987). Because a child is in a developing state, a return to a previous level of functioning is not the same as recovery if the child has not returned to the same trajectory of developmental progress.

Neuropsychological Deficits

There is general agreement on the shortterm neuropsychological effects of pediatric traumatic brain injury, but less consensus exists regarding longterm effects. Severity of injury interacts with other factors influencing neurobehavioral recovery from traumatic brain injury. These factors include age at which the injury was sustained, extent of injury (focal vs. diffuse lesions), and time since injury.

Specific Age Factors Contributing to Outcome and Recovery

Both animal and human studies of brain injury suggest that the age at which the injury was sustained is a major contributor to eventual outcome. This set of research data provides a conceptual framework for understanding the effects of traumatic brain injury in children. In contrast to a commonly held belief, recent evidence does not support the notion that the young brain is less vulnerable to insult or recovers better than the mature brain. Emerging evidence suggests that there are cognitive effects that can occur late, which are attributed to patients' "growing into their deficits," especially executive function deficits (Grattan and Eslinger 1991; Kolb 1995; Slomine et al. 2002).

The assumption that the immature CNS affords greater plasticity was based in part on the view that different brain regions could support the function subserved by the damaged region. The basis for this view was the relative sparing of language in young children who experience significant left-hemisphere damage, including hemispherectomy. However, although children resume the capacity to speak, they may also manifest more subtle communication dysfunction. It is likely that the age limit for hemispheric transfer of function may be lower than was commonly believed (Kolb 1995). In addition, sparing of communication skills may occur at a price, such as lowered overall IQ (Boll and Barth 1981).

Language recovery may be unique in childhood simply because the etiology and pathophysiology of the injury differ from that in adults. Much of the research on recovery from aphasia was obtained from studies on adults who suffered vascular lesions, which are rare in childhood. When vascular lesions are present in childhood, deficits appear more similar to those in adults (Dennis 1980). This point signals that one must be cautious when contrasting adult and childhood recovery from traumatic brain injury, because pediatric cases differ from adult cases in common mechanisms of injury, severity of injury, and medical complications.

Studies of recovery from focal damage indicate that some functions, such as language, may recover better than others. Woods (1980) did not find evidence of compensation of visuospatial function after right-hemisphere damage in early infancy. Relevant to outcome in pediatric traumatic brain injury is the research considering recovery of executive function after early insult. Goldman (1971, Goldman et al. 1970) found that orbitofrontal lesions produced similar deficits in young and mature monkeys but that there was relative sparing of function following dorsolateral lesions.

The extent of injury may influence recovery, with less recovery expected when an entire functional area is affected. With diffuse cerebral injury, residual cognitive deficit may be more severe when the injury occurs in early infancy rather than in later childhood. However, we now know that the relationship between age at injury, lesion site and size, and cognitive outcome is complex (summarized in Kolb 1995). IQ is particularly vulnerable to early brain damage (Boll and Barth 1981).

Fletcher and Levin (1988), in a review of research on age factors in traumatic brain injury, found evidence for greater compromise in children younger than 6 years of age. However, the findings from earlier studies that show worse outcome in the younger sample may have been colored by a high rate of traumatic brain injury from abuse. It is now known that abused children may suffer more severe injuries, may differ from nonabused children prior to the injury, and have a worse general outcome after traumatic brain injury (Goldstein et al. 1993, Michaud et al. 1992; Trickett et al. 1991). When a subsample of physically abused children was removed from analyses, younger and older children with severe injury were equally compromised from traumatic brain injury (Kriel et al. 1989). Nevertheless, age effects noted in other studies that did not include abuse as a confound suggest somewhat worse outcome in younger children when severity of injury is equated with that in older children (Ewing-Cobbs et al. 1987; Gulbrandsen 1984, Levin et al. 1982). This is especially true for the preschool age group (Michaud et al. 1993; Wrightson et al. 1995). Slomine and associates (2002) found evidence that children injured at a young age where more likely to demonstrate executive function deficits than those injured later.

There is increasing evidence that skills in a rapid state of development at the time of injury may be more vulnerable to the effects of traumatic brain injury. Preschoolers are likely to demonstrate compromise in motor and expressive language skills (Ewing-Cobbs et al. 1989), and school-age children may be more compromised in reading (Barnes 1999; Shaffer et al. 1975) as well as written language (Ewing-Cobbs et al. 1987).

Time Since Injury

Adults and children differ in the time it takes to reach a stable point in recovery. The severity of injury is also a factor. In adults, the Glasgow Outcome Scale reliably predicts the amount of disability in 90% of victims within the first 6 months after the event (Jennett 1983). In children younger than 14 years of age, motor and sensory deficits recovered within 3 months, at which point the recovery was considered stable (Black et al. 1971). However, neurocognitive recovery can be more prolonged, particularly after more severe injuries. After milder injuries, neurocognitive recovery takes place within the first 6 to 12 months after the injury and slows after 12 months (Brooks and Aughson 1979; Jones 1990). Plateaus may be reached after 1 year in moderate to severe injuries as well (Yeates et al. 2002). The recovery gradient may remain steep through the second year for very severe injuries and may continue into the third year (Chadwick et al. 1981). Simple information-processing deficits present 3 years after injury can be considered permanent, and compromise in more complex intellectual skills can be considered permanent after 5 years (Long et al. 1984). Lingering sequelae can be observed after traumatic brain injury of any degree of severity, even after mild injury.

Neurocognitive Deficits Related to Severity of Injury

Mild traumatic brain injury commonly results in reduced information-processing capacity. In the early posttraumatic phase, the patient may process information more slowly, be inattentive and distractible, and appear forgetful (Gronwall 1989). Memory, attentional, and information-processing deficits form the core cognitive constellation known as *postconcussion syndrome* (Table 24.8). Postconcussion syndrome also includes a number of physical and emotional complaints. Studies in which groups of adult patients with mild traumatic brain injury were paired with orthopedic control groups indicate that certain somatic complaints and patterns of cognitive dysfunction may be specific to traumatic brain injury, whereas pain and emotional distress may be a nonspecific response to trauma in general. Postconcussion syndrome frequently resolves 1 to 3 months after the injury, but a subgroup of mildly injured patients may suffer more lingering neuropsychological deficits and/or subjective discomfort. Cognitive performance follows a predictable recovery curve, but subjective complaints do not (Alexander 1992; Cicerone and Kalmar 1995; Gerber and Schraa 1995).

The incidence and source of postconcussion syndrome in adults, particularly persistent subjective complaints, have been the focus of considerable controversy in recent years (see, e.g., Bohnen et al. 1994). Postconcussion syndrome is easily and reliably feigned (Mittenberg et al. 1992) and is subject to considerable secondary gain from litigation compensation (Youngjohn et al. 1995). Personality factors, such as somatization, also play a role (Karzmark et al. 1995). On the other hand, positron- emission tomography (PET) and neuropsychological test data, and even histological examination provide support for neuropathology of postconcussion syndrome even in the absence of abnormalities on MRI or CT (Bigler 2003). These findings are unrelated to history of loss of consciousness. The most pronounced neuropathology is found in frontal and anteriotemporal regions (Ruff et al. 1994).

Thus, although malingering or somatization may indeed be factors, there is strong evidence for an organic etiology in certain cases of persistent postconcussion syndrome, particularly when neuropsychological deficits are present. High-speed motor vehicle accident, age over 30 years at time of injury, and early presentation of cognitive dysfunction are relatively more common among patients with persistent postconcussion syndrome (Leininger et al. 1990). Factors that may make adjustment more difficult in the period following the injury include immediate return to school or work, emotional reactions to the accident, and preexisting obsessive-compulsive disorder or other anxiety disorders (Ruff et al. 1986). Symptoms common to post-traumatic stress disorder do not occur in mild traumatic brain injury (Sbordone and Liter 1994).

Information-processing deficits occur in children and adolescents following mild traumatic brain injury, particularly in the acute stages (Bassett and Slater 1990; Levin and Eisenberg 1979a, 1979b). Although initial cognitive deficit is apparently a common sequela of pediatric head injuries of mild severity, there is little evidence of sustained neurocognitive or learning deficit in the majority of children (Asarnow et al. 1995; Bawden et al. 1985; Bijur and Haslum 1995; Chadwick et al. 1980; Gulbrandsen 1984; Levin et al. 1988). Research on traumatic brain injury in preschoolers is quite limited and inconsistent. Shortterm prospective studies suggest preschoolers recover much the same as older children after mild traumatic brain injury (Anderson et al. 2000; Arffa and Goldstrum 2003a). Other studies suggest that preschoolers may be especially vulnerable to mild head injury, and it may take years for the deficit to become fully apparent (Gronwall et al. 1997; Wrightson et al. 1995). For example, Roberts and colleagues (1995) described a young child who sustained whiplash injury in a motor vehicle accident without loss of consciousness. Staring spells, brief confusional episodes, and emotional outbursts were noted 2 years after injury, and epileptiform activity was documented on the electroencephalogram (EEG) 4 years

TABLE 24.8
POSTCONCUSSION COMPLAINTS

Cognitive Complaints	Emotional Symptoms	Somatic Symptoms
Poor concentration	Depression	Fatigue
Forgetfulness	Anxiety	Dizziness
Slowness in thinking	Irritability	Blurred vision
Indecisiveness	Reduced tolerance for frustration	Oversensitivity to light and noise
	Low self-confidence	Tinnitus
		Sleep problems
		Poor coordination

after injury. PET scan revealed hypometabolism in both temporal lobes, and neuropsychological testing documented verbal and visual memory deficits. The outcome for children sustaining multiple concussion has not been adequately addressed in the pediatric literature (Bijur and Haslum 1995), although there is emerging literature from sports medicine indicating greater neurocognitive compromise with multiple concussions.

There is comparatively little research on reported postconcussion complaints in children and adolescents. Casey and colleagues (1987) reported minimal reporting of physical and emotional symptoms in children with "minor" traumatic brain injury (i.e., no loss of consciousness or altered level of consciousness); headache was more frequently reported following mild traumatic brain injury in children (Farmer et al. 1987; Klonoff et al. 1977; Lanser et al. 1988) and preschoolers (Arffa and Goldstrum, 2003c). Children with moderate traumatic brain injury showed significantly more postconcussion complaints than did children with other injuries both acutely and after 6 months (Barry et al. 1994). Persistent postconcussion syndrome has received little attention, and the frequency with which it occurs (or even whether it occurs) in pediatric samples is not known.

More severe injuries in childhood result in persisting neurocognitive compromise (Table 24.9). Excellent reviews are available on this subject (Dalby and Obrzut 1991; Fletcher and Levin 1988; Fletcher et al. 1987; Levin et al. 1995, Yeates et al. 2002). There is a moderate correlation between length of coma and both psychometrically assessed IQ (Brink et al. 1970; Chadwick et al. 1981; Johnston and Mellitz 1980; Klonoff and Paris 1974; Levin and Eisenberg 1979b; Levin et al. 1982; Winogren et al. 1984) and school achievement (Shaffer et al. 1980). Persistent problems in school achievement are common (Berger-Gross and Shackelford 1985; Brink et al. 1970; Ewing-

Cobbs et al. 1998; Fuld and Fisher 1977; Heiskanen and Kaste 1974; Klonoff et al. 1977).

Language deficits do not conform to any particular dysphasic pattern, and receptive language function is relatively spared (Ewing-Cobbs et al. 1985, 1987; Levin and Eisenberg 1979a). Language problems at the discourse level may be particularly persistent (Chapman 1995; Dennis and Barnes 1990), and the role of the frontal lobes in this type of communication disorder has been highlighted in both adults (Alexander et al. 1989) and children (Chapman 1995).

Attention and memory deficits are common after severe pediatric traumatic brain injury. They tend to persist for at least 1 year and may lead to academic failure marked by problems in assimilating new information (Gaidolfi and Vignolo 1980; Kaufman et al. 1993; Levin and Eisenberg 1979a, 1979b; Levin et al. 1982, 1988). Immediate or short-term memory deficits may be common in developmental disorders such as attention-deficit/hyperactivity disorder (ADHD) and dyslexia, but longterm memory deficits in these disorders are uncommon. The anatomic regions responsible for the transfer of verbal and visual information into longterm storage are discrete and localized and thus vulnerable to damage from traumatic brain injury. Memory deficits, therefore, appear to be unique to acquired brain injury in children, although it is possible that mental retardation with or without autism may be another manifestation of a developmental amnesia (Pennington 1991).

Visuomotor and visuospatial deficits are present in some patients (Bawden et al. 1985; Chadwick et al. 1981; Hannay and Levin 1984; Klonoff et al. 1977; Levin and Eisenberg 1979a, 1979b; Levin et al. 1982).

The impact of traumatic brain injury on executive function in children is an evolving and promising area of research. Executive deficits are cognitive processes that include voluntary initiation and inhibition of behavior; selective attention; planning; organization; and ability to switch sets. These deficits result from damage to the prefrontal regions or their connections, as well as diffuse injury. Although the advanced organizing functions of the frontal lobes may not be functional until adolescence (12 to 15 years) or adulthood (see, e.g., Golden 1981), there is evidence for an evolving functional state of the frontal lobes. Animal and human studies provide support for the development of core frontal lobe skills as early as 6–9 months in humans and at parallel ages in monkeys (Diamond and Goldman–Rakic 1989). Developmental researchers (Chelune and Baer 1986; Dennis 1991; Levin et al. 1991; Mateer and Williams 1991; Passler et al. 1985; Welsh and Pennington 1988) have documented the expected ages for mastery in a wide range of executive functions, with continued development noted at least through age 15 years. In adults and children, neuropsychological evidence of executive function deficits secondary to traumatic brain injury has been identified that correlates with the CT and MRI findings (Goldstein and Levin 1991; Levin et al. 1995; Slomine et al. 2002).

TABLE 24.9

NEUROCOGNITIVE DEFICITS SECONDARY TO SEVERE TRAUMATIC BRAIN INJURY IN CHILDREN

Intelligence	Intellectual level depressed with longer periods of unconsciousness
Achievement	Persistent academic problems noted in reading, math, and other areas of school achievement
Language	Dysnomia, dysgraphia, reduced verbal fluency, problems in writing to dictation, problems in discourse (i.e., misinterpretation of ambiguous messages)
Attention/memory	Persistent deficits common
Visuomotor	Problems on tasks of speeded performance and reaction time; visuospatial deficits noted
Executive function	Problems in planning, strategy development

Finally, there has been some support for "cognitive reserve" theory (Ropacki & Elias, 2003) suggesting that a previous brain insult (or other conditions that diminish cognitive reserve such as substance abuse), potentate the cognitive sequelae that adults experience after mild to moderate traumatic brain injury.

Behavioral and Psychiatric Disorder Secondary to Traumatic Brain Injury

Early uncontrolled research identified high rates of psychiatric disturbance in groups of patients with brain damage of multiple etiology (Gudmunsson 1966; Holdsworth and Whitmore 1974; Pond and Bidwell 1960). More recent controlled studies confirmed that brain injury increases the likelihood of psychiatric disturbance (Brown et al. 1981; Rutter et al. 1970; Seidel et al. 1975; Shaffer et al. 1975; Weiland et al. 1992). Psychiatric disorder is twice as likely to be found in children with cerebral damage from multiple causes than in children with physical disabilities or chronic illnesses or healthy control children. Increased rates of psychiatric disorder have been correlated with more severe brain injury, greater cognitive impairment, and complicating psychosocial difficulties (Breslau 1985, Kirkwood et al 2000; Rutter et al. 1970; Seidel et al. 1975; Schwartz et al. 2003; Taylor et al. 2002).

Behavioral morbidity may be more common with early bilateral damage than with unilateral damage (Chelune and Edwards 1981). Behavioral disturbance is also greater if seizure or EEG disturbance occurs at younger ages. Disturbance of functioning like that present in epilepsy may be more harmful than actual removal or decay of tissue, since beneficial neuroplasticity may not occur. However, these findings may simply reflect a greater degree of brain pathology or effects of longterm anticonvulsant treatment (O'Leary et al. 1983).

Although brain damage increases the likelihood of psychiatric disturbance, it does not predispose one to a specific disorder or symptom cluster (Rutter et al. 1970). The pattern of psychiatric disorder in individuals with brain damage is similar to that seen in the general population (Bijur and Haslum 1995; Shaffer 1985). The effect of early brain injury may be to increase the variability of behavioral response (O'Leary and Boll 1984), a hypothesis that is consistent with the fact that psychiatric disturbance results from an interplay of direct and indirect effects of brain damage, secondary emotional responses, and family and environmental contingencies.

Injury Severity

In traumatic brain injury, a specific interaction between behavioral disturbance of recent onset and head injury severity/neurocognitive sequelae has been found. Findings from studies of this phenomenon vary considerably depending on what criteria were used to describe behavior problems or change (e.g., Brink et al. 1980; Fletcher et al. 1990; Rivara et

al. 1994). In studies by Rutter and colleagues (Brown et al. 1981; Rutter et al. 1983), the rate of new-onset psychiatric disorder in children with severe head injury was three times that in orthopedically injured control patients. In a recent study (Schwartz et al. 2003), behavioral dysfunction was recognized in 36% of severely injured, in 22% of moderately injured children with traumatic brain injury, compared to a 10% occurrence in the orthopedic control group. Behavioral disposition may actually worsen over time in persons with severe injury (Fletcher et al. 1995; Schwartz et al. 2003). A severity threshold was proposed; the risk of psychiatric disorder is much higher in very severe injury (defined as posttraumatic amnesia lasting 22 days or longer) than in severe (posttraumatic amnesia lasting 7 to 21 days) or mild injuries. Threshold effects noted in other studies (e.g., Levin and Eisenberg 1979b) were lower than those found by Brown and colleagues. No significant difference in rate of new psychiatric disorder was observed in children with mild injuries and orthopedic control groups (Brown et al. 1981; Fletcher et al. 1990; Rutter et al. 1983). Preinjury behavior was related to behavioral outcome in Rutter and colleagues' studies; more than half of the children with a doubtful disorder developed a definable disorder, and all had symptoms.

Psychiatric disorder was found to be related to length of posttraumatic amnesia, presence of neurological abnormalities, and degree of intellectual impairment, but persisting neurocognitive dysfunctions were less predictive of behavioral disturbance after 1 year. These findings suggest that other factors, such as noncompliance with treatment recommendations, presence of litigation, deviant patterns of relating in the family, and psychosocial adversity, were instrumental in causing later behavioral dysfunction (Brown et al. 1981; Fletcher and Levin 1988; Fletcher et al. 1990; Rutter et al. 1970; 1983; Shaffer et al. 1975, 1980; Schwartz et al. 2003; Taylor et al. 2002).

Age at Injury

In comparison to neurocognitive morbidity, there is less support for increased risk of behavioral problems in younger age groups (Fletcher et al. 1990; Klonoff and Paris 1974; Shaffer et al. 1975). Johnston and Mellitz (1980) suggested that age was not a good predictor of behavioral outcome once length of coma was controlled. Preschoolers have not been extensively studied. In one retrospective study (Michaud et al. 1993), children injured as preschoolers showed increased behavioral morbidity at school age. The authors suggested that injury during the preschool years may cause more behavioral disturbance than does injury later. However, Arffa and Goldstrum (2003b) found a very high initial base rate but no evidence of new behavioral disorder in mildly to moderately injured preschoolers at a 6 month follow-up.

However, age at injury may affect the manifestation of the behavioral disturbance. Klonoff (1971) reported that the most common complaints in the postacute period of traumatic brain injury in preschoolers were irritability and personality change and in school-age children headache and dizziness. Brink and colleagues (1970) found that children age 10 years and younger had symptoms of hyperactivity, destructiveness, decreased attention, impulsivity, and aggression, whereas children older than 10 years of age showed affective disturbance and poor judgment.

Symptoms/Disorders

After severe traumatic brain injury, a large variety of psychiatric symptoms can be found (Black et al. 1971; Brink et al. 1980; Shaffer 1995), and disinhibited, socially inappropriate behavior is more common than other behaviors (Brown et al. 1981). Insensitivity to emotional cues, even the misreading of positive emotions as negative, may be a factor leading to social compromise (L. Peterson 1991). Even with cognitive recovery, children with severe head injuries had more behavioral problems, were more socially inept, and had poorer adaptive living skills than their sibling control (Perrott et al. 1991). Two of five children manifesting disinhibition in the study by Brown and colleagues (1981) later received a diagnosis of ADHD. Depression has recently been identified after moderate-to-severe pediatric traumatic brain injury, on clinicians and family reports. The child or adolescent did not self-report depressive symptoms, but this may be a failure of self-awareness. Depressive symptoms correlate with family pathology but not cognitive dysfunction (Kirkwood et al. 2000; Viguier et al. 2001). Depressive symptoms resolve faster than externalizing symptoms (Bloom et al. 2001).

Overall, the risk of later-developing schizophrenia is increased in a head-injured population (2 to 3% risk) compared with the neuropsychiatrically normal population (0.8% risk) (Davidson and Bagley 1969; Wilcox and Nasrallah 1987). It is uncertain, however, whether brain injury raises the threshold for schizophrenia or whether the familial characteristics of children at risk for schizophrenia are the same as those for children at risk for head injury (i.e., impaired caretakers who also suffer schizophrenic disturbance).

Lesion Location

Lesion location has been tied to certain psychiatric disorders in adults with traumatic brain injury. For instance, depression and mania have been tied to right frontal lobe damage. Mania is a rare complication of traumatic brain injury and may require focal right-hemisphere lesions and a genetic predisposition for affective disorder. Acute-onset depression is thought to be lesion-related, whereas depression of later onset may be mediated by psychosocial factors. Paranoid delusional syndromes have been reported in both right and left frontal lesions, sometimes coupled with lesions elsewhere (Guze and Gitlin 1994; Jorge et al. 1993; Malloy and Duffy 1994; Starkstein et al. 1990).

There is comparatively less research involving pediatric traumatic brain injury samples. Shaffer and colleagues (see Shaffer 1995) found increases in affective symptomatology in children with lesions localized to the right frontal and left temporoparietal regions. Sollee and Kindlon (1987) found a lateralized effect in a pediatric group with brain injury of mixed etiology. Externalizing symptoms were correlated with dominant hemisphere lesion, and internalizing symptoms, excluding neurovegetative symptoms, were related to right-hemisphere damage. In an epileptic sample followed throughout childhood, a schizophrenia-like psychosis was recognized in 13 children with lesions bilateral or localized to the left hemisphere (Lindsay et al. 1979).

The frontal lobes have recently been implicated in numerous psychiatric symptoms, but, again, more is known about the adult than the child in this regard (Barkley et al. 1992). Although subdivisions of the frontal lobes are highly interconnected, there do appear to be symptom patterns tied to the different regions. Orbitofrontal damage leads to distractibility, stimulus-bound behavior, disinhibition, and dyscontrol behaviors. Dorsolateral lesions cause syndromes of executive dysfunction such as the inability to shift sets, to plan, and to organize. Mesial damage has been related to apathy and lack of spontaneity (Duffy and Campbell 1994; Malloy and Duffy 1994; Malloy and Richardson 1994). Sophisticated neuroimaging has helped to document the vulnerability of the frontal regions, most commonly the orbitofrontal region, in adults with traumatic brain injury (Ichise et al. 1994).

Our understanding of the effects of frontal damage in childhood has been limited by the paucity of knowledge about the normal development of executive functions, the relatively low incidence of focal frontal lesions in children, the relatively recent development of neurodiagnostic imaging to the point that it is possible to identify frontal pathology, and the limited amount of extended follow-up. However, several case studies of perinatal and childhood frontal lobe damage suggest syndromes similar to those seen in adulthood. Cognitive inflexibility, social disability, reduced empathic ability, self-regulatory deficits, and problems in deploying attention are observed. As in adults, frontal lobe damage in children does not lead to significant reduction in overall IQ, although pervasive dementia may follow severe early frontal lobe damage with subcortical involvement. Functional subdivisions develop during childhood, and variants of the frontal lobe syndrome, including lateralized effects, are reported in children. For example, one child who sustained right frontal damage was able to use verbal mediation to guide behavior, whereas another with left frontal damage was not. In another child, a mesial frontal lobe syndrome marked by aspontaneity was diagnosed at age 9 years (Benton 1991; Grattan and Eslinger 1991).

A delay in the onset of symptoms has been reported with all types of brain injury, but particularly with frontal injury in childhood. One case discussed by Grattan and Eslinger (1991) involved a youth who sustained frontal damage at age 7 years and who appeared spared from behavioral effects until adolescence, when progressive social and emotional deterioration was evidenced. There is some support for delayed onset of symptoms in animal models as well (Goldman and Alexander 1977).

Although frontal lobe syndromes bear some similarity to ADHD, and there is evidence linking frontal lobe function to this disorder (Chelune et al. 1986; Lou et al. 1984); children with ADHD do not grow up to show cardinal features of these syndromes. In addition, although hyperactivity does occur with frontal lobe pathology, it is certainly not a prominent feature (Benton 1991; Grattan and Eslinger 1991).

Psychosocial Factors

The ultimate expression of psychiatric symptoms depends on personality and psychosocial factors predating the injury, as well as the family's ability to cope afterward (Fig. 24.10). In one study, more than half of the children with adjustment problems following traumatic brain injury had a history of adjustment problems premorbidly (Brown et al. 1981). Longer-lasting behavioral problems are associated with family distress, including marital discord, parental psychiatric disturbance, and single-parent households (Brown et al. 1981, Fletcher et al. 1990; Perrott et al. 1991; Yeates et al. 1997).

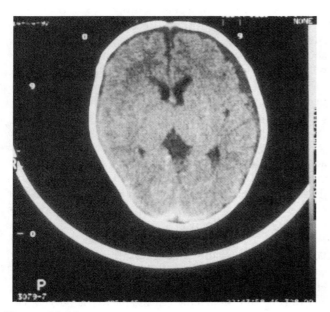

Figure 24.10 Psychosocial adversity and the development of "new" psychiatric disorders after traumatic brain injury. Numbers along vertical axis correspond to likelihood of development of psychiatric disorders (1 = as likely, 2 = two times more likely, etc.). Under conditions of high adversity, even control subjects developed psychiatric disturbance. Psychiatric disturbance was two to three times more likely in individuals with severe injury under conditions of high psychosocial adversity. Mild injury was defined as posttraumatic amnesia of at least 1 hour but no more than 7 days, limits that exceed those currently used. Reprinted from Rutter M, Chadwick O, Shaffer D. Head injury, in *Developmental Neuropsychiatry*. Edited by Rutter M. New York: Guilford, 1983, pp. 83–111. Used with permission of Guilford Press.

Severe head injury in children places significant stress on the parent–child relationship. Children with severe head injury are significantly more demanding than their siblings (Perrott et al. 1991). One study of abused children with neurocognitive dysfunction found that in 50% of the children the neurological impairment was a consequence of the abuse, whereas in the other 50% it was a contributory factor. Failure of the family members to move through a grieving process can lead to poor adaptation and unrealistic expectations, as well as conflict with doctors and caregivers (Birmaher and Williams 1994).

DIAGNOSIS

Unlike the situation that the clinician faces in dealing with the adult patient with traumatic brain injury, with children, a parent or caretaker is usually available to provide history unencumbered by the neurocognitive limitations that result from the injury. Parental report of the injury and subsequent behavioral change is likely to be most valid when obtained in proximity to the event. It is not uncommon, however, for neuropsychiatric evaluation and treatment to be pursued years after a traumatic brain injury, when specific details of the injury and immediate aftermath have faded from memory. It is also apparent that some parents, at a loss to explain their child's behavioral problems, may retrospectively attribute them to an identifiable past event. Other parents, uncomfortable with the prospect of an organic etiology, may highlight situational or other environmental factors.

Because neurobehavioral symptoms have multiple causes, a comprehensive history should be obtained, including developmental, academic, medical, social, and psychiatric histories. Hospital records of acute treatment provide critical data on injury severity and medical complications and should be reviewed (Taylor and Price 1994). As many as 32% of children with head injuries may have a preexisting learning disorder or history of school failure (Rutter et al. 1970). An important source of collateral information in these cases can be school records and yearly standardized achievement test scores. When available, previous psychological or psychiatric evaluations can be indispensable in defining baseline level of disturbance. Even with memories clouded by time and personal attributions, the parent is, in all likelihood, the best source for a history of behavioral change following traumatic brain injury in children. Specific details, including the exact behaviors or symptoms exhibited and the age at onset and the duration or frequency of symptoms, should be elicited.

Thus, comprehensive medical, neurological, and neuropsychiatric assessments are essential in evaluating the behavior problems of a child or adolescent with a history of traumatic brain injury. Behavioral rating scales are an efficient and inexpensive way to gather large amounts of information on behavioral adjustment, although none has been developed specifically for the pediatric head-injured population. A broad focus instrument, such as the Child Behavior Checklist (Achenbach and Edelbrock 1983), can be used along with scales that highlight certain cluster symptoms. Structured interviews for children may be selectively tapered after initial screening with a behavior checklist. Taylor and colleagues (1995) recently developed a structured interview to identify behavioral changes and maladaptive family reactions secondary to traumatic injury.

Finally, diagnosis is limited by the classification systems we use. A child may display multiple symptoms, but these symptoms may not meet the DSM-IV criteria for a specific disorder. Cataloguing and rating the severity of behavioral symptoms, independent of psychiatric diagnosis, can be useful in designing treatments. Prigatano (1992) discusses the need to distinguish between primary and secondary behavioral symptoms. For example, aggression may be considered a "side effect" of frontal damage since such damage limits the repertoire of behavioral response and the ability to process complex social interchanges.

Neurodiagnostic Studies

Defining the relationship between neurobehavioral assessments and structural and functional neurodiagnostics is an area of rapidly evolving research. As sophistication in both technologies grow, our ability to diagnose traumatic brain injury in children and provide treatment will greatly improve. Currently, neuroimaging plays a major role in both acute and postacute assessments of traumatic brain injury.

CT scanning is the procedure of choice in the acute setting in cases of traumatic brain injury, as it is quicker and less expensive than MRI, relatively less affected by motion artifact, and contributes information necessary for surgical management (Taylor and Price 1994). Because it visualizes bone better, CT is superior to MRI in the diagnosis of skull fracture. However, MRI is superior to CT in visualizing areas of contusion next to the skull, because bone artifact does not interfere, and is better for identifying diffuse axonal injury involving the deep white matter, corpus callosum, or brain stem. MRI (Levin et al.1987a; Akhtar 2003) identified abnormalities up to four times more often in patients with mild and moderate traumatic brain injuries than CT. Gennarelli and colleagues (1982) found MRI to be ten times more sensitive than CT in visualizing deep white matter shearing, which is the injury correlated with depth and duration of coma in primates. MRI is also superior to CT in identifying certain intracranial hemorrhages, especially isodense subdural hematomas, in determining the ages of intracranial hemorrhages, and in estimating the overall extent of brain damage in the early postacute period (Alavi 1989; Shores et al. 1990). MRI can be used at later times to identify deep white matter lesions and ventricular enlargement, both of which correlate with clinical outcome and some parameters of neuropsychological study (Verger

et al. 2001; Wilson and Wyper 1992). For these reasons, MRI is the instrument of choice starting 3 days after injury (Taylor and Price 1994).

Functional neuroimaging techniques, such as single-photon emission computed tomography (SPECT), PET, and fMRI, have a demonstrated role in identifying brain abnormalities that correlate with neuropsychological deficit and neurobehavioral symptoms (Ichise et al. 1994; Shores et al. 1990). This kind of imaging is not frequently utilized in the routine care of patients with traumatic brain injuries, although Johnston and colleagues (2001) suggest that fMRI may be useful in return to play decisions in athletes. PET and SPECT can be used to measure cerebral blood flow, cerebral blood volume, oxygen utilization, glucose or protein metabolism, and specific neurotransmitter function and has good spatial resolution. However, it is not available in most hospital settings because it requires expensive equipment and highly trained personnel. Although SPECT has poorer spatial resolution, it is more readily available than PET and, coupled with structural imaging and neuropsychological data, can help in understanding the functional correlates of structural lesions (Wilson and Wyper 1992). The fMRI can be used to detect changes in cerebral blood flow or blood volume, although oxygenation is most common (Johnston et al. 2001).

Neuropsychological testing is the most sensitive method of detecting subtle brain disturbances affecting cognition and behavior, especially after milder injuries (Taylor and Price 1994). Neurocognitive function can be impaired even when the MRI scan is normal (Levin et al. 1993). Recent developments in understanding the normal development of various neurocognitive functions (e.g., Welsh and Pennington 1988), and sophistication in test development and norms (e.g., Heaton et al. 1993), promise to enhance the utility of neuropsychological testing in pediatric traumatic brain injury.

MANAGEMENT

Management in the Acute Setting

In the acute setting, the neuropsychiatrist may be called on to rule out alternative and treatable causes of delirium in patients with traumatic brain injury (e.g., medication toxicity) and to establish the role of prior psychiatric disturbance in current presentation, as well as to assess functional capacity and the ability to benefit from rehabilitation. Environmental manipulation, such as minimizing environmental noise, establishing predictability in routine, and utilizing sitters or Naugahyde padded room enclosures, has been useful in controlling agitation that occurs during recovery from coma (Trzepacz 1994). Educating the patient and family about the aftereffects of mild traumatic brain injury may reduce the incidence of emotional and functional sequelae (Mittenberg et al. 1993).

Neuroleptics use is controversial. The sedative effects can increase confusion and lengthen posttraumatic amnesia, lower seizure threshold, and result in anticholinergic toxicity or extrapyramidal reactions (Birmaher and Williams 1994; Smeltzer et al. 1994). There is some experimental evidence that dopaminergic antagonists may impede neuronal recovery (Gualtieri 1991); this is supported by animal study (Feeney et al. 1982, 1990; Goldstein 1993; Hovda and Feeney 1985). However, Elovic and colleagues (2003) note that much of the caution is centered upon typical antipsychotics such as haloperidol, and that the atypical antipsychotics such as clozapine, olanzapine, quetiapine, risperidone, and ziprasidone, target serotonergic neurons and hold considerable promise in the treatment of patients with traumatic brain injury. Neuroleptics are frequently prescribed for agitation. When prescribed for psychosis, it is important to ascertain whether the behavior is psychosis, delirium, or a confabulatory process. The author recalls the case of a 54-year-old nurse hospitalized on a psychiatric unit after rupture of an anterior communicating artery. This woman was initially called delusional as she tried to lead the group therapy sessions on the unit. However, she suffered a dense amnesia after her lesion, and in the absence of ongoing memory, assumed her work role in what appeared to be her work environment. Symptoms were responsive to reality therapy and ultimately transfer from the hospital setting.

Research on psychopharmacology in the acute setting is limited, and most is conducted with adult patients. Two case of methylphenidate to minimally conscious patients, led to one positive response, indicating a role for single subject drug trials (Laborde and Whyte, 1997). Cholinomimetic agents in the promotion of cognitive recovery in the acute period is promising. Citicoline led to decreased length of coma and hospitalization and fostered better rehabilitation potential (Lorenzo 1991). Amantadine may promote faster cognitive recovery when used in the first 3 months (Meythaler et al. 2002), and clinical trials in the pediatric population are currently under way. The neuropsychiatrist practicing primarily in the acute setting may want to explore the research on neuroprotective agents, prominent in the animal literature. Cop-1, a synthetic polymer used in multiple sclerosis, was shown to counteract the loss of neurons from glycolysis in mice (Kipnis et al. 2003).

Psychopharmacological Management

The current role of psychopharmacology in the postacute setting is to control certain emotional and cognitive target symptoms. To date, there have been few double-blind, placebo-controlled clinical trials specifically aimed at children with traumatic brain injury, and guidelines must be borrowed from the literature on developmental disorder and adults with traumatic brain injury (see, e.g., reviews by Gadow 1992; Ross 1992; Wroblewski and Glenn 1994).

Several caveats are indicated:

1. Monotherapy is better than polypharmacy.
2. Start the medication at low doses and increase gradually.
3. Reassess often.
4. Carefully monitor side effects.
5. Monitor drug-drug interactions.

Psychopharmacological treatment for arousal and attention deficits has gained popularity (Wroblewski and Glenn 1994; Whyte et al. 2002). Stimulants have been effective in reducing distractibility, inattention, and hyperactivity in children and adults with ADHD (Gualtieri 1988); in improving hypersomnia, hypoarousal, and apathy in patients with narcolepsy or Kleine-Levin syndrome (Lemire 1993); and in improving all these symptoms in children with autism or mental retardation (Birmaher and Williams 1994; Birmaher et al. 1988). Because stimulants appear to effect change by modulating dopaminergic and noradrenergic neurotransmitters, especially in the frontal neocortex, they are a rational choice for the treatment of the cognitive sequelae of traumatic brain injury. There is also support from animal research that stimulants may foster cortical recovery (Feeney et al. 1982; Levin and Kraus 1994). Methylphenidate can be used safely in populations of brain-injured individuals who are at high risk for seizures (Wroblewski et al. 1992). The clinical research in traumatic brain injury samples has been inconsistent, especially in children. In 10 controlled studies, psychostimulants led to improved speed of mental processing and observational ratings of mood and behavior (Whyte et al. 2002). However, in the two pediatric samples, one was positive (Mahalick et al. 1998) and the other disappointing (Williams et al. 1998). In a carefully controlled study with adults, there does appear to be some advantage in increasing initial, but not sustained attention (Whyte et al. 2002).

Cholinomimetic agents, many originally developed to treat cognitive disorders in adults suffering from Alzheimer's disease, may be useful in enhancing cognitive recovery after traumatic brain injury in adults (Blount et al. 2002). Small scale clinical studies demonstrated benefits of citicoline (Levin et al. 1991). Physostigmine effectiveness has been inconsistent (Cardenas et al. 1994; Levin et al. 1986). Donepezil led to benefits in two patients (Taverni et al. 1998), three of seven patients (Whitlock 1999), and four patients (Masanic et al. 2001). A retrospective study of 53 patients showed benefits on subjective ratings but not cognitive testing (Whelan et al. 2000). However, only IQ tests were used, and these are not the most sensitive to posttraumatic brain injury cognitive dysfunction.

The neuropsychiatrist must consider medication-induced depression and emotional lability in the differential diagnosis of traumatic brain injury patients with affective symptoms (Silver and Yudofsky 1994). Antidepressants and mood stabilizers have been utilized in the treatment of posttraumatic affective symptoms. Antiepileptic drugs such as carbamazepine have been helpful in stabilizing mood in adults with traumatic brain injury and have recently been utilized for treatment of behavior disorders in children both with and without epileptic seizures (Evans et al. 1987; Gilberg 1995). Although carbamazepine may be particularly helpful in managing episodic/explosive behaviors associated with EEG abnormalities (Kuhn-Gebhart 1976), worsening of symptoms can occur in some children (Birmaher and Williams 1994). Recently, there has been an explosion of novel anticonvulsants, all of which appear equally effective in seizure control (Hoch and Daly, 2003), although some have more favorable cognitive effects. For example, Galopentin and Lamotrigine were superior to carbamazepine and topiramate (Meador et al. 1999, 2001; Showalter et al. 2000). Tricyclic antidepressants may potentiate seizure potential after severe traumatic brain injury (Wroblewski et al. 1990).

The treatment of aggressive behaviors calls for careful analysis of the behavior and environmental contingencies, diurnal characteristics, and baseline history. Lithium, carbamazepine, propranolol, stimulants, and neuroleptics (especially atypical) have been used in the treatment of aggressive behaviors (Campbell et al. 1984; Elovic et al 2003; Evans et al. 1987; Gadow 1992).

Behavioral Management Strategies

A multidisciplinary and multimodal approach to behavioral management is best for pediatric traumatic brain injury patients. Specific treatments are selected according to the age, cognitive level, and psychiatric presentation of the child or adolescent and the resources in the home and school. Environmental treatment strategies, recently advocated for adults with traumatic brain injury (Campbell et al. 1994; Mateer and Williams 1991; Sohlberg et al. 1993), are probably easier to apply in pediatric samples, since special educators and mental health providers are often skilled in behavioral treatment.

Traditional behavioral management strategies, such as contingency-reward, response cost, or time-out, may be effectively applied in the environment of the pediatric patient with traumatic brain injury. Children with brain injury respond optimally to a consistent, predictable routine in an environment where sensory stimulation is kept to a minimum. These patients often cannot tolerate multiple options or complex contingency contracts. Providing clear, uncomplicated instructions and breaking multistage problems into steps is advised. Modeling may not be effective without instruction identifying the behavior to change and the target behavior. Some patients may respond to cueing techniques such as "memory books" and cue cards that prompt the desired behavior.

Self-control and other metacognitive techniques are popular in the treatment of children and adolescents with behavior problems (Kendall and Braswell 1993) and can be adopted for use in some traumatic brain injury patients

(Feeney and Ylvisaker 2003; Sohlberg et al. 1993). Teaching systematic problem solving, social skills or conversation training, and verbal rehearsal is suggested for individuals with higher-level executive dysfunctions (see Stuss 1987). Cognitive rehabilitation of related neurocognitive deficit, such as attentional training and memory cueing systems, might augment response to metacognitive techniques (Sohlberg and Mateer 1987).

Emotional reactions to the loss of function may occur in pediatric traumatic brain injury patients who are aware of their deficits (Cicerone 1991). The "sense of self" can be disrupted, particularly in adolescents, for whom identity issues are prominent. The utility of more traditional psychotherapies for brain-injured individuals has been realized only relatively recently (Prigatano 1992). Group therapy is advocated, particularly for adolescents (Barin et al. 1985).

Family involvement is critical to the success of other treatments. Interventions with the family may involve psychoeducational and supportive therapy and grief therapy, as well as cognitive behavior therapy, to increase coping abilities (Barin et al. 1985). Parents of brain-injured children have more stress and psychological distress than parents of orthopedically-injured children (Wade et al. 1998). Family members benefit from education about brain injury sequelae (i.e., attributing amotivational syndromes to frontal pathology and not to recalcitrance). Family patterns that were previously adaptive (i.e., flexibility in rules or routine, tolerance of a high level of emotion) may become devastating to a brain-injured child or adolescent. Dysfunctional patterns present before the injury may be compounded in its aftermath (Wade et al. 2003). Thus, parent effectiveness training may prove to be of merit. Caring for a brain-injured child or adolescent places considerable stress on the parents and siblings in the family. Support and stress management training for, and in some cases psychiatric treatment of, family members may be indicated.

Rehabilitation and Education

Comprehensive rehabilitation is frequently recommended after significant traumatic brain injury and is designed to correct the physical, speech, and cognitive dysfunction that can follow such injury. Other goals include increasing the child's capacity for self-care and returning to school or vocational training. Neuropsychiatric consultation in the rehabilitation environment is often integral to maximizing benefit from this setting. Control of aggressive and impulsive behaviors and dysphoria, for example, sets the stage for progress in therapies. Judiciously eliciting the family's involvement in the rehabilitation process may foster both the child's recovery and the family's adaptation to the child's limitations (Novack et al. 1992).

Children with traumatic brain injury must ultimately return to school and the care of educators. Unlike adults, who may be able to return to a job that offers predictability and routine, children are returned to an environment that constantly calls for new learning and adaptation to novel settings. At the same time, educational settings may be ill equipped to manage the head-injured child.

Children with head injuries are entitled to special education services under the category of "other health impaired" in the Education for All Handicapped Children Act (PL 94–142) (1976). School districts differ in policy and orientation; some consider augmentation of academic subjects as their sole purpose, whereas others see physical therapy, occupational therapy, speech, and even cognitive therapy as prerequisite treatments to learning. School districts typically only recognize as special-needs students children who sustained severe injury. The child with mild or even moderate injury may return to school without special attention, and sometimes teachers may be unaware of the head injury. Designing the correct educational placement is essential for optimal postacute recovery, even for children with mild injuries. For example, a child with attention and memory problems may adjust best with short homebound instruction followed by a modified program (less demanding course load, alternative test approaches, and/or in-school tutoring). With children who sustained severe injury, school reentry should be approached gradually, with frequent consultation and collaboration with rehabilitation providers and family. Children with severe injury should not be returned to school until a readiness to learn has been established (Cohen et al. 1985).

Children with traumatic brain injury have unique educational needs. Because they are quite different from children with learning disabilities (e.g., memory deficits are unique to acquired brain injury), their needs are often misunderstood by educators. Neuropsychiatric consultation may be helpful both for behavioral difficulties directly caused by cranial trauma and for those that evolve from a mismatch of the child's needs and educational approach.

REFERENCES

Achenbach TM, Edelbrock C. *Manual for the Child Behavior Checklist and Revised Child Behavior Profile*. Burlington, VT: University of Vermont, Department of Psychiatry, 1983.

Adams JH, Doyle D, Ford I, et al. Diffuse axonal injury in head injury: definition, diagnosis, and grading. Histopathology 15:49–59, 1989.

Akhtar JI, Spear RM, Senac MO. Detection of traumatic brain injury with MRI and S-100B protein in children, despite normal computed tomography of the brain. Pediatr Crit Care Med, 4:322–326, 2003.

Alavi A. Functional and anatomic studies of head injury. J Neuropsychiatry Clin Neurosci 1:S45–S50, 1989.

Alberico AM, Ward JD, Choi SC, et al. Outcome after severe head injury: relationship to mass lesions, diffuse injury, and ICP course in pediatric and adult patients. J Neurosurg 67:648–656, 1987.

Albright JP, McAuley E, Martin RK, et al. Head and neck injuries in college football: an eight-year analysis. Am J Sports Med 13:147–152, 1985.

Alexander MP. Neuropsychiatric correlates of persistent postconcussive syndrome. Journal of Head Trauma Rehabilitation 7:60–69, 1992.

Alexander MP, Benson DF, Stuss DT. Frontal lobes and language. Brain Lang 37:656–691, 1989.

American Psychiatric Association. *Diagnostic and Statistical Manual of Mental Disorders*, 4th Ed. Washington, DC: American Psychiatric Association, 1994.

Anderson VA, Catroppa C, Rosenfeld J, et al. Recovery of memory function following traumatic brain injury in preschool children. Brain Injury 14:679–692, 2000.

Annegars JF. The epidemiology of head trauma in children, in *Pediatric Head Trauma*. Edited by Shapiro K. Mt Kisco, NY: Futura Publishing, 1983, pp 1–10.

Annegars JF, Grabow JD, Kurland IT, et al. The incidence, causes, and secular trend of head trauma in Olmstead County, Minnesota, 1935–1974. Neurology 30:912–919, 1980.

Arffa S. Pediatric head injury. Presentation at symposium "Head Injury Through the Life Span" (Fields R, Arffa S, Lovell M, moderators) at the National Meeting for Neuropsychologists, San Francisco, November 1–4, 1995.

Arffa S, Goldstrum S. Preschool Children with Mild to Moderate Traumatic Brain Injury: Pre-existing Developmental Dysfunction and Recovery Patterns. Arch Clin Neuropsychol 18:714, 2003a.

Arffa S, Goldstrum S. A study of behavioral and familial function in preschool aged children hospitalized for mild to moderate traumatic brain injury Arch Clin Neuropsychol 18:714, 2003b.

Arffa S, Goldstrum S. Post concussion symptoms in preschool aged children with mild to moderate traumatic brain injury. Submitted 2003c.

Asarnow RF, Satz P, Light R, et al. Behavior problems and adaptive functioning in children with mild and severe closed head injury. J Pediatr Psychol 16:543–555, 1991.

Asarnow RF, Satz P, Light R, et al. The UCLA Study of Mild Closed Head Injury in Children, in *Traumatic Head Injury in Children*. Edited by Broman SH, Michel ME. New York: Oxford University Press, 1995, pp 117–146.

Ashwal S, Bale JF, Coulter DL, et al. The persistent vegetative state in children: report of the Child Neurology Society Ethics Committee. Ann Neurol 32:570–576, 1992.

Bach Y Rita P. Theoretical basis for brain plasticity after a TBI. Brain Inj 17:643–651, 2003.

Baker SP, O'Neill B, Haddon W, et al. The Injury Severity Score: a method for describing patients with multiple injuries and evaluating emergency care, J Trauma 143: 187–196,1974a.

Baker SP, Robertson LS, O'Neill B. Fatal pedestrian collisions: driver negligence. Am J Public Health 64:318–325,1974b.

Barin JJ, Hanchctt JM, Jacob WL, et al. Counseling the head injured patient, in *Head Injury Rehabilitation: Children and Adolescents*. Edited by Ylvisaker M. San Diego, CA: College-Hill, 1985, pp 359–380.

Barkley RA, Grodzinsky G, DuPaul GJ. Frontal lobe functions in attention deficit disorder with and without hyperactivity: a review and research report. J Abnorm Child Psychol 20:163–188, 1992.

Barlow B, Niemirska M, Gandhi R, et al. Ten years of experience with falls from a height in children. J Pediatr Surg 18:509–511, 1983.

Barnes MA, Dennis M, Wilkinson M. Reading after closed head injury in childhood: Effects on accuracy, fluency, and comprehension. Developmental Neuropsychology 15:1–24, 1999.

Barry CT, Klein SK, Taylor HG. Validity of postconcussion symptoms in children with traumatic brain injury (abstract). Ann Neurol 36: 519, 1994.

Bassett SS, Slater E. Neuropsychological function in adolescents sustaining closed head injury. J Pediatr Psychol 15:225–237, 1990.

Bawden HN, Knights RM, Winogren HW. Speeded performance following head injury in children. J Clin Exp Neuropsychol 7:39–54, 1985.

Benton A. Prefrontal injury and behavior in children. Developmental Neuropsychology 7:275–282, 1991.

Berger-Gross P, Shackelford M. Closed-head injury in children: neuropsychological and scholastic outcomes. Percept Mot Skills 61: 254, 1985.

Bigler E. *Diagnostic Clinical Neuropsychology*. Austin, TX: University of Texas Press, 1991.

Bigler E. Response to commentary-Neurobiology and neuropathology underlie the neuropsychological deficits associated with traumatic brain injury. Arch Clin Neuropsych 18:595–622, 2003.

Bijur PE, Haslum M. Cognitive, behavioral, and motoric sequelae of mild head injury in a national birth cohort, in *Traumatic Head Injury in Children*. Edited by Broman SH, Michel ME, New York: Oxford University Press, 1995, pp 147–164.

Billmire ME, Myers PA. Serious head injury in infants: accidents or abuse? Pediatrics 75:340–342, 1985.

Birmaher B, Williams DT. Children and adolescents, in *Neuropsychiatry of Traumatic Brain Injury*. Edited by Silver JM, Yudofsky SC, Hales RE. Washington, DC: American Psychiatric Press, 1994, pp 393–412.

Birmaher B, Quintana H, Greenhill L. Methylphenidate for the treatment of hyperactive autistic children. J Am Acad Child Adolesc Psychiatry 27:248–251, 1988.

Black P, Blumer D, Wellner A, et al. The head injured child: time-course of recovery, with implications for rehabilitation, in Head Injuries: Proceedings of the International Symposium. Edinburgh: Churchill Livingstone, 1971.

Bloom DR, Levin HS, Ewing-Cobbs, et al. Lifetime and novel psychiatric disorders after pediatric traumatic brain injury. J Am Acd Child Adolesc Psychiatr 40:572–579, 2001.

Blount PJ, Nguyen CD, McDeavitt JT. Clinical use of cholinomimetic agents: A review J Head Trauma Rehabil 17:314–321, 2002.

Bohnen N, Van Zutphen W Twijnstra A, et al. Late outcome of mild head injury: results from a controlled postal survey. Brain Inj 8:701–708, 1994.

Boll TJ, Barth JT. Neuropsychology of brain damage in children, in *Handbook of Clinical Neuropsychology*, Vol 1. Edited by Filsov SB, Boll TJ. New York: Wiley, 1981, pp 418–452.

Breslau N. Psychiatric disorder in children with physical disabilities. J Am Acad Child Psychiatry 24:87–94, 1985.

Brink JD, Garrett AL, Hale AR, et al. Recovery of motor and intellectual function in children sustaining severe head injuries. Dev Med Child Neurol 12:565–571, 1970.

Brink JD, Imbus C, Woo-Sam J. Physical recovery after severe closed head trauma in children and adolescents. J Pediatr 97:721–727, 1980.

Brooks DN, Aughson ME: Psychological consequences of blunt head injury. Int Rehabil Med 1:160–165, 1979.

Brown CL, Chadwick O, Shaffer D, et al. A prospective study of children with head injuries, III: psychiatric sequelae. Psychol Med 11:63–78, 1981.

Bruce DA. Outcome following head trauma in childhood, in *Pediatric Head Trauma*. Edited by Shapiro K. Mt Kisco, NY: Futura Publishing, 1983, pp 213–223.

Bruce DA. Head trauma, in *Pediatric Trauma: Prevention, Acute Care, and Rehabilitation*. Edited by Eichelberger MR. Baltimore, MD: Mosby Year Book, 1993, pp 353–361.

Bruce DA. Pathophysiological responses of the child's brain following trauma, in *Traumatic Head Injury in Children*. Edited by Broman SH, Michel ME. New York: Oxford University Press, 1995, pp 40–51.

Bruce DA, Zimmerman RA. Shaken impact syndrome. Pediatr Ann 18:482–484, 1989.

Bruce DA, Schut L, Bruno LA, et al. Outcome following severe head injury in children. J Neurosurg 48:679–688, 1978.

Bruce DA, Raphaely RC, Goldberg AI, et al. Pathophysiology, treatment and outcome following severe head injury in children. Childs Brain 5:174–191, 1979.

Bruce DA, Schut L, Sutton LN. Brain and cervical spine injuries occurring during organized sports activities in children and adolescents. Clin Sports Med 1:495–514, 1982.

Caffey J. On the theory and practice of shaking infants. American Journal of Diseases of Children 124:161–169, 1972.

Campbell JJ, Duffy JD, Salloway SP. Treatment strategies for patients with dysexecutive syndromes. J Neuropsychiatry Clin Neurosci 6:411–418, 1994.

Campbell M, Perry R, Green WH. The use of lithium in children and adolescents. Psychosomatics 25:95–106, 1984.

Cantu RC. Guidelines for return to contact sports after a c Guidelines for return to contact sports after a cerebral concussion. Phys Sports Med, 14:75–83, 1986.

Cantu RC, Voy R. Second impact syndrome: A risk in any contact sport. Phys Sportsmed 23:27–34, 1995.

Cardenas DD, McLean A, Farrell-Roberts L et al. Oral physostigmine & impaired memory in adults with brain injury. Brain Inj 8:579–587, 1994.

Casey R, Ludwig S, McCormick MC. Morbidity following minor head trauma in children. Pediatrics 80:159–164, 1987.

Chadwick O, Rutter M, Brown G, et al. A prospective study of children with head injuries, II: cognitive sequelae. Psychol Med 11:49–61, 1980.

Chadwick O, Rutter M, Shaffer D, et al. A prospective study of children with head injuries, TV: specific cognitive deficits. J Clin Neuropsychol 3:101–120, 1981.

Chapman SB. Discourse as an outcome measure in pediatric head-injured populations, in *Traumatic Head Injury in Children*. Edited by Broman SH, Michel ME. New York: Oxford University Press, 1995, pp 95–116.

Chelune GJ, Baer RA. Developmental norms for the Wisconsin Card Sorting Test. J Clin Exp Neuropsychol 8:219–228, 1986.

Chelune GL, Edwards P. Early brain lesions: ontogenetic environmental considerations. J Clin Consult Psychol 49:777–790, 1981.

Chelune GJ, Ferguson W Koon R, et al. Frontal lobe disinhibition in attention deficit disorder. Child Psychiatry Hum Dev 16:221–234, 1986.

Christman CW Grady MS, Walker SA, et al. Ultrastructural studies of diffuse axonal injury in humans. J Neurotrauma 11:173–186, 1994.

Cicerone KD. Psychotherapy after mild traumatic brain injury: relation to the nature and severity of subjective complaints. J Head Trauma Rehabil 6:30–43, 1991.

Cicerone KD, Kalmar K. Persistent postconcussion syndrome: the structure of subjective complaints after mild traumatic brain injury. J Head Trauma Rehabil 10:1–17, 1995.

Cohen S, Joyce C, Rhodes D, et al. Educational programming for head injured students, in *Head Injury Rehabilitation: Children and Adolescents*. Edited by Ylvisaker M. San Diego, CA: College-Hill, 1985, pp 383–409.

Cohn AH. An approach to preventing child abuse. Chicago, IL: National Committee for Prevention of Child Abuse, 1983.

Collins MW, Lovell MR, Iverson GL. Cumulative effects of concussion in high school athletes. Neurosurg 51:1175–9, 2002.

Conn JM, Annest JL, Gilchrist J. Sports and recreation related injury episodes in the US population, 1997–99, Inj Prev 9:117–123, 2003.

Dalby PR, Obrzut JE. Epidemiologic characteristics and sequelae of closed head-injured children and adolescents: a review. Dev Neuropsychol 7:35–68, 1991.

Davidson K, Bagley CR. Schizophrenia–like psychosis associated with organic disorders of the central nervous system: a review of the literature. Br J Psychiatry Special Publ 4, 1969, pp 113–184.

Dennis M. Stroke in childhood, I: communicative intent, expression, and comprehension after left hemisphere arteriopathy in a right-handed 9-year-old, in *Language Development and Aphasia in Children*. Edited by Reiher RW New York: Academic Press, 1980, pp 45–67.

Dennis M. Frontal lobe function in childhood and adolescence: a heuristic for assessing attention regulation, executive control, and the intentional states important for social discourse. Dev Neuropsychol 7:327–358, 1991.

Dennis M, Barnes MA. Knowing the meaning, getting the point, bridging the gap, and carrying the message: aspects of discourse following closed head injury in childhood and adolescence. Brain Lang 3:203–229, 1990.

Denny-Brown D, Russell WR. Experimental cerebral concussion. Brain 64:93–163, 1941.

Diamond A, Goldman-Rakic PS. Comparison of human infants and rhesus monkeys on Piaget's AB task: evidence for dependence on dorsolateral prefrontal cortex. Exp Brain Res 74:24–40, 1989.

Diamond LJ, Jaudes PK. Child abuse in a cerebral palsied population. Dev Med Child Neurol 25:169–174, 1983.

Donders J. Premorbid behavioral and psychosocial adjustment of children with traumatic brain injury. J Abnorm Child Psychol 20:233–246, 1992.

Duffy JD, Campbell JJ. The regional prefrontal syndromes: a theoretical and clinical overview. J Neuropsychiatry Clin Neurosci 6:379–386, 1994.

Duhaime AC, Alario AJ, Lewander WJ, et al. Head injury in very young children: mechanisms, injury types, and ophthalmologic findings in 100 hospitalized patients younger than 2 years of age. Pediatrics 90:179–185, 1992.

Education for All Handicapped Children Act (PL 94-142). Federal Register 42:42496–7, 1976.

Eiben CF, Anderson TP, Lockman L, et al: Functional outcome of closed head injury in children and young adults. Arch Phys Med Rehabil 65:168–170, 1984.

Eisenberg HM. Outcome after head injury: general considerations and neurobehavioral recovery, Part I: general considerations, in Central Nervous System Trauma Status Report 1985. Edited by Becker DP Povlishock JT. Bethesda, MD: National Institute of Neurological and Communicative Disorders and Stroke, 1985, pp 271–280.

Eisenberg HM, Werner RL. Input variables: how information from the acute injury can be used to characterize groups of patients for studies of outcome, in *Neurobehavioral Consequences of Closed Head Injury.* Edited by Levin HS, Grafman J, Eisenberg HM. New York: Oxford University Press, 1987, pp 13–29.

Elovic EP, Lansang R, Li Y et al. The use of atypical antipsychotics in traumatic brain injury. J Head Trauma Rehabil 18:177–195, 2003.

Evans RW, Clay TH, Gualtieri CT. Carbamazepine in pediatric psychiatry. J Am Acad Child Adolesc Psychiatry 26:2–8, 1987.

Ewing-Cobbs L, Fletcher JM, Levin HS. Neuropsychological sequelae following pediatric head injury, in *Head Injury Rehabilitation: Children and Adolescents.* Edited by Ylvisaker M. San Diego, CA: College-Hill, 1985, pp 71–89.

Ewing-Cobbs L, Levin HS, Eisenberg HM, et al. Language functions following closed head injury in children and adolescents. J Clin Exp Neuropsychol 9:575–592, 1987.

Ewing-Cobbs L, Miner ME, Fletcher JM, et al. Intellectual, motor, and language sequelae following closed head injury in infants and preschoolers. J Pediatr Psychol 14:531–547, 1989.

Ewing-Cobbs L, Levin HS, Fletcher JM, et al. The Children's Orientation and Amnesia Test: relationship to severity of acute head injury and to recovery of memory. Neurosurgery 27:683–691, 1990.

Ewing-Cobbs L, Duhaime AC, Fletcher JM. Inflicted and non-inflicted traumatic brain injury in infants and preschoolers. J Head Trauma Rehabil 10:13–24, 1995.

Ewing-Cobbs L, Fletcher JM, Levin HS et al. Academic achievement and academic placement following traumatic brain injury in children and adolescents: a two-year longitudinal study. J Clin Exp Neuropsychol 20:769–781, 1998.

Farmer MY, Singer HS, Mellitis ED, et al. Neurobehavioral sequelae of minor head injuries in children. Pediatr Neurosci 13:304– 308, 1987.

Feeney DM, Gonzales A, Law WA. Amphetamine, haloperidol and experience interact to affect rate of recovery after motor cortex injury. Science 217:855–857, 1982.

Feeney DM, Westerberg VS. Norepinephrine and brain damage: alpha noradrenergic pharmacology alters functional recovery after cortical trauma. Can J Psychol 44:233–252, 1990.

Feeney TJ, Ylvisaker M. Context-sensitive behavioral supports for young children with TBI: Short term effects and long term outcome. J Head Trauma Rehabil 18:33–51, 2003.

Field M, Collins MW, Lovell MR, et al. Does age play a role in recovery from sports related concussion? A comparison of high school and collegiate athletes. J. Pediatr 142:546–53, 2003.

Fife D, David J, Tate L, et al. Fatal injuries to bicyclists: the experience of Dade County, Florida. J Trauma 23:745–755, 1983.

Fife D, Faich G, Hollinshead WI, et al. Incidence and outcome of hospital treated head injury in Rhode Island. Am J Public Health 76: 773–778, 1986.

Fletcher JM, Levin HS. Neurobehavioral effects of brain injury in children, in *Handbook of Pediatric Psychology.* Edited by Routh D. New York: Guilford, 1988, pp 258–294.

Fletcher JM, Miner ME, Ewing-Cobbs L. Age and recovery from head injury in children, in *Neurobehavioral Recovery From Head Injury.* Edited by Levin HS, Grafman J, Eisenberg HM. New York: Oxford University Press, 1987, pp 279–291.

Fletcher JM, Ewing-Cobbs L, Miner ME, et al. Behavioral changes after closed head injury in children. J Consult Clin Psychol 58:93–98, 1990.

Fletcher JM, Ewing-Cobbs I., Francis DJ, et al. Variability in outcomes after traumatic brain injury, in *Traumatic Head Injury in Children.* Edited by Broman SH, Michel ME. New York: Oxford University Press, 1995, pp 3–21.

Frankowski RF. Head injury mortality in urban populations and its relation to the injured child, in *The Injured Child.* Edited by Brooks BF. Austin, TX: University of Texas Press, 1985, pp 20–29.

Frankowski RF, Annegars JF, Whitman S. Epidemiological and descriptive studies, Part I: the descriptive epidemiology of head trauma in the United States, in *Central Nervous System Trauma Status Report 1985.* Edited by Becker DP, Povlishock JT. Bethesda, MD: National Institute of Neurological and Communicative Disorders and Stroke, 1985, pp 33–44.

Friede AM, Azzara CV, Gallagher SS, et al. The epidemiology of injuries to bicycle riders. Pediatr Clin North Am 32:141–151, 1985.

Fuld PA, Fisher P. Recovery of intellectual ability after closed head injury. Dev Med Child Neurol 25:495–502, 1977.

Gadow KG. Pediatric psychopharmocology: a review of recent research. J Child Psychol Psychiatry 33:153–195, 1992.

Gaidolfi E, Vignolo LA. Closed head injuries of schoolaged children: neuropsychological sequelae in early adulthood. J Neurol Sci 1: 65–73, 1980.

Gennarelli TA, Thibault LE, Adams JH, et al. Diffuse axonal injury and traumatic coma in primates. Ann Neurol 12:564–574, 1982.

Genuardi FJ, King WD. Inappropriate discharge instructions for youth athletes hospitalized for concussion. Pediatr 95:216–8, 1995.

Gerber DJ, Schraa JC. Mild traumatic brain injury: searching for the syndrome. J Head Trauma Rehabil 10:28–40, 1995.

Gerberich SG, Priest JD, Boen JR, et al. Concussion incidences and severity in secondary school varsity football players. Am J Publ Health 73:1370–1375, 1983.

Ghosh A, DiScala C, Drew C et al. Horse related injuries in pediatric patients J Pediatr Surg 35:1766–70, 2000.

Gilberg C. *Interventions and Treatments in Clinical Child Neuropsychiatry.* Cambridge, UK: Cambridge University Press, 1995, pp 326–343.

Goethe KE, Levin HS. Behavioral manifestations during the early and long-term stages of recovery after closed head injury. Psychiatr Ann 14:540–546, 1984.

Golden CJ. The Luria-Nebraska Children's Battery: theory and formulation, in *Neuropsychological Assessment of the School-Aged Child.* Edited by Hynd GW, Obrzut JE. New York: Grune & Stratton, 1981, pp 277–302.

Goldman PS. Functional recovery of the prefrontal cortex in early life and the problem of neuronal plasticity. Exp Neurol 32:366–387, 1971.

Goldman PS, Alexander GE. Maturation of prefrontal cortex in the monkey revealed by local reversible cryogenic depression. Nature 267:613–615, 1977.

Goldman PS, Rosvold HE, Mishkin M. Selective sparing of function following prefrontal lobectomy in infant monkeys. Exp Neurol 29: 222–226, 1970.

Goldstein B, Kelly MM, Bruton D, et al. Inflicted versus accidental head injury in critically injured children. Crit Care Med 21:328–332, 1993.

Goldstein IB. Basic and clinical studies of pharmacological effects on recovery from brain injury. N Neural Transplant Plast 4:175–192, 1993.

Goldstein FC, Levin HS. Epidemiology of pediatric closed head injury: incidence, clinical characteristics, and risk factors. J Learn Disabil 20:518–525, 1987.

Goldstein FC, Levin HS. Question-asking strategies after severe closed head injury. Brain Cogn 17:23–30, 1991.

Goodman D, Gaetz M, Meichenbaum D. Concussions in hockey: there is cause for concern. Med Sci Sports Exerc 33:2004–9, 2001.

Gottschall CS. Epidemiology of childhood injury, in *Pediatric Trauma: Prevention, Acute Care, and Rehabilitation.* Edited by Eichelberger MR. Chicago: Mosby Year Book, 1993, pp 16–19.

Grattan LM, Eslinger PJ. Frontal lobe damage in children and adults: a comparative review. Dev Neuropsychol 7:283–326, 1991.

Gronwall D. Cumulative and persisting effects of concussion on attention and cognition, in *Mild Head Injury.* Edited by Levin HS, Eisenberg HM, Benton AL. New York: Oxford University Press, 1989, pp 153–162.

Growall D, Wrightson P, McGinn V. Effect of mild head injury during the preschool years. Int Neuropsychol Soc 3:592–597, 1997.

Gualtieri CT. Pharmocotherapy and the neurobehavioral sequelae of traumatic brain injury. Brain Inj 2:101–129, 1988.

Gualtieri CT. *Neuropsychiatry and Behavioral Pharmacology.* New York: Springer-Verlag, 1991.

Gudmunsson G. Epilepsy in Iceland: a clinical literature review. Clinl Child Hosp 15:153–172, 1966.

Gulbrandsen GB. Neuropsychological sequelae of light head injury in older children 6 months after trauma. J Clin Neuropsychol 6:257–268, 1984.

Guthkelch AN. Assessment of outcome: post-traumatic amnesia, post-concussional symptoms, and accident neurosis. Acta Neurochir Suppl (Wien) 28:120–133, 1979.

Guze BH, Gitlin M. The neuropathologic basis of major affective disorders: neuroanatomic insights. J Neuropsychiatry Clin Neurosci 6: 114–121, 1994.

Hackam D, Kreller M, Pearl R. Snow related recreational injuries in children: assessment of morbidity and management strategies. J Pediatr Surg 33:65–69, 1999.

Hagen C, Makmus D, Durham P. *Levels of Cognitive Functioning.* Downey, CA: Ranchos Los Amigos Hospital, 1972.

Hahn YS, Raimondi AJ, McLone DG, et al. Traumatic mechanisms of head injury in child abuse. Child's Brain 10:229–241, 1983.

Hannay HJ, Levin HS. Visual continuous recognition memory in normal and closed head injured adolescents. J Clin Exp Neuropsychol 1:444–460, 1984.

Harwood-Nash DC, Hendrick EB, Hudson AR. The significance of skull fracture in children: a study of 1,187 patients. Radiology 101: 151–155, 1971.

Hauser WA. Post-traumatic epilepsy in children, in *Pediatric Head Trauma*, Edited by Shapiro K. Mt Kisco, NY: Futura Publishing, 1983, 271–287.

Heaton RK, Chelune GJ, Talley JL, et al. *Wisconsin Card Sorting Test Manual*, Revised and Expanded. San Antonio, TX: Psychological Corporation, 1993.

Heiskanen O, Kaste M. Late prognosis of severe brain injury in children. Dev Med Child Neurol 16:11–14, 1974.

Helfer RE, Kempe RS (eds). *The Battered Child*, 4th Ed. Chicago: University of Chicago Press, 1987.

Hettler J, Greenes DS. Can the initial history predict whether a child with a head injury has been abused? Pediatrics 111:602–607, 2003.

Hoch DB, Daly L. Anticonvulsants. J Head Trauma Rehabil 18:383–386, 2003.

Holdsworth L, Whitmore K. A study of children with epilepsy attending ordinary schools, I: their seizure patterns, progress, and behavior in school. Dev Med Child Neurol 21:333–342, 1974.

Honig LS, Albers GW. Neuropharmacological treatment for acute brain injury, in *Neuropsychiatry of Traumatic Brain Injury*. Edited by Silver JM, Yudofsky SC, Hales RE. Washington, DC: American Psychiatric Press, 1994, pp 771–803.

Hovda D, Lee S, Smith M, et al. The neurochemical and metabolic cascade following brain injury:moving from animal models to man. J Neurotrauma 12:903–906, 1995.

Howard A, KcKeag AM, Rothman L, et al. Ejections of young chi1drern in motor vehicle crashes. J Trauma-Inj Inf Crit Care 55:126–129, 2003.

Ichise M, Chung D, Wang P, et al. Technetium-99m–HMPAO SPECT, CT, and MRI in the evaluation of patients with chronic traumatic brain injury: a correlation with neuropsychological performance. J Nucl Med 35:217–226, 1994.

Janda DH, Bir CA, Cheney AL. An evaluation of the cumulative effect of soccer heading in the youth population. Inj Control Saf Promot 9:25–31, 2002.

Jennett B. Pathology and natural history of head injury, in *An Introduction to Neurosurgery*, 4th Ed. Edited by Jennett B, Lindsay KW Oxford: Butterworth–Heinemann, 1983, pp 189–211.

Jennett B, Bond MR. Assessment of outcome after severe head injury: a practical scale. Lancet 1:480–484, 1975.

Jennett B, Teasdale G. *Management of Head Injuries*. Philadelphia: FA Davis, 1981.

Jennett B, Teasdale G, Fry J, et al. Treatment for severe head injury. J Neurol Neurosurg Psychiatry 43:289–295, 1980.

Johnston KM, Prito A, Chankowsky J, et al. New frontiers in diagnostic imaging in concussive head injury. Clin J Sports Med 11:166–175, 2001.

Johnston RB, Mellitz EP. Pediatric coma: prognosis and outcome. Dev Med Child Neurol 72:3–12, 1980.

Joint Committee on Injury Scaling. *The Abbreviated Injury Scale (AIS)*, *1980 Revision*. Arlington Heights, IL: American Association for Automotive Medicine, 1980.

Jones CL. Recovery from head trauma: a curvilinear process? in *Handbook of Head Trauma: Acute Care to Recovery*. Edited by Long CJ, Ross LK. New York: Plenum, 1990, pp 247–267.

Jorge RE, Robinson RG, Arndt S, et al. Comparison between acute- and delayed-onset depression following traumatic brain injury. J Neuropsychiatry Clin Neurosci 5:43–49, 1993.

Kalsbeek WD, McLaurin RL, Harris BSH, et al. The National Head and Spinal Cord Injury Survey: major findings. J Neurosurg 53:519–531, 1980.

Karzmark P, Hall K, Englander J. Late-onset post-concussion symptoms after mild brain injury: the role of premorbid, injury-related, environmental, and personality factors. Brain Inj 9:21–26, 1995.

Kaufman PM, Fletcher JM, Levin HM, et al. Attentional disturbance after pediatric closed head injury. J Child Neurol 8:348–353, 1993.

Keenan HT, Runyan DK, Marshall SW. A population-based study of inflicted traumatic brain injury in young children. JAMA 290:621–626, 2003.

Kelly JP. Concussion, in *Current Therapy in Sports Medicine*, 3rd Ed. Edited by Torg JS, Shephard RJ. Philadelphia: CV Mosby, 1995, pp 21–24.

Kelly JP, Nichols JS, Filley CM, et al. Concussion, in sports: Guidelines for the prevention of catastrophic outcome. JAMA, 266:2867–2869, 1991.

Kendall PC, Braswell L. *Cognitive-Behavioral Therapy for Impulsive Children*, 2nd Ed. New York: Guilford, 1993.

Kipnis, J, Nevo U, Panikashvili, et al. Therapeutic vaccination for closed head injury. J Neurotrauma 20:559–569, 2003.

Kirkwood M, Janusz J, Yeates KO, et al. Prevalence and correlates of depressive symptoms following traumatic brain injury in children. Child Neuropsychol 6:195–208, 2000.

Klonoff H. Head injuries in children: predisposing factors, accident conditions, accident proneness and sequelae. Am J Public Health 61:2405–2417, 1971.

Klonoff H, Paris R. Immediate short-term and residual effects of acute head injuries in children, in *Clinical Neuropsychology: Current Status and Applications*. Edited by Reitan R, Davison IA. Washington, DC: Winston, 1974, pp 179–210.

Klonoff H, Low MD, Clark C. Head injuries in children: a prospective five-year follow-up. J Neuro Neurosurg Psychiatry 40:1211–1219, 1977.

Kolb B. *Brain Plasticity and Behavior*. Hillsdale, NJ: Lawrence Erlbaum, 1995.

Kottmeier PK. Falls from heights, in *Management of Pediatric Trauma*. Edited by Buntain WL. Philadelphia: WB Saunders, 1995, pp 450–458.

Kountakis SE, Rafie JJ, Ghorayeb B, et al. Pediatric gunshot wounds to the head and neck. Otolaryngol Head Neck Surg 114:756–60, 1996.

Kraus JF. Epidemiological features of brain injury in children: occurrence, children at risk, causes and manner of injury, severity, and outcomes, in *Traumatic Head Injury in Children*. Edited by Broman SH, Michel ME. New York: Oxford University Press, 1995, pp 22–39.

Kraus JF, Sorenson SB. Epidemiology, in *Neuropsychiatry of Traumatic Brain Injury*. Edited by Silver JM, Yudofsky SC, Hales RE. Washington, DC: American Psychiatric Press, 1994, pp 3–42.

Kraus JF, Black MA, Hessol N, et al. The incidence of acute brain injury and serious impairment in a defined population. Am J Epidemiol 119:186–201, 1984.

Kraus JF, Fife D, Cox P, et al. Incidence, severity, and external causes of pediatric brain injury. Am J Dis Child 140:687–693, 1986.

Kraus JF, Fife D, Conroy C. Pediatric brain injuries: the nature, clinical course, and early outcomes in a defined United States population. Pediatrics 79:501–507, 1987.

Kraus JF, Rock A, Hemyari P. Brain injuries among infants, children, adolescents, and young adults. Am J Dis Child 144:684–691, 1990.

Kriel RL, Krach LE, Panser LA. Closed head injury: comparison of children younger and older than 6 years of age. Pediatr Neurol 5:296–300, 1989.

Kuhn-Gebhart V. Behavioral disorders in non-epileptic children and their treatment with carbamazepine, in *Epileptic Seizures-Behavior-Pain*. Edited by Birkmayer W. Bern: Hans Huber, 1976, pp 72–97.

Kushner DS. Concussion in sports: Minimizing the risk for complications. Amer Fam Phy 64:1007–1014, 2001.

Laborde A, Whyte J. Two dimensional quantitative data analysis: assessing the functional utility of psychostimulants. J Head Trauma Rehabil 12:90–92, 1997.

Langburt W, Cohen B, Akhthar N. Incidence of concussion in high school football players of Ohio and Pennsylvania. J Child Neurol 16:83–5, 2001.

Lanser JB, Jenkens-Schinkel A, Peters AC. Headache after closed head injury in children. Headache 28:176–179, 1988.

Lehr E. *Psychological Management of Traumatic Brain Injuries in Children and Adolescents*. Rockville, MD: Aspen, 1990.

Leininger BE, Gramling SE, Farrell AD, et al. Neuropsychological deficits in symptomatic minor head injury patients after concussion and mild concussion. J Neurol Neurosurg Psychiatry 53:293–296, 1990.

Lemire I. Revue de syndrome de Kleine-Levin: vers une aproche integree [Review of Kleine-Levin syndrome: toward an integrated approach]. Can J Psychiatry 38: 277–284, 1993.

Levin HS, Eisenberg HM. Neuropsychological impairment after closed head injury in children and adolescents. J Pediatr Psychol 4:389–402, 1979a.

Levin HS, Eisenberg HM. Neuropsychological outcome after closed head injury in children and adolescents. Childs Brain 5:281–292, 1979b.

Levin HS, Eisenberg HM, Wigg NR, et al. Memory and intellectual ability after head injury in children and adolescents. Neurosurgery 22:1043–1052, 1982.

Levin HS, Peters BH, Kalisky Z, et al. Effects of oral physostigmine and lecithin on memory and attention in the closed head injured patient. Cent Nerv Syst Trauma 3:333–342, 1986.

Levin HS, Amparo E, Eisenberg HM, et al. Magnetic resonance imaging and computerized tomography in relation to the neurobehavioral sequelae of mild and moderate head injuries. J Neurosurg 66:706–713, 1987a.

Levin HS, High W Goethe KE, et al. The Neurobehavioral Rating Scale: assessment of the behavioral sequelae of closed head injury by the clinician. J Neurol Neurosurg Psychiatry 50:183–193, 1987b.

Levin HS, High WM, Ewing-Cobbs L, et al. Memory functioning during the first year after closed head injury in children and adolescents. Neurosurgery 22:1043–1052, 1988.

Levin HS, Hamilton WJ, Grossman RG. Outcome after head injury, in *Handbook of Clinical Neurology*. Edited by Braakman R. New York: Elsevier, 1990, pp 367–395.

Levin HS. Treatment of postconcussional symptoms with CDP-Choline. J Neurol Sci 103:S39–S42, 1991.

Levin HS, Culhane KA, Hartmann J. Developmental changes in performance on tests of purported frontal lobe functioning. Dev Neuropsychol 7:377–395, 1991.

Levin HS, Culhane KA, Mendelsohn D. Cognition in relation to magnetic resonance imaging in head-injured children and adolescents. Arch Neurol 50:897–905, 1993.

Levin HS, Kraus MF. The frontal lobes and traumatic brain injury. J Neuropsychiatry Clin Neurosci 6:443–454, 1994.

Levin HS, Ewing-Cobbs L, Eisenberg HM. Neurobehavioral outcome of pediatric closed head injury in *Traumatic Head Injury in Children*. Edited by Broman SH, Michel ME. New York: Oxford University Press, 1995, pp 70–94.

Lezak MD. *Neuropsychological Assessment*. New York: Oxford University Press, 1994.

Lindsay J, Ounsted C, Richards P. Long-term outcome in children with temporal lobe seizures, III: psychiatric aspects in childhood and adult life. Dev Med Child Neurol 21:630–636, 1979.

Long CJ, Gouvier WD, Cole JC. A model of recovery for the total rehabilitation of individuals with head trauma. J Rehab 50:39–45, 1984.

Lorenzo R. CDP-choline in the treatment of craniencephalic traumata. J Neurol Sci 103:S43–S47, 1991.

Lou HC, Henriksen L, Bruhn P. Focal cerebral hypoperfusion in children with dyslexia and/or attention deficit disorder. Arch Neurol 41:825–829, 1984.

Luerssen TG, Klauber MR, Marshall LF. Outcome from head injury related to patient's age: a longitudinal prospective study of adult and pediatric head injury J Neurosurg 68:409–416, 1988.

MacGregor DM. Golf related head injuries in children. Emerg Med J 19: 576–7, 2002.

MacKay M. Mechanisms of injury and biomechanics: vehicle design and crash performance. World J Surg 16:420–427, 1992.

Mahalick D, Carmel P, Greenberg J, et al. Psychopharmacologic treatment of acquired attention disorders in children with brain injury. Pediatr Neurosurg 29:121–126, 1998.

Malloy PF, Duffy J. The frontal lobes in neuropsychiatric disorders, in *Handbook of Neuropsychology*, Vol 9. Edited by Boller F, Grafman J. New York: Elsevier, 1994, pp 203–232.

Malloy PF, Richardson ED. The frontal lobes and content specific delusions. J Neuropsychiatry Clin Neurosci 6:455–466, 1994.

Mankovsky AB, Mendoza–Sagaon M, Cardinaux C, et al. Evaluation of soccer related injuries in children. J Pediatr Surg 37:755–9, 2002.

Marshall LF, Marshall SB, Klauber MR, et al. A new classification of head injury based on computerized tomography. J Neurosurg 75:S14–S20, 1991.

Masanic CA, Bayley MT, VanReekum R, et al. Open-label study of donepezil in traumatic brain injury Arch Phys Med Rehabil 82:896–901, 2001.

Mateer C, Williams D. Effects of frontal lobe injury in childhood. Dev Neuropsychol 7:359–376, 1991.

Matheny AP. Injuries among toddlers: contributions from child, mother, and family, in *Annual Progress in Child Psychiatry and Child Development*. Edited by Chess S, Thomas A, Hertzig M. New York: Brunner/Mazel, 1987, pp 35–42.

McCrory P. Does second impact syndrome exist? Clin J Sports Med 11:144–149, 2001.

McCullagh S, Oucherlony D, Protzner A, et al. Prediction of neuropsychiatric outcome following mild traumatic brain injury: an examination of the Glascow Coma Scale. Brain Inj 15:489–497, 2001.

Meador KJ, Loring DW, Moore EE, et al. Comparative studies of phenobarbital, phenytoin, and valproate in healthy adults. Neurol 45:1494–1499, 1995.

Meythaler JM, Bruner RC, Johnson A, et al. Amantadine to improve neurorecovery in traumatic brain injury-Associated diffuse axonal injury: A double-blind randomized trial J Head Trauma Rehabil 17:300–313, 2002.

Michaud LJ, Rivara FP, Grady MS, et al. Predictors of survival and severity of disability after severe brain injury in children. Neurosurgery 31:254–264, 1992.

Michaud LJ, Rivara FP Jaffe KM, et al. Traumatic brain injury as a risk factor for behavioral disorders in children. Arch Phys Med Rehabil 74:368–375, 1993.

Miller JD, Becker DP. General principles and pathophysiology of head injury, in *Neurological Surgery*. Edited by Youmans JR. Philadelphia, PA: WB Saunders, 1982, pp 292–298.

Miller JD, Jennett WB. Complications of depressed skull fractures. Lancet 2:215–218, 1968.

Mittenberg W DiGuilio DV Perrin S, et al. Symptoms following mild head injury: expectation as aetiology. J Neurol Neurosurg Psychiatry 55:200–204, 1992.

Mittenberg W Zielinski R, Fichera S. Recovery from mild head injury: a treatment manual for patients. Psychotherapy in Private Practice 12:37–53, 1993.

Mueller F, Blythe C. Fatalities from head and cervical spine injuries occurring in tackle football 40 years' experience. Clin Sports Med 6:185–196, 1987.

Nguyen D, Letts M. In-line skating injuries in children: a 10 year review. J Pediatr Orthop 21:613–8, 2001.

Novack TA, Bergquist TF, Bennett G. Family involvement in cognitive recovery following traumatic brain injury, in *Handbook of Head Trauma: Acute Care to Recovery*. Edited by Long CJ, Ross LK. New York, Plenum, 1992, pp 330–355.

O'Leary DS, Boll TJ. Neuropsychological correlates of early generalized brain dysfunction in children, in *Early Brain Damage*, Vol 1: *Research Orientations and Clinical Observations*. Edited by Almli CR, Finger S. London, Academic Press, 1984, pp 215–228.

O'Leary DS, Lovell MR, Sackellares C, et al. The effects of age of onset of partial and generalized seizures on neuropsychological performance in children. J Nerv Ment Dis 171:624–629, 1983.

Ommaya AK. Mechanisms of cerebral concussion and traumatic unconsciousness, in *Neurological Surgery*. Edited byYoumans JR. Philadelphia: WB Saunders, 1982, pp 1877–1895.

Pang D. Pathophysiologic correlations of neurobehavioral syndromes following closed head injury, in *Head Injury Rehabilitation: Children and Adolescents.* Edited by Ylvisaker M. San Diego, CA: College-Hill, 1985, pp 3–70.

Passler MA, Isaac W, Hynd GW. Neuropsychological development of behavior attributed to frontal lobe functioning in children. Developmental Neuropsychology 1: 349–370, 1985.

Pautle NM, Henning J, Buntain WL. Mechanisms and biomechanics of traffic injuries, in *Management of Pediatric Trauma.* Edited by Buntain WL. Philadelphia: WB Saunders, 1995, pp 10–27.

Pelco L, Sawyer M, Duffield G, et al. Premorbid emotional and behavioral adjustment in children with mild head injuries. Brain Inj 6: 29–37, 1992.

Pennington BF. *Diagnosing Learning Disorders: A Neuropsychological Framework.* NewYork: Guilford, 1991.

Perrott SB, Taylor HG, Montes JL. Neuropsychological sequelae, familial stress, and environmental adaptation following pediatric head injury. Dev Neuropsychol 7:69–86, 1991.

Peterson L. Sensitivity to emotional cues and social behavior in children and adolescents after head injury. Percept Mot Skills 73:1139–1150, 1991.

Peterson TD, Royer K. Motor vehicle crash injury: mechanism and prevention. Am Fam Physician 44:1307–1323, 1991.

Peterson TD, Royce K. Motor vehicle crash injury: mechanisms and prevention. Am Fam Physician 44:1307–1312, 1995.

Plum F, Posner JB. *The Diagnosis of Stupor and Coma,* 3rd Edition. Philadelphia: FA Davis, 1980.

Poirier MP, Wadsworth MR. Sports-related concussion. Pediatr Emer care, 16:278–283, 2000.

Pond DA, Bidwell BH. A survey of epilepsy in 14 general practices, II: social and psychological aspects. Epilepsia 1:258–299, 1960.

Povlishock JT. Traumatically induced axonal injury: pathogenesis and pathobiological implications. Brain Pathol 2:1–12, 1992.

Povlishock JT. Pathobiology of traumatically induced axonal injury in animals and man. Ann Emerg Med 22:41–47, 1993.

Povlishock JT. Neuroanatomical findings and pathological changes in mild traumatic brain injury. Symposium presented at Allegheny General Hospital, September 1994.

Povlishock JT, Coburn TH. Morphopathological change associated with mild head injury, in *Mild Head Injury.* Edited by Levin HS, Eisenberg HM, Benton AL. New York: Oxford University Press, 1989, pp 37–53.

Powell EC, Tanz RR, DiScala C. Bicycle related injuries among preschool children Ann Emerg Med 30:260–265, 1997.

Powell JW, Barber-Foss K. Traumatic brain injury in high school athletes. JAMA 282:958–963, 1999.

Prigatano GP. Personality disturbances associated with traumatic brain injury. J Consult Clin Psychol 60:360–368, 1992.

Raimondi AJ, Hirschauer J. Head injury in the infant and toddler: Coma Outcome Scale. Childs Brain 11:12–35, 1984.

Reece RM, Sege R. Childhood head injuries: accidental or inflicted? Arch Pediatr Adolesc Med 154:9–10, 2000.

Reitan R, Wolfson D. *Traumatic Brain Injury,* Vol I: *Pathophysiology and Neuropsychological Evaluation.* Tucson, AZ: Neuropsychology Press, 1986.

Reynolds BM, Balsano NA, Reynolds FX. Falls from heights: a surgical experience of 200 consecutive cases. Ann Surg 174:304–308, 1971.

Rice DP, MacKenzie EJ. Cost of injury in the United States: a report to Congress, 1989.

Rieder MJ, Schwartz C, Newman J. Patterns of walker use and walker injury. Pediatrics 78:408–493, 1986.

Rimel RW Giordani B, Barth JT, et al. Disability caused by minor head injury. Neurosurgery 9:221–228, 1981.

Rivara JB, Jaffe KM, Polissar NL, et al. Family functioning and children's academic performance and behavior problems in the year following traumatic brain injury. Arch Phys Med Rehabil 75:369–379, 1994.

Rivera FP, Barber M. Demographic analysis of childhood pedestrian injuries. Pediatrics 76:375–381, 1985.

Rivera FP, Mueller BA. The epidemiology and prevention of pediatric head injury. J Head Trauma Rehabil 1:7–15, 1986.

Roberts MA, Manshadi FF, Bushnell DL, et al. Neurobehavioral dysfunction following mild traumatic brain injury in childhood: a case report with positive findings on positron emission tomography (PET). Brain Inj 9:427–436, 1995.

Ropacki MT, Elias JW. Preliminary examination of cognitive reserve theory in closed head injury Arch Clin Neuropsych 18:643–654, 2003.

Ross LK. The use of pharmacology in the treatment of head-injured patients, in *Handbook of Head Trauma: Acute Care to Recovery.* Edited by Long CJ, Ross LK. New York: Plenum, 1992, pp 137–163.

Ruff RM, Levin HS, Marshall LF. Neurobehavioral methods of assessment and the study of outcome in minor head injury. J Head Trauma Rehab 1:43–52, 1986.

Ruff RM, Crouch JA, Troster AT, et al. Selected cases of poor outcome following a minor brain trauma: comparing neuropsychological and positron emission tomography assessment. Brain Inj 8:297–308, 1994.

Russell WR, Smith A. Post-traumatic amnesia in closed head injury. Arch Neurol 5:4–17, 1961.

Rutter M, Graham P, Yule W. *A Neuropsychiatric Study in Childhood.* London: SIMP/Heinemann Medical, 1970.

Rutter M, Chadwick O, Shaffer D. Head injury, in *Developmental Neuropsychiatry.* Edited by Rutter M. New York: Guilford, 1983, pp 83–111.

Salcman M. The unconscious patient, in *Neurologic Emergencies,* 2nd Edition. Edited by Salcman M. New York: Raven, 1990, pp 17–38.

Sato Y, Yuh WIC, Smith WL, et al. Head injury in child abuse: evaluation with MR imaging. Radiology 173: 653–657, 1989.

Sbordone RJ, Liter JC. Mild traumatic brain injury does not produce post-traumatic stress disorder. Brain Inj 9:405–412, 1994.

Schwatz L, Taylor HG, Drotar D, et al. Long-term behavior problems following pediatric traumatic brain injury: Prevalence, predictors and correlates. J Pediatr Psychol 28:251–263, 2003.

Seidel VP, Chadwick O, Rutter M. Psychological disorders in crippled children: a comparative study of children with and without brain damage. Dev Med Child Neurol 17:563–573, 1975.

Shaffer D. Brain damage, in *Child and Adolescent Psychiatry: Modern Approaches,* 2nd Ed. Edited by Rutter M, Hersov L. Oxford: Blackwell Scientific, 1985, pp 129–151.

Shaffer D. Behavioral sequelae of serious head injury in children and adolescents: the British studies, in *Traumatic Head Injury in Children.* Edited by Broman SH, Michel ME. New York: Oxford University Press, 1995, pp 55–69.

Shaffer D, Chadwick O, Rutter M. Psychiatric outcome of localized head injury in children, in *Outcome of Severe Damage to the Central Nervous System.* Edited by Porter R, Fitzsimons DW. New York: Guilford, 1975, pp 191–214.

Shaffer D, Bijur P, Chadwick O, et al. Head injury and later reading disability. J Am Acad Child Psychiatry 19:592–610, 1980.

Shaffer D, Schonfeld IS, O'Connor PA, et al. Neurological soft signs and their relationship to psychiatric disorder and intelligence in childhood and adolescence. Arch Gen Psychiatry 42:342–351, 1985.

Sheslow D, Adams W. *Wide Range Assessment of Memory and Learning.* San Antonio, TX: Psychological Corporation, 1990.

Shetter A, Demakis J. The pathophysiology of concussion: a review. Adv Neurol 22:5–14, 1979.

Shores EA. Comparison of the Westmead Post-Traumatic Amnesia Scale and the Glasgow Coma Scale as predictors of neuropsychological outcome following extremely severe blunt head injury. J Neurol Neurosurg Psychiatry 52:126–127, 1989.

Shores EA, Krajuhin C, Zurynski Y, et al. Neuropsychological assessment and brain imaging technologies in evaluation of the sequelae of blunt head injury. Aust NZ J Psychiatry 24:133–138, 1990.

Showalter PEC, Kimmel DN. Stimulating consciousness and cognition following severe brain injury: a new potential clinical use for lamotrigine Brain Inj 14:997—1001, 2000.

Sieban RL, Leavitt JD, French JH. Falls as childhood accidents: an increasing urban risk. Pediatrics 47:886–892, 1971.

Silver JM, Yudofsky SC. Pharmocological approaches to the patient with affective and psychotic features. J Head Trauma Rehab 9:61–77, 1994.

Skokan EG, Junkins EP, Kadish H. Serious winter sport injuries in children and adolescents requiring hospitalization. Am J Emerg Med 21:95–99, 2003.

Slomine BS, Gerring JP, Grados MA, et al. Performance on measures of 'executive function' following pediatric traumatic brain injury. Brain Inj 16:759–772, 2002.

Smeltzer DJ, Nasrallah HA, Miller SC. Psychotic disorders, in *Neuropsychiatry of Traumatic Brain Injury*. Edited by Silver JM, Yudofsky SC, Hales RE. Washington, D.C.: American Psychiatric Press, 1994, pp 251–283.

Smith DH, Meaney DF, Shull WH. Diffuse axonal injury in head injury. J Head Trauma Rehabil 18:307–316, 2003.

Sohlberg MM, Mateer CA. Effectiveness of an attentional training program. J Clin Exp Neuropsychol 9:117–130, 1987.

Sohlberg MM, Mateer CA, Stuss D. Contemporary approaches to the management of executive control dysfunction. J Head Trauma Rehab 8:45–58, 1993.

Sollee ND, Kindlon DJ. Lateralized brain injury and behavior problems in children. J Abnorm Child Psychol 15:479–490, 1987.

Sosin DM, Sacks JJ, Webb KW. Pediatric head injuries and deaths from bicycling in the United States. Pediatr 98:868–870, 1996.

Spaite DW, Murphy M, Criss EA, et al. A prospective analysis of injury severity among helmeted and nonhelmeted bicyclists involved in collisions with motor vehicles. J Trauma 31:1510–1516, 1991.

Spiegel CN, Lindaman FC. Children can't fly: a program to prevent childhood morbidity and mortality from window falls. Am J Public Health 67:1143–1147, 1977.

Starkstein SE, Mayberg HS, Berthier ML, et al. Mania after brain injury: neuroradiological and metabolic findings. Ann Neurol 27:652–659, 1990.

Stevenson MR, Lo SK, Laing BA, et al. Childhood pedestrian injuries in the Perth metropolitan area. Med J Aust 156:234–238, 1992.

Still A, Roberts I, Koelmeyer L, et al. Child passenger fatalities and restraints used in Auckland. NZ Med J 105: 449–452, 1992.

Stiller JW, Weinberger DR. Boxing and chronic brain damage. Psychiatr Clin North Am 8:339–356, 1985.

Stuss DT. Contributions of frontal lobe injury to cognitive impairment after closed head injury, in *Neurobehavioral Recovery From Head Injury*. Edited by Levin HS, Grafman J, Eisenberg HM. New York: Oxford University Press, 1987, pp 166–177.

Tanz RR, Christoffel KK. Pedestrian injury, the next motor vehicle injury challenge. Am J Dis Child 139:1187–1190, 1985.

Taverni JP, Selinger G, Lichtman SW. Donezepil-mediated memory improvement in traumatic brain injury during post acute rehabilitation. Brain Inj 12:77–80, 1998.

Taylor CT, Price TRP. Neuropsychiatric assessment, in *Neuropsychiatry of Traumatic Brain Injury*. Edited by Silver JM, Yudofsky SC, Hales RE. Washington, DC: American Psychiatric Press, 1994, pp 81–132.

Taylor DA. Traumatic brain injury: outcome and predictors of outcome, in *Handbook of Head Trauma: Acute Care to Recovery*. Edited by Long CJ, Ross LK. New York: Plenum, 1992, pp 294–306.

Taylor HG, Yeates KO, Wade SL, et al. A prospective study of short- and long-term outcomes after traumatic brain injury in children: behavior and achievement. Neuropsychology 16:15–27, 2002.

Taylor HG, Drotar D, Wade S, et al. Recovery from traumatic brain injury in children: the importance of the family, in *Traumatic Head Injury in Children*. Edited by Broman SH, Michel ME, New York: Oxford University Press, 1995, pp 188–216.

Teasdale G, Jennett B. Assessment of coma and impaired consciousness: a practical scale. Lancet 2:81–84, 1974.

Teasdale G, Mendelow D. Pathophysiology of head injury, in *Closed Head Injury: Psychological, Social, and Family Consequences*. Edited by Brooks N. Oxford: Oxford University Press, 1984, pp 4–36.

Thurman DJ, Branche CM, Sniezek JE. The epidemiology of sports-related traumatic brain injuries in the United States: recent developments. J Head Trauma Rehabil 13:1–8, 1998.

Trickett PK, Aber JL, Carlson V, et al. Relationship of socioeconomic status to the etiology and developmental sequelae of physical child abuse. Dev Psychol 27:148–158, 1991.

Trzepacz PT. Delirium, in *Neuropsychiatry of Traumatic Brain Injury*. Edited by Silver JM, Yudofsky SC, Hales RE. Washington, DC: American Psychiatric Press, 1994, pp 189–217.

Tysvaer A, Storli O. Association football injuries to the brain: A preliminary report. Br J Sp Med 15:163–166, 1981.

U.S. Department of Health and Human Services. *Child Abuse and Neglect: A Shared Community Concern (Interagency Task Force Report)*. Chicago, IL, March 1989.

Verger K, Junque' C, Levin HS. Correlation of atrophy measures on MRI with neuropsychological sequelae in children and adolescents with traumatic brain injury. Brain Inj 15:211–221, 2001.

Viguier D, Dellatolas G, Gasquet I, et al. A psychological assessment of adolescent and young adult inpatients after traumatic brain injury. Brain Injury 15:263–271, 2001.

Wade SL, Taylor HG, Drotar D, et al. Family burden and adaptation during the initial year after traumatic brain injury in children. Pediatrics 1:110–116, 1998.

Wade SL, Taylor HG, Drotar D, et al. Parent-adolescent interactions after traumatic brain injury: Their relationship to family adaptation and adolescent adjustment. J Head Trauma Rehabil 18:164–176, 2003.

Waller JA. Recreational activities, in *Injury Control*. Edited by Waller JA. Lexington, MA: DC Heath, 1985, pp 361–404.

Wang MY, Kim KA, Griffith PM, et al. Injuries from falls in the pediatric population: an analysis of 729 cases. J Pediatr Surg 36:1528–1534, 2001.

Ward JD. Craniocerebral injuries, in *Management of Pediatric Trauma*. Edited by Buntain WL. Philadelphia: WB Saunders, 1995a, pp 178–188.

Ward JD. The prospect of pediatric clinical trials: experience with adult trials, in *Traumatic Head Injury in Children*. Edited by Broman SH, Michel ME. New York: Oxford University Press, 1995b, pp 258–267.

Wechsler D. *Manual for the Wechsler Intelligence Scale for Children*, 3rd Ed. San Antonio, TX: Psychological Corporation, 1991.

Weiland SK, Pless IB, Roghmann KJ. Chronic illness and mental health problems in pediatric practice: results from a survey of primary care providers. Pediatrics 89:445–449, 1992.

Weinstein EA, Lyerly OG. Confabulation following brain injury. Arch Gen Psychiatry 18:348–354, 1968.

Welsh MC, Pennington BF. Assessing frontal lobe functioning in children: views from developmental psychology. Dev Neuropsychol 4:199–230, 1988.

Wesson DE, Rieder MJ, Spence LJ. Sports and recreation injuries, in *Management of Pediatric Trauma*. Edited by Buntain WL. Philadelphia, PA: WB Saunders, 1995, pp 541–552.

Whelan FJ, Walker MS, Schultz SK. Donezepil in the treatment of cognitive dysfunction associated with traumatic brain injury. Ann Clin Psychiatry 12:131–135, 2000.

Whitman S. Coonley-Hoganson R, Desai BT. Comparative head trauma experiences in two socioeconomically different Chicago-area communities-a population study. Am J Epidemiol 119:570–580, 1984.

Whitlock JA. Brain injury, cognitive impairment, and donepezil. J Head Trauma Rehabil 14:424–427, 1999.

Whyte J, Vaccaro M, Grieb-Neff P, et al. Psychostimulant use in the rehabilitation of individuals with traumatic brain injury. J Head Trauma Rehabil 17:284–299, 2002.

Wilcox JA, Nasrallah HA. Childhood head trauma and psychosis. Psychiatry Res 21:303–306, 1987.

Williams JM. Neuropsychological assessment of traumatic brain injury in the intensive care and acute care environment, in *Handbook of Head Trauma: Acute Care to Recovery*. Edited by Long CJ, Ross LK. New York: Plenum, 1992, pp 271–293.

Williams S, Ris M, Ayyanger R et al. Recovery in pediatric brain injury: Is psychostimulant medication beneficial? J Head Trauma Rehabil 13:73–81, 1998.

Wilson T, Wyper D. Neuroimaging and neuropsychological functioning following closed head injury: CT, MRI, and SPECT. J Head Trauma Rehab 7:29–39, 1992.

Winogren HW, Knights RM, Bawden HN. Neuropsychological deficits following head injury in children. J Clin Neuropsychol 6:269–186, 1984.

Wolfe AC, O'Day J. Pedestrian accidents in the U.S. Health Services Research Institute Research Review 12:1–16, 1982.

Woods BT. The restricted effects of right hemisphere lesions after age one: Wechsler test data. Neuropsychologia 18:65–70, 1980.

Wrightson P, McGinn V, Gronwall D. Mild head injury in preschool children: evidence that it can be associated with a persisting cognitive defect. J Neurol Neurosurg Psychiatry 59:375–380, 1995.

Wroblewski BA, Glenn MB. Pharmacological treatment of arousal and cognitive deficits. J Head Trauma Rehab 9:19–41, 1994.

Wroblewski BA, McClogan K, Smith K, et al. The incidence of seizures during tricyclic antidepressant drug treatment in a brain-injured population. J Clin Psychopharmacol 10:124–128, 1990.

Wroblewski BA, Leary JM, Phelan AM, et al. Methylphenidate and seizure frequency in brain-injured patients with seizure disorders. J Clin Psychiatry 53:86–89, 1992.

Yager JY, Johnston B, Seshia SS. Coma scales in pediatric practice. Am J Dis Child 144:1088–1091, 1990.

Yeates KO, Taylor HG, Drota D, et al. Preinjury family environment as a determinant of recovery from traumatic brain injury in school-aged children. Int J Neuropsychol Soc 3:617–630, 1997.

Yeates KO, Taylor HG, Wade SL, et al. A prospective study of short and long term neuropsychological outcomes after traumatic brain injury in children. Neuropsychology 16:514–523, 2002.

Youngjohn JR, Burrows L, Erdal K. Brain damage or compensation neurosis? The controversial postconcussion syndrome. Clin Neuropsychol 9:112–123, 1995.

Spina Bifida and Hydrocephalus

25

Gregory S. Liptak, MD, MPH

SPINA BIFIDA AND MENINGOMYELOCELE

The term *spina bifida*, which means split spine, refers to a group of disorders that are in the family of neural tube defects. Figure 25.1 shows the most common types of spina bifida. Meningomyelocele (or myelomeningocele) refers to the most serious form of spina bifida in which the covering of the spinal cord (meninges) and the spinal cord itself (myelon) are abnormal. The "cele" refers to the fluid-filled sac that herniates through the opening in the back. The overlying skin, vertebrae, and soft tissue are abnormal as well. The major focus of this chapter will relate to meningomyelocele.

In meningocele, the spinal cord is normal but the meninges and overlying structures are not. In occult spinal dysraphism, the overlying skin is intact, although usually a hyperpigmented spot, hairy patch, mass (lipoma) or sinus tract overlying the defect is present. Abnormalities of the spinal cord, such as tethering, a split cord, diastematomyelia (cartilaginous or boney spicule dividing the cord) and/or fibrous bands or tumors (such as lipomas) are common in occult spinal dysraphism and are often asymptomatic in early life but become symptomatic as the child grows. In spina bifida occulta, which occurs in up to 20% of otherwise healthy individuals (Fidas et al. 1987), the posterior arch of the vertebral body is abnormal, but no other abnormalities occur. This condition is benign (Boone et al. 1985), produces no symptoms, and appears to be genetically unrelated to the other forms of spina bifida.

Epidemiology, Etiology, and Prevention

In the United States, the prevalence of meningomyelocele is approximately 60 per 100,000 births (Olney and Mulinare 1998). It has been described as "the most common severely disabling birth defect in North America" (Fletcher et al. 2002).

The embryonic events resulting in meningomyelocele occur very early in gestation, during the period of neurulation (26 days after fertilization) (Copp, Fleming, and Greene 1998). During neurulation, the neural plate is transformed into a hollow tube. The neural groove folds over to become the neural tube, which develops into the spinal cord and vertebral arches, as well as the ventricular system in the brain. This finely regulated sequence of cell specification and proliferation involves multiple signaling systems. If a portion of the neural groove does not close completely, a neural tube defect results, and the spinal cord is malformed. Although the mechanism of neural tube closure is not fully understood, it does not simply close like a zipper but rather has multiple sites of closure, each of which is under separate genetic and environmental influences (Golden and Chernoff 1995; Urui and Oi 1995; Van Allen et al. 1993).

The causes of neural tube defects remain uncertain. Although both environmental and genetic factors play a role, their interaction is complex (Hall and Solehdin 1998; Volcik et al. 2003). For example, in mice, mutations of over 50 different genes (Juriloff and Harris, 2000) as well as multiple environmental factors can result in neural tube defects (Juriloff and Harris 1998). Men and women with meningomyelocele who can reproduce have a 4% chance of having an infant with a neural tube defect. Specific factors associated with increased risk for the development of neural tube defects include chromosomal disorders (trisomy 13 and 18), advanced maternal age, as well as exposure to a variety of drugs during pregnancy, such as valproic acid (Depakene, Depakote) (Davis, Peters, and McTavish 1994), carbamazepine (Tegretol) (Yerby 2003), and isotretinoin (retinoic acid, Accutane). Other factors include maternal hyperther-

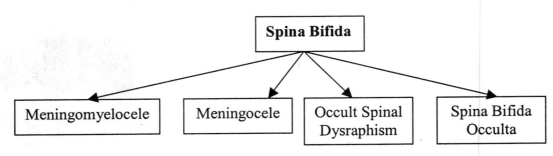

Figure 25.1 The most common types of spina bifida.

mia (e.g., saunas or high fever) (Sandford, Kissling, and Joubert 1992). Maternal diabetes (Sadler, Robinson, and Msall 1995), malnutrition (Gross et al. 2001), and obesity during pregnancy have also been identified as risk factors (Shaw et al. 2003).

Gender and socioeconomic factors have also been implicated as risk factors. Girls are three to seven times more likely to have meningomyelocele than boys, except for sacral level neural tube defects where the occurrence is equal (Hall et al. 1988). The birth prevalence is greater with lower socioeconomic status and is more common in certain racial and ethnic groups. Thus, obese Latina women who have daughters are eight times more likely to have a child with meningomyelocele than nonobese white women who have sons (Shaw et al. 2000).

The prevalence of meningomyelocele is decreasing as a result of a several factors. Developed countries are now using maternal alpha-fetoprotein serum testing for prenatal screening for neural tube defects (Roberts et al. 1995). Approximately 50% of couples, upon learning that they are carrying an affected fetus, choose to terminate the pregnancy (Forrester and Merz, 2000). Since 1998, the folic acid fortification program has been in effect in the United States and certain foods such as bread, cereals, flour, and rice have been supplemented with synthetic folic acid. However, the amount of folic acid in a typical diet, even with fortification, is not sufficient to prevent neural tube defects. Most obstetricians place women on supplemental folic acid (0.4 mg per day) as soon as pregnancy is diagnosed.

Studies have shown that daily supplemental doses of folic acid can reduce the incidence of new cases of neural tube defects in the general population by more than 50% (Bower and Stanley 1992; Werler, Shapiro, and Mitchell 1993). In a prospective study conducted in China, women who received daily folic acid, 0.4 mg (400 µg) given periconceptionally (from just before conception through the first trimester), had a rate of neural tube defects of 1 per 1,000 births compared with a rate of 4.8 per 1,000 in the control group (Berry et al. 1999). As a result, it is now recommended that all women who are contemplating a pregnancy take 0.4 mg of supplemental folic acid per day while they are trying to conceive and during the first 12 weeks of pregnancy (American Academy of Pediatrics 1999; Manning, Jennings, and Mad-

sen 2000). Yet, only about one third of women who are planning a pregnancy take folic acid around the time of conception (Schader and Corwin, 1999) and half of all pregnancies in the United States are unplanned.

Hydrocephalus

The prevalence of hydrocephalus is about 1 in 2,000 children. Hydrocephalus occurs as a result of an imbalance between the production and absorption of cerebrospinal fluid in the ventricular system so that cerebrospinal fluid accumulates within the cerebral ventricles. The ventricular system is made up of four ventricles connected by narrow pathways. Normally, cerebrospinal fluid is secreted by the choroid plexus in the lateral ventricles, flows through the ventricles, exits into cisterns (closed spaces that serve as reservoirs) at the base of the brain, then over the surfaces of the brain and spinal cord, where it is absorbed into the bloodstream. As cerebrospinal fluid is accumulated in the ventricles, the ventricles enlarge. In the fetus and newborn infant with patent sutures, the head expands. After the sutures are closed, increased intracranial pressure is more severe and can be potentially life-threatening.

The majority of children with meningomyelocele (75%) also have hydrocephalus. However, hydrocephalus often occurs in the absence of meningomyelocele. Hydrocephalus can either be present at birth (congenital hydrocephalus) or can be acquired. In general, most congenital cases of hydrocephalus are multifactorial with a recurrence risk of 4%. Congenital hydrocephalus has a prevalence of 10:1,000 in preterm infants and 1:1,000 in term infants. It is higher in preterm infants because of the higher incidence of intraventricular hemorrhage in small premature infants. A rare (1/30,000 males) X-linked recessive form of congenital hydrocephalus is associated with congenital stenosis of aqueduct of Sylvius (Rosenthal, Joulet, and Kenwrick 1992.) This form of X-linked hydrocephalus is the result of mutations in the L1CAM gene, which encodes the L1 protein, a protein involved in neuronal cell adhesion. Patients with this mutation have hydrocephalus, agenesis or hypoplasia of corpus callosum and corticospinal tracts, mental retardation, spastic paraplegia, and adducted thumbs. (Weller and Gartner 2001).

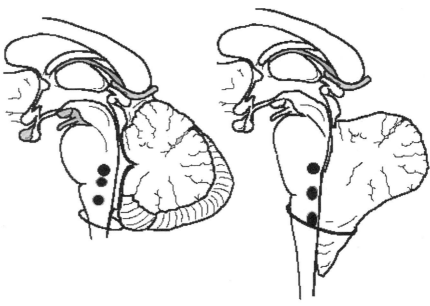

Figure 25.2 Illustration of Chiari II malformation

Normal

Chiari II Malformation

Hydrocephalus can be classified as communicating or obstructive. Causes of communicating hydrocephalus include obstruction of the subarachnoid space (following intracranial hemorrhage or infections), developmental failure of arachnoid villi, and excessive CSF production (from a choroid plexus tumor). Obstructive hydrocephalus results from aqueductal stenosis, mass lesions that block the flow of cerebrospinal fluid (neoplasms, cysts, hematomas, aneurysms), or obstruction of the fourth ventricle (Dandy Walker malformation, arachnoiditis).

The Chiari II (previously known as Arnold-Chiari) malformation is frequently associated with meningomyelocele above the sacral level (Griebel, Oakes, and Worley 1991; Rauzzino and Oakes 1995) (Fig. 25.2). This malformation involves the downward displacement of the medulla and cerebellar tonsils through the foramen magnum. Three different types varying in severity have been identified. Type II is typically associated with meningomyelocele and involves the herniation of the medulla, cerebellar tonsils, and vermis through the foramen magnum. The fourth ventricle is at the level of the foramen magnum. In the Type II Chiari malformation, aqueductal stenosis is also present and results in hydrocephalus. In the most severe type of Chiari malformation (type III), the fourth ventricle is displaced below the foramen magnum. Type II and III Chiari malformations result in dysfunction of the medullary outflow cranial nerves.

Using folic acid to prevent meningomyelocele and its associated hydrocephalus and preventing germinal matrix–intraventricular hemorrhage in the premature newborn [which leads to communicating hydrocephalus (Volpe 1989)] (See Chapter 23 on Prematurity) are two strategies to prevent the occurrence of hydrocephalus in newborns. Strategies to prevent germinal matrix–intraventricular

hemorrhage include prevention of premature delivery, antenatal corticosteroids, avoidance of prolonged labor, avoidance of hemodynamic disturbances, prevention of respiratory distress syndrome and its complications (Roland and Hill 2003), and drainage, irrigation, and fibrinolytic therapy after intraventricular hemorrhage occurs (Whitelaw et al. 2003)

Neurosurgical repair of the meningomyelocele in utero has been shown to decrease the severity of the Chiari malformation and the need for shunting for hydrocephalus (Tulipan et al. 2003). However, no effect on lower extremity functioning or bowel and bladder impairments has been found (Tubbs et al. 2003). The National Institutes of Health currently is conducting a randomized study of prenatal surgery in three sites to evaluate the effects of this intervention (NICHD 2004). Earlier attempts at prenatal treatment of hydrocephalus by shunting the fetus were disappointing. Newer technologies such as prenatal magnetic resonance imaging may improve this intervention, however (von Koch et al. 2003).

Neurological Impairments Associated With Meningomyelocele

The primary neurological abnormalities of meningomyelocele are paralysis, loss of sensation, variable bladder and bowel dysfunction, and Chiari II malformation with associated hydrocephalus. Although most people think only of the spine when they hear the term "spina bifida," the malformation leading to meningomyelocele affects the entire CNS (Dahl et al. 1995; Gilbert et al. 1986).

A variety of malformations of the brain are associated with meningomyelocele. These include defective myelinization of the brainstem, and neuromigrational anomalies of the cortex and cerebellum (Gilbert et al. 1986). Subcortical abnormalities, including beaking of the colliculi and complete or near-complete fusion of the thalami, are also commonly observed (Gilbert et al.). Agenesis of the corpus callosum commonly occurs in meningomyelocele and can be complete or partial (Barkovich, 2000). This is believed to be a manifestation of the underlying defect in neuronal migration that is associated with spina bifida. In one neuropathological study (Gilbert et al.), 92% of children with meningomyelocele had abnormal migration of cortical neurons, 72% had cerebellar dysplasia, 20% had hypoplasia or aplasia of cranial nerve nuclei, 16% had fusion of the thalami, and 12% had agenesis of the corpus callosum. In a series of MRI studies, Kawamura and colleagues (2001, 2002) found partial agenesis of the corpus callosum, hypoplasia of the cerebral hemispheres, polymicrogyria, heterotopic gray matter, as well as cervicomedullary anomalies, such as herniation of the cerebellar tonsils through the foramen magnum. Other areas of the spinal cord may be involved above the site of the meningomyelocele (for example, syringomyelia), resulting in additional motor and sensory impairment (Dias and Pang 1995).

Not surprisingly, these cerebral anomalies are likely to result in an array of cognitive impairments. Abnormalities of the corpus callosum are negatively related to intelligence (Barf et al. 2003). The corpus callosum provides an important pathway for communication across different parts of the brain. It also contributes to the development of cerebral specialization of language, nonverbal skills (e.g., spatial cognition), and other cognitive skills (Hannay et al. 1999). Children with meningomyelocele who have abnormalities of the corpus callosum have been found to have impaired nonverbal skills (Hannay et al.).

Involvement of the cranial nerve nuclei controlling ocular movements results in strabismus, which is observed in 20% of children with meningomyelocele (Griebel 1991; Lennerstrand, Gallo, and Samuelsson, 1990). Related to the Chiari malformation is an array of symptoms reflecting compromise of the medulla and cranial nerves at that level—difficulty swallowing, choking, hoarseness, breath-holding spells, apnea, stridor and disordered breathing during sleep, upper extremity spasticity, and opisthotonos. Rare sudden deaths from cardiorespiratory arrest related to the Chiari malformation have been reported (Charney et al. 1987; Kirk, Morielli, and Brouillette 1999).

It is important to screen children with meningomyelocele for sleep problems. Disordered breathing during sleep, including apnea, occurs in individuals with meningomyelocele, and has been called "the missed diagnosis" by some (Kirk et al. 1999). It can be the result of obstructive sleep apnea, central apnea, or central hypoventilation (Kirk et al. 2000). Disordered sleep can cause children to be tired during the day, and interfere with their ability to function in school. A formal sleep study can help differentiate between the many problems a child may be having that can cause disordered breathing during sleep (e.g., upper airway obstruction from enlarged tonsils and adenoids).

Children with meningomyelocele exhibit impairments of many of the functions associated with abnormalities of the cerebellum. Cerebellar dysfunction results in impairments of balance, coordination, motor performance, and sequential motor learning (Van Mier and Petersen 2002). However, it is now recognized that the cerebellum plays an important role in a broad range of cognitive functions (Leiner et al. 1991). The neocerebellum projects to and receives projections from dorsolateral prefrontal cortex (Middleton and Strick 1994). These structures are activated simultaneously during performance of different types of cognitive tasks (Berman 1995; Nagahama 1996). Cerebellar dysfunction appears to result in dysregulation (dysmetria) of response in both the cognitive and emotional realm (Schmahmann 1998). Gao and colleagues (1996) demonstrated that the cerebellum is engaged during the acquisition and discrimination of sensory information. The right posterolateral cerebellar hemisphere assists the left cerebral hemisphere in generating specific types of spoken word associations (Gebhart et al. 2002). Individuals who have had resection of part of the cerebellum secondary to brain tumors have been identified as having a unique syndrome called *cerebellar cognitive affective syndrome*, characterized by impairments in executive function (including planning and sequencing), visual–spatial function, expressive language, verbal memory, and modulation of affect (Levisohn et al. 2000; Riva et al. 2000).

Hydrocephalus affects a number of brain functions. As cerebrospinal fluid accumulation increases, the ventricles increase in size, leading to thinning of the cerebral mantle. This mainly affects white matter and disrupts myelinization in the young child, particularly in the posterior regions (Del Bigio 1993). The pathway containing the motor fibers to the legs arises from the medial area of the frontal lobes and descends along the lateral margins of the lateral ventricles. As the ventricles become increasingly dilated, these fibers are stretched and result in spastic paraparesis. In severe, untreated hydrocephalus, the child may be quadriplegic.

Paralysis of upward gaze may also occur with increased intracranial pressure. If the child is shunted promptly (often in the newborn period), there is often dramatic improvement in the spastic paraparesis and ocular abnormalities. In the older child with closed sutures, shunt failure may result in the typical symptoms of increased intracranial pressure—headache, visual dysfunction, spastic paraparesis, and disturbance of consciousness. Tables 25.1 and 25.2 list some abnormalities of the brain and associated findings in children with meningomyelocele.

Epilepsy develops in approximately 15% of individuals with meningomyelocele (Noetzel 1989; Talwar, Baldwin, and Horbatt 1995). The seizures usually are generalized tonic–clonic and respond well to antiepileptic medication. Rarely, a blocked shunt or shunt infection may precipitate seizures.

TABLE 25.1
DISORDERS OF THE CENTRAL NERVOUS SYSTEM ASSOCIATED WITH MENINGOMYELOCELE

Disorder	Associated Conditions
Brain	
Chiari II malformation	Abnormal swallowing
	Vocal cord paralysis
	Apnea, hypoventilation
	Spasticity of upper extremities
	Hydrocephalus
	Sudden death
Hydrocephalus	Stretching of periventricular corticospinal fibers
	Thinning of corpus callosum
	Complications of shunting (e.g., ventriculitis)
	Disruption of myelination
	Disruption of optic tracts
	Impaired visuomotor dexterity and visuospatial skills
	Precocious puberty
Dysgenesis of corpus callosum	Impaired nonverbal skills
	Disordered pragmatic language skills
Dysgenesis of cerebellum	Impaired balance, coordination, motor performance and sequential motor learning
	Decreased discrimination of sensory information
	Cerebellar cognitive affective syndrome (see text)
Abnormal cranial nerve nuclei	Strabismus
Unknown	Epilepsy
Spinal Cord	
Primary Lesion	Motor paralysis
	Sensory loss
	Bowel and bladder dysfunction
	Tethered spinal cord
Split cord lesions (including diastematomyelia)	Neurological deterioration
Spinal cord atrophy	Neurological deterioration
Syrinx (syringomyelia, syringobulbia, hydromyelia)	Neurological deterioration

Associated Medical Conditions

Motor Paralysis and Sensory Loss

Some of the associated impairments that occur with meningomyelocele are shown in Figure 25.3. Motor paralysis and sensory loss occur below the level of the defect in the spinal cord. For example, children with lesions at the thoracic or high lumbar (L1 or L2) level have paralysis of the legs and weakness and sensory loss below the waist, while children with sacral lesions usually have only mild weakness of their ankles or toes and loss of sensation in the perineum and on their feet. The motor paralysis leads to problems with mobility, contractures, and osteoporosis with pathological fractures. More serious impairment of mobility occurs in children who have meningomyelocele above the sacral level. The higher the level of the meningomyelocele, the greater the muscle weakness, the more ambulation will be impaired (McDonald 1995). For example, children with L3 level often require crutches and bracing up to the hip. Children with thoracic or high-lumbar paralysis may eventually stand upright and walk, but only with support of the hips, knees, and ankles. This support may be provided by extensive bracing and/or mobility devices such as a parapodium (Liptak et al. 1992), reciprocal gait orthosis (Guidera et al. 1993), or hip-knee-ankle-foot orthosis used in combination with crutches or a walker (Mazur et al. 1989). As children approach adolescence and their center of gravity and relative strength change, even those with mid-lumbar level lesions will increasingly rely on wheelchairs for mobility. Paralysis and muscle imbalance around a joint can lead to contractures. For instance, clubfoot and other deformations, such as calcaneus deformity, are commonly noted at birth and are related to the lack of normal innervation and resultant fetal immobility. Hip flexion contractures and acquired deformities around the knee, ankle, and foot are common in older children.

Almost 90% of children with meningomyelocele above the sacral level have scoliosis and/or kyphosis. Scoliosis and kyphosis may be congenital or acquired, and may be related to abnormalities of the vertebral bodies, such as hemivertebrae or butterfly vertebrae, to abnormal muscle balance (the muscles act like guy wires on a telephone pole), or to tethering of the spinal cord (see subsequent discussion). The higher the lesion, the more likely the deformity. If untreated, spinal deformities may eventually interfere with sitting and walking and decrease vital capacity. Kyphosis is usually located in the lumbar spine and may be severe at birth. Like scoliosis, it is more common with higher lesions and may progress over time.

Lacking normal sensory input and the ability to shift position when pressure over a bony prominence becomes uncomfortable, decubitus ulcers are likely to develop in individuals with meningomyelocele. Insensate skin often leads to injuries that would not happen if pain perception was normal (e.g., cutting the bottom of the foot while swimming) and can also lead to lesions that are hard to heal. Individuals who use wheelchairs for extended periods may develop pressure sores on the buttocks or coccyx. Problems with skin breakdown become more frequent during adolescence. The ulcers often resist healing and require extensive treatment because of impaired circulation, continued pressure, contamination by stool and urine, and secondary bacterial infections. Deep decubiti may lead to osteomyelitis of underlying bones.

TABLE 25.2
SELECT CONDITIONS ASSOCIATED WITH MENINGOMYELOCELE, THEIR EVALUATION AND TREATMENT

Urogenital System

Age	Conditions	Possible Tests	Possible Treatments
Newborn/Infant	Hydronephrosis	Renal ultrasound	Intermittent catheterization Vesicostomy
	Urinary reflux	Voiding cystourethrogram	Prophylactic antibiotics Intermittent catheterization Vesicostomy
	Elevated intravesical pressure	Urodynamics	Intermittent catheterization Vesicostomy
	Urinary tract infection	Urine culture DMSA renal scan	Antibiotics
	Renal dysfunction Renal dysgenesis (e.g., horseshoe kidney)	Serum BUN, creatinine, urinalysis Renal ultrasound	Any of the above
Preschool School Age	Infancy issues + continence Preschool issues + hypertension	Above + urodynamics Same as above + blood pressure monitoring	Same as above Urinary diversion (e.g., appendicovesicostomy)
	Female precocious puberty	Serum FSH, LH testing Bone age determination	Leuprolide
Adolescence	School age + Male sexual function Female sexual function	Same as above	Same as above + sildenafil and others Birth control

Musculoskeletal System

Age	Conditions	Possible Tests	Possible Treatments
Newborn/Infant	Foot/ankle deformities (e.g., club foot)	Radiograms	Serial casting Surgery
	Hip dislocation	Hip ultrasound or radiogram	Abduction orthosis surgery
	Kyphosis	Radiograms	TLSO Surgery
Preschool	Above + hip and knee contractures or rotational deformities	Radiograms	Above + lower extremity bracing (e.g., HKAFO or RGO, or parapodium)
	Impaired mobility		Mobility device
	Diminished range of motion		Therapy, orthotics
School age	Above + scoliosis	Above + MRI scan	TLSO Surgery
Adolescence	Same as above	Same as above	Same as above

Neurological System

Age	Conditions	Possible Tests	Possible Treatments
Newborn/Infant	Open lesion on back		Antibiotics Closure of lesion
	Hydrocephalus	MRI or CT scan Cranial ultrasound	Ventricular-peritoneal or subgaleal shunt
	Chiari malformation	Cranial MRI or ultrasound Sleep study Pharyngogram (swallow study) Visualization of vocal cords	Posterior fossa decompression
	Spinal cord malformations	Spinal MRI	Surgery
	Epilepsy	EEG	Anticonvulsants
Preschool	Above + spinal cord tethering (minus open lesion)	Cystometrogram Spinal MRI Manual muscle strength testing	Surgical untethering
	Ventricular shunt malfunction	Cranial CT, ultrasound or MRI Shunt tap Neuropsychological testing	Shunt revision
School age	Same as above	Same as above	Same as above
Adolescence	Same as above	Same as above	Same as above

BUN, blood urea nitrogen; CT, computed tomography; DMSA, dimercaptosuccinic acid; EEG, electroencephalogram; FSH, follicle-stimulating hormone; HKAFO, hip-knee-ankle-foot orthosis; LH, luteinizing hormone; MRI, magnetic resonance imaging; RGO, reciprocating gait orthosis; TLSO, thoraco-lumbar-sacral orthosis.

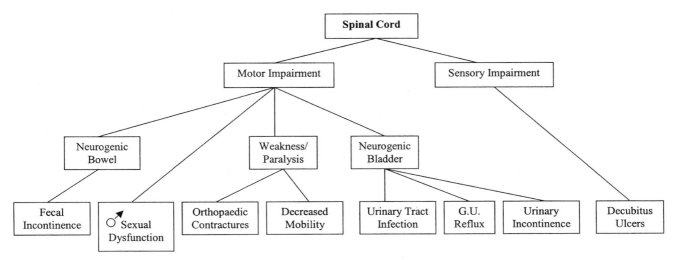

Figure 25.3   Impairments found in meningomyelocele

Genitourinary and Bowel Dysfunction

Because the bladder, urethra, external rectal sphincter, and perineal sensation are all controlled by sacral nerves, bladder and bowel dysfunction are present in virtually all children with meningomyelocele. Even children with sacral lesions and normal leg movement typically have bladder and bowel problems. Neurogenic bowel causes fecal incontinence and is associated with constipation. Neurogenic bladder is associated with numerous urological and medical problems. Not infrequently, these children also have malformations of the kidneys, including horseshoe and absent kidney (Hulton et al. 1990). There are different patterns of bladder dysfunction; some children with meningomyelocele have patulous sphincters and are chronically incontinent. Others have tight sphincters and develop large, distended bladders with increased intravesicular pressure, leading to ureteral reflux, hydronephrosis, and kidney stones, and recurrent bouts of infection. If untreated, irreversible renal damage can result. The management of urinary incontinence depends on the specific type of bladder dysfunction, which cannot be predicted by the level of lesion. Urinary tract infections are extremely common in this population. Bladder augmentation surgery, which is one of the surgical treatments, is associated with a small risk for bladder cancer (Game et al. 1999; Shaw and Lewis 1999). Although most children with meningomyelocele are born with normal kidneys, careful urological evaluation and continuous monitoring is required to prevent damage to the kidneys. Renal failure is not uncommon in adults with meningomyelocele who have not received adequate urological management (Muller, Arbeiter, and Aufricht 2002).

Although 75% of postpubertal males with meningomyelocele are able to have erections (Diamond, Rickwood, and Thomas 1986), most are achieved reflexively by stimulation rather than in response to psychogenic stimuli (Dik et al. 1999; Sandler et al. 1996). Erections are related to level of sensory deficit, with males who have affected sacral level having more erections than those with affected thoracic or lumbar levels. Therefore, their ability to have unaided sexual intercourse from sexual stimulation is limited. In addition, males frequently have retrograde ejaculation, which further limits their reproductive capacity. Cryptorchidism occurs in 15 to 25% of boys with spina bifida (Greene et al. 1985; Meyer and Landau 1984). Many postpubertal women with meningomyelocele are able to experience orgasm during sexual intercourse. However, they typically have decreased genital sensation and less sexually stimulated lubrication. As a result, intercourse without adequate lubrication can lead to vaginal sores.

Precocious puberty (defined as Tanner stage 2 breast or pubic hair development before age 9.2 years) is common in females who have meningomyelocele with hydrocephalus, and less common in females with isolated hydrocephalus (Elias and Sadeghi-Nejad 1994). This is likely due to hypothalamic dysfunction (Perrone et al. 1994). In one study, the incidence of precocious puberty in girls with meningomyelocele was at least 52%. Girls with precocious puberty appeared to have a history of increased intracranial pressure in the perinatal period, greater motor and urological dysfunction, and more shunt revisions than girls in whom precocious puberty did not develop (Proos et al. 1996).

Tethered Cord

Tethering of the spinal cord may be present at birth in children with little external evidence of spinal dysraphism or can occur after closure of the primary meningomyelocele defect. As the child grows, the spinal cord, which is bound down by adhesions or congenital fibrous bands, becomes increasingly stretched which results in progressive ischemic damage to the cord. Lower extremity weakness, new contractures, sensory deficits, pain, and bowel and bladder function can occur quite insidiously and ambulation and daily living skills may deteriorate. There may be a rapid progression of scoliosis. Tethered cord syndrome occurs in 3 to 15% of patients with a history of repaired meningomyelocele (Phuong, Schoeberl, and Raffel 2002). Even after surgical repair of the tethering, a significant percent of children will have recurrent or new symptoms consistent with tethering.

Other Medical Issues

Individuals with meningomyelocele with thoracic to L2 lesions are at increased risk for obesity in part as a result of their decreased activity and energy expenditure (Polito, et al. 1995; Littlewood et al. 2003). However, Fiore and colleagues conducted a study of anthropometric measurements and dietary adequacy in a group of 100 children. Forty of the 100 children and adolescents were classified as markedly overweight (body mass index above the 95th percentile). Five were classified as malnourished or at risk for malnutrition. Most of the obese subjects took in less than the expected recommended daily energy intake; only 25% had an energy intake appropriate for age and gender. The expected correlation between obesity and motor impairment was not found, whereas energy intake was correlated with body mass index. They concluded that obesity in this population resulted from a complex set of factors (Fiore et al. 1998). Obesity is unquestionably one of the several factors that adversely affect mobility and social opportunities, which may in turn contribute to increased inactivity and further weight gain. The medical complications of chronic obesity are an additional problem.

About one third of children with meningomyelocele are short as a result of growth hormone deficiency (Fiore et al. 1998). Untreated children with meningomyelocele and short stature achieve an adult recumbent height falling one standard deviation or more below the mean. Treatment with growth hormone results in an increase of recumbent height into the average range as well as reducing body mass index significantly, thus diminishing the problems associated with obesity (Rotenstein and Breen 1996; Rotenstein and Bass 2004).

An allergy to latex, including anaphylaxis, develops in between 40 and 60% of children with meningomyelocele (Pearson, Cole, and Jarvis 1994; Dormans et al. 1995). The risk of latex allergy increases with age (Mazon et al., 2000) and frequency of surgical procedures (Ellsworth et al., 1993).

Cognition

Early studies of children with meningomyelocele born before routine ventricular shunting for hydrocephalus showed a high rate of mental retardation among survivors (Foltz and Shurtleff 1963; Laurence and Coates 1962; Shurtleff, Foltz, and Loeser 1973). As ventricular shunting

became more widespread, the occurrence of mental retardation decreased (Brookshire et al. 1995; Fletcher et al. 1992b, Wills et al. 1990). However, even today, children with meningomyelocele who have had an episode of shunt infection (ventriculitis) have significantly lower scores on intelligence tests, often in the mentally retarded range, have more seizures, higher future risks of shunt infection and malfunction, and perform more poorly in school (McLone 1992; Kanev and Sheehan 2003). Some studies have found that frequent shunt revisions have a negative effect on IQ (Mazur et al. 1988; Holler et al. 1995; Hunt et al. 1999; Dennis and Barnes 2002), although others have not replicated this finding (Ralph et al. 2000).

On standard tests of intelligence, children with meningomyelocele and shunted hydrocephalus typically perform worse on performance than on verbal scales, with a verbal performance gap of 0.5 to 1.5 standard deviations (Hurley et al. 1983; Wills et al. 1990; Brookshire et al. 1995; Casari and Fantino 1998). Most studies of cognition in children with meningomyelocele have involved school-aged children. The cognitive profile of preschool children and adults with meningomyelocele are not well understood. Some studies of young adults have shown the same pattern of higher verbal than performance scores on intelligence tests (Dennis and Barnes 2002; Hommet et al. 1999). There is significant variability in intellectual status of children with meningomyelocele, which may be related to genetic as well as medical factors, including the severity of the hydrocephalus, the number of shunt revisions, and the extent of cerebellar dysfunction. As is true of children without meningomyelocele, socioeconomic status is a factor affecting performance on cognitive tests (Bier et al. 1997).

Yeates and colleagues (2003) found that about half of children with meningomyelocele have a cognitive and behavioral profile typical of nonverbal learning disability, described by Myklebust (1975) and Rourke (1989). Children with this syndrome have deficits in tactile and visual perception, complex psychomotor skills, and in dealing with novel circumstances (Rourke et al. 2002). They demonstrate strengths in verbal and auditory abilities (although they have difficulty grasping the pragmatic aspects of language), but have weaknesses in nonverbal areas. Impairment in motor coordination, visual attention, visual–spatial perception, flexibility, abstract thinking, executive function, organizational skills, and generalizing what they have learned (Fletcher et al. 2002).

Children with meningomyelocele have impairments in executive functioning that are similar to those with nonverbal learning disabilities. (Dise and Lohr 1998; Brewer et al. 2001; Fletcher et al. 1996; Mahone et al. 2002). Executive function skills include planning future activities, organizing, inhibiting competing (inappropriate) responses, self-regulation, remembering rules, initiating tasks, and remembering to remember an activity. These children do better thinking in a linear fashion rather than in gestalt terms, and have difficulty with context. Children with nonverbal learning disabilities have difficulty learning new concepts, especially in novel situations; they rely extensively on previously learned rote information; and adapt poorly to new situations, which affects their ability to learn. Their information processing tends to be unimodal rather than intermodal (Rourke et al. 2002). Metacognitve skills (e.g., mental flexibility, mental efficiency, learning from experience, and conceptual sophistication) are more affected than behavioral inhibition (Mahone et al.).Executive function impairment may make it very difficult for the individual with meningomyelocele to reliably perform necessary daily self-care activities. They may not consistently remember what daily self-care tasks must be performed in what sequence (e.g., understanding the importance of catheterizing on time and the importance of checking for and preventing pressure sores as well as understanding the consequences of failure to do so) (Russel 2004).

Associations between nonverbal skills and MRI findings have been found. For instance, Fletcher and colleagues (1996) found that children with hydrocephalus who had proportionately greater posterior than anterior cerebrospinal fluid percentages had significantly poorer visuomotor dexterity and visuospatial skills than those who had normal percentages of cerebrospinal fluid. Some children with meningomyelocele may have only a few of the features of nonverbal learning disabilities while others may have many severe deficits in the nonverbal learning disability spectrum.

Attention Deficit–Hyperactivity Disorder

Davidovitch and colleagues (1999) reported that 39% of children with meningomyelocele have some form of attention deficit disorder (most commonly the inattentive type) and about 30% of these children showed a clinical response to methylphenidate; although a small sample, double-blind placebo-controlled study was not informative. Other children may be inattentive and have poor organizational skills, but not have true attention deficit–hyperactivity disorder (ADHD) (Shaffer et al. 1985). In one study (Loss et al. 1996), children with myelomeningocele showed deficits across all four elements of attention (encode, focus/execute, sustain, and shift) compared to their siblings. It can be difficult to differentiate primary ADHD from attention deficits that are secondary to other neurological impairments in children with meningomyelocele, which result in problems with alertness and arousal (Brewer et al. 2001). Their inability to integrate, organize, and interpret information, especially when they try to accomplish unfamiliar tasks, may reflect impaired executive function.

Language

Children who survived severe, unshunted hydrocephalus were often described as having "cocktail party syndrome" (Tew 1979; Tew and Laurence 1979; Hurley et al. 1990). This refers to the tendency of these children to chatter on about topics in a superficial, nonmeaningful or inappropriate way. They may use and repeat memorized common phrases, such as, "Hello, how are you today?" or, "What's up?" They may be able to repeat parts of a story that they have heard without really understanding what the story means. Typically, the content of these verbal expressions is absent or trivial at best. Thus, these children, as well as those who are less affected by hydrocephalus, have difficulty deriving meaning from context (Barnes and Dennis 1998).

Children with meningomyelocele often demonstrate adequate linguistic skills, with appropriate form and structure; yet they too frequently display deficits in semantic-pragmatic skills. As a result, their expressive language often lacks substance and is poorly matched to the communicative context as in the cocktail party syndrome. Studies of school-age children with meningomyelocele have shown that although they use and understand single words, they have difficulty using language in a flexible and adaptive manner (Dennis and Barnes 1993; Dennis et al. 1994; Fletcher et al. 2002). Thus, many children with meningomyelocele have problems with the construction of meaning and in pragmatic communication. They may have deficits in several different aspects of oral discourse, including establishing alternative meanings to ambiguous sentences, understanding figurative expressions, making inferences, and producing speech acts (Dennis and Barnes 1993). In a study of narrative discourse in 100 children with hydrocephalus, Dennis and colleagues (1994) noted that their narratives tend to be less coherent and cohesive than a control group. They conveyed less content, included more ambiguous or implausible material, and were more verbose and less economical in quality.

Academic Achievement

Children with meningomyelocele often meet discrepancy criteria for learning disability (defined as low academic achievement that is unexpected based on the child's overall cognitive abilities). Of course, in some cases, the lower level of academic achievement is in line with the IQ.

Several studies have shown that children and adolescents with meningomyelocele perform more poorly than their typically developing peers on measures of intelligence and/or achievement, and are more likely to receive special services, or repeat a grade (Appleton et al. 1994; Fowler et al. 1985; Friedrich et al. 1991; Jacobs et al. 2001; Tew and Laurence 1984). Their learning difficulties often are not particularly apparent in the earlier grades (Rowley-Kelly and Reigel 1993). However, fine motor skill deficits often impair the child's performance in the early years of elementary school because of their difficulty using scissors, holding a pencil, tying shoelaces, and buttoning buttons. In the later school years, writing is a challenge (Barnes et al. 2002; Dennis and Barnes 2002; Pearson et al. 1988).

A fairly consistent finding in school-age children is deficient performance in arithmetic, which is again reminiscent of a nonverbal learning disorder. They typically perform more poorly on standardized math tests than do children without spina bifida, and perform more poorly in arithmetic than in language-based tasks, such as reading and spelling. Weak number skills, delays in the ability to count or seriate, can be observed as early as 36 months of age and persist into adulthood (Wills et al. 1990; Dennis and Barnes 2002). The presence of a shunt has been associated with lower IQ scores and lower mathematics scores in some studies (Kalucy, Bower, and Stanley 1996).

Visual–spatial difficulties can make learning certain aspects of mathematics such as geometry a major challenge. Similarly, problems with estimation and the ability to solve word problems are associated with problems in visual–spatial integration (Barnes et al. 2002). These students also have short-term memory impairment, manifested in difficulty with list learning (Cull and Wyke 1984; Yeates et al. 1995; Scott et al. 2003). Children with meningomyelocele also evidence impaired procedural skills that persist to adulthood (Dennis and Barnes 2002). They also have diminished speed of retrieval (efficiency).

The difficulty that children with meningomyelocele experience in academic environments increases as they progress through school. Although they have relatively good mechanical reading skills and, therefore, do not appear to have as much difficulty in this area as they do in arithmetic, when the academic tasks begin to require the ability to comprehend text and make inferences, their difficulty in reading comprehension interferes with their ability to perform (Barnes and Dennis 1992). Moreover, the language difficulties described previously make it hard for them to adequately formulate abstract and coherent verbal responses and written material. They are less likely to advance to postsecondary education than children without meningomyelocele. In one study, 34% of affected children involved in postsecondary education compared to 47% of the general population and were 1 to 2 years delayed in educational attainment compared to age-matched peers (Bomalaski et al. 1995). In another study of 48 adults with meningomyelocele, only seven were attending college. Achievement and IQ scores as well as measures of language and visual–spatial ability differentiated those who attended college from those who did not (Hurley and Bell 1994).

Meningomyelocele may affect academic performance in several ways. First, it has an obvious direct effect on cognition. Second, it is associated with increased absences from school for reasons that may include acute illnesses, visits to health professionals, inappropriate health beliefs and perceptions of vulnerability, and worsening of chronic symptoms. Medical and neurological problems may contribute directly to poor performance in school. Shunt malfunction may present with subtle symptoms including worsening academic performance. Anticonvulsants and anticholinergic medications (used to help manage bladder function) can lead to lethargy and adversely affect school performance. The young child may be absent because of frequent hospitalizations and elective and emergency surgeries. Children with meningomyelocele are pulled out of regular classroom academic sessions for physical therapy and occupational therapy, and for catheterization and other medical procedures. Even today, some children experience restricted or delayed school attendance because of inaccessible school facilities (lack of handicapped access); they often cannot negotiate a flight of stairs or walk with braces and crutches rapidly enough to get to their next class on time (Wasson et al. 1992). They may have to go to another building for therapy, losing significant time from classroom activities. School facilities often do not provide adequate privacy for toileting and self-catheterization and in some settings, trained personnel to assist younger children with catheterization are lacking.

Social Abilities

Children with meningomyelocele have been found to be socially immature and passive, more isolated, more dependent on adults, and less likely to make independent decisions than children without meningomyelocele (Blum et al. 1991; Holmbeck et al. 2003). Successful social interactions require abilities in verbal pragmatics, social-problem-solving skill, social memory, as well as the ability to predict consequences. For an individual with a nonverbal learning disability, the interpretation of social cues such as facial expressions and body language can become a major problem and lead to confusion and social rejection. Difficulty with visual attention and failure to understand nonverbal cues lead to difficulty interpreting behavior. Although children with meningomyelocele may be talkative, they often interrupt and have difficulty entering conversations correctly.

Neuropsychiatric Aspects of Meningomyelocele

Studies of self-concept in children with meningomyelocele are equivocal. Some (MacBriar 1983; Murch and Cohen 1989) failed to show a difference between children with meningomyelocele and controls. Others, however, have found significant differences (King et al. 1993; Kazak and Clark 1986; Appleton et al. 1994; Zurmohle et al. 1998). In a recent study, children with spina bifida were found to have lower self-concept than controls. This was particularly true for girls. Furthermore, urinary continence was associated with a more normal self-concept (Moore, Kogan, and Parekh 2004). In a related study, children who had a Malone antegrade colonic enema implanted surgically reported increased self-reliance, independence and a feeling of security, which led to significant improvement in self-esteem (Aksnes et al. 2002.) These results suggest that better continence is associated with better self-concept.

Many children with myelomeningocele face a daunting challenge in terms of having any control over their environment. In the preschool years, they are often required to undergo repeated surgery (orthopedic, urological, and neurosurgical, when a shunt revision is required). They may spend months in a cast, which effectively immobilizes them. They must deal with pain and the preoccupation with symptoms that often accompany spina bifida. In elementary school, they are notably "different" from the other children, and often must deal with their inability to participate in games with peers and understand academics at the level of their peers. This in turn leads to diminished expectations and lower self-esteem. When a child is able to ambulate with crutches and braces, their energy expenditure is substantial and they must struggle with fatigue. Moreover, their impaired executive function often makes the world appear even more complex. All of this results in a decreased sense of self-efficacy (Mobley, Harless, and Miller 1996) and these children often develop "learned helplessness," believing that their efforts to change the environment are ineffective. This limits their willingness trying to perform academically or to reach out socially (Peterson, Maier, and Seligman 1993). In adolescence, the awareness of their potentially impaired sexual functioning becomes an issue. Not surprisingly, children with meningomyelocele, particularly girls, are at increased risk for depressive mood, low self-esteem, self-blame, and suicidal ideation. Effective parental support tends to be a moderating variable, especially in girls (Appleton et al. 1997).

MANAGEMENT OF THE INFANT AND CHILD WITH MENINGOMYELOCELE

The birth of an infant with meningomyelocele requires a very rapid assessment by a team of physicians. Within 2 days after birth, assuming that the infant is medically stable, the neurosurgeon repairs the back lesion, and in many cases if there is any evidence of hydrocephalus, a shunting procedure is performed at the same time or shortly thereafter. If a shunting procedure is not required at that point, the baby will be closely monitored because of the high probability that hydrocephalus will develop. The baby is also evaluated by the urologist and the orthopedic surgeon. When the infant is being managed in a center with a meningomyelocele team a team member meets with the parents and reviews the implications of a meningomyelocele, explains the surgical procedures and the need for close monitoring. Parents need a great deal of support during this period and it is helpful to them to have a trusting relationship with the physicians and nurses who care for the infant.

Developmental Interventions

Because children with meningomyelocele have multiple impairments that affect development, and are at increased risk for developmental disabilities, they are likely to benefit from an Early Intervention program (typically from birth to age 3 years). Interventions include physical and occupational therapies, speech therapy, and special educational services. No scientific evaluations of the effectiveness of these early interventions in this population have been conducted to determine the optimal combination of therapies. When the child turns 3 years of age, other programs, typically through the local school district become available. They also should have a formal psychoeducational evaluation before school entry to identify their capabilities, strengths, and weaknesses. This will allow modifications of the school environment and the development of an individualized education program (IEP) (Rowley-Kelly and Reigel 1993).

The Individuals with Disabilities Education Act (IDEA), Public Law 102–119, provides children with meningomyelocele with improved access to educational services in the least restrictive environment. IDEA entitles children with disabilities ages 3 to 21 to a free, appropriate education. Related services must be paid for by the school. A related service is any additional service that is needed to allow the child to benefit from instruction, and includes transportation, audiology, recreation, school health services, psychological services, physical therapy, occupational therapy, speech and language therapy, catheterization, assistive technology, and social work services. Parents have the right to question placement decisions and the right to due process to settle differences. Two criteria have to be met for a child to qualify under IDEA: (1) that the child has a disability, and (2) that special education services are necessary to address the disability. Children who have meningomyelocele can be classified as having a disability under IDEA in several different ways, including the categories "learning disabled," "orthopaedically impaired," or "other health impaired." The second criterion can be met if any aspect of the disability has a negative impact on any aspect of participation in the general curriculum, including academic, behavior, communication, vocational skills, basic life skills, social skills, and physical needs.

If a child with meningomyelocele does not qualify under IDEA, then Section 504 of the Rehabilitation Act of 1973 can provide access to services. This regulation states that no qualified person with a handicap shall be excluded from participation in any program or activity that receives benefits from federal financial assistance. Under this legislation, a child does not have to be enrolled in special education or eligible under IDEA to receive related services from a school. However, parents have fewer rights and children receive fewer services under Section 504.

Strategies to address disorders of cognition in school include remediation (additional instructional time or different instructional approaches to "fix" a certain area of weakness and build strength in a particular area to facilitate potential learning) and compensation (alternative approaches [e.g., assistive technology] to offset, or counterbalance, a learning disability and produce the desired level of performance). For example, in a child who has problems with executive function, remediation methods could include the following: develop the child's self-awareness of his or her impairments, model the desired behavior (e.g., talking quietly to oneself to solve a problem), review tasks to be completed, use organizers, and outline materials to be learned. Compensatory strategies include providing routine, using checklists, timetables, and teaching coping strategies, such as asking the teacher to slow down or explain a topic again (Tanguay, 2002).

Strategies have been developed to improve social skills, which are as important for well-being as academic and other skills. A number of strategies that have been used include: interventions for parents (Duke et al. 1996), social skills curriculum (McAfee 2002), in vivo coaching, social stories (comic strip conversations), didactic teaching about social skills and emotions, group-based interventions, and peer mentorship (e.g., circle of friends).

In the "circle of friends," children are put in a structured peer network with scheduled time and shared activities. There they can practice various activities together; for example, observing a movie or television show with the sound muted while they try to determine what emotions the actors are portraying. They then practice showing those emotions. They can also play games like liar's bluff, act out specific characters and practice telling jokes. These complex social interactions are broken down by their coach into more discrete activities like eye contact, tone of voice, body language, choice of words, turn-taking, transitions from subject to subject, and so on.

Many references are available to help with social skills training, including the Skill-Streaming series (McGinnis and Goldstein 2000). These books emphasize classroom survival skills, friendship-making skills, dealing with feelings, alternatives to aggression, and dealing with stress. A few case series have examined the effectiveness of these interventions (Minskoff 1980a, 1980b; Loomis et al. 1994; King 1997; Barnhill 2002). However, few, if any, studies have scientifically evaluated these techniques for children who have meningomyelocele.

REFERENCES

Aksnes, G., Diseth, T. H., Helseth, A., Edwin, B., Stange, M., Aafos, G. et al. (2002). Appendicostomy for antegrade enema: effects on somatic and psychosocial functioning in children with myelomeningocele. Pediatrics, 109, 484—9.

American Academy of Pediatrics. Committee on Genetics. (1999). Folic acid for the prevention of neural tube defects. Pediatrics, 104, 325–7.

Appleton, P. L., Minchom, P. E., Ellis, N. C., Elliott, C. E., Boll, V., & Jones, P. (1994). The self-concept of young people with spina bifida: A population-based study. Dev Med Child Neurol, 36, 198–215.

Barf, H. A., Verhoef, M., Jennekens-Schinkel, A., Post, M. W., Gooskens, R. H., & Prevo, A. J. (2003). Cognitive status of young adults with spina bifida. Dev Med Child Neurol, 45(12), 813–20.

Barkovich, A. J. (2000). Pediatric Neuroimaging. 3rd Ed. Philadelphia: Lippincott Williams and Wilkins.

Barnes, M. A., & Dennis, M. (1992). Reading in children and adolescents after early onset hydrocephalus and in normally developing age peers: Phonological analysis, word recognition, word compre-

hension, and passage comprehension skills. J Pediatr Psychol, 17, 445–465.

Barnes, M. A., & Dennis, M. (1998). Discourse after early-onset hydrocephalus: core deficits in children of average intelligence. Brain Lang, 61, 309–334.

Barnes, M., Pengelly, S., Dennis, M., Wilkinson, M., Rogers, T., & Faulkner, H. (2002). Mathematics skills in good readers with hydrocephalus. J Int Neuropsychol Soc, 8, 72–82.

Barnhill, G. P. (2002). The effectiveness of social skills intervention targeting nonverbal communication for adolescents with Asperger syndrome and related pervasive developmental delays. Focus on Autism & Other Developmental Disabilities, 17, 112–118.

Berman, K., Ostrem, J., Randolph, C., Gold, J., et al. (1995). Physiological activation of a cortical network during performance of the Wisconsin Card Sorting Test: A positron emission tomography study. Neuropsychologia, 33, 1027–1046.

Berry, R. J., Li, Z., Erickson, J. D., et al. (1999). Prevention of neural-tube defects with folic acid in China. China-U.S. Collaborative Project for Neural Tube Defect Prevention. N Engl J Med, 341, 1485–90.

Bier, J. A., Morales, Y., Liebling, J., Geddes, L., & Kim, E. (1997). Medical and social factors associated with cognitive outcome in individuals with myelomeningocele. Dev Med Child Neurol 39, 263–266.

Blum, R. W., Resnick, M. D., Nelson, R., & St. Germaine, A. (1991). Family and peer issues among adolescents with spina bifida and cerebral palsy. Pediatrics, 88, 280–285.

Bomalaski, M. D., Teague, J. L., & Brooks, B. (1995). The long-term impact of urological management on the quality of life of children with spina bifida. J Urol, 154, 778–781.

Boone, D., Parsons, D., Lachman, S. M., & Sherwood, T. (1985). Spina bifida occulta: lesion or anomaly? Clin Radiol, 36, 159–61.

Bower, C., & Stanley, F. J. (1992). Periconceptional vitamin supplementation and neural tube defects: Evidence from a case-control study in Western Australia and a review of recent publications. J Epidemiol Commun Health, 46, 157–161.

Brewer, V. R., Fletcher, J. M., Hiscock, M., & Davidson, K. C. (2001). Attention processes in children with shunted hydrocephalus versus attention deficit-hyperactivity disorder. Neuropsychology, 15, 185–198.

Brookshire, B. L., Fletcher, J. M., Bohan, T. P., Landry, S. H., Davidson, K. C., & Francis, D. J. (1995). Verbal and nonverbal skill discrepancies in children with hydrocephalus: a five-year longitudinal follow-up. J Pediatr Psychol, 20, 785–800.

Casari, E. F., & Fantino, A. G. (1998). A longitudinal study of cognitive abilities and achievement status of children with myelomeningocele and their relationship with clinical types. Eur J Pediatr Surg, 8, 52–54.

Charney, E. B., Rorke, L. B., Sutton, L. N., et al. (1987). Management of Chiari II complications in infants with MM. J Pediatr, 111, 364–371.

Copp, A. J., Fleming, A., & Greene, N. D. E. (1998). Embryonic mechanisms underlying the prevention of neural tube defects. Ment Retard Dev Disabilities Res Rev, 4, 264–68.

Cull, C., & Wyke, M. A. (1984). Memory function of children with spina bifida and shunted hydrocephalus. Dev Med Child Neurol, 26, 177–183.

Dahl, M., Ahlsten, G., Carlson, H., et al. (1995). Neurological dysfunction above cele level in children with spina bifida cystica: A prospective study to three years. Dev Med Child Neurol, 37, 30–40.

Davidovitch, M., Manning-Courtney, P., Hartmann, L. A., Watson, J., Lutkenhoff, M., & Oppenheimer, S. (1999). The prevalence of attentional problems and the effect of methylphenidate in children with myelomeningocele. Pediatr Rehabil, 3, 29–35.

Davis, R., Peters, D. H., & McTavish, D. (1994). Valproic acid: A reappraisal of its pharmacological properties and clinical efficacy in epilepsy. Drugs, 47, 332–372.

Del Bigio, M. R. (1993). Neuropathological changes caused by hydrocephalus. Acta Neuropathol, 85, 573–585.

Dennis, M., & Barnes, M. (1993). Oral discourse skills in children and adolescents after early-onset hydrocephalus: Linguistic ambiguity, figurative language, speech acts, and script-based inferences. J Pediatr Psychol, 18, 639–652.

Dennis, M., & Barnes, M. (2002). Math and numeracy in young adults with spina bifida and hydrocephalus. Dev Neuropsychol, 21(2), 141–155.

Dennis, M., Jacennik, B., & Barnes, M. (1994). The content of narrative discourse in children and adolescents after early-onset hydrocephalus and in normally-developing age peers. Brain Lang, 46, 129–165.

Diamond, D. A., Rickwood, A. M., & Thomas, D.G. (1986). Penile erections in myelomeningocele patients. Br J Urol, 58, 434–5.

Dias, M. S., & Pang, D. (1995). Split cord malformations. Neurosurg Clin North Am, 6, 339–358.

Dik, P., Van Gool, J. D., & De Jong, T. P. (1999). Urinary continence and erectile function after bladder neck sling suspension in male patients with spinal dysraphism. Br J Urol Int, 83, 971–5.

Dise, J. E., & Lohr, M. E. (1998). Examination of deficits in conceptual reasoning abilities associated with spina bifida. Am J Phys Med Rehabil, 77, 247–251.

Dormans, J. P., Templeton, J., Schreiner, M. S., et al. (1995). Intraoperative latex anaphylaxis in children: Early detection, treatment, and prevention. Contemp Orthop, 30, 342–347.

Duke, M. P., Martin, E. A., & Nowicki, S. Jr (1996). Teaching Your Child the Language of Social Success. Atlanta, GA: Peachtree.

Elias, E. R., & Sadeghi-Nejad, A. (1994). Precocious puberty in girls with myelodysplasia. Pediatrics, 93, 521–522.

Ellsworth, P. I., Merguerian, P. A., Klein, R. B., et al. (1993). Evaluation and risk factors of latex allergy in spina bifida patients: Is it preventable? J Urol, 150, 691–693.

Fidas, A., MacDonald, H. L., Elton, R. A., Wild, S. R., Chisholm, G. D., & Scott, R. (1987). Prevalence and patterns of spina bifida occulta in 2707 normal adults. Clin Radiol, 38, 537–42.

Fiore, P., Picco, P., Castagnola, E., Palmieri, A., Levato, L., Gremmo, M., Tramalloni, R., & Cama, A. (1998). Nutritional survey of children and adolescents with myelomeningocele (MMC): overweight associated with reduced energy intake. Eur J Pediatr Surg, 8, 34–6

Fletcher, J. M., Barnes, M., & Dennis, M. (2002). Language development in children with spina bifida. Semin Pediatr Neurol, 9, 201–208.

Fletcher, J. M., Bohan, T. P., Brandt, M. E., et al. (1992a). Cerebral white matter and cognition in hydrocephalic children. Arch Neurol, 49, 818–824.

Fletcher, J. M., Francis, D. J., Thompson, N. M., et al (1992b). Verbal and nonverbal skill discrepancies in hydrocephalic children. J Clin Exp Neuropsychol, 14:593–609.

Fletcher, J. M., McCauley, S. R., Brandt, M. E., Bohan, T. P., Kramer, L. A., Francis, D. J., Thorstad, K., et al., (1996). Regional brain tissue composition in children with hydrocephalus. Relationships with cognitive development. Arch Neurol, 53, 549–557.

Foltz, E., & Shurtleff, D. (1963). Five-year comparative study of hydrocephalus in children with and without operations (113 cases). J Neurosurg, 20, 1064–1079.

Forrester, M. B., & Merz, R. D. (2000). Prenatal Diagnosis and Elective Termination of Neural Tube Defects in Hawaii, 1986–1997. Fetal Diagn Ther, 15, 146–151.

Fowler, M. G., Johnson, M. P., & Atkinson, S. S. (1985). School achievement and absence in children with chronic health conditions. J Pediatr, 106, 683–687.

Friedrich, W. N., Lovejoy, M. C., Shaffer, J., Shurtleff, D. B., & Beilke, R. L. (1991). Cognitive abilities and achievement status of children with myelomeningocele: a contemporary sample. J Pediatr Psychol, 16, 23–428.

Game, X., Villers, A., Malavaud, B., & Sarramon, J. (1999). Bladder cancer arising in a spina bifida patient. Urology (Online), 54, 923.

Gao, J. H., Parsons, L. M., Bower, J. M., Xiong, J., Li, J., & Fox, P. T. (1996). Cerebellum implicated in sensory acquisition and discrimination rather than motor control. Science, 272, 545–547.

Gebhart, A. L., Petersen, S. E., & Thach, W. T. (2002). Role of the posterolateral cerebellum in language. Ann NY Acad Sci, 978, 318–333.

Gilbert, J. N., Jones, K. L., Rorke, L. B., et al. (1986). Central nervous system anomalies associated with meningomyelocele, hydrocephalus, and the Arnold-Chiari malformation: Reappraisal of theories regarding the pathogenesis of posterior neural tube closure defects. Neurosurgery, 18, 559–564.

Golden, J., & Chernoff, G. F. (1995). Multiple sites of anterior neural tube closure in humans: Evidence from anterior neural tube defects (anencephaly). Pediatrics, 95, 506–510.

Greene, S. A., Frank, M., Zachmann, M., & Prader, A. (1985). Growth and sexual development in children with meningomyelocele. Eur J Pediatr, 144, 146–148.

Griebel, M. L., Oakes, W. J., & Worley, G. (1991). The Chiari malformation associated with meningomyelocele. In H. L. Rekate (ed.), Comprehensive Management of Spina Bifida (pp. 67–92). Boca Raton, FL: CRC Press.

Gross, S. M., Caufield, L. A., Kinsman, S. L., & Ireys, H. T. (2001). Inadequate folic acid intakes are prevalent among young women with neural tube defects. J Am Diet Assoc, 101, 342–5.

Guidera, K. J., Smith, S., Raney, E., et al. (1993). Use of the reciprocating gait orthosis in myelodysplasia. J Pediatr Orthogr, 13, 341–348.

Hall, J. G., Friedman, J. M., Kenna, B. A., et al. (1988). Clinical, genetic, and epidemiological factors in neural tube defects. Am J Hum Genet, 43, 827–37.

Hall, J. G., & Solehdin, F. (1998). Genetics of neural tube defects. Ment Retard Dev Disab Res Rev, 4, 269–81.

Hannay, H. J., Fletcher, J. M., & Brandt, M. (1999). Role of the corpus callosum in the cognitive development of children with congenital brain malformations. In S. H. Broman, & J. M. Fletcher (eds.). The Changing Nervous System: Neurobehavioral Consequences of Early Brain Disorders. New York: Oxford University Press, 149–171.

Holler, K. A., Fennell, E. B., Crosson, B., Boggs, S. R., & Mickle, J. P. (1995). Neuropsychological and adaptive functioning in younger versus older children shunted for early hydrocephalus. Child Neuropsychol, 1, 63–73.

Holmbeck, G. N., Westhoven, V. C., Phillips, W. S., Bowers, R., Gruse, C., Nikolopoulos, T., Totura, C. M., & Davison, K. (2003). A multimethod, multi-informant, and multidimensional perspective on psychosocial adjustment in preadolescents with spina bifida. J Consult Clin Psychol, 71, 782–96.

Hommet, C., Billiard, C., Gillet, P., Barthez, M., Lourmiere, J., Santini, J. J., de Toffol, B., Corcia, P., & Autret, A. (1999). Neuropsychologic and adaptive functioning in adolescents and young adults shunted for congenital hydrocephalus. J Child Neurol, 14, 144–150.

Hulton, S. A., Thomson, P. D., Milner, L. S., et al. (1990). The pattern of congenital renal anomalies associated with neural tube defects. Pediatr Nephrol 4, 491–2.

Hunt, G. M., Oakeshott, P., & Kerry, S. (1999). Link between the CSF shunt and achievement in adults with spina bifida. J Neurol Neurosurg Psychiatry, 67, 591–595.

Hurley, A. D., & Bell, S. (1994). Educational and vocational outcome of adults with spina bifida in relationship to neuropsychological testing. Eur J Pediatr Surg, 4, 17–8.

Hurley, A. D., Dorman, C., Laatsch, L., Bell, S., & D'Avignon, J. (1990). Cognitive functioning in patients with spina bifida, hydrocephalus, and the "cocktail party" syndrome. Dev Neuropsychol, 6, 151–172.

Hurley, A. D., Laatsch, L. K., & Dorman, C. (1983). Comparison of spina bifida, hydrocephalic patients and matched controls on neuropsychological tests. Z.Kinderchir, 38, 116–118.

Jacobs, R., Northam, E., & Anderson, V. (2001). Cognitive outcome in children with myelomeningocele and perinatal hydrocephalus: A longitudinal perspective. J Dev Physical Disabil, 13, 389–405.

Juriloff, D. M., & Harris, M. J. (2000). Mouse models for neural tube closure defects. Hum Mol Genet, 9, 993–1000.

Juriloff, D. M., & Harris, M. J. (1998). Animal models of neural tube defects. Ment Retardation and Developmental Disabilities Research Reviews, 4, 254–63.

Kalucy, M., Bower, C., & Stanley, F. (1996). School-aged children with spina bifida in western Australia: Parental perspectives on functional outcome. Dev Med Child Neurol, 38, 325–334.

Kanev, P. M., & Sheehan, J. M. (2003). Reflections on shunt infection. Pediatr Neurosurg., 39, 285–90.

Kawamura, T., Morioka, T., Nishio, S., Mihara, F., & Fukui, M. (2001). Cerebral abnormalities in lumbosacral neural tube closure defect: MR imaging evaluation. Childs Nerv Syst, 17, 405–410.

Kawamura, T., Nishio, S., Morioka, T., & Fukui, K. (2002). Callosal anomalies in patients with spinal dysraphism: correlation of clinical and neuroimaging features with hemispheric abnormalities. Neurol Res, 24, 463–467.

Kazak, A. E., & Clark, M. W. (1986). Stress in families of children with myelomeningocele. Dev Med Child Neurol, 28, 220–8.

King, G. A. (1997). Social skills training for withdrawn unpopular children with physical disabilities: A preliminary evaluation. Rehab Psychol, 42, 47–60.

King, G. A., Shultz, I. Z., Steel, K., Gilpin, M., & Cathers, T. (1993). Self-evaluation and self-concept of adolescents with physical disabilities. Am J Occup Ther, 47, 132–40.

Kirk, V. G., Morielli, A., & Brouillette, R. T. (1999). Sleep-disordered breathing in patients with myelomeningocele: the missed diagnosis. Dev Med Child Neurol, 41, 40–3.

Kirk, V. G., Morielli, A., Gozal, D., et al. (2000). Treatment of sleep-disordered breathing in children with myelomeningocele. Pediatr Pulmonol, 30, 445–52.

Laurence, K. M., & Coates, S. (1962). The natural history of hydrocephalus. Arch Dis Child 37:345–362.

Leiner, H. C., Leiner, A. L., & Dow, R. S. (1991). The human cerebro-cerebellar system: its computing, cognitive, and language skills. Behav Brain Res, 44, 113–128.

Lennerstrand, G., Gallo, J.E., & Samuelsson, L. (1990). Neuro-ophthalmological findings in relation to CNS lesions in patients with myelomeningocele. Dev Med Child Neurol, 32, 423–431.

Levisohn, L., Cronin-Golomb, A., & Schmahmann, JD. (2000). Neuropsychological consequences of cerebellar tumour resection in children: cerebellar cognitive affective syndrome in a paediatric population. Brain, 123, 1041–50.

Liptak, G. S., Shurtleff, D. B., Bloss, J. W., et al. (1992). Mobility aids in children with high-level meningomyelocele: Parapodium versus wheelchair. Dev Med Child Neurol, 34, 787–796.

Littlewood, R. A., Trocki, O., Shepherd, R. W., Shepherd, K., & Davies, P. S. (2003). Resting energy expenditure and body composition in children with myelomeningocele. Pediatr Rehabil, 6, 31–7.

Loomis, J. W., Lindsey, A., Javornisky, J. G., & Monahan, J. J. (1994). Measures of cognition and adaptive behavior as predictors of adjustment outcomes in young adults with spina bifida. Eur J Pediatr Surg, 4, 35–36.

Loss, N., Yeates, K. O., & Enrile B. (1996). Attention in children with myelomeningocele (abstract). Clin Neuropsychol, 10, 347.

MacBriar, B. R. (1983). Self-concept of preadolescent and adolescent children with a meningomyelocele. Issues Compr Pediatr Nurs, 6, 1.

Mahone, E. M., Zabel, T. A., Levey, E., Verda, M., & Kinsman, S. (2002). Parent and self-report rating of executive function in adolescents with myelomeningocele and hydrocephalus. Child Neuropsychol, 8, 258–270.

Manning, S. M., Jennings, R., & Madsen, J. R. (2000). Pathophysiology, prevention and potential treatment of neural tube defects. Ment Retard Dev Disabil Res Rev, 6, 6–14.

Mazon, A., Nieto, A., Linana, J. J., Montoro, J., Estornell, F., & Garcia-Ibarra, F. (2000). Latex sensitization in children with spina bifida: follow-up comparative study after two years. Ann Allergy Asthma Immunol, 84, 207–10.

Mazur, J. M., Aylward, G. P., Colliver, J., Stacey, J., Menelaus, M. (1988). Impaired mental capabilities and hand function in myelomeningocele patients. Z Kinderchir, 43, 24–27.

Mazur, J. M., Shurtleff, D., Menelaus, M., Colliver, J. (1989). Orthopaedic management of high-level spina bifida. Early walking compared with early use of a wheelchair. J Bone Joint Surg Am., 71, 56–61.

McAfee, J. (2002). *Navigating the Social World: A Curriculum for Individuals with Asperger's Syndrome, High Functioning Autism and Related Disorders.* Arlington, TX: Future Horizons.

McDonald, C. M. (1995). Rehabilitation of children with spinal dysraphism. Neurosurg Clin North Am, 6, 393.

McGinnis, E. & Goldstein, A. P. (2000). *Skillstreaming the Elementary School Child. New Strategies and Perspectives for Teaching Prosocial Skills.* Champaign, IL: Research Press. Classroom Survival Skills, Friendship-Making Skills, Dealing with Feelings, Alternatives to Aggression, and Dealing with Stress.

McLone, D. G. (1992). Continuing concepts in the management of spina bifida. Pediatr Neurosurg, 18, 254–256.

Meyer, S. & Landau, H. (1984). Precocious puberty in myelomeningocele patients. J Pediatr Orthop, 4, 28–31.

Middleton, F. A., & Strick, P. L. (1994) Anatomical evidence for cerebellar and basal ganglia involvement in higher cognitive function. Science, 266, 458–461

Minskoff, E. (1980a). Teaching approach for developing nonverbal communication skills in students with social perception deficits, Part 1: The basic approach and body language cues. J Learning Disabil, 13, 118–124.

Minskoff, E. (1980b). Teaching approach for developing nonverbal communication skills in students with social perception deficits, Part 2: Proxemic, vocalic, and artifactual cues. J Learning Disabil, 13, 203–208.

Mobley, C. E., Harless, L. S., & Miller, K. L. (1996). Self-perceptions of preschool children with spina bifida. J Pediatr Nurs, 11, 217–224.

Moore, C., Kogan, B. A., & Parekh, A. (2004). Impact of urinary incontinence on self-concept in children with spina bifida. J Urol, 171, 1659–62.

Muller, T., Arbeiter, K., & Aufricht, C. (2002). Renal function in meningomyelocele: risk factors, chronic renal failure, renal replacement therapy and transplantation. Curr Opin Urol, 12, 479–84.

Murch, R. L. & Cohen, L. H. (1989). Relationships among life stress, perceived family environment, and the psychological distress of spina bifida adolescents. J Pediatr Psychol, 14, 193–214.

Myklebust, H. R. (1975). Nonverbal learning disabilities: Assessment and intervention. In H. R. Myklebust (ed.), *Progress in Learning Disabilities* (pp. 85–121). New York: Grune & Stratton.

Nagahama, Y., Fuykuyama, H., Yamauchi, H., Matsuzaki, S., et al. (1996) Cerebral activation during performance of a card sorting test. Brain, 119, 1667–1775.

NICHD, Management of Myelomeningocele Study (MOMS). Available at: http://www.clinicaltrials.gov/show/NCT00060606. Retrieved March 9, 2004.

Noetzel, M. J. (1989). Meningomyelocele: Current concepts of management. Clin Perinatol, 16, 311–329.

Olney, R., & Mulinare, J. (1998). Epidemiology of neural tube defects. Ment Retard Dev Disabil Res Rev, 4, 241–46.

Pearson, A. M., Carr, J., & Hallwell, M. D. (1988). The handwriting of children with spina bifida. Z Kinderchir, 43, 40–42.

Pearson, M. L., Cole, J. S., & Jarvis, W. R. (1994). How common is latex allergy? A survey of children with myelodysplasia. Dev Med Child Neurol, 36, 64–69.

Perrone, L., De Gaizo, D., D'Angelo, E., Rea, L., Di Manso, G., Del Gado, R. (1994) Endocrine studies in children with myelomeningocele. J Pediatr Endocrinol, 7, 219–23.

Peterson, C., Maier, S. F., & Seligman, M. (1993). Learned helplessness: a theory for the age of personal control. New York: Oxford University Press.

Phuong, L. K., Schoeberl, K. A., & Raffel, C. (2002). Natural history of tethered cord in patients with meningomyelocele. Neurosurgery, 50, 989–93.

Polito, C., DelGaizo, G., DiManso, D., et al. (1995). Children with myelomeningocele have shorter stature, greater body weight, and lower bone mineral content than healthy children. Nutr Res, 15, 161–162.

Proos, L. A., Dhal, M., Ahlsten, G., Tuvemo, T., & Gustafsson, J. (1996) Increased perinatal intracranial pressure and prediction of early puberty in girls with myelomeningocele. Arch Dis Child, 75, 42–45.

Ralph, K., Moylan, P., Canady, A., & Simmons, S. (2000). The effects of multiple shunt revisions on neuropsychological functioning and memory. Neurol Res, 22, 131–136.

Rauzzino, M., & Oakes, W. J. (1995). Chiari II malformation and syringomyelia. Neurosurg Clin North Am, 6, 293–309.

Riva, D., & Giorgi, C. (2000). The cerebellum contributes to higher functions during development: evidence from a series of children surgically treated for posterior fossa tumours. Brain, 123, 1051–1061.

Roberts, H. E., Moore, C. A., Cragan, J. D., et al. (1995). Impact of prenatal diagnosis on the birth prevalence of neural tube defects, Atlanta, 1990–1991. Pediatrics, 96, 880–883.

Roland, E. H., & Hill, A. (2003). Germinal matrix-intraventricular hemorrhage in the premature newborn: management and outcome. Neurol Clin, 21, 833–51.

Rosenthal, A., Joulet, M., & Kenwrick, S. (1992). Aberrant splicing of neural cell adhesion molecule L1 mRNA in a family with X-linked hydrocephalus. Nature Genet, 2, 107–112.

Rotenstein, D., & Bass, A.N. (2004). Treatment to near adult stature of patients with myelomeningocele with recombinant human growth hormone. J Pediatr Endocrinol Metab, 17, 1195—1200.

Rotenstein, D., & Breen, T. J. (1996). Growth hormone treatment of children with myelomeningocele. J Pediatr, 128, S28–31.

Rourke, B. P. (1989). *Nonverbal Learning Disabilities: The Syndrome and the Model*. New York: Guilford.

Rourke, B. P., Ahmad, S. A., Collins, D. W., Hayman-Abello, B. A., Hayman-Abello, S. E., & Warriner, E. M. (2002). Child clinical/pediatric neuropsychology: some recent advances. Annu Rev Psychol, 53, 309–339.

Rowley-Kelly, F. L., & Reigel, D. H. (eds.). (1993). *Teaching the Student With Spina Bifida*. Baltimore: Paul H Brookes.

Russel, C. L. (2004). Understanding nonverbal learning disorders in children with spina bifida. Teaching Exceptional Children, 36, 8–13.

Sadler, L. S., Robinson, L. K., & Msall, M. E. (1995). Diabetic embryopathy: Possible pathogenesis. Am J Med Genet, 55, 363–366.

Sandford, M. K., Kissling, G. E., & Joubert, P. E. (1992). Neural tube defect etiology: new evidence concerning maternal hyperthermia, health and diet. Dev Med Child Neurol, 34, 661–75.

Sandler, A. D., Worley, G., Leroy, E. C., Stanley, S. D., & Kalman, S. (1996). Sexual function and erection capability among young men with spina bifida. Dev Med Child Neurol, 38, 823–829.

Schader, I., & Corwin, P. (1999). How many pregnant women in Christchurch are using folic acid supplements in early pregnancy? N Z Med J, 112, 463–5.

Schmahmann, J. D. (1998) Dysmetria of thought: clinical consequences of cerebellar dysfunction on cognition and affect. Trends Cogn Sci, 25, 362–371.

Scott, M. A., Fletcher, J. M., Brookshire, B. L., Davidson, K. C., Landry, S. H., Bohan, T. C., & Kramer, L. A., et al. (2003). Memory functions in children with early hydrocephalus. Neuropsychology, 4, 578–589.

Shaffer, J., Friedrich, W. N., Shurtleff, D. B., & Wolf, L. (1985). Cognitive and achievement status of children with myelomeningocele. J Pediatr Psychol, 10, 325–336.

Shaw, G. M., Quach, T., Nelson, V., Carmichael, S. L., Schaffer, D. M., Selvin, S., & Yang W. (2003). Neural tube defects associated with maternal periconceptional dietary intake of simple sugars and glycemic index. Am J Clin Nutr, 78, 972–8.

Shaw, G. M., Todoroff, K., Finnell, R. H., & Lammer, E. J. (2000). Spina bifida phenotypes in infants or fetuses of obese mothers. Teratology, 61, 376–381.

Shaw, J., & Lewis, M. A. (1999). Bladder augmentation surgery - what about the malignant risk? Eur J Pediatr Surg, 9, 39–40.

Shurtleff, D. B., Foltz, E., & Loeser, J. (1973). Hydrocephalus: a definition of its progression and relationship to intellectual function diagnosis, and complications. Am J Dis Child, 125, 688–693.

Talwar, D., Baldwin, M. A., & Horbatt, C. I. (1995). Epilepsy in children with meningomyelocele. Pediatr Neurol, 13, 29–32.

Tanguay, P. B. (2002). *Nonverbal Learning Disabilities at School: Educating Students with NLD, Asperger Syndrome, and Related Conditions*. London: Jessica Kingsley Publishers.

Tew, B. J. (1979). The "cocktail party syndrome" in children with hydrocephalus and spina bifida. Br J Disord Commun, 14, 89–101.

Tew, B. J., & Laurence, K. M. (1979). The clinical and psychological characteristics of children with "cocktail party" syndrome. Zeitschrift für Kinderchirurgie, 28, 360–367.

Tew, B. J., & Laurence, K. M. (1984). The relationship between intelligence and academic achievements in spina bifida adolescents. Z Kinderchir, 39, 122–124.

Tubbs, R. S., Chambers, M. R., Smyth, M. D., Bartolucci, A. A., Bruner, J. P., Tulipan, N., & Oakes, W. J. (2003). Late gestational intrauterine myelomeningocele repair does not improve lower extremity function. Pediatr Neurosurg, 38, 128–32.

Tulipan, N., Sutton, L. N., Bruner, J. P., Cohen, B. M., Johnson, M., & Adzick, N. S. (2003). The effect of intrauterine myelomeningocele repair on the incidence of shunt-dependent hydrocephalus. Pediatr Neurosurg, 38, 27–33.

Urui, S., & Oi, S. (1995). Experimental study of embryogenesis of open spinal dysraphism. Neurosurg Clin North Am, 6, 195–202.

Van Allen, M. I., Kalousek, D. K., Chernoff, G. F., et al. (1993). Evidence for multi-site closure of the neural tube in humans. Am J Med Genet, 47, 723–743.

Van Mier, H. I., & Petersen, S. E. (2002). Role of the cerebellum in motor cognition. Ann NY Acad Sci, 978, 334–53.

Volcik, K. A., Shaw, G. M., Zhu, H., Lammer, E. J., & Finnell, R. H. (2003). Risk factors for neural tube defects: associations between uncoupling protein 2 polymorphisms and spina bifida. Birth Defects Res Part A Clin Mol Teratol, 67, 158–61.

Volpe, J. L. (1989). Intraventricular hemorrhage in the premature infant-current concepts, Part I. Ann Neurol, 25, 3–11.

von Koch, C. S., Gupta, N., Sutton, L. N., & Sun, P. P. (2003). In utero surgery for hydrocephalus. Child's Nerv Syst, 19, 574–86.

Wasson, C. M., Bannister, C. M., & Ward, G. S. (1992). Factors affecting the school placement of children with spina bifida. Eur J Pediatr Surg, 2, 29–34.

Weller, S., & Gartner, J. (2001). Genetic and clinical aspects of X-linked hydrocephalus (L1 disease): mutations in the L1CAM gene. Hum Mutat, 18, 1–12.

Werler, M. M., Shapiro, S., & Mitchell, A. A. (1993). Periconceptional folic acid exposure and risk of occurrent neural tube defects. JAMA, 269, 1257–1261.

Whitelaw, A., Pople, I., Cherian, S., Evans, D., & Thoresen, M. (2003). Phase 1 trial of prevention of hydrocephalus after intraventricular hemorrhage in newborn infants by drainage, irrigation, and fibrinolytic therapy. Pediatrics, 111, 759–65.

Wills, K. E., Holmbeck, G., Dillon, K., et al. (1990). Intelligence and achievement in children with myelomeningocele. J Pediatr Psychol, 15, 161–176.

Yeates, K. O., Enrile, B. G., Loss, N., Blumenstein, E., & Delis, D. C. (1995). Verbal learning and memory in children with myelomeningocele. J Pediatr Psychol, 20, 801–815.

Yeates, K. O., Loss, N., Colvin, A. N., & Enrile, B. G. (2003). Do children with myelomeningocele and hydrocephalus display nonverbal learning disabilities? An empirical approach to classification. J Int Neuropsychol Soc, 9, 653–62.

Yerby, M. S. (2003). Management issues for women with epilepsy: neural tube defects and folic acid supplementation. Neurology, 61, S23–6.

Zurmohle, U. M., Homann, T., Schroeter, C., Rothgerber, H., Hommel, G., & Ermert, J. A. (1998). Psychosocial adjustment of children with spina bifida. J Child Neurol, 13, 64–70.

Pediatric Brain Tumors

David L. Kaye, MD   *Patricia K. Duffner, MD*

Brain tumors are the most common solid malignancy of childhood, second only to the leukemias in overall incidence. Most cases are diagnosed before patients are the age of 10 years, although over one third of cases are diagnosed in adolescence. The incidence of childhood and primary brain tumors both benign and malignant is 3.9 cases per 100,000 person-years. The rate is somewhat higher in males (4.2 per 100,000 person-years) than females (3.8 per 100,000 person-years). The Central Brain Tumor Registry of the United States estimated that 3,260 new cases of pediatric brain tumors would be diagnosed in 2004, more than two thirds of which are malignant (Central Brain Tumor Registry of the United States 2002). More than 26,3000 children were living with the diagnosis of a primary brain tumor in the United States in the year 2000; over 80% of these children have malignant brain tumors. The chance of survival of children with brain tumors has increased dramatically over the past 30 years. In the 1960s, a child diagnosed with a brain tumor had approximately a 15% 5-year survival rate. By 1975, 5-year survival rates approached 50%. The most recent 5-year survival rate for children diagnosed before 19 with a primary malignant brain tumor was 64% (Central Brain Tumor Registry of the United States 2002–3).

Most of the changes in survival from 1960 to 1975 were primarily due to advances in surgery, intensive care treatment, and radiation techniques. Further improvements in these areas, as well as the advent of chemotherapy for certain tumors, have led to continued increases in longevity. In addition, there has been a philosophical change in the approach to many children with brain tumors. When the anticipated survival rate was only 15%, concerns over the potential adverse longterm effects of therapy were meaningless. Now that many children will be longterm survivors, attention has been increasingly directed toward quality-of-life issues. As such, today, pediatric neurologists, oncologists, radiation therapists, neurosurgeons, neuropathologists, pediatricians, psychologists, psychiatrists, and endocrinologists are all an integral part of the team approach to the child with a central nervous system (CNS) malignancy.

CLASSIFICATION OF BRAIN TUMORS

The classification of brain tumors has evolved throughout this century. Currently, the most widely accepted classification is that of the World Health Organization (WHO) (Kleihues et al. 2002). It is a complicated schema that is based primarily on cell type (e.g., astrocytes, embryonal cells, oligodendroglia, ependymal, mixed), with multiple variants based on histological features. The most common types of brain tumors in children are astrocytoma, medulloblastoma, ependymoma, brainstem glioma, and craniopharyngioma (Table 26.1). Glioma is a general term referring to any neoplasm deriving from interstitial tissue cells of the nervous system (e.g. astrocytes, ependymal cells, oligodendrocytes). As such, ependymomas would be a type of glioma. Glioblastoma multiforme, a particularly devastating tumor, is synonymous with grade IV astrocytoma. While most adult brain tumors are metastatic and supratentorial, pediatric brain tumors are typically primary and more varied in location. Often, the literature will refer to the grading of the tumor based on the degree of anaplasia (i.e., "low grade" vs. "high grade," or grades 1 to 4, with 4 being most anaplastic). Location may also be specified. For example, astrocytomas can originate in the cerebral hemispheres, brainstem, or cerebellum. Although medulloblastomas almost always are located in the cerebellum, histologically similar tumors are occasionally seen in other locations. To describe these latter tumors, it has been proposed by some that medulloblastomas and other histologically similar tumors be referred to as primitive neuroectodermal tumors (Dehner 1986; Fung and Trojanowski 1995; Yachnis 1997). However, the most recent WHO classification distinguishes medulloblastoma from supratentorial primitive neuroectodermal tumors.

TABLE 26.1

INCIDENCE AND 5-YEAR, 10-YEAR SURVIVAL RATES FOR SELECTED PEDIATRIC (0-19) BRAIN TUMORS

Tumor Type	Incidence (as % of all PBT's)	5-yr Survival	10-yr Survival
Pilocytic astrocytoma	26	95	92
Embryonal/medulloblastoma	20	55	48
Astrocytoma, NOS	8	77	73
Ependymoma	8	55	47
Glioblastoma	4	19	16
Craniopharyngioma*	4	90+	85
Anaplastic astrocytoma	3	52	47
TOTAL	100	64	60

Source: Central Brain Tumor Registry of the United States 2004-2005
*Van Effenterre R, Bach AL (2002)

PRESENTING SIGNS AND SYMPTOMS

Neuropsychiatric symptoms rarely bring the child with an unsuspected brain tumor to a psychiatrist as the first medical contact. The child with symptoms of brain tumor much more commonly will present with either nonlocalizing signs and symptoms reflecting increased intracranial pressure, or localizing signs reflecting either compression or infiltration of surrounding brain. Typically, the parents report coincident personality and/or cognitive deterioration. Diagnosis is commonly delayed for a number of months after parents note presenting symptoms. Three studies have documented that the mean time to diagnosis of a pediatric brain tumor is 20 to 28 weeks (Flores et al. 1986; Edgeworth et al. 1996; Mehta et al. 2002) with infratentorial tumors being recognized earlier than supratentorial ones.

Nonlocalizing Neurological Symptoms

Symptoms associated with increased intracranial pressure are headache, nausea and vomiting, and personality change (Child Brain Tumor Consortium, Keene 1999, Mehta 2002). Nearly 80% of children with a brain tumor will present with headache or nausea/vomiting; typically all three symptoms appear together. Unlike children with migraine, in whom there is a crescendo/decrescendo pattern to the headaches with symptom-free intervals, the child with a brain tumor will frequently complain of a steady increase in both the frequency and the intensity of the headaches over time. The exception to this is the very young child with a brain tumor. The typical history is of a 2- or 3-year-old child who repeatedly wakes in the morning with severe headache and vomiting. The pediatrician may suggest that this is due to a flulike syndrome and that the child should be observed. Indeed, the symptoms are evanescent and resolve after 1 or 2 weeks. Unfortunately, several weeks later the symptoms recur with increased intensity, and the diagnosis of an intracranial mass lesion is made. This biphasic pattern reflects the ability of the

young child's skull to expand to accommodate the increasing intracranial pressure. The ability of the sutures of the skull to separate occurs in young children but is not often seen after the age of 5 years.

Warning headache symptoms, according to Medina et al. (1997, 2003), that should raise the index of suspicion of a mass lesion are those that:

1. wake the child from sleep or occur first thing in the morning;
2. are associated with confusion, disorientation, or abnormal neurological findings;
3. are consistently focal in location;
4. increase with Valsalva maneuvers;
5. less than 6 months' duration that do not respond to medical treatment;
6. are associated with nausea and vomiting, especially if family history is negative for migraine.

Nausea and vomiting are also important symptoms of the child with a brain tumor. The vomiting either tends to occur secondary to increased intracranial pressure or may reflect direct involvement of the floor of the fourth ventricle. Projectile vomiting is relatively uncommon.

Personality change and worsened school performance are sensitive indicators of structural CNS disease and occur with tumors in all locations. Lethargy, apathy, irritability, or depression are commonly reported. At times, these symptoms may be the first sign of a mass lesion (see subsequent discussion).

Nonlocalizing Neurological Signs

Nonlocalizing signs of increased intracranial pressure include papilledema, sixth nerve palsy, and an expanding head circumference. Although it is often difficult to evaluate the young child's optic fundus, such evaluation is an essential part of the examination of the child who presents with headache. Papilledema is associated with normal visual acuity, but longstanding papilledema will lead to optic atrophy and a consequent decline in vision. At times, papilledema must be differentiated from papillitis. The child with papillitis will have visual loss and a central scotoma, whereas the child with papilledema will have normal central vision but an enlarged blind spot.

Diplopia in children with brain tumors is usually secondary to an abducens nerve palsy. Cranial nerve VI has a very long free intracranial course. Therefore, when a mass lesion increases the intracranial contents of the brain, cranial nerve VI may be compressed against various bony prominences, with the pressure causing a paralysis of abduction. This is a nonlocalizing sign and does not necessarily suggest the true location of the tumor. Diplopia may also occur in children with palsies of cranial nerve III and cranial nerve IV, but these occur less frequently.

The young child will rarely complain of double vision. If the child enters the office closing one eye or turning the head, the physician must be suspicious that diplopia is present. As the image moves into the involved field, the images will separate. The child will close one eye to eliminate the double image or will turn the head such that the nose will obscure the image of the other eye.

Localizing Neurological Signs and Symptoms

Other than the nonspecific signs of increased intracranial pressure, children with brain tumors will present with signs and symptoms referable to the location of the mass lesion (i.e., cerebral hemispheres, midline, and posterior fossa).

Cerebral Hemispheric Location

The most common supratentorial hemispheric tumors are astrocytomas, anaplastic astrocytomas, and glioblastoma multiforme. Other tumors occurring in this region include oligodendrogliomas, meningiomas, and cerebral primitive neuroectodermal tumors. Children with hemispheric tumors typically present late with increased intracranial pressure, because pressure symptoms tend to occur secondary to tumor bulk rather than to obstruction of cerebrospinal fluid (CSF) pathways. Localizing signs and symptoms of tumors in this location include headache, seizures, hemiparesis, hemisensory loss, and hemianopsia. When present, a focal headache is highly correlated with tumor localization, although generalized headaches are more common.

Supratentorial tumors are often epileptogenic in nature. Seizures tend to occur more frequently with slower-growing tumors such as oligodendrogliomas and low-grade astrocytomas than with higher-grade tumors such as glioblastoma multiforme. In those cases of children with seizures in whom an initial evaluation has been negative for a mass lesion, if after several years there is a change in the frequency or the quality of the seizures, a change on electroencephalogram (EEG) pattern from spike to slow wave, or a change in neurological examination and/or change in behavior or school performance, the child must

be reevaluated. A previously unrecognized hamartoma may have dedifferentiated into a malignant lesion. It should be emphasized, however, that most children with seizures do not have an underlying malignancy.

Other signs of hemispheric mass lesions further reflect the site of involvement (e.g., hemiparesis, hemisensory loss, and/or hemianopsias). Hemipareses in this context are usually more subtle than those occurring following a stroke; a drift of the arm, a pronator sign, or a slight dragging of the leg may be all that is identified on careful neurological examination. Indeed, one of the most striking characteristics of some children with large supratentorial mass lesions is the relative lack of symptoms.

Midline Location

Midline tumors include optic pathway and hypothalamic tumors (typically pilocytic astrocytomas), as well as craniopharyngiomas and pineal region tumors. This latter group ranges from the highly malignant pineoblastoma to the radiosensitive and chemosensitive germinoma. Children whose tumors involve the optic pathway present with visual loss, visual field abnormalities, or, in the case of tumor involving the optic chiasm, nystagmus. The last-mentioned symptom may at times be confused with congenital nystagmus or spasmus nutans. Hypothalamic and pituitary involvement may produce a variety of endocrinopathies, including precocious or delayed puberty, diabetes insipidus, hypothyroidism, weight loss or gain, and growth failure. Children with tumors in the pineal region typically present with increased intracranial pressure, as well as Parinaud's sign (i.e., failure of upward gaze and disorders of accommodation and convergence secondary to compression of the quadrigeminal plate). Precocious puberty may occur in boys who have tumors in this location.

Posterior Fossa Location

Posterior fossa tumors include medulloblastomas, cerebellar astrocytomas, ependymomas, and brainstem gliomas. Most children with posterior fossa tumors present early with signs and symptoms of increased intracranial pressure due to obstruction of the aqueduct of Sylvius or the fourth ventricle. In addition, children with cerebellar tumors present with disorders of coordination that vary in character depending on location of the tumor. Children whose tumors are located in the midline of the cerebellum (vermis) present with truncal ataxia, whereas those children whose tumors are located more laterally in the cerebellar hemispheres present with dysmetria and dysdiadochokinesia. Nystagmus reflects brain-stem involvement. Other cerebellar signs include scanning speech, hypotonia, pendular reflexes, and skew deviation of the eyes.

Children with brain-stem tumors have ataxia, corticospinal tract signs, and cranial neuropathies, but increased intracranial pressure occurs either late or not at all. For example, depending on the location of the mass in the brain stem, the child may have an ipsilateral palsy of cranial nerve VI or cranial nerve VII with ataxia and contralateral hemiparesis. Lesions of the lower brain stem tend to be associated with hypernasal speech, difficulty with swallowing, and dysarthria. Increased tone in the lower extremities with hyperactive reflexes and extensor plantar responses is commonly seen in children with pontine and medullary lesions. Personality changes are also typical.

Neuropsychiatric Symptoms as Presenting Signs of Brain Tumors in Children

Despite the critical clinical importance of the pattern of presenting symptoms, research data on this question are limited. Psychiatrists especially would like to know how often children with brain tumors present with neuropsychiatric signs and symptoms only and a normal neurological history and examination. Furthermore, what patterns of symptoms are most likely suggestive of a brain tumor?

In one of the few studies, Keschner and coworkers (1938) reviewed 530 cases of brain tumors in adults and noted that an early clinical indication of a tumor was a neuropsychiatric symptom in 18% of their patients with supratentorial tumors and in 5% with infratentorial tumors. A more recent study (Zaki et al. 1993) reviewed the presenting symptoms in 1,111 cases (mostly adults) with primary brain tumors. A "mental defect" was the sole presenting sign in 8% of the patients, and, overall, 19% of the patients had a normal neurological examination on presentation.

In the pediatric literature, Flores and coworkers (1986) reviewed the records of 79 children with primary brain tumors. In their series, 9% of the patients presented with a single symptom (including headache, vomiting, weight loss, or mood or behavioral changes) and normal neurological findings. No further description of the neuropsychiatric status was offered. The remainder of the patients had signs and symptoms of increased intracranial pressure or focal neurological deficits. Edgeworth and colleagues (1996) reviewed in more detail the presentations of 74 children with primary tumors. Although vomiting (65%) and headache (64%) were the most common presenting symptoms, neuropsychiatric symptoms were also common (52%), as was deterioration in school function (20%). It was not clear how frequently neuropsychiatric or neurocognitive symptoms were the sole presenting complaint, although on initial consultation the symptoms of 17% of the children were thought to have a psychological etiology. Keene (1999) reported that more than 50% of their series of 74 pediatric brain tumor patients exhibited behavioral changes. Mehta (2002) found that, in their Canadian series of 104 pediatric patients, 66% had nausea/vomiting, 63% headaches, and 50% had behavioral changes at presentation. Nearly 80% of their series presented with either headaches, nausea, or vomiting. Only one had behavioral changes as their sole presenting finding without other symptoms or neurological signs This was a case presenting as anorexia nervosa but without the body image distortion and fear of gaining weight so characteristically seen, much like the case series reported by Chipkevitch (1994).

Taken together, this literature would suggest that a significant but very small minority of patients present with broad neuropsychiatric symptoms and no other neurological findings.

The types of symptoms and psychopathology reported in association with brain tumors in children range widely. Although there are no large studies of the incidence of specific neuropsychiatric disorders in this population, there are case reports that describe psychosis (Caplan et al. 1991; Carson et al. 1997; Mordecai et al. 2000), depressive disorders, anorexia nervosa (Chipkevitch 1994; Weller 1982; Heron 1976), aggression (Nakaji 2003; Weissenberger 2001), obsessive-compulsive behaviors and obsessive-compulsive disorder (Caplan et al. 1992; Peterson et al. 1996; Shuren et al. 1995), school refusal (Overmeyer et al .1992; Stein et al. 1996), learning disabilities, and deteriorations in school performance. In addition, in the adult literature, there are descriptions of mania (Binder 1983; Bourgeois et al. 1992; Starkstein et al. 1988), panic disorder (Filley and Kleinschmidt-DeMasters 1995), other anxiety disorders (Bristow 1991), and schizophrenia (Kan et al. 1989). Taken together, these cases demonstrate a wide variety of psychopathology associated with brain tumors in children and adults.

Relationship of Tumor Type and Location to Symptoms

There are no data to suggest that the type of brain tumor has any relationship to specific symptoms, although many authors suggest that there is a relationship between the location of the tumor and the type of symptoms. The sparse literature that does exist on this issue relates primarily to adults and was reviewed by Price and coworkers (1992).

Affective syndromes and psychotic symptoms are not uncommon in frontal lobe tumors.

Temporal lobe tumors are often associated with psychosis or schizophrenia-like illnesses, nonspecific personality changes, anxiety symptoms, or mood disorders. Parietal and occipital lobe tumors are generally less likely to cause behavioral changes. Parietal lobe tumors appear to be more likely to result in neuropsychological difficulties (e.g., astereognosis, agraphesthesia, apraxias, dysgraphia, acalculia, finger agnosia, and right/left confusion). Occipital tumors are associated with visual hallucinations in a minority of patients. These hallucinations tend to be unformed images and only rarely are more complex and sustained. Diencephalic tumors typically involve regions that are part of or close to the limbic system. Consequently, neuropsychiatric symptoms are common. Schizophrenia-like illnesses, depression, nonspecific personality changes, and hyperphagia and/or anorexia nervosa (typically associated with hypothalamic tumors) have all been reported. Pituitary tumors generally present with endocrine abnormalities, but neuropsychiatric symptoms are common as well. Posterior fossa tumors reportedly present less frequently with neuropsychiatric symptoms, although some series report otherwise. The symptoms are highly variable and do not differ from those of supratentorial tumors.

All in all, although tumor location plays a role in presenting symptoms, it is not a major factor. This is probably due to the widespread and complex connections - between different areas of the brain disrupted by tumors. Other factors thought to be of greater significance in symptom generation include the extent of the mass, rapidity of growth, presence of increased intracranial pressure, premorbid neuropsychiatric symptoms, and psychological defenses.

GUIDELINES FOR NEUROIMAGING

Although it is unusual for children to present with clear-cut neuropsychiatric syndromes and no neurological signs and symptoms, this does occur rarely. Typically these cases present in complex ways making it difficult to separate out effects of the tumor per se from life stress, family effects, genetic loading for neuropsychiatric disorders, other medical problems associated with the tumor (e.g., seizures, endocrine abnormalities), and treatment effects.

So where does this leave the clinician? What kind of neurological workup should be carried out on children with neuropsychiatric disorders? Very little has been written about this subject, and major textbooks generally do not address the issue. There is some discussion of this subject in the adult literature (Filley et al 1995; Weinberger 1984), but findings in adults have limited utility for children and adolescents. We are in agreement with Ron (1989), who states that "to perform costly investigations for every psychiatric patient because of the rare chance of finding a brain tumour is unnecessary and wasteful. In this age of advanced technology, a detailed clinical history and a careful physical examination are still the best predictors of brain pathology" (p. 738).

This perspective is supported by the findings from two studies. Ghaziuddin and colleagues (1993) reviewed the CT scans of 122 child and adolescent psychiatric inpatients. Whereas 22% of these patients' scans were abnormal, the vast majority were categorized as nonspecific or mildly abnormal. In only two patients were the findings grossly abnormal, and both of these patients had previously diagnosed brain tumors. In no patient was a change in the diagnosis or management made as a result of the CT findings. Adams and colleagues (1996) assessed the value of neuroimaging tests in 111 consecutively admitted adolescent inpatients with first-onset psychosis. None of the patients had abnormal EEGs, and 12% had abnormal CT scans. None of these positive test results identified an unsuspected medical disorder or made a difference in any patient's clinical management. The authors concluded that neuroimaging screening tests in first-onset adolescent psychosis have neither demonstrated diagnostic utility nor positive predictive value.

Ryan (1996), in a discussion of Adams and colleagues' findings, concurs with and modestly expands their recommendations, as does Zametkin in his ten year review of the role of the laboratory (1998). The neurological literature also supports judicious use of neuroimaging (Lewis et al. 2002; Medina et al. 2003; Sudlow 2002). Combining all of these conclusions with our clinical experience, we suggest that neuroimaging screening to rule out brain tumors in the pediatric population be considered in the following situations:

1. New-onset neuropsychiatric disorder with focal neurological signs.
2. New-onset neuropsychiatric disorder with concomitant history of seizures, nausea and vomiting, visual disturbances, motor abnormalities, altered consciousness, or high-risk headaches (see subsection on nonlocalizing neurological symptoms earlier in this chapter).
3. New-onset neuropsychiatric disorder with positive family history of heritable medical condition or stigmata of known medical illness (e.g., neurofibromatosis).
4. First-onset psychosis with uncertain or unreliable medical history.
5. New-onset neuropsychiatric disorder associated with confusion or clear signs of neuropsychological deterioration.

MEDICAL–SURGICAL TREATMENT OF BRAIN TUMORS

Surgery is the primary treatment approach to the child with a brain tumor. The goals of surgery are to remove the tumor, obtain a tissue diagnosis, reopen CSF pathways, and reduce mass effect. Advances in surgery, including development of the operating microscope, laser, and microsurgical techniques, have allowed the surgeon access to previously inaccessible parts of the nervous system. Even tumors located in the pineal region, brain stem, and midline can be surgically approached in most cases. Some tumors can be cured with surgical excision alone. These include cystic cerebellar astrocytomas, meningiomas, choroid plexus papillomas, and, in cases with severe visual loss, optic nerve tumors. Even if surgery alone is not curative, there is strong evidence to suggest that a gross total resection will measurably improve survivals in certain tumor types, most notably medulloblastoma and ependymoma.

Radiation is administered postoperatively in cases where surgical excision will not provide a cure. The volume of radiation (i.e., whole brain, local, or craniospinal) in these cases is determined by the tendency of the tumor to spread both locally and throughout the CSF pathways. As such, the child with a low-grade supratentorial astrocytoma will receive local radiation, the child with a medulloblastoma (a tumor that tends to seed the CSF pathways) will receive craniospinal radiation, and the child with a glioblastoma will receive either whole-brain radiation or local radiation with wide ports. Newer techniques to reduce the volume of radiation include three-dimensional conformal radiotherapy. The dose of radiation varies. Children with medulloblastomas typically receive 3,600 centi-Gray units to the neuraxis and 5,500 centi-Gray units to the posterior fossa, whereas children with brainstem gliomas receive 5,500 centi-Gray units to the posterior fossa alone. In recent years, longterm effects of radiation on intelligence, learning abilities, and endocrine function have been described. These studies have led to modifications of both the dose and the volume of radiation for children with brain tumors, especially the very young. Even in older children, current national treatment protocols for medulloblastoma are reducing the amount of radiation to the brain and spinal cord while maintaining high-dose radiation to the primary tumor site. To do this safely, adjuvant chemotherapy is added. It is hoped that a reduction in radiation dose will be associated with comparable survival rates but fewer and less severe adverse effects on intelligence and learning. Whether this is true remains controversial (see section on Neuropsychological Functioning).

Over the past decade, chemotherapy has played an increasingly important role in the treatment of children with brain tumors. Chemotherapeutic agents have primarily been given postoperatively along with radiation, or alone at the time of tumor recurrence. The drugs are typically administered either intravenously or orally. Intrathecal therapy, such as methotrexate, may be associated with severe untoward side effects, and hence this route has been less popular in recent years. The most promising drugs to date include cyclophosphamide, *cis*- platinum and its analogues, etoposide, the nitrosoureas, and vincristine.

Chemotherapy has been the primary postoperative treatment modality for infants and very young children with malignant brain tumors, in whom issues of radiation toxicity have been of the greatest concern. Although results with chemotherapy are generally no better than those achieved with radiation, survival rates in certain tumor types appear to be comparable. It is hoped that the longterm effects of chemotherapy will be fewer and less severe than those associated with radiation to the infant brain.

NEUROPSYCHIATRIC AND PSYCHOSOCIAL COMPLICATIONS OF BRAIN TUMORS AND THEIR TREATMENT

Psychiatric Perspectives

As noted, there are numerous case reports and small case series documenting neuropsychiatric disorders in children presenting with brain tumors. We could find no study that

systematically documented neuropsychiatric disorders subsequent to presentation in the pediatric brain tumor (PBT) population. Although some studies do address the general issue of the psychosocial adjustment of children, specific definitions of disorder, dysfunction, or disability are generally lacking. Virtually all of the data from these studies are of a dimensional, as opposed to categorical, nature, and do not use Diagnostic and Statistical Manual of Mental Disorders (DSM) (or comparable) criteria for evaluation of the children. These studies used parent questionnaires and/or nonstandardized interview schedules to assess psychosocial adjustment. Standardized clinical or semistructured interview protocols have not been used.

As a backdrop to further discussion of this topic, it is worthwhile to remind readers of Rutter's Isle of Wight study (Rutter et al. 1970). Although Rutter did not look specifically at the impact of brain tumors on neuropsychiatric disorder, he did look at correlates of neurological disorders in general. In his large population sample of older latency-age children, he found the prevalence of neuropsychiatric disorder to be 7%. This contrasted with a prevalence of 12% in children who had nonneurological, chronic illness and 44% in children with a chronic illness involving the CNS. When these findings were further broken down on the basis of presence or absence of epilepsy, the results were even more striking. Nearly 60% of children with CNS involvement plus epilepsy had a neuropsychiatric disorder. Rates in those without epilepsy approached 40%. Overrepresented were cases of hyperactivity and pervasive developmental disorder in the children with neurological involvement. Thus, we know that CNS disease in general is associated with excess rates of neuropsychiatric disorder, and we might expect that this would also, or even especially, be so for children with brain tumors.

While there is no study that has addressed a population of children with brain tumors in this manner, there recently have been a few reports that take more of a psychiatric perspective. Meyer and Kieran (2002) retrospectively studied 34 "surgery-only" survivors of pediatric malignancies. These children had completed treatment from 2 weeks to 5 years prior to the study. The authors reviewed the data from clinical interviews done as part of their overall medical care and DSM criteria were used to establish whether or not a disorder existed. They found that 46% of their shortterm follow-up (less than 1 year) patients, and 29% of the longterm follow-up (more than 1 year), met criteria for dysthymia or major depression; similar numbers met criteria for a "disruptive disorder"; for anxiety disorders, less than 10% of both groups had a disorder (no different from population expectations). No patients reported suicidal ideation or acts. They concluded that large percentages of pediatric brain tumor patients show psychiatric morbidity in the short and long term. While there have been no other studies in children using DSM criteria, Wellisch (2002) also reported high rates (28%) of major depression in an adult sample of 88 consecutive brain tumor patients. With respect to suicidal ideation and acts only a few studies have mentioned this, almost always reporting its striking absence. However, these studies typically report this as an incidental finding, and no studies have systematically investigated this issue. It would appear that suicidal ideation and acts are rare in this population but this remains to be confirmed. In another relevant study Ross and colleagues (2003) reviewed the records of all 3,710 Danes who had been diagnosed before the age of 20 and survived any type of cancer for more than 3 years. Using the files of the Danish Cancer Registry and the Danish National Psychiatric Central Register, they observed all cases for a mean of 15 years or until death. Of the entire cohort, 978 were survivors of brain malignancies. They found that while there was no increase in rates of psychiatric hospitalization for cancer survivors as a whole, the brain tumor survivors had over a twofold increase in expected rates of hospitalization (nearly 9% of them had been hospitalized). Exposure to radiation treatment did not increase the risk for hospitalization, although the psychiatric discharge diagnoses suggested elevated rates of schizophrenia and psychotic disorders. This echoes the findings of Loganovsky and Lganovskaja (2000) who, in a population sample study, suggested increasing rates of schizophrenia in those exposed to the Chernobyl accident. The possibility that brain tumors or its treatments might further compromise a genetically vulnerable individual has been suggested by these studies. Aside from these few studies there is no literature that has documented rates of psychiatric disorders or morbidity in the pediatric brain tumor population. While it can be speculated that survivors of pediatric brain tumors would have elevated rates of attention deficit-hyperactivity disorder, mood disorders, and schizophrenia among others, these studies have not been done.

Psychological and Health-Related Quality of Life Perspectives

Although there are few studies of pediatric brain tumors from a neuropsychiatric perspective, there is a substantial literature addressing "psychosocial" or "health-related quality of life" issues for this population (Fuemmeler et al. 2002). Psychosocial studies generally use standardized parent or teacher questionnaires such as the Child Behavior Checklist (CBCL) or PIC to measure levels of emotional distress, "at risk" or clinical status. These measures have typically been included in broader evaluations of the overall status of survivors, and few studies have queried or observed the children directly. Health related quality of life studies use brief (e.g. 15 question) interview schedules that tap into overall impairment in multiple domains or attributes (e.g. sensory, mobility, emotion/mental health, cognition, self-care, pain). These are complementary perspectives and will be discussed together in this section. These studies are summarized in Table 26.2.

In a study addressing the acute reactions of children with cancer, Mulhern and colleagues (1993) compared the psychosocial status of 81 children with brain tumors and, as a control, 31 children with other types of cancer (mostly acute lymphocytic leukemia). The children in the two groups were 9 and 12 years of age, respectively, and were evaluated within 3 months of their diagnosis. Psychosocial adjustment was measured with the CBCL list. They found that approximately 75% of each group had clinical elevations on at least one subscale of the CBCL and that approximately 20% of both groups scored above the clinical cut-off for total behavior scores on this instrument. There were no differences between the two groups. In this acute phase, the authors noted that 70% of the children with brain tumors had significant cosmetic disfigurement, compared with 23% of those with other types of cancer. They also noted that nearly half of the children with brain tumors had substantial neurological deficit (vs. 4% of those in the control group). Stuber and colleagues (1998) suggested that the acute response to pediatric cancer can be understood from a perspective of post traumatic stress disorder (PTSD) symptoms. These authors suggest that while a full PTSD syndrome is not normative, many children respond to cancer as a repeated trauma and report PTSD symptoms. The model may also apply to parents' responses. In the only study in patients with pediatric brain tumors to date, Fuemmeler and colleagues (2001) evaluated the families of 19 pediatric brain tumor survivors for PTSD symptoms. They found that 43% of the parents, 7 years after diagnosis of the disease in their child, met criteria for PTSD. Their symptoms were deemed to be in the moderate to severe range, somewhat lower than for other acute stressors (e.g. rape, combat, accident/fire). In summary, this work suggests that in the immediate aftermath of diagnosis, the majority of children with brain tumors show considerable psychological distress. It also suggests that the rate of psychological disorder is elevated, but no more so than in children with other types of cancer. Posttraumatic stress models may help to explain the child's and parents' emotional experiences in the short and perhaps long term.

Other studies have addressed longer-term psychosocial adjustment and quality of life of children with brain tumors. A number of studies have examined these issues in the intermediate term (less than 5 years follow-up), generally using the CBCL or PIC. Earlier studies of mixed tumor types found rates of psychological/behavioral morbidity of 42 to 64% (Kun and Mulhern 1983; Mulhern and Kun 1985; LeBaron and colleagues 1988). More recent studies (Mulhern et al. 1994; Slavc et al. 1994; Fossen et al. 1998) found rates of clinical emotional problems in 25 to 62% of school-age survivors. Three other studies used mean CBCL scores to measure psychological adjustment but did not report numbers of patients meeting clinical cutoff scores. Radcliffe and colleagues (1996) evaluated 38 children 2 to 5 years after diagnosis using CBCL (parent and teacher reports) and selected additional self- and parent-report questionnaires. They

TABLE 26.2
PSYCHOSOCIAL OUTCOME IN SURVIVORS OF PEDIATRIC BRAIN TUMORS

Study	N	Mean Age Dx/F-U [a]	Tumor Type [b]	Treatment [c]	Measures [d]	Behavioral/ Emotional* [e]	Cognitive [f]	Academic [g]	Employment/ Marital Status [h]	Neurological [i]	Comments [j]
						Intermediate-term Studies (≤5 yr)					
Kun et al. 1983	30	6/8	50% ST 50% IT 30% No RT	67% RT 10% CMT	WISC/MC, PIAT, PIC	62%	10% MR FSIQ 97	60% SEd	—	20% Mod-Sev	Lower risk for posterior fossa
Mulhern and Kun 1985	26	8/8.5	57% ST 43% IT	96% RT	WISC/MC, LBC or PIC, WRAT	42%	4% MR FSIQ 103	24% SEd	—	15% Sz	No relation to gender, age at diagnosis, tumor location Hc, RT
LeBaron et al. 1988	15	8.4/10.10	PF	73% RT	WISC, PIAT, NP, CBCL	64%	2% MR FSIQ 77	47% SEd	—	20% Mod-Sev	
Mulhern et al. 1994	16	4.1/6.5	BSAC	56% RT	WISC/MC, WRAT, CBCL, Vineland	62.5%	12% MR FSIQ 94	30% SEd	—	39% Mod-Sev 7% Sz	
Slavc et al. 1994	48	7.6/10.2	54% ST 46% IT	60% RT 50% CMT	CBCL, Lansky, WISC	25%	5% MR 38% BIF FSIQ 89	22% SEd	—	15% Mod-Sev 19% Sz	Prospective follow-up of consecutive patients
Carlson-Green et al. 1995	63	7/11	48% AC 33% PNET 6% CP	63% RT; 30% surg	CBCL, S-B, VL, WRAT	CBCL mean 58	IQ 92, VL 85, WRAT 86				Family stress, not RT, a/w behavior problems
Radcliffe et al. 1996	38	7.5/11	53% ST 47% IT	64% RT 36% CMT	CBCL, CDI, CMAS, SPP, TRF, Vineland	—	—	41% SEd	—	—	—
Fossen et al. 1998	16	6/11	63% MB 19% AC 12% Epend.	100% RT	CBCL (P,T), WISC, VMI	31%	FSIQ 78; 25% MR	87% SEd			ALL/MTX control group
Meyer and Kieran 2002	34	9/9.5	75% AC 41% IT	Surgery only 0% RT	NSI	56% disorder; 35% depressive d/o; 35% disruptive d/o		35% academic problems			Used DSM-IV criteria

Longterm Studies (>5 yr)

Study	N	Mean[a] Age Dx/F-U	Tumor[b] Type	Treatment[c]	Measures[d]	Behavioral/[e] Emotional*	Cognitive[f]	Academic[g]	Employment/[h] Marital Status	Neurological[i]	Comments[j]
Follow-up into Adolescence											
Spunberg et al. 1981	14	<2/13	43% ST 57% IT	100% RT 0 CMT	WISC/Mc, WRAT, TAT, CAT, NSI	35%	64% MR	46% SEd	—	64% Mod-Sev 36% Sz	All patients diagnosed before age 2 years; minimum 5-year survival
Danoff et al. 1982	38	8/17	68% ST 32% IT	100% RT 0 CMT	WISC, WRAT, NSI	39%	17% MR	40% "Special school"	33% Unemp	11% Mod-Sev	31 refused to participate No evaluation of psychosocial status
Packer et al. 1987	24	7.9/12	PNET	100% RT 30% CMT	WISC, WRAT, Vineland, NP-	—	13% MR FSIQ 97	54% SEd	—	11% Mod-Sev	
Hoppe-Hirsch et al. 1990	120	6/11	MB	81% RT 60% CMT	Not described	47% at 5 years; 78% at 10 years	18% MR at 5 years; 46% MR at 10 years	26% "Special school" at 5 years; 62% at 10 years	36% Unemp CompEmp	11% Sz	Only 13 patients participated in 10-year follow-up
Seaver et al. 1994	18	6/15	66% MB 33% PFE	100% RT 77% CMT	WRAT, WISC/Mc, WSPR, API, SCL-90 CBCL	25%-40%	N/A	83% SEd	—	N/A	Relation to greater time from diagnosis; no relation to treatment or dose
Foley et al. 2000	29	6.5/12.5	HT/optic chiasm	Unclear	CBCL (P), FAD	38% internalizing; 24% ext.		63% SEd; 22% repeated grade		21%	Control 29 mixed PBT; no statistical difference between groups. No relationship between function family and psychosocial problems.
Carpentieri et al. 2003	32	9.5/14.5	44% AC 13% MB 16% CP	30% surg only; 70% RT	BASC (P, T, C)	P: attention, somatization, leadership; T: learning, somatization					Children report no problems. Only mean scores reported, compared to standardization norms.
Follow-up into Adulthood											
Lannering et al. 1990	56	9/19	48% ST 52% IT	38% RT 29% CMT	WISC, NSI	14%	13% MR 17% BIF	46% HS grad (vs. 88%), 17% Ma (vs. 45%)	66% Emp (vs. 80%)	34% Mod-Sev 10% Sz	Minimum 5-year survival; random control group

(continued)

TABLE 26.2 (continued)

Study	N	Mean Age Dx/F-U[a]	Tumor[b] Type	Treatment[c]	Measures[d]	Behavioral/ Emotional[e]	Cognitive[f]	Academic[g]	Employment/ Marital Status[h]	Neurological[i]	Comments[j]
Mostow et al. 1991	342	11/32	18% ST 39% IT	54% RT 3% CMT 36% NOS	NSI	12%	8% mentally incompetent	12th grade (vs. 13th)	15% Unemp (vs. 1%) Ma: 44% ? 75% /	N/A	Minimum 5-year survival; no relation to age, tumor type; males fared worse; matched sibling control
Hays et al. 1992	22	NA/33	N/A	60% RT	NSI	N/A	N/A	91% HS grad	54% Emp (vs. 86%), 36% Ma (vs. 63%), 23% Div (vs. 8%)	N/A	NonCNS tumor group as control
Syndikus et al. 1994	67	2.8/16.5 (26 > age 18)	53% ST 47% IT	100% RT 15% CMT	WISC, WRAT, NSI	33%	39% MR	58% SEd	61.5% adults Emp 3.8% adults Ma	48% Mod-Sev 15% Sz	All < age 3 years at treatment; minimum 6-year survival; defined.
Zebrack et al. 2003	1101	Dx ,19; F/U 26	65% AC 18% PNET 17% mixed	72% RT; 21% CMT	BSI-18	11% "at risk"; primarily due to elevated depression					Control group 2,916 siblings. Mean scores WNL and no diff. vs. sibs. although only 5% sibs. "at risk". No rel. to age of dx, RT, CMT

Note. N/A = not applicable

[a]Dx =diagnosis; F-U = follow-up. Values not expressed as decimals are in years and months.

[b]BSAC = brainstem astrocytoma; IT = infratentorial; MB = medulloblastoma; NOS = not otherwise specified; PF = posterior fossa; PFE = posterior fossa ependymoma; PNET = primitive neuroectodermal tumors; ST = supratentorial.

[c]CMT = chemotherapy; RT = radiotherapy

[d]API = Adolescent Psychosocial Inventory; CAT = Child Apperception Test; CBCL = Child Behavior Checklist; CPI = Child Depression Inventory; CMAS = Child Manifest Anxiety Scale; Lansky = Lansky Play Scale; LBC = Louisville Behavior Checklist; MC = McCarthy Scales of Children's Abilities; NP = neuropsychological battery; NSI = nonstandardized interview; PIAT = Peabody Individual Achievement Test; PIC = Personality Inventory for Children; SCL–90 = Symptom Checklist–90; SPP = Self-Perception Profile for Children; TAT = Thematic Apperception Test; TRF = Teachers Report Form; Vineland = Vineland Adaptive Behavior Scales; WISC = Wechsler Intelligence Scale for Children; WRAT = Wide Range Achievement Test; WSPR = Washington Structured Psychosocial Review; YSR = Youth Self-Report (of CBCL).

[e]Percentages given are those of sample meeting study criteria for "behavior problem or disturbance," "emotional problem," "psychological dysfunction," and so forth.

[f]BIF = borderline intellectual functioning; FSIQ = Full Scale IQ; MR = mental retardation.

[g]SEd = special education; HS = high school.

[h]Div = divorced; Emp = employed; Ma = married; Unemp = unemployed; CompEmp = competitively employed.

[i] Mod-Sev = moderate to severe neurological sequellae as defined by study; Sz = seizures.

[j]Hc = hydrocephalus.

found that mean scores did not differ significantly from test norms. In distinction, Mabbott (2005) obtained CBCL and TRF scores for 53 pediatric brain tumor subjects 3 years after diagnosis. All subjects had posterior fossa tumors and had received radiotherapy. They found that scores for internalizing, social, and attentional problems were elevated 0.5–1 standard deviation above the norm. Carlson-Green (1995) used a similar strategy reporting mean CBCL results for 63 pediatric brain tumor cases 4 years after diagnosis (age 11). Even though the mean scores represented almost one standard deviation above population norms, the results did not reach statistical significance. They noted that family dysfunction, but not illness or treatment factors, predicted clinical emotional/behavioral problems. In summary most, but not all, studies of younger children a few years postdiagnosis report high percentages of survivors with emotional problems.

From a different vantagepoint, a number of researchers have taken a health related quality of life perspective. Barr (1999), using the Health Utilities Index, evaluated 44 patients with pediatric brain tumors at 9.5 years of age (diagnosed at 6). They found that 27% had an emotional disability. In a parallel study using the HUI, Glaser and colleagues (1999) found that 60% of the 30 survivors (age 6 at diagnosis; 10.5 when evaluated) had an emotional disability. In a slightly longer follow-up, Foreman (1999) used the HUI to evaluate 52 patients with pediatric brain tumors at 16 years of age, 8 years after diagnosis. Thirty-five percent had an emotional disability. These health related quality of life studies, as well as that of Jenkin (1999), have reported that relatively few children (4 to 20%) have no deficits in any areas evaluated and that the majority have problems in two or more attribute areas, most notably in the areas of cognition and emotional health. Surprisingly, these studies noted that many (20 to 35%) of the children also experienced significant pain; many (roughly 20%) had sensory deficits, ambulation difficulties, and cosmetic problems. Up to one third had significant neurological sequelae. Taken together, these studies suggest that in the intermediate run, the majority of children face multiple difficulties, especially in cognitive and emotional realms.

Numerous studies have examined longer-term follow-up of patients with pediatric tumors into adolescence (Danoff et al. 1982; Hoppe-Hirsch et al. 1990; Packer et al. 1987; Seaver et al. 1994; Spunberg et al. 1981). Rates of emotional/behavior disorder ranged from 35 to 47%. Hoppe-Hirsch and colleagues (1990) reported that 78% of their patients were disturbed at 10-year follow-up, but there was large attrition, and only 13 patients were included in that analysis. In a study using more detailed psychosocial evaluation, Seaver and colleagues (1994) evaluated 18 patients with posterior fossa tumors. Mean age at diagnosis was 6 years; mean age at follow-up was 15 years. The study used a variety of self-report and parent-report measures (i.e., CBCL, Youth Self Report [of the CBCL], Symptom Checklist–90, and Adolescent Psychosocial Inventory) and a structured clinical interview

(Washington Structured Psychosocial Review). On each individual measure, scores for 25 to 40% of the survivors were in a clinical range, and only 56% of the cohort had normal psychosocial adjustment. Foley and colleagues (2000) compared CBCL results in 29 patients with hypothalamic or optic chiasm tumor with 29 other pediatric brain tumor patients. Results were obtained at 12.5 years old, 6 years after diagnosis. While the two groups did not differ in their scores, 38% of the entire cohort scored in a clinical range for an internalizing disorder and 24% for an externalizing disorder. Unlike Carlson-Green (1995), they found no relationship between family functioning and behavior problems. Syndikus and colleagues (1994) reviewed 156 cases of children diagnosed with a variety of different types of brain tumors diagnosed at a mean age of just under 3 years. Mean age at follow-up was 16 years. Of the 57 survivors, nonspecific emotional or behavioral problems were reported by the parents in 33% of the cases. Generally, these difficulties appeared to be of a depressive nature, but no standardized measures or diagnostic approaches were utilized. In distinction to these reports, Carpentieri (2003) studied 32 pediatric brain tumor patients 5 years after treatment. At a patient mean age of 14.5 years, the Behavioral Assessment System for Children (BASC) was administered to the children, parents, and teachers. While 5 to 15% of the children reported themselves to be in an "at risk" range, this was not significantly different from the standardization sample. Parents and teachers rated problem areas much higher (10 to 20% scoring in an at risk range), and this was especially true for attentional problems and somatization. This discrepancy between informants may reflect neurologically based cognitive deficits, emotionally based denial, situational differences, or other factors. Regardless, when evaluating the literature it is critical to note the informant used.

A few studies have observed survivors of pediatric brain tumor into adulthood, but few have looked at psychological functioning. Mostow and colleagues (1991) followed up 342 pediatric brain tumor survivors at a mean age of 32 years and found that 23% of survivors with supratentorial tumors and 10% of those with infratentorial tumors had an emotional problem. This represented an odds ratio of 19.8 and 2.5, respectively, as compared with matched sibling controls. Lannering and colleagues (1990) described the follow-up status, at a mean age of 19 years, of a group of mixed tumor patients who had survived for a mean of 10 years. The patients in the group had received relatively little radiotherapy. Using a nonstandardized interview, the authors found that 14% had an emotional disorder. In by far the largest study, Zebrack and colleagues (2003), as part of the Childhood Cancer Survivor Study, administered the Brief Symptom Inventory to over 1,100 pediatric brain tumor survivors and 2,817 sibling controls. Unfortunately, this instrument asks about symptoms in the past 7 days only. Study participants were 26 years old at the time. Mean scores were found to be within normal limits, although 11% scored "at risk" versus 5% of sibling controls.

Social Functioning

Some investigators have addressed the social functioning and difficulties of children with brain tumors. In the immediate aftermath of diagnosis, children's lives are highly disrupted with frequent absence from school and other social activities. Over the next years many have observed changes in social relationship patterns. Earlier studies utilized parent-report CBCL as the measure of social competence and did find a decrease in social competence (Carpentieri et al. 1993; Fossen et al. 1998; Radcliffe et al. 1996). In two of these studies (Carpentieri, Fossen), pediatric brain tumor patients were compared to children with other, nonCNS cancers and found to be functioning significantly worse. Two other studies using parent report measures have confirmed social difficulties. Carpentieri (2003) studied 32 adolescents and young adults diagnosed between 2 and 15 years of age. At a mean age of 14.5, they administered the BASC to parents, teachers, and the youth. While the survivors reported no social problems, the parents endorsed significant problems in leadership. Foreman (1999) evaluated 52 pediatric brain tumor patients with a modified Health Utilities Index completed by mothers. In their study 67% showed evidence of a social impairment. All of these studies are consistent with the review of social competency of neurologically impaired children by Nassau and Drotar (1997). In this review of relevant studies of children with epilepsy, cerebral palsy, and spina bifida, they concluded that there was evidence that these children had lowered social competence compared with healthy children and with chronically (nonCNS affected) ill children. Like the above studies, however, the nature of the social difficulty was unclear. The findings could reflect cognitive deficits (i.e., nonverbal learning disability), sensory deficits, emotional impairments, cosmetic or physical infirmities, or fewer social opportunities.

In an effort to address the mediators of this social deficit, Noll and colleagues (1992) compared results of the Revised Class Play in 15 pediatric brain tumor survivors with 26 children with nonCNS cancer patients, and 16 with sickle cell disease. In the Revised Class Play, children and teachers "cast" classmates in an imaginary play to tap social reputation. While the sickle cell and nonCNS tumor patients were rated similarly to their healthy classmates, the brain tumor sample was described as significantly more sensitive-isolated. In more recent work, this same group (Vannatta et al. 1998) tried to further delineate the nature of the social difficulties. They studied 28 pediatric brain tumor survivors and compared them with 28 matched nonchronically ill classmate-controls. They evaluated these children 3 years after diagnosis (at mean age 14) using multiple teacher, peer, and self-rated sociometric measures. The measures included the Revised Class Play, Three Best Friends, in which children are asked to nominate their three best friends; and the Liking Rating Scale, which generates an average "liking" scale for each child in the class. Results revealed that the brain tumor survivors were significantly more socially isolated and sensitive, missed more school, and were less frequently nominated as a "best friend." These studies suggest that the social deficit is not merely due to fewer opportunities. One group (Barakat et al. 2003) has attempted to provide a social skills training intervention for pediatric brain tumor survivors and found that a small to medium effect size was attained. More approaches like this can be expected in the future.

School Functioning and Educational Attainment

Because of concerns about cognitive decline (see subsequent section), it has been assumed that pediatric brain tumor survivors would have widespread school and academic problems. Four studies have looked at school behavior and three (Radcliffe et al. 1996; Glaser et al. 1997; Carpentieri et al. 2003) found that pediatric brain tumor survivors do not show excess behavioral problems in the school setting when compared to age mates. In a smaller study Fossen (1998) used the same Teacher Report Form to compare 16 children with brain tumors and 15 nonirradiated children with acute lymphocytic leukemia. They found that the children with brain tumors had higher total problem scores, although less than 20% were rated in a clinical range.

Many children with brain tumors require special educational services. Early studies (Kun and Mulhern 1983; Mulhern and Kun and Mulhan 1985; LeBaron et al. 1988; Mulhern et al. 1994; Radcliffe et al. 1996; Slavc et al. 1994) used small numbers and documented figures from 22 to 60% requiring these services. Recently, as part of the Childhood Cancer Survivor Study, Mitby and colleagues (2003) surveyed 12,430 survivors (at least 5 years) of childhood cancer and 3,410 sibling controls for utilization of special education services. Among this group were 1,637 brain tumor survivors. While the study showed elevated rates of special education for all cancer survivors (23%), the rates for brain tumor survivors was over 50%, nearly a sevenfold increase versus siblings (8%). Seventy percent of those diagnosed before the age of 5 years required services. Radiotherapy, and the combination of radiotherapy with intrathecal methotrexate, elevated risk substantially. Females were more vulnerable than males.

With respect to educational attainment, a number of longterm studies have documented lesser achievement for survivors of pediatric brain tumors. Earlier and smaller studies showed that most survivors graduate high school, although at lower rates than expected (Hays et al. 1992; Lannering et al. 1990; Mostow et al. 1991; Syndikus et al. 1994). Kelaghan (1988) retrospectively interviewed 2,283 longterm survivors (mean age of 33) of childhood cancer, 338 of whom were survivors of brain tumors. While the cohort as a whole graduated high school at the same rate as sibling controls (86%), the brain tumor patients did so at a significantly lower rate (77%). They were also much less likely to enter college. Survivors with supratentorial tumors and those receiving radiotherapy fared worse, although nonCNS tumor patients who received radiotherapy did not differ from siblings suggesting a dose effect. In the large study previously cited, Mitby (2003) reported that 18% of 1,637 brain tumor survivors did not graduate high school as compared with 9% of sibling controls. Radiotherapy survivors had lower rates of high school graduation, although this was not statistically significant.

Employment and Marital Status

Based on longterm follow-up studies into adulthood, it appears that many pediatric brain tumor survivors have deficits in these areas. Mostow and colleagues (1991) reviewed the quality of life in 342 cases of children who survived brain tumors a minimum of 5 years as compared with 479 sibling control subjects. The children were 11 years of age at the time of diagnosis, and the mean age at follow-up was 32 years. Fifteen percent of the brain tumor group had never been employed (vs. 1% of the control group). A majority of the men (56%) and 25% of the women had never married (compared with 9% of the male and 15% of the female sibling control subjects). Cranial radiotherapy increased the risk of never having been employed (21%). Syndikus and colleagues (1994) reviewed 156 cases of children diagnosed with a variety of different types of brain tumors at a mean age of just under 3 years. Of the 26 individuals who reached adulthood, 16 (61.5%) were able to work. Most were unable to live independently, and only one was married. Lannering and colleagues (1990) found that, compared with the control group subjects, survivors had a lower rate of employment (66 vs. 80%) and of marriage (17 vs. 45%). Hays and colleagues (1992) studied a large number of childhood cancer patients (mean age at follow-up was 33 years), of which 22 had had CNS tumors. Rates of employment and marriage were lower in the survivors who had had brain tumors than in those who had not had tumors affecting the CNS. As part of the Childhood Cancer Survivor Study, more recently Rauck and colleagues (1999) tracked over 10,000 childhood cancer survivors to a mean age of 26. Pediatric brain tumor survivors accounted for 1,403 of these survivors. Compared to the general population, rates of marriage were slightly lower for all cancer survivors but were much lower for the brain tumor survivors across the age span. In their early 20s the rate is 50% that of the general population. As survivors grow older, their rates slowly approach the norm, but even over age 40 the rates are lower (77 vs. 88%). Interestingly divorce rates are lower until over age 40 when survivors' rates surpass those of the general population (27 vs. 18%). Like earlier studies, this study found that the marriage deficit was larger for males than females. Langeveld and colleagues (2003) tracked 500 Dutch longterm survivors of childhood cancer. Results were compared with a reference group of 1,092 persons with no cancer history. Substantially lower rates of employment and marriage were found in the group as a whole, but particularly for those with a history of CNS tumors. They were also more likely to live with their parents.

Summary of Psychiatric and Psychosocial Literature

As described, many of the studies cited have had significant limitations (e.g., small numbers, large attrition, nonstandardized instruments, lack of a clinical or psychiatric perspective, cross sectional and retrospective in nature, and so forth) and are constructed so differently that it is difficult to compare studies and pool data. Despite these limitations, we can tentatively conclude the following regarding the psychiatric and psychosocial sequelae of pediatric brain tumors:

1. In the immediate aftermath, a large percentage of children with brain tumors show elevated levels of distress, but these levels appear to be no more than those for children in the midst of other catastrophic illness. Posttraumatic stress disorder may be a viable model for understanding patient and family experiences.
2. In the intermediate run (3 to 5 years), although a substantial minority of children with brain tumors have emotional or behavioral problems, the vast majority appear to be functioning adequately. In the longer term, difficulties continue, although still the majority appears to be without disorder. The majority of survivors have diminished quality of life and often have cognitive and emotional deficits; sensory, ambulation, self-care, neurological, and motor impairments are also common.
3. In adulthood, 12 to 33% develop significant psychological or emotional problems. Symptoms frequently mentioned are passivity, immaturity, withdrawal, shyness, depression, and anxiety.
4. Although there is sporadic mention of psychiatric disorders (rare cases of suicidal ideation Lannering et al. 1990; Seaver et al. 1994; "psychotic symptomatology", Kun et al. 1983, ADHD, Mulhern et al. 1994), little is known about rates or types of psychiatric disorder in the short or longterm. These issues have not been systematically investigated, although it appears that longterm survivors are at increased risk for psychiatric hospitalization.
5. While pediatric brain tumor survivors are not behavior problems at school they frequently require special education services. Need for these services is common, at roughly 50% of pediatric brain tumor survivors.
6. Whereas the majority of childhood brain tumor survivors, as adults, are able to work, a significant minority are unable to do so, and a larger number experience substantial interference at work as a result of associated neurological, cognitive, emotional, sensory, and motor deficits. There is a suggestion that many, as adults, are unable to live independently, but this is less clear.

7. It would appear that many survivors of childhood brain tumors, especially men, do not marry.

8. Elevated risk for psychosocial difficulties may be associated with the extent of the tumor (Mulhern and Kun 1985), neuroendocrine abnormalities (Syndikus et al. 1994), male gender (Mostow et al. 1991), physical disfigurement (Mostow et al. 1991), and a greater time from diagnosis to evaluation (Seaver et al. 1994). Although exposure to cranial radiotherapy is associated with significant decrements in cognitive functioning, it is less clear that such exposure is associated with psychosocial morbidity. Younger age at diagnosis and treatment is associated with an increased psychosocial morbidity in at least one study (Mostow et al. 1991), but other studies found no correlation.

LONGTERM EFFECTS ON NEUROPSYCHOLOGICAL FUNCTIONING

The neuropsychological functioning of pediatric brain tumor patients has been the focus of more than 100 research and ten review articles (Anderson et al. 2001; Dennis et al. 1996; Duffner et al. 1995, 2004; Gamis and Nesbit 1991; Glauser and Packer 1991; Moore et al. 2005; Mulhern et al. 1983, 1992, 2003; Mulhern and Butler 2004; Mulhern, Merchant et al. (2004); Ris and Noll 1994) in the past 15 years. Clearly, there is a deterioration of cognitive function in longterm survivors of PBTs as suggested by these studies. Numerous risk factors have been considered to explain this decline and are discussed later in this section. The effects of radiotherapy have been the most intensely studied. Because much of the literature on the effects of radiotherapy has focused on patients with leukemia, we include this topic in the following discussion.

Overall Functioning

The impact of CNS therapy on the IQ of children with leukemia and brain tumors has been extensively studied since the mid-1970s. Most of the early research focused on those children with leukemia who did not have meningeal disease so that the effects of therapy could be assessed in otherwise neurologically intact children. Rowland and colleagues (1984) evaluated 106 children with acute lymphoblastic leukemia. The three treatment arms for CNS prophylaxis were (1) cranial radiotherapy, (2) intravenous plus intrathecal methotrexate, or (3) intrathecal methotrexate. Detailed neuropsychological testing revealed in this study, as well as in others, that children who had received radiation had significantly lower scores on both IQ tests and the Wide Range Achievement Test than did children who had not received radiation. Distractibility and memory deficits have also been identified in children with acute lymphoblastic leukemia who received radiation, particularly those treated in the first decade of life (Goff et al.

1980). Others have found that children who received radiation for leukemia have significantly worse IQ scores compared with their siblings, whereas children who did not receive radiation tend to score approximately the same as do sibling control subjects (Moss et al. 1981). Thus, although, superficially, many children who received radiation for acute lymphoblastic leukemia seem to function well in regular classes, more detailed evaluations reveal significant areas of weakness in intellectual function. The reader is referred to the review by Moleski (2000). Because of the consistency of these findings standard treatment of children with acute lymphoblastic leukemia without CNS disease no longer includes cranial radiotherapy. Instead they are treated with chemotherapy prophylaxis achieving similar survival rates. Although these chemical agents are not benign, it appears that they have less neurocognitive toxicity than cranial radiotherapy. In contrast, radiation remains an integral part of the treatment of children with brain tumors. Evaluating the effects of CNS treatment is much more difficult in children with brain tumors, because surgery, the presence of hydrocephalus, the neurological deficits caused by the tumor, the effects of chemotherapy, and associated seizure disorders and anticonvulsant therapy complicate interpretation of the results. In an attempt to focus on as homogeneous a group as possible, several investigators retrospectively evaluated children with posterior fossa tumors. It was found that 30 to 50% of the children who had received postoperative radiation (with or without chemotherapy) had IQs below 70 and that approximately 10 to 20% had IQs above 90 (Duffner et al. 1983; Hirsch et al. 1979; Raimondi and Tomita 1979). In our study of ten children with posterior fossa tumors, 50% of the patients had IQs below 80, and only 20% had IQs above 100. Of perhaps more concern, in the four children who had had intelligence testing in school prior to the diagnosis and treatment of the tumor, declines in IQ of at least 25 points were found following therapy. Even those children with IQs in the normal range required special educational help because of learning disabilities and attentional problems (Duffner).

Prospective analyses have produced somewhat different results than did the earlier studies. Carpentieri (2003) studied 106 mixed tumor patients at a mean age of 9.5 years, following surgery but before CRT. They found that in this window the group did show cognitive deterioration, especially on performance IQ subtests, reflecting slowed motor output, poor visuo-spatial processing, and decreased verbal memory. Interestingly the FS IQ was 105, VIQ 107, while PIQ 99. Although baseline testing was not available, this study suggests that cognitive changes occur prior to CRT but they appear to be mild. Beebe (2005) prospectively evaluated 103 children with cerebellar astrocytomas who received surgery only. Three months postoperatively the group showed a 4-point loss on FS IQ scores, suggesting that even without radiotherapy there is risk. In an early, longer follow-up study, Hoppe-Hirsch and colleagues (1990) sequentially evaluated children with medulloblastoma at both 5 and 10 years posttreatment. Five years following treatment 58% of the 120 children had IQs above 80, whereas 10 years after treatment only 15% had IQs above 80. In a smaller, long term followup study, Maddrey evaluated 16 10-year survivors of medulloblastoma. All had received radiotherapy and 60% chemotherapy. At age 22 the mean estimated IQ was 75. Thus, the changes associated with CNS therapy appear to be progressive over a period of at least 10 years after treatment. These findings were confirmed in more recent studies (Ris et al. 2001; Palmer et al. 2001, 2003; Spiegler, 2004) that found that FSIQ decreased 2 to 4 points per year and that the declines continued for a number of years. In the long term, total decreases were typically in the 15- to 20-point range; 10 to 20% tested in a mentally retarded range. Interestingly these studies did not find discrepancies between verbal and performance IQ scores.

In summary, the CNS treatment for both leukemia and brain tumors is associated with progressive decline in general intellectual function as well as learning abilities. On average, patients lose the equivalent of, roughly, 10 to 20 FSIQ points, although many suffer little or no loss (especially older children and adolescents who did not receive radiation), and some suffer catastrophic deterioration. Rates of mental retardation appear to be in the 10 to 20% range, although some older studies showed higher rates especially with longer follow-up.

Risk Factors for Cognitive Loss

Much of the research in the past several years has focused on risk factors for treatment-induced cognitive decline. Risk factors identified in children with leukemia include having received radiotherapy, early age at diagnosis (particularly age under 4 years), presence of CNS leukemia at diagnosis, and at least one CNS relapse (Meadows et al. 1981; Picard and Rourke 1995). Children with meningeal disease are at particular risk because they tend to have an increased number of radiation courses and a higher incidence of epilepsy, and are most prone to develop leukoencephalopathy, all of which are potent risk factors (Longeway et al. 1990).

Children with brain tumors have also been studied in an effort to identify risk factors, with the ultimate goal of modifying treatment. Studies of risk factors in pediatric brain tumor patients are summarized in Table 26.3.

In the pediatric brain tumor population, the most important risk factor for treatment-induced decline is exposure to radiation, especially at young ages. Although the "safe" age to radiate the brain has not been determined, children younger than 3 to 5 years of age appear to suffer the brunt of intellectual deterioration following CNS therapy. Mulhern and colleagues (1989a) showed that babies with brain tumors may be developmentally delayed even before they receive radiation. They found that at baseline, prior to either radiation or chemotherapy, fewer than 25% had develop-

mental quotients within the normal range! More recent studies (Ris et al. 2001; Reimers et al. 2003) have further confirmed the risk of young age at irradiation. In a large, population-based study, Reimers and colleagues (2003) studied a consecutive sample of 133 irradiated PBT survivors. Performing multivariate statistical analysis, they identified that radiotherapy exposure was by far the biggest risk factor (FS IQ mean for the nonirradiated group was 97; the irradiated group scored 79). Younger age at diagnosis was also a significant risk. They found that the amount of radiation had a significant effect on performance, but not FS or verbal IQ.

In an effort to clarify whether lower dose irradiation lowers the neurocognitive risk, Mulhern and colleagues (1998) studied a small sample of medulloblastoma survivors assigned to either standard or reduced dose CRT. Although they estimated that the reduced dose CRT group scored 10 to 15 points higher on FS IQ the number of subjects was quite small. Ris and colleagues (2001) studied a slightly larger group of similar patients, who all received reduced dose CRT, and found that their FS IQ dropped 4.3 points per year and continued to drop throughout the study period (4 years). Although there was no control group, it was thought that this represented less of a decrement than the 8 points per year loss estimated for standard dose radiotherapy (Silber et al. 1992). Grill and colleagues (1999) followed 31 pediatric brain tumor survivors exposed to varying amounts of irradiation and also found that higher exposure was a significant risk factor. On the other hand Mulhern (2005) prospectively reported on 38 children with medulloblastoma and found that those who received low dose radiotherapy did not appear to score better on a WISC than those who received standard dose. Thus, although some data supports the benefits of reduced dose radiotherapy, other studies have confirmed that lower dose irradiation in the absence of chemotherapy is associated with worse survival rates (Thomas et al. 2000) and therefore is less of an option than had been hoped.

The volume of radiation also appears to be a major risk factor. Thus, the child treated with whole-brain radiation is more at risk than the child who receives either local or no radiation. Of interest, in Ellenberg and colleagues' (1987) study, only those children who had whole-brain radiation had a decline in IQ, whereas those children who had either local or no radiation had no deterioration. Findings from the studies of Kun and Mulhern (1983), Danoff and colleagues (1982), and Grill and colleagues (1999) support the conclusions that wider exposure (i.e., whole brain or craniospinal irradiation) leads to worse outcomes.

Another risk factor is the location of the tumor. Children whose tumors are located in the supratentorial region have intellectual difficulties more often than those whose tumors are located in the posterior fossa (Ellenberg et al. 1987). There is contradictory evidence as to whether children with midline tumors are also at increased risk. In one study, patients whose tumors involved the hypothalamus were 2.5

TABLE 26.3
RISK FACTORS FOR COGNITIVE DEFICIT IN PATIENTS WITH PEDIATRIC BRAIN TUMORS

Risk Factor	Association With Adverse Outcome	
	Yes	**No**
Patient Characteristics		
Younger age at diagnosis	Chapman et al. 1995, Danoff et al. 1982; Duffner et al. 1988; Ellenberg et al. 1987; Garcia-Perez et al. 1993; Ilveskoski et al. 1996; Maddrey 2005; Moore et al. 1992; Mulhern and Kun 1985; Mulhern et al. 1988, 1989a; Mulhern 2005; Packer et al. 1987; Radcliffe et al. 1992; Ris et al. 2001; Seaver et al. 1994; Silverman et al. 1984; Spunberg et al. 1981	Grill et al. 1999; Kun and Mulhern 1983; Mulhern et al. 1994; Syndikus et al. 1994
Gender	Mulhern and Kun 1985; Ris et al. 2001	Kao et al. 1994; Jannoun and Bloom 1990; Reimers et al. 2003; Silber et al. 1992
Pretreatment Characteristics		
Location of tumor	Clopper et al. 1977; Danoff et al. 1982; Dennis et al. 1991a, 1991b, 1992; Ellenberg et al. 1987; Hirsch et al. 1979; Reimers et al. 2003; Slavc et al. 1994	Carpentieri et al. 2003; Jannoun and Bloom 1990; Mulhern and Kun 1985; Radcliffe et al. 1994; Syndikus et al. 1994
Extent/stage	——	Kao et al. 1994; Radcliffe et al. 1992
Hydrocephalus	Bamford et al. 1976; Bloom et al. 1969; Reimers et al. 2003	Danoff et al. 1982; Ellenberg et al. 1987; Jannoun and Bloom 1990; Kao et al. 1994; Kun and Mulhern 1983; Mulhern and Kun 1985; Silber et al. 1992
Treatment Characteristics		
Extent of resection	Packer et al. 1987	Cavazzuti et al. 1983; Ellenberg et al. 1987; Mulhern et al. 1994; Syndikus et al. 1994
Radiotherapy (RT)	Dennis et al. 1992; Duffner et al. 1983, 1988; Ellenberg et al. 1987; Garcia-Perez et al. 1994; Grill et al. 1999; Hirsch et al. 1979; Jannoun and Bloom 1990; Kun and Mulhern 1983; Lannering et al. 1990; Moore et al. 1992; Mulhern et al. 1989a; Packer et al. 1989; Reimers et al. 2003; Riva et al. 1989; Silber et al. 1992; Silverman et al. 1984; Spunberg et al. 1981	Bloom et al. 1969; Bordeaux et al. 1988; Cavazzuti et al. 1983; LeBaron et al. 1988; Mulhern et al. 1994
Whole-brain RT	Ellenberg et al. 1987; Kun and Mulhern 1983	Jannoun and Bloom 1990; Mulhern and Kun 1985; Syndikus et al. 1994
Restricted field RT	——	Danoff et al. 1982; Ellenberg et al. 1987
Dose of RT	Goldwein et al. 1993; Grill et al. 1999; Ilveskoski et al. 1996; Mulhern et al. 1998; Palmer et al. 2001; Ris et al. 2001; Silber et al. 1992	Danoff et al. 1982; Kao et al. 1994; Spunberg et al. 1981; Syndikus et al. 1994
Age at RT	Dennis et al. 1992; Ellenberg et al. 1987; Grill et al. 1999; Jannoun and Bloom 1990; Lannering et al. 1990; Moore et al. 1992; Mulhern et al. 1998; Palmer et al. 2001; Silber et al. 1992	—
Chemotherapy (CMT)	Duffner et al. 1988, Grill et al. 1999, Mulhern et al. 1989a, Riva et al. 1989	Ellenberg et al. 1987; Kao et al. 1994; Packer et al. 1989; Radcliffe et al. 1994; Reimers et al. 2003
RT plus CMT	Duffner et al. 1983, 1988	Syndikus et al. 1994
Post-treatment Characteristics		
Perioperative complications	Chapman et al. 1995; Ilveskoski et al. 1996; Kao et al. 1994; Maddrey 2005; Mulhern et al. 1988, 1994; Packer et al. 1987; Silber et al. 1992	Ellenberg et al. 1987; Radcliffe et al. 1994
Seizures	Mulhern et al. 1988; Syndikus et al. 1994	——
Tumor recurrence	Mulhern et al. 1988	Cavazzuti et al. 1983
Sensory–motor impairment	Mulhern and Kun 1985	Cavazzuti et al. 1983
Long interval after treatment	Duffner et al. 1988; Ellenberg et al. 1987; Hoppe-Hirsch et al. 1990; Maddrey 2005; Moore et al. 1992; Mulhern and Kun 1985; Mulhern et al. 1989a; Packer et al. 1989	Cavazzuti et al. 1983; Kun and Mulhern 1983a; Radcliffe et al. 1992

times more likely to have a lower IQ than were those whose tumors did not involve the hypothalamus (Jannoun and Bloom 1990). In contrast, Ellenberg and colleagues (1987) did not find that children with third-ventricle tumors had significantly lower IQs compared with children whose tumors were either supratentorial or infratentorial in location. Children whose tumors were in the anterior third ventricle seemed to have the most impairment. Reimers and colleagues (2003), on the other hand, found that those with third-ventricle tumors scored higher than survivors with either supratentorial or infratentorial tumors.

Although one of the putative risk factors for intellectual impairment was believed to be hydrocephalus, it has been shown by several investigators that hydrocephalus does not have an adverse impact on intelligence. Hirsch and colleagues (1979) compared the IQs of children treated for cerebellar astrocytomas with those of children treated for medulloblastomas. The children with cerebellar astrocytomas received surgery alone, whereas the children with medulloblastomas received postoperative radiation and chemotherapy. Children with medulloblastomas were found to have more intellectual impairment than did those with cerebellar astrocytomas: 62% of children with cerebellar astrocytomas, but only 11% of the children with medulloblastomas, had IQs above 90. Since both groups of patients had posterior fossa tumors associated with obstructive hydrocephalus, Hirsch and colleagues concluded that it was the postoperative treatment rather than either the posterior fossa location or the hydrocephalus that produced the learning difficulties. A number of other studies failed to confirm a link, although two studies (Parker 1987; Reimers et al. 2003) have supported an association between hydrocephalus with shunt and lower IQ.

Another important risk factor in children with brain tumors is perioperative morbidity. Although the degree of surgical resection does not appear to influence intelligence directly, children with posterior fossa syndrome and other perioperative complications tend to have much more severe neurological and intellectual sequelae (Kao et al. 1994).

Although chemotherapy is not generally considered to adversely influence intelligence, the development of methotrexate-induced leukoencephalopathy is associated with dementia and other neurological complications. The diagnosis of methotrexate (MTX) leukoencephalopathy was first made in children irradiated for leukemia who had also been treated with intrathecal methotrexate. CT scans of 53% of those children revealed calcification in the basal ganglia, hypodense areas, and widened subarachnoid spaces. This finding was termed methotrexate leukoencephalopathy (Peylan-Ramu et al. 1978). The abnormality appeared to develop primarily in those children with leukemia treated with MTX who had received radiation as part of CNS prophylaxis or those who had leptomeningeal disease. In contrast, the child who did not have CNS leukemia and had been treated with MTX but without radiotherapy did not seem to be at

significant risk (Ochs et al. 1980). As higher and more frequent doses of MTX have been utilized, increasing concern has developed about the effects of MTX. A Pediatric Oncology Group (Mahoney 1998) study of children with acute lymphoblastic leukemia who did not receive radiotherapy nor have CNS leukemia demonstrated a high incidence of acute neurotoxicity and abnormal neuroimaging findings.

MTX has also been used in the treatment of children with brain tumors. When this agent was used via the intraventricular route in patients with obstructive hydrocephalus, profound necrotizing leukoencephalopathy occurred. Even in the absence of such a catastrophic complication, MTX leukoencephalopathy may develop in children with brain tumors treated with intrathecal MTX and radiation.

Another important influence on neuropsychological functioning is the presence of seizures and the use of anticonvulsants. Long interval after treatment (i.e., lengthier follow-up) has generally been associated with increased cognitive deficits. This association has usually been attributed to a latency in the full effect of radiotherapy. Other factors, such as gender effects, tumor recurrence, and sensory/motor impairment, have been less well investigated, and their importance is unclear.

In summary, the patients at greatest risk for neuropsychological complications appear to be those who receive radiation (especially higher dose and larger volume), are younger at the time of treatment, receive concomitant intrathecal MTX, and have seizures.

Mechanisms of damage and specific deficits

A number of studies have documented white matter abnormalities and demyelination as a result of CNS irradiation (Steen et al. 2001; Reddick 2003). It is thought that these findings result from damage to oligodendrocytes, with consequent axonal demyelination, or microvascular damage to endothelial cells, which compromises the blood-brain barrier. This leukoencephalopathy appears to occur subsequent to both cranial radiotherapy and CNS chemotherapy exposure, although more so to the former. These changes have, in turn, been associated with IQ loss.

The specific types of neuropsychological deficits associated with brain tumors have been studied, although a clearly defined composite has not emerged. This should not be surprising given the widely varying locations of tumors. Nevertheless, a number of studies suggest that the greatest difficulties are in attention, memory, sequential processing, processing speed, and visuospatial/perceptual organization. Mathematics skills are frequently mentioned as problematic, as are performance subtests on the WISC (or an equivalent test), although many studies show no difference between verbal and performance subtests (Ris et al. 2001; Palmer et al. 2001). Palmer (2001) has suggested that the IQ deficits result from a difficulty in assimilating new knowledge as opposed to a loss of acquired information.

Treatment of Neurocognitive Deficits

Few studies have addressed treatment of the neurocognitive deficits associated with pediatric brain tumors, although Butler (2005) recently reviewed this area. Both pharmacologic and educational interventions for the cognitive deficits associated with pediatric brain tumors have been reported. One uncontrolled trial of methylphenidate (DeLong 1992) yielded promising results, while another (Torres 1996) was negative. Recently Thompson (2001) reported a randomized, double-blind, placebo-controlled study of 32 pediatric cancer survivors (acute lymphoblastic leukemia and pediatric brain tumors). During this one-day laboratory study, subjects receiving methylphenidate showed significantly greater improvement on the continuous performance test. Mulhern (2004) extended this investigation to a 3-week placebo-controlled, double-blind trial of low and moderate dose methylphenidate in 83 long term survivors of acute lymphoblastic leukemia and pediatric brain tumors with attentional and academic deficits. Modest but significant improvement was seen in the treated group, although higher dose conferred no advantage. Other investigators have taken a cognitive remediation approach. A seven-member consortium group is currently investigating the efficacy of using a 20 session cognitive rehabilitation program in pediatric brain tumor and acute lymphoblastic leukemia survivors (Butler 2002).

SUMMARY

Brain tumors are the second most common malignancy, and the most common solid malignancy, in the pediatric population. Because of improved treatments, survival rates have improved substantially in the past 30 years, and as a consequence the population of longterm survivors has grown. The child and adolescent psychiatrist faces two issues in this population. One is diagnosis and its potential for neuropsychiatric presentation. The other is the need for comprehensive treatment frequently required by long-term survivors, who often have psychological, cognitive, and academic difficulties as well as endocrinological and neurological complications.

Although there are few data on neuropsychiatric disorders in survivors, there is a literature on the psychosocial functioning of these patients. As their lives unfold, most appear to be functioning adequately, although not at their premorbid level. Often they are described as immature, shy, lacking confidence, withdrawn, depressive, and anxious. Although most appear physically normal, many have noticeable neurological impairment, have hearing or visual problems, and are shorter than age mates.

Cognitively, most children with brain tumors function in a normal range, although IQs are low average, which represents a decrement from premorbid functioning. Wechsler Full Scale IQs in these children as a group probably drop 10 to 20 points on average. Attention and memory functions appear to be especially vulnerable and are associated with white matter changes. Older children and those not requiring radiotherapy appear to suffer substantially less in this regard. Younger age and exposure to radiotherapy appear to be the major risk factors for serious loss of cognitive abilities. Of the group of children with brain tumors who become mentally retarded (10 to 20%), most were diagnosed at young ages and had received or were receiving radiotherapy. Most child survivors require special educational services and/or have had to repeat grades because of cognitive loss and extended absences from school.

Little is known about the effects on families and levels of family functioning, although PTSD may be a useful conceptual frame for understanding their experiences and needs. As adults, most survivors of pediatric brain tumors are employed in some capacity and are able to drive. Limitations commonly require that these individuals receive assistance to support work and independent living. They marry, although at much lower rates than in the general population.

In the future, increasing numbers of survivors of pediatric brain tumors can be expected. Child and adolescent psychiatrists can be valuable members of the multidisciplinary teams needed to care for these patients. Although narrowly defined neuropsychiatric needs are not well delineated, currently psychiatrists are uniquely able to integrate neurological, psychosocial, cognitive, and psychiatric approaches and perspectives.

REFERENCES

Achenbach, TM. *Manual for the Teacher's Report Form and 1991 Profile.* Burlington, VT: University Associates in Psychiatry, 1991

Achenbach, TM. *Manual for the Youth Self-Report and 1991 Profile.* Burlington VT: University Associates in Psychiatry, 1991

Adams M, Kutcher S, Antoniw E, et al: Diagnostic utility of endocrine and neuroimaging screening tests in first-onset adolescent psychosis. J Am Acad Child Adolesc Psychiatry 35:67–73, 1996.

Anderson DM, Rennie KM, Ziegler RS, et al: Medical and neurocognitive late effects among survivors of childhood central nervous system tumors. Cancer 92:2709–2719, 2001.

Anderson VA, Godber T, Smibert E, et al: Cognitive and academic outcome following cranial irradiation and chemotherapy in children: a longitudinal study. Br J Cancer 82:255–262, 2000.

Armstrong CL. Gyato K. Awadalla AW. Lustig R. Tochner ZA. A critical review of the clinical effects of therapeutic irradiation damage to the brain: the roots of controversy. Neuropsychology Review. 14(1):65-86, 2004 Mar.

Bamford FN, Jones PM, Pearson D, et al: Residual disabilities in children treated for intracranial space-occupying lesions. Cancer 37:1149–1151, 1976.

Barakat LP, Hetzke JD, Foley B, et al: Evaluation of a social-skills training group intervention with children treated for brain tumors: a pilot study. J Pediatr Psychol 28:299–307, 2003.

Barr RD, Simpson T, Whitton A, et al: Health-related quality of life in survivors of tumours of the central nervous system in childhood- a preference-based approach to measurement in a cross-sectional study. Eur J Cancer 35:248–255, 1999.

Beebe DW, Ris MD, Armstrong FD, Fontanesi J, Mulhern R, Holmes E, Wisoff JH. Cognitive and adaptive outcome in low-grade pediatric cerebellar astrocytomas: evidence of diminished cognitive and adaptive functioning in National Collaborative Research Studies (CCG 9891/POG 9130). Journal of Clinical Oncology. 23(22):5198–204, 2005 Aug 1.

Bellak L , Bellak S. Children's Apperception Test (CAT). Psychological Assessment Resources, Inc., 1987

Binder RL: Neurologically silent brain tumors in psychiatric hospital admissions: three cases and a review. J Clin Psychiatry 44:94–97, 1983.

Bloom HJG, Wallace ENK, Hank JM, et al: The treatment and prognosis of medulloblastoma in children: a study of 82 verified cases. AJR 105:43–62, 1969.

Bordeaux JD, Dowell RE, Copeland DR, et al: A prospective study of neuropsychological sequelae in children with brain tumors. J Child Neurol 3:63–68, 1988.

Bourgeois JA, Nisenbaum J, Drexler KG, et al: A case of subcortical grey matter heterotopia presenting as bipolar disorder. Compr Psychiatry 33:407–410, 1992.

Bristow MF: Posterior fossa tumors presenting to psychiatrists. Behav Neurol 4:249–253, 1991.

Butler R, Copeland DR: Attentional processes and their remediation in children treated for cancer: a literature review and the development of a therapeutic approach. J Int Neuropsychol Soc 8: 115–124; 2002.

Butler RW, Mulhern RK. Neurocognitive interventions for children and adolescents surviving cancer. Journal of Pediatric Psychology. 30(1):65–78, 2005 Jan-Feb.

Caplan R, Shields WD, Mori L, et al: Middle childhood onset of interictal psychosis. J Am Acad Child Adolesc Psychiatry 30:893–896, 1991.

Caplan R, Comair Y, Shewmon DA, et al: Intractable seizures, compulsions and coprolalia: a pediatric case study. J Neuropsychiatry Clin Neurosci 4:315–319, 1992.

Carlson-Green B, Morris R, Krawiecki. Family and illness predictors of outcome in pediatric brain tumors. J Pediatr Psychol 20:769–784, 1995.

Carpentieri SC, Meyer EA, Delaney BL, et al: Psychosocial and behavioral functioning among pediatric brain tumor survivors. J Neuro-Oncol 63:279–287, 2003.

Carpentieri SC, Waber DP, Pomeroy SL, et al: Neuropsychological functioning after surgery in children treated for brain tumor. Neurosurgery 52:1348–1357, 2003.

Carson BS, Weingart JD, Guarnieri M, et al: Third ventricular choroid plexus papilloma with psychosis. case report. Journal of Neurosurgery 87:103–5, 1997.

Cavazzuti V, Fischer EG, Welch K, et al: Neurological and psychophysiological sequelae following different treatments of craniopharyngioma in children. J Neurosurg 59:409–417, 1983.

Central Brain Tumor Registry of the United States. Statistical report: primary brain tumors in the United States 1997–2001. Central Brain Tumor Registry of the United States. 2004–2005.

Chapman CA, Waber DP, Bernstein JH, et al: Neurobehavioral and neurologic outcome in long-term survivors of posterior fossa brain tumors: role of age and perioperative factors. J Child Neurol 10:209–212, 1995.

Chipkevitch E: Brain tumors and anorexia nervosa syndrome. Brain Dev 16:175–179, 1994.

Clopper RR, Meyer WJ, Udvarhelyi GB, et al: Postsurgical IQ and behavioral data on 20 patients with a history of childhood craniopharyngioma. Psychoneuroendocrinology 2:365–372, 1977.

Cohen ME, Duffner PK: Brain Tumors in Children, 2nd ed. New York, Raven, 1994.

Costello A, Shallice T, Gullan R, Beaney R. The early effects of radiotherapy on intellectual and cognitive functioning in patients with frontal brain tumours: the use of a new neuropsychological methodology. Journal of Neuro-Oncology. 67(3):351–9, 2004 May.

Cummings JL: Frontal-subcortical circuits and human behavior. Arch Neurol 50:873–880, 1993.

Danoff BF, Cowchock FS, Marquette C, et al: Assessment of the long-term effects of primary radiation therapy for brain tumors in children. Cancer 49:1580–1586, 1982.

Dehner LP: Peripheral and central primitive neuroectodermal tumors. A nosologic concept seeking a consensus. Arch Pathol Lab Med 110:997–1005, 1986.

DeLong R, Friedman H, Friedman N, Gustafson K, Oakes J. Methylphenidate in neuropsychological sequelae of radiotherapy and chemotherapy of childhood brain tumors and leukemia. Journal of Child Neurology. 7(4):462–3, 1992 Oct.

Dennis M, Spiegler BJ, Fitz CR, et al: Brain tumors in children and adolescents, II: the neuroanatomy of deficits in working, associative and serial-order memory. Neuropsychologia 29:829–847, 1991a.

Dennis M, Hetherington CR, Spiegler BJ: Memory and attention after childhood brain tumors. Med Pediatr Oncol Suppl 1:25–33,1998.

Dennis M, Spiegler BJ, Hoffman HJ, et al: Brain tumors in children and adolescents, I: effects on working, associative and serial-order memory of IQ, age at tumor onset and age of tumor. Neuropsychologia 29:813–827, 1991b.

Dennis M, Spiegler BJ, Obonsawin MC, et al: Brain tumors in children and adolescents, III: effects of radiation and hormone status on intelligence and on working, associative and serial-order memory. Neuropsychologia 30:257–275, 1992.

Dennis M, Spiegler BJ, Hetherington CR, et al: Neuropsychological sequelae of the treatment of children with medulloblastoma. J Neurooncol 29:91–101, 1996.

Derogatis LR. SCL-90-R (Symptom Checklist-90-Revised). Pearson Assessments.

Duffner PK: Long-term effects of radiation therapy on cognitive and endocrine function in children with leukemia and brain tumors. The Neurologist, 10:293–310, 2004.

Duffner PK, Cohen ME, Thomas PRM: Late effects of treatment on the intelligence of children with posterior fossa tumors. Cancer 51:233–237, 1983.

Duffner PK, Cohen ME, Myers MH, et al: Survival of children with brain tumors: SEER Program, 1973–1980. Neurology 36:597–601, 1986.

Duffner PK, Cohen ME, Parker MS: Prospective intellectual testing in children with brain tumors. Ann Neurol 23:575–579, 1988.

Duffner PK, Jackson LA, Cohen M: Neurobehavioral abnormalities resulting from brain tumors and their therapy, in Y. Frank (ed.). Pediatric Behavioral Neurology. New York, CRC Press, 1995:289–308.

Edgeworth J, Bullock P, Bailey A, et al: Why are brain tumors still being missed? Arch Dis Child 74:148–151, 1996.

Ellenberg L, McComb JG, Siegel SE, et al: Factors affecting intellectual outcome in pediatric brain tumor patients. Neurosurgery 21: 638–644, 1987.

Filley CM, Kleinschmidt-DeMasters BK: Neurobehavioral presentations of brain neoplasms. West J Med 163: 19–25, 1995.

Flores L, Williams D, Ragab BM: Delay in the diagnosis of pediatric brain tumors. Am J Dis Child 140:684–686, 1986.

Foley B, Barakat LP, Herman-Liu A, et al: The impact of childhood hypothalamic/chiasmatic brain tumors on child adjustment and family functioning. Child Health Care 29:209–233, 2000.

Fossen A, Abrahamsen TG, Storm-Mathisen I: Psychological outcome in children treated for brain tumor. Pediatr Hematol Oncol 15:479–488, 1998.

Frishberg BM: The utility of neuroimaging in the evaluation of headache in patients with normal neurologic examinations. Neurology 44:1191–1197, 1994.

Fuemmeler BF, Mullins LL, Marx BP: Posttraumatic stress and general distress among parents of children surviving a brain tumor. Child Health Care 30:169–182, 2001.

Fuemmeler BF, Elkin T D, Mullins LL: Survivors of childhood brain tumors: Behavioral, emotional, and social adjustment. Clin Psychol Rev 22:547–585, 2002.

Fung KM, Trojanowski JQ: Animal models of medulloblastomas and related primitive neuroectodermal tumors. A review. J Neuropathol Exp Neurol 54:285–296, 1995.

Gamis AS, Nesbit ME: Neuropsychologic (cognitive) disabilities in long-term survivors of childhood cancer. Pediatrician 18:11–19, 1991.

Garcia-Perez A, Narbona Garcia J, Sierrasesumaga L, et al: Neuropsychological outcome of children after radiotherapy for intracranial tumors. Dev Med Child Neurol 35:139–148, 1993.

Garcia-Perez A, Sierrasesumaga L, Narbona Garcia J, et al: Neuropsychological evaluation of children with intracranial tumors: impact of treatment modalities. Med Pediatr Oncol 23:116–123, 1994.

Ghaziuddin R, Tsai LY, Ghaziuddin N, et al: Utility of the head computerized tomography scan in child and adolescent psychiatry. J Am Acad Child Adolesc Psychiatry 32:123–126, 1993.

Glaser AW, Nik Abdul Rashid NF, CL U, et al: School behaviour and health status after central nervous system tumours in childhood. Br J Cancer 76:643–650, 1997.

Glaser AW, Kennedy C, Punt J, et al: Standardized quantitative assessment of brain tumor survivors treated within clinical trials in childhood. Int J Cancer Suppl 12:77–82, 1999.

Glaser AW, Furlong W, Walker DA, et al: Applicability of the health utilities index to a population of childhood survivors of central nervous system tumours in the U.K. Eur J Cancer 35:256–261, 1999.

Glauser TA, Packer RJ: Cognitive deficits in long-term survivors of childhood brain tumors. Childs Nerv Syst 7:2–12, 1991.

Goff JR, Anderson HR, Cooper PF: Distractibility and memory deficits in long-term survivors of acute lymphoblastic leukemia. Dev Behav Pediatr 1:158–163, 1980.

Goldwein JW, Radcliffe J, Packer RJ, et al: Results of a pilot study of low-dose craniospinal radiation therapy plus chemotherapy for children younger than 5 years with primitive neuroectodermal tumors. Cancer 71:2647–2652, 1993.

Grill J, Kieffer Renaux V, Bultheau C, et al: Long-term intellectual outcome in children with posterior fossa tumors according to radiation doses and volumes. Int J Radiation Oncology Biol Phys 45:137–145, 1999.

Hays DM, Landsverk J, Sallan SE, et al: Educational, occupational, and insurance status of childhood cancer survivors in their fourth and fifth decades of life. J Clin Oncol 10:1397–1406, 1992.

Harter S. Self-Perception Profile for Children: Manual. Denver: University of Denver, 1985.

Heron GB, Johnston DA: Hypothalamic tumor presenting as anorexia nervosa. Am J Psychiatry 133:580–582, 1976.

Hirsch JF, Reiner D, Czernichow P, et al: Medulloblastoma in childhood: survival and functional results. Acta Neurochir (Wien) 48:1–15, 1979.

Hoppe-Hirsch E, Renier D, Lellouch-Tubiana C, et al: Medulloblastoma in childhood: progressive intellectual deterioration. Childs Nerv Syst 6:60–65, 1990.

Ilveskoski I, Pihko H, Wiklund T, et al: Neuropsychologic late effects in children with malignant brain tumors treated with surgery, radiotherapy and "8 in 1" chemotherapy. Neuropediatrics 27:124–129, 1996.

Jannoun L, Bloom HJG: Long-term psychological effects in children treated for intracranial tumors. Int J Radiat Oncol Biol Phys 18:747–753, 1990.

Jenkin D, Danjoux C, Greenberg M : Subsequent quality of life for children irradiated for a brain tumor before age four years. Med Pediatr Oncol 31:506–511, 1998.

Kan R, Mori Y, Suzuki S, et al: a case of temporal lobe astrocytoma associated with epileptic seizures and schizophrenia-like psychosis. Jap J Psychiatry Neurol 43:97–103, 1989.

Kao GD, Goldwien JW, Schultz DJ, et al: The impact of perioperative factors on subsequent intelligence quotient deficits in children treated for medulloblastoma/posterior fossa primitive neuroectodermal tumors. Cancer 74:965–971, 1994.

Keschner M, Bander MB, Straus I, et al: Mental symptoms associated with brain tumor: a study of 530 verified cases. JAMA 110:714–718, 1938.

Kleihues P, Louis DN, Scheithauer BW, Rorke LB: The WHO classification of tumours of the nervous system. J Neuropathol Exp Neurol 61:215–225, 2002.

Kovacs M. Children's Depression Inventory Manual. Los Angeles: Western Psychological Services, 1992.

Kun LE, Mulhern RK: Neuropsychologic functioning in children with brain tumors, II: serial studies of intellect and time after treatment. Am J Clin Oncol 6: 651–656, 1983.

Kun LE, Mulhern RK, Crisco JJ: Quality of life in children treated for brain tumors. J Neurosurg 58:1–6, 1983.

Langeveld NE, Ubbink MC, Last BF, Grootenhuis MA, Voute PA, DeHaan RJ: Educational achievement, employment and living situation in long-term young adult survivors of childhood cancer in the Netherlands. Psychooncology 12:213–225, 2003.

Lannering B, Marky I, Lundberg A, et al: Long-term sequelae after pediatric brain tumors: their effect on disability and quality of life. Med Pediatr Oncol 18:304–310, 1990.

Lansky LL, List MA, Lansky SB, Cohen ME, Sinks LF. Toward the development of a play performance scale for children (PPSC). Cancer. 1985 Oct 1;56(7 Suppl):1837–40.

LeBaron S, Zeltzer PL, Zeltzer LK, et al: Assessment of quality of survival in children with medulloblastoma and cerebellar astrocytoma. Cancer 62:1215–1222, 1988.

Lewis DW, Ashwal S, Dahl G, et al: American Academy of Neurology Practice parameter: Evaluation of children and adolescents with recurrent headaches. Neurology 59:490–498, 2002.

Loganovsky KN, Lganovskaja TK: Schizophrenia spectrum disorders in persons exposed to ionizing radiation as a result of the Chernobyl accident. Schizophr Bull 26:751–773, 2000.

Longeway J, Mulhern RK, Crisco JJ, et al: Treatment of meningeal relapse in childhood acute lymphoblastic leukemia, II: a prospective study of intellectual loss specific to CNS relapse and therapy. Am J Pediatr Hematol Oncol 12:45–50, 1990.

Mabbott DJ, Spiegler BJ, Greenberg ML, Rutka JT, Hyder DJ, Bouffet E. Serial evaluation of academic and behavioral outcome after treatment with cranial radiation in childhood. Journal of Clinical Oncology. 23(10):2256–63, 2005 Apr 1.

Maddrey AM, Bergeron JA, Lombardo ER, McDonald NK, Mulne AF, Barenberg PD, Bowers DC. Neuropsychological performance and quality of life of 10 year survivors of childhood medulloblastoma. Journal of Neuro-Oncology. 72(3):245–53, 2005 May.

Mahoney DH, Shuster JJ, Nitschke R, et al. Acute neurotoxicity in children with B-precursor acute lymphoid leukemia; an association with intermediate-dose intravenous methotrexate and intrathecal triple therapy—a Pediatric Oncology Group study. J Clin Oncol 16:1712–1722, 1998.

Markwardt FC. Peabody Individual Achievement Test-Revised (PIAT-R). Circle Pines, MN: American Guidance Service, 1989.

McCarthy DA. Manual for the McCarthy Scales of Children's Abilities. San Antonio TX: The Psychological Corporation, 1972.

Miller LC. Louisville Behavior Checklist-Revised. Los Angeles: Western Psychological Services, 1984.

Meadows AT, Gordon J, Massari DJ, et al: Declines in IQ scores and cognitive dysfunctions in children with acute lymphocytic leukemia treated with cranial irradiation. Lancet 2:1015–1018, 1981.

Medina LS, Pinter JD, Zurakowski D, et al: Children with headache: clinical predictors of surgical space-occupying lesions and the role of neuroimaging. Radiology 202:819–824, 1997.

Medina LS, D'Souza B, Vasconcellos E. Adults and children with headache: evidence-based diagnostic evaluation. Neuroimag Clin North Am 13:225–235, 2003.

Mehta V, Chapman A, McNeely, PD, et al: Latency between symptom onset and diagnosis of pediatric brain tumors: An eastern canadian geographic study. Neurosurgery, 51:365–373, 2002.

Merchant TE, Kiehna EN, Miles MA, et al: Acute effects of irradiation on cognition: changes in attention on a computerized continuous performance test during radiotherapy in pediatric patients with localized primary brain tumors. Int J Radiat Oncol Biol Phys 53(5):1271–1278, 2002.

Meyer EA, Kieran MW: Psychological adjustment of "surgery-only" pediatric neuro-oncology patients: a retrospective analysis. Psychooncology 11:74–49, 2002.

Meyers CA, Weitzner MA, Valentine AD, et al: Methylphenidate therapy improves cognition mood, and function of brain tumor patients. J Clin Oncol 16:2522–2527, 1998.

Moore BD 3rd. Neurocognitive outcomes in survivors of childhood cancer. Journal of Pediatric Psychology. 30(1):51–63, 2005 Jan–Feb.

Moore BD, Ater JL, Copeland DR: Improved neuropsychological outcome in children with brain tumors diagnosed during infancy and treated without cranial irradiation. J Child Neurol 7:281–290, 1992.

Mordecai D, Shaw RJ, Fisher PG, et al: Case study: suprasellar germinoma presenting with psychotic and obsessive-compulsive symptoms. J Am Acad Child Adolesc Psychiatry 39:1, 2000.

Moss HA, Nannis ED, Poplack DG: The effects of prophylactic treatment of the central nervous system on the intellectual functioning of children with acute lymphocytic leukemia. Am J Med 71:47–52, 1981.

Mostow EN, Byrne J, Connelly RR, et al: Quality of life in long-term survivors of CNS tumors of childhood and adolescence. J Clin Oncol 9:592–599, 1991.

Mulhern RK: Neuropsychological late effects, in DJ Bearison, RK Mulhern (eds.). *Pediatric Psychooncology*. New York: Oxford University Press, 1994:99–121.

Mulhern RK, Butler RW. Neurocognitive sequelae of childhood cancers and their treatment. Pediatric Rehabilitation. 7(1):1-14; discussion 15-6, 2004 Jan–Mar.

Mulhern RK, Khan RB, Kaplan S, Helton S, Christensen R, Bonner M, Brown R, Xiong X, Wu S, Gururangan S, Reddick WE. Short-term efficacy of methylphenidate: a randomized, double-blind, placebo-controlled trial among survivors of childhood cancer. Journal of Clinical Oncology. 22(23):4795–803, 2004 Dec 1.

Mulhern RK, Kun LE: Neuropsychologic functioning in children with brain tumors, III: interval changes in the six months following treatment. Med Pediatr Oncol 13:318–324, 1985.

Mulhern RK, Crisco JJ, Kun LE: Neuropsychological sequelae of childhood brain tumors: a review. J Clin Child Psychol 12:66–73, 1983.

Mulhern RK, Merchant TE, Gajjar A, Reddick WE, Kun LE. Late neurocognitive sequelae in survivors of brain tumours in childhood. Lancet Oncology. 5(7):399–408, 2004 Jul.

Mulhern RK, Ochs J, Fairclough D, et al: Intellectual and academic achievement status after CNS relapse: a retrospective analysis of 40 children treated for ALL. J Clin Oncol 5:933–940, 1987.

Mulhern RK, Palmer SL, Merchant T, Wallace D, et al. Neurocognitive Consequences of Risk-Adapted Therapy for Childhood Medulloblastoma. J Clinical Oncology Aug 20 2005: 5511–5519.

Mulhern RK, Kovnar EH, Kun LE, et al: Psychologic and neurologic function following treatment of childhood temporal astrocytoma. J Child Neurol 3:47–53, 1988.

Mulhern RK, Horowitz ME, Kovnar EH, et al: Neurodevelopmental status of infants and young children treated for brain tumors with preirradiation chemotherapy. J Clin Oncol 7:1660–1666, 1989a.

Mulhern RK, Wasserman AL, Friedman AG, et al: Social competence and behavioral adjustment of children who are long-term survivors of cancer. Pediatrics 83:18–25, 1989b.

Mulhern RK, Hancock J, Fairclough D, et al: Neuropsychological status of children treated for brain tumors: a critical review and integrative analysis. Med Pediatr Oncol 20:181–191, 1992.

Mulhern RK, Carpentieri S, Shema S, et al: Factors associated with social and behavioral problems among children recently diagnosed with brain tumor. J Pediatr Psychol 18:339–350, 1993.

Mulhern RK, Heideman RL, Khatib Z, et al: Quality of survival among children treated for brain stem glioma. Pediatr Neurosurg 20:226–232, 1994.

Mulhern RK, Kepner JL, Thomas PRR, et al. Neuropsychologic functioning of survivors of childhood medulloblastoma randomized to receive conventional or reduced-dose craniospinal irradiation: a Pediatric Oncology Group study. J Clin Oncol 16:1723–1728, 1998.

Mulhern RK, Reddick WE, Palmer SL, et al: Neurocognitive deficits in medulloblastoma survivors and white matter loss. Ann Neurol 46(6):834–41, 1999.

Mulhern RK, Palmer S: Neurocognitive late effects in pediatric cancer. Curr Probl Cancer 27(4): 177–197, 2003.

Murray, MA. *Thematic Apperception Test*. Cambridge: Harvard University Press, 1943.

Nakaji P, Meltzer HS, Singel SA, et al: Improvement of aggressive and antisocial behavior after resection of temporal lobe tumors. Pediatrics 112:430–433, 2003.

Nassau JH, Drotar D: Social competence among children with central nervous system-related chronic health conditions. Rev J Pediatr Psychol 22:771–793, 1997.

Noll RB, Ris MD, Davies WH, Butkowski WM, Koontz K. Social interactions between children with cancer or sickle cell disease and their peers: teacher ratings. Dev Behav Pediatr 13:187–193, 1992.

Ochs JJ, Berger P, Brecher ML, et al: Computed tomography brain scans in children with acute lymphocytic leukemia receiving methotrexate alone as central nervous system prophylaxis. Cancer 45:2274–2278, 1980.

Overmeyer S, Rothenberger A, Koelfen W: Psychiatric disturbances in children with hamartomas: a neglected somatopsychic issue. Acta Paedopsychiatr 55: 243–249, 1992.

Packer RJ, Gurney JG, Punyko JA, et al: Long-term neurologic and neurosensory sequelae in adult survivors of a childhood brain tumor: Childhood cancer survivor study. J Clin Oncol 21:3255–3261, 2003.

Packer RJ, Sposto R, Atkins TE, et al: Quality of life in children with primitive neuroectodermal tumors (medulloblastoma) of the posterior fossa. Pediatr Neurosci 13:169–175, 1987.

Packer RJ, Sutton LN, Atkins TE, et al: A prospective study of cognitive function in children receiving whole-brain radiotherapy and chemotherapy: 2-year results. J Neurosurg 70:707–713, 1989.

Palmer SL, Goloubeva O, Reddick WE, et al: Patterns of intellectual development among survivors of pediatric medulloblastoma; A longitudinal analysis. J Clin Oncol 19:2302–2308, 2001.

Peterson BS, Bronen RA, Duncan CC: Three cases of symptom change in Tourette's syndrome and obsessive-compulsive disorder associated with paediatric cerebral malignancies. J Neurol Neurosurg Psychiatry 61:497–505, 1996.

Peylan-Ramu N, Poplack DG, Pizzo PA, et al: Abnormal CT scans of the brain in asymptomatic children with acute lymphocytic leukemia after prophylactic treatment of the central nervous system with radiation and intrathecal chemotherapy. N Engl J Med 298:815–818, 1978.

Picard EM, Rourke BP: Neuropsychological consequences of prophylactic treatment for acute lymphocytic leukemia, in BP Rourke (ed.). *Syndrome of Nonverbal Learning Disabilities*. New York: Guilford, 1995:282–330.

Poggi G, Liscio M, Galbiati S, Adduci A, Massimino M, Gandola L, Spreafico F, Clerici CA, Fossati-Bellani F, Sommovigo M, Castelli E. Brain tumors in children and adolescents: cognitive and psychological disorders at different ages. Psycho-Oncology. 14(5): 386–95, 2005 May.

Price TR, Goetz KL, Lovell MR: Neuropsychiatric aspects of brain tumors. In Yudofsky SC, Hales RE (eds.). *The American Psychiatric Press Textbook of Neuropsychiatry*, 2nd Ed. Washington, DC: American Psychiatric Press, 1992:473–497.

Radcliffe J, Packer RJ, Atkins TE, et al: Three- and four-year cognitive outcome in children with noncortical brain tumors treated with whole-brain radiotherapy. Ann Neurol 32:551–554, 1992.

Radcliffe J, Bunin GR, Sutton LN, et al: Cognitive deficits in long-term survivors of childhood medulloblastoma and other noncortical tumors: age-dependent effects of whole brain radiation. Int J Dev Neurosci 12: 327–334, 1994.

Radcliffe J, Bennett D, Kazak AE, et al: Adjustment in childhood brain tumor survival: child, mother and teacher report. J Pediatr Psychol 21:529–539, 1996.

Raimondi AJ, Tomita T: Advantages of "total" resection of medulloblastoma and disadvantages of full head post-operative radiation therapy. Childs Brain 5:550–551, 1979.

Rauck AM, Green DM, Yasui Y, et al: Marriage in the survivors of childhood cancer: A preliminary description from the childhood cancer survivor study. Med Pediatr Oncol 33:60–63, 1999.

Reddick WE, Whit HA, Glass JO, et al: Developmental model relating white matter volume to neurocognitive deficits in pediatric brain tumor survivors. Cancer 97: 2512–2519, 2003.

Reimers T, Ehrenfels S, Lykke Mortensen E, et al: Cognitive deficits in long-term survivors of childhood brain tumors: Identification of predictive factors. Med Pediatr Oncol 40:26–34, 2003.

Reynolds, C , Kamphaus RC. *Behavior Assessment System for Children (BASC)*. Circle Pines, MN: American Guidance Service Publishing, 1992.

Reynolds CR, Richmond BO. Revised Children's Manifest Anxiety Scales (RCMAS) Manual. Los Angeles: Western Psychological Services.

Ris MB, Packer R, Goldwein J, et al: Intellectual outcome after reduced-dose radiation therapy plus adjuvant chemotherapy for medulloblastoma: A children's cancer group study. J Clin Oncol 19:3470–3476, 2001.

Ris MB, Noll R: Long-term neurobehavioral outcome in pediatric brain tumor patients: review and methodological critique. J Clin Exp Neuropsychol 16:21–42, 1994.

Riva D, Pantaleoni C, Milani N, et al: Impairment of neuropsychological functions in children with medulloblastomas and astrocytomas in the posterior fossa. Childs Nerv Syst 5:107–110, 1989.

Ron MA: Psychiatric manifestations of frontal lobe tumors. Br J Psychiatry 155:735–738, 1989.

Ross L, Johansen C, Oksbjerg D, et al: Psychiatric hospitalizations among survivors of cancer in childhood or adolescence. N Engl J Med 349:650–657, 2003.

Rowland JH, Glidewell OJ, Sibley RF, et al: Effects of different forms of central nervous system prophylaxis on neuropsychologic function in childhood leukemia. J Clin Oncol 2:1327–1335, 1984.

Rutter M, Graham P, Yule W, et al: *A Neuropsychiatric Study in Childhood (Clinics in Developmental Medicine 35/36)*. London: Heinemann, 1970.

Ryan ND: Discussion of "Diagnostic utility of endocrine and neuroimaging screening tests in first-onset adolescent psychosis." J Am Acad Child Adolesc Psychiatry 35:73, 1996.

Seaver E, Geyer R, Sulzbacher S, et al: Psychosocial adjustment in long-term survivors of childhood medulloblastoma and ependymoma treated with craniospinal irradiation. Pediatr Neurosurg 20:248–253, 1994.

Shuren JE, Flynn R, Fennell E, et al: Insula and obsessive-compulsive disorder (letter). Can J Psychiatry 40:112, 1995.

Silber JH, Radcliffe J, Peckham V, et al: Whole-brain irradiation and decline in intelligence: the influence of dose and age on IQ score. J Clin Oncol 10:1390–1396, 1992.

Silverman CL, Palkes H, Talent B, et al: Late effects of radiotherapy on patients with cerebellar medulloblastoma. Cancer 54:825–829, 1984.

Slavc I, Salchegger C, Hauer C, et al: Follow-up and quality of survival of 67 consecutive children with CNS tumors. Childs Nerv Syst 10:433–443, 1994.

Sparrow SS, Balla DA, Cicchetti DV. *Vineland Adaptive Behavior Scales*. Circle Pines, MN: American Guidance Service, 1984.

Spiegler BJ, Bouffet E, Greenberg ML, Rutka JT, Mabbott DJ. Change in neurocognitive functioning after treatment with cranial radiation in childhood. Journal of Clinical Oncology. 22(4):706–13, 2004 Feb 15.

Spunberg JJ, Chang CH, Goldman M, et al: Quality of long-term survival following irradiation for intracranial tumors in children under the age of two. Int J Radiat Oncol Biol Phys 7:727–736, 1981.

Starkstein SE, Boston JD, Robinson RG: Mechanisms of mania after brain injury: 12 case reports and review of the literature. J Nerv Ment Dis 176:87–100, 1988.

Steen RG, Spence D, Wu S, et al: Effect of therapeutic ionizing radiation on the human brain. Ann Neurol 50:787–795, 2001.

Steen RG, Koury BSM, Granja CI, et al: Effect of ionizing radiation on the human brain: white matter and gray matter T1 in pediatric brain tumor patients treated with conformal radiation therapy. Int J Radiat Oncol Biol Phys 49:79–91, 2001.

Stein M, Duffner PK, Werry JS, et al: School refusal and emotional lability in a 6-year-old boy. Dev Behav Pediatr 17:187–190, 1996.

Stuber ML, Kazak AE, Meeske K, et al: Is posttraumatic stress a viable model for understanding responses to childhood cancer? Rev Child Adolesc Psychiatr Clin North Am 7:169–82, 1998.

Syndikus I, Tait D, Ashley S, et al: Long-term follow-up of young children with brain tumors after irradiation. Int J Radiat Oncol Biol Phys 30:781–787, 1994.

Thomas PR, Deutsch M, Kepner JL, et al. Low-stage medulloblastoma: final analysis of trial comparing standard-dose with reduced-dose neuraxis irradiation. J Clin Oncol 18:3004–3011, 2000.

Thompson SJ, Leigh L, Christensen R, et al: Immediate neurocognitive effects of methylphenidate on learning-impaired survivors of childhood cancer. J Clin Oncol 19:1802–8, 2001.

Torres C, Korones D, Palumbo D et al. Effect of methylphenidate in the post-radiation attention and memory deficits in children. Ann Neurol 40 (1996), pp. 331–332.

VanEffenterre R, Boch AL: Craniopharyngioma in adults and children: a study of 122 surgical cases. J Neurosurg 97:3–11, 2002.

Vannatta K, Gartstein MA, Short A, et al: A controlled study of peer relationships of children surviving brain tumors: Teacher, peer, and self ratings. J Pediatr Psychol 23:279–287, 1998.

Wechsler, D. *Wechsler Intelligence Scale for Children-Fourth Edition*. San Antonio, TX: The Psychological Corporation, 2004

Wilkinson, GS. *The Wide Range Achievement Test-3 (WRAT-3)*, Baltimore, MD: Wide Range, Inc., 1993.

Weinberger DR: Brain disease and psychiatric illness: when should a psychiatrist order a CT scan? Am J Psychiatry 141:1521–1527, 1984.

Weller RA, Weller EB: Anorexia nervosa in a patient with an infiltrating tumor of the hypothalamus. Am J Psychiatry 139:824–829, 1982.

Wirt 2001 Wirt, RD, Lacher D, Seat PD, et al. *Personality Inventory for Children -2nd Edition*. Los Angeles: Western Psychological Services, 2001.

Yachnis AT: Neuropathology of pediatric brain tumors. Semin Pediatr Neurol 4:282–291, 1997.

Zaki A, Natarajan N, Mettlin CJ: Patterns of presentation in brain tumors in the United States. J Surg Oncol 53:110–112, 1993.

Zametkin AJ, Ernst M, Silver R. Laboratory and diagnostic testing in child and adolescent psychiatry: a review of the past 10 years. J Am Acad Child Adol Psychiatry 37:468, 1998.

Zebrack BJ, Gurney JG, Oeffinger K, Whitton J, Packer RJ, Mertens A, Turk N, Castleberry R, Dreyer Z, Robison LL, Zeltzer LK. Psychological outcomes in long-term survivors of childhood brain cancer: a report from the childhood cancer survivor study. Journal of Clinical Oncology. 22(6):999–1006, 2004 Mar 15.

Principles of
Treatment In Pediatric
Neuropsychiatry

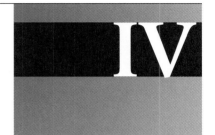

Pediatric Psychopharmacology

27

Daniel A. Geller, MBBS, FRACP   *Paul Hammerness, MD*

Since the first edition of this text, there have been important advances in our knowledge of pediatric psychopharmacology. Since the mid-1990s, our understanding and appreciation of both the neurobiological underpinnings of childhood psychiatric disorders as well as neuropsychopharmacology have increased (1), the randomized controlled trials literature has continued to expand, novel agents have come to market, and, in support of pediatric pharmacology research, the president signed the Pediatric Research Equity Act into law on December 3, 2003. This law codifies the protections of the 1998 Pediatric Rule, a Food and Drug Administration (FDA) regulation requiring drug manufacturers to test their products for use in children, which provided incentives to industry to study investigational new drugs (INDs) in children, gave an impetus to the field, and doubled the evidence base for pediatric psychopharmacology. While enactment of this legislation supports the continuation of pediatric clinical psychopharmacology trials, industry as well as federal and other efforts are needed to bridge the large gaps in our knowledge of pediatric psychopharmacology. Indeed, because of the ethical and methodological difficulties in conducting pharmacological research in minors (2), many new medications are used "off-label" after being studied and approved in adults only.

Psychopharmacology may be divided into two broad domains: pharmacokinetics, which refers to the actions of the body upon the drug, and pharmacodynamics, which refers to the actions of the drug on the body at its target site(s). It is now understood that children are not simply small adults and that treatment practices used for adults may not translate well into safe or effective treatments for children. Changes with age in both pharmacokinetic and pharmacodynamic parameters may lead to differences in

clinical response and adverse effect profiles in children versus adults (2). A number of relevant physiological changes occur during growth and development (3). For example, height and weight increase markedly during childhood and adolescence (4). The proportion of total body water and extracellular water decreases from birth, reaching adult values by 12 years of age (5). The percentage of body fat doubles through infancy and then decreases with an increase in lean body mass during early childhood (2), which increases again in later life.

PHARMACOKINETICS

Pharmacokinetics refers to the body's actions on a drug. Unique properties of the drug such as pH, fat solubility, protein binding, and molecular weight will affect its absorption from the gastrointestinal (GI) tract or elsewhere, its distribution (especially in the brain), and its metabolism and eventual excretion (4). Compared with adults, children have more rapid metabolism and excretion of many drugs due to a greater relative liver mass and greater renal clearance. Such factors may produce shorter half-lives of drugs compared with adults, necessitating more frequent dosing schedules to yield steady plasma levels and avoid withdrawal effects. Pharmacokinetic differences between children and adults lessen by late puberty.

Absorption

Although studies examining differences in drug absorption among children, adolescents, and adults are limited, gastrointestinal absorption rates are generally faster in children compared with adults (6). Since younger children have decreased gastric acidity (higher pH), weak bases are preferentially absorbed and weak acids more slowly absorbed (5). By adolescence, gastric pH and emptying time are similar to adults. Disturbances in bowel flora, from the frequent use of antibiotics, for example, may lead to changes in intestinal motility and bile acid function in ways not yet studied. The effect of probiotic supplementation on drug absorption, though popular, is also unknown.

Distribution

Drug distribution is affected by several factors, including extracellular water volume, serum albumin concentration, and percentage of body fat (5). Children have a greater relative, but smaller absolute, extracellular water volume (volume of distribution) compared with adults. Since free drug is distributed into the extracellular volume, the smaller absolute volumes in children will lead to faster equilibration and half-life and higher drug concentration compared to the higher volumes of adults. Because many drugs are highly protein bound, the variable serum albumin concentrations of children may lead to inter- and intraindividual differences in the proportion of drug that is protein bound and consequently the concentration of free and active drug in plasma (5). Any condition that causes a reduction in serum protein concentration, such as nephrotic syndrome, will lead to decreased binding and increased free drug concentration and possible toxicity (4). Because obesity in children has reached epidemic proportions in North America, variability in proportion of body fat is an important factor for drugs that are fat soluble. In addition to having better blood-brain barrier penetration, fat-soluble drugs are stored in fat and redistributed to plasma and brain over time. Morbidly obese subjects may require higher doses of such drugs for these reasons.

For the purposes of psychopharmacology, the brain is the target organ of interest, yet the in vivo study of drugs in the brain is severely hampered by the difficulty of assaying the drug at this site. New techniques in noninvasive imaging, especially magnetic resonance spectroscopy may, however, permit repeated in vivo sampling of chemicals in the brain at specific sites of interest and offer promise for significant breakthroughs in psychopharmacology. While the permeability of the blood-brain barrier is thought to be compromised in children with neurological insult such as perinatal ischemia, little is known about this important property in children with more subtle developmental disabilities.

Metabolism and Excretion

As noted earlier, children have greater *relative* liver volume and weight-adjusted mass compared with adults as well as more rapid kidney filtration that may lead to shorter drug half-lives and the need for higher weight-based dosages (2, 7, 8). Of the four primary hepatic pathways for drug metabolism, oxidation, reduction, hydrolysis, and conjugation(5), oxidative pathways appear to be more rapid in children compared with adults (2). Further, changes in binding capacity of cytochrome P450 enzymes (4) lead to greater oxidation in males compared to females after puberty. Drugs that are primarily excreted via the kidney (for example, lithium) may have a shorter half-life in older children compared with adults, although the clinical significance of this finding is uncertain (7).

PHARMACODYNAMICS

The mechanism of a drug's action at its target site, in this case the nervous system, and the secondary and tertiary events that lead to a drug's desired activity are termed *pharmacodynamic* actions. While the primary event is frequently at the neuronal membrane such as a receptor or uptake site, it may also be intracellular such as with the highly soluble drug lithium. Secondary and tertiary cascades of effects such as changes in energy metabolism or conformational shape and permeability of ion channels ensue, leading often to intranuclear effects that are translated via transcription and protein synthesis leading to altered neuronal function. We do not know how and whether age-related developmental changes in these pharmacodynamic processes occur and what effects in turn such changes have on the expression of drug actions in humans. Childhood and adolescence are characterized by rapid anatomic and functional changes in the brain that persist into adulthood. While animal data indicate developmental differences in the ontogeny of both serotonergic and noradrenergic systems, which could affect response to psychotropics (9), human studies suggest more stability in serotonergic systems but significant changes in both dopaminergic and noradrenergic systems over the course of development. For example, striatal dopamine receptor density decreases rapidly in the second decade of life. The spontaneous resolution of many chronic tic disorders in adolescence may be a reflection of these changes. This decrease, however, continues throughout life (10) and may result in decreased dopaminergic activity (11) and an increased risk for Parkinson's disease or depression in the elderly. In contrast, noradrenergic activity increases after puberty (12, 13). This finding could explain in part the differential efficacy of the tricyclic antidepressants in adults compared with children.

Lastly, the serotonergic system is a phylogenetically ancient transmitter system that is developed during early fetal life and appears relatively mature in humans at birth. It may be for this reason that serotonergic drugs appear to affect even young children, in contrast to noradrenergic drugs. Serotonin synthesis in preschool children may even reach a 200% increase over adult rates, until near school age when it may drop to adult levels (14).

Attention has focused on serotonin, dopamine, and norepinephrine systems largely because it is these systems that are targeted by our common armementarium of medications. However, many other neurotransmitter systems that are of interest and may yield important advances in psychopharmacology have yet to be well studied, especially developmentally. Examples include increased acetylcholine concentration in the cortex during adolescence (theoretically leading to improved memory and retention) and the important roles of glutamate and GABA (gamma-aminobutyric acid) over time. Like looking for a lost coin under a street lamp because that is where the light is to be found, our knowledge of developmental changes in pharmacodynamics, outside the halo provided by drugs that serve as pharmacological probes, is extremely limited. It remains unknown whether psychotropics administered to youth can produce changes in the neuroanatomy or neurophysiology of the developing brain that persist after the drug is discontinued; that is, whether permanent changes occur (2). This issue is clearly of great concern as there is at least some animal data suggesting that this is possible (15).

Compliance

The magnitude of *noncompliance*, that is, of *not* taking medication as prescribed in pediatric medicine, is a clinically significant issue in all populations and at all ages. In youth with psychological and emotional disorders, rates of noncompliance as a limiting factor in treatment efficacy are likely to be even greater. Further, children rarely self-administer, relying on parents to remember and give medications (16). In traditional pediatric settings, noncompliance rates are at least 50% (16). In addition, physicians do a poor job in assessing noncompliance in their patients (17). As in most areas of medicine, the therapeutic relationship is an essential element in drug compliance, but adequate education (*informed* consent), frequent supervision, simplified drug regimens, and peer support can also be helpful (16).

Special Populations

Psychopharmacological agents may have radically different effects in patients who are neurologically compromised compared to nonneurologically impaired individuals. For example, in patients with perinatal injuries leading to mental retardation, seizures, or cerebral palsy, atypical and unexpected responses may occur so that caution and vigilance are necessary when introducing psychoactive medication into this population. Clearly, a host of illnesses and pathophysiology are represented in these children so that no general rules may be generated for practitioners other than "start low and go slow."

Because neurologically compromised children are usually excluded from clinical studies and research protocols, the existing literature provides little guidance on their

management. Existing data on drug characteristics and treatment recommendations are therefore derived from neurologically "healthy" subjects.

Drug Monitoring

Therapeutic drug monitoring in pediatric psychopharmacology has a limited role. First and most important, the correlation between plasma levels and therapeutic effects are often poor and unhelpful, providing no useful information to the clinician. One example is monitoring stimulant plasma levels in the treatment of the child with attention deficit hyperactivity disorder (ADHD) where the correlation between plasma and brain levels is poor and tremendous intraindividual variability occurs. Therapeutic ranges are guidelines only, frequently derived from adult dose titration studies of efficacy and tolerability, and may not apply closely to children. For drugs with a low margin of safety or with potential serious adverse events (such as lithium and the antiepileptic drugs), serum levels are clearly important. By convention, drugs are measured at their trough levels; that is, at the lowest plasma levels obtained just prior to next dosing after steady state is achieved, or about five half-lives.

For off-label dosing in youth, strategies based simply on age, weight, or even body surface area and derived from adult studies may not be correct (5, 8). Body surface area calculations are feasible based on weight and height, but routine measurement of these parameters among child psychiatrists is still not widespread, and their use in clinical settings is not practical because dose guidelines based on body surface area are usually not provided. At a minimum, however, practitioners should endeavor to obtain weight at baseline and regular intervals, since weight-based dosing provides at least some guidance. Ultimately, practitioners must rely on a mix of the evidence-based medical literature that is summarized in this chapter, practice guidelines where available, expert clinical opinion, and individual clinical experience.

AN EVIDENCE-BASED APPROACH

Treatment decisions are increasingly being made on research-based evidence rather than on expert opinion or clinical experience alone. In 1999, Congress directed the Agency for Healthcare Research and Quality (AHRQ) to undertake a systematic examination of approaches to assess the strength of scientific evidence. Such systems allow evaluation of either individual articles or entire bodies of research on a particular subject for use in making evidence-based health care decisions and to provide some guidance as to "best practices" in the field. Several generic systems were identified that fully addressed key quality domains for systematic reviews, randomized controlled trials (RCTs), observational studies, and diagnostic test studies. For example, a description of the study population (including inclusion and exclusion criteria), randomization, blinding, interventions, outcomes (including "last observation carried forward" data and description of dropouts), and statistical analysis were key domains for RCTs. Of note, sources of sponsorship or funding were considered key elements for each type of study (e.g., industry sponsored). Systems for grading the strength of a body of evidence, including the quality, quantity, and consistency of studies, are also included in this report (18). These methods have been applied to trials evaluating newer pharmacotherapies for depression as well the treatment of ADHD, where 78 RCTs were included.

A simpler quality rating system was devised by the Texas Consensus Conference Panel on Medication Treatment of Childhood Major Depressive Disorder. This widely imitated system categorizes data into three levels: Level A data consist of both child and adult randomized controlled clinical trials, Level B data consist of open trials and retrospective analyses, and Level C data are based on case reports and expert panel consensus as to recommended clinical practices.

At its best, evidence-based medicine is the conscientious, explicit, and judicious use of current best evidence in making individual patient-care decisions. The practice of evidence-based medicine means integrating individual clinical expertise with the best available external evidence from systematic research (18). Despite the obvious premise of evidence-based medicine, the great variability by region and discipline in current practice in child psychiatry argues against the notion that it is already in widespread use. Following the lead from other disciplines, efforts have been made to present an evidence-based approach in pediatric psychiatry (19, 20). These authors concluded that "although the number of evidence based treatments in child psychiatry is growing, much of clinical practice remains based on the adult literature and traditional models of care" (19, p. 1388). In this chapter, we use an evidence-based approach to clinical pediatric psychopharmacology by attending to the quality of individual studies as well as the strength of the entire body of evidence. Limitations in such an approach abound and include the numerous exclusion criteria used in clinical trials (especially industry sponsored trials) that affect the representativeness of study samples (21), high placebo response rates in child subjects, frequent comorbidity in many if not all child psychiatric disorders and lack of validity of current diagnostic nosology in pediatric subjects.

Finally, in view of the great responsibility involved in prescribing psychoactive agents to minors, diligence is needed in disseminating evidence-based efficacy information as well as accurate safety data to practicing clinicians. A special section of the *Journal of the American Academy of Child and Adolescent Psychiatry* dedicated to a review of safety assessments in pediatric psychopharmacology found inconsistency in safety ascertainment as a major limitation

in identifying drug-induced adverse events (22). In the following section of the edition, Vitiello et al. (2003) (23) described methods for more rigorous, standardized drug safety evaluation. Since we lack a well defined "standard of care" for much of child psychopharmacology practice, the dictum *non nocere* ("do no harm") is especially relevant.

OVERVIEW OF PEDIATRIC PSYCHOPHARMACOLOGY

In this chapter, we review the clinical pharmacology and the psychotherapeutic use of psychotropics used to manage and treat neuropsychiatric disorders in children and adolescents. The primary agents used in pediatric psychopharmacology, antidepressants, anxiolytics, mood stabilizers, antipsychotics, and stimulants, will be discussed in separate sections, integrating psychopharmacology and clinical application. Pharmacokinetic and pharmacodynamic information relevant to each class is discussed, followed by an evidence-based review of the supporting literature, safety data, and, finally, guidelines regarding initiation and maintenance of clinical treatment and monitoring. For many common applications in pediatric psychopharmacology, there is a dearth of controlled data and limited FDA approval in pediatric populations. As such, clinical use, which covers a broad spectrum of juvenile psychiatric illness, is primarily "off-label" (see Table 27.1), creating a dilemma for clinicians who, in good faith, seek to relieve symptomatic distress in their young patients.

ANTIDEPRESSANTS

This section reviews the neuropsychopharmacology and the psychotherapeutic use of antidepressants used to manage and treat a variety of neuropsychiatric disorders in children and adolescents, not just depression. Selective serotonin reuptake inhibitors (SSRIs) and mixed action agents, including Nefazadone, Buproprion, Venlafaxine, Mirtazapine, and tricyclic antidepressants (TCAs), will be reviewed separately.

SELECTIVE SEROTONIN REUPTAKE INHIBITORS (SSRIs)

Neuropsychopharmacology

Although usually considered as a single homogeneous class of agents, SSRI medications do differ in their pharmacology and clinical application. The pharmacokinetics and pharmacodynamics of SSRIs is briefly discussed here; more detailed reviews of the neurotransmitter serotonin and the pharmacology of SSRIs can be found elsewhere (24–27). SSRIs available in the United States include citalopram (Celexa), fluoxetine (Prozac), fluvoxamine (Luvox), parox-

TABLE 27.1

COMMON MEDICATIONS USED IN PEDIATRIC PSYCHOPHARMACOLOGY RANKED BY LEVEL OF SUPPORTING EVIDENCE

Trade Name	Generic Name	Level of Support	Indication	FDA Approved Age (Years)
SSRIs				
Celexa	Citalopram	A, B, C	MDD[A] anxiety[B] OCD[B] PTSD[B] impulse control disorders[C]	N/A
Luvox	Fluvoxamine	A, C	OCD[A] anxiety[A] PTSD[C]	≥8
Paxil	Paroxetine	A, B, C	MDD[A] OCD[A] panic[B] PTSD[C] impulse control disorders[C]	N/A
Prozac	Fluoxetine	A, B, C	OCD[A] MDD[A] anxiety[B] panic[B] bulimia[B] PTSD[C] impulse control disorders[C] Anorexia[C]	≥7
Zoloft	Sertraline	A, B, C	OCD[A] MDD[Aα] anxiety[A] PTSD[C] impulse control disorders[C] ED[C]	≥6
Other Mood Medications				
Wellbutrin	Bupropion	A, B	ADHD[A] MDD[B]	N/A
Remeron	Mirtazapine	B, C	MDD[B] autism[C]	N/A
Desyrel	Trazodone	B, C	Sleep disturbances[B] PTSD[C]	N/A
Effexor	Venlafaxine	B	MDD OCD autism	N/A
Tricyclic Antidepressants				
Elavil	Amitriptyline	C	Severe MDD[C]	N/A
Anafranil	Clomipramine	A, B, C	OCD[A] PDD[B] MDD[C]	≥10
Norpramin	Desipramine	A, B, C	Tics[A] ADHD[A] anxiety[B] MDD[C]	N/A
Sinequan	Doxepin	A, C	Anxiety[A] MDD[C]	≥12
Tofranil	Imipramine	A, B	Enuresis[A] anxiety[B] ADHD[B]	≥6
Pamelor	Nortritptyline	B, C	Tics[B] ADHD[B] severe MDD[C]	N/A
Stimulant Medications				
Adderall	Amphetamine	A	ADHD	≥3
Adderall XR (extended release)	Amphetamine	A	ADHD	≥6
Concerta	Methylphenidate	A	ADHD	≥6
Cylert	Pemoline	A	ADHD	≥6
Dexedrine	Dextroamphetamine	A	ADHD	≥3
Dextrostat	Dextroamphetamine	A	ADHD	≥3
Focalin	Dexmethylphenidate	A	ADHD	≥6
Metadate ER	Methylphenidate	A	ADHD	≥6
Metadate CD	Methylphenidate	A	ADHD	≥6
Ritalin	Methylphenidate	A	ADHD	≥6
Ritalin LA	Methylphenidate	A	ADHD	≥6
Nonstimulant for ADHD				
Strattera	Atomoxetine	A	ADHD	≥6
Antipsychotic Medications				
Thorazine	Chlorpromazine	A	Schizophrenia	N/A
Clozaril	Clozapine	A	Schizophrenia	N/A
Haldol	Haloperidol	A	Tics/Tourette's, psychosis/schizophrenia	≥3
Loxitane	Loxepine	A[α]	Schizophrenia	N/A
Zyprexa	Olanzapine	B, C	Psychosis[B] ED[B] autism/PDD[B] bipolar disorder[C]	N/A
Orap	Pimozide	A	Tourette's syndrome	≥2
Seroquel	Quetiapine	A,[α] B, C	Bipolar disorders[AαC] psychosis[B] autism/PDD[B]	N/A
Risperdal	Risperidone	A, B, C	Tourette's syndrome[A] autism[A] severe behavioral disturbance[A] psychosis/schizophrenia bipolar disorder[C] OCD[C]	N/A
Mellaril	Thioridazine	A	Severe behavioral disturbance and hyperactivity	≥2
Geodon	Ziprasidone	B	Psychosis, autism/PDD	N/A

(continued)

TABLE 27.1
(continued)

Trade Name	Generic Name	Level of Support	Indication	FDA Approved Age (Years)
Lithium				
CibalithNAS	Lithium citrate	A,B	Bipolar disorder[A] dysphoric Conduct disorder[B]	≥12
Eskalith	Lithium carbonate	A,B	Bipolar disorder[A] dysphoric Conduct disorder[B]	≥12
Lithobid	Lithium carbonate	A,B	Bipolar disorder[A] dysphoric Conduct disorder[B]	≥12
Antiepileptic Medications				
Tegretol	Carbamazepine	A, B, C	Seizures[A] aggression[B] bipolar disorder[C]	≥6
Depakote	Divalproex Sodium	A, B	Seizures[A] aggression[B] bipolar disorder[B]	≥2
Neurontin	Gabapentin	C	Mood anxiety	N/A
Lamictal	Lamotrigine	C	MDD bipolar disorder	N/A
Trileptal	Oxcarbazepine	C	Bipolar disorder	N/A
Gabitril	Tiagabine	C	Mood disorder	N/A
Topamax	Topiramate	C	Bipolar disorder weight control	N/A

[a]Adolescents only.
N/A, Not approved for pediatric use; ADHD: Attention-deficit/hyperactivity disorder; ED: Eating disorder; OCD: Obsessive-compulsive disorder; TS: Tourette's disorder.
Level A data consist of pediatric randomized controlled clinical trials.
Level B data consist of open trials and retrospective analyses.
Level C data are based on case reports or panel consensus as to recommended current clinical practice.

etine (Paxil), and sertraline (Zoloft). At this time only fluoxetine (depression and obsessive-compulsive disorder [OCD]), fluvoxamine (OCD), and sertraline (OCD) are FDA approved for use in children.

Pharmacokinetics

After ingestion, SSRIs are all well absorbed from the gut but differ in their subsequent bioavailability, metabolism, degree of protein binding, presence of metabolites, and elimination (24, 28) (Table 27.2).

In general, recommended weight-adjusted doses of SSRIs have been similar in children and adolescents compared with adults. Although limited, some information regarding the pharmacokinetic properties of the SSRIs in children have emerged, including studies of sertraline (29–32), fluoxetine (33), and paroxetine (34).

When normalized for body weight, pediatric pharmacokinetic studies have demonstrated many similarities compared to adults, including interindividual pharmacokinetic variation. For example, Strauss et al. (2002) (35) conducted a fluorine magnetic resonance spectroscopy study of

TABLE 27.2
SSRI PHARMACOKINETIC PARAMETERS

	Citalopram	Fluoxetine	Sertraline	Paroxetine	Fluvoxamine
Percentage protein bound	80	94	99	95	77
T-Max (hours)	3–4	6–8	6–8	2–8	2–8
Half-life hours(♦)	35	24–72*(120)	25	11*(20)	11*(15)
Half-life of active metabolite (days)	N/A	7	2.5–4.5	N/A	N/A
Linear kinetics	Yes	No	Yes	No	No
Dose range (mg/d)	5–60	5–80	25–200	5–60	25–300
Absorption altered by fast or fed status	No	No	Yes	No	No
GI absorption (%)	~100	80	≥44	≥64	≥94

* Single dose.
♦ Steady-state hours.
T-Max: Time to peak plasma level.
N/A: Not applicable.
Sources: Van Harten (1993) (610); Preskorn (1997) (611); data on file, Forest Laboratories; Preskorn (1993) (612). Notations in parentheses indicate alternate metabolic pathways for the substrate listed.
Source: Adapted from Oesterheld and Shader (1998) (626).

brain fluvoxamine and fluoxetine in pediatric pervasive developmental disorders and demonstrated that SSRI brain concentrations were not different from adult subjects when corrected for body mass. Enhanced metabolic activity may occur, however, in part due to a greater liver-to-body mass ratio in children (36). Findling et al. (1999) (34), for example, demonstrated a T1/2 of 11 hours for paroxetine, compared to twice that duration observed in adults.

Paroxetine, fluoxetine, and fluvoxamine have demonstrated nonlinear kinetics in adults (24, 28), meaning that clearance or half-life is a function of blood levels. This effect is typically due to the drug's inhibition of its own clearance via inhibition of its enzymatic metabolism, leading to increased half-life with multiple dosing. In a pharmacokinetic study of paroxetine in youth, Findling et al. (1999) (34) reported a 6.9-fold increase in serum drug concentration following a dose increase from 10 to 20 mg. The clinical relevance of this effect may also be seen in "discontinuation syndromes" as blood levels fall and drug clearance speeds up, leading to exponential decline. As such, children taking SSRIs with a short half-life (14-hour) may benefit from twice-a-day administration to avoid withdrawal effects (37). Enteric-coated formulations may in part modify these kinetic characteristics and enhance tolerability (38). Examples include paroxetine-controlled release (Paxil CR), which offers a reduction in absorption rate compared to paroxetine (GlaxoSmithKline, Paxil prescribing information).

Fluoxetine and citalopram possess a chiral center that permits existence of stereoisomeric forms of the molecule, and they were originally marketed as racemic mixtures of enantiomers with different kinetics and dynamics. While (R) and (S) enantiomers of fluoxetine are similar in 5HT activity, (S) fluoxetine is more potent in its p450 inhibition yet has a more potent metabolite (28). Conversely, the newest member of the SSRI class, Lexapro (approved by the FDA in August 2002), the pure (S) isomer of citalopram, displays at least 100-fold 5HT activity compared to the (R) isomer (Forest Pharmaceuticals, Lexapro prescribing information).

Knowledge of SSRI metabolism is clinically useful, as it relates to potential drug interactions and overall drug safety. Although SSRI medications have fewer drug interactions than their predecessors, drug interactions may occur, primarily via the metabolic cytochrome p450 (CYP450) system, such as CYP450 2D6.

Paroxetine and fluoxetine show the most potent CYP450 2D6 inhibition, followed by sertraline, fluvoxamine, and citalopram (39). For paroxetine and fluoxetine, plasma concentrations and dosage have been shown to influence the magnitude of enzyme inhibition (40). Awareness of CYP450 interactions must include clinically significant interactions with herbals or supplements, such as St. John's wort and unwanted pregnancy with concomitant birth control pills (41). Increasingly, controlled studies are including pharmacokinetic sampling to assess the impact of CYP450 genetic polymorphisms on efficacy, safety, and tolerability, particularly

when CYP450-2D6 is the main enzymatic pathway, as 7% of the Caucasian population is naturally deficient in this enzyme. Other mechanisms of drug-drug interaction may also include UDP-glucuronyltransferase inhibition, as described in a case report of a citalopram interaction with clomipramine (42) (Table 27.3).

Pharmacodynamics

Both the absolute potency of serotonergic uptake inhibition as well as their relative serotonin:norepinephrine uptake inhibition ratio (selectivity) may be important in the action of SSRIs, both of which are far greater than in the predecessor tricyclic antidepressants (TCAs), with the exception of clomipramine. In general, the SSRIs have low affinity for other receptors, such as adrenergic, cholinergic, or histaminic sites. Table 27.4 displays in vitro potency of serotonin uptake inhibition for the SSRIs.

Paroxetine and sertraline show the most potent absolute 5HT reuptake inhibition, while citalopram is most selective (i.e., has the greatest 5HT/NE ratio) (43). With doses commonly used in adult controlled trials, such as 20 mg fluoxetine and 50 mg sertraline, serotonin uptake inhibition has been found to be in the range of 60 to 80% (24). The transmission of synaptic serotonin increases with acute administration of SSRI medications is likely due to reduced sensitivity of 5HT (1A) inhibitory autoreceptors. Desensitization of 5-HT (1A) autoreceptors in the dorsal and median raphe may be due to changes at or distal to receptor-G protein interaction (44). Over time, postsynaptic 5HT2 receptors are probably also down-regulated (45). While the SSRIs are primarily serotonergic in their actions, ongoing neuropharmacological studies have described paroxetine's marked NE transporter inhibition at doses >40 mg/day (46) and sertraline's potency at the dopamine reuptake site (47).

TABLE 27.3

CYP450 ISOENZYME INHIBITION BY SSRIs

Drug	CYP Isoenzymes (in vitro)				
	1A2	2C9	2C19	2D6	3A4
Citalopram	+	0	0	0	0
Fluoxetine	+	++	+/++	+++	+/++
Norfluoxetine	+	++	+/++	+++	++
Fluvoxamine	+++	++	+++	+	++
Paroxetine	+	+	+	+++	+
Sertraline	+	+	+/++	+	+

The clinical significance of in vitro data is unknown. In vitro enzyme inhibition data did not reveal an inhibitory effect of citalopram in CYP3A4, and citalopram would be expected to have little inhibitory effect on in vivo metabolism by this enzyme.
0, minimal or no inhibition; +, mild; ++, moderate; +++, strong.
Source: From Greenblatt et al. (1993) (613); data on file, Forest Laboratories.

TABLE 27.4

SRI INHIBITION OF [³H]-MONOAMINE UPTAKE INTO RAT BRAIN SYNAPTOSOMES IN VITRO

Compound	$K_i(nM)$			
	[³H]-5-HT	[³H]-NE	[³H]-DA	NE/5HT
Paroxetine	1.1	350	2,000	318
Citalopram	1.8	8,800	>10,000	4,888
Fluvoxamine	6.2	1,100	>10,000	177
Sertraline	7.3	1,400	230	192
Clomipramine	7.4	96	9,100	13
Fluoxetine	25	500	4,200	20
Amitriptyline	87	79	4,300	0.9

Source: Relative values from a series of related trials from Boyer & Feighner (614–617).
5-HT, serotonin; NE, norepinephrine; DA, dopamine.
NE/5HT is a measure of serotonin selectivity.
K_i, inhibitory constant; nM, nanomolar.

Pharmacotherapy

This discussion of SSRI pharmacotherapy is organized according to primary clinical applications supported by controlled trials, although for many common SSRI applications, there is a dearth of controlled data. Despite widespread use, SSRI medications are certainly not universally effective.

Randomized Controlled Trials (Level A) Evidence

Mood Disorders

Contrary to the adult mood disorder literature, the only controlled evidence demonstrating efficacy in pediatric unipolar depressive disorders is found in studies with SSRI medications. Open-label studies suggest variable response rates to SSRIs in children and adolescents with major depressive disorder (MDD), yet higher than rates observed in controlled studies (40 to 70%). Placebo response rates are also high (30 to 60%) in controlled trials, indicating that overall effect sizes are modest and that underpowered studies are unlikely to demonstrate statistically significant efficacy (type 2 errors). There is no controlled evidence targeted at pharmacological treatment of suicidality in depressed youth (48–50) (Table 27.5).

Several RCTs have demonstrated efficacy of SSRIs for the acute management of major depression. Emslie and colleagues demonstrated significant benefit, in both acute and maintenance fluoxetine treatment, in children and adolescents with depression (51–53). In addition, a multicenter controlled trial of adolescent MDD sponsored by the National Institute of Mental Health (NIMH) demonstrated efficacy of fluoxetine (10 to 40 mg/day) and fluoxetine plus cognitive behavior therapy (CBT) compared to placebo (49). Studies have demonstrated a 40 to 65% response rate to 10 to 40 mg of fluoxetine daily, compared to a 20 to 50% placebo response rate (depending on outcome variable). A

multivariate post-hoc analysis did not identify any variables that might predict a positive response to fluoxetine in this study (54). Fluoxetine has been shown to be beneficial for maintenance treatment in children and adolescents with MDD (48), addressing the uncertainty regarding the impact of SSRIs on recurrence of depressive episodes.

Paroxetine (mean daily dose, 28 mg) demonstrated superiority over placebo (55) and comparability to the serotonergic TCA clomipramine in one randomized multicenter trial of adolescent major depression (56). Although in two prior RCTs, paroxetine did not achieve significant superiority over placebo (57), treatment response stratified by age showed a significant difference in outcome, in that a greater proportion of older youth (>16 years old) were responders (www.gsk.com/media/paroxetine.htm). Combined controlled and open trials with sertraline 25 to 200 mg daily have demonstrated significant superiority across multiple measures in adolescents (58) and global improvement measures in children (59) compared to placebo. One 8-week controlled trial of citalopram in pediatric MDD demonstrated significant superiority in change from baseline compared to placebo (60), but a similar study from the UK did not (57).

The 1999 Report of the Texas Consensus Conference Panel on Medication Treatment of Childhood Major Depressive Disorder recommended fluoxetine, sertraline, or paroxetine as first-line agents (61). However, a more recent review of the efficacy and safety of SSRI medications in pediatric depression by the FDA led to the endorsement of fluoxetine only (62). This FDA review followed concerns regarding the safety and efficacy of SSRIs in pediatric populations (see the "Safety" section, presented later).

Expert panels, including a task force convened by the American College of Neuropsychopharmacology in response to these concerns, identified *several* SSRIs (fluoxetine, sertraline, paroxetine, and citalopram) as significantly more effective than placebo in at least one controlled trial.

TABLE 27.5
A SUMMARY OF RANDOMIZED CONTROLLED TRIALS IN PEDIATRIC DEPRESSION

Author (Year)	Drug	N (Act/PBO)	Length of Tx (Weeks)	Dose Mean mg/day (Range)	Percentage Completers		Mean Age in Years (Range)		Measure	Outcome
					Act	PBO	Act	PBO		
Braconnier et al. (2003) (56)	Clomipramine	58	8	92 (75 or 150)	68	N/A	16.2	N/A	MADRS	p = 0.062
	Paroxetine	63		23 (20 or 40)	58	N/A	15.9 (12–20)	N/A	· GAF HSCL58 CGI	p = 0.57 p = 0.47 p = 0.71
Wagner et al. (2003) (78)	Sertraline	376 (189/187)	10	131 (50–200)	76	83	NR (6–17)	NR	CDRS-R† CGI-I♦ CGI-S♦	p = 0.05 p = 0.009 p = 0.005
Emslie et al. (2002) (51)	Fluoxetine	219 (109/110)	9	20 (20)*	83	62	12.7 (8–17)	12.7	CDRS-R§ CGI-I† CGI-S§ BDI CDI GAF MADRS†	p < 0.001 p = 0.028 p < 0.001 p = 0.700 p = 0.822 p = 0.176 p = 0.023
Keller et al. (2001) (55)	Imipramine Paroxetine Placebo	95 93 87	8	206 (200–300) 28 (20–40)	60 72 76	N/A N/A N/A	14.9 14.8 15.1 (12–18)	N/A N/A N/A	HAM-D K-SADS-L CGI-I HAM-D K-SADS-L CGI-I†	p = 0.87 p = 0.98 p = 0.64 p = 0.13 p = 0.07 p = 0.02
Wagner (2001) (60)	Citalopram	174 (89/85)	8	23.3yo (7–11) 24.4yo (12–17) (20–40)	75	86	NR (7–17)	NR	CDRS-R	p = 0.05
Emslie et al. (1997) (52)	Fluoxetine	96 (48/48)	8	20(20)*	71	54	12.2 (7–17)	12.5	CDRS-R§ CGI-I†	p = 0.002 p = 0.02
Mandoki et al. (1997) (160)	Venlafaxine	40 (20/20)	6	8–12yo: 12.5 qd-tid 13–17yo: 25 qd-tid	80	85	NR (13–18)	NR	CDI CDRS CBCL HAM-D	p = 0.37 p = 0.48 p = 0.08 p = 0.50
Simeon et al. (1990) (58)	Fluoxetine	40	7	(40–60)	NR	NR		NR	HAM-D CGI	NS NS

§ p < 0.001, ♦ p <0.01, † p ≤ 0.05, * fixed dose.
Act, Active; PBO, Placebo; N/A, Not applicable; NR, Not reported; NS, Not significant; BDI, Beck Depression Inventory; BPRS-C, Brief Psychiatric Rating Scale-Children; CBCL, Child Behavior Checklist; CDI, Children's Depression Inventory; CDRS-R, Children's Depression Rating Scale-Revised; CGI-I, Clinical Global Impressions-Improvement; CGI-S, Clinical Global Impressions-Severity; GAF, Global Assessment of Functioning; HAM-D, Hamilton Rating Scale for Depression; HSCL58, Hopkins Symptom Checklist; K-SADS-L, Kiddie Schedule for Affective Disorders and Schizophrenia-Lifetime Version; MADRS, Montgomery and Asberg Depression Rating Scale; WSAS, Weinberg Screening Affective Scale.

This panel did acknowledge that paroxetine and citalopram have also registered negative findings (57). While the data regarding SSRI use in youth are growing, clinicians face the difficult task of interpreting the extant literature, particularly when negative trials may not be presented in scientific forums (file drawer effect), when drug trials use weak methodology, when faced with high placebo response rates, and when safety and tolerability are presented in a limited manner (63–65) .

Anxiety Disorders

Extensive evidence from many randomized controlled trials supports the efficacy of SSRIs in adults in virtually all of the anxiety disorders including posttraumatic stress disorder (PTSD). Similarly, but with a less strong evidence base, this class of medications has also been shown to be effective in placebo-controlled studies of pediatric anxiety, primarily in obsessive-compulsive disorder and mixed anxiety cohorts.

Obsessive-Compulsive Disorder (OCD)

Pediatric OCD pharmacotherapy has been studied more than other anxiety disorders; multiple randomized placebo-controlled studies (mostly industry sponsored) have been conducted in cohorts of children and adolescents with obsessive-compulsive disorder (66, 67). This body of evidence, including more than 19 studies representing more than a thousand children and adolescents, indisputably supports the short- and medium-term efficacy of serotonergic medications (74, 75), including fluoxetine (68, 69), fluvoxamine (70), paroxetine (71–73), and sertraline (29, 74–77) (Table 27.6). Cumulatively, these data constitute the highest level (Level 1) using AHRQ strength of evidence criteria of quality, quantity, and consistency of scientific studies. Five of these studies also report on the longterm efficacy (>12 months) of the SSRIs for OCD in youth showing continuing benefit from treatment without any evidence of loss of efficacy. In fact, in a longterm study reporting on a 12-month extension study of sertraline in youth with OCD, Wagner et al. (2003) (78) found that Children's Yale-Brown Obsessive Compulsive Scales (CY-BOCS) scale scores *continued to improve* throughout the duration of treatment. Overall responder rates, defined by ≥25% reduction in the CY-BOCS, are around 50% and are shown for each SSRI in Table 27.6.

In a meta-analysis of this literature, Geller et al. (2003) (21) (Table 27.7) found that the pooled standardized mean difference (SMD) for results of all studies was 0.46 (95% confidence intervals [CI] = 0.37−0.55), showing a highly significant difference between drug and placebo treatment (z = 9.87, p<0.001). Multivariate regression of the drug effect controlled for other variables showed that clomipramine was significantly superior to each of the SSRIs (chi-square = 16.49, df = 4, p = 0.002) but that the other SSRIs were comparably effective.

As noted later, informed consent for the use of SSRIs for OCD must include some discussion of the value of non-pharmacological treatment, particularly CBT. A federally funded pediatric OCD treatment study (POTS) compared combined CBT and medication to either treatment alone and found that combined treatment had an additive effect on outcome with the greatest overall effect size (79). This approach is likely to become the gold standard for OCD treatment in the future (Table 27.8).

Mixed Anxiety Disorders

Randomized controlled studies have been conducted on mixed samples of anxiety disorders, reflecting the frequent comorbidity found within childhood anxiety disorders. Following positive earlier open studies (80–82), the first large, multicenter randomized controlled shortterm trial of an SSRI in mixed pediatric anxiety demonstrated significant improvements in the Pediatric Anxiety Rating Scale (PARS) and Clinical Global Impression (CGI) in the actively treated group using fluvoxamine (maximum dose, 300 mg) compared to placebo (83). A further 6-month open treatment extension in this sample demonstrated continued improvement. More recently, Birmaher (2003) (84) demonstrated the benefit of fluoxetine for the treatment of the childhood anxiety disorders social phobia (SP), separation anxiety disorder (SAD), and generalized anxiety disorder (GAD). Only one controlled trial using low-dose sertraline for treatment of pediatric generalized anxiety disorder has been reported to date (85) (Tables 27.9 and 27.10).

Other Sanctioned Uses (Level B Evidence)

Eating Disorders

Despite anecdotal reports of positive outcomes, randomized controlled studies of fluoxetine have *not* demonstrated efficacy in underweight adult anorexia nervosa (AN) inpatients (86). However, it appears that SSRIs *do* have a place in treatment of AN *following* weight restoration (and repletion of neuronal 5HT stores), including treatment of associated depressive symptoms. In one small 12-month controlled study, placebo-treated subjects with anorexia nervosa showed a greater rate of relapse compared to fluoxetine-treated subjects (87). More recently, restrictor-type pediatric-onset anorexia nervosa subjects showed reduction in obsessional thinking and improvement in depression scores with fluoxetine compared to placebo (63 versus 16%) at 1-year follow-up (88). Case reports and open trials document efficacy with other SSRI agents in binge eating and purging disorders using sertraline and fluoxetine combined with psychotherapy. (89).

Other Anxiety Disorders

Open studies have shown efficacy of SSRIs in anxiety disorders, including panic disorder (90), social phobia (91), and selective mutism (92). Based on their efficacy for other anxiety disorders, SSRIs are also commonly used in PTSD both for core symptoms as well as comorbid conditions

TABLE 27.6
A SUMMARY OF RANDOMIZED CONTROLLED TRIALS IN PEDIATRIC OBSESSIVE-COMPULSIVE DISORDER

Author (Year)	Drug	N (Act/PBO)	Length of Tx (Weeks)	Dose Mean mg/day (Range)	% Completers Act	% Completers PBO	Mean Age in Years (Range) Act	Mean Age in Years (Range) PBO	Measure	% Responders on CY-BOCS Act	% Responders on CY-BOCS PBO
Liebowitz et al. (2002) (68)	Fluoxetine	43 (21/22)	16	65.5 (20–80)	52	32	13.0 (6–18)	12.3	CY-BOCS NIMH-GOCS CGI-S	NR[f]	NR
Geller (2002) (73)	Paroxetine	203 (98/105)	10	23.0 (10–50)	65	75	11.3 (7–17)	11.3	CY-BOCS	65♦	41
Geller (2003) (67)	Paroxetine	193 (95/98)	16	32.2 (10–60)	44	34	11.8 (8–17)	11.6	CY-BOCS	30♦	14
Geller et al. (2001) (69)	Fluoxetine	103 (71/32)	13	24.6 (20–60)	69	63	11.4 (7–17)	11.4	CY-BOCS NIMH-GOCS♦ CGI-S♦	49[f]	25
Riddle et al. (2001) (70)	Fluvoxamine	120 (57/63)	10	165 (50–200)	67	57	13.4 (8–17)	12.7	CY-BOCS NIMH-GOCS[f] CGI-S[f]	42[f]	26
March et al. (1998) (74)	Sertraline	187 (92/95)	12	167 (25–200)	80	86	12.6[1] (6–17)	12.6[1]	CY-BOCS NIMH-GOCS[f] CGI-S[f]	53♦	37
Riddle et al. (1992) (618)	Fluoxetine	13 (7/6)	8	20 (20)*	86	83	11.8[1] (8–15)	11.8[1]	CY-BOCS CGI-S♦ LOI-CV	NR	NR
DeVeaugh-Geiss et al. (1992) (619)	Clomipramine	60 (31/29)	8	NR (75–200)	87	93	14.5 (10–17)	14.0	CY-BOCS NIMH-GOCS[f]	50[f]	10
Leonard et al. (1991) (234)	Clomipramine Desipramine	11 (N/A) 9(N/A)	8	143 (50–225) 123 (50–250)	100 90	N/A	14.7[1] (8–19)	14.7[1]	NIMH-GOCS[f] LOI-CV	N/A	N/A
March et al. (1990) (620)	Clomipramine	16 (8/8)	10	190 (50–200)	75	100	15.0[1] (10–18)	15.0[1]	CY-BOCS NIMH-GOCS[f]	NR	NR
Leonard et al. (1989) (235)	Clomipramine Desipramine	23(N/A) 25(N/A)	10	50 (25–250) 153 (25–250)	92[1] 92[1]	N/A	13.9[1] (7–19)	13.9[1]	NIMH-GOCS♦ LOI-CV	N/A	N/A
Flament et al. (1985) (236)	Clomipramine	38 (19/19)	10	141 (50–200)	91[1]	91[1]	14.5[1] (10–18)	14.5[1]	NIMH-GOCS[f] LOI-CV[f]	N/A	N/A

*Fixed dose; [1]Pooled data provided for drug and placebo; [2]Desipramine used as comparator; [f]p < 0.05 ♦p < 0.01; Act, Active; CGI-S, Clinical Global Impressions Scale: Severity; CY-BOCS, Children's Yale-Brown Obsessive Compulsive Scale; LOI-CV, Leyton Obsessional Inventory-Child Version; NIMH-GOCS, National Institute of Mental Health Global Obsessive Compulsive Scale; NR, Not reported; N/A: not applicable; PBO: placebo.
CMI data supplied by the neuroscience department at Novartis Pharmaceuticals Corporation; responders defined as ≥25% reduction on CY-BOCS.

TABLE 27.7
META-ANALYSIS OF EFFECT SIZES OF SSRIs IN PEDIATRIC OCD

	SMD*	95% Confidence Interval	p value versus placebo
Paroxetine	.405	.204–.606	p < .001
Fluoxetine	.546	.353–.738	p < .001
Fluvoxamine	.375	.167–.584	p < .001
Sertraline	.327	.160–.493	p < .001
Clomipramine	.693	.475–.910	p < .001

*SMD refers to standardized mean difference of CY-BOCS scalar scores before and after treatment.
Source: Adapted from Geller et al. (2003) (21).

(93), and open-label trials have supported this practice (94). SSRIs have been proven effective in the treatment of adult PTSD in multiple controlled trials (95–97).

Pervasive Development Disorders/Autism

Only one controlled trial of fluvoxamine in children with autism and pervasive development disorders (PDDs) has been reported. This placebo-controlled 12-week trial of fluvoxamine demonstrated only limited efficacy and poor tolerability (98). Only one child experienced improvement, while 14 of 18 subjects randomized to fluvoxamine experienced adverse effects, including insomnia, hyperactivity, agitation, aggression, *increased* rituals, and anxiety.

Novel Uses (Level C Evidence)

Disruptive Behavior and Impulse Control Disorders

Open-label reports suggest benefit from treatment with the SSRIs for a variety of disruptive and impulse control symptoms including impulsive aggression (99, 100), self-scratching, self-mutilation, trichotillomania, and sexual behaviors (101–107). SSRIs may have utility in

addressing the comorbid symptoms frequently present in children with oppositional defiant disorder (ODD) and conduct disorder, including dysphoria and anxiety symptoms.

Initiating and Maintenance of Medication

Standard informed consent with parents or guardians and assent by the child or adolescent are the first steps in initiating medication. Informed consent includes, at a minimum, a discussion of potential risks and benefits of the proposed treatment, common adverse effects, and alternatives to the proposed treatment (*including no treatment and nonpharmacological treatment*). This discussion should be documented in the medical record. SSRI medication guides for families and clinicians are now available from the FDA (www.fda.gov/cder/drug/antidepressants/MG_template.pdf) and jointly from the American Psychiatric Association and the American Academy of Child and Adolescent Psychiatry (www.aacap.org/Announcements/pdfs/parentsmedguide.pdf; www.aacap.org/Announcements/pdfs/physicians-medguide.pdf).

In the case of a patient with OCD, informed consent should also include a discussion on the value and availability of cognitive behavioral treatments that are recommended as first-line interventions by the American Academy of Child and Adolescent Psychiatry for mild to moderate OCD. The presence of comorbid depression, more severe OCD, lack of intact family, or lack of available skilled CBT therapists all argue for an earlier introduction of medications. When initiating SSRI medications, several variables should be considered, including age, body weight, pubertal status, neurological status, and family history of drug response. The lowest available dose should be used for initiating medication in children or those with neurological insult or developmental delay, while adolescents can begin with dosages intermediate to those used in adult practice. Currently, there is no indica-

TABLE 27.8
RECOMMENDED DOSE RANGES FOR SSRIs IN PEDIATRIC OCD

Drug	Starting Dose (mg) Preadolescent	Adolescent	Typical Dose Range (mg) (Mean Dose)*
Clomipramine**	6.25–25	25	50–200
Fluoxetine***	2.5–10	10–20	10–80 (25)
Sertraline***	12.5–25	25–50	50–200 (178)
Fluvoxamine**	12.5–25	25–50	50–300 (165)
Paroxetine****	2.5–10	10	10–60 (32)
Citalopram***	2.5–10	10–20	10–60

*Mean daily doses used in published controlled trials.
**Doses <25 mg/day may be administered by compounding 25 mg into 5 ml suspension.
***Oral concentrate commercially available.
****Oral suspension available.

TABLE 27.9
SUMMARY OF OPEN-LABEL SSRI TRIALS IN PEDIATRIC ANXIETY DISORDERS

Author (year)	Drug	Diagnosis	N	Length of Treatment (Weeks)	Dose Range (mg/day)	Age Range (Years)	Results
Chavira & Stein (2002) (621)	Citalopram	General social anxiety	12	12	10–40 Mean: 35	8–17	83% improved; 42% very much on CGI
Compton et al. (2001) (91)	Sertraline	Social phobia	14	8	Mean: 123 Max: 200	10–17	36% CGI responders
Masi et al. (2001) (622)	Paroxetine	Panic and other anxiety diagnosis	18	2–24	10–40 Mean: 24	7–16	83% CGI responders
Mancini et al. (1999) (623)	Nefazodone Paroxetine Sertraline	GAD, social phobia w/ anxiety or MDD	7	Up to 28	400 50–80 175	7–18	All responded with functional improvements
Renaud et al. (1999) (90)	Fluoxetine Paroxetine Sertraline	Panic w/ comorbid MDD, anxiety	12	6–8 follow-up: 36	20–60 20 125 +/– BZD	8–18	75% showed much or very much improvement on CGI-I
Fairbanks et al. (1997) (81)	Fluoxetine	GAD, SAD, multiple anxiety	16	6–9	Max: 24	9–18	100% CGI responders; SAD and social phobia had best response
Dummit et al. (1996) (92)	Fluoxetine	Selective mutism	21	9	10–60	5–14	76% improved on CGI-I, with more speech in public and at school; social anxiety improved
Birmaher et al. (1994) (80)	Fluoxetine	OAD, SAD, social phobia	21	40	10–60 Mean: 26	Not reported	81% CGI responders
Manassis & Bradley (1994) (82)	Fluoxetine	SAD, avoidant, mutism, OAD	5	6	10–20	Not reported	100% improved on parent and self-reports

BZD, Benzodiazepine; CGI, Clinical Global Impressions Scale; GAD, Generalized anxiety disorder; MDD, Major depressive disorder; OAD, Overanxious disorder; SAD, Separation anxiety disorder.

tion for baseline laboratory tests (hematological, thyroid, hepatic or renal function tests) before and during the administration of SSRIs (108). Titration schedules should be conservative, with modest increases every 3 weeks or so to allow for improvement to manifest before aggressively increasing doses. An exception may be the treatment of inpatients where more control and supervision is available. Especially for treatment of anxiety disorders, *patience is key to successful outcomes*, since it may take a full 12 weeks for benefits to occur.

Common transient somatic side effects include gastrointestinal upset and headache. Parents should be aware of possible behavioral activation as well as the possibility of manic irritability, euphoria, and explosiveness in unusual and severe reactions, as discussed in the safety section that follows. Severe mood dysregulation on SSRI medications is not necessarily pathognomonic of underlying juvenile bipolar disorder. Clinical experience suggests that children with PDD spectrum disorders may be

particularly sensitive to serotonergic agents. As such, low dosage and slow titration is indicated in this population as well.

Maintenance/Monitoring
National psychiatric associations (the American Psychiatric Association [APA] and the American Academy of Child and Adolescent Psychiatry [AACAP]) concur with the need for close monitoring of children and adolescents on antidepressants. The FDA suggests monitoring to include weekly face-to-face contact with patients, family members, or caregivers during the first 4 weeks of treatment, then every other week for the next 4 weeks, then at 12 weeks, and as clinically indicated beyond 12 weeks, but this schedule is more frequent than common current clinical practice and may not be practical in all settings. The APA and AACAP suggest individualized monitoring; clinicians and families should watch for clinical worsening, agitation, irritability, suicidality, insomnia, or any unusual change in behavior,

TABLE 27.10

SUMMARY OF RANDOMIZED CONTROLLED TRIALS OF SSRIs IN PEDIATRIC ANXIETY DISORDERS

Author (Year)	Drug	Diagnosis	N	Length of Treatment (Weeks)	Dose Range (mg/day)	Age Range (Years)	Results
Birmaher et al. (2003) (84)	Fluoxetine	GAD, SAD, social phobia	74	12	10–20	7–17	61 versus 35% showed much to very much improvement on CGI, p = 0.03; pts with SOC and GAD showed better response for med than placebo; severity of anxiety at baseline and positive family history predicted poorer response
Rynn et al. (2001) (85)	Sertraline	GAD	22	9	Up to 50	5–17	90% CGI improvement in active group, 10% in placebo, p < 0.001
Walkup et al. (2001) (83)	Fluvoxamine	GAD, SAD, social phobia	128	8	25–300 (mean:110)	6–18	76% responders among active, 29% among placebo on CGI-I, p < 0.01
Carlson et al. (1999) (624)	Sertraline	Elective Mutism	5	16	50–100	5–11	All much or very much improved on CGI-I up to 20 weeks
Black & Udhe (1994) (625)	Fluoxetine	Elective Mutism	15	12	12–27	6–12	Fluoxetine was better, although most still impaired; no significant difference between groups on CGI scales

CGI-I, Clinical Global Impressions Scale–Improvement; GAD, Generalized anxiety disorder; SAD, Separation anxiety disorder; SOC, Social phobia.

especially during the initial few months of drug therapy or at times of dose changes (www.fda.gov/cder/drug/antidepressants/MG_template.pdf).

The limited study of blood plasma levels and clinical response, primarily with fluoxetine, does *not* support routine use of therapeutic drug monitoring (28). Some exceptions may apply, for example, in combined pharmacotherapy or in overdose situations. A study of citalopram presented information on plasma levels in a naturalistic treatment of adolescents with depression (109). Multiple RCTs have not found any clinically significant changes in laboratory parameters such as complete blood count with differential, liver, renal, and thyroid function, or lipid and glucose metabolism nor in electrocardiographic (ECG) parameters (84), precluding the necessity for routine evaluation.

Optimal antidepressant maintenance therapy, discontinuation, and therapy failure are still being studied in adults with mood disorder (110, 111). Limited information can be found for pediatric populations (112). AACAP guidelines suggest continuing antidepressant treatment for

at least 6 to 12 months following clinical response, depending on the patient's clinical status, functioning, support systems, environmental stressors, motivation for treatment and compliance, and the presence of comorbid disorders (108). In those with no response, treatment with adequate and tolerable doses should continue for at least 4 to 6 weeks before considering other treatment options. Overall, allowing sufficient time to achieve clinical response is likely more important than aggressive titration, due to a flatter dose response curve at higher doses (26). These recommendations are generally consistent with the adult literature. Certain factors, such as recurrent, frequent, or severely disabling episodes, suggest the need for longer-term maintenance treatment.

Gradual taper and discontinuation should be timed appropriately, taking into account the impact of psychosocial stressors on clinical condition, such as the beginning and end of the school year. SSRI medications with short half-lives, such as paroxetine, should be tapered more gradually to avoid discontinuation effects (113, 114).

Safety

In general, SSRIs are well-tolerated medications, and they are safer than their predecessor TCAs, especially in the setting of misuse or overdose. Side effects are usually mild and often dose dependent. Acute effects such as gastrointestinal upset, decreased appetite, headache, restlessness, insomnia, and fatigue may occur, as well as behavioral or mood changes. There are no *known* longterm adverse effects of the use of SSRI medications in pediatric populations.

Suicidality. After the UK Department of Health statement in the summer of 2003 alerting the public of a 1.5- to 3-fold increased risk of self-harm or suicidal thinking in youth taking paroxetine, the FDA (Dr. Mosholder, Division of Drug Risk Evaluation) and expert panels conducted an extensive review of SSRI medications in all shortterm pediatric clinical trials.

Although Dr. Mosholder reported a statistically significant association of "suicidality" adverse events (N = 78) with antidepressant drug treatment in shortterm pediatric clinical trials, due to concerns regarding misclassification of cases and prior to a definitive analysis, the FDA contracted Columbia University in the summer of 2004 to perform an independent and blinded review of adverse events. Using original narratives, the panel redefined adverse events from pediatric antidepressant trials as (1) suicidal events (attempts, aborted attempts, interrupted attempts, and suicidal ideation–related events), (2) nonsuicidal events (self-injury or mutilation without suicidal intent, events attributable to other psychiatric symptoms, medical or accidental injuries), (3) and indeterminate events (nonconsensus or unable to classify due to limited data) (www.fda.gov/cder/drug/antidepressants/classification-Project.htm).

Following the Columbia classification, Dr. Hammad (FDA, Division of Neuropharmacological Drug Products) performed a new meta-analysis of 95 adverse event cases across 23 pediatric trials. *No individual trial* showed a statistically significant signal for suicidality. However, many trials had a relative risk of 2 or more, and some of the *overall estimates*, across various trial groupings, were statistically significant. Most events were in trials in which the highest proportion of patients had a history of suicide attempt or ideation *at baseline*. Dr. Mosholder concluded that the Columbia reclassification did not materially affect his prior conclusions. Yet the overall risk estimate for "all trials" analysis decreased with the Columbia University reclassification from 1.89 to 1.78, and the risk estimate for SSRI *MDD-only* trials decreased and lost statistical significance. However, for individual drugs, the risk estimates for paroxetine and venlafaxine increased.

Based on these analyses of 24 pediatric antidepressant trials involving more than 4,400 patients, in October 2004, the FDA issued a black box warning on all pediatric antidepressants (www.fda.gov/cder/drug/antidepressants/ SSRIlabelChange.htm), as well as a public health advisory (www.fda.gov/cder/drug/antidepressants/ SSRIPHA200410.htm). The FDA concluded there was a greater risk of suicidality during the first few months of treatment in those receiving antidepressants; 4% average risk of such events on drug, and twice the placebo risk of 2%. *No suicides* occurred in these trials. In February 2005, the FDA made an important alteration to its black box labeling language from "antidepressants *increase* the risk of suicidal thinking and behavior (suicidality) in children and adolescents with major depressive disorder (MDD) and other psychiatric disorders" to "antidepressants *increased* the risk of suicidal thinking and behavior (suicidality) *in short-term studies.*"

Although there was a 4% average risk of *spontaneously reported (parent or youth)* suicidal thinking or suicidality on drug versus 2% on placebo, in 17 of these 23 trials, a direct assessment *(standardized youth self-assessment)* of suicidality demonstrated a slight *reduction* in suicidality (http://www.aacap.org/Announcements/pdfs/physiciansmedguide.pdf). Consistent with this evidence, in the most recent multicenter trial of SSRI in pediatric depression (49), the number of youth reporting suicidal ideation declined from 29% at baseline to 10% at week 12. Suicidal thinking declined in the fluoxetine + CBT group compared to placebo (p = 0.02), fluoxetine alone (p = 0.002), and CBT alone (p = 0.05). There were no completed suicides, and the number of attempts (7 patients; 1.6%) was too small to analyze.

In addition to the evaluation of clinical trial data just described, toxicological and epidemiological data support a favorable risk-benefit ratio of SSRIs in the treatment of depression in youth (115). The Task Force on SSRIs and Suicidal Behavior in Youth (January 2004) posted by the American College of Neuropsychopharmacology (http://acnp.org) described toxicological analysis in adults and youth noting that, in those completing suicide, the majority had *not* been taking the antidepressant prior to death. Further, the task force cited international epidemiological data in support of *declining* rates of suicide in youth over the previous decade, coincident with increasing antidepressant prescription rates. The Center for Disease Control (CDC) concurs the overall rate of suicide among youth has declined slowly since 1992 (116).

In an examination of 1996–1998 U.S. suicide rate data from the CDC, with county-level prescription data (ages 5 and older) from a random sample of 20,000 pharmacies, increases in SSRI prescriptions were associated with lower suicide rates (117). These findings were consistent with a similar U.S. analysis in youth from 1990 to 2000; a 1% increase in adolescent use of antidepressants was associated with a decrease of 0.23 suicide per 100,000 adolescents per year (P < 0.001) (118). In addition, a retrospective longitudinal cohort study of managed care enrollees aged 12 to 18 years found that antidepressant treatment for at least 6 months reduced the likelihood of suicide attempt compared with antidepressant treatment for just 8 weeks (hazard ratio = 0.34; CI 0.21, 0.55) (119).

Clearly there is need for ongoing study in this area, to provide a better delineation of risk for a given child or adolescent treated with an SSRI. However, the following risk estimate is offered based on a 4% average risk of spontaneously reported suicide thinking or suicidality on the drug versus 2% on placebo; if a clinician prescribes an SSRI for 200 *new* patients, 8 patients may express increased suicidal thinking or behavior. Of these 8 patients, increased suicidality may be attributed to the underlying depression in 4 patients and attributed to the SSRI in 4 patients (AACAP letter to clinicians, October 31, 2004).

Paroxetine's short half-life, nonlinear pharmacokinetics, and CYP450 2D6 inhibition and metabolism are likely relevant to its side effect profile (63). In a pediatric pharmacokinetic (PK) study of paroxetine, the subject with the poorest 2D6 metabolic activity was the first subject to develop hypomania, at week 3 of treatment (34). Paxil CR, which contains a degradable matrix designed to control release of paroxetine over 4 to 5 hours using an enteric coating to delay release (GlaxoSmithKline, 2004), may provide a useful alternative.

Activation/Switching. Activation implies an alteration in mood, anxiety, or behavioral state (such as restlessness) induced by a medication, such as an SSRI. Activation does not signify the presence of hypomania or mania or necessarily herald bipolar disorder. These relatively mild adverse events may be dose related and may resolve with reduction of dose without discontinuation. Contrary to activation, treatment-emergent affective (mood) switching (TEAS) implies a switch from one mood state (depression) to another (hypomania or mania) in the context of an antidepressant, such as an SSRI. While TEAS has been described in the adult bipolar disorder literature, there has been little study in the pediatric literature regarding the phenomenon of switching on antidepressant medications. Martin et al. (120) examined a national database (1997–2000) of 7 million mental health users 5 to 29 years old to assess the risk of mood switching (manic conversion) by age and antidepressant class. The authors found manic conversion in 4,786 patients (5%), with the lowest risk in the SSRI class (hazard ratio 2.1) versus other antidepressant classes (hazard ratio 3.8–3.9). In this review, peripubertal children (10 to 14 years old) were at highest risk of conversion.

In his analysis, Dr. Hammad examined 90 events in all pediatric MDD trials characterized by emergent symptoms of hostility or agitation. No individual trial had a statistically significant result, yet the overall RRs for all drugs, for all SSRIs, and for Paxil were statistically significant, showing an increase in the risk of developing these symptoms compared to placebo.

As depression may be the (unknown or unexpected) index episode of a bipolar disorder, clinicians must monitor for switching into a hypomanic or manic state. True manic conversion precludes the further use of SSRIs without first achieving adequate mood stabilization. Case reports of treatment-emergent mania or hypomania in children or adolescents treated with SSRI medications have been described across numerous diagnostic categories (121–124). Such SSRI-induced mania or hypomania may require treatment with mood stabilizers beyond discontinuation of the antidepressant.

Other. Serious adverse effects, including the serotonin syndrome, have been described in children taking SSRIs (125). Numerous case reports also document the emergence of extrapyramidal symptoms (EPS) as well as tics and myoclonus in children and adolescents treated with SSRI medications (121, 126–131), as well as in adults (132). Hyperreflexic tendon reflexes are common on neurological exam. Animal studies have suggested that SSRIs possess tonic inhibitory properties within the central dopamine system, but it is unknown if this is the cause for motoric adverse effects since their dopaminergic effects are clinically insignificant (45). The amotivational syndrome, previously described in adults taking SSRIs, has been described in several children and adolescents and could also reflect dopamine inhibition (133).

Concerns have been expressed regarding possible decreased growth (101, 134), and increased bleeding rates (135, 136) in SSRI-treated patients. In a population-based cohort study in Denmark and the Netherlands, serotonergic antidepressants increased the risk of gastrointestinal adverse effects in adults, including upper GI bleeding, which was increased in turn by nonsteroidal anti-inflammatory drugs (NSAIDS) and low-dose aspirin (137, 138). Disruption in sleep architecture along with sleep disturbance and subjective accounts of vivid dreaming has also been described with SSRIs, although infrequently in children (139).

Drug Interactions

Mono-amine oxidase inhibitors (MAOIs) should not be given within 5 weeks after discontinuation of fluoxetine or within 2 weeks after other SSRIs. Conversely, SSRIs should not be administered within 2 weeks after discontinuing MAOI treatment. Inappropriate combination with MAOIs may induce potentially serious adverse effects, including the serotonin syndrome. Interactions with medications that utilize or inhibit various CYP450 pathways may occur, as described in the pharmacokinetic section presented earlier. Clinical effects may reflect 2D6 and 1A2 (TCA, antipsychotics), 2C (TCA), and 3A4 (TCA, erythromycin) enzyme interactions (see Table 27.10). In addition, the SSRIs are protein bound to varying degrees and can displace other protein-bound medications and increase their effects (Table 27.11).

SSRI medications are widely used in part due to their wide therapeutic margin of safety (140, 141). Overdoses do occur, such as a life-threatening overdose of fluvoxamine in

TABLE 27.11

HEPATIC CYTOCHROME 450 DRUG INTERACTIONS WITH COMMONLY USED AGENTS IN PEDIATRIC PSYCHOPHARMACOLOGY

CYP	1A1/2	2C9	2C19	2D6	3A4/5
Clinically relevant inhibitors	Cimetidine Ciprofloxacin Fluvoxamine	Cimetidine Fluconazole Fluoxetine Fluvoxamine Mephenytoin Ritonavir	Fluoxetine Fluvoxamine Ritonavir	Dextropropoxyphene Fluoxetine Norfluoxetine Isoniazid Paroxetine Quinidine Ritonavir Thioridazine	Cimetidine Diltiazem Erythromycin Fluconazole Grapefruit juice Indinavir Itraconazole Ketoconazole Nefazodone Norfluoxetine Propoxyphene Ritonavir
Clinically relevant inducers	Broccoli Charbroiled food Cigarettes	Carbamazepine Phenobarbital Rifampin	Rifampin S-Mephenytoin	Phenobarbital	Carbamazepine Phenylbutazone Phenobarbital Primidone Rifampin

Substrates	Aminophylline
	Caffeine
	  (3A4/5, 2E1)
	Clomipramine
	  (2C19, 3A4/5,
	  2D6)
	Clozapine
	  (3A4/5, 2C19)
	Metoclopramide
	  (2D6)
	Mirtazepine
	  (2D6, 3A4/5)
	Olanzapine (2D6)
	Theophylline
	  (3A4/5, 2E1)
		Amitriptyline
		  (2C19, 3A4/5, 2D6)
		Fluoxetine
		NSAIDs
		Phenytoin
		  (1A1/2, 2D6)
		Propanolol
		  (1A1/2, 2C19, 2D6)
		S-Warfarin
			Amitriptyline
			  (2C9, 3A4/5, 2D6)
			Clozapine
			  (3A4/5, 1A1/2)
			Diazepam (3A4/5)
			Imipramine
			  (1A1/2, 2D6,
			  3A4/5)
			S-Mephenytoin
				Amphetamines
				Antiarrhythmics
				Antidepressants
				Desipramine
				Mirtazepine
				  (1A1//2, 3A4/5)
				Nortriptyline
				Venlafaxine (3A4/5)
				Antipsychotics
				Aripriprazole (3A4)
				Atomoxetine
				β-Blockers
				Chlorpheniramine
				Codeine
				Dextromethorphan
				Isoniazid
				(Methylphenidate)
				  (esterases)
					Antibiotics
					  Doxycycline
					  Macrolides
					  Rifampin
					Anticonvulsants
					  Carbamazepine
					  Ethosuximide
					  Trimethadione
					Antidepressants
					  Bupropion (2B6)
					  Citralopam (2C19)
					  Mirtazepine
					  (1A1/2, 2D6)
					Nefazodone
					  Trazodone
					  Tertiary TCAs
					Antipsychotics
					  Clozapine
					  (1A1/2, 2C19)
					  Pimozide
					Benzodiazepines/
					  zolpidem
					  (1A1/2, 2D6)
					  Alprazolam
					  Clonazepam
					  Diazepam (2C19)
					  Midazolam
					Cisapride
					Hormones/steroids
					Anticancer
					Nonsedating
					  antihistamines
					  Astermizole
					  Loratadine
					Opioids
					  Alfentanil

Notations in parentheses indicate alternate metabolic pathways for the substrate listed.
Source: Adapted from Oesterheld and Shader (1998) (626).

a 4-year-old child (142), sertraline (143), and paroxetine (144), and one fluoxetine-related death in a child with cytochrome P-450 2D6 genetic deficiency (145).

NOVEL ANTIDEPRESSANTS

Bupropion/Venlafaxine/Mirtazapine/Trazodone

Pharmacokinetics

Pharmacokinetic studies in pediatric populations are extremely limited. For example, Stewart et al. (2001) (146) examined the moderating effects of smoking status and gender on single-dose pharmacokinetic parameters of bupropion in adolescents and found that plasma levels of bupropion and its metabolite hydroxybupropion did not differ between smokers and nonsmokers. However, the mean area under the curve (AUC) ratio of hydroxybupropion to bupropion was lower than reported in adults. Both bupropion and venlafaxine are available in controlled release formulations, which may have pharmacokinetic advantages, such as lower peak drug levels and smaller fluctuations between peak and trough plasma levels, resulting in better tolerability (147). Bupropion XL, an even longer-acting formulation, is now available. One 300 mg XL capsule provides comparable equivalence in peak plasma and AUC to 100 mg three times a day immediate-release tablets (GlaxoSmithKline, 2003); this formulation may also have superior tolerability (148). Marked inter- and intra-individual variability was observed in one study of the pharmacokinetics of nefazodone with children showing greater absorption and faster clearance compared with adults (149) (Table 27.12)

TABLE 27.12

CLINICAL PHARMACOLOGY OF NOVEL ANTIDEPRESSANTS

	Bupropion	Mirtazapine	Trazodone	Venlafaxine
Pharmacokinetic Parameters				
T-Max (hours)	6 h for sustained release 2 h for immediate release	2 h	1–2 h	2 h (immediate release) 5.5 h (extended release)
Half-life (T 1/2) (hours)	21 h ±9	20–40 h	3–9 h	5 ±2 h
Mechanism of excretion	Renal+ Hepatic CYP 2B6	Hepatic CYP 3A4 and 2D6	Renal	Renal
Pharmacodynamic Parameters				
Mechanism of action	Agonist: Indirect dopamine agonist; relatively weak inhibitor of the neuronal uptake of NE, 5HT, and DA	Antagonist: Presynaptic alpha 2 adrenergic 5HT2 5HT3 Net increase in N/A and 5HT1A activity	Inhibits 5HT uptake	Potent inhibitor of neuronal 5HT and NE reuptake and weak inhibitor of DA reuptake
Clinical Parameters				
Dose range (mg/day)	75–300 (children) 75–450 (adolescents)	7.5–15 (children) 15–45 (adolescents)	50–100 (children) 100–300 (adolescents)	25–300 (children) 37.5–375 (adolescents)
Common side effects	Irritability, anxiety, anorexia, and insomnia, and rarely, edema, rashes, and nocturia	Sedation, increase appetite, weight gain; serotonergic effects minimal, minimal anticholinergic effects, little CVS effects, potent H1 blockade	Mental clouding, sedation, orthostasis, priapism, nausea, rare arrhythmias	Weakness, sweating, nausea, constipation, anorexia, vomiting, somnolence, dry mouth, dizziness, nervousness, anxiety, tremor, and blurred vision, abnormal ejaculation/ orgasm, and impotence in men

5HT, Serotonin; CVS, Cardiovascular system; CYP, Cytochrome; P450 DA, dopamine; H1, Histamine; NE, Norepinephrine; T-Max, Time to peak plasma level.

Pharmacodynamics

This group of antidepressants possesses mixed actions on several neurotransmitter sites, including Norepinephrine (NE), dopamine (DE), and 5HT. Mirtazapine is an antagonist of presynaptic alpha 2-adrenergic autoreceptors as well as presynaptic norepinephrine and serotonin (5-HT) heteroreceptors. It is also a potent antagonist of postsynaptic 5-HT2 and 5-HT3 receptors. Net effects of treatment include greater noradrenergic and serotonergic activity, especially at the 5-HT1A (auto) receptor (150, 151). Venlafaxine exhibits mixed NE and 5HT activity; 5HT reuptake inhibition predominates at lower doses, while NE reuptake inhibition increases with higher doses, and some dopamine reuptake inhibition occurs at high dose (25, 152). Bupropion exerts its effects via an alternate mechanism with inhibition of both NE and DA reuptake, although its occupancy of the DA transporter (DAT) is low (153). Trazodone possesses 5HT reuptake inhibition and 5HT2 antagonism, as well as alpha-1 antagonism and antihistamine effects (25). One of the more common uses of trazodone exploits the potential adverse effect of sedation produced by this receptor activity by employing it at night as a hypnotic agent.

Pharmacotherapy

Mixed neurotransmitter antidepressants may possess special therapeutic utility, such as in conditions refractory to common SSRI agents. Yet even in the extant adult literature, there is little controlled trial evidence available that can guide subsequent treatment for those individuals with no response or partial response to a first-line agent such as an SSRI. Therapeutic strategies may include switching agents within the same class, using another class of agents, or using augmentation with a second drug that has differing pharmacodynamic actions, such as adding noradrenergic or dopaminergic activity to a primary serotonergic drug (154). Bupropion's proposed NE activity, limited CYP-450 interactions, and infrequent sexual side effects has made it a popular augmentation agent in depressed adult partial responders to SSRIs or venlafaxine, and this strategy is supported by efficacy in open trials (155).

In addition, the adult literature suggests that medications affecting multiple neurochemical systems, such as venlafaxine, may achieve higher rates of remission relative to other agents (156, 157). Mirtazapine's increased neuronal cell firing, due to its mixed actions on NE (alpha(2) antagonism) and 5-HT (alpha(1)-stimulation by NE), may result in faster onset of action than more selective antidepressants as suggested by clinical evidence (158).

Mood Disorders

Despite frequent use in clinical settings of mixed activity antidepressants in youth, very limited data exists regarding their safety and efficacy. Controlled trials in youth have been conducted with bupropion, showing a significant advantage for depression symptoms in a small cohort (N = 24) (159) and with low-dose venlafaxine (160). In the latter trial, venlafaxine was not superior to placebo for the treatment of depression in children and adolescents, possibly due to the low doses and short duration of this trial. Open-label studies suggest benefit from these agents as monotherapy, as well as in combination treatment, such as venlafaxine combined with lithium in adolescent depression (161).

Trazodone has been used for insomnia in adolescents with depression (162). Such use is well supported by adult practice, in which trazodone is uniquely utilized in the management of insomnia associated with mood disorder or SSRI treatment (163, 164), as well as PTSD, and primary sleep disorders (165, 166). In these adults, trazodone has been shown to have positive effects on sleep without altering normal sleep architecture (167–169). Mirtazapine has demonstrated similar improvement on objective sleep parameters in depressed adults (170) and because of its sedating properties may be useful in agitated depression.

Anxiety Disorders

There is some rationale for using mixed or dual action agents in pediatric anxiety disorders. For example, individuals with generalized anxiety disorder may benefit from drug activity in both 5HT systems as well as normalization of a presumptive overactive NE system (171). In fact, venlafaxine XR was the *first* antidepressant approved by the FDA for the treatment of GAD (172). Unfortunately, there are no controlled studies of mixed action antidepressants for anxiety disorders in pediatric populations.

The use of trazodone has been recommended by "Expert Consensus Guidelines" for PTSD, when sleep improvement does not improve with first-line agents (173). Open reports also cite improvements in symptoms of mood disturbance and hyperarousal, anger, aggression, restlessness, insomnia, and concentration in youth with PTSD (174).

Attention Deficit Hyperactivity Disorder

Clinical trials of bupropion for ADHD have included a single site placebo-controlled study (175), a multicenter controlled trial (176), a crossover trial with methylphenidate (MPH) (177), and a study of bupropion sustained release formulation in adolescents with attention deficit hyperactivity disorder and comorbid depression (159). Collectively, these studies show that bupropion is an effective agent for the treatment of ADHD in youth, albeit with a more modest effect size than traditional stimulants. Furthermore, bupropion may have clinical value for youth with ADHD and comorbid substance abuse or dependence, as well as mood disorder (178).

PDD Disorders/Autism

A small retrospective clinical study with venlafaxine in children with DSM-IV autism spectrum disorder showed some improvement in repetitive behaviors and restricted interests, social deficits, communication and language function, inattention, and hyperactivity at a very low mean dose of 24 mg daily (179).

Disruptive Behavior, Impulse Control, and TIC Disorders

Trazodone has been used to treat aggression, including cases with neurological injury, and hydrocephalus in youth (180). Case reports suggest efficacy in reducing refractory aggression, hyperactivity, and self-injurious behavior in children with frontal lobe atrophy (181) or treatment refractory hospitalized aggressive children (182).

Initiating and Maintenance of Medication

Initiation. The principles in initiating this group of medications are similar to those outlined in the SSRI section including obtaining informed consent and consideration of age, body weight, pubertal status, neurological status, and family history of drug response. Medication guides for families and clinicians are now available from the FDA (www.fda.gov/cder/drug/antidepressants/MG_template.pdf) and jointly from the American Psychiatric Association and the American Academy of Child and Adolescent Psychiatry (www.aacap.org/Announcements/pdfs/parentsmedguide.pdf; www.aacap.org/Announcements/pdfs/physiciansmedguide.pdf).

The lowest available dose should be used for initiating medication treatment in children or those with neurological insult or developmental delay, and titration schedules should be conservative, with modest increases each 3 to 4 weeks to allow improvement to manifest before increasing doses. Prior to initiating bupropion treatment, one should assess for factors that increase risk for seizures (head trauma, prior history of seizure, concomitant medications that lower seizure threshold). Doses greater than 450 mg daily increase the risk of seizures compared to other antidepressants. Baseline cardiovascular parameters (heart rate, blood pressure) should be obtained, particularly when using bupropion and venlafaxine, which can cause diastolic hypertension.

Monitoring. As discussed in the SSRI section presented earlier, national psychiatric associations (the American Psychiatric Association and the American Academy of Child and Adolescent Psychiatry) concur with the need for close monitoring of children and adolescents on antidepressants.

Monitoring and maintenance use of this group of medications is according to the principles outlined in the SSRI section; that is, routine serum level assays are not clinically helpful and routine liver, renal, thyroid, glucose, lipid, and hematological monitoring studies are not generally required. However, assessment of cardiovascular parameters (blood pressure, heart rate) is recommended with this group of medications.

Safety

Adverse Effects. In general, these medications are well tolerated clinically in youth. Side effects tend to be mild and dose dependent. In the short term, gastrointestinal upset, constipation, decreased appetite, headache, dry mouth, restlessness, insomnia, fatigue, and sedation may occur. Adverse effects with this group reflect their various pharmacological profiles; histamine blockade with agents such as trazodone and mirtazapine cause more sedation than bupropion and venlafaxine, which possess little such activity.

In adult studies, mirtazapine has been associated with somnolence, increased appetite, and weight gain that are attributed to its antihistaminic (H1) activity at low doses (183). Adult case reports have also described glucose deregulation, weight gain (184), hepatoxicity (185), hypertriglyceridemia, pancreatitis, and diabetic ketoacidosis with mirtazapine (186). Nicholas et al. (2003) (187) reported significantly increased total cholesterol at week 4 in one controlled study of otherwise healthy adults treated with mirtazapine.

In adults, venlafaxine may be associated with small, but statistically significant, dose-dependent increases in systolic and diastolic blood pressure during acute and continuation therapy. This effect is more frequent at doses at or above 300 mg daily (188). In another study, no differential effect on blood pressure in young (13 to 56 years) versus old (65 to 86 years) depressed patients treated with dosages of 50 to 250 mg daily were found, despite a higher mean weight-adjusted daily dosage in younger patients. No significant changes in systolic blood pressure were noted in either group. In the older group only, there was a 4.7 mm Hg mean increase in diastolic blood pressure (p = ns) (189).

Trazodone-associated priapism has been well described in adults and in adolescents (190), although scattered cases also have been reported with use of other medications, including venlafaxine (191). This effect appears related to trazodone's alpha-adrenoreceptor-blocking properties and interference of sympathetic control of penile detumescence (192).

The risk of seizures with bupropion is dose dependent, estimated at 0.1% at 300 mg daily of slow-release formulation compared to 0.4% at doses from 300 to 450 mg of –immediate-release drug. Seizure risk may increase 10-fold in dosages greater than 450 mg daily (GlaxoSmithKline). Since its introduction, bupropion has been believed empirically to have fewer cardiovascular adverse effects than other treatments, including in adults with preexisting cardiac disease (193–196). Adverse sexual effects are also uncommon. There are no known longterm adverse effects of using mixed-action antidepressants in pediatric populations; however, controlled longitudinal data are lacking.

Suicidality. As described earlier in detail in the SSRI section, the FDA has performed meta-analyses of adverse event cases across antidepressant pediatric trials, including bupropion, mirtazapine, and venlafaxine. The FDA has instituted the following black box labeling: "antidepressants *increased* the risk of suicidal thinking and behavior (suicidality) *in short-term studies.*"

Activation/Switching. As described in detail in the SSRI section, activation implies an alteration in mood, anxiety, or behavioral state (such as restlessness) induced by a medication, such as an antidepressant (197). Activation does not signify the presence of hypomania or mania, nor does it necessarily herald bipolar disorder. These relatively mild adverse events may be dose related and may resolve with reduction of dose without discontinuation. Contrary to activation, treatment-emergent affective (mood) switching (TEAS) implies a switch from one mood state (depression) to another (hypomania or mania) in the context of a treatment, such as with an antidepressant. As depression may be the (unknown or unexpected) index episode of a bipolar disorder, clinicians must monitor for switching into a hypomanic or manic state. True manic conversion precludes the further use of an antidepressant without first achieving adequate mood stabilization.

Overdose

Retrospective studies of overdose exposure to these agents are available for both adult and pediatric samples. Overdose with bupropion is primarily associated with neurological, rather than cardiac effects. A retrospective review of 7,348 bupropion-only pediatric overdose exposures reported clinical adverse effects in 2,247 exposures overall, but in only 8% of children younger than 6 years old compared to 46% of teenagers (198). Similarly, in a prospective study of bupropion, adverse effects of poisoning in 59 adults and 10 children included tachycardia (83%), hypertension (56%), dose-dependent seizures (37%), gastrointestinal symptoms (37%), and agitation (32%). Only one out of eight children with accidental ingestion had symptoms (vomiting and hallucinations) (199). Bupropion overdose (mean 3.8 g) has been associated with tachycardia, hypertension, and prolongation of QTc of 461 +/− 34 msec (200). Rarely death with massive ingestion has been reported; a 26-year-old man ingested 23 g of bupropion, with seizures and cardiac arrest (201).

The relative toxicity of SSRIs and venlafaxine was reviewed and found to be generally similar (140). Seizures occurred in 7 out of 51 venlafaxine overdoses with greater than 900 mg. SSRIs were less likely to prolong the QRS interval and intensive care unit (ICU) admissions were also less likely (140). Venlafaxine's potential for cardiac and neurotoxicity may be dependent on whether the individual is an extensive or poor metabolizer (deficient CYP2D6 enzyme phenotype) (202). Overdose with 30 and 50 times a normal daily dose of mirtazapine has resulted in full recovery (203); case reports of ingestions including a 3-year-old child did not observe serious sequelae (204). In addition, the clinical trial development program of mirtazapine,

performed in Europe and the United States, evaluated its safety based on data from all patients who took at least one dose of study medication during studies comparing mirtazapine with placebo or other comparators. The only adverse symptom in patients taking an overdose of mirtazapine alone or in combination with other drugs was excessive but transient somnolence (205).

Seizures, hyponatremia, torsades de pointes, prolonged QT, and complete atrio-ventricular (AV) block have all been reported with trazodone overdose (206–209).

Drug Interactions

Interactions based on pharmacokinetics, specifically the CYP450 system, are shown in Table 27.10. Venlafaxine has modest effect on CYP 2D6 substrates (210). While mirtazapine does not itself substantially inhibit CYP450 enzymes in vitro (211), induction or inhibition of CYP450 enzymes by other agents may cause significant increases or decreases in concentration as demonstrated by a 46% reduction in mirtazapine plasma concentration with the addition of phenytoin, a CYP3A34 inducer (212). Mirtazapine and lithium appear to be safe in combination (213).

Few drug interactions are described with bupropion. However, Shad and Preskorn (1997) (214) described an approximately fourfold increase in levels of imipramine and desipramine after the addition of bupropion. Popli et al. (1995) (215) reported that coadministration with carbamazepine may reduce bupropion levels, while valproate levels may increase with concomitant bupropion.

Pharmacodynamic interactions may cause additive degrees of sedation when sedating antidepressants such as trazodone and mirtazapine are taken with other CNS-active depressants. In addition, trazodone may potentiate hypotension when taken with other agents with similar effect.

TRICYCLIC ANTIDEPRESSANTS

Until the emergence of fluoxetine in 1987, tricyclic antidepressants were mainstay agents in both general and child and adolescent neuropsychopharmacology. Agents include tertiary (imipramine, clomipramine) and secondary amines (desipramine, nortriptyline).

Pharmacokinetics

Absorption is rapid from the gastrointestinal tract, reaching peak levels in 2 to 4 hours. TCAs are highly protein-bound and lipophilic agents. In animals, brain penetration of amitriptyline is enhanced when the blood-brain barrier is deficient, a finding that may have some importance in neurologically compromised children (216). TCAs undergo metabolism via the CYP450 system; the primary metabolic enzyme is 2D6, yet other pathways may be involved, such as CYP2C19 (217). TCAs have a shorter half-life in children compared to adults (218), and linear pharmacokinetics. Excretion is primarily renal as the inactive metabolite.

Research regarding TCA pharmacokinetics has found an effect of variable CYP2C19 and CYP2D6 genotypes on the metabolism of clomipramine (219). In another study, the duplication of CYP2D6 genes predicted higher clearance of desipramine (220). Novel formulations are under investigation, such as a sustained-release dosage form of clomipramine and osmotic-release (OROS) amitriptyline (221).

Pharmacodynamics

In addition to inhibition of NE and 5HT reuptake, other putative mechanisms of TCA action include decreasing the density of postsynaptic B-adrenoreceptors and 5HT receptors with chronic administration. However, the final pathway of action is likely to involve modulation of a biochemical chain of events and altered genomic expression (222). Secondary amines such as nortriptyline (NT) and desipramine (DMI) have greater relative effect on NE transmission (and little or no 5HT effect), compared to tertiary amines which usually have both NE and 5HT effects. In addition, secondary amine TCAs have less anticholinergic and antihistaminic activity and consequently fewer such side effects.

Neuroimaging studies include work by Suhara et al. (2003) (223). Using positron emission tomography, the authors showed a high degree of serotonin transporter occupancy with low-dose clomipramine in a comparative occupancy study with fluvoxamine.

Pharmacotherapy

For children and adolescents, TCAs have proven efficacy in the treatment of enuresis, OCD, and ADHD, with second-line utility in a variety of other neuropsychiatric conditions (224). FDA indications for this class are limited to enuresis (imipramine) and OCD (clomipramine).

Mood Disorder

Despite an approximately 80% response rate in adults with major depressive disorder (222), TCAs have not been shown to be significantly effective in juvenile depressive disorders (225, 226). According to a *Cochrane Systematic Review* (227) of 13 trials (506 participants), no overall improvement with TCA treatment compared to placebo was seen for children or adolescents. Subgroup analyses suggested a larger benefit among adolescents (effect size [ES] = −0.47, 95% confidence interval −0.92 to −0.02) and no benefit among children (ES = 0.15, 95% confidence interval −0.34 to 0.64). Interpretation of individual trial results is limited by numerous methodological shortcomings. However, TCAs may be otherwise appropriate in specific pediatric populations, such as treatment-resistant or severe MDD (56, 228).

Anxiety Disorders

Despite comparable efficacy to the SSRIs in adult panic disorder (229), with the exception of pediatric OCD, there are limited controlled data in pediatric anxiety disorders. Four double-blind, placebo-controlled studies, evaluating TCAs for the treatment of anxiety-based school refusal produced conflicting results (230–233).

Clomipramine (CMI) may have unique properties among the TCAs as the parent compound has potent serotonergic activity before being metabolized to a secondary amine. Early studies and subsequent multisite industry-sponsored RCTs demonstrated its superiority over placebo and desipramine in both shortterm and longer-term RCTs for pediatric OCD (234–236). Meta-analyses in both adults (237–239) and children (21) have suggested that it is significantly more effective than the SSRIs for OCD at all ages. In the latter study, the effect size for CMI was 0.69, which was significantly higher than for each of the SSRIs (21). However, head-to-head studies in adults have failed to show this superiority and also found that SSRIs are better tolerated. Such studies have not been done in youth.

Attention Deficit Hyperactivity Disorder (ADHD)

Expert opinion is that tricyclic antidepressants have positive efficacy comparable to that of stimulants (240–242). However, their adverse effect profile limits their utility (240, 241). Agents with efficacy demonstrated in RCTs include imipramine, desipramine, and amitriptyline. In the largest controlled trial of desipramine (DMI) in children, Biederman et al. (1989) observed a robust response in 62 children with ADHD. Four trials comparing TCAs with MPH indicated either no differences in response or slightly better results with stimulants (244).

Tic Disorders

Following observation in open reports that the TCA desipramine improved tics as well as ADHD symptoms, Spencer (2003) (243) conducted a 6-week, double-blind, placebo-controlled, parallel trial of desipramine (to 3.5 mg/kg per day) versus placebo. Desipramine significantly reduced tic symptoms by about 30% from baseline relative to placebo using the Yale Global Tic Severity Scale with equal response in both motor and vocal tics.

Enuresis

Imipramine has an FDA indication for treatment of enuresis, and until the emergence of the newer pharmacological treatments such as desmopressin acetate (DDAVP) (244), TCAs had a primary role in the management of enuresis. A 2002 Cochrane systematic review of 54 RCTs (N = 3379) of TCAs or related drugs for nocturnal enuresis in children showed that treatment with tricyclic drugs (imipramine, amitriptyline, nortriptyline, clomipramine, and desipramine) was associated with a reduction of approximately one wet night per week. About 20% of the children became dry while on treatment, but this effect was not sustained after treatment stopped. Overall, these reviewers concluded that although tricyclics and desmopressin are effective in reducing the number of wet nights, most children relapse after stopping active treatment, compared to about 50% relapse after alarm treatment (245).

Pervasive Developmental Disorders

Clomipramine (CMI) showed improvement on standardized ratings of stereotypic and self-injurious behaviors, anger and aggression, impulsivity, and social relatedness in autistic children (246). Efficacy of the serotonergic CMI was superior to the noradrenergic TCA desipramine in another controlled study (247). In a shortterm trial, individuals with autistic disorder were randomly assigned to placebo, clomipramine, or haloperidol. Fewer individuals receiving clomipramine were able to complete the trial due to side effects and lack of efficacy or behavioral problems. In the intent-to-treat sample, only haloperidol showed significant improvement from baseline on global measure of autistic severity, as well as specific measures for irritability and hyperactivity (248).

Initiating and Maintenance of Medication

Initiation

Medication guides for families and clinicians are now available from the FDA (www.fda.gov/cder/drug/anti depressants/MG_template.pdf) and jointly from the American Psychiatric Association and the American Academy of Child and Adolescent Psychiatry (www.aacap.org/Announcements/pdfs/parentsmedguide.pdf; www.aacap.org/Announcements/pdfs/physiciansmedguide.pdf).

In addition to general principles that apply to all medications, the unique side effect profile, particularly suppression of cardiac conductivity, mandates a careful evaluation of baseline physical health, cardiovascular parameters, and ECG prior to initiating TCAs in children. A family history of cardiac illness, such as conduction deficits or early sudden death (as distinct from late-onset coronary atherosclerotic disease), should be elicited. Blood count and liver enzyme assays are often suggested as baseline evaluation. Ideally, initiation of a TCA should be done in cooperation with a child or adolescent's primary care physician. Guidelines have been published regarding the use of TCAs in children and adolescents (249, 250). TCAs are typically begun in the range of 1.0 mg/kg daily, with gradual titration (e.g., q 7 to 14 days). Maximum dosing is 3 mg/kg daily for CMI and NT or 5 mg/kg daily for DMI.

Monitoring

As discussed in the SSRI section presented earlier, national psychiatric associations (the American Psychiatric Association and the American Academy of Child and Adolescent Psychiatry) concur with the need to closely monitor children and adolescents on antidepressants.

Pulse and blood pressure measurement should be performed at office visits intermittently, as well as an ECG with dosage increases and upon reaching target dose, and then periodically during maintenance therapy at three to six monthly intervals. TCA serum levels are monitored to guide treatment, as well as to assess for potential toxicity. It should also be noted that laboratory reference ranges are broad guides only and that some children may benefit from maintenance at serum levels that are above the upper limit of the reference range. In these cases, close attention to ECG parameters is necessary.

Safety and Side Effects

Adverse effects of TCAs can be attributed to the multiple receptor activity of these agents; antimuscarinic (anticholinergic), antiadrenergic (alpha-1, alpha-2), and antihistaminic. Tertiary amines have greater affinities for these sites and therefore produce more adverse effects. Anticholinergic effects include dry mouth, constipation, blurred vision, and sinus tachycardia. Antiadrenergic effects include orthostatic hypotension, dizziness (alpha-1), and blockade of alpha agonists such as clonidine. Antihistaminic effects include weight gain and sedation.

Clinical trials with TCAs in youth cite frequent adverse effects such as dizziness, headache, tremor, nausea, insomnia, dry mouth, and anxiety (56). According to a *Cochrane Systematic Review* (227) of 13 TCA trials (506 participants), only vertigo, orthostatic hypotension, tremor, and dry mouth occurred more often than with placebo. Dry mouth in children may increase risk for dental caries. Extrapyramidal symptoms have been described in adults using TCAs (251).

TCAs exert a quinidine-like (class 1A antiarrhythmic) effect, which can result in slowed cardiac conduction. Specific electrocardiogram (ECG) changes may occur, such as prolonged PR intervals, increased QRS duration, and increased rate-corrected QT intervals (QTc). In a study evaluating desipramine effects up to 5 mg/kg/day, Schroeder et al. (1989) (252) reported a 21% increase in heart rate and a 2.5% increase in QTc intervals at 4 weeks and 8 weeks, yet no dysrhythmias or clinically significant changes in blood pressure occurred. However, in the following years there were cases of sudden death in children treated with desipramine and imipramine (253–258). Potential contributing factors were noted in each case, including exercise prior to death, history of paroxysmal atrial tachycardia, cardiac vascular anomaly, and family history of early-onset cardiac disease, including sudden death (259). Members of the Work Group on Research and Office of Research of the American Academy of Child and Adolescent Psychiatry (1992) concluded that the rate of deaths during DMI treatment was not clearly statistically increased over the background incidence of sudden deaths in the pediatric population generally. Guidelines regarding *un*acceptable electrocardiographic indices for the use (or increase) of TCAs have been recommended by the FDA as follows: (1) PR interval >200 ms, (2) QRS interval >30% increased over baseline or >120 ms, (3) blood pressure

>140 systolic or 90 diastolic, and (4) heart rate >130 bpm at rest (260, 261). Finally, a prolonged QTc (corrected QT interval >450 ms) is associated with an increased risk of ventricular tachyarrythmias and is a contraindication for TCA use (or further increase). TCAs may also lower the threshold for seizures, and brain-injured children may be more prone to this serious adverse effect (262).

Suicidality

As described earlier in detail in the SSRI section, the FDA has performed meta-analyses of adverse event cases across nonTCA antidepressant pediatric trials. The FDA has instituted the following black box labeling: "antidepressants *increased* the risk of suicidal thinking and behavior (suicidality) *in short-term studies.*"

Activation/Switching

As described earlier in detail in the SSRI section, activation implies an alteration in mood, anxiety, or behavioral state (such as restlessness) induced by a medication, such as an antidepressant (197). Activation does not signify the presence of hypomania or mania, or necessarily herald bipolar disorder. These relatively mild adverse events may be dose related and may resolve with reduction of dose without discontinuation. Contrary to activation, treatment-emergent affective (mood) switching (TEAS) implies a switch from one mood state (depression) to another (hypomania or mania) in the context of treatment, such as with an antidepressant.

As depression may be the (unknown or unexpected) index episode of a bipolar disorder, clinicians must monitor for switching into a hypomanic or manic state. True manic conversion precludes the further use of an antidepressant without first achieving adequate mood stabilization.

Overdose

Glauser (2000) (263) has reviewed the associated electrocardiographic abnormalities seen with TCA poisoning; ventricular dysrhythmias, hypotension, heart block, bradyarrhythmias, or asystole can occur. Hypotension, seizures, coma, and death may result. Treatments such as sodium bicarbonate, activated charcoal (which binds TCAs), and hypertonic saline may be helpful. A QRS interval > 100 ms appears to be a predictor of serious complications.

Drug Interactions

TCA interactions may be based on their pharmacokinetic or pharmacodynamic properties. Concomitant medications that may alter TCA levels include phenothiazines, haloperidol, SSRIs (29), mirtazapine (264), bupropion (214), and venlafaxine (210). Aspirin (ASA) may displace protein bound TCA, increasing the number and severity of adverse events (265). Carbemazepine (CBZ) affects both metabolism and protein binding of TCAs (266). Oesterheld (1996) (267) noted a risk in concomitant medications

that also lengthen QTc, as well as agents that alter the levels of TCAs or their metabolites. Cohen et al. (1999) (268) found no effect of stimulants on the phamacokinetics of desipramine in children.

TCAs, especially the 5HT-active clomipramine, are not recommended within 2 weeks of discontinuing or starting an MAO-I. The anticholinergic effects of the TCAs provide a relative contraindication for their use in poorly controlled asthmatics on multiple asthma medications (269).

STIMULANTS

Neuropsychopharmacology

Since the previous edition of this text, new stimulant formulations have arrived on the market. A summary of methylphenidate (MPH), amphetamine (AMPH; d-AMPH), and magnesium pemoline will be presented.

Pharmacokinetics

Overall, stimulants are rapidly absorbed and metabolized, and they possess little protein binding. Although individual and comparison drug profiles can be found in the literature, there is tremendous interindividual variability, which precludes direct extrapolation of these concentration-over-time profiles to an individual child or adolescent.

Stimulants are available in several formulations; standard immediate release (IR), first-generation sustained release (SR), and second-generation extended release (ER) compounds, representing novel mechanisms of drug liberation. Products differ in their drug delivery mechanisms and in their proportions of immediate versus extended release drug.

Methylphenidate comprises 4 stereoisomers, d- and l-threo- and d- and l-erythro-MPH; the CNS active threo isomers are found in marketed preparations. Absorption is rapid from the GI tract. Bioavailability of the d-threo isomer is approximately 23%, due to a significant first pass (hepatic extraction) effect. Protein binding is approximately 15%. A primary metabolic site is within the intestinal wall, to inactive ritalinic acid. Time to peak plasma levels is about 1.5 to 2.5 hours, with plasma half-life of about 2 to 3.5 hours (270, 271). The presence of food may delay or reduce peak levels.

Development of SR formulations followed immediate release preparations, yet they were not fully embraced in clinical practice due to an apparent lack of comparative efficacy; in comparison to IR products, plasma concentration over time showed a flatter curve (270). More recently, oral osmotic release system (OROS) technology has led to the marketing of the third generation of MPH drugs such as Concerta, with its unique ascending dose curve (272). Comparisons of mean-concentration-over-time profiles demonstrate pair-wise differences between Concerta and other drug formulations such as Metadate CD (273) and

Ritalin LA (274), and between extended-release agents (271). Swanson et al. (1999) (272) reported pharmacokinetic and pharmacodynamic data in support of the efficacy of OROS technology. An ascending DA release-curve maintained efficacy for ADHD symptoms throughout the day, whereas IR MPH lost 40% of its benefit in the afternoon hours. Another advance is represented by the purified d-threo MPH isomer, Focalin. Phase 2 studies demonstrated pharmacokinetic activity comparable to IR MPH, yet with superior efficacy to placebo up to 6 hours postdose (275).

Adderall and Adderall XR are compositions of mixed salts of l-AMPH and d-AMPH. Absorption of AMPH from the GI tract is rapid. Amphetamine metabolism occurs via several pathways such as hydroxylation and de-amination in the liver (276). However, the majority is excreted renally, unchanged (277). The half-life of its behavioral effects is 3 to 6 hours, although clearance or serum half-life is 12 to 20 hours. Due to the mixed nature of the compounded formulation, variable pharmacokinetic curves are likely. Ingestion of acid, such as ascorbic acid in juices, will enhance renal clearance and possibly reduce efficacy (276). Absorption of Adderall XR may be slowed in the presence of food, unlike Concerta (278). Only minor differences in Cmax and Tmax have been found in Adderall XR absorption following fasting, sprinkled on food or with a high-fat breakfast (279). Dexedrine is the d-AMPH form of this molecule, and the behavioral half-life is 2 to 6 hours, with a clearance or serum half-life of 12 to 20 hours (Fig. 27.1).

The pharmacokinetics of pemoline produce maximum plasma concentrations 2 to 5 hours after a single, 2 mg/kg oral dose, followed by a slow decline in plasma concentration over time. Marked interindividual variation in elimination half-life and clearance may explain the unpredictable nature of its pharmacodynamic effects (280). In children, the mean elimination half-life of pemoline is considerably shorter than the 11 to 13 hours reported in adults (281). Pemoline undergoes hepatic metabolism, with the remainder excreted renally (280); half is excreted as unchanged drug.

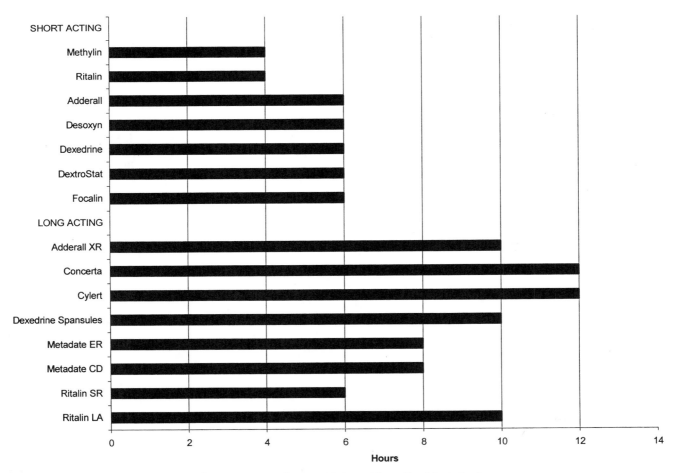

Figure 27.1 Stimulants: Duration of action. (Adapted from Physician's Desk Reference, 2002.)

FIG AQ1

Pharmacodynamics

Stimulants' putative mechanism of action is due to increased synaptic concentration of catecholamines. Increased activity of catecholamines in frontal-striatal pathways is implicated in the mechanism of action in ADHD.

MPH increases striatal DA via blockade of the dopamine transporter (DAT). DAT blockade is followed by increase in DA and DA receptor activation (282). Dose-dependent blockade has been observed; 78% DAT inhibition occurs at a dose of 0.5 mg/kg IV, and 50% DAT inhibition at a dose of 0.25 mg/kg orally (282). Several reports have described reductions in striatal DAT density with MPH treatment (283, 284). In addition, there is significant interindividual variability of DA response to MPH, perhaps reflecting an individual's DA neuron and receptor density (282) as well as pharmacokinetic variability.

Positron emission tomography (PET) scans following administration of the d-threo MPH isomer compared with the l-threo MPH isomer (285), and animal studies demonstrated no therapeutic activity of the l-MPH isomer lending support to efforts to purify the d-threo MPH isomer as found in Focalin. d-MPH was found to have more than three times the potency of l-MPH (286), with both greater DA and NE uptake inhibition (287).

Amphetamine's mechanism of action is slightly different from that of MPH. In addition to DAT blockade, AMPH is taken up into the terminal neuron, causing DA release from storage vesicles within the neuron as well as release into the synapse. Amphetamines also promote NE and 5HT release during in vivo studies (288), as well as having peripheral adrenergic effects (for example, on heart rate and blood pressure), but the clinical significance of any 5HT activity is unknown.

Animal models suggest that the central stimulant effects of pemoline may be due to catecholamine-uptake inhibition, causing indirect DA agonism similar to other stimulants. For example, pemoline inhibited uptake of DA (competitively) and NE (noncompetitively) from striatum and hypothalamus (289). The pharmacodynamic effects of pemoline in youth have been described by Sallee et al. (1992) (290), who correlated plasma pemoline concentration with psychometric measures and analyzed plasma prolactin response to determine the physiological effect of pemoline on dopaminergic transmission.

Pharmacotherapy

The primary application of stimulants in pediatric psychopharmacology is in the treatment of childhood attention deficit hyperactivity disorder (ADHD). Stimulants may also offer benefit in other neuropsychiatric syndromes, such as mental retardation, chronic fatigue syndrome, chronic depression, multiple sclerosis, and traumatic brain injury.

Attention Deficit Hyperactivity Disorder (ADHD)

The strength of evidence of this body of literature regarding efficacy of stimulants in ADHD is Level, the highest, using AHRQ criteria of quality, quantity, and consistency of scientific studies. Until the approval of atomoxetine (Strattera), stimulants were the only FDA-approved class of medications indicated for treatment of ADHD.

Randomized Controlled Trials in ADHD

An extensive body of literature supports the shortterm efficacy of stimulant medications in ADHD. The majority of clinical trials involve Caucasian, latency-age boys treated with stimulants (primarily MPH) for a short duration (291, 292). Improvement typically occurs in 65 to 75% of stimulant treated subjects, compared to a 5 to 30% placebo response (291).

Findings from the NIMH-sponsored Collaborative Multisite Multimodal Treatment Study of Children With Attention-Deficit/Hyperactivity Disorder (MTA) suggest that school-age children with ADHD who received higher and more frequent stimulant doses experienced better outcomes than those children treated with lower and less frequent doses (293, 294). Previously, however, others (295) have noted a *curvilinear* response to stimulants; lower doses produced improvements, with declines in performance at higher doses. Dose-dependent efficacy has been shown in core ADHD symptoms, cognitive function, disruptive behavior, and, more recently, in broader aspects of social-emotional well-being in ADHD youth (296).

Efficacy of the different stimulants shows great individuality in response rates. In one meta-analysis, Greenhill et al. (1996) (297) found equal response to MPH and d-amphetamine in 40%, a greater response to MPH in 26%, and a greater response to d-amphetamine in 35% of subjects tested. An evidence-based review by the Agency for Healthcare Research and Quality (AHRQ) of 78 ADHD studies found 23 studies that compared MPH, DEX, and pemoline, and these studies showed few differences between these drugs (292). However, another meta-analysis of four clinical trials using Adderall and MPH in 188 children with ADHD found a small, but statistically significant advantage of Adderall over MPH (298).

Novel extended-release agents have demonstrated bioequivalence to the IR products (299, 300) as well as superiority over placebo (301, 302). In a multicenter study comparing Metadate CD and Concerta with placebo in children with ADHD, three different patterns of effectiveness across the day were described, consistent with plasma MPH concentrations: (1) Metadate > Concerta > placebo in the morning, (2) Metadate = Concerta > placebo in the afternoon, and (3) Concerta > Metadate = placebo in the evening (301). These differences in clinical effect reflect the differing proportions of immediate- and extended-release drug in each proprietary formulation, indicating that attention to drug formulation in order to target specific times of the day is worthwhile.

Pemoline has considerably less scientific support compared to MPH and AMPH products. However, a comparison of pemoline to MPH and d-AMPH suggested similar efficacy in childhood ADHD (303), but with a longer duration of action. Behavioral effects last up to 7 hours postingestion (304). Randomized controlled trials have demonstrated efficacy in both adolescent (2.88 mg/kg/day in two divided doses) (305) and adult (2.2 mg/kg/day) populations (306).

Tics With Comorbid ADHD
Despite concerns about the potential for stimulants to exacerbate or even cause tics, longitudinal and naturalistic studies show that stimulants have little impact on the *long-term* course of tic disorders (307–309) and remain effective in those children with ADHD comorbid with tic disorders and Tourette's (310). Tics are therefore no longer considered an absolute contraindication for the use of stimulants, but rather a relative contraindication, especially considering that many children with chronic tic disorders will have comorbid ADHD and could benefit considerably from their use.

Mood Disorders
Stimulants have a role in the management of adult and geriatric unipolar depression, especially in the medically compromised, such as persons suffering from poststroke depression and prominent apathy. However, there is no known controlled evidence for the use of stimulants in depressed youth. Studies to evaluate stimulant effects in bipolar youth with comorbid ADHD are proceeding. One systematic chart review of bipolar youth found greater efficacy in treating ADHD symptoms *following prior mood stabilization* (311) supporting clinical judgment to address the primary mood symptoms before ADHD symptoms.

Autism/Pervasive Developmental Disorders With Comorbid ADHD
Symptoms of ADHD are prevalent in children with autism and pervasive developmental disorders, yet there is little controlled evidence to support the efficacy of stimulants in this population. A small placebo-controlled trial of methylphenidate (0.3 to 0.6 mg/kg/day) conducted in children with autism and symptoms of attention deficit hyperactivity disorder (312) found MPH to be beneficial, but poorly tolerated at the higher dose range.

Mental Retardation Syndromes with Comorbid ADHD
ADHD symptoms are frequently manifest in children with mild to moderate mental retardation (MR) and appear phenomenologically similar to ADHD outside the context of MR. Yet, while expert consensus opinion supports the use of psychostimulants as the first-line treatment for ADHD in MR (313), low-IQ children with ADHD may respond to psychostimulants with lower or more variable rates, as well as experience increased rates of adverse effects compared to normal-IQ children. Lower-functioning children (314) and children with genetic syndromes, such as fragile X, may be the most vulnerable (315–317).

Seizures With Comorbid ADHD
The prevalence of ADHD symptoms in patients with epilepsy ranges from 40 to 80% (318). Seizures, epileptiform discharges, antiepileptic drugs (AEDs), and underlying brain disease may all contribute to the presence of inattention in these children (319–321). Open and retrospective study has demonstrated relative safety and efficacy of stimulants in small samples of children with ADHD and seizures (320). Like those with MR, children with seizures are generally excluded from controlled drug trials, along with other physically ill youth. However, two controlled trials report on the benefit of stimulants in ADHD children with epilepsy (322, 323).

Traumatic Brain Injury
ADHD-like symptoms and mood disorders have been described as the most common lifetime and new-onset difficulties associated with traumatic brain injury (TBI) in children (324). A controlled trial in pediatric neurosurgical subjects cites efficacy of MPH in a small cohort of children with *acquired* attentional disorders secondary to brain injury (325). Whyte et al. (2002) (326) reviewed the use of stimulants in adults with TBI that describes their role.

Uses in Other Neuropsychiatric Conditions
Psychiatric illness in children and adolescents with neurological or other general medical illness may represent a primary coincident diagnosis, illness secondary to a primary brain or other organ system disease, or some complex interplay of these factors. Effective management of ADHD symptoms in children who are deaf or hard of hearing requires comprehensive and coordinated services (327). Stimulant efficacy in adult narcolepsy has been established, but there are no known applications in pediatric primary sleep disorders.

Initiation and Maintenance of Psychostimulants
Initiation
Standard informed consent with parents or guardians is the first step in initiating treatment. Common, mild, and dose-related side effects should be anticipated. As always, clinicians should conduct a thorough medical history in the context of a comprehensive psychiatric evaluation. As promulgated by the American Heart Association in large part to screen for those at risk for sudden death, clinical history should include assessment of family history of heart defects, sudden early death, or child history of congenital

or acquired cardiac problems. At intake and with treatment, practitioners should query for syncope, palpitations, or chest pain whether associated with exertion, postexertion, or at rest (328). ECGs are not recommended in routine patients either at baseline or with active stimulant treatment. With any concerning family or patient history, clinicians should consult with primary care physicians and consider cardiology consultation. Due to potential serious liver injury and failure, pemoline is not considered a first-line agent.

Using a stimulant medication involves consideration of practical matters such as time of onset and duration of action. In those children with prominent schoolday symptoms, IR or SR products may be indicated, whereas children with symptomatic impairment throughout the day and into early evening hours may benefit from the newer 8- to 12-hour ER formulations. A combination of IR and SR or ER products is also possible and commonly employed to obtain individually tailored symptom coverage. MPH and AMPH differ in potency by a ratio of about 2:3. As such, appropriate dosing for MPH is 0.5 mg/kg/day to 2 mg/kg/day and AMPH 0.5 mg/kg/day to 1 mg/kg/day. *Optimal dosing is the lowest effective dose.* Children with organic brain disease may be more sensitive to CNS active psychotropic drugs and the general rule of "start low, go slow" applies.

Maintenance and Monitoring

As suggested by the AACAP and American Academy of Pediatrics, the use of stimulants for ADHD should involve collaboration with families, schools, primary care providers, and other mental health professionals in order to achieve targeted outcomes and to monitor other comorbid conditions and psychosocial stressors. Education and behavioral management combined with pharmacotherapy may offer optimal results for an individual child (294).

In monitoring ADHD symptom response, those with intolerable adverse effects or lack of efficacy with an adequate trial of a first agent should receive a trial of an alternate stimulant. Combination treatment with SR or ER agents may be helpful, such as addition of a small, late afternoon dose of IR drug for management of evening symptoms. Clinical experience suggests that mood lability and rebound phenomena may be less problematic with SR or ER agents, which provide slower fluctuations in blood levels, avoiding the plasma peaks and rapid troughs produced by IR products.

No routine laboratory studies are indicated in maintenance MPH or AMPH stimulant therapy. Vital signs and growth parameters should be routinely monitored (see safety section below). Routine monitoring of pemoline concentration is not useful due to the wide variation in optimum serum concentration and the linear relationship between dose and serum concentration (281). However, monitoring of liver function is advised.

Safety

Mild and dose-related side effects include insomnia, GI upset and abdominal pain, reduced appetite, headache, and behavioral or mood changes, such as irritability or heightened anxiety. In the Agency for Healthcare Research and Quality evidence-based review of 29 ADHD studies evaluating adverse effects of therapy, side effects were generally mild and dose related (292).

Concern about the longterm effects of psychostimulants on growth followed several decades of the use of stimulants in children. Spencer et al. (1996) reported that the modest height deficits (2 cm) in a large sample of ADHD boys were *unrelated* to stimulant treatment. This finding was similar to prior reports of height deficits of 1 to 3 cm (329). Minimal deficits in height and weight have also been reported with once-daily products, including Concerta (243) and Adderall XR (330). In a thorough review of the evidence, Spencer et al. (2003) (331) suggested that observed height deficits could represent disorder-specific developmental delays. In a 9-month study of OROS MPH, adolescents demonstrated greater than expected growth in height during stimulant treatment, possibly representing catch-up growth (332). A temporary retardation in the rate of growth in weight and height with later catch-up growth has also been observed in children treated with pemoline (333).

In one review, Spencer (2003) (243) found that stimulants transiently exacerbate tics in some children. However, because ADHD typically has its onset several years earlier than tic disorders and many children are already taking stimulants at the time of peak risk for tic onset, a cause–effect relationship is difficult to ascertain. Animal studies have found that stereotypic and self-injurious behaviors may be enhanced in the setting of underlying cortical damage (334) as may be found in certain pediatric neurological syndromes. Nonetheless, as noted earlier in the treatment section, stimulants may be very helpful for some children with tics and ADHD symptoms.

Children with poorly stabilized mania could experience explosive outbursts with methylphenidate (335). One review discusses the risk of stimulants in those at risk, (i.e., those with vulnerability for psychosis) and in situations of stimulant abuse (336).

In one sample, comorbid anxiety did not influence either the tolerability or the efficacy of MPH (up to 0.7 mg/kg/day) upon ADHD symptoms (Diamond et al., 1999) (337).

Modest yet statistically significant elevations in systolic, diastolic blood pressure and heart rate were demonstrated in a review of five RCTs of stimulants and nonstimulants in adults with ADHD (41). Similar minor and clinically insignificant adverse cardiovascular effects have been noted with both methylphenidate and Adderall in samples of children and adolescents (338). Cardiac conduction effects with stimulant use have been infrequently reported, but their clinical importance is uncertain (339).

In February 2005, Health Canada suspended the market authorization of Adderall XR based on safety information concerning the association of sudden deaths, heart-related deaths, and strokes in children and adults taking Adderall and Adderall XR. A public health advisory by FDA followed this report (www.fda.gov). The FDA advisory describes important complicating factors in sudden unexplained deaths (SUDs) in persons taking Adderall. In 5 of 12 cases, underlying structural heart defects were found, such as abnormal arteries, valves, and thickened walls. Several of the remaining cases included other variables, such as a family history of ventricular tachycardia or association of death with dehydration, near-drowning, rigorous exercise, heat exhaustion, or liver or metabolic (diabetes) disease. Duration of treatment varied widely in these cases, from 1 day to as many as 8 years. In considering these reports, it is important to recognize the background population rate for sudden unexplained death (SUD) in children and adolescents varies from 1 to 6/100,000; higher in competitive athletes and in adolescence (340). With 20 cases of SUD per 4 million patient Adderall exposures (adjusted per year), the rate of SD is 0.5/100,000. While the rate of underreporting of SD in children and adolescents is unknown, if one-tenth are reported, the SD rate associated with Adderall administration would remain less than or equal to the population rate of SD. According to the FDA, the number of cases of sudden deaths reported for Adderall is only slightly greater, per million prescriptions, than the number reported for methylphenidate products. It is also important to remember that the stimulants (including Adderall) have relatively benign cardiovascular effects and have no effects on the QTc duration of the ECG.

Reports of pemoline hepatotoxic drug reactions sent to the FDA between 1975 and 1996 were reviewed by Safer et al. (341). In premarketing trials of the early 1970s, hepatic enzyme abnormalities were noted in 1 to 3% of youth receiving maintenance treatment, with some abnormalities confirmed by biopsies. Between 1975 and 1989, 12 cases of jaundice and 6 deaths in youths ascribed to pemoline hepatotoxicity were reported to the FDA. However, the first report in the medical literature of a serious adverse drug reaction ascribed to pemoline did not appear until 1989, and physicians did not generally became aware of potentially serious pemoline hepatotoxicity until the mid-1990s, by which time there had been 13 cases of liver failure, with 11 resulting in death (342, 343). Although the majority of cases of pemoline-associated hepatic injury have been in youth under 12 years of age (344), adult cases of liver failure exist as well (345). An idiosyncratic metabolic process (344) and an autoimmune process (346) have been proposed as pathogenetic mechanisms.

Concerns about abuse of stimulants have been long-standing and drawn considerable attention from some organizations that are philosophically opposed to the use of psychoactive medications. Without question, isolated cases of stimulant abuse do occur, predominantly in adolescents and often in school settings where stimulants may be readily available. Mood disturbance and nasal septum necrosis (from snorting) are possible results. However, orally administered MPH has a considerably slower rate of uptake centrally, compared with intravenous MPH, and PET studies show that although intravenous MPH has rapid central uptake, this is followed by slow clearance from the brain. These characteristics interfere with the mood elevation produced by frequent administration, unlike cocaine, which is rapidly cleared from the brain (347). Newer and longer-acting agents are much less likely to be abused due to the nature of their formulations. Despite concerns regarding abuse, it should be noted that nonmedicated ADHD patients are at much higher risk for substance abuse than controls *and* medicated ADHD patients due to their impulse-control deficits and novelty-seeking behaviors (348). Therefore, withholding psychostimulant medication from genuine cases of ADHD for fear of stimulant abuse is not supported by the scientific evidence. In cases where abuse is a concern, careful monitoring is nevertheless required.

In those with a seizure disorder, some reports suggest a lowering of the seizure threshold with stimulants (349, 350).

Drug Interactions

Following an extensive review, Markowitz et al. (351) concluded that the only true contraindication to the use of stimulants is coadministration of MAOIs; their combination may result in serious hypertension. Notably, stimulants do not increase serum levels of TCAs (268), nor do there appear to be serious side effects in combining these treatments (352). However, isolated reports of drug interactions can be found in the literature, such as grand mal seizures with bupropion and methylphenidate combined or pharmacokinetic interactions between cyclosporine and bupropion or methylphenidate (353, 354). From a clinical standpoint, such interactions are rarely a concern.

Despite isolated concerns stemming from reported possible cases of pediatric sudden death with combination MPH and clonidine (355), the FDA could not cite a causal link after investigating this matter. Hypotension was found in all cases, but it was not clearly due to a drug interaction. Subsequent studies found no EKG changes with clonidine treatment (356), though one small sample showed slight increased PR interval with combination MPH and clonidine therapy (357). Current expert consensus opinion supports continued combined use of stimulant and clonidine as an appropriate treatment option (358).

Markowitz (359) reviewed the risks of drug interactions between MPH and antiepileptic drugs (AEDs). In general the risks were considered negligible, but there are case reports of MPH inhibition of phenytoin and primidone metabolism as well as carbamazepine lowering MPH plasma levels.

Overdose

Klein-Schwartz (2003) (360) reviewed 7 years of pediatric MPH exposures across U.S. poison centers and found tachycardia, agitation, and hypertension to be the most common events. In only 0.9% of 759 cases were outcomes considered severe. Nakamura et al. (2002) (361) described five pediatric cases of excessive pemoline ingestion. Overall, patients experienced a relatively benign course. Symptoms of pemoline toxicity occurred within 6 hours, lasted up to 48 hours, and were related to CNS and cardiovascular pharmacological effects, with tachycardia, hypertension, choreoathetoid movements, and hallucinations. Elevation of serum creatine phosphokinase (CPK) was also observed in 3 of 4 patients.

ATOMOXETINE

Atomoxetine, approved by the FDA in January of 2003, is inherently interesting for a number of reasons. It is the first medication approved for the treatment of ADHD that is not a stimulant, the first medication specifically approved for the treatment of ADHD in adults, the first psychiatric medication that has been approved for use in children before adults, and the first of a new generation of selective noradrenergic reuptake inhibitors. The rapid increase in prescriptions written over its first year (more than 4 million written and more than 1 million children initiated into treatment) testifies to the many gaps and frustrations that practitioners face in the pharmacological treatment of youth and adults with ADHD, despite the long history and success of the stimulants. It is increasingly likely to be used as a first-line agent for newly diagnosed children with ADHD. The research into atomoxetine is far and away the most robust in pediatric psychopharmacology, as the number of children studied through industry-sponsored trials and the duration of longterm safety and tolerability trials are an order of magnitude greater than with any previous drug. At least 10 different RCTs of atomoxetine using multisite design have been done, and the comulative number of children studied is around 5,000, some studied over 3 years.

Pharmacokinetics

Atomoxetine is rapidly absorbed following oral administration and peaks in 1 to 2 hours. High-fat meals slow absorption slightly so that peak levels are delayed by an hour or 2, and the peak serum levels are about 10% lower. However, the total AUC and extent of absorption is unaffected by food. The serum half-life of this agent is relatively short, about 5 hours. Based on this observation, it was originally conceived that atomoxetine would

be administered as a twice-daily dose, hence the limited dosing formulations available currently. Later observations led to further single daily dose studies and in general, single daily administration is equally effective for the majority of patients. Atomoxetine is a substrate for the CYP2D6 hepatic enzyme and demonstrates linear pharmacokinetics. It does not itself inhibit or induce any hepatic enzymes, but CYP2D6 deficiency or inhibition will substantially increase its serum levels and extend half-life (362), though even poor metabolizers tolerate atomoxtine extremely well. The parent drug is hydroxylated to a metabolically active compound, which circulates at very low levels and is not clinically significant, before being excreted in the urine. Neither renal nor hepatic deficiency substantially increase risk of its administration.

Pharmacodynamics

Inhibition of monoamine transporters for NE, serotonin (5 HT), and DA with dissociation constants (Ki) of 5, 77, and 1,451 nanomolar, respectively, suggests good NE selectivity as well as potency. There is little to no activity at receptors of the serotonin, norepinephrine, dopamine, histamine, adrenergic or muscarinic type, and the adverse effect profile reflects this characteristic. Animal studies have suggested that extracellular dopamine is increased in prefrontal cortex (but not nucleus accumbens or striatum) via nonspecific monoamine uptake inhibition or stimulation of ventral tegmental NE neurons projecting to the cortex (363).

Clinical Pharmacology

The impetus to study atomoxetine came from studies of secondary amine tricyclics in ADHD (see tricyclic section presented earlier). Spencer et al. (1998) (364) first explored atomoxetine in double-blind fashion in 22 adults with ADHD and found a robust response. Two subsequent early identical proof-of-concept 12-week studies (365) in 291 children randomized to either placebo, atomoxetine, or methylphenidate found highly significant effects ($p < 0.001$) for atomoxetine over placebo on the clinician-scored parent-reported ADHD symptom rating scale. The study was not powered to detect differences in effect sizes between the drugs, but in this study no differences in primary outcomes measures were detected between them (366). Once-daily treatment was seen to be as effective as twice-daily dosing studies with an effect size of 0.71 as reported by parents, teachers, and clinicians. Further, parent diary ratings suggested that drug-specific effects were sustained late in the day following morning dosing (367). Many practitioners have found, however, that the overall effect size of atomoxetine is less than that of the stimulants in uncomplicated ADHD subjects. Preliminary evidence indicates that atomoxetine does not exacerbate tics and may even be helpful in decreasing tics in those with comorbid tics and ADHD (368).

Initiating and Maintenance

Dose response studies found that, in the pooled sample, 1.2 mg/kg/d and 1.8 mg/kg/d of atomoxetine were consistently associated with superior outcome in ADHD symptoms versus placebo, but they were not significantly different from each other (369, 370). Dose response curves are linear between zero and the target dose of 1.2 to 1.4 mg/kg/d, however. Thus, the recommended daily dose follows these guidelines with initiation at 0.5 to 0.8 mg/kg/d and increasing to target dose over several days to several weeks depending on tolerance. Because weight-adjusted doses provide reliable and similar blood level profiles at different weights and ages, weight-based dosing is an appropriate strategy at all ages. Abrupt discontinuation in both children and adults pooled from four large studies of atomoxetine did not appear to be associated with any acute discontinuation syndrome and was well tolerated although symptoms of ADHD worsened (371).

Safety

All clinical studies have demonstrated good tolerability and safety with discontinuation rates due to adverse events generally very low (<5%) (367, 369). Cardiovascular effects were evaluated in a large group of children and adolescents and showed statistically significant but modest increases in diastolic blood pressure and heart rates consistent with its noradrenergic profile. These increases usually occurred early in treatment, stabilized, and returned to normal levels upon drug discontinuation. Corrected QT intervals (QTc) did not change from baseline, and routine EKG monitoring is not required (372). Routine laboratory monitoring of hematological, renal, hepatic, or thyroid indices and serum levels is not required, avoiding any need for blood tests.

While more than 2 million patients have taken Strattera since its approval, there have been two postmarketing cases (one adolescent, one adult) of severe liver injury. Based on these reports, the FDA issued a warning (December 2004) that is also included in the package insert. In both cases, liver function returned to normal after Strattera was stopped. Because of the rarity of this event, routine liver function assays are *not* recommended, but any sign of possible injury such as jaundice or malaise should be reported.

Common adverse events include sedation (the commonest side effect), abdominal discomfort, and decreased appetite. Other adverse events did not separate from placebo in pediatric studies but included insomnia, urinary retention, and dizziness in adults. Mood lability has also been observed anecdotally but is less common than with the stimulants. The apparent absence of dopaminergic activity in the nucleus accumbens and striatum predict little abuse liability and adverse effects of tics, consistent

with clinical experience. Based on baseline percentiles, there is an initial slight decrease in expected weight gain with a return to predicted growth rates with longer-term treatment. Effects on growth rates for height were even smaller (373).

MOOD STABILIZERS: LITHIUM AND ANTICONVULSANTS

Neuropsychopharmacology

This group of medications includes lithium, the older anticonvulsants sodium valproic acid (VPA), and carbamazepine (CBZ) and some relatively novel agents, including gabapentin, lamotrigine, tiagabine, oxcarbazepine, and topiramate. The anticonvulsants are used in the management of pediatric seizure disorders (374). While increasingly used for pediatric bipolar disorder, there is little controlled scientific evidence for anticonvulsant use in children with mental disorders, and their application stems largely from extrapolating evidence from the literature on adult mood disorders, which, in contrast, is extensive. Efficacy of the anticonvulsants in adults is reflected by several FDA indications for adults with bipolar disorder.

Lithium/Valproic Acid/Carbamazepine

Lithium

Lithium is absorbed from the gastrointestinal tract at variable rates depending on the formulation of the tablet or capsule (IR versus extended release preparations). As a simple ion, lithium is distributed widely in body fluid and tissue and is not protein bound. The intracellular regulation of lithium is complex. Lithium does not undergo metabolism and is excreted renally. Because children and adolescents have higher relative body water volume and renal glomerular filtration rates compared with adults (375), studies show that lithium in children has a shorter elimination half-life and higher total clearance despite generally similar pharmacokinetics to adults (376). Moore et al. (2002) (377) used ^{7}lithium magnetic resonance spectroscopy (MRS) to measure in vivo brain lithium levels in nine children and adolescents and 18 adults with bipolar disorder. While serum and brain lithium concentrations were positively correlated, younger subjects had lower brain-to-serum concentration ratios than adults: 0.58 versus 0.92. Therefore it was suggested that children and adolescents may extrude lithium more effectively from neurons; therefore youth may require higher serum lithium concentrations than adults to achieve therapeutic brain lithium concentrations. Many formulations of lithium are available, including Lithium, Lithobid, and Eskalith CR, which vary in Cmax and AUC (378, 379).

Valproic Acid and Carbamazepine

VPA is readily absorbed after oral ingestion, is significantly protein bound, and undergoes hepatic metabolism via mitochondrial beta-oxidation and CYP450 glucoronidation. Its metabolism may be accelerated with coadministration of CYP450-inducing agents (380). The clearance of valproic acid correlates with concentration of the unbound fraction and is age dependent, decreasing progressively from infancy to 14 years. For these reasons, the correlation between weight-adjusted dose, plasma concentrations, and efficacy is poor. Time to peak plasma concentration (Tmax) occurs within 3 to 4 hours after ingestion of Divalproex sodium delayed-release (DR), while the half-life (T1/2) is relatively short at 8 to 17 hours. These pharmacokinetic properties require that divalproex sodium DR be administered in a twice-daily dosing regimen. The FDA approved an extended-release (ER) formulation of divalproex sodium, and this once-daily formulation offers 89% bioavailability and 10 to 20% less plasma fluctuation compared to divided dose divalproex with maximum plasma concentrations (Cmax) occuring at 7 to 14 hours. In pediatric studies, Depakote ER produced plasma concentration-time profiles similar to those observed in adults (Abbott, Depakote prescribing information).

Absorption of carbamazepine is gradual and erratic following oral ingestion. CBZ is highly protein bound and is extensively metabolized in the liver, generating multiple metabolites including the toxic epoxide. Autoinduction (induction of CYP450 enzymes for which it is a substrate) occurs with continued use, with a subsequent reduction in half-life and doubling of clearance rate over the first 2 to 3 months (380). Both metabolic conversion of carbamazepine, as well as renal clearance, are much higher in younger children than in adults, so that its half-life is shorter. Oxcarbazepine (Trileptal) (OXC) is a closely related but different molecule from CBZ that yields different metabolites via primary reduction with no epoxide metabolite, reducing potential toxicity. Autoinduction does not occur, protein binding is low, and OXC pharmacokinetics are linear. Although the agent has minimal CYP450 activity, oxcarbazepine may induce CYP3A4/5 at a higher dose and inhibit CYP2C19 (Novartis, Trileptal prescribing information).

Pharmacodynamics

Lithium

Molecular studies suggest that lithium affects neurotransmitter systems by altering intracellular signal transduction mechanisms such as phosphoinositide hydrolysis, adenylyl cyclase, G protein, glycogen synthase kinase-3 beta, and protein kinase C. Such mechanisms produce longterm changes in signaling patterns and levels of cytoskeletal protein phosphorylation, leading to neuroplastic changes (381). Longterm neurotrophic and neuroprotective effects of lithium are indicated by increases in human gray matter,

N-acetyl-aspartate concentrations, and other markers of neuronal viability. (382).

Valproic Acid and Carbamazepine

Direct neuronal effects of valproic acid (VPA) include blockade of voltage-dependent sodium channels and increased calcium-dependent potassium conductance (374). Indirectly, metabolically mediated increases in GABA levels and altered DA and N-methyl D-aspartate (NMDA) activity may underlie its activity (380). Carbamazepine also blocks sodium-dependent channels but decreases depolarization-dependent calcium uptake (374). Inhibition of sodium channel activity appears to be the primary mechanism of anticonvulsant action for both CBZ and OXC (383) (Table 27.13).

Pharmacotherapy

Mood Disorders

There is an extensive literature for lithium, VPA, and CBZ in adult mood disorders. Although anticonvulsant agents are increasingly being used in the management of juvenile bipolar disorder, controlled studies in this population are difficult to conduct. However, controlled trials are emerging, and treatment algorithm have been presented in an attempt to offer consensus guidelines to clinicians. Monotherapy with lithium, divalproex, and carbamazepine (in addition to atypical antipsychotics) are among first-line treatments for juvenile bipolar disorder (384).

Child psychiatrists should be aware of adult endeavors, such as the NIMH Systematic Treatment Enhancement Program for Bipolar Disorder (STEP-BD), a longterm outpatient project that aims to discover which treatments are most effective for depression and mania, as well as prevention of recurrent episodes (www.stepbd.org). Although these agents are generally studied individually in RCTs, monotherapy is the exception and not the rule. The propensity for pharmacotherapy that combines anticonvulsants or anticonvulsants and atypical antipsychotics has been similarly observed in pediatric bipolar samples (385, 386).

Lithium

In adults, lithium has shown efficacy in multiple controlled trials of acute mania, acute bipolar depression, and prophylaxis of adult bipolar disorder, and it is also the only psychotropic to demonstrate decreased suicidality (387–389). A pooled analysis on episode recurrence from 24 studies over 30 years found recurrence rates for those not on lithium averaged 18 times greater than those on lithium. In addition, recurrence rates for patients on lithium decreased fivefold from the 1970s to 1990s (390). Unfortunately, lithium is often inadequate as maintenance monotherapy; only 14% of 247 bipolar persons remaining on lithium achieved euthymia at 5 years, and approximately half achieved only partial improvement (391). Yet adjunctive antidepressant therapy in bipolar disorder

TABLE 27.13

CLINICAL PHARMACOLOGY OF ANTICONVULSANTS

	Carbamazepine	Gabapentin[1]	Lamotrigine	Oxcarbazepine	Topiramate	Valproic Acid
Pharmacokinetic Parameters						
T-Max (hours)	1.5 h (suspension) 4–5 h (tablet) 3–12 h (XR tablet)	2–3 h	2.2 h (single dose) 1.7 (multiple dose) 1.8 (single dose + VPA) 1.9 (multiple dose + VPA)	4.5 h (tablet) 6 h (suspension)	2 h	4 h without food, 8 h with food tablet); 3.3 h without food, 4.8 h with food (sprinkle capsule)
Steady state	Initiation: 3–5 wk; After induction: 2–4 d	1–2 d (normal renal function)	3–15 d	2–3 d	4–5 d (normal renal function)	2–5 d
Half-life (T 1/2)	25–65 h (initially) 12–17 h (chronic)	Renal-function-dependent; 5–7 h (normal renal function)	25 h (mean, monotherapy); 12.6 h (mean, LTG + enzyme inducer); 70. h (mean, LTG + VPA)	2 h (parent) 9 h (metabolite)	18–30 h (normal renal function) 59 h (impaired renal function)	5–13 h
Mechanism of excretion	>85% hepatic; major pathway: CYP3A4; active metabolite: CBZ epoxide	>95% renal excretion as unchanged drug	10% renal unchanged; >85% hepatic, major pathway: N-glucuronidation	>95% renal	70% renal unchanged (monotherapy)	>95% hepatic: glucuronidation (30–50%), β-oxidation (40%), CYP (minor)
Pharmacodynamic Parameters						
Mechanism of action	Blocks voltage-dependent sodium channels but decreases depolarization-dependent calcium uptake	GABA binds to neuronal membranes glutamate synapse	Blocks voltage-dependent sodium channels, antiglutamatergic and neuroprotective actions	Blocks voltage-dependent sodium channels	Modulates voltage-dependent sodium channels, potentiates GABA evoked potentials, and blocks the kainate/AMPA subtype of the glutamate receptor	GABA (to a lesser extent), blockade of voltage-dependent sodium channels and increased calcium-dependent potassium conductance
Dose range (mg/day)	10–35 mg/kg/day	30–60 mg/kg/d (t.i.d)[1]	LTG+enzyme-inducing AED w/o VPA: 0.6 mg/ kg/d (initial), 5–15 mg/kg/d (maintenance); LTG+ AED regimin w/VPA: 0.15 mg/kg/d (initial), 1–5 mg/kg/d (maintenance)	Adjunctive Rx: 20–30 kg: 900 mg 30–40 kg: 1200 >40 kg: 1800 Monotherapy: 20–70 kg: 30–45 mg >70 kg: 23–30 mg increase by 10 mg/kg//wk	1–9 mg/kg/d[1] (b.i.d)	15–60 mg/kg/d (b.i.d-q.i.d)

(continued)

TABLE 27.13
(continued)

Clinical Parameters	Carbamazepine	Gabapentin[1]	Lamotrigine	Oxcarbazepine	Topiramate	Valproic Acid
Common side effects	Drowsiness, dizziness, diplopia, ataxia, blurring of vision peripheral neuropathy, water rentention, hyponatremia	Fatigue, somnolence, dizziness, ataxia	Dizziness, ataxia, somnolence, diplopia, nausea	Dizziness, somnolence, diplopia, fatigue nausea, vomiting, ataxia, abnormal vision, abdominal pain, tremor, dyspepsia, abnormal gait	Somnolence, fatigue, psychomotor slowing, difficulty with concentration, confusion, paresthesias, kidney stones (1.5%)	Nausea, vomiting, drowsiness, tremor, dizziness, hair loss/thinning, weight gain, thrombocytopenia
Prevalent idiosyncratic side effects	Skin rash, hepatotoxicity, blood dyscrasias	None reported to date	Skin rash (including Stevens-Johnson syndrome and toxic epidermal necrolysis), hepatotoxicity	Hyponatremia	Abnormal vision Narrow angle glaucoma	Hepatotoxicity, pancreatitis, blood dyscrasias
Therapeutic serum level range (µg/mL)	4–12	Not established	Not established	10–35	Not established	50–125
Interactions ON drug	↑CBZ: fluoxetine, propoxyphene, erythromycin, cimetidine ↓CBZ: FBM, PB, PHT	↓GBP 20%: aluminum hydroxide/magnesium hydroxide	↓LTG: PHT, CBZ, PB, PRM ↑LTG: VPA	OXC↓: CBZ, PB, PHT, VPA	↓TPM: PHT (48%); CBZ (40%); VPA (14%)	↑VPA: FBM, salicylates (increase free); ↓VPA: CBZ, LTG, PB, PHT
Interactions BY drug	↓doxycycline, FBM, LTG, oral contraceptives, TGB, theophyline, TPM, VPA	None	↓VPA 25%	↑PB 14%; ↑PHT (up to 40%)	↑PHT 25%; ↓VPA 11%, oral contraceptives	↑CBZ epoxide, FBM, LTG, PB, zidovudine

[1]Approval in United States is limited to adjunctive therapy in adults.
AED, Antiepileptic drug; CBZ, Carbamazepine; CYP, Cytochrome; P450 D, Days; FBM, Felbamate; GBP, Gabapentin; H, Hour; LTG, Lamotrigine; PB, Phenobarbital; PHT, Phenytoin; PRM, Primidone; T-Max, Time to peak plasma level; TGB, tiagabine; TPM, Topiramate; VPA, Valproic acid; Wks, Weeks.

depressive episodes has never been more effective than lithium monotherapy.

In pediatric populations, there are limited published controlled data in bipolar disorder to date. Several early studies of lithium demonstrating benefits in mood, aggression, and psychosis were methodologically limited, including small sample size and crossover design (392). These studies in pediatric bipolar disorder (393–395) reported findings similar to a larger open trial for acute mania in adolescents with bipolar disorder I (396), where approximately 50 to 55% of subjects met criteria for remission using the Young Mania Rating Scale (YMRS). In the only published RCT lithium trial, Geller et al. (1998) (397) completed a small, double-blind parallel group trial of lithium for adolescents with bipolar spectrum disorder and substance dependence. Using global measures, significant improvement was evident in 46% of the lithium-treated sample compared to 8% of the placebo-treated group. The mean serum lithium drug level for completing responders was 0.88 mEq/L.

Valproic Acid and Carbamazepine

There have been no randomized controlled trials published to date using VPA or CBZ for pediatric bipolar disorder. Several open reports describe efficacy of VPA in bipolar youth, such as that by Papatheodorou (398). Oxcarbazepine and CBZ use in bipolar youth has also been reported, including case reports of efficacy in refractory childhood mania (399, 400). Comparative treatment trials using open-label lithium versus divalproex sodium (401) and randomized lithium versus divalproex versus CBZ but without placebo control (402) have been reported. The latter study suggested effect sizes of 1.06 for lithium (38% response), 1.63 for divalproex (53% response), and 1.00 for CBZ (38% response) in children and adolescents with bipolar I or II disorder. The majority of responders at the end of the continuation phase were on combination therapy (either a stimulant or a second anticonvulsant). Supporting this, a retrospective chart review of hospitalized bipolar preadolescents (403) found that by week 2, both lithium and VPA may be more efficacious than CBZ.

Multiple open and controlled trials of VPA in *adult* bipolar disorder show efficacy similar to lithium. Bowden et al. (2000) (404) compared the 1-year outcome of prophylaxis treatment with lithium, VPA, and placebo showing that VPA but not lithium was significantly better than placebo in preventing relapse. In a meta-analysis, Hirschfeld et al. (2003) (405) reported that oral loading of VPA leads to a more rapid antimanic effect compared with standard titration of divalproex, lithium, or placebo. Gyulia et al. (2003) (406) reported that divalproex-treated adults on maintenance therapy had less worsening of depressive symptoms than lithium-treated patients and reduced depressive episodes relapse. Rapid cycling or mixed mania has been suggested to be predictive of a good VPA response (380). Carbamazepine has demonstrated efficacy in RCTs in adults with mania, comparable to lithium, but there is less evidence supporting its usefulness in treatment of bipolar depressive episodes and in maintenance therapy (380). Oxcarbazepine may be useful for adults with mood disorders as well. Open studies demonstrate mild to moderate improvement in refractory bipolar disorder, including decreased irritability and improvement in depressive symptoms (407–410).

Aggression and Conduct Disorder

Expert consensus opinion supports the use of VPA, CBZ, and lithium in the management of aggressive adults with mental retardation (313). There are case reports (411), but no controlled trials of these agents in youth with MR. However, anticonvulsants, particularly VPA, have been found effective in the management of a range of neurobehavioral symptoms in patients with a history of brain injury (412–414).

Biederman et al. (1999) (415) presented compelling data in defining a dysphoric subtype of conduct disorder, noting that a positive response to mood stabilizers in levels of aggression in conduct-disordered children could be due to their antimanic effects, suggesting a comorbid bipolar disorder in some children with conduct disorder (CD).

There have been multiple shortterm controlled trials of mood stabilizers, primarily with lithium, in inpatient and outpatient youth with CD, with mixed results overall (416, 417). For example, Malone et al. (418, 419), examined the effectiveness of lithium for aggressive conduct-disordered inpatients showing a significantly superior response in the lithium group (16/20) compared to the placebo group (6/20). More recently, Steiner et al. (2003) (417) completed a randomized controlled trial of VPA in youth with conduct disorder, demonstrating dose-dependent effects (53% response with high dose versus 8% response with low-dose VPA). The one published controlled trial of CBZ in aggressive youth did not find significant benefit compared to placebo (420).

Pervasive Developmental Disorders

Anticonvulsants are commonly used in autistic spectrum disorders, due to the increased prevalence of epilepsy in these children. Open reports suggest improvement in social and behavioral domains in autistic subjects with epileptic discharges (421). They may also target underlying associated affective disorders (422).

Initiating and Maintenance of Medication

Standard informed consent with parents or guardians and assent by the child or adolescent is the first step in initiating medication. A medical history of cardiac disease, thyroid disease (lithium), renal impairment, psoriasis (lithium, CBZ), liver disease (VPA, CBZ), blood dyscrasia (VPA, lithium, CBZ), and pregnancy (VPA, lithium, CBZ) are *potential* contraindications to initiation of a mood stabilizer. Baseline laboratory studies including complete blood count (CBC), liver function tests (LFTs), electrolytes, thyroid stimulating hormone (TSH), urine, and, where indicated, pregnancy test, are recommended. An EKG to assess baseline intervals may be appropriate as well. Sexually active female patients should be counseled about the relationship between anticonvulsants and teratogenicity, and they should be assessed for baseline menstrual irregularities (VPA). Although rarely utilized as pharmacotherapy in infants and toddlers in child psychiatry, before initiating VPA, clinicians may perform screening tests, such as serum ammonium, amino acids, blood gases, lactate-pyruvate ratio, urinary organic acids, and free and total serum carnitine to rule out underlying metabolic disorders in children under the age of 2 years in order to decrease risk of fatal hepatotoxicity.

Lithium should be initiated at the lowest possible dose in children, and at 300 mg qhs in adolescents, depending on weight. Dosages are increased every 2 to 4 days, in increments of the starting dose, reaching the target dose in 2 to 4 weeks. Rapid titration could increase the incidence of adverse effects. Patients should be advised to maintain good hydration and cautioned regarding use of NSAIDs, such as ibuprofen, which may elevate lithium levels.

VPA should be initiated at the lowest possible dose in younger children (125 mg/d) and at 250 mg qhs in older children and adolescents, depending on weight. Dosages may be increased every 2 to 4 days, in increments of the starting dose, reaching a target dose in 2 to 4 weeks. Depakote sprinkle capsules (sodium valproate and valproic acid) are useful for children who are unable to tolerate valproate suspension, tablets, or capsules.

Carbamazepine should be initiated at the lowest possible dose in children, and at 200 to 300 mg/day in divided doses in adolescents, depending on weight (adult dose may be 200 to 600 mg divided twice a day). Dosages may be increased every 2 to 4 days, in increments of the starting dose, reaching a target dose in 2 to 4 weeks. Carbatrol is a new formulation composed of 25% IR beads, 40% ER beads, and 35% Enteric release beads (Shire Pharmaceuticals). Oxcarbazepine should be initiated at the lowest possible dose in children, and at 300 mg qhs in adolescents, depending on weight. The dose target is based on weight (900 mg/d in 20 to 29 kg; 1200 mg/d in 30 to 39 kg; 1800 mg/d in >40 kg).

Maintenance/Monitoring

Practice guidelines and expert reviews in the adult and pediatric psychiatry literature provide guidance on the complex issues of medication monitoring and maintenance. APA guidelines for lithium monitoring suggest checking renal function every 2 to 3 months and thyroid function every 3 to 6 months in the first 6 months, and then every 6 to 12 months thereafter (423). Monitoring of lithium blood levels is indicated to achieve the narrow therapeutic and safety window of 0.5 to 1.2 meq/L. The range of 0.6 to 0.8 meq/L may be most commonly utilized in adult practice (423). However, maintenance at a constant blood level may be more important than the level itself. By convention, lithium levels are drawn 12 hours after last dose, after reaching steady state or about 5 days after dose adjustment.

As most serious adverse effects with anticonvulsants occur in the initial 2 to 3 months, monthly blood screening (CBC, LFT) for the first 3 months has been recommended, followed by monitoring at three to six monthly intervals or as clinically indicated. Indications for anticonvulsant monitoring in children include: (1) at beginning of therapy to confirm serum levels are in the therapeutic range, (2) to monitor for noncompliance, (3) during growth spurts when serum levels may change unexpectedly, (4) during combined pharmacotherapy due to potential drug interactions, (5) symptoms and signs of toxicity, (6) patients with liver or kidney disease, and (7) disabilities that make evaluation of drug effect difficult (374).

Standard practice with VPA in adults typically includes safety monitoring of hematological parameters and liver function at a minimum every 6 months (423). Blood level monitoring in VPA is indicated to achieve the therapeutic and safety window of 50 to 125 ug/ml. Blood for VPA levels is usually drawn at trough, prior to next dose, and after steady state is reached or about 5 days after dose adjustment. Free plasma carnitine levels may be monitored and l-carnitine supplementation may be given if clinical symptoms suggest carnitine deficiency (e.g., weakness, lethargy, hypotonia).

APA guidelines for safety monitoring of CBZ suggest that CBC and liver function tests be drawn every 2 weeks in the first 2 months, and every 3 months thereafter (423). Blood level monitoring in CBZ is indicated to achieve the safe therapeutic window of 4 to 12 ug/ml. Carbamazepine levels are typically drawn at trough, prior to next dose, after steady state is reached or about 5 days after dose adjustment. Unlike carbamazepine, oxcarbazepine carries no black box warning regarding hematological adverse effect such as bone marrow suppression, and therefore no monitoring of hematological indices is indicated. Serum drug levels may be assayed to monitor compliance or make dose adjustments but have a lesser role than with CBZ. However, measurement of serum sodium may be appropriate if clinically significant adverse effects appear due to isolated reports of hyponatremia (424).

Safety
Side Effects

Side effect profiles reported are based largely on adult experience with these agents. Side effects are common with lithium. Transient side effects such as gastrointestinal upset and tremor related to peak levels may be predicted, and may be noted more often if beginning treatment during a depressed state versus a manic phase. Dose-related adverse effects include weight gain, gastrointestinal upset, benign increase in white blood count (WBC), lethargy, cognitive dulling, and impaired memory, acne, hair loss, edema, polydipsia, and polyuria. Lithium citrate may be better tolerated than the carbonate salt with respect to gastrointestinal upset. Benign EKG changes associated with repolarization may occur (423) such as T wave inversion or flattening. Cardiac toxicity (sinus node dysfunction) has been described in children receiving longterm lithium therapy (425). Longer-term effects include thyroid (hypothyroidism, hypoparathyroidism), kidney (impaired concentrating capacity), or bone (morphologic changes) disturbances with chronic use (423). Impaired thyroid function manifested by lower T4 levels has been associated with increased affective episodes, relapse, and depression (426, 427).

Dose-related adverse effects with VPA include sedation, weight gain, tremor, benign decrease in WBC and platelets, and gastrointestinal upset. Greater weight gain than that seen with lithium treatment (23 versus 16%) has been demonstrated with valproic acid treatment of bipolar adults at 1 year. In addition, rates of sedation, tinnitus, and hair loss were increased compared to lithium (404). VPA therapy may be associated with a transient elevation in liver enzymes in 15 to 30% of patients and rarely with fatal hepatotoxicity. Clinically significant and persistent gastrointestinal symptoms necessitate careful evaluation during the initial few months of valproate therapy (374). The majority of VPA hepatotoxicity has been observed in children younger than 2 years of age with prior neurological or medical conditions. Mitochondrial or metabolic diseases, such as blocks in carnitine metabolic pathways (leading to increased serum ammonia), VPA inhibition of beta-oxidation, and toxicity from VPA metabolites, may all be causative (428). However, Hirose et al. (1998) (429) reported that carnitine levels are unaffected by VPA in patients with epilepsy, without severe neurological or nutritional problems, and that a regular childhood diet provides sufficient amounts of carnitine. Pancreatitis has also been described in multiple case reports. Among 36 VPA-associated cases of pancreatitis (430), 9 patients (25%) were under 10 years old and 12 (33%) were between 10 and 20 years old. The association between VPA and polycystic ovarian syndrome (weight gain, hyperandrogenemia, and hyperinsulinemia) remains unclear (423), although Nelson-DeGrave et al. (2004) (431) reported a link between VPA and increased ovarian androgen biosynthesis. Adults using extended-release (ER) divalproex sodium reported significantly less frequent and severe adverse events when switched from divalproex sodium delayed-release (DR) formulations (432), perhaps due to smaller diurnal fluctuations and decreased formation of minor toxic metabolites (433).

Adverse effects of carbamazepine include reversible dose-related neurological symptoms such as fatigue, dizziness, ataxia, blurred vision, and cognitive dulling. In addition, rash, weight gain, mild reductions in WBC, platelets, sodium and thyroid hormones, and elevation in liver enzymes may all occur. Rare serious adverse effects include aplastic anemia, agranulocytosis, thrombocytopenia, liver or renal failure, cardiac conduction effects, and Stevens-Johnson syndrome, most often in the initial 3 to 4 months of therapy (374, 423).

Oxcarbazepine causes fewer overall adverse effects compared to carbamazepine, with the exception of hyponatremia (<125 mmol/L) (434), observed in about 2.5% of adults (Novartis). Although Holtman et al. (2002) (424) reported hyponatremia in 26% of a sample of 75 children with epilepsy, clinically relevant hyponatremia occurred in only one child. Adverse effects of oxcarbazepine include drowsiness,and neurological symptoms such as ataxia. About 25 to 30% of subjects with hypersensitivity to carbamazepine may experience adverse reactions to oxcarbazepine (Novartis, 2002).

Overdose/Intoxication

Although lithium toxicity may occur at elevated serum levels, intoxication has also been described within the normal range of values. Neurological signs of toxicity include tremor, confusion, seizure, and coma. Cardiac dysrhythmia can also occur. In contrast, VPA possesses a wider margin of safety. In overdose, however, sedation, cardiac conduction block, and coma can occur, and deaths have been reported. CBZ toxicity presents with neurological effects, such as sedation, ataxia, seizure, and coma, as well as cardiac conduction disturbances (423).

Drug Interactions

An extensive review of the safety and efficacy of mood stabilizers (VPA, Li, CBZ, Lamotrigine) in various combinations concluded that the safest and most efficacious mood stabilizer combinations appear to be anticonvulsants with lithium, particularly valproate plus lithium (435).

Agents that affect lithium clearance such as diuretics and NSAIDs may increase serum levels. Isolated case reports describe lithium neurotoxicity when administered with concomitant neuroleptics, CBZ, and calcium channel blockers (435). VPA drug interactions are related to its hepatic metabolism and protein binding. Coadministration of aspirin may decrease clearance of the unbound fraction of VPA and necessitate a decrease in the daily dose (436). VPA is unique in that it inhibits rather than induces hepatic enzymes and may therefore cause elevations in levels of concomitant medications, such as TCAs and CBZ. Notably, lamotrigine levels may be doubled with concurrent VPA administration (423), and skin rashes may occur with greater frequency or severity, so that great care is required when combining these agents.

Conversely, CBZ may increase the rate of VPA metabolism and reduce VPA levels (380). Isolated reports since 2002 also suggest an interaction between risperidone and VPA in youth, with protein-binding displacement yielding increased free VPA levels or alterations in VPA via cytochrome P450 2D6 interaction (437–439). However, Good et al. (2003) (440) found no significant difference in trough VPA drug levels with combination VPA and olanzapine or risperidone treatment in 45 subjects. Combined treatment with olanzapine and divalproex has also been associated with greater elevations of hepatic enzymes than with VPA monotherapy (441).

Carbamazepine can cause numerous potential drug interactions, due to its potent hepatic enzyme induction. Serum levels of concomitant medications, including neuroleptics, birth control pills, TCAs, lamotrigine, benzodiazepines, VPA, and prednisone, may be lowered, as well as CBZ itself, via autoinduction. CBZ has been shown not only to alter the metabolism of imipramine and its metabolites, but also its protein binding so that despite reductions in total TCA serum levels, the unchanged free fraction concentration is maintained (266). In addition, CBZ levels may be increased by concomitant medications, such as erythromycin, calcium channel blockers, fluoxetine, and VPA, via inhibition of CBZ metabolism (380). Notably, the CBZ epoxide/CBZ ratio (and toxicity) may be increased by metabolic inducers or by inhibition of carbamazepine epoxide conversion to carbamazepine diol (such as with VPA). Carbamazepine-epoxide, an active metabolite, may produce toxicity even at therapeutic carbamazepine levels (374). The effect of VPA on CBZ-E metabolism may be age dependent; in preschoolers, VPA is an inhibitor of CBZ-E metabolism (442). Finally, CBZ-associated hematological adverse effects must be considered when CBZ is used with concomitant medications. Oxcarbazepine may induce CYP3A4/5 at high dose and may inhibit CYP2C19; concurrent birth control pills may be less effective.

LAMOTRIGINE/TOPIRAMATE/ GABAPENTIN

Neuropsychopharmacology

There is a dearth of data regarding the efficacy of these agents in children and adolescents. Although information from adult studies may not directly extrapolate to pediatric populations, they may nevertheless inform our understanding of clinical use and safety.

Pharmacodynamics

Ion channel effects (sodium channel blockade), antiglutamatergic, and neuroprotective actions may all contribute to the underlying mechanism of action of lamotrigine. Although lamotrigine does not have robust GABA or monoaminergic actions, longterm lamotrigine treatment has been associated with significant elevations in central GABA concentrations (443).

Gabapentin is structurally related to the inhibitory neurotransmitter GABA, although it does not act directly at the GABA site. Studies of healthy adults have demonstrated acute increases in cerebral GABA concentrations following single doses of gabapentin (443). Gabapentin binds to neuronal membranes' glutamate synapse as well (374).

Topiramate modulates voltage-dependent sodium conductance, potentiates GABA evoked potentials, and blocks the kainate/AMPA subtype of the glutamate receptor (443). Like gabapentin, acute increases in cerebral GABA concentrations follow single doses of topiramate (443).

Pharmacokinetics

Lamotrigine (LTG) is completely absorbed and undergoes hepatic metabolism and renal elimination. Metabolism is accelerated by drugs that induce CYP450 enzymes and inhibited by valproate. Although lamotrigine itself does not significantly affect the metabolism of other agents, increased CYP450 metabolism of LTG could increase formation of its reactive metabolite and increase the risk of rash (428).

Gabapentin is rapidly absorbed, but its absorption pathway becomes saturated at higher doses so that increasing the dose further may not yield a further increase in plasma levels. Clinical trials reported dose-dependent bioavailability ranging from 74 to 36% when the dose was increased from 100 to 1600 mg (444). Peak plasma levels occur in 1 to 3 hours. Gabapentin is not bound to plasma proteins and has a large volume of distribution, an elimination half-life (T 1/2) of 5 to 7 hours, linear kinetics, and renal elimination.

Topiramate has low protein binding, little hepatic metabolism, and is excreted primarily unchanged by the kidney, with a half-life of around 24 hours.

Pharmacotherapy

Mood Disorders

Lamotrigine may "stabilize mood from below" in that it may improve depressive symptoms in bipolar disorder, as demonstrated by its efficacy in controlled studies of *adult* bipolar disorder (445, 446). The US FDA has approved Lamictal for maintenance treatment of adults with bipolar I disorder; the first FDA-approved therapy since lithium for longterm maintenance therapy of bipolar I disorder. In youth, open studies in small samples of adolescents with refractory mood disorders have been positive (447).

Two 18-month, controlled trials compared lamotrigine, lithium, and placebo in the maintenance treatment of 1,315 manic or depressed adults with bipolar I disorder. Compared with placebo, lamotrigine and lithium significantly prolonged the time to intervention for a mood episode. Lamotrigine was mostly effective for depressive symptoms, whereas lithium was primarily effective against mania (448).

Gabapentin was not effective in two controlled trials of adult mania (423). In adults, the controlled data do not support the use of gabapentin either as an antimanic medication or as a mood stabilizer (449). However, numerous open-label studies and limited controlled trial data suggest an adjunctive role in the treatment of comorbid anxiety disorder or substance abuse (450). Only isolated case reports of gabapentin use in pediatric mood disorders can be found, and no conclusions regarding its potential benefit may be drawn at this time (451).

In adults, preliminary evidence from open trials of topiramate for acute and refractory mania is promising, but controlled evidence is lacking (449). Likewise, there are open-label reports of topiramate treatment of bipolar spectrum youth. One retrospective review of 26 patients with bipolar disorder treated for a mean duration of 4 months at a mean topiramate dose of 104 mg/day showed a response rate of 73% for mania (452). Pavuluri et al. (2002) (453) reported that topiramate plus risperidone controlled both weight gain and symptoms in preschoolers with mania.

Anxiety Disorder

Gabapentin has been found effective in adults with anxiety disorder, with a meta-analysis showing an overall effect size of 0.78 (95% CI, 0.29 to 1.27) in social anxiety disorder (454), improvement in panic symptoms in severely ill patients in a RCT (455) case reports of benefit for generalized anxiety disorder (456), and insomnia in patients with PTSD (457).

Miscellaneous Uses

Because of its effect in reducing weight, topiramate has been studied as an agent for weight loss (458) or stabilization in several populations including eating disorders such as bulimia (459). An open-label study of topiramate in patients with Prader–Willi syndrome reported weight loss or a reduction in weight gain, as well as improvements in mood, aggression, and obsessive-compulsive behaviors (460). Topiramate is *not* approved by the FDA as a weight loss treatment.

Gabapentin has been used successfully in multiple pain syndromes in adults, including trigeminal neuralgia, neuropathic pain, and postoperative pain. Analgesia has also been observed in open reports in pediatric patients (461, 462).

Initiating and Maintenance of Medication

Initiation

Prior to initiation of treatment with lamotrigine, patients and their parents should be instructed that a rash or other signs or symptoms of hypersensitivity (e.g., fever, lymphadenopathy) may herald a serious medical event and that the patient should immediately confer with their physician. Due to an increased risk of rash, the recommended initial dosing and dose increase guidelines should not be exceeded. With careful dose adjustments, the incidence of serious rash in youth given LTG has been reduced to about 1% (463). Nearly all cases of life-threatening rash have occurred within 2 to 8 weeks of initiation.

Dose increase regimens depend on whether lamictal is used as monotherapy or as adjunctive therapy, and on the particular second anticonvulsant being used (VPA or another). For adult patients not taking other anticonvulsants or other enzyme-inducing drugs, 25 mg daily for 2 weeks, followed by 50 mg daily for 2 weeks, followed by 100 mg daily for 1 week, and then 200 mg daily is recommended by the manufacturer (GlaxoSmithKline). In pediatric patients, lamotrigine should be initiated at 2 mg/kg/d as monotherapy or at 0.2 mg/kg/d if used with VPA and then titrated slowly at about monthly intervals (464).

Gabapentin should be initiated at the lowest possible dose in children (100 mg/daily), and doses intermediate to adult dosage in adolescents (initial adult dose of 300 mg twice a day is recommended), and then may be increased every 3 to 7 days, in increments of the starting dose, reaching a target dose in 4 to 6 weeks. Topiramate should be initiated at the lowest possible dose in children and doses intermediate to adult dosage in adolescents.

Maintenance/Monitoring

Lamotrigine and gabapentin require neither baseline nor medical monitoring, other than diligence regarding emergence of a lamotrigine rash. Lamotrigine should be discontinued at the first sign of rash, unless the rash is clearly not drug related. Maintenance dose ranges from 1 to 5 mg/kg/d when used as adjunctive therapy with valproate, to 5 to 15 mg/kg/d when given as monotherapy (464).

With topiramate, baseline and periodic monitoring of HCO3 levels are recommended, especially in youth with conditions that may predispose to acidosis. Evidence of hematuria and hypercalciuria should also be checked before and during topiramate therapy in these children (465).

Safety

Side Effects

The most common (≥5% incidence) side effects associated with lamotrigine in pediatric epilepsy trials were vomiting, nonserious rash, nausea, somnolence, dizziness, diarrhea, abdominal pain, ataxia, tremor, weakness, infection, and diplopia. Serious rashes requiring hospitalization have been reported, including Stevens-Johnson syndrome. In adult mood disorder trials, the incidence of these rashes was 0.08% (fewer than 1 per 1,000) in patients receiving lamotrigine as initial monotherapy and 0.13% (1.3 per 1,000) in patients receiving lamotrigine as adjunctive therapy. However, in epilepsy trials the incidence of rashes with lamotrigine used as *adjunctive* therapy was 0.3% (3/1,000) in adult and 0.8% (8/1,000) in pediatric patients. In a cohort of about 2,000 pediatric epilepsy patients taking lamotrigine as *adjunctive* therapy, there was one rash-related death. Rash may be increased by concurrent administration of VPA or by exceeding the recommended initial dose or dose increase parameters.

In children with epilepsy, gabapentin (20 to 100 mg/kg/d) has been well tolerated as an anticonvulsant agent. The most common side effects associated with gabapentin therapy are somnolence, dizziness, fatigue, ataxia, nystagmus, and weight gain. There have been a few case reports of behavioral changes at higher doses consisting of tantrums, hyperexcitability, and outbursts of anger (464).

Adverse effects of topiramate include somnolence, dizziness, fatigue, nervousness, headache, diplopia, ataxia, speech difficulties, psychomotor slowing, nystagmus, paresthesia, impaired concentration, anorexia, sleep disorders, and anorexia with or without weight loss (466). Davanzo et al. (2001) (467) reported a child with refractory juvenile-onset bipolar disorder treated with topiramate (TPM) who experienced cognitive and academic deterioration 4 months after mood symptoms remitted. In adults, most of the commonly reported adverse effects were related to the central nervous system and observed with greater frequency at dosages of greater than 200 to 600 mg/day (468). No clinically significant abnormalities were observed in laboratory parameters or in neurological, electrocardiographic, ophthalmologic, or audiological tests (469). Chronic topiramate use may result in a distal tubular acidification defect, leading to an elevated risk of calcium phosphate nephrolithiasis (465). Others have reported that a metabolic acidosis (typically mild) may develop in adult patients over time (465, 470, 471). There is no apparent correlation between dose and acidosis. In December 2003, the prescribing information for topiramate was revised to include a warning that it may cause hyperchloremic nonanion gap metabolic acidosis (decreased serum bicarbonate). The incidence of markedly low bicarbonate in clinical trials ranges from 3 to 11%, compared to 0 to 1% for placebo.

Drug Interactions

Lamotrigine's total daily dose and titration regimens vary according to whether it is used as monotherapy or as adjunctive treatment. Interactions with VPA were discussed earlier.

Topiramate has no significant effect on plasma levels of other anticonvulsants including carbamazepine and valproic acid. However, topiramate's inhibition of carbonic anhydrase and glutamine synthetase may cause hyperammonemia and encephalopathy (472). In addition, when topiramate is used concurrently with hepatic enzyme-inducing agents, its plasma concentrations are approximately 50% lower than when administered as monotherapy (473).

ANTIPSYCHOTICS

Neuropsychopharmacology

The use of antipsychotics in both adult and pediatric psychiatry has increased greatly since the introduction of the atypical antipsychotic agents. Goals for development of these atypical agents included equivalence in antipsychotic efficacy, less EPS and prolactin elevation, and broader efficacy for cognitive and "negative" symptoms. This section focuses mainly on the class of atypical antipsychotic drugs, which are increasingly utilized for more severe and treatment refractory conditions as well as first-line agents in juvenile bipolar disorder. Despite the broader scope of action and enhanced tolerability of the "atypicals," standard typical antipsychotics also retain clear indications in pediatric neuropsychiatry.

Pharmacokinetics

There has been little study of the pharmacokinetics of antipsychotic medications in children. Studies on the typical agent chlorpromazine and the atypical agent risperidone suggested faster metabolic rates compared to adults (473, 474). However, more recent studies found similar pharmacokinetics for olanzapine, quetiapine (475, 476), and ziprasidone (477) across age groups. Sallee et al. (2003) (478) performed a single-dose, open study of ziprasidone (0.2 to 0.3 mg/kg) in 24 youths with Tourette's or chronic tic disorder; mean AUC ranged between 457 and 247 ngh $-1mL-1$, with peak serum concentrations at 4 hours postdose.

Frazier et al. (2003) (479) studied clozapine (CLZ) (3 mg/kg) and its metabolites, norclozapine (NOR) and clozapine-N-oxide (NOX), in six youth with childhood-onset schizophrenia. NOR concentrations (410 ng/ml) exceeded CLZ (289 ng/ml) and NOX (63 ng/ml). In adults, NOR serum concentrations on average are 10 to 25% < CLZ. This difference between children and adults in the ratio of metabolites to parent compound may reflect greater activity of hepatic CYP450 isoenzymes 1A2 and 3A4. In addition, clearance varied up to 17-fold among individuals. Dose normalized concentrations of CLZ (mg/kg/d) did not vary with age and were similar to adult values.

Pharmacodynamics

While traditional antipsychotics primarily cause dopamine type 2 (D2) receptor blockade to produce clinical effects, atypical antipsychotics possess mixed neurotransmitter effects, including 5HT receptor blockade and greater limbic selectivity. Within this class, 5HT/DA blockade ratio is greatest with clozapine, quetiapine, and olanzapine, followed by risperidone. The mixed neurotransmitter selectivity that distinguishes the atypical agents from more typical agents is likely responsible for both fewer adverse effects (EPS) and their clinical efficacy including reduced negative symptoms and improved mood regulation.

The newest of the atypical agents (e.g., aripiprazole) may be considered dopamine system stabilizers. By interacting with multiple dopamine receptors, they enhance dopamine activity where levels are low (e.g., mesocortical region) and reduce activity where dopamine levels are in excess (e.g., mesolimbic region), while maintaining normal dopamine levels elsewhere (e.g., nigrostriatal region) (480). Dopamine type 1 (D1) receptor blockade in mesocortical regions may provide beneficial cognitive effects.

Two agents in the atypical antipsychotic class are ziprasidone and aripiprazole. The in vitro 5-HT2A/D2 receptor affinity ratio of ziprasidone is higher than that of the other first-line atypical agents, and it has moderate affinity for both serotonin and norepinephrine reuptake sites (481). Clinically, this characteristic may be responsible for its antidepressant effects at lower doses and the activation sometimes seen in bipolar patients. At higher doses, the D2 blockade is more apparent, so that moving up more rapidly to target doses will effect its antipsychotic properties more quickly. In animal models, ziprasidone also increases prefrontal cortical dopamine (482). Sallee et al. (2003) (478) performed an open study of ziprasidone (0.2 to 0.3 mg/kg) in 24 youths with Tourette's syndrome or chronic tics. This was the first human study to indicate that ziprasidone may cause both dopamine antagonism, supported by prolactin increase, and agonism, supported by an increase in spontaneous eye blink rates. Aripiprazole also displays properties of an agonist and antagonist in animal models of dopaminergic hypoactivity and hyperactivity, respectively. Given its partial agonism at 5-HT1A receptors (presynaptic) and antagonism at 5-HT2A receptors (postsynaptic), aripiprazole may be thought of as a dopamine-serotonin system *stabilizer* (483).

In addition to their DA and 5HT actions, atypical agents have varying antiadrenergic, anticholinergic and antihistaminergic effects. Alpha-adrenergic blockade causes hypotension, cholinergic blockade is responsible for side effects such as constipation, sinus tachycardia, blurred vision and dry mouth, and histamine blockade may cause weight gain and sedation (Table 27.14).

Pharmacotherapy

Discussion of the therapeutic use of the antipsychotic medications is organized according to the primary clinical applications that are supported by controlled clinical trials. However, the clinical applications of atypical antipsychotics have become quite broad in pediatric care.

Psychotic Disorders

Antipsychotic agents are recommended for treatment of the acute and stabilization phase of schizophrenia. The adult literature suggests that atypical agents may also enhance neurocognitive function (484, 485) and improve negative symptoms associated with psychosis, although the effect size advantage over more typical agents may be small (486). Available studies, case reports, and clinical experience all suggest that patterns of response in youth are similar to that found in adults (487). Ongoing research efforts include the NIMH study of childhood-onset schizophrenia. Although little controlled data on the treatment of primary psychotic disorders in young children exists, the use of antipsychotic drugs is considered justified in early onset schizophrenia (487). Frazier et al. (2003) (479) reported the efficacy and safety of clozapine in youth with DSM-IV schizophrenia, during both open and double-blind trials of clozapine and haloperidol. These and other authors demonstrated that clozapine plasma concentrations may be positively correlated with response (488). An 8-week pilot study comparing the acute antipsychotic effect size of risperidone and olanzapine to that of haloperidol found that a majority of subjects treated with olanzapine (88%), risperidone (74%), and haloperidol (53%) all met criteria for positive response (489). Randomized controlled trails of antipsychotic drugs in psychotic disorders in youth include the more typical agents loxapine and haloperidol (490, 491).

Open trials of atypical agents have also demonstrated efficacy for olanzapine in the shortterm treatment of adolescents with schizophrenia, schizoaffective, or schizophreniform disorders (492) and in a 1-year prospective open-label trial of childhood-onset schizophrenia (493), for risperidone in adolescents with schizophrenia (494) and for quetiapine in adolescents with selected psychotic disorders (495).

Mood Disorders

RCTs of atypical agents have also shown benefit for adults with bipolar disorder. Unlike the typical neuroleptics, atypical agents show benefit for *maintenance* of treatment response and as adjunctive agents for depressive symptoms (496) in addition to controlling acute mania. Rigorous studies in this severely disturbed and likely heterogeneous pediatric population are hindered by ethical (placebo control) and nosological dilemmas. Despite this, controlled studies of juvenile bipolar disorder are under way, mostly with the atypical antipsychotic agents. In addition, treatment algorithms have been presented in an attempt to offer consensus guidelines to clinicians. Monotherapy with olanzapine, risperidone, and quetiapine (in addition to lithium, divalproex, and carbamazepine) are among the first-line treatments for juvenile bipolar disorder (384).

In a double-blind, placebo-controlled study of quetiapine in adolescent mania (452), 30 adolescent inpatients with bipolar I disorder received VPA with either adjunctive quetiapine or placebo for 6 weeks. The combination VPA + quetiapine treated subjects had significantly greater reduction in YMRS scores compared to VPA + placebo treated

TABLE 27.14

CLINICAL PHARMACOLOGY OF ATYPICAL ANTIPSYCHOTICS

	Aripiprazole	Olanzapine	Quetiapine	Risperidone	Ziprasidone
Pharmacokinetic Parameters					
T-Max (hours)	3–5 h	6 h	1.5 h	1 h	6–8 h
Half-life (T 1/2)	75 h (parent) 94 h (active metabolite)	30 h	6 h	20 h	7 h
Mechanism of excretion	Hepatic	Hepatic	Hepatic	Hepatic	Hepatic
	CYP2D6 and 3A4	CYP1A2 and 2D6	CYP3A4	CYP2D6	CYP3A4 +/−1A2
Pharmacodynamic Parameters					
Mechanism of action	Antagonist: 5HT2A D2 in *hyperdo-paminergic* environment Agonist: Partial 5HT1A D2 in *hypodo-paminergic* environment	Antagonist: D1–4 5HT2 M1–5 alpha 1 H1	Antagonist: D1 D2 5HT2 adrenergic alpha 1 and 2 H1	Antagonist: D2 5HT2 alpha 1 and 2 adrenergic H1 5HT1D	Agonist: 5HT1A Antagonist: D2 5HT2A 5HT1D
Clinical Parameters					
Dose range (mg/day)	5–30 (q.d. or b.i.d.)	1.25–15 (q.d. or b.i.d)	25–100 (prepubertal) 25–300 (adolescents) (q.d. or b.i.d.)	0.125–12 (qd or b.i.d)	20–160 (b.i.d)
Common side effects	Headache, weight gain, anxiety, insomnia, nausea/vomiting, lightheadedness, somnolence, akathenia, constipation, asthenia, rash, blurred vision, tremor, cough fever	Drowsiness, orthostasis, weight gain, seizures, cognitive impairment; EPS uncommon, elevates prolactin	Drowsiness, orthostasis, weight gain; EPS uncommon	Weight gain, drowsiness, orthostasis, (prolonged QTc); EPS uncommon, elevates prolactin	Somnolence, EPS, respiratory disorder, orthostatic hypotension, weight gain, rash
Serious side effects	Tardive dyskinesia and NMS rare but possible	Tardive dyskinesia and NMS rare but possible	Tardive dyskinesia and NMS rare but possible; lenticular changes possible; seizures, hypothyroidism	Tardive dyskinesia and NMS rare but possible	Increase in QTc interval and risk of sudden death

5HT, Serotonin; CYP, Cytochrome P450; D, Dopamine; EPS, Extrapyramidal symptoms; H, Histamine; M, Muscarine; NMS, Neuroleptic malignant syndrome QTc. The beginning of the depolarization of the left ventricle is labeled Q (wave), and the ventricular repolarization is labeled T (wave). QTc is the interval corrected by a mathematical formula for heart rate. T-Max: time to peak plasma level.

subjects. Adjunctive augmentation trials include open-label olanzapine in manic children (497) and open-label olanzapine augmentation of lithium in bipolar psychosis (386). In the latter study, 43% of manic, psychotic adolescents relapsed when they discontinued the antipsychotic after 4 weeks of stabilization with adjunctive treatment. These studies followed preliminary reviews of pharmacotherapy in childhood mania (498) and case reports of open-label atypical antipsychotic monotherapy in juvenile bipolar disorder. Rapid, robust improvement has been observed with risperidone and olanzapine (451, 499, 500) as well as quetiapine (476), including longterm safety and efficacy (501).

In adults, olanzapine has an FDA indication for both acute *and maintenance* bipolar monotherapy and may produce greater remission rates in acute manic or mixed episodes compared to standard agents, such as divalproex (502). In December 2003, the FDA approved the use of risperidone as monotherapy, or in combination with lithium or valproate, for the treatment of acute manic or mixed episodes of bipolar I disorder. Atypical antipsychotics may possess broad efficacy beyond their antimanic effects and have use in depressed phase bipolar disorder or even unipolar depression. Efficacy for quetiapine in psychotic depression has already been described in one report (503).

Anxiety Disorders

The sum of evidence at this time points to the benefits of atypical antipsychotic augmentation of SSRIs for treatment resistant OCD in adults (504). In children, however, this subject is confusing. One case series on pediatric OCD found that symptoms progressively diminished with increase in dose of risperidone used for augmentation (505). However, there have been case reports of worsening of obsessive-compulsive symptoms with the atypical antipsychotic in adults (506–509) and children (510). Several authors also noted rapid resolution of OCD symptoms upon discontinuation of risperidone (510, 511). Others did not see OCD symptoms reemerge with risperidone rechallenge, yet others found that obsessions gradually diminished with continued treatment. Risperidone has greater relative dopamine blocking activity at higher doses (512). These observations add to a number of others that dopamine may be involved in the pathogenesis of OCD in some way (513, 514). At this time there is insufficient evidence to support the routine use of the atypicals in pediatric OCD unless there are comorbid tics.

Pervasive Developmenta Disorder/Mental Retardation

Following several decades of using the typical antipsychotics in children with pervasive developmental disorders and intellectual disabilities, atypical antipsychotics are now commonly used for behavioral problems in these children (515). Of the neuroleptics, haloperidol has been the most thoroughly studied with efficacy shown in both shortterm (516) and longterm (517) studies. Open trials have compared atypicals to typical agents, such as a parallel-group study of 12 children with autism treated with olanzapine or haloperidol (518). Five of six subjects in the olanzapine group and three of six in the haloperidol group were rated as responders.

The National Institute of Mental Health funded Research Units on Pediatric Psychopharmacology (RUPP) Autism Network completed an 8-week, double-blind, placebo-controlled study of risperidone in 101 children and adolescents with autism (519). In the risperidone group, 69% achieved a positive response for serious behavioral problems compared to just 12% in the placebo group (P < 0.001). Besides risperidone, other atypical antipsychotics with demonstrated efficacy in open trials of autism or PDD include clozapine, olanzapine, quetiapine, and ziprasidone (520). A 3-year naturalistic study described 47% improvement in a sample of preschool children with PDD treated with risperidone monotherapy (521).

The efficacy of risperidone has also been demonstrated in children with subaverage IQs and severe disruptive behaviors in controlled trials (522, 523). In a follow-up extension study, risperidone was safe and well tolerated with positive effect maintained over 1 year (524).

Tic Disorders/Tourette's Disorder

Atypical antipsychotics have been shown comparable to typical neuroleptics for tic supression in studies in adolescents and adults. Two placebo-controlled studies and two randomized trials with active comparators have shown that risperidone is effective for the supression of moderate to severe tics in children and adolescents with Tourette's syndrome (525, 526). Sallee et al. (2003) (478) suggested that ziprasidone may act primarily on the neocortex to dampen excitatory glutamatergic overdrive.

Eating Disorders

Several reports describe open-label efficacy of olanzapine in the treatment of anorexia nervosa (527–529). In these medically and psychiatrically compromised populations, olanzapine may assist in mood regulation, distorted thinking, and ego function, as well as provide a shortterm boost in weight gain that often accompanies its use.

Initiating and Maintenance of Medication

Initiation

Use of antipsychotic agents requires adequate informed consent from the parent or the youth (depending on the legal age requirements or legal status). Special regulations may govern the prescribing of antipsychotics in children who are in state custody or foster care. In addition, documentation of target symptoms, baseline and follow-up laboratory monitoring, documentation of treatment response and side-effects—including EPS (Abnormal Involuntary Movement Scale) and weight gain—and adequate therapeutic trials of sufficient dosages over 4 to 6 weeks are all important (487).

The smallest dosage should generally be used for initiating antipsychotic medication in youth. Minimum effective doses for newer atypical antipsychotic medications across fixed-dose placebo-controlled studies in *adults*, defined by their equivalency to 100 mg/day of chlorpromazine, are 2 mg/day for risperidone, 5 mg/day for olanzapine, 75 mg/day for quetiapine, 60 mg/day for ziprasidone, and 7.5 mg/day for aripiprazole (530).

They should be used with caution in youth with a personal or family history of diabetes or hyperlipidemia due to metabolic adverse effects, as highlighted by the FDA. In 2004, the American Diabetes Association published a consensus statement recommending a baseline weight, height, waist circumference, blood pressure, fasting glucose, and lipid profile.

Clinical experience suggests that children with PDD spectrum disorders may be particularly sensitive to serotonergic agents. As such, low dosage and slow titration of atypical agents is indicated in this population, as with SSRI medications.

Maintenance/Monitoring

Although clinical practice may vary, practice guidelines and expert reviews provide some guidance on the complex issues of medication monitoring and maintenance. The decision to lower dosages (to minimize side effects) or undergo medication-free trials must be balanced by the increased risk for relapse, particularly in psychotic disorders. In general, first-episode psychotic patients should receive maintenance psychopharmacological treatment for 1 to 2 years following an initial episode, due to risk for relapse (487). For mood disorders, treatment for 9 to 12 months beyond time to achieve remission is usual.

In 2004, the American Diabetes Association published a consensus statement suggesting follow-up monitoring of weight (4 weeks, 8 weeks, 12 weeks, quarterly), waist circumference (annually), blood pressure (12 weeks, annually), fasting glucose (12 weeks, annually), and lipid profile (every 5 years), noting that more frequent assessment may be warranted according to clinical status. For example, fasting serum insulin levels and HbA1C could be checked if morbid obesity is present to assess risk for type 2 diabetes. Melkersson and Dahl (2004) (531), in an extensive review, discuss preventative strategies for weight gain.

ECG monitoring is not routinely required, but in children QTc intervals should be checked for prolongation if other drugs that may also alter QTc are used concurrently or in overdose situations.

Clozapine is unique in the class of atypical agents, due to a "therapeutic window" and potentially severe hematological adverse effects such as bone marrow suppression. Based on emerging data for pediatric populations, it has been suggested that CLZ serum assays in youth be standardized to include CLZ + NOR metabolite rather than to CLZ alone (typically used in adults) due to their combined contribution to the overall effectiveness and side effect profile of CLZ in youth (479).

Safety

There are ongoing efforts to acquire longterm safety data on the antipsychotic medications in youth, as they are applied increasingly in mood and other psychiatric disorders. Although well tolerated in shortterm use, significant weight gain, extrapyramidal symptoms, and cardiac and metabolic effects may negatively skew the risk-benefit ratio of atypical agents over the medium to longterm.

For traditional antipsychotics, potency measured by degree of DA blockade correlates with adverse effects; high-potency agents such as haloperidol tend to produce EPS, whereas low-potency agents such as thioridazine and chlorpromazine have more anticholinergic side effects and sedation.

Weight Gain

A review of an FDA postmarketing surveillance database on olanzapine found that the risk of complaints of weight gain was 4.3 times higher for children and 3.2 times higher for adolescents than for adults. Similarly, complaints of increased appetite were 24 times higher in childhood compared to adults (532). Increased weight gain may involve serotoninergic, histaminergic, and adrenergic mechanisms (533) and, in reviews of adults, may be increased two- to threefold with administration of concomitant lithium or valproate (534). Management of this adverse event includes switching atypical agents or the discontinuation or addition of a targeted treatment. For example, Molindone may be uniquely weight neutral. Overall, treatment-induced obesity is a particularly challenging issue for practitioners. Familiarity with other management options, such as local weight-control behavioral programs for youth, may be helpful and associated with less frequent relapse than in adult populations (535).

Metabolic

Thorough reviews of metabolic adverse effects such as hyperglycemia and hyperlipidemia may be found elsewhere (531). After the appearance of clozapine, the first atypical agent, reports of metabolic adverse effects, primarily on glucose and lipid regulation, are found in the adult literature. Noninsulin-dependent hyperglycemia has been observed with several of the atypical antipsychotics, primarily olanzapine and clozapine. Initially, elevated rates of diabetes (36% of 82 patients over 5 years) were described in small samples of adult patients treated with clozapine (536). In a 4-month study comparing the prevalence of diabetes in adults with schizophrenia (N = 38,000), atypical antipsychotic treated patients showed a greater prevalence than those treated with a typical neuroleptic (9% versus 6%). However, these authors suggested that atypical antipsychotics may hasten onset rather than cause the diabetes (537). On March 1, 2004, the FDA has asked manufacturers of atypical antipsychotic medications to add a warning statement to package inserts describing hyperglycemia, rarely extreme and associated with ketoacidosis or hyperosmolar coma and even death in patients treated with atypical antipsychotics (www.fda.gov/medwatch).

Studies in pediatric populations (N = 175) have also demonstrated significant weight gain with atypical agents (olanzapine, risperidone, quetiapine), as well as insulin resistance in children taking olanzapine. Insulin resistance was predicted by weight gain. Putative risk factors include increased premorbid weight and personal or family history of diabetes (538). However, impaired glucose tolerance and diabetes have also been found in certain psychiatric populations, such as schizophrenia compared to the general population (536, 539). In certain refractory cases, targeted drugs such as metformin to increase insulin sensitivity may have benefit. In one study, 15 of 19 children responded with weight loss (540).

Hyperlipidemia has also been observed with atypical agents, primarily olanzapine and clozapine. In a 2002, 4-year UK study of adult schizophrenics (N = 18,000), a three-fold increase in triglycerides and cholesterol was found with olanzapine compared to more typical neuroleptics (541).

Endocrine

Antipsychotic agents' dopamine blockade releases dopamine-induced tonic inhibition of prolactin secretion. Transient, dose-related increases in serum prolactin have been reported in adult schizophrenia (542), although serum effects may not be correlated significantly with adverse effects, such as acne, estrogen deficiency, galactorrhea, or decreased libido (543). The clinical significance of hyperprolactinemia outside of these adverse effcets is unknown. Open-label treatment with numerous typical and atypical agents such as haloperidol, risperidone, and olanzapine has caused hyperprolactinemia in children (499, 544). A review of an FDA postmarketing surveillance database on the agent olanzapine found the risk of prolactin increase-related complaints to be 4.8 times higher for adolescents than adults (532). In one study, serum prolactin levels were shown to rise in the shortterm and then steadily decrease (545). Others have also demonstrated hyperprolactinemia in youth appearing within 4 weeks of beginning risperidone treatment and declining over time to within the normal range (524). Some of the newer agents in the class, ziprasidone and aripiprazole, have minimal chronic effect on prolactin concentrations in healthy adult males (546).

Expert opinion suggests that management of hyperprolactinemia includes assay of levels every 3 to 6 months, since serum prolactin often decreases over time. In refractory or symptomatic cases, medication may be considered if the atypical cannot be discontinued. Cohen and Biederman (2001) (547) successfully reversed hyperprolactinemia in four males (ages 6 to 11) with risperidone-induced increases (serum prolactin 57 to 129 ng/mL) with the dopamine agonist cabergoline. An alternative option is to switch drugs; for example, olanzapine reversed hyperprolactinemia in risperidone-treated females with schizophrenia (548).

Motor

Extrapyramidal symptoms occur commonly in people taking antipsychotic medications, albeit less frequently with the atypical class. Meta-analysis (486) of data from more than 7,000 adult patients found the effect size of the difference to be 0.30 (i.e., 30% more extrapyramidal side effects with typical than atypical antipsychotics). Although there is little information, a review of the FDA postmarketing surveillance database on the agent olanzapine found a relatively low risk of EPS complaints across age groups, similar to prior reports (532). However, this same review found a fourfold increased risk of dyskinesia in children compared with adults. In a prospective, longitudinal study of haloperidol in 118 children with autism, Campbell et al. (1997) (549) reported that withdrawal dyskinesias (WD) developed in 40 (34%) children; 20 had more than one dyskinetic episode. A subgroup that remained longer in the study with a higher cumulative haloperidol dose evidenced a significantly higher WD incidence. Occurrence rates of tardive dyskinesia (TD) and multiple episodes of TD/WD were higher among girls. In an analysis of long-term risperidone treatment (0.02 to 0.06 mg/kg/day), 18% of a sample of 700 youth experienced at least one symptom of EPS during a 12-month period (545).

Cardiac

Prolonged ECG QTc intervals have been associated with various medications, including the antipsychotics. The QTc interval reflects time occupied for combined depolarization and repolarization of the ventricles. Prolongation of the QTc via potassium channel blockade and delayed repolarization shortens the time that the heart is electrically at rest (isoelectric) and has been shown to be associated with torsade de pointes, a polymorphic ventricular tachycardia, and sudden death. QTc lower than 440 msec are considered normal, with values >500 associated with significantly greater risk (550). The typical neuroleptic thioridazine, which blocks the potassium channel, has been found to cause torsade de pointes and sudden death, in contrast to tricyclic antidepressants, which block sodium channels associated with depolarization and thus increase QTc via another mechanism. A large retrospective cohort study of adult typical antipsychotic users (N = 481,744) found a 2.4-fold increase in sudden death with doses greater than 100 mg thioridazine daily or the equivalent (551). Of the atypical agent class, several block potassium channels, primarily ziprasidone, although risperidone, olanzapine, and quetiapine also do to a lesser degree (550). ECG monitoring should be performed at maximum daily (peak) blood levels to best observe for cardiac conduction effects (550). Automated computer interpretations of ECGs should be followed by a cardiologist's review.

Ocular

Beyond such risk factors as old age and diabetes, medications, particularly antipsychotics, have been associated with the development of cataracts. Although the typical antipsychotics thioridazine and perphenazine have been associated with cataracts, no causal relationship has been determined. In preclinical studies, quetiapine was associated with increased rates of cataracts in puppies at doses four times the maximum human dose (prescribing information, quetiapine). However, in a survey of 620,000 persons taking quetiapine, a lower rate (0.005%) of cataracts was found than in the general population (552).

Hematological Clozapine

Clozapine is available only through a distribution system that ensures appropriate WBC monitoring (Novartis). Clinical studies of clozapine in youth are limited. However, sialorrhea, tachycardia, sedation, enuresis, weight gain, and elevated hepatic transaminase concentrations have been reported. Side effects, including weight gain, have been shown to correlate positively with serum concentrations (479). Of more concern are potentially serious hematological adverse effects such as reduced neutrophil count. In the Frazier et al. trial (2003) (479), one 9-year-old female experienced moderate neutropenia. The higher NOR/CLZ ratio observed in these youth may increase vulnerability due to possible marrow toxicity of NOR (553). Alvir and Lieberman reported that patients younger than 21 years of age (and females) may be at higher risk for agranulocytosis (554).

Neurological

Electroencephalographic (EEG) abnormalities have been demonstrated in adults using the typical antipsychotics. Among the new atypical class, the commonest abnormalities (47%) have been found with clozapine, while olanzapine and risperidone had lesser effects (555).

Drug Interactions

Clozapine is metabolized primarily by CYP1A2, with additional pathways via CYP2C19, CYP2D6, and CYP3A4. Risperidone is metabolized primarily by CYP2D6 and to a lesser extent by CYP3A4. Olanzapine is metabolized primarily by CYP1A2 and to a lesser extent by CYP2D6. Quetiapine and ziprasidone are metabolized by CYP3A4. Although substrates for the CYP450 enzymes, at usual clinical doses these drugs appear not to significantly affect the metabolism of other medications (556).

Several case reports have appeared since 2002 regarding a possible interaction between risperidone and valproic acid in youth, suggesting protein-binding displacement to yield increased serum valproic acid levels or alterations in valproic acid levels mediated by a cytochrome 2D6 interaction (437–439). In response, Good et al. (2003) (440) retrospectively described their pediatric data (N = 45) using combination divalproex sodium with atypical antipsychotics finding no significant difference in trough divalproex levels with combination divalproex sodium and olanzapine or risperidone.

Overdose

Scattered cases of antipsychotic overdose have been reported in youth. In a review of the current literature, Catalono et al. (2001) (557) suggested that special care may be indicated with pediatric cases of atypical antipsychotic overdose including intensive monitoring of potential respiratory or cardiac difficulties. Olanzapine overdose in a 12-year-old boy presented as opioid-like and was followed by complete recovery (558). Catalono et al. (2002) (474) presented the case of a 15-year-old girl who ingested 1,250 mg of quetiapine (21.6 mg/kg) in a suicide attempt and developed symptoms including tachycardia, agitation, hypotension, and unconsciousness. James et al. (2000) (559) described the epidemiology, clinical presentation, management, and outcome of phenothiazine and butyrophenone ingestions in children. Depressed levels of consciousness (91%) and dystonia (51%) were most common.

MISCELLANEOUS AGENTS

Benzodiazepines

Although possessing similar pharmacodynamic actions at GABA receptors, benzodiazepines (BZD) differ in their pharmacokinetics and metabolism, such as hepatic metabolic pathways, presence of active metabolites, Tmax, and half-life.

The study of benzodiazepines has been limited in pediatric populations and consists primarily of open-label small case reports or studies with variable or mixed samples of anxiety disorders. Open-label studies have demonstrated efficacy in overanxious disorder (560) and panic disorder (561, 562) using alprazolam (0.5 to 1.5 mg/day) and clonazepam (0.5 to 3.0 mg/day). Although controlled studies of alprazolam in overanxious youth (563) and clonazepam in mixed anxiety (564) disorders did not demonstrate significant differences over placebo, these were methodologically limited by small sample sizes. In one small, placebo-controlled study of alprazolam and imipramine in children with school refusal, Bernstein et al. (1990) (231) found no significant differences following treatment between groups in either anxiety or depressive symptoms. However, another placebo-controlled study found clonazepam effective for neuroleptic-induced akathisia, suggesting utility beyond primary anxiety disorders (565).

Adverse effects of BZDs such as sedation and behavioral changes may be particularly pronounced in neurologically vulnerable populations, as well as at either age extreme. For example, based on a literature review (566), behavioral side effects occurred in 13% of 446 individuals with mental retardation using benzodiazepines for psychiatric conditions, epilepsy, or other medical conditions. Children, including those with pervasive developmental delays or autism, may be vulnerable to paradoxical behavioral agitation as well (567). Children hospitalized for accidental or deliberate benzodiazepine ingestion (568) experienced the following transient adverse effects: ataxia (87%), lethargy (57%), coma (35%), and respiratory depression (9%). BZDs should be initiated at the lowest available dosage, with gradual titration, particularly with agents with a longer half-life, such as clonazepam, allowing for its accumulation over several days. Adverse effects such as sedation tend to peak as steady state is being reached, and this may take a week or longer with clonazepam. Physiological tolerance may occur with the BZD class necessitating careful and gradual withdrawal. Withdrawal from short-acting agents such as alprazolam may be best achieved by switching to a longer-acting formulation such as clonazepam and then weaning gradually to enhance tolerance of discontinuation (Table 27.15).

Buspirone

Buspirone, an azaspirone, may exert its effect via the dopaminergic or serotonergic system. The drug is rapidly absorbed with time to reach peak levels under 1 hour. It is extensively metabolized, with an elimination half-life of 2.5 hours and linear pharmacokinetics (569).

Adult-controlled studies have demonstrated efficacy in generalized anxiety disorder (570). Efficacy and safety of buspirone in pediatric samples have primarily been observed in open studies of social anxiety (571) and anxiety disorders in children with PDD (572). In a sample of prepubertal psychiatric inpatients, it had limited benefit and caused increased aggression, agitation, and euphoria (573). Preliminary reports of benefit have also been presented in small open samples of ADHD (574, 575) and comorbid ODD (576).

In addition buspirone may facilitate antidepressant response, as suggested in the adult literature, via activation of presynaptic and postsynaptic 5-HT1A receptors and modulation of serotonin release (577). Only limited reports of SSRI augmentation with buspirone (for OCD) may be found in the pediatric literature (578).

Alpha-2 Agonists

Clonidine, an imidazoline-derived agent, has agonist effects on central alpha-2-adrenergic receptors. Guanfacine is a longer-acting and more selective agonist than clonidine. Research in animal models demonstrates that too little alpha-2-receptor stimulation or too much alpha-1-receptor stimulation can impair prefrontal cortical function. Thus, agents that normalize NE prefrontal transmission may reduce impulsivity and enhance attention by improving prefrontal cortical behavioral control (579).

The alpha-2-receptor clonidine has been shown to be superior to placebo in ADHD in a number of randomized controlled trials, though methodological weakness limit

TABLE 27.15

USUAL DOSE RANGES FOR MEDICATIONS IN PEDIATRIC ANXIETY DISORDERS

Drug	Starting Dose (mg)	Typical Dose Range (mg)
First-Line Treatment		
Citalopram	5–20 QD	5–60
Fluoxetine	5–20 QAM	5–80
Fluvoxamine	12.5–50 QHS	25–300
Paroxetine	5–10 QPM	5–60
Sertraline	12.5–25 QAM	25–200
Buspirone	5 BID	5–60
Second-Line Treatment		
Clomipramine	12.5–25 HS	25–150 (2–5 mg/kg/day)
Desipramine	10–25 QHS	10–250 (2–5 mg/kg/day)
Imipramine	10–25 QHS	10–200 (2–5 mg/kg/day)
Nortriptyline	10 QHS	10–150 (1–3 mg/kg/day)
Protriptyline	5–10 QHS	5–50 (0.5–2 mg/kg/day)
Clonazepam	0.125–0.5	0.125–3.0
Diazepam	1–2 HS	0.25–5.0
Lorazepam	0.125–0.5 BID	0.125–3.0
Third-Line Treatment		
Mirtazapine	7.5–15 HS	15–45
Venlafaxine	12.5–37.5 BID	25–300

their interpretation (588, part 1). Connor et al. (1999) (580) conducted a meta-analysis of 11 trials utilizing clonidine (0.10 to 0.24 mg/day) in children with ADHD. Across parent, teacher, and clinician ratings, positive findings were observed, with an overall moderate effect size of 0.58 and great variability depending on the methodology of individual studies. In one shortterm controlled trial, clonidine was modestly effective in reducing irritability and hyperactivity in eight male children with autism (581). Two uncontrolled studies (1.5 to 3.2 mg guanfacine/day) found scattered and limited improvement in hyperactivity and inattention (582, 583). Open studies of alpha-2 agonists in a small sample of aggressive youth with childhood disruptive behavior disorders demonstrated improvement in opposition and conduct (584).

Clonidine (CLON) or guanfacine are considered first-line agents in tic disorders and Tourette's syndrome due to their modest efficacy and relatively benign profile compared to the antipsychotic agents. A multicenter, randomized, double-blind, 16-week clinical trial conducted in 136 children with ADHD and a chronic tic disorder (CLON alone, MPH alone, combined CLON + MPH, or placebo) showed efficacy of clonidine in tic disorders. Compared with placebo, the greatest benefit for comorbid children occurred with combined CLON + MPH ($p < 0.0001$). Compared with placebo, tic severity lessened in all treatment groups in the following order: CLON + MPH, CLON alone, MPH alone (310). In addition, in an 8-week placebo controlled study of guanfacine (0.5 mg to 3 mg divided) in ADHD and tic disorder, Scahill et al. (2001) (585) found significant superiority of active drug over placebo in both ADHD symptoms *and* tic reduction. Based on open-label studies suggesting benefit for anxiety, arousal, and impulsivity, an ongoing RCT of clonidine for posttraumatic stress disorder is under way (586, 587).

Clonidine may be started as a single bedtime dose (0.05 mg) and titrated over 2 to 4 weeks to a total daily divided dose of 0.05 mg to 0.4 mg/day, with dose adjustments every 3 to 5 days. Clonidine's half-life is very short (3 to 4 hours) so that divided doses may be needed. It is often sedating and finds one of its most widespread uses as a hypnotic in hyperactive youth. Guanfacine has lower potency and a longer duration of action. Daily doses range from 0.5 to 4 mg/day, given on a schedule similar to that used for clonidine (588). Guanfacine and clonidine in children and adolescents have the common adverse events of sedation/lethargy and irritability (580, 589). Mood disturbances with longer-term use may also be noted. Sleep disturbances associated with ADHD may be improved with clonidine (590, 591), although clinical trials report sleep disturbance, such as awakening in the middle of the night (580).

Cardiac side effects (dysrhythmia, bradycardia, hypotension, first-degree heart block, nonspecific intraventricular conduction delay) associated with the use of clonidine in children have been reported (592, 593). Following the cases of four children who died, presumably while receiving

clonidine in combination with methylphenidate (MPH), Wilens and Spencer (1999) (358) critically summarized the literature. The authors acknowledged that clonidine can be associated with cardiovascular side effects in the context of coadministered sympatholytic agents or in the face of pre-existing myocardial impairment. Yet there were mitigating circumstances surrounding each of these cases, and there were insufficient data to declare any causal relationship. The American Heart Association has stated that ECG monitoring is not routinely required for clonidine treatment (328).

Physiological tolerance may occur, necessitating careful and gradual withdrawal to avoid rebound hypertension. A reasonable taper schedule could be reduction by 0.05 mg clonidine or 0.5 mg guanfacine each 5 to 7 days.

Beta-Blockers

Beta-blockers, agents that block beta-adrenergic receptors, may be useful for adults in states of hyperarousal, such as panic, performance anxiety, aggression, and posttrauma. Beta-blockers differ in pharmacology, such as beta-selectivity and solubility; propanolol readily crosses the blood-brain barrier due its lipid solubility. According to a *Cochrane Database of Systematic Reviews*, the best evidence for efficacy of beta-blockers is in the management of aggression in acquired brain injury (ABI) (594). Only one controlled trial of children with ADHD and comorbid conduct disorder has been reported (595), demonstrating modest efficacy for pindolol compared to MPH. A study of beta-blockers (propranolol) in adults with trauma suggests that they could mitigate or perhaps even prevent PTSD symptoms (596). Beta-blockers have anecdotally been usefully combined with stimulants to reduce systemic adrenergic adverse events such as tremor, for example, nadolol at 20 mg/daily. Lastly, there are case reports of pindolol used for treatment resistant OCD.

Beta-blockers are generally well tolerated. In addition to bradycardia, adverse effects may include fatigue and bronchoconstriction, so that asthma may be a relative contraindication for their use. In these situations, using a selective beta-1 antagonist, such as atenolol or betaxolol, is recommended. Physiological tolerance may occur, necessitating careful and gradual withdrawal to avoid rebound hypertension.

Novel Anticonvulsants

Tiagabine, a nipecotic acid derivative that enhances GABAergic activity by inhibiting GABA reuptake, is approved for adjunctive treatment of partial seizures in adults and children older than 12 years (597). Zonisamide, a sulfonamide derivative that blocks calcium channels and prolongs sodium channel inactivation, is approved as adjunctive therapy for partial seizures in patients aged 16 years and older (597). Both agents have only preliminary data in adult bipolar disorder (449) and none at all in pediatric psychiatry.

Modafinil

Modafinil, an alerting agent that targets the hypothalamus and other sleep-regulating areas of the brain, is approved for the treatment of adult narcolepsy. Its pharmacokinetic properties have been reviewed (598). Modafinil may have utility for daytime somnolence in youth, suggested by a systematic chart review of 13 children (599). Care should be taken not to use modafinil for somnolence that may be the result of a sleep disorder such as obstructive apnea to avoid masking an underlying problem that requires a more specific intervention. According to commercial sales figures, sleep experts, psychiatrists, and generalists are increasingly prescribing modafinil for somnolence not caused by narcolepsy, such as found in depression and multiple sclerosis, as well as for ADHD (600). In one randomized, double-blind, placebo-controlled study of 24 children, Conners' Rating Scales ADHD total T scores for the modafinil group improved compared to control subjects (P = 0.04). Ten of 11 treatment patients were reported as "significantly" improved, whereas 8 of 11 control subjects were reported as manifesting "no" or only "slight" improvement (P < 0.001) (601).

Nicotine/Acetylcholine

Nicotinic interactions with dopaminergic and glutaminergic systems may be important in cognitive function (602). Further, there may be genetically distinct subtypes of ADHD, so that attention problems could be responsive to receptor subtype selective nicotine agonists (603). Cholinesterase inhibitors may also be useful in ADHD. For example, five youth aged 8 to 17 years demonstrated improvement in ADHD with the acetylcholinesterase inhibitor donepezil (Aricept) (604).

Opiate Antagonists

The opioid antagonist naltrexone has been studied in autism and specifically for self-injurious behaviors. This data suggest some positive effect on motoric overactivity but not on the core social deficits associated with autism (605). In a trial of 32 adults (7 with autism, 16 with autism and self-injurious behavior, and 9 nonautistic individuals with self-injurious behavior), naltrexone did not demonstrate efficacy for either self-injurious behavior or core autism symptoms. In fact, naltrexone increased the incidence of stereotypic behaviors, and at 50 mg/d, naltrexone-treated subjects were rated significantly globally worse than those on placebo (606).

Alternative Medicines

Although widespread in their use, including in pediatric populations, studies of herbals, supplements, and other alternative medicine agents or techniques have significant methodological limitations, including a general lack of standardization. Potentially useful agents such as omega-3/6 fatty acids, St John's wort, melatonin, and others are being studied with sponsorship by the National Center for Complimentary and Alternative Medicine (NCCAM) (nccam.nih.gov). As our knowledge base slowly expands regarding the efficacy of these agents, we are also increasingly aware of adverse effects and potentially clinically significant drug interactions (41), despite the public (and clinician) perception that these "natural" alternative remedies possess a benign safety profile.

Calcium Channel Blockers

Many mood-disordered patients show increased intracellular calcium alterations during, and even between, depressive episodes, leading to the hypothesis that blockade of calcium influx may be clinically helpful. Hollister and Trevino (1999) (607) reviewed the literature for the use of calcium channel blockers (CCBs) in psychiatry and found 61 reports, including 17 controlled trials, all in adults. Most studies involved treatment of mania using verapamil but also included nimodipine. Results were mixed, but typically lithium and even placebo fared better than verapamil. Treatment for depression, schizophrenia, tardive dyskinesia, and dementia has largely failed to show justification for the use of CCBs. At this time, this class of drug has no indication in pediatric psychopharmacology.

CONCLUSION AND FUTURE DIRECTIONS

In summary, we have seen an exponential growth in our evidence-based knowledge of pediatric psychopharmacology. The strongest evidence supports the use of stimulants in ADHD and SSRIs in OCD in children. Support for SSRIs in major depressive disorder and other anxiety disorders is substantial. The improved methodology, greater statistical power, and sheer number of psychopharmacology studies under way at this time should add greatly to our knowledge over the next decade. Areas of special interest are in the use of glutamate and NMDA receptor antagonists that promise to yield benefits over a range of clinical disorders. Neurobiological studies have implicated an intimate role for glutamate in the pathogenesis of OCD symptoms, mediated through glutamatergic inervation of caudate from prefrontal cortex as part of a cortico-frontal-striatal-thalamic loop (608). As such, the clinical value of glutamate antagonists in the treatment of OCD is being actively explored.

One possible etiological subtype of early-onset OCD, that is pediatric autoimmune neuropsychiatric disorder associated with streptococcus (PANDAS), has garnered much attention for its implication that antibiotic treatment may alleviate symptoms of tics and OCD through suppression of antibody-stimulating streptococci that indirectly cause immune-mediated inflammation of basal ganglia structures (609). However, definitive evidence that antibody prophylaxis can reduce symptoms of OCD or prevent relapse is still lacking, despite some empirical evidence supporting this approach.

In the future, the use of sophisticated molecular genetic as well as functional, structural, and spectroscopic magnetic resonance imaging studies could lead to the development of pharmacogenetic and endophenotype studies to better craft pharmacotherapeutic interventions for children.

REFERENCES

1. Coyle JT: Disorders of Development, in The Fifth Generation of Progress. Edited by Davis KL, Charney D, Coyle JT, Nemeroff C. Nashville, TN: American College of Neuropsychopharmacology, 2002.
2. Vitiello B, Jensen PS: Developmental perspectives in pediatric psychopharmacology. Psychopharmacology Bulletin 1995; 31:(1)75–81.
3. Kauffman RE: Drug therapeutics in the infant and child, in Pediatric Pharmacology: Therapeutic Principles in Practice. Edited by Yaffe SJ, Aranda JV. Philadelphia: WB Saunders, 1992, pp. 212–19.
4. Hein K: The use of therapeutics in adolescence. Journal of Adolescent Health Care 1987; 8(1):8–35.
5. Milsap RL, Hill MR, Szefler SJ: Special pharmacokinetic considerations in children, in Applied Pharmacokinetics: Principles of Therapeutic Drug Monitoring. Edited by Evans WE, Schentag JJ, Jusko WJ. Vancouver, WA: Applied Therapeutics, 1992.
6. Bourin M, Couetoux du Tertre A: Pharmacokinetics of psychotropic drugs in children. Clinical Neuropharmacology 1992; 15(Suppl 1):224A–225A.
7. Geller B: Psychopharmacology of children and adolescents: pharmacokinetics and relationships of plasma/serum levels to response. Psychopharmacology Bulletin 1991; 27(4):401–9.
8. Murry DJ, Crom WR, Reddick WE, Bhargava R, Evans WE: Liver volume as a determinant of drug clearance in children and adolescents. Drug Metabolism and Disposition: The Biological Fate of Chemicals 1995; 23(10):1110–16.
9. Carrey NJ, Dursun S, Clements R, Renton K, Waschbusch D, MacMaster FP: Noradrenergic and serotonergic neuroendocrine responses in prepubertal, peripubertal, and postpubertal rats pretreated with desipramine and sertraline. Journal of the American Academy of Child and Adolescent Psychiatry 2002; 41(8):999–1006.
10. Seeman P, Bzowej NH, Guan HC, Bergeron C, Becker LE, Reynolds GP, Bird ED, Riederer P, Jellinger K, Watanabe S, et al.: Human brain dopamine receptors in children and aging adults. Synapse 1987; 1(5):399–404.
11. Cohen DJ, Shaywitz BA, Johnson WT, Bowers MJ: Biogenic amines in autistic and atypical children: cerebrospinal fluid measures of homovanillic acid and 5-hydroxyindoleacetic acid. Archives of General Psychiatry 1974; 31(6):845–53.
12. Freedman L, Ohuchi T, Goldstein M, Axelrod F, Fish I, Dancis J: Changes in human serum dopamine-hydroxylase activity with age. Nature 1972; 236(535):310–11.
13. Ziegler MG, Lake CR, Kopin IJ: Plasma norepinephrine increases with age. Nature 1976; 261(558):333–335.
14. Chugani D, Muzik O, Chakraborty P, Mangner T, Chugani H: Human brain serotonin synthesis capacity measured in vivo with alpha-[C-11]methyl- l -tryptophan. Synapse 1998; 28(1):33–43.
15. Hill HF, Engblom J: Effects of pre- and postnatal haloperidol administration to pregnant and nursing rats on brain catecholamine levels in their offspring. Developmental Pharmacological Therapy 1984; 7(2):188–97.
16. Litt IF: Compliance with pediatric medication regimens, in Pediatric Pharmacology: Therapeutic Principles in Practice. Edited by J. YS, Aranda JV. Philadelphia: WB Saunders, 1992, pp. 45–54.
17. Charney E, Bynum R, Eldredge D, Frank D, MacWhinney J, McNabb N, Scheiner A, Sumpter E, Iker H: How well do patients take oral penicillin? A collaborative study in private practice. Pediatrics 1967; 40(2):188–95.
18. West S, King V, Carey TS, Lohr KN, McKoy N, Sutton SF, Lux L: Systems to Rate the Strength of Scientific Evidence. Rockville, MD: Agency for Healthcare Research and Quality (AHRQ), 2002, pp. 1–195.
19. McClellan JM, Werry JS: Evidence-based treatments in children and adolescent psychiatry: An inventory. Journal of the American Academy of Child and Adolescent Psychiatry 2003; 42(12):1388–1400.
20. Coghill D: Evidence based psychopharmacology for children and adolescents. Current Opinions in Psychiatry 2002; 15(4):361–68.
21. Geller DA, Biederman J, Stewart ES, Mullin B, Martin A, Spencer T, Faraone SV: Which SSRI? A meta-analysis of pharmacotherapy trials in pediatric obsessive compulsive disorder. American Journal of Psychiatry 2003; 160(11):1919–28.
22. Greenhill L, Vitiello B, Riddle M, Fisher P, Shockey E, March J, Levine J, Freid J, Abikoff H, Zito JM, JT M, Findling RL, Robinson J, Cooper TB, Davies M, Varipatis E, Labellarte M, Scahill L, Walkup J, Capasso L, Rosengarten J: Review of safety assessment methods used in pediatric psychopharmacology. Journal of the American Academy of Child and Adolescent Psychiatry 2003; 42(6):627–33.
23. Vitiello B, Riddle M, Greenhill L, March J, Levine J, Schachar R, Abikoff H, Zito JM, McCracken J, Walkup J, Findling RL, Robinson J, Cooper HM, Davies M, Varipatis E, Labellarte M, Scahill L, Capasso L: How can we improve the assessment of safety in child and adolescent psychopharmacology? Journal of the American Academy of Child and Adolescent Psychiatry 2003; 42(6):634–41.
24. Preskorn SH: Clinical pharmacology of selective serotonin reuptake inhibitors. Professional Communications, 1996.
25. Stahl SM: Psychopharmacology of antidepressants. London: Dunitz, 1997.
26. Leonard H, March J, Rickler K, Allen A: Pharmacology of the selective serotonin reuptake inhibitors in children and adolescents. Journal of the American Academy of Child and Adolescent Psychiatry 1997; 36(6):725–36.
27. Aghajanian GK, Sanders-Bush E: Serotonin, in The Fifth Generation of Progress. Edited by Davis KL, Charney D, Coyle JT, Nemeroff C. Nashville, TN: American College of Neuropsychopharmacology, 2002.
28. DeVane CL: Metabolism and pharmacokinetics of selective serotonin reuptake inhibitors. Cellular and Molecular Neurobiology 1999; 19(4):443–66.
29. Alderman J, Wolkow R, Chung M, Johnston H: Sertraline treatment of children and adolescents with obsessive-compulsive disorder or depression: pharmacokinetics, tolerability, and efficacy. Journal of the American Academy of Child and Adolescent Psychiatry 1998; 37(4):386–94.
30. Axelson DA, Perel JM, Birmaher B, Rudolph GR, Nuss S, Bridge J, Brent DA: Sertraline pharmacokinetics and dynamics in adolescents. Journal of the American Academy of Child and Adolescent Psychiatry 2002; 41(9):1037–44.
31. DeVane CL, Liston HL, Markowitz JS: Clinical pharmacokinetics of sertraline. Clinical Pharmacokinetics 2002; 41(15):1247–66.
32. Ronfeld RA, Wilner KD, Baris BA: Sertraline: chronopharmacokinetics and the effect of coadministration with food. Clinical Pharmacokinetics 1997; 32 (Suppl.):50–55.
33. Wilens TE, Cohen L, Biederman J, Abrams A, Neft D, Faird N, Sinha V: Fluoxetine pharmacokinetics in pediatric patients. Journal of Clinical Psychopharmacology 2002; 22(6):568–75.
34. Findling RL, Reed MD, Myers C, O'Riordan MA, Fiala S, Branicky L, Waldorf B, Blumer JL: Paroxetine pharmacokinetics in depressed children and adolescents. Journal of the American Academy of Child and Adolescent Psychiatry 1999; 38(8):952–59.
35. Strauss WL, Unis AS, Cowan C, Dawson G, Dager SR: Fluorine magnetic resonance spectroscopy Measurement of Brain Fluvoxamine and Fluoxetine in Pediatric Patients Treated for Pervasive Developmental Disorders. American Journal of Psychiatry 2002; 159(5):755–60.

36. DeVane CL: Metabolism and pharmacokinetics of selective serotonin reuptake inhibitors. Cellular and Molecular Neurobiology 1999; 19(4): 443–66.

37. Birmaher B, Brent D: Depression Disorder, in Pediatric Psychopharmacology: Principles and Practice. Edited by Martin A, Scahill L, Charney DS, Leckman JF. Oxford, UK: Oxford University Press, 2003, pp. 466–83.

38. DeVane CL: Pharmacokinetics, drug interactions, and tolerability of paroxetine and paroxetine CR. Psychopharmacology Bulletin 2003; 37 (Suppl.):29–41.

39. Crewe HK, Lennard MS, Tucker GT, Woods FR, Haddock RE: The effect of selective serotonin reuptake inhibitors on the cytochrome P45002D6 activity in human liver microsomes. British Journal of Clinical Pharmacology 1992; 34(3):262–65.

40. Lam YW, Gaedigk A, Ereshefsky L, Alfaro CL, Simpson J: CYP2D6 inhibition by selective serotonin reuptake inhibitors: analysis of achievable steady-state plasma concentrations and the effect of ultrarapid metabolism at CYP2D6. Pharmacotherapy 2002; 22(8):1001–6.

41. Hammerness P, Basch E, Ulbricht C, Barrette EP, Foppa I, Basch S, Bent S, Boon H, Ernst E, Collaboration NSR: St John's wort: a systematic review of adverse effects and drug interactions for the consultation psychiatrist. Psychosomatics 2003; 44(4):271–82.

42. Haffen E, Vandel P, Bonin B, Vandel S: Citalopram pharmacokinetic interaction with clomipramine. UDP-glucuronosyltransferase inhibition? A case report. Therapie 1999; 54(6):768–70.

43. Sanchez C, Hyttel J: Comparison of the effects of antidepressants and their metabolites on reuptake of biogenic amines and on receptor binding. Cellular & Molecular Neurobiology 1999; 19(4):467–89.

44. Hensler JG: Differential regulation of 5-HT1A receptor-G protein interactions in brain following chronic antidepressant administration. Neuropsychopharmacology 2002; 26(5):565–73.

45. Tollefson GD, Rosenbaum JF: Selective Serotonin Reuptake Inhibitors, in Essentials of Clinical Psychopharmacology. Edited by Schatzberg AF, Nemeroff CB. Washington, DC: American Psychiatric Publishing, 2001.

46. Nemeroff CB, Owens MJ: Neuropharmacology of Paroxetine. Psychopharmacology Bulletin 2003; 37 (Suppl.):8–18.

47. Hyttel J: Comparative pharmacology of selective serotonin reuptake inhibitors (SSRIs). Nordic Journal of Psychiatry 1993; 47 (Suppl. 30):5–12.

48. Emslie GJ, Heiligenstein JH, Hoog SL, Wagner KD, Findling RL, McCracken JT, et al.: Fluoxetine treatment for prevention of relapse of depression in children and adolescents: a double-blind, placebo-controlled study. Journal of the American Academy of Child and Adolescent Psychiatry 2004; 43(11):1397–1405.

49. Treatment for Adolescents With Depression Study Team (TADS): Treatment for adolescents with depression study: rationale, design and methods. Journal of the American Academy of Child and Adolescent Psychiatry 2003; 42(5):531–42.

50. Gould MS, Greenberg T, Velting DM, Shaffer D: Youth suicide risk and preventive interventions: a review of the past 10 years. Journal of the American Academy of Child and Adolescent Psychiatry 2003; 42(4):386–405.

51. Emslie GJ, Heiligenstein JH, Wagner KD, Hoog SL, Ernest DE, Brown E, Nilsson M, Jacobsen JG: Fluoxetine for acute treatment of depression in children and adolescents: a placebo-controlled, randomized clinical trial. Journal of the American Academy of Child Adolescent Psychiatry 2002; 41(10):1205–15.

52. Emslie G, Rush J, Weinberg W, Kowatch R, Hughes C, Carmody T, Rintelmann J: A double-blind, randomized, placebo-controlled trial of fluoxetine in children and adolescents with depression. Archives of General Psychiatry 1997; 54(11):1031–37.

53. Emslie GJ, Rush AJ, Weinberg WA, Kowatch RA, Carmody T, Mayes TL: Fluoxetine in child and adolescent depression: acute maintenance and treatment. Depression and Anxiety 1998; 7(1):32–39.

54. Kowatch RA, Carmody TJ, Emslie GJ, Rintelmann JW, Hughes CW, Rush AJ: Prediction of response to fluoxetine and placebo in children and adolescents with major depression: a hypothesis generating study. Journal of Affective Disorders 1999; 54(3):269–76.

55. Keller MB, Ryan ND, Strober M, Klein RG, Kutcher SP, Birmaher B, Hagino OR, Koplewicz H, Carlson GA, Clarke GN, Emslie G, Feinberg D, Geller B, Kusumakar V, Papatheodorou G, Sack WH, Sweeney M, Wagner KD, Weller EB, Winters NC, Oakes R, McCafferty JP: Efficacy of paroxetine in the treatment of adolescent major depression: a randomized, controlled trial. Journal of the American Academy of Child and Adolescent Psychiatry 2001; 40(7):762–72.

56. Braconnier A, Le Coent R, Cohen D, Group DS: Paroxetine versus clomipramine in adolescents with severe major depression: a double-blind, randomized, multicenter trial. Journal of the American Academy of Child and Adolescent Psychiatry 2003; 42(1):22–29.

57. American College of Neuropsychopharmacology: Executive Summary: preliminary report of the task force on SSRIs and suicidal behavior in youth. Nashville, TN: American College of Neuropsychopharmacology, 2004, pp. 1–88.

58. Simeon J, Dinicola V, Ferguson B, Copping W: Adolescent depression: a placebo-controlled fluoxetine treatment study and follow-up. Progress in Neuro-Psychopharmaclogy and Biological Psychiatry 1990; 14(5):791–795.

59. Donnelly CL: A comparison of the response to sertraline in children and adolescents with major depressive disorder, in American Academy of Child and Adolescent Psychiatry. Miami Beach, FL, 2003.

60. Wagner K: Citalopram in pediatric major depression, in American College of Neuropsychopharmacology. Waikoloa, Hawaii, 2001.

61. Hughes CW, Emslie GJ, Crismon ML, Wagner K, Birmaher B, Geller B, Pliszka SR, Ryan ND, Strober M, Trivedi MH, Toprac MG, Sedillo A, Llana ME, Lopez M, Rush AJ, Disorder: The Texas children's medication algorithm project: report of the Texas consensus conference panel on medication treatment of childhood major depressive disorder. Journal of the American Academy of Child and Adolescent Psychiatry 1999; 38(11):1442–54.

62. FDA: www.fda.gov/bbs/topics/ANSWERS/2003/ANS01256.html, Food and Drug Administration, 2003.

63. Riddle MA: Letter to the editor: paroxetine and the FDA. Journal of the American Academy of Child and Adolescent Psychiatry 2004; 43(2):128–30.

64. Brent DA: Letter to the editor: paroxetine and the FDA. Journal of the American Academy of Child and Adolescent Psychiatry 2004; 43(2):127–28.

65. Connor DF: Letter to the editor: paroxetine and the FDA. Journal of the American Academy of Child and Adolescent Psychiatry 2004; 43(2):127.

66. Geller D, Spencer T: Obsessive-Compulsive Disorder, in Pediatric Psychopharmacology: Principles and Practice. Edited by Martin A, Scahill L, Charney DS, Leckman JF. Oxford, UK: Oxford University Press, 2002.

67. Geller DA, Biederman J, Stewart SE, Mullin B, Farrell C, Wagner KD, Emslie G, Carpenter D: Impact of comorbidity on treatment response to paroxetine in pediatric obsessive compulsive disorder: is the use of exclusion criteria empirically supported in randomized clinical trials? Journal of Child and Adolescent Psychopharmacology 2003; 13 (Suppl. 1):S19–29.

68. Liebowitz MR, Turner SM, Piacentini J, Beidel DC, Clarvit SR, Davies SO, Graae F, Jaffer M, Lin SH, Sallee FR, Schmidt AB, Simpson HB: Fluoxetine in children and adolescents with OCD: a placebo-controlled trial. Journal of the American Academy of Child and Adolescent Psychiatry 2002; 41(12):1431–38.

69. Geller DA, Hoog SL, Heiligenstein JH, Ricardi RK, Tamura R, Kluszynski S, Jacobsen JG, Team TFPOS: Fluoxetine treatment for obsessive-compulsive disorder in children and adolescents: a placebo-controlled clinical trial. Journal of the American Academy of Child and Adolescent Psychiatry 2001; 40(7):773–79.

70. Riddle MA, Reeve EA, Yaryura-Tobias JA, Yang HM, Claghorn JL, Gaffney G, Greist JH, Holland D, McConville BJ, Pigott T, Walkup JT: Fluvoxamine for children and adolescents with obsessive-compulsive disorder: a randomized, controlled, multicenter trial. Journal of the American Academy of Child and Adolescent Psychiatry 2001; 40(2):222–29.

71. Emslie G, Wagner K, Birmaher B, Geller D, Riddle M, Carpenter D: Safety and Efficacy of Paroxetine in the Treatment of Children and Adolescents with OCD, in 153rd annual meeting of the American Psychiatric Association. Chicago, IL, 2000.

72. Geller D, Biederman J, Emslie G, Carpenter D, Gallagher D, Wagner K: Comorbid Psychiatric Illness and Response to Treatment in Pediatric OCD, in 154th annual meeting of the American Psychiatric Association. New Orleans, LA, 2001.

73. Geller DA, Wagner KD, Emslie GJ, Murphy TK, Gallagher D, Gardiner C, Carpenter DJ, Group PPOS: Efficacy of Paroxetine in Pediatric OCD: Results of a Multicenter Study, in 155th annual meeting of the American Psychiatric Association Annual Meeting. Philadelphia, 2002.

74. March JS, Biederman J, Wolkow R, Safferman A, Mardekian J, Cook EH, Cutler NR, Dominguez R, Ferguson J, Muller B, Riesenberg R, Rosenthal M, Sallee FR, Wagner KD: Sertraline in children and adolescents with obsessive-compulsive disorder: a multicenter randomized control trial. Journal of the American Medical Association 1998; 280(20):1752–56.

75. Cook EH, Wagner K, March JS, Biederman J, Landau P, Wolkow R, Messig M: Long-term sertraline treatment of children and adolescents with obsessive-compulsive disorder. Journal of the American Academy of Child and Adolescent Psychiatry 2001; 40(10):1175–81.

76. March JS: Cognitive-behavioral psychotherapy for children and adolescents with OCD: A review and recommendations for treatment. Journal of the American Academy of Child and Adolescent Psychiatry 1995; 34(1):7–18.

77. Wagner KD, Cook EH, Chung H, Messig M: Remission status after long-term sertraline treatment of pediatric obsessive-compulsive disorder. Journal of Child and Adolescent Psychopharmacology 2003; 13 (Suppl. 1):S53–60.

78. Wagner KD, Ambrosini P, Rynn M, Wohlberg C, Yang R, Greenbaum MS, Childress A, Donnelly C, Deas D: Efficacy of sertraline in the treatment of children and adolescents with major depressive disorder: two randomized controlled trials. Journal of the American Medical Association 2003; 290(8):1033–41.

79. March JS: Pediatric OCD Treatment Study (POTS), in 156th annual meeting of the American Academy of Child and Adolescent Psychiatry. San Francisco, 2003.

80. Birmaher B, Waterman GS, Ryan N, Cully M, Balach L, Ingram J, Brodsky M: Fluoxetine for childhood anxiety disorders. Journal of the American Academy of Child and Adolescent Psychiatry 1994; 33(7):993–99.

81. Fairbanks JM, Pine DS, Tancer NK, Dummit ES, Kentgen LM, Martin J, Asche BK, Klein RG: Open fluoxetine treatment of mixed anxiety disorders in children and adolescents. Journal of Child and Adolescent Psychopharmacology 1997; 7(1):17–29.

82. Manassis K, Bradley S: Fluoxetine in anxiety disorders. Journal of the American Academy of Child and Adolescent Psychiatry 1994; 33:761–62.

83. Walkup JT, Labellarte M, Riddle MA, Pine DS, Greenhill L, Klein R, Davies M, March JS, Compton S, Robinson J, O'Hara T, Baker S, Vitiello B, Ritz L, Roper M: Fluvoxamine for the Treatment of Anxiety Disorders in Children and Adolescents. New England Journal of Medicine 2001; 344(17):1279–85.

84. Birmaher B, Axelson DA, Monk K, Kalas C, Clark DB, Ehmann M, Bridge J, Heo J, Brent DA: Fluoxetine for the treatment of childhood anxiety disorders. Journal of the American Academy of Child and Adolescent Psychiatry 2003; 42(4):415–23.

85. Rynn MA, Siqueland L, Rickels K: Placebo-Controlled Trial of Sertraline in the Treatment of Children with Generalized Anxiety Disorder. American Journal of Psychiatry 2001; 158(12):2008–14.

86. Attia E, Haiman C, Walsh BT, Flater SR: Does fluoxetine augment the inpatient treatment of anorexia nervosa? American Journal of Psychiatry 1998; 155(4):548–51.

87. Kaye W: The Use of Fluoxetine to Prevent Relapse in Anorexia Nervosa, in Eating Disorder Research Society. Pittsburgh, 1996.

88. Kaye WH, Nagata T, Weltzin TE, Hsu LK, Sokol MS, McConaha C, Plotnicov KH, Weise J, Deep D: Double-blind placebo-controlled administration of fluoxetine in restricting- and restricting-purging-type anorexia nervosa. Biological Psychiatry 2001; 49(7):644–52.

89. Kotler LA, Devlin MJ, Davies M, Walsh BT: An open trial of fluoxetine for adolescents with bulimia nervosa. Journal of Child and Adolescent Psychopharmacology 2003; 13(3):329–35.

90. Renaud J, Birmaher B, Wassick SC, Bridge J: Use of selective serotonin reuptake inhibitors for the treatment of childhood panic disorder: a pilot study. Journal of Child and Adolescent Psychopharmacology 1999; 9(1):73–83.

91. Compton SN, Grant PJ, Chrisman AK, Gammon PJ, Brown VL, March JS: Sertraline in children and adolescents with social anxiety disorder: an open trial. Journal of the American Academy of Child and Adolescent Psychiatry 2001; 40(5):564–71.

92. Dummit ESr, Klein RG, Tancer NK, Asche B, Martin J: Fluoxetine treatment of children with selective mutism: an open trial. Journal of the American Academy of Child and Adolescent Psychiatry 1996; 35(5):615–21.

93. Donnelly C: Pharmacologic treatment approaches for children and adolescents with posttraumatic stress disorder. Child & Adolescent Psychiatric Clinics of North America 2003; 12(2):251–69.

94. Seedat S, Stein DJ, Ziervogel C, Middleton T, Kaminer D, Emsley RA, Rossouw WC: Comparison of response to a selective serotonin reuptake inhibitor in children, adolescents, and adults with posttraumatic stress disorder. Journal of Child and Adolescent Psychopharmacology 2002; 12(1):37–46.

95. Stein D, Davidson J, Seedat S, Beebe K: Paroxetine in the treatment of post-traumatic stress disorder: pooled analysis of placebo-controlled studies. Expert Opinion on Pharmacotherapy 2003; 4(10):1829–38.

96. Davidson J: Long-term treatment and prevention of posttraumatic stress disorder. Journal of Clinical Psychiatry 2004; 65 (Suppl. 1):44–48.

97. Davidson J, Rothbaum B, van der Kolk B, Sikes C, Farfel G: Multicenter, double-blind comparison of sertraline and placebo in the treatment of posttraumatic stress disorder. Archives of General Psychiatry 2001; 58(5):485–92.

98. McDougle CJ: Current and emerging therapeutics of autistic disorder and related pervasive developmental disorders, in Neuropsychopharmacology: The Fifth Generation of Progress. Edited by Davis KL, Charney D, Coyle JT, Nemeroff C. Nashville, TN: American College of Neuropsychopharmacology, 2002.

99. Armenterose JL, Lewis JE: Citalopram treatment for impulsive aggression in children and adolescents: an open pilot study. Journal of the American Academy of Child and Adolescent Psychiatry 2002; 41(5):522–29.

100. Constantino JN, Liberman M, Kincaid M: Effects of serotonin reuptake inhibitors on aggressive behavior in psychiatrically hospitalized adolescents: results of an open trial. Journal of Child and Adolescent Psychopharmacology 1997; 7(1):31–44.

101. Weintrob A: Paxil and self-scratching. Journal of the American Academy of Child and Adolescent Psychiatry 2001; 40(1):5.

102. Velazquez L, Ward-Chene L, Loosigian SR: Fluoxetine in the treatment of self-mutilating behavior. Journal of the American Academy of Child and Adolescent Psychiatry 2000; 39(7):812–14.

103. Dwivedi S, Pavuluri M, Heidenreich J, Wright T: Response to fluvoxamine augmentation for obsessive and compulsive symptoms in schizophrenia. Journal of Child and Adolescent Psychopharmacology 2002; 12(1):69–70.

104. Aguirre B: Fluoxetine and compulsive sexual behavior. Journal of the American Academy of Child and Adolescent Psychiatry 1999; 38(8):943.

105. Palmer CJ, Yates WR, Trotter L: Childhood trichotillomania: successful treatment with fluoxetine following an SSRI failure. Psychosomatics 1999; 40(6):526–28.

106. Block C, West SA, Baharoglu B: Paroxetine treatment of trichotillomania in an adolescent. Journal of Child and Adolescent Psychopharmacology 1998; 8(1):69–71.

107. Galli VB, Raute NJ, McConville BJ, McElroy SL: An adolescent male with multiple paraphilias successfully treated with fluoxetine. Journal of Child and Adolescent Psychopharmacology 1998; 8(3):195–97.

108. Birmaher B, Brent DA, Benson RS: Summary of the practice parameters for the assessment and treatment of children and adolescents with depressive disorders. Journal of the American Academy of Child and Adolescent Psychiatry 1998; 37(10S):63S–83S.

109. Reis M, Olsson G, Carlsson B, Lundmark J, Dahl ML, Walinder J, Ahlner J, Bengtsson F: Serum levels of citalopram and its main metabolites in adolescent patients treated in a naturalistic clinical setting. Journal of Clinical Psychopharmacology 2002; 22(4):406–13.

110. Byrne SE, Rothschild AJ: Loss of antidepressant efficacy during maintenance therapy: possible mechanisms and treatments. Journal of Clinical Psychiatry 198; 59(6):279–88.

111. Quitkin FM, Petkova E, McGrath PJ, Taylor B, Beasley C, Stewart J, Amsterdam J, Fava M, Rosenbaum J, Reimherr F, Fawcett J, Chen Y, Klein DN: When should a trial of fluoxetine for major depression be declared failed? American Journal of Psychiatry 2003; 160(4):734–40.

112. Pine DS: Treating children and adolescents with selective serotonin reuptake inhibitors: how long is appropriate? Journal of Child and Adolescent Psychopharmacology 2002; 12(3): 189–203.

113. Diler RS, Tamam L, Avci A: Withdrawal symptoms associated with paroxetine discontinuation in a nine-year-old boy. Journal of Clinical Psychopharmacology 2000; 20(5):586–87.

114. Manassis K, Menna R: Depression in anxious children: possible factors in comorbidity. Depression and Anxiety 1999; 10(1): 18–24.

115. American College of Neuropsychopharmacology: Executive Summary: Preliminary report of the task force on SSRIs and suicidal behavior in youth. Nashville, TN: American College of Neuropsychopharmacology; 2004 01/21/04.

116. Lubell KM, Swahn MH, Crosby AE, Kegler SR: Methods of suicide among persons aged 10–19 years—United States, 1992–2001. MMWR 2004; 53:471–73. Available online from URL: www.cdc.gov/mmwr/PDF/wk/mm5322.pdf.

117. Gibbons RD, Hur K, Bhaumik DK, Mann JJ: The relationship between antidepressant medication use and rate of suicide. Archives of General Psychiatry 2005; 62(2):165–72.

118. Olfson M, Shaffer D, Marcus SC, Greenberg T: Relationship between antidepressant medication treatment and suicide in adolescents. Archives of General Psychiatry 2003; 60(10): 978–82.

119. Valuck RJ, Libby AM, Sills MR, Giese AA, Allen RR: Antidepressant treatment and risk of suicide attempt by adolescents with major depressive disorder: a propensity-adjusted retrospective cohort study. CNS Drugs 2004; 18(15):1119–32.

120. Martin A, Young C, Leckman JF, Mukonoweshuro C, Rosenheck R, Douglas L: Age effects of antidepressant-induced manic conversion. Archives in Pediatrics and Adolescent Medicine 2004; 158(8):773–80.

121. Bates G, Willson SW: Use of selective serotonin reuptake inhibitors in children with pervasive developmental disorder: risk of treatment emergent mania. Developmental Medicine and Child Neurology 2003; 45(5):359.

122. Storch DD: Medication-induced hypomania in Asperger's disorder. Journal of the American Academy of Child and Adolescent Psychiatry 1999; 38(2):110–11.

123. Damore J, Stine J, Brody L: Medication-induced hypomania in Asperger's disorder. Journal of the American Academy of Child and Adolescent Psychiatry 1998; 37(3):248–49.

124. Diler RS, Avci A: SSRI-induced mania in obsessive-compulsive disorder. Journal of the American Academy of Child and Adolescent Psychiatry 1999; 38(1):6–7.

125. Pao M, Tipnis T: Serotonin syndrome after sertraline overdose in a 5-year-old girl. Archives of Pediatrics and Adolescent Medicine 1997; 151(10):1064–67.

126. Diler RS, Yolga AY, Avci A: Fluoxetine-induced extrapyramidal symptoms in an adolescent: a case report. Swiss Medical Weekly 2002; 132(9–10):125–26.

127. Ghaziuddin N, Iqbal A, Khetarpal S: Myoclonus during prolonged treatment with sertraline in an adolescent patient. Journal of Child and Adolescent Psychopharmacology 2001; 11(2):199–202.

128. Oldroyd J: Paroxetine-induced mania. Journal of the American Academy of Child and Adolescent Psychiatry 1997; 36(6): 721–22.

129. Wilkinson D: Loss of anxiety and increased aggression in a 15-year-old boy taking fluoxetine. Journal of Psychopharmacology 1999; 13(4):420–21.

130. Heimann SW, March JS: SSRI-induced mania. Journal of the American Academy of Child and Adolescent Psychiatry 1996; 35(1):4.

131. Jones-Fearing KB: SSRI and EPS with fluoxetine. Journal of the American Academy of Child and Adolescent Psychiatry 1996; 35(9):1107–8.

132. Baldassano CF, Truman CJ, Nierenberg A, Ghaemi SN, Sachs GS: Akathisia: a review and case report following paroxetine treatment. Comprehensive Psychiatry 1996; 37(2):122–24.

133. Garland EJ, Baerg EA: Amotivational syndrome associated with selective serotonin reuptake inhibitors in children and adolescents. Journal of Child and Adolescent Psychopharmacology 2001; 11(2):181–86.

134. Frank GK: Sertraline in underweight binge eating/purging-type eating disorders: Five case reports. International Journal of Eating Disorders 2001; 29:495–98.

135. Lake MB, Birmaher B, Wassick S, Mathos K, Yelovich AK: Bleeding and selective serotonin reuptake inhibitors in childhood and adolescence. Journal of Child and Adolescent Psychopharmacology 2000; 10(1):35–8.

136. Calhoun JW, Calhoun DD: Prolonged bleeding time in a patient treated with sertraline. American Journal of Psychiatry 1996; 153(3):443.

137. Dalton S, Johansen C, Mellemkjaer L, Norgard B, Sorensen H, Olsen J: Use of selective serotonin reuptake inhibitors and risk of upper gastrointestinal tract bleeding: a population-based cohort study. Archives of Internal Medicine 2003; 163:59–64.

138. de Jong J, van den Berg P, Tobi H, de Jong L: Combined use of SSRIs and NSAIDS increases the risk of gastrointestinal adverse effects. British Journal of Clinical Pharmacology 2003; 55:591–95.

139. Armitage R, Emslie G, Rintelmann J: The effect of fluoxetine on sleep EEG in childhood depression: a preliminary report. Neuropsychopharmacology 1997; 17(4):241–45.

140. Whyte I, Dawson A, Buckley N: Relative toxicity of venlafaxine and selective serotonin reuptake inhibitors in overdose compared to tricyclic antidepressants. Quarterly Journal of Medicine 2003; 96(5):369–74.

141. Phillips S, Brent J, Kulig K, Heiligenstein J, Birkett M: Fluoxetine versus tricyclic antidepressants: a prospective multicenter study of antidepressant drug overdoses. The Antidepressant Study Group. Journal of Emergency Medicine 1997; 15(4):439–45.

142. Fraser J, South M: Life-threatening fluvoxamine overdose in a 4-year-old child. Intensive Care Medicine 1999; 25(5):548.

143. Catalano G, Cooper D, Catalano M, Guttman J: Pediatric sertraline overdose. Clinical Neuropharmacology 1998; 21(1):59–61.

144. Myers L, Krenzelok E: Paroxetine (Paxil) overdose: a pediatric focus. Veterinary and Human Toxicology 1997; 39(2):86–88.

145. Sallee F, DeVane C, Ferrell R: Fluoxetine-related death in a child with cytochrome P-450 2D6 genetic deficiency. Journal of Child and Adolescent Psychopharmacology 2000; 10(1):27–34.

146. Stewart J, Berkel H, Parish R, Simar M, Syed A, Bocchini JJ, Wilson J, Manno JE: Single-dose pharmacokinetics of bupropion in adolescents: effects of smoking status and gender. Journal of Clinical Pharmacology 2001; 41(7):770–78.

147. DeVane C: Immediate-release versus controlled-release formulations: pharmacokinetics of newer antidepressants in relation to nausea. Journal of Clinical Psychiatry 2003; 64 (Suppl. 18): 14–19.

148. Wilens T, Horrigan J, Haight B, Hampton K: The Safety and Tolerability of Extended-Release Bupropion in Adult ADHD, in the 50th Annual Meeting of the American Academy of Child and Adolescent Psychiatry. Miami, Fl, 2003.

149. Findling RL, Preskorn SH, Marcus RN, Magnus RD, D'Amico F, Marathe P, Reed MD: Nefazodone pharmacokinetics in depressed children and adolescents. Journal of the American Academy of Child Adolescent Psychiatry 2000; 39(8):1008–16.

150. Puzantian T: Mirtazapine, an antidepressant. American Journal of Health-System Pharmacy 1998; 55(1):44–49.

151. Stimmel GL, Dopheide JA, Stahl SM: Mirtazapine: an antidepressant with noradrenergic and specific serotonergic effects. Pharmacotherapy 1997; 17(1):10–21.

152. Harvey A, Rudolph R, Preskova SH: Evidence of the dual mechanisms of action of venlafaxine. Archives of General Psychiatry 2000; 57(5):503–9.

153. Meyer J, Goulding V, Wilson A, Hussey D, Christensen B, Houle S: Bupropion occupancy of the dopamine transporter is low during clinical treatment. Psychopharmacology 2002; 163(1):102–5.

154. Rush A, Trivedi M, Fava M: Depression, IV: STAR*D treatment trial for depression. American Journal of Psychiatry 2003; 160(2):237.

155. DeBattista C, Solvason H, Poirier J, Kendrick E, Schatzberg A: A prospective trial of bupropion SR augmentation of partial and non-responders to serotonergic antidepressants. Journal of Clinical Psychopharmacology 2003; 23(1):27–30.

156. Thase M: Effectiveness of antidepressants: comparative remission rates. Journal of Clinical Psychiatry 2003; 64 (Suppl. 2):3–7.

157. Mallick R, Chen J, Entsuah A, Schatzberg A: Depression-free days as a summary measure of the temporal pattern of response and remission in the treatment of major depression: a comparison of venlafaxine, selective serotonin reuptake inhibitors, and placebo. Journal of Clinical Psychiatry 2003; 64(3):321–30.

158. Schatzberg A: Pharmacological principles of antidepressant efficacy. Human Psychopharmacology 2002; 17 (Suppl. 1):S17–22.

159. Daviss W, Bentivoglio P, Racusin R, Brown K, Bostic J, Wiley L: Bupropion sustained release in adolescents with comorbid attention-deficit/hyperactivity disorder and depression. Journal of the American Academy of Child & Adolescent Psychiatry 2001; 40(3):307–14.

160. Mandoki M, Tapia M, Tapia M, Sumner G, Parker J: Venlafaxine in the treatment of children and adolescents with major depression. Psychopharmacology Bulletin 1997; 33(1):149–54.

161. Walter G, Lyndon B, Kubb R: Lithium augmentation of venlafaxine in adolescent major depression. Australian and New Zealand Journal of Psychiatry 1998; 32(3):457–59.

162. Kallepalli B, Bhatara V, Fogas B, Tervo R, Misra L: Trazodone is only slightly faster than fluoxetine in relieving insomnia in adolescents with depressive disorders. Journal of Child and Adolescent Psychopharmacology 1997; 7(2):97–107.

163. Dording C, Mischoulon D, Petersen T, Kornbluh R, Gordon J, Nierenberg A, Rosenbaum J, Fava M: The pharmacologic management of SSRI-induced side effects: a survey of psychiatrists. Annals of Clinical Psychiatry 2002; 14(3):143–47.

164. Nierenberg A, Adler L, Peselow E, Zornberg G, Rosenthal M: Trazodone for antidepressant-associated insomnia. American Journal of Psychiatry 1994; 151(7):1069–72.

165. Balon R: Sleep terror disorder and insomnia treated with trazodone: a case report. Annals of Clinical Psychiatry 1994; 6(3):161–63.

166. Warner M, Dorn M, Peabody C: Survey on the usefulness of trazodone in patients with PTSD with insomnia or nightmares. Pharmacopsychiatry 2001; 34(4):128–31.

167. Ware J, Pittard J: Increased deep sleep after trazodone use: a double-blind placebo-controlled study in healthy young adults. Journal of Clinical Psychiatry 1990; 51 (Suppl.):18–22.

168. Saletu-Zyhlarz G, Abu-Bakr M, Anderer P, Gruber G, Mandl M, Strobl R, Gollner D, Prause W, Saletu B: Insomnia in depression: differences in objective and subjective sleep and awakening quality to normal controls and acute effects of trazodone. Progress in Neuro-Psychopharmacology & Biological Psychiatry 2002; 26(2):249–60.

169. Scharf M, Sachais B: Sleep laboratory evaluation of the effects and efficacy of trazodone in depressed insomniac patients. Journal of Clinical Psychiatry 1990; 51 (Suppl.):13–17.

170. Winokur A, DeMartinis Nr, McNally D, Gary E, Cormier J, Gary KA: Comparative effects of mirtazapine and fluoxetine on sleep physiology measures in patients with major depression and insomnia. Journal of Clinical Psychiatry 2003; 64(10):1224–29.

171. Gorman J, Hirschfeld R, Ninan P: New developments in the neurobiological basis of anxiety disorders. Psychopharmacology Bulletin 2002; 36 (Suppl.):49–67.

172. Meoni P, Hackett D: Characterization of the longitudinal course of long-term venlafaxine XR treatment of GAD. International Journal of Neuropsychopharmacology 2000; 3(S282).

173. Foa EB, Davidson JRT, Frances A: Treatment of posttraumatic stress disorder: the expert consensus guidelines series. Journal of Clinical Psychiatry 1999; 60 (Suppl. 16):1–76.

174. Domon S, Andersen M: Nefazodone for PTSD. Journal of the American Academy of Child & Adolescent Psychiatry 2000; 39(8):942–43.

175. Casat CD, Pleasants DZ, Van Wyck Fleet J: A double-blind trial of bupropion in children with attention deficit disorder. Psychopharmacology Bulletin 1987; 23(1):120–22.

176. Conners C, Casat C, Gualtieri C, Weller E, Reader M, Reiss A, Weller R, Khayrallah M, Ascher J: Bupropion hydrochloride in attention deficit disorder with hyperactivity. Journal of the American Academy of Child & Adolescent Psychiatry 1996; 35(10):1314–21.

177. Barrickman LL, Perry PJ, Allen AJ, Kuperman S, Arndt SV, Herrmann KJ, Schumacher E: Bupropion versus methylphenidate in the treatment of attention-deficit hyperactivity disorder. Journal of the American Academy of Child and Adolescent Psychiatry 1995; 34(5):649–57.

178. Solhkhah R, Wilens T, Prince JB, Daly J, Biederman J: Bupropion Sustained, in 48th Annual meetings of the American Academy of Child and Adolescent Psychiatry. Honolulu, HI, 2001.

179. Hollander E, Kaplan A, Cartwright C, Reichman D: Venlafaxine in children, adolescents, and young adults with autism spectrum disorders: an open retrospective clinical report. Journal of Child Neurology 2000; 15(2):132–35.

180. Mashiko H, Yokoyama H, Matsumoto H, Niwa S: Trazodone for aggression in an adolescent with hydrocephalus. Psychiatry & Clinical Neurosciences 1996; 50(3):133–36.

181. Nguyen M, Myers W: Trazodone for symptoms of frontal lobe atrophy. Journal of the American Academy of Child & Adolescent Psychiatry 2000; 39(10):1209–10.

182. Zubieta J, Alessi N: Acute and chronic administration of trazodone in the treatment of disruptive behavior disorders in children. Journal of Clinical Psychopharmacology 1992; 12:346–51.

183. Fawcett J, Barkin R: Review of the results from clinical studies on the efficacy, safety and tolerability of mirtazapine for the treatment of patients with major depression. Journal of Affective Disorders 1998; 51(3):267–85.

184. Fisfalen M, Hsiung R: Glucose dysregulation and mirtazapine-induced weight gain. American Journal of Psychiatry 2003; 160(4):797.

185. Hui CK, Yuen MF, Wong WM, Lam SK, Lai CL: Mirtazapine-induced hepatotoxicity. Journal of Clinical Gastroenterology 2002; 35(3):270–71.

186. Chen JL, Spinowitz N, Karwa M: Hypertriglyceridemia, acute pancreatitis, and diabetic ketoacidosis possibly associated with mirtazapine therapy: a case report. Pharmacotherapy 2003; 23(7):940–44.

187. Nicholas LM, Ford AL, Esposito SM, Ekstrom RD, Golden RN: The effects of mirtazapine on plasma lipid profiles in healthy subjects. Journal of Clinical Psychiatry 2003; 64(8):883–89.

188. Thase M: Effects of venlafaxine on blood pressure: a meta-analysis of original data from 3744 depressed patients. Journal of Clinical Psychiatry 1998; 59(10):502–8.

189. Zimmer B, Kant R, Zeiler D, Brilmyer M: Antidepressant efficacy and cardiovascular safety of venlafaxine in young vs. old patients with comorbid medical disorders. International Journal of Psychiatry in Medicine 1997; 27(4):353–64.

190. Kem D, Posey D, McDougle C: Priapism associated with trazodone in an adolescent with autism. Journal of the American Academy of Child & Adolescent Psychiatry 2002; 41(7):758.

191. Samuel R: Priapism associated with venlafaxine use. Journal of the American Academy of Child & Adolescent Psychiatry 2000; 39(1):16–7.

192. Saenz de Tejada I, Ware J, Blanco R, Pittard J, Nadig P, Azadzoi K, Krane R, Goldstein I: Pathophysiology of prolonged penile erection associated with trazodone use. Journal of Urology 1991; 145(1):60–64.

193. Kiev A, Masco HL, Wenger TL, Johnston JA, Batey SR, Holloman LC: The cardiovascular effects of bupropion and nortriptyline in depressed outpatients. Annals of Clinical Psychiatry 1994; 6(2):107–15.

194. Roose SP, Glassman AH, Giardina EG, Johnson LL, Walsh BT, Bigger JTJ: Cardiovascular effects of imipramine and bupropion in depressed patients with congestive heart failure. Journal of Clinical Psychopharmacology 1987; 7(4):247–51.

195. Wenger TL, Stern WC: The cardiovascular profile of bupropion. Journal of Clinical Psychiatry 1983; 44(5 Pt 2):176–82.

196. Roose SP, Dalack GW, Glassman AH, Woodring S, Walsh BT, Giardina EG: Cardiovascular effects of bupropion in depressed patients with heart disease. American Journal of Psychiatry 1991; 148(4):512–16.

197. Marshall B, Napolitano D, McAdam D, Dunleavy III J, Tessing J, Varrell J: Venlafaxine and increased aggression in a female with autism. Journal of the American Academy of Child & Adolescent Psychiatry 2003; 42(4):383–84.

198. Belson M, Kelley T: Bupropion exposures: clinical manifestations and medical outcome. Journal of Emergency Medicine 2002; 23(3):223–30.

199. Balit C, Lynch C, Isbister G: Bupropion poisoning: a case series. Medical Journal of Australia 2003; 178(2):61–63.

200. Isbister G, Balit C: Bupropion overdose: QTc prolongation and its clinical significance. Annals of Pharmacotherapy 2003; 37(7–8):999–1002.

201. Harris C, Gualtieri J, Stark G: Fatal bupropion overdose. Journal of Toxicology—Clinical Toxicology 1997; 35(3):321–24.

202. Blythe D, Hackett L: Cardiovascular and neurological toxicity of venlafaxine. Human & Experimental Toxicology 1999; 18(5):309–13.

203. Holzbach R, Jahn H, Pajonk F, Mahne C: Suicide attempts with mirtazapine overdose without complications. Biological Psychiatry 1998; 44(9):925–26.

204. Bremner J, Wingard P, Walshe T: Safety of mirtazapine in overdose. Journal of Clinical Psychiatry 1998; 59(5):233–35.

205. Montgomery S: Safety of mirtazapine: a review. International Clinical Psychopharmacology 1995; 10 (Suppl. 4):37–45.

206. Vanpee D, Laloyaux P, Gillet J: Seizure and hyponatraemia after overdose of trazodone. American Journal of Emergency Medicine 1999; 17(4):430–31.

207. Levenson J: Prolonged QT interval after trazodone overdose. American Journal of Psychiatry 1999; 156(6):969–70.

208. Balestrieri G, Cerudelli B, Ciaccio S, Rizzoni D: Hyponatraemia and seizure due to overdose of trazodone. British Medical Journal 1992; 304(6828):686.

209. de Meester A, Carbutti G, Gabriel L, Jacques JM: Fatal overdose with trazodone: case report and literature review. Acta Clinica Belgica 2001; 56(4):258–61.

210. Albers L, Reist C, Vu R, Fujimoto K, Ozdemir V, Helmeste D, Poland R, Tang S: Effect of venlafaxine on imipramine metabolism. Psychiatry Research 2000; 96(3):235–43.

211. Stormer E, von Moltke L, Shader R, Greenblatt D: Metabolism of the antidepressant mirtazapine in vitro: contribution of cytochromes P-450 1A2, 2D6, and 3A4. Drug Metabolism & Disposition 2000; 28(10):1168–75.

212. Spaans E, van den Heuvel MW, Schnabel PG, Peeters PA, Chin-Kon-Sung UG, Colbers EP, Sitsen JM: Concomitant use of mirtazapine and phenytoin: a drug-drug interaction study in healthy male subjects. European Journal of Clinical Pharmacology 2002; 58(6):423–29.

213. Sitsen J, Voortman G, Timmer C: Pharmacokinetics of mirtazapine and lithium in healthy male subjects. Journal of Psychopharmacology 2000; 14(2):172–76.

214. Shad M, Preskorn S: A possible bupropion and imipramine interaction. Journal of Clinical Psychopharmacology 1997; 17(2):118–19.

215. Popli AP, Tanquary J, Lamparella V, Masand PS: Bupropion and anticonvulsant drug interactions. Annals of Clinical Psychiatry 1995; 7:99–101.

216. Uhr M, Steckler T, Yassouridis A, Holsboer F: Penetration of amitriptyline, but not of fluoxetine, into brain is enhanced in mice with blood-brain barrier deficiency due to mdr1a P-glycoprotein gene disruption. Neuropsychopharmacology 2002; 22(4):380–87.

217. Shin JG, Park JY, Kim MJ, Shon JH, Yoon YR, Cha IJ, Lee SS, Oh SW, Kim SW, Flockhart DA: Inhibitory effects of tricyclic antidepressants (TCAs) on human cytochrome P450 enzymes in vitro: mechanism of drug interaction between TCAs and phenytoin. Drug Metabolism & Disposition 2002; 30(10):1102–7.

218. Geller B, Cooper TB, Graham DL, Marsteller FA, Bryant DM: Double-blind placebo-controlled study of nortriptyline in depressed adolescents using a "fixed plasma level" design. Psychopharmacology Bulletin 1990; 26(1):85–90.

219. Yokono A, Morita S, Someya T, Hirokane G, Okawa M, Shimoda K: The effect of CYP2C19 and CYP2D6 genotypes on the metabolism of clomipramine in Japanese psychiatric patients. Journal of Clinical Psychopharmacology 2001; 21(6):549–55.

220. Bergmann TK, Bathum L, Brosen K: Duplication of CYP2D6 predicts high clearance of desipramine but high clearance does not predict duplication of CYP2D6. European Journal of Clinical Pharmacology 2001; 57(2):123–27.

221. Gupta SK, Shah JC, Hwang SS: Pharmacokinetic and pharmacodynamic characterization of OROS and immediate-release amitriptyline. British Journal of Clinical Pharmacology 1999; 48(1):71–78.

222. Potter WZ, Manji HK, Rudorfer MV: Tricyclics and Tetracyclics, in Essentials of Clinical Psychopharmacology. Edited by Schatzberg AF, Nemeroff CB. Washington, DC, 2001.

223. Suhara T, Takano A, Sudo Y, Ichimiya T, Inoue M, Yasuno F, Ikoma Y, Okubo Y: High levels of serotonin transporter occupancy with low-dose clomipramine in comparative occupancy study with fluvoxamine using positron emission tomography. Archives of General Psychiatry 2003; 60(4):386–91.

224. Daly J, Wilens T: The use of trycyclic antidepressants in children and adolescents. Child and Adolescent Psychopharmacology 1998; 45(5):1123–35.

225. Geller B, Reising D, Leonard HL, Riddle M, Walsh TB: Critical review of tricyclic antidepressant use in children and adolescents. Journal of the American Academy of Child and Adolescent Psychiatry 1999; 38(5):513–16.

226. Coyle JT, Pine DS, Charney DS, Lewis L, Nemeroff CB, GA, Carlson PT, Joshi D, Reiss RD, Todd M, Hellander, Panel. DaBSACD: Depression and bipolar support alliance consensus statement on the unmet needs in diagnosis and treatment of mood disorders in children and adolescents. Journal of the American Academy of Child and Adolescent Psychiatry 2003; 42(12):1494–1503.

227. Hazell P, O'Connell D, Heathcote D, Henry D: Tricyclic drugs for depression in children and adolescents. Cochrane Database of Systematic Reviews 2002; 2:CD002317.

228. Sallee FR, Nesbitt L, Jackson C, Sine L, Sethuraman G: Relative efficacy of haloperidol and pimozide in children and adolescents with Tourette's disorder. American Journal of Psychiatry 1997; 154(8):1057–62.

229. Bakker A, van Balkom AJ, Spinhoven P: SSRIs vs. TCAs in the treatment of panic disorder: a meta-analysis. Acta Psychiatrica Scandinavica 2002; 106(3):163–67.

230. Berney T, Kolvin I, Bhate SR, Garside RF, Jeans J, Kay B, Scarth L: School phobia: a therapeutic trial with clomipramine and short-term outcome. British Journal of Psychiatry 1981; 138( ):110–18.

231. Bernstein GA, Garfinkel BD, Borchardt CM: Comparative studies of pharmacotherapy for school refusal. Journal of the American Academy of Child and Adolescent Psychiatry 1990; 29(5):773–81.

232. Gittelman-Klein R, Klein DF: Controlled imipramine treatment of school phobia. Archives of General Psychiatry 1971; 25(3):204–7.

233. Klein RG, Koplewicz HS, Kanner A: Imipramine treatment of children with separation anxiety disorder. Journal of the American Academy of Child and Adolescent Psychiatry 1992; 31(1):21–28.

234. Leonard HL, Swedo SE, Lenane MC, Rettew DC, Cheslow DL, Hamburger SD, Rapoport JL: A double-blind desipramine substitution during long-term clomipramine treatment in children and adolescents with obsessive-compulsive disorder. Archives of General Psychiatry 1991; 48(10):922–27.

235. Leonard H, Swedo S, Rapoport J, Koby E, Lenane M, Cheslow D, Hamburger S: Treatment of obsessive-compulsive disorder with clomipramine and desipramine in children and adolescents. Archives of General Psychiatry 1989; 46(12):1088–92.

236. Flament MF, Rapoport JL, Berg CJ, Sceery W, Kilts C, Mellstrom B, Linnoila M: Clomipramine treatment of childhood obsessive-compulsive disorder: A double-blind controlled study. Archives of General Psychiatry 1985; 42(10):977–83.

237. Greist J, Jefferson J, Kobak K, Katzelnick D, Serlin R: Efficacy and tolerability of serotonin transport inhibitors in obsessive-compulsive disorder. Archives of General Psychiatry 1995; 52(1):53–60.

238. Stein DJ, Spadaccini E, Hollander E: Meta-analysis of pharmacotherapy trials for obsessive-compulsive disorder. International Clinical Psychopharmacology 1995; 10(1):11–18.

239. Ackerman DL, Greenland S: Multivariate meta-analysis of controlled drug studies for obsessive-compulsive disorder. Journal of Clinical Psychopharmacology 2002; 22(3):309–17.

240. Spencer T, Biederman J, Wilens T, Faraone S: Novel treatments for attention-deficit/hyperactivity disorder in children. Journal of Clinical Psychiatry 2002; 63 (Suppl. 12):16–22.

241. Biederman J, Spencer T: Non-stimulant treatments for ADHD. European Child & Adolescent Psychiatry 2000; 9 (Suppl. 1):I51–59.

242. Jadad AR, Boyle M, Cunningham C: Treatment of Attention Deficit/Hyperactivity Disorder. Evidence Report/Technology Assessment No. 11. Rockville, MD, Agency for Healthcare Research and Quality (AHRQ), 1999.

243. Spencer TJ: The long-term safety of stimulant treatment. New York, Mt. Sinai School of Medicine Reports on ADHD, 2003.

244. Mikkelsen E: Enuresis and encopresis: ten years of progress. Journal of the American Academy of Child & Adolescent Psychiatry 2001; 40(10):1146–58.

245. Glazener C, Evans J, Peto R: Tricyclic and related drugs for nocturnal enuresis in children. Cochrane Database of Systematic Reviews 2003; 3:CD002117.

246. Gordon C, State R, Nelson J, Hamburger S, Rapoport J: A double-blind comparison of clomipramine, desipramine, and placebo in the treatment of autistic disorder. Archives of General Psychiatry 1993; 50(6):441–47.

247. McDougle CJ, Price LH, Volkmar FR, Goodman WK, Ward-O'Brien D, Nielsen J, Bregman J, Cohen DJ: Clomipramine in autism: preliminary evidence of efficacy. Journal of the American Academy of Child and Adolescent Psychiatry 1992; 31(4):746–50.

248. Remington G, Sloman L, Konstantareas M, Parker K, Gow R: Clomipramine versus haloperidol in the treatment of autistic disorder: a double-blind, placebo-controlled, crossover study. Journal of Clinical Psychopharmacology 2001; 21(4):440–44.

249. Wilens T, Biederman J, Prince J, Spencer T, Faraone S, Warburton R, Schleifer D, Harding M, Linehan C, Geller D: Six-week, double-blind, placebo-controlled study of desipramine for adult attention deficit hyperactivity disorder. American Journal of Psychiatry 1996; 153(9):1147–53.

250. Gutgessell H, Atkins D, Barst R, Buck M, Franklin W, Humes R, Ringel R, Shaddy R, Taubert K: AHA scientific statement: cardiovascular monitoring of children and adolescents receiving psychotropic drugs. Journal of the American Academy of Child and Adolescent Psychiatry 1999; 38(8):1047–50.

251. Gill H, DeVane L, Risch C: Extrapyramidal symptoms associated with cyclic antidepressant treatment: a review of the literature and consolidating hypotheses. Journal of Clinical Psychopharmacology 1997; 17(5):377–89.

252. Schroeder JS, Mullin AV, Elliott GR, Steiner H, Nichols M, Gordon A, Paulos MJ: Cardiovascular effects of desipramine in children. Journal of the American Academy of Child and Adolescent Psychiatry 1989; 28(6):376–79.

253. Abramowicz MS (ed): Sudden death in children treated with tricyclic antidepressant. The Medical Letter, 1990.

254. Riddle MA, Nelson JC, Kleinman CS, Rasmussen A, Leckman JF, King RA, Cohen DJ: Case Study: Sudden death in children receiving norpramin: A review of three reported cases and commentary. Journal of the American Academy of Child and Adolescent Psychiatry 1991; 30(1):104–8.

255. Riddle MA, Geller B, Ryan N: Case study: another sudden death in a child treated with desipramine. Journal of the American Academy of Child and Adolescent Psychiatry 1993; 32(4):792–797.

256. Popper CW, Ziminitzky B: Sudden death putatively related to desipramine treatment in youth: a fifth case and a review of speculative mechanisms. Journal of Child and Adolescent Psychopharmacology 1995; 5:283–300.

257. Ziminitzky B, Popper CW: A Fifth Case of Sudden Death in a Child Taking Desipramine, in American Psychiatric Association. Philadelphia, 1994.

258. Varley CK: Sudden death of a child treated with imipramine. Case study. Journal of Child and Adolescent Psychopharmacology 2000; 10(4):321–25.

259. Biederman J, Baldessarini R, Goldblatt A, Lapey K, Doyle A, Hesslein P: A naturalistic study of 24-hour electrocardiographic recordings and echocardiographic finding in children and adolescents treated with desipramine. Journal of the American Academy of Child and Adolescent Psychiatry 1993; 32(4):805–13.

260. Puig-Antich J, Perel JM, Lupatkin W, Chambers WJ, Shea C, Tabrizi M, Stiller RL: Plasma levels of imipramine (IMI) and desmethylimipramine (DMI) and clinical response in prepubertal major depressive disorder. Journal of American Academy of Child Psychiatry 1979; 18(4):616–27.

261. Puig-Antich J, Perel JM, Lupatkin W, Chambers WJ, Tabrizi MA, King J, Goetz R, Davies M, Stiller RL: Imipramine in prepubertal major depressive disorders. Archives of General Psychiatry 1987; 44(1):81–89.

262. Wroblewski BA, McColgan K, Smith K, Whyte J, Singer WD: The incidence of seizures during tricyclic antidepressant drug treatment in a brain-injured population. Journal of Clinical Psychopharmacology 1990; 10(2):124–28.

263. Glauser J: Tricyclic antidepressant poisoning. Cleveland Clinic Journal of Medicine 2000; 67(10):704–6, 709–13, 717–19.

264. Sennef C, Timmer C, Sitsen J: Mirtazapine in combination with amitriptyline: a drug-drug interaction study in healthy subjects. Human Psychopharmacology 2003; 18(2):91–101.

265. Juarez-Olguin H, Jung-Cook H, Flores-Perez J, Asseff IL: Clinical evidence of an interaction between imipramine and acetylsalicylic acid on protein binding in depressed patients. Clinical Neuropharmacology 2002; 25(1):32–36.

266. Szymura-Oleksiak J, Wyska E, Wasieczko A: Pharmacokinetic interaction between imipramine and carbamazepine in patients with major depression. Psychopharmacology 2001; 154(1):38–42.

267. Oesterheld J: TCA cardiotoxicity: the latest. Journal of the American Academy of Child and Adolescent Psychiatry 1996; 35(6):701–2.

268. Cohen LG, Prince J, Biederman J, Wilens T, Faraone SV, Whitt S, Mick E, Spencer T, Meyer MC, Polisner D, Flood JG: Absence of effect of stimulants on the pharmacokinetics of desipramine in children. Pharmacotherapy 1999; 19(6):746–52.

269. Wamboldt MZ, Yancey AGJ, Roesler TA: Cardiovascular effects of tricyclic antidepressants in childhood asthma: a case series and review. Journal of Child and Adolescent Psychopharmacology 1997; 7(1):45–64.

270. Patrick KS, Straughn AB, Jarvi EJ, Breese GR, Meyer MC: The absorption of sustained-release methylphenidate formulations compared to an immediate-release formulation. Biopharmaceutics Drug Dispositions 1989; 10(2):165–71.

271. Markowitz JS, Straughn AB, Patrick KS: Advances in the pharmacotherapy of attention-deficit-hyperactivity disorder: focus on methylphenidate formulations. Pharmacotherapy 2003; 23(10):1281–99.

272. Swanson J, Gupta S, Lam A, Shoulson I, Lerner M, Modi N, Lindemulder E, Wigal S: Development of a new once-a-day formulation of methylphenidate for the treatment of attention-deficit/hyperactivity disorder: proof-of-concept and proof-of-product studies. Archives of General Psychiatry 2003; 60(2):204–11.

273. Gonzalez MA, Pentikis HS, Anderl N, et al.: Methylphenidate bioavailability from two extended-release formulations. International Journal of Clinical Pharmacology and Therapeutics 2002; 40(4):175–84.

274. Markowitz JS, Straughn AB, Patrick KS, DeVane CL, Pestreich L, Lee J, Wang Y, Muniz R: Pharmacokinetics of methylphenidate after oral administration of two modified-release formulations in healthy adults. Clinical Pharmacokinetics 2003; 42(4):393–401.

275. Srinivas NR, Hubbard JW, Quinn D, Midha KK: Enantioselective pharmacokinetics and pharmacodynamics of dl-threo-methylphenidate in children with attention deficit hyperactivity

disorder. Clinical Pharmacology and Therapeutics 1992; 52(5):561–68.

276. Caldwell J, Sever PS: The biochemical pharmacology of abused drugs. Clinical Pharmacology and Therapeutics 1974; 16(5 Part 1):625–38.

277. Caldwell J: The metabolism of amphetamines in mammals. Drug Metabolism Reviews 1976; 5(2):219–80.

278. Auiler JF, Liu K, Lynch JM, Gelotte CK: Effect of food on early drug exposure from extended release stimulants. Current Medical Research and Opinions 2002; 18(5):311–18.

279. Tulloch SJ, Zhang Y, McLean A, Wolf KN: SLI381 (Adderall XR), a two-component, extended-release formulation of mixed amphetamine salts: bioavailability of three test formulations and comparison of fasted, fed, and sprinkled administration. Pharmacotherapy 2002; 22(11):1405–15.

280. Sallee F, Stiller R, Perel J, Bates TCPT: Oral pemoline kinetics in hyperactive children. Clinical Pharmacology and Therapeutics 1985; 37(6):606–9.

281. Collier CP, Soldin SJ, Swanson JM, MacLeod SM, Weinberg F, Rochefort JG: Pemoline pharmacokinetics and long term therapy in children with attention deficit disorder and hyperactivity. Clinical Pharmacokinetics 1985; 10(3):269–78.

282. Volkow ND, Wang G, Fowler JS, Logan J, Gerasimov M, Maynard L, Ding Y, Gatley SJ, Gifford A, Franceschi D: Therapeutic doses of oral methylphenidate significantly increase extracellular dopamine in the human brain. Journal of Neuroscience: The Official Journal of the Society of Neuroscience 2001; 21(2):RC121.

283. Krause KH, Dresel SH, Krause J, Kung HF, Tatsch K: Increased striatal dopamine transporter in adult patients with attention deficit hyperactivity disorder: effects of methylphenidate as measured by single photon emission computed tomography. Neuroscience Letters 2000; 285(2):107–10.

284. Vles JS, Feron FJ, Hendriksen JG, Jolles J, van Kroonenburgh MJ, Weber WE: Methylphenidate down-regulates the dopamine receptor and transporter system in children with attention deficit hyperkinetic disorder (ADHD). Neuropediatrics 2003; 34(2):77–80.

285. Ding YS, Fowler JS, Volkow ND, Dewey SL, Wang GJ, Logan J, Gatley SJ, Pappas N: Chiral drugs: comparison of the pharmacokinetics of [11C]d-threo and L-threo-methylphenidate in the human and baboon brain. Psychopharmacology 1997; 131(1):71–78.

286. Davids E, Zhang K, Tarazi FI, Baldessarini RJ: Stereoselective effects of methylphenidate on motor hyperactivity in juvenile rats induced by neonatal 6-hydroxydopamine lesioning. Psychopharmacology 2002; 160(1):92–98.

287. Patrick KS, Caldwell RW, Ferris RM, Breese GR: Pharmacology of the enantiomers of threo-methylphenidate. Journal of Pharmacology and Experimental Therapeutics 1987; 241(1):152–58.

288. Kuczenski R, Segal DS: Effects of methylphenidate on extracellular dopamine, serotonin, and norepinephrine: comparison with amphetamine. Journal of Neurochemistry 1997; 68(5):2032–37.

289. Molina VA, Orsingher OA: Effects of Mg-pemoline on the central catecholaminergic system. Archives Internationales de Pharmacodynamie et de Therapie 1981; 251(1):66–79.

290. Sallee F, Stiller R, Perel J: Pharmacodynamics of pemoline in attention deficit disorder with hyperactivity. Journal of the American Academy of Child and Adolescent Psychiatry 1992; 31(2):244–51.

291. Spencer T, Biederman J, Harding M, O'Donnell D, Faraone S, Wilens T: Growth deficits in ADHD children revisited: Evidence for disorder-associated growth delays? Journal of the American Academy of Child and Adolescent Psychiatry 1996; 35(11):1460–69.

292. Agency for Healthcare Research and Quality: A Treatment of ADHD. Rockville, MD: Department of Health and Human Services, 1999.

293. Jensen PS, Hinshaw SP, Kraemer HC, Lenora N, Newcorn JH, Abikoff H, March JS, Arnold E, Cantwell D, Conners K, Elliott G, Greenhill L, Hechtman L, Hoza B, Pelham WE, Severe J, Swanson J, Wells K, Wigal T, Vitiello B: ADHD comorbidity findings from the MTA study: comparing comorbid subgroups. Journal of the American Academy of Child Adolescent Psychiatry 2001; 40(2):147–58.

294. The MTA Cooperative Group: A 14-month randomized clinical trial of treatment strategies for attention-deficit/hyperactivity disorder. Archives of General Psychiatry 1999; 56(12):1073–86.

295. Gan J, Cantwell DP: Dosage effects of methylphenidate on paired associate learning: positive/negative placebo responders. Journal of the American Academy of Child and Adolescent Psychiatry 1982; 21(3):237–42.

296. Wilens TE, Spencer TJ: The stimulants revisited. Child and Adolescent Psychiatric Clinics of North America 2000; 9(3):573–603, viii.

297. Greenhill LL, Abikoff HB, Arnold LE, Cantwell DP, Conners CK, Elliott G, Hechtman L, Hinshaw SP, Hoza B, Jensen PS, March JS, Newcorn J, Pelham WE, Severe JB, Swanson JM, Vitiello B, Wells K: Medication treatment strategies in the MTA Study: relevance to clinicians and researchers. Journal of the American Academy of Child and Adolescent Psychiatry 1996; 35(10):1304–13.

298. Faraone SV, Biederman J, Roe CM: Comparative efficacy of adderall and methylphenidate in attention-deficit/ hyperactivity disorder: a meta-analysis. Journal of Clinical Psychopharmacology 2002; 22(5):468–73.

299. Wolraich M, Greenhill LL, Pelham W, Swanson J, Wilens T, Palumbo D, Atkins M, McBurnett K, Bukstein O, August G: Randomized controlled trial of OROS methylphenidate qd in children with attention deficit/hyperactivity disorder. Pediatrics 2001; 108(4):883–92.

300. Pelham WE, Gnagy EM, Burrows-Maclean L, Williams A, Fabiano GA, Morrisey SM, Chronis AM, Forehand GL, Nguyen CA, Hoffman MT, Lock TM, Fielbelkorn K, Coles EK, Panahon CJ, Steiner RL, Meichenbaum DL, Onyango AN, Morse GD: Once-a-day Concerta methylphenidate versus three-times-daily methylphenidate in laboratory and natural settings. Pediatrics 2001; 107(6):E105.

301. Hatch SJ, Swanson JM: The COMACS study: was it fair and does it matter? in American Academy of Child and Adolescent Psychiatry. Miami, FL, 2003.

302. Biederman J, Lopez FA, Boellner SW, Chandler MC: A randomized, double-blind, placebo-controlled, parallel-group study of SLI381 in children with attention deficit hyperactivity disorder. Pediatrics 2002; 110(2):258–66.

303. Pelham WEJ, Greenslade KE, Vodde-Hamilton M, Murphy DA, Greenstein JJ, Gnagy EM, Guthrie KJ, Hoover MD, Dahl RE: Relative efficacy of long-acting stimulants on children with attention deficit-hyperactivity disorder: a comparison of standard methylphenidate, sustained-release methylphenidate, sustained-release dextroamphetamine, and pemoline. Pediatrics 1990; 86(2):226–37.

304. Pelham W, Swanson J, Furman M, Schwindt H: Pemoline effects on children with ADHD: A time-response by dose-response analysis on classroom measures. Journal of the American Academy of Child and Adolescent Psychiatry 1995; 34(11):1504–13.

305. Bostic JQ, Biederman J, Spencer TJ, Wilens TE, Prince JB, Monuteaux MC, Sienna M, Polisner DA, Hatch M: Pemoline treatment of adolescents with attention deficit hyperactivity disorder: a short-term controlled trial. Journal of Child and Adolescent Psychopharmacology 2000; 10(3):205–16.

306. Wilens T, Biederman J, Spencer T, Frazier J, Prince J, Bostic J, Rater M, Soriano J, Hatch M, Sienna M, Millstein R, Abrantes A: Controlled trial of high doses of pemoline for adults with attention-deficit/hyperactivity disorder. Journal of Clinical Psychopharmacology 1999; 19(3):257–64.

307. Spencer T, Biederman J, Coffey B, Geller D, Wilens T, Faraone S: The 4-year course of tic disorders in boys with attention-deficit/hyperactivity disorder. Archives of General Psychiatry 1999; 56(9):794–847.

308. Law SF, Schachar RJ: Do typical clinical doses of methylphenidate cause tics in children treated for attention-deficit hyperactivity disorder? Journal of the American Academy of Child and Adolescent Psychiatry 1999; 38(8):944–51.

309. Palumbo D: Impact of ADHD Treatment Once-Daily OROS Formulation of MPH on Tics, in Pediatric Academic Societies Annual Meeting. Seattle, WA, 2003.

310. Tourette's Syndrome Study Group: Treatment of ADHD in children with tics: A randomized controlled trial. Neurology 2002; 58(4):527–36.

311. Biederman J, Mick E, Prince J, Bostic JQ, Wilens TE, Spencer T, Wozniak J, Faraone SV: Systematic chart review of the pharmacologic treatment of comorbid attention deficit hyperactivity disorder in youth with bipolar disorder. Journal of Child and Adolescent Psychopharmacology 1999; 9(4):247–56.

312. Handen BL, Johnson CR, Lubetsky M: Efficacy of methylphenidate among children with autism and symptoms of attention-deficit hyperactivity disorder. Journal of Autism and Developmental Disorders 2000; 30(3):245–55.

313. Rush AJ, Frances A: Expert Consensus Guideline Series. Treatment of psychiatric and behavioral problems in mental retardation. American Journal on Mental Retardation 2000; 105(3):159–228.

314. Handen BL, Feldman H, Gosling A, Breaux AM, McAuliffe S: Adverse side effects of methylphenidate among mentally retarded children with ADHD. Journal of the American Academy of Child and Adolescent Psychiatry 1991; 30(2):241–45.

315. Hagerman RJ, Murphy MA, Wittenberger MD: A controlled trial of stimulant medication in children with the fragile X syndrome. American Journal of Medical Genetics 1988; 30(1–2):377–92.

316. Power TJ, Blum NJ, Jones SM, Kaplan PE: Brief report: response of methylphenidate in two children with Williams syndrome. Journal of Autism & Developmental Disorders 1997; 27(1):79–87.

317. Riley K, Ikle LO, Hagerman RJ: A Randomized, Double-Blind Comparative Trial of Adderall in the Treatment of Attention Deficit Disorder in Children with Fragile X, in the Seventh International Fragile X Conference, Los Angeles, CA, 2000.

318. Dunn DW, Austin JK, Huster GA: Behaviour problems in children with new-onset epilepsy. Seizure 1999; 6(4):283–87.

319. Aldenkamp AP, Arends J, Overweg-Plandsoen TC, van Bronswijk KC, Schyns-Soeterboek A, Linden I, Diepman L: Acute cognitive effects of nonconvulsive difficult-to-detect epileptic seizures and epileptiform electroencephalographic discharges. Journal of Child Neurology 2001; 16(2):119–23.

320. Semrud-Clikeman M, Wical B: Components of attention in children with complex partial seizures with and without ADHD. Epilepsia 1999; 40(2):211–15.

321. Perrine K, Kiolbasa T. Cognitive deficits in epilepsy and contribution to psychopathology. American Academy of Neurology 1999; 53 (Suppl.):S39–S48.

322. Feldman H, Crumrine P, Handen BL, Alvin R, Teodori J: Methylphenidate in children with seizures and attention-deficit disorder. American Journal of Diseases of Children 1989; 143(9):1081–86.

323. Gross-Tsur V, Manor O, van der Meere J, Joseph A, Shalev RS: Epilepsy and attention deficit hyperactivity disorder: Is methylphenidate safe and effective? Pediatrics 1997; 130(4):670–74.

324. Bloom DR, Levin HS, Ewing-Cobbs L, Saunders AE, Song J, Fletcher JM, RA. K: Lifetime and novel psychiatric disorders after pediatric traumatic brain injury. Journal of the American Academy of Child and Adolescent Psychiatry 2001; 40(5):572–79.

325. Mahalick DM, Carmel PW, Greenberg JP, Molofsky W, Brown JA, Heary RF, Marks D, Zampella E, Hodosh R, von der Schmidt ER: Psychopharmacologic treatment of acquired attention disorders in children with brain injury. Pediatric Neurosurgery 1998; 29(3):121–26.

326. Whyte J, Vaccaro M, Grieb-Neff P, Hart T: Psychostimulant use in the rehabilitation of individuals with traumatic brain injury. Journal of Head Trauma Rehabilitation 2002; 17(4):284–99.

327. Kelly D, Forney J, Parker-Fisher S, Jones M: Evaluating and managing attention deficit disorder in children who are deaf or hard of hearing. American Annals of the Deaf 1993; 138(4):349–57.

328. Gutgesell H, Atkins D, Barst R, et al.: AHA scientific statement: Cardiovascular monitoring of children and adolescents receiving psychotropic drugs. Journal of the American Academy of Child and Adolescent Psychiatry 1999; 38(8):1047–50.

329. Spencer T, Biederman J, Wilens T, Harding M, O'Donnell D, Griffin S: Pharmacotherapy of attention-deficit hyperactivity disorder across the life cycle. Journal of the American Academy of Child and Adolescent Psychiatry 1996; 35(4):1–24.

330. Biederman J, Spencer T, Faraone SV: Extended-release mixed amphetamine salts in ADHD: Growth Parameter Analysis, in 156th Annual Meeting of the American Psychiatric Association. Edited by Randell D. San Francisco, CA, American Psychiatric Association, 2003.

331. Spencer and Group: Long term once daily OROS Methylphenidate treatment for ADHD: Evaluating Effect on Growth, in Annual Meeting of the American Psychiatric Association. San Francisco, CA, American Psychiatric Association, 2003.

332. Lynch JM, et al.: OROS methylphenidate ADHD therapy: height and weight effects, in 50th anniversary meeting of American Association of Child and Adolescent Psychiatry. Miami, FL, 2003.

333. Friedmann N, Thomas J, Carr R, Elders J, Ringdahl I, Roche A: Effect on growth in pemoline-treated children with attention deficit disorder. American Journal of Diseases of Children 1981; 135(4):356–60.

334. Cromwell HC, Levine MS, King BH: Cortical damage enhances pemoline-induced self-injurious behavior in prepubertal rats. Pharmacology, Biochemistry and Behavior 1999; 62(2):233–37.

335. Adrian N: Explosive outbursts associated with methylphenidate. Journal of the American Academy of Child and Adolescent Psychiatry 2001; 40(6):618–19.

336. Cherland E, Fitzpatrick R: Psychotic side effects of psychostimulants: a 5-year review. Canadian Journal of Psychiatry—Revue Canadienne de Psychiatrie 1999; 44(8):811–13.

337. Diamond IR, Tannock R, Schachar RJ: Response to methylphenidate in children with ADHD and comorbid anxiety. Journal of the American Academy of Child and Adolescent Psychiatry 1999; 38(4):402–9.

338. Wilens T, Pelham W, Stein M, Conners KC, Abikoff H, Atkins M, August G, Greenhill L, McBurnett K, Palumbo D, Swanson J, Wolraich M: ADHD treatment with once daily OROS methylphenidate: interim 12-month results from long-term open-label study. Journal of the American Academy of Child and Adolescent Psychiatry 2003; 42(4):424–33.

339. Gracious BL: Atrioventricular nodal re-entrant tachycardia associated with stimulant treatment. Journal of Child and Adolescent Psychopharmacology 1999; 9(2):125–28.

340. Berger S, Kugler JD, Thomas JA, Friedberg DZ: Sudden cardiac death in children and adolescents: Introduction and overview. Pediatric Clinics of North America 2004; 51(5):1201–9.

341. Safer DJ, Zito JM, Gardner JE: Pemoline hepatotoxicity and post-marketing surveillance. Journal of the American Academy of Child and Adolescent Psychiatry 2001; 40(6):622–29.

342. Berkovitch M, Pope E, Phillips J, Koren G: Pemoline-associated fulminant liver failure: testing the evidence for causation. Clinical Pharmacology and Therapeutics 1995; 57(6):696–98.

343. Pratt DS, Dubois RS: Hepatoxicity due to pemoline (Cylert): a report of two cases. Journal of Pediatric Gastroenterology 1990; 10(2):239–41.

344. Nehra A, Mullick F, Ishak KG, Zimmerman HJ: Pemoline-associated hepatic injury. Gastroenterology 1990; 99(5):1517–19.

345. Abbiati C, Vecchi M, Rossi G, Donata MF, de Franchis R: Inappropriate pemoline therapy leading to acute liver failure and liver transplantation. Digestive and Liver Disease 2002; 34(6):447–51.

346. Rosh JR, Dellert SF, Narkewicz M, Birnbaum A, Whitington G: Four cases of severe hepatotoxicity associated with pemoline: possible autoimmune pathogenesis. Pediatrics 1998; 101(5):921–23.

347. Volkow ND, Wang GJ, Fowler JS, Gatley SJ, Logan J, Ding YS, Dewey SL, Hitzemann R, Gifford AN, Pappas NR: Blockade of striatal dopamine transporters by intravenous methylphenidate is not sufficient to induce self-reports of "high." Journal of Pharmacology and Experimental Therapeutics 1999; 288(1):14–20.

348. Biederman J, Wilens T, Mick E, Spencer T, Faraone SV: Pharmacotherapy of attention-deficit/hyperactivity disorder reduces risk for substance use disorder. Pediatrics 1999; 104(2):e20.

349. Hemmer SA, Pasternak JF, Zecker SG, Trommer BL: Stimulant therapy and seizure risk in children with ADHD. Pediatric Neurology 2001; 24(2):99–102.

350. Tavakoli SA, Gleason OC: Seizures associated with venlafaxine, methylphenidate, and zolpidem. Psychosomatics 2003; 44(3):262–64.

351. Markowitz JS, Morrison SD, DeVane CL: Drug interactions with psychostimulants. International Clinical Psychopharmacology 1999; 14(1):1–18.

352. Rapport M, Carlson G, Kelly K, Pataki C: Methylphenidate and desipramine in hospitalized children: I. Separate and combined effects on cognitive function. Journal of the American Academy of Child and Adolescent Psychiatry 1993; 32(2):333–42.

353. Ickowicz A: Bupropion-methylphenidate combination and grand mal seizures. Canadian Journal of Psychiatry—Revue Canadienne de Psychiatrie 2002; 47(8):790–91.

354. Lewis BR, Aoun SL, Bernstein GA, Crow SJ: Pharmacokinetic interactions between cyclosporine and bupropion or methylphenidate. Journal of Child and Adolescent Psychopharmacology 2001; 11(2):193–98.

355. Popper CW, Elliot GR: Sudden death and tricyclic antidepressants: Clinical considerations for children. Journal of Child and Adolescent Psychopharmacology 1990; 1(2):125–32.

356. Kofoed L, Tadepalli G, Oesterheld JR, Awadallah S, Shapiro R: Case series: clonidine has no systematic effects on PR or QTc intervals in children. 1999; 38(9):1193–96.

357. Connor DF, Barkley RA, Davis HT: A pilot study of methylphenidate, clonidine, or the combination in ADHD comorbid with aggressive oppositional defiant or conduct disorder. Clinical Pediatrics 2000; 39(1):15–25.

358. Wilens TE, Spencer TJ: Combining methylphenidate and clonidine: A clinically sound medication option. Journal of the American Academy of Child and Adolescent Psychiatry 1999; 38(5):614–19.

359. Markowitz JS, Patrick KS: Pharmacokinetic and pharmacodynamic drug interactions in the treatment of attention-deficit hyperactivity disorder. Clinical Pharmacokinetics 2001; 40(10): 753–72.

360. Klein-Schwartz W: Pediatric methylphenidate exposures: 7-year experience of poison centers in the United States. Clinical Pediatrics 2003; 42(2):159–64.

361. Nakamura H, Blumer JL, Reed MD: Pemoline ingestion in children: a report of five cases and review of the literature. Journal of Clinical Pharmacology 2002; 42(3):275–82.

362. Sauer JM, Ponsler GD, Mattiuz EL, Long AJ, Witcher JW, Thomasson HR, Desante KA: Disposition and metabolic fate of atomoxetine hydrochloride: the role of CYP2D6 in human disposition and metabolism. Drug Metabolism and Disposition 2003; 31(1):98–107.

363. Bymaster FP, Katner JS, Nelson DL, Hemrick-Luecke SK, Threlkeld PG, Heiligenstein JH, Morin SM, Gehlert DR, Perry KW: Atomoxetine increases extracellular levels of norepinephrine and dopamine in prefrontal cortex of rat: a potential mechanism for efficacy in attention deficit/hyperactivity disorder. Neuropsychopharmacology 2002; 27(5):699–711.

364. Spencer T, Biederman J, Wilens T, Prince J, Hatch M, Jones J, Harding M, Faraone SV, Seidman L: Effectiveness and tolerability of tomoxetine in adults with attention deficit hyperactivity disorder. American Journal of Psychiatry 1998; 155(5): 693–95.

365. Spencer T, Heiligenstein JH, Biederman J, Faries DE, Kratochvil CJ, Conners CK, Potter WZ: Results from 2 proof-of-concept, placebo-controlled studies of atomoxetine in children with attention-deficit/hyperactivity disorder. Journal of Clinical Psychiatry 2002; 63(12):1140–47.

366. Kratochvil CJ, Heiligenstein JH, Dittman R, Spencer TJ, Biederman J, Wernicke J, Newcorn JH, Casat C, Milton D, Michelson D: Atomoxetine and methylphenidate treatment in children with ADHD: a prospective, randomized, open-label trial. Journal of the American Academy of Child Adolescent Psychiatry 2002; 41(7):776–84.

367. Michelson D, Allen AJ, Busner J, Casat C, Dunn D, Kratochvil C, Newcorn J, Sallee FR, Sangal RB, Saylor K, West S, Kelsey D, Wernicke J, Trapp NJ, Harder D: Once-daily atomoxetine treatment for children and adolescents with attention deficit hyperactivity disorder: a randomized, placebo-controlled study. American Journal of Psychiatry 2002; 159(11):1896–1901.

368. McCracken JT, Sallee FR, Leonard HL, Dunn DW, Budman CL, Geller DA, Milton DR, Layton LL, Feldman PD, Spencer T, Allen AJ: Improvement of ADHD by Atomoxetine in Children with Tic

369. Michelson D, Faries D, Wernicke J, Kelsey D, Kendrick K, Sallee FR, Spencer T, Group tAS: Atomoxetine in the treatment of children and adolescents with attention-deficit/hyperactivity disorder: a randomized, placebo-controlled, dose-response study. Pediatrics 2001; 108(5):E83.

370. Spencer T, Biederman J, Heiligenstein J, Wilens T, Faries D, Prince J, Faraone SV, Rea J, Witcher J, Zervas S: An open-label, dose-ranging study of atomoxetine in children with attention deficit hyperactivity disorder. Journal of Child and Adolescent Psychopharmacology 2001; 11(3):251–65.

371. Wernicke JF, Adler L, Spencer T, West SA, Allen AJ, Heiligenstein J, Milton D, Ruff D, Brown WJ, Kelsey D, Michelson D: Changes in symptoms and adverse events after discontinuation of atomoxetine in children and adults with attention deficit/hyperactivity disorder: a prospective, placebo-controlled assessment. Journal of Clinical Psychopharmacology 2004; 24(1): 30–35.

372. Wernicke JF, Faries D, Girod D, Brown J, Gao H, Kelsey D, Quintana H, Lipetz R, Michelson D, Heiligenstein J: Cardiovascular effects of atomoxetine in children, adolescents, and adults. Drug Safety 2003; 26(10):729–40.

373. Spencer TJ, Ruff DR, Feldman PD, Michelson D: Long-Term Effects of Atomoxetine on Growth in Children and Adolescents With ADHD, in American Academy of Child and Adolescent Psychiatry. Miami Beach, FL, Eli Lilly and Company, 2003.

374. Johnston MV: Seizures in childhood, in Behrman: Nelson Textbook of Pediatrics. Edited by Behrman R, Kliegman R, Jenson H. St. Louis, MO: Mosby, 2004.

375. Tueth MJ, Murphy TK, Evans DL: Special considerations: use of lithium in children, adolescents, and elderly populations. Journal of Clinical Psychiatry 1998; 59 (Suppl. 6):66–73.

376. Vitiello B, Behar D, Malone R, Delaney MA, Ryan PJ, Simpson GM: Pharmacokinetics of lithium carbonate in children. Journal of Clinical Psychopharmacology 1988; 8(5):355–59.

377. Moore CM, Demopulos CM, Henry ME, Steingard RJ, Zamvil L, Katic A, Breeze JL, Moore JC, Cohen BM, Renshaw PF: Brain-to-serum lithium ratio and age: an in vivo magnetic resonance spectroscopy study. American Journal of Psychiatry 2002; 159(7): 1240–42.

378. Kirkwood CK, Wilson SK, Hayes PE, Barr WH, Sarkar MA, Ettigi PG: Single-dose bioavailability of two extended-release lithium carbonate products. American Journal of Hospital Pharmacology 1994; 51(4):486–89.

379. Reischer H, Pfeffer CR: Lithium pharmacokinetics. Journal of the American Academy of Child and Adolescent Psychiatry 1996; 35(2):130–31.

380. Keck PEJ, McElroy SL: Definition, evaluation, and management of treatment refractory mania. Psychological Bulletin 2001; 35(4):130–48.

381. Lenox RH, Hahn CG: Overview of the mechanism of action of lithium in the brain: fifty-year update. Journal of Clinical Psychiatry 2000; 61 (Suppl. 9):5–15.

382. Moore GJ, Bebchuk JM, Hasanat K, Chen G, Seraji-Bozorgzad N, Wilds IB, Faulk MW, Koch S, Glitz DA, Jolkovsky L, Manji HK: Lithium increases N-acetyl-aspartate in the human brain: in vivo evidence in support of bcl-2's neurotrophic effects? Biological Psychiatry 2000; 48(1):1–8.

383. Ambrosio AF, Soares-Da-Silva P, Carvalho CM, Carvalho AP: Mechanisms of action of carbamazepine and its derivatives, oxcarbazepine, BIA 2-093, and BIA 2-024. Neurochemical Research 2002; 27(1–2):121–30.

384. Kowatch RA, Fristad M, Birmaher B, Wagner KD, Findling RL, Hellander M: Treatment guidelines for children and adolescents with bipolar disorder. Journal of the American Academy of Child and Adolescent Psychiatry 2005; 44(3):213–35.

385. Kowatch RA, Sethuraman G, Hume JH, Kromelis M, Weinberg WA: Combination pharmacotherapy in children and adolescents with bipolar disorder. Biological Psychiatry 2003; 53(11):978–84.

386. Kafantaris V, Coletti DJ, Dicker R, Padula G, Kane JM: Adjunctive antipsychotic treatment of adolescents with bipolar psychosis. Journal of the American Academy of Child and Adolescent Psychiatry 2001; 40(12):1448–56.

387. Thies-Flechtner K, Weigel I, Muller-Oerlinghausen B: 5-HT uptake in platelets of lithium-treated patients with affective disorders and of healthy controls. Pharmacotherapy 1994; 27 (Suppl. 1):4–6.

388. Tondo L, Baldessarini RJ: Reduced suicide risk during lithium maintenance treatment. Journal of Clinical Psychiatry 2000; 61(9):97–104.

389. Geddes JR, Burgess S, Hawton K, Jamison K, Goodwin GM: Long-term lithium therapy for bipolar disorder: systematic review and meta-analysis of randomized controlled trials. American Journal of Psychiatry 2004; 161(2):217–22.

390. Baldessarini RJ, Tondo L: Does lithium treatment still work? Evidence of stable responses over three decades. Archives of General Psychiatry 2000; 57(2):187–90.

391. Maj M, Pirozzi R, Magliano L, Bartoli L: Long-term outcome of lithium prophylaxis in bipolar disorder: a 5-year prospective study of 402 patients at a lithium clinic. American Journal of Psychiatry 1998; 155(1):30–35.

392. DeLong GR, Nieman GW: Lithium-induced behavior changes in children with symptoms suggesting manic-depressive illness. Psychopharmacology Bulletin 1983; 19(2):258–65.

393. Geller B, Cooper TB, Watts HE, Cosby CM, Fox LW: Early findings from a pharmacokinetically designed double-blind and placebo-controlled study of lithium for adolescents comorbid with bipolar and substance dependency disorders. Progress in Neuro-psychopharmacology and Biological Psychiatry 1992; 16(3):281–99.

394. Carlson GA, Rapport MD, Kelly KL, Pataki CS: The effects of methylphenidate and lithium on attention and activity level. Journal of the American Academy of Child and Adolescent Psychiatry 1992; 31(2):262–70.

395. Strober M, Morrell W, Lampert C, Burroughs J: Relapse following discontinuation of lithium maintenance therapy in adolescents with bipolar I illness: a naturalistic study. American Journal of Psychiatry 1990; 147(4):457–61.

396. Kafantaris V, Coletti DJ, Dicker R, Padula G, Kane JM: Lithium treatment of acute mania in adolescents: a large open trial. Journal of the American Academy of Child and Adolescent Psychiatry 2003; 42(9):1038–45.

397. Geller B, Cooper TB, Sun K, Zimerman B, Frazier J, Williams M, Heath J: Double-blind and placebo-controlled study of lithium for adolescent bipolar disorders with secondary substance dependency. Journal of the American Academy of Child and Adolescent Psychiatry 1998; 37(2):171–78.

398. Papatheodorou G, Kutcher SP, Katic M, Szalai JP: The efficacy and safety of divalproex sodium in the treatment of acute mania in adolescents and young adults: an open clinical trial. Journal of Clinical Psychopharmacology 1995; 15(2):110–16.

399. Teitelbaum M: Oxcarbazepine in bipolar disorder. Journal of the American Academy of Child and Adolescent Psychiatry 2001; 40(9):993–94.

400. Woolston JL: Case study: carbamazepine treatment of juvenile-onset bipolar disorder. Journal of the American Academy of Child and Adolescent Psychiatry 1999; 38(3):335–38.

401. Findling RL, McNamara NK, Gracious BL, Youngstrom EA, Stansbrey RJ, Reed MD, Demeter CA, Branicky LA, Fisher KE, Calabrese JR: Combination lithium and divalproex sodium in pediatric bipolarity. Journal of the American Academy of Child and Adolescent Psychiatry 2003; 42(8):895–901.

402. Kowatch RA, Suppes T, Carmody TJ, Bucci JP, Hume JH, Kromelis M, Emslie GJ, Weinberg WA, Rush AJ: Effect size of lithium, divalproex sodium, and carbamazepine in children and adolescents with bipolar disorder. Journal of the American Academy of Child and Adolescent Psychiatry 2000; 39(6):713–20.

403. Davanzo P, Gunderson B, Belin T, Mintz J, Pataki C, Ott D, Emley-Akanno C, Montazeri N, Oppenheimer J, Strober M: Mood stabilizers in hospitalized children with bipolar disorder: a retrospective review. Psychiatry and Clinical Neurosciences 2003; 57(5):504–10.

404. Bowden CL, Calabrese JR, McElroy SL, Gyulai L, Wassef A, Petty F, Pope HGJ, Chou JC, Keck PEJ, Rhodes LJ, Swann AC, Hirschfeld RM, Wozniak PJ, Group DMS: A randomized, placebo-controlled 12-month trial of divalproex and lithium in treatment of outpatients with bipolar I disorder. Archives of General Psychiatry 2000; 57(5):481–89.

405. Hirschfeld RM, Baker JD, Wozniak P, Tracy K, Sommerville KW: The safety and early efficacy of oral-loaded divalproex versus standard-titration divalproex, lithium, olanzapine, and placebo in the treatment of acute mania associated with bipolar disorder. Journal of Clinical Psychiatry 2003; 64(7):841–46.

406. Gyulia L, Bowden CL, McElroy SL, Calabrese JR, Petty F, Swann AC, Chou JC, Wassef A, Risch CS, Hirschfeld RM, Nemeroff CB, Keck PEJ, Evans DL, Wozniak PJ: Maintenance efficacy of divalproex in the prevention of bipolar depression. Neuropsychopharmacology 2003; 28(7):1374–82.

407. Ghaemi N, Ko JY, Katzow JJ: Oxcarbazepine treatment of refractory bipolar disorder: a retrospective chart review. Bipolar Disorders 2002; 4(1):70–74.

408. Suhayl N: Oxcarbazepine for mood disorder. American Journal of Psychiatry 2002; 159(10):1793.

409. Hummel B, Walden J, Stampfer R, Dittmann S, Amann B, Sterr A, Schaefer M, Frye MA, Grunze H: Acute antimanic efficacy and safety of oxcarbazepine in an open trial with an on-off-on design. Bipolar Disorders 2002; 4(6):412–17.

410. Wagner KD: Safety and efficacy of Divalproex in childhood bipolar disorder, in American Academy of Child and Adolescent Psychiatry. Washington DC, 2000.

411. Whittier MC, West SA, Galli VB, Raute NJ: Valproic acid for dysphoric mania in a mentally retarded adolescent. Journal of Clinical Psychiatry 1995; 56(12):590–91.

412. Kim E, Humaran TJ: Divalproex in the management of neuropsychiatric complications of remote acquired brain injury. Journal of Neuropsychiatry and Clinical Neuroscience 2002; 14(2):202–5.

413. Kennedy R, Burnett DM, Greenwald BD: Use of antiepileptics in traumatic brain injury: a review for psychiatrists. Annals of Clinical Psychiatry 2001; 13(3):163–71.

414. Wroblewski BA, Joseph AB, Kupfer J, Kalliel K: Effectiveness of valproic acid on destructive and aggressive behaviours in patients with acquired brain injury. Brain Injury 1997; 11(1):37–47.

415. Biederman J, Faraone SV, Chu MP, Wozniak J: Further evidence of a bidirectional overlap between juvenile mania and conduct disorder in children. Journal of the American Academy of Child and Adolescent Psychiatry 1999; 38(4):468–76.

416. Gerardin P, Cohen D, Mazet P, Flament MF: Drug treatment of conduct disorder in young people. European Neuropsychopharmacology: Journal of the European College of Neuropsychopharmacology 2002; 12(5):361–70.

417. Steiner H, Petersen ML, Saxena K, Ford S, Matthews Z: Divalproex sodium for the treatment of conduct disorder: a randomized controlled clinical trial. Journal of Clinical Psychiatry 2003; 64(10):1183–91.

418. Malone RP, Luebbert JF, Delaney MA, Biesecker KA, Blaney BL, Rowan AB, Campbell M: Nonpharmacological response in hospitalized children with conduct disorder. Journal of the American Academy of Child and Adolescent Psychiatry 1997; 36(2):242–47.

419. Malone RP, Delaney MA, Luebbert JF, Cater J, Campbell M: A double-blind placebo-controlled study of lithium in hospitalized aggressive children and adolescents with conduct disorder. Archives of General Psychiatry 2000; 57(7):649–54.

420. Cueva JE, Overall JE, Small AM, Armenteros JL, Perry R, Campbell M: Carbamazepine in aggressive children with conduct disorder: a double-blind and placebo-controlled study. Journal of the American Academy of Child and Adolescent Psychiatry 1996; 35(4):480–90.

421. Di Martino A, Tuchman RF: Antiepileptic drugs: affective use in autism spectrum disorders. Pediatric Neurology 2001; 25(3):199–207.

422. Hollander E, Dolgoff-Kaspar R, Cartwright C, Rawitt R, Novotny S: An open trial of divalproex sodium in autism spectrum disorders. Journal of Clinical Psychiatry 2001; 62(7):530–34.

423. Hirschfeld RM, Bowden CL, Gitlin MJ, Keck PE, Perlis RH, Suppes T, Thase ME, Wagner KD: Practice guideline for the treatment of patients with bipolar disorder (revision). American Psychiatric Association Practice Guidelines, 2002.

424. Holtmann M, Krause M, Opp J, Tokarzewski M, Korn-Merker E, Boenigk HE: Oxcarbazepine-induced hyponatremia and the regulation of serum sodium after replacing carbamazepine with Oxcarbazepine in children. Neuropediatrics 2002; 33(6): 298–300.

425. Moltedo JM, Porter GA, State MW, Snyder CS: Sinus node dysfunction associated with lithium therapy in a child. Texas Heart Institute Journal from the Texas Heart Institute of St. Luke's Episcopal Hospital, Texas Children's Hospital 2002; 29(3):200–2.

426. Frye MA, Denicoff KD, Bryan AL, Smith-Jackson EE, Ali SO, Luckenbaugh D, Leverich GS, Post RM. Association between lower serum free T4 and greater mood instability and depression in lithium-maintained bipolar patients. American Journal of Psychiatry 1994; 156(12):1909–14.

427. Hatterer JA, Kocsis JH, Stokes PE: Thyroid function in patients maintained on lithium. Psychiatry Research 1988; 26(3):249–57.

428. Anderson GD: Children versus adults: pharmacokinetic and adverse-effect differences. Epilepsia 2002; 43 (Suppl. 3):53–59.

429. Hirose S, Mitsudome A, Yasumoto S, Ogawa A, Muta Y, Tomoda Y: Valproate therapy does not deplete carnitine levels in otherwise healthy children. Pediatrics 1998; 101(5):E9.

430. Yazdani K, Lippmann M, Gala I: Fatal pancreatitis associated with valproic acid: review of the literature. Medicine (Baltimore) 2002; 81(4):305–10.

431. Nelson-DeGrave VL, Wickenheisser JK, Cockrell JE, Wood JR, Legro RS, Strauss JF, McAllister JM: Valproate potentiates androgen biosynthesis in human ovarian theca cells. Endocrinology 2004; 145(2):799–808.

432. Horne RL, Cunanan C: Safety and efficacy of switching psychiatric patients from a delayed-release to an extended-release formulation of divalproex sodium. Journal of Clinical Psychopharmacology 2003; 23(2):176–81.

433. Kondo T, Tokinaga N, Suzuki A, Ono S, Yabe H, Kaneko S, Hirano T: Altered pharmacokinetics and metabolism of valproate after replacement of conventional valproate with the slow-release formulation in epileptic patients. Pharmacology and Toxicology 2002; 90(3):135–38.

434. LaRoche SM, Helmers SL: The new antiepileptic drugs: scientific review. Journal of the American Medical Association 2004; 291(5):605–14.

435. Freeman MP, Stoll AL: Mood stabilizer combinations: a review of safety and efficacy. American Journal of Psychiatry 1998; 155(1):12–21.

436. Battino D, Estienne M, Avanzini G: Clinical pharmacokinetics of antiepileptic drugs in pediatric patients. Part II. Phenytoin, carbamazepine, sulthiame, lamotrigine, vigabatrin, oxcarbazepine and felbamate. Clinical Pharmacokinetics 1995; 29 (5):341–69.

437. Bertoldo M: Valproic acid and risperidone. Journal of the American Academy of Child and Adolescent Psychiatry 2002; 41(6):632.

438. Van Wattum PJ: Valproic acid and risperidone. Journal of the American Academy of Child and Adolescent Psychiatry 2001; 40(8):866.

439. Vitiello B: Valproic acid and risperidone. Journal of the American Academy of Child and Adolescent Psychiatry 2001; 40(8):867.

440. Good CR, Petersen CA, Krecko VF: Valproic Acid and risperidone. Journal of the American Academy of Child and Adolescent Psychiatry 2003; 42(1):2–3.

441. Gonzalez-Heydrich J, Raches D, Wilens TE, Leichtner A, Mezzacappa E: Retrospective study of hepatic enzyme elevations in children treated with olanzapine, divalproex, and their combination. Journal of the American Academy of Child and Adolescent Psychiatry 2003; 42(10):1227–33.

442. Minkova GD, Getova DP: Influence of carbamazepine-10,11-epoxide on the serum level of valproic acid in epileptic patients on combined treatment with carbamazepine and valproic acid. Folia Medica 2000; 42(3):16–19.

443. Kuzniecky R, Ho S, Pan J, Martin R, Gilliam F, Faught E, Hetherington H: Modulation of cerebral GABA by topiramate, lamotrigine, and gabapentin in healthy adults. Neurology 2002; 58(3):368–72.

444. Stewart BH, Kugler AR, Thompson PR, Bockbrader HN: A saturable transport mechanism in the intestinal absorption of gabapentin is the underlying cause of the lack of proportionality between increasing dose and drug levels in plasma. Pharmaceutical Research 1993; 10(2):276–87.

445. Calabrese JR, Bowden CL, Sachs GS, Ascher JA, Monaghan E, Rudd GD, Group LS: A double-blind placebo-controlled study of lamotrigine monotherapy in outpatients with bipolar I depression. Journal of Clinical Psychiatry 1999; 60(2):79–88.

446. Ketter TA, Calabrese JR: Stabilization of mood from below versus above baseline in bipolar disorder: a new nomenclature. Journal of Clinical Psychiatry 2002; 63(2):146–51.

447. Carandang CG, Maxwell DJ, Robbins DR, Oesterheld JR: Lamotrigine in adolescent mood disorders. Journal of the American Academy of Child and Adolescent Psychiatry 2003; 42(7): 750–51.

448. Calabrese JR, Bowden CL, Sachs G, Yatham LN, Behnke K, Mehtonen OP, Montgomery P, Ascher J, Paska W, Earl N, DeVeaugh-Geiss J, Group LS: A placebo-controlled 18-month trial of lamotrigine and lithium maintenance treatment in recently depressed patients with bipolar I disorder. Journal of Clinical Psychiatry 2003; 64(9):1013–24.

449. Evins AE: Efficacy of newer anticonvulsant medications in bipolar spectrum mood disorders. Journal of Clinical Psychiatry 2003; 64 (Suppl. 8):9–14.

450. Carta MG, Hardoy MC, Hardoy MJ, Grunze H, Carpiniello B: The clinical use of gabapentin in bipolar spectrum disorders. Journal of Affective Disorders 2003; 75(1):83–91.

451. Soutello CA, Casuto LS, Keck PEJ: Gabapentin in the treatment of adolescent mania: a case report. Journal of Child and Adolescent Psychopharmacology 1998; 8(1):81–85.

452. Delbello MP, Schwiers ML, Rosenberg HL, Strakowski SM: A double-blind, randomized, placebo-controlled study of quetiapine as adjunctive treatment for adolescent mania. Journal of the American Academy of Child and Adolescent Psychiatry 2002; 41(10):1216–23.

453. Pavuluri MN, Janicak PG, Carbray J: Topiramate plus risperidone for controlling weight gain and symptoms in preschool mania. Journal of Child and Adolescent Psychopharmacology 2002; 12(3):271–73.

454. Blanco C, Schneier FR, Schmidt A, Blanco-Jerez CR, Marshall RD, Sanchez-Lacay A, Liebowitz MR: Pharmacological treatment of social anxiety disorder: a meta-analysis. Depress Anxiety 2003; 18(1):29–40.

455. Pande AC, Pollack MH, Crockatt J, Greiner M, Chouinard G, Lydiard RB, Taylor CB, Dager SR, Shiovitz T: Placebo-controlled study of gabapentin treatment of panic disorder. Journal of Clinical Psychopharmacology 2000; 20(4):467–71.

456. Pollack MH, Otto MW, Worthington JJ, Manfro GG, Wolkow R: Sertraline in the treatment of panic disorder: A flexible-dose multicenter trial. Archives of General Psychiatry 1998; 55(11): 1010–15.

457. Hamner MB, Brodrick PS, Labbate LA: Gabapentin in PTSD: a retrospective, clinical series of adjunctive therapy. Annals of Clinical Psychiatry 2001; 13(3):141–46.

458. Bray GA, Hollander P, Klein S, Kushner R, Levy B, Fitchet M, Perry BH: A 6-month randomized, placebo-controlled, dose-ranging trial of topiramate for weight loss in obesity. Obesity Research 2003; 11(6):722–33.

459. Barbee JG: Topiramate in the treatment of severe bulimia nervosa with comorbid mood disorders: a case series. International Journal of Eating Disorders 2003; 33(4):468–72.

460. Smathers SA, Wilson JG, Nigro MA: Topiramate effectiveness in Prader-Willi syndrome. Pediatric Neurology 2003; 28(2): 130–33.

461. Behm MO, Kearns GL: Treatment of pain with gabapentin in a neonate. Pediatrics 2001; 108(2):482–84.

462. McGraw T, Stacey BR: Gabapentin for treatment of neuropathic pain in a 12-year-old girl. Clinical Journal of Pain 1998; 14(4): 354–56.

463. Messenheimer J: Efficacy and safety of lamotrigine in pediatric patients. Journal of Child Neurology 2002; 17 (Suppl. 2): 2S34–2S42.

464. Pellock JM, Appleton R: Use of new antiepileptic drugs in the treatment of childhood epilepsy. Epilepsia 1999; 40 (Suppl. 6):S29–S38.

465. Izzedine H, Launay-Vacher V, Deray G: Topiramate-induced renal tubular acidosis. American Journal of Medicine 2004; 116(4):281–82.

466. Coppola G, Caliendo G, Terracciano MM, Buono S, Pellegrino L, Pascotto A: Topiramate in refractory partial-onset seizures in children, adolescents and young adults: a multicentric open trial. Epilepsy Research 2001; 43(3):255–60.

467. Davanzo P, Cantwell E, Kleiner J, Baltaxe C, Najera B, Crecelius G, McCracken J: Cognitive changes during topiramate therapy. Journal of the American Academy of Child and Adolescent Psychiatry 2001; 40(3):262–63.

468. Martin R, Kuzniecky R, Ho S, Hetherington H, Pan J, Sinclair K, Gilliam F, Faught E: Cognitive effects of topiramate, gabapentin, and lamotrigine in healthy young adults. Neurology 1999; 52(2):321–27.

469. Shorvon SD: Safety of topiramate: adverse events and relationships to dosing. Epilepsia 1996; 37 (Suppl. 2):S18–S22.

470. Stowe CD, Bollinger T, James LP, Haley TM, Griebel ML, Farrar HC: Acute mental status changes and hyperchloremic metabolic acidosis with long-term topiramate therapy. Pharmacotherapy 2000; 20(1):105–09.

471. Wilner A, Raymond K, Pollard R: Topiramate and metabolic acidosis. Epilepsia 1999; 40(6):792–95.

472. Hamer HM, Knake S, Schomburg U, Rosenow F: Valproate-induced hyperammonemic encephalopathy in the presence of topiramate. Neurology 2000; 54(1):230–32.

473. Rosenfeld WE, Sachdeo RC, Faught RE, Privitera M: Long-term experience with topiramate as adjunctive therapy and as monotherapy in patients with partial onset seizures: retrospective survey of open-label treatment. Epilepsia 1997; 38 (Suppl. 1):S34–S36.

474. Catalano G, Catalano MC, Agustines RE, Dolan EM, Paperwalla KN: Pediatric quetiapine overdose: a case report and literature review. Journal of Child and Adolescent Psychopharmacology 2002; 12(4):355–61.

475. Grothe DR, Calis KA, Jacobsen L, Kumra S, DeVane CL, Rapoport JL, Bergstrom RF, Kurtz DL: Olanzapine pharmacokinetics in pediatric and adolescent inpatients with childhood-onset schizophrenia. Journal of Clinical Psychopharmacology 2000; 20(2):220–225.

476. McConville BJ, Arvanitis LA, Thyrum PT, Yeh C, Wilkinson LA, Chaney RO, Foster KD, Sorter MT, Friedman LM, Brown KL, Heubi JE: Pharmacokinetics, tolerability, and clinical effectiveness of quetiapine fumarate: an open-label trial in adolescents with psychotic disorders. Journal of Clinical Psychiatry 2000; 61(4):252–60.

477. Murray S, Micelli JJ: Pharmacokinetics of Ziprasidone in Pediatric Versus Adult Subjects, in Annual Meeting of the American Academy of Child and Adolescent Psychiatry, Miami, FL, 2003.

478. Sallee FR, Gilbert DL, Vinks AA, Miceli JJ, Robarge L, Wilner K: Pharmacodynamics of ziprasidone in children and adolescents: impact on dopamine transmission. Journal of the American Academy of Child and Adolescent Psychiatry 2003; 42(8):902–907.

479. Frazier JA, Cohen LG, Jacobsen L, Grothe D, Flood J, Baldessarini RJ, Piscitelli S, Kim GS, Rapoport JL: Clozapine pharmacokinetics in children and adolescents with childhood-onset schizophrenia. Journal of Clinical Psychopharmacology 2003; 23(1):87–91.

480. Stahl SM: Dopamine system stabilizers, aripiprazole, and the next generation of antipsychotics, part 1. Journal of Clinical Psychiatry 2001; 62(11):841–42.

481. Stahl SM, Shayegan DK: The psychopharmacology of ziprasidone: receptor-binding properties and real-world psychiatric practice. Journal of Clinical Psychiatry 2003; 64 (Suppl. 19):6–12.

482. Rollema H, Lu Y, Schmidt AW, Sprouse JS, Zorn SH: 5-HT(1A) receptor activation contributes to ziprasidone-induced dopamine release in the rat prefrontal cortex. Biological Psychiatry 2000; 48(3):229–37.

483. Burris KD, Molski TF, Xu C, Ryan E, Tottori K, Kikuchi T, Yocca FD, Molinoff PB: Aripiprazole, a novel antipsychotic, is a high-affinity partial agonist at human dopamine D2 receptors. Journal of Pharmacology and Experimental Therapeutics 2002; 302(1):381–89.

484. Bilder RM, Goldman RS, Volavka J, Czobor P, Hoptman M, Sheitman B, Lindenmayer JP, Citrome L, McEvoy J, Kunz M, Chakos M, Cooper TB, Horowitz TL, Lieberman JA: Neurocognitive effects of clozapine, olanzapine, risperidone and haloperidol in patients with chronic schizophrenia, or schizoaffective disorder. American Journal of Psychiatry 2002; 159(6):1018–28.

485. Miyamoto S, Duncan GE, Goff DC, Lieberman JA: Therapeutics of schizophrenia, in Neuropsychopharmacology: The Fifth Generation of Progress. Edited by Davis KL, Charney D, Coyle JT, Nemeroff C. Nashville, TN: American College of Neuropsychopharmacology, 2002.

486. Leucht S, Pitschel-Walz G, Abraham D, Kissling W: Efficacy and extrapyramidal side-effects of the new antipsychotics olanzapine, quetiapine, risperidone, and sertindole compared to conventional antipsychotics and placebo: a meta-analysis of randomized controlled trials. Schizophrenia Research 1999(1); 35:51–68.

487. McClellan J, Werry J: Practice Parameter for the Assessment and Treatment of Children and Adolescents With Schizophrenia. Washington, DC: American Academy of Child and Adolescent Psychiatry, 2000.

488. Piscitelli SC, Frazier JA, McKenna K, Albus KE, Grothe DR, Gordon CT, Rapoport JL: Plasma clozapine and haloperidol concentrations in adolescents with childhood-onset schizophrenia: association with response. Journal of Clinical Psychiatry 1994; 55(Suppl B):94–97.

489. Sikich L, Hamer RM, Bashford RA, Sheitman BB, Lieberman JA: A pilot study of risperidone, olanzapine, and haloperidol in psychotic youth: a double-blind, randomized, 8-week trial. Neuropsychopharmacology 2004; 29(1):133–45.

490. Pool D, Bloom W, Mielke DH, Roniger JJJ, Gallant DM: A controlled evaluation of loxitane in seventy-five adolescent schizophrenia patients. Current Therapeutic Research Clinical and Experimental 1976; 19(1):99–104.

491. Spencer EK, Kafantaris V, Padron-Gayol MV, Rosenberg C, Campbell M: Haloperidol in schizophrenic children: early findings from a study in progress. Psychopharmacology Bulletin 1992; 28(2):183–86.

492. Findling RL, McNamara NK, Youngstrom EA, Branicky LA, Demeter CA, Schulz SC: A prospective, open-label trial of olanzapine in adolescents with schizophrenia. Journal of the American Academy of Child and Adolescent Psychiatry 2003; 42(2):170–75.

493. Ross RG, Novins D, Farley GK, Adler LE: A 1-year open-label trial of olanzapine in school-age children with schizophrenia. Journal of Child and Adolescent Psychopharmacology 2003; 13(3):301–9.

494. Armenterose JL, Whitaker AH, Welikson M, Stedge DJ, Gorman J: Risperidone in adolescents with schizophrenia: an open pilot study. Journal of the American Academy of Child and Adolescent Psychiatry 1997; 36(5):694–700.

495. McConville B, Arvanitis L, Thyrum P, Smith K: Pharmacokinetics, tolerability, and clinical effectiveness of quetiapine in adolescents with selected psychotic disorders. European Neuropsychopharmacology: Journal of the European College of Neuropsychopharmacology 1999; 9 (Suppl. 5):S267.

496. Ghaemi SN, Soldani F, Hsu DJ: Commentary. International Journal of Neuropsychopharmacology 2003; 6(3):303–8.

497. Chang H, Berman I: Treatment issues for patients with schizophrenia who have obsessive-compulsive disorder. Psychiatric Annals 1999; 29(9):529–32.

498. Biederman J, Mick E, Bostic JQ, Prince J, Daly J, Wilens TE, Spencer TJ, Garcia-Jetton J, Russell R, Wozniak J, Faraone SV: The naturalistic course of pharmacologic treatment of children with maniclike symptoms: a systematic chart review. Journal of Clinical Psychiatry 1998; 59(11):628–37.

499. Frazier JA, Meyer MC, Biederman J, Wozniak J, Wilens TE, Spencer TJ, Kim GS, Shapiro S: Risperidone treatment for juvenile bipolar disorder: a retrospective chart review. Journal of the American Academy of Child and Adolescent Psychiatry 1999; 38(8):960–65.

500. Biederman J: Risperidone and Affective Symptoms in Children With Disruptive Behavior Disorders, in Society of Biological Psy-

chiatry: 58th Annual Convention and Scientific Program. San Francisco, CA, Society of Biological Psychiatry, 2003, p. 24.

501. McConville B, Carrero L, Sweitzer D, Potter L, Chaney R, Foster K, Sorter M, Friedman L, Browne K: Long-term safety, tolerability, and clinical efficacy of quetiapine in adolescents: an open-label extension trial. Journal of Child and Adolescent Psychopharmacology 2003; 13(1):75–82.

502. Tohen M, Baker RW, Altshuler LL, Zarate CA, Suppes T, Ketter TA, Milton DR, Risser R, Gilmore JA, Breier A, Tollefson GA: Olanzapine versus divalproex in the treatment of acute mania. American Journal of Psychiatry 2002; 159(6):1011–17.

503. Padla D: Quetiapine resolves psychotic depression in an adolescent boy. Journal of Child and Adolescent Psychopharmacology 2001; 11(2):207–8.

504. McDougle CJ, Scahill L, McCracken JT, Aman MG, Tierney E, Arnold LE, Freeman BJ, Martin A, McGough JJ, Cronin P, Posey DJ, Riddle MA, Ritz L, Swiezy NB, Vitiello B, Volkmar FR, Votolato NA, Walson P, Network RUoPPRA: Background and rationale for an initial controlled study of risperidone. Child and Adolescent Psychiatric Clinics of North America 2000; 9(1):201–24.

505. Fitzgerald KD, Stewart CM, Tawile V, Rosenberg DR: Case report: risperidone augmentation of serotonin reuptake inhibitor treatment of pediatric obsessive compulsive disorder. Journal of Child and Adolescent Psychopharmacology 1999; 9(2):115–23.

506. McDougle CJ, Epperson CN, Price LH: Obsessive-compulsive symptoms with neuroleptics. Journal of the American Academy of Child and Adolescent Psychiatry 1996; 35(7):837.

507. Morrison D, Clark D, Goldfarb E, McCoy L: Worsening of obsessive-compulsive symptoms following treatment with olanzapine. American Journal of Psychiatry 1998; 155(6):855.

508. Pfanner C, Marazziti D, Dell'Osso L, Presta S, Gemignani A, Milanfranchi A, Cassano GB: Risperidone augmentation in refractory obsessive-compulsive disorder: an open-label study. International Clinical Psychopharmacology 2000; 15(5):297–301.

509. Toren P, Samuel E, Weizman R, Golomb A, Eldar S, Laor N: Case study: emergence of transient compulsive symptoms during treatment with clothiapine. Journal of the American Academy of Child and Adolescent Psychiatry 1995; 34(11):1469–72.

510. Diler RS, Yolga A, Avci A, Scahill L: Risperidone-induced obsessive-compulsive symptoms in two children. Journal of the American Academy of Child and Adolescent Psychiatry 2003; 13 (Suppl. 1):S89–92.

511. Alevizos B, Lykouras L, Zervas IM, Christodoulou GN: Risperidone-induced obsessive-compulsive symptoms: a series of six cases. Journal of Clinical Psychopharmacology 2002; 22(5):461–67.

512. Kapur S, Remington G, Zipursky RB, Wilson AA, Houle S: The D2 dopamine receptor occupancy of risperidone and its relationship to extrapyramidal symptoms: a PET study. Life Sciences 1995; 57(10):PL103–7.

513. Austin LS, Lydiard RB, Ballenger JC, Cohen BM, Laraia MT, Zealberg JJ, Fossey MD, Ellinwood EH: Dopamine blocking activity of clomipramine in patients with obsessive-compulsive disorder. Biological Psychiatry 1991; 30(3):225–32.

514. McDougle CJ, Goodman WK, Price LH: Dopamine antagonists in tic-related and psychotic spectrum obsessive compulsive disorder. Journal of Clinical Psychiatry 1994; 55 (Suppl. 3):24–31.

515. Aman MG, Madrid A: Atypical antipsychotics in persons with developmental disabilities. Mental Retardation and Developmental Disabilities Research Review 1999; 5( ):253–63.

516. Campbell M, Anderson LT, Meier M, Cohen IL, Small AM, Samit C, Sachar EJ: A comparison of haloperidol and behavior therapy and their interaction in autistic children. Journal of the American Academy of Child and Adolescent Psychiatry 1978; 17(4):640–55.

517. Perry R, Campbell M, Adams P, Lynch N, Spencer EK, Curren EL, Overall JE: Long-term efficacy of haloperidol in autistic children: continuous versus discontinuous drug administration. Journal of the American Academy of Child and Adolescent Psychiatry 1989; 28(1):87–92.

518. Malone RP, Maislin G, Choudhury MS, Gifford C, Delaney MA: Risperidone treatment in children and adolescents with autism: short- and long-term safety and effectiveness. Journal of the American Academy of Child and Adolescent Psychiatry 2002; 41(2):140–47.

519. McCracken JT, McGough J, Shah B, Cronin P, Hong D, Aman MG, Arnold LE, Lindsay R, Nash P, Hollway J, McDougle CJ, Posey D, Swiezy N, Kohn A, Scahill L, Martin A, Koenig K, Volkmar F, Carroll D, Lancor A, Tierney E, Ghuman J, Gonzalez NM, Grados M, Vitiello B, Ritz L, Davies M, Robinson J, McMahon D, Network RUoPPA: Risperidone in children with autism and serious behavioral problems. New England Journal of Medicine 2002; 347(5):314–21.

520. McDougle CJ, Kem DL, Posey DJ: Case series: use of ziprasidone for maladaptive symptoms in youths with autism. Journal of the American Academy of Child and Adolescent Psychiatry 2002; 41(8):921–27.

521. Masi G, Cosenza A, Mucci M, Brovedani P: A 3-year naturalistic study of 53 preschool children with pervasive developmental disorders treated with risperidone. Journal of Clinical Psychiatry 2003; 64(9):1039–47.

522. Snyder R, Turgay A, Aman M, Binder C, Fisman S, Carroll A, Group RCS: Effects of risperidone on conduct and disruptive behavior disorders in children with subaverage IQs. Journal of the American Academy of Child and Adolescent Psychiatry 2002; 41(9):1026–36.

523. Aman MG, De Smedt G, Derivan A, Lyons B, Findling RL, Group RDBS: Double-blind, placebo-controlled study of risperidone for the treatment of disruptive behaviors in children with subaverage intelligence. American Journal of Psychiatry 2002; 159(8):1337–46.

524. Turgay A, Binder C, Snyder R, Fisman S: Long-term safety and efficacy of risperidone for the treatment of disruptive behavior disorders in children with subaverage IQs. Pediatrics 2002; 110(3):e34.

525. Bruggeman R, van der Linden C, Buitelaar JK, Gericke GS, Hawkridge SM, Temlett JA: Risperidone versus pimozide in Tourette's disorder: a comparative double-blind parallel-group study. Journal of Clinical Psychiatry 2001; 62(1):50–56.

526. Dion Y, Annable L, Sandor P, Chouinard G: Risperidone in the treatment of Tourette's syndrome: a double-blind, placebo-controlled trial. Journal of Clinical Psychopharmacology 2002; 22(1):31–39.

527. Boachie A, Goldfield GS, Spettigue W: Olanzapine use as an adjunctive treatment for hospitalized children with anorexia nervosa: case reports. International Journal of Eating Disorders 2003; 33(1):98–103.

528. Malina A, Gaskill J, McConaha C, Frank GK, LaVia M, Scholar L, Kaye WH: Olanzapine treatment of anorexia nervosa: a retrospective study. International Journal of Eating Disorders 2003; 33(2):234–37.

529. Powers PS, Santana CA, Bannon YS: Olanzapine in the treatment of anorexia nervosa: an open label trial. International Journal of Eating Disorders 2002; 32(2):146–54.

530. Woods SW: Chlorpromazine equivalent doses for the newer atypical antipsychotics. Journal of Clinical Psychiatry 2003; 64(6):663–67.

531. Melkersson K, Dahl ML: Adverse metabolic effects associated with atypical antipsychotics: literature review and clinical implications. Drugs 2004; 64(7):701–23.

532. Woods SW, Martin A, Spector SG, McGlashan TH: Effects of development on olanzapine-associated adverse events. Journal of the American Academy of Child and Adolescent Psychiatry 2002; 41(12):1439–46.

533. Nasrallah H: A review of the effect of atypical antipsychotics on weight. Psychoneuroendocrinology 2003; 28 (Suppl. 1):83–96.

534. Meyer JM: A Retrospective Comparison of Lipid, Glucose, and Weight Changes at One Year Between Olanzapine and Risperidone Treated Inpatients, in 39th Annual Meeting of the American College of Neuropsychopharmacology. Puerto Rico, 2000.

535. Devlin MJ, Yanovski SZ, Wilson GT: What mental health practitioners need to know. American Journal of Psychiatry 2000; 157:854–66.

536. Henderson DC, Cagliero E, Gray C, Nasrallah RA, Hayden DL, Schoenfeld DA, Goff DC: Clozapine, diabetes mellitus, weight gain, and lipid abnormalities: a five-year naturalistic study. American Journal of Psychiatry 2000; 157(6):975–81.

537. Sernyak MJ, Leslie DL, Alarcon RD, Losonczy MF, Rosenheck R: Association of diabetes mellitus with use of atypical neuroleptics in the treatment of schizophrenia. American Journal of Psychiatry 2002; 159(4):561–66.

538. Lindenmayer JP, Nathan AM, Smith RC: Hyperglycemia associated with the use of atypical antipsychotics. Journal of Clinical Psychiatry 2001; 62 (Suppl. 2):30–38.

539. Dixon L, Adams C, Lucksted A: Update on family psychoeducation for schizophrenia. Schizophrenia Bulletin 2000; 26(26):1.

540. Morrison JA, Cottingham EM, Barton BA: Metformin for weight loss in pediatric patients taking psychotropic drugs. American Journal of Psychiatry 2002; 159(4):655–57.

541. Koro CE, Fedder DO, L'Italien GJ, Weiss S, Magder LS, Kreyenbuhl J, Revicki D, Buchanan RW: An assessment of the independent effects of olanzapine and risperidone exposure on the risk of hyperlipidemia in schizophrenic patients. Archives of General Psychiatry 2002; 59(11):1021–26.

542. Turrone P, Kapur S, Seeman MV, Flint AJ: Elevation of prolactin levels by atypical antipsychotics. American Journal of Psychiatry 2002; 159(1):133–35.

543. Kleinberg DL, Davis JM, de Coster R, Van Baelen B, Brecher M: Prolactin levels and adverse events in patients treated with risperidone. Journal of Clinical Psychopharmacology 1999; 19(1):57–61.

544. Wudarsky M, Nicolson R, Hamburger SD, Spechler L, Gochman P, Bedwell J, Lenane MC, Rapoport JL: Elevated prolactin in pediatric patients on typical and atypical antipsychotics. Journal of Child and Adolescent Psychopharmacology 1999; 9(4):239–45.

545. Findling RL: Normalization of prolactin levels in children after long-term treatment with risperidone, in American Academy of Child and Adolescent Psychiatry. San Francisco, CA, 2002.

546. Miceli JJ, Wilner KD, Hansen RA, Johnson AC, Apseloff G, Gerber N: Single- and multiple-dose pharmacokinetics of ziprasidone under non-fasting conditions in healthy male volunteers. British Journal of Clinical Pharmacology 2000; 49 (Suppl. 1):5S–13S.

547. Cohen LG, Biederman J: Treatment of risperidone induced hyperprolactinemia with a dopamine agonist in children. Journal of Child and Adolescent Psychopharmacology 2001; 11(4):435–40.

548. Kim KS, Pae CU, Chae JH, Bahk WM, Jun TY, Kim DJ, Dickson RA: Effects of olanzapine on prolactin levels of female patients with schizophrenia treated with risperidone. Journal of Clinical Psychiatry 2002; 63(5):408–13.

549. Campbell M, Armenteros JL, Malone RP, Adams PB, Eisenberg ZW, Overall JE: Neuroleptic-related dyskinesias in autistic children: a prospective, longitudinal study. Journal of the American Academy of Child and Adolescent Psychiatry 1997; 36(6): 835–43.

550. Glassman AH, Bigger Jr. JT: Antipsychotic drugs: Prolonged QTC interval, torsade de pointes, and sudden death. American Journal of Psychiatry 2001; 158(11):1774–82.

551. Ray WA, Meredith S, Thapa PB, Meador KG, Hall K, Murray KT: Antipsychotics and the risk of sudden cardiac death. Archives of General Psychiatry 2001; 58(12):1161–67.

552. Shahzad S, Suleman MI, Shahab H, Mazour I, Kaur A, Rudzinskiy P, Lippmann S: Cataract occurrence with antipsychotic drugs. Psychosomatics 2002; 43(5):354–59.

553. Gerson SL, Arce C, Meltzer HY: N-desmethylclozapine: a clozapine metabolite that suppresses hemapoiesis. British Journal of Haemotology 1994; 86(3):555–61.

554. Alvir JM, Lieberman JA: Agranulocytosis: incidence and risk factors. Journal of Clinical Psychiatry 2001; 55 (Suppl. B):137–38.

555. Centorrino F, Price BH, Tuttle M, Bahk WM, Hennen J, Albert MJ, Baldessarini RJ: EEG abnormalities during treatment with typical and atypical antipsychotics. American Journal of Psychiatry 2002; 159(1):109–15.

556. Prior TI, Baker GB: Interactions between the cytochrome P450 system and the second-generation antipsychotics. Journal of Psychiatry and Neuroscience 2003; 28(2):99–112.

557. Catalano G, Catalano MC, Nunez CY, Walker SC: Atypical antipsychotic overdose in the pediatric population. Journal of Child and Adolescent Psychopharmacology 2001; 11(4): 425–34.

558. Kochhar S, Nwokike JN, Jankowitz B, Sholevar EH, Abed T, Baron DA: Olanzapine overdose: a pediatric case report. Journal of Child and Adolescent Psychopharmacology 2002; 12(4):351–53.

559. James LP, Abel K, Wilkinson J, Simpson PM, Nichols MH: Phenothiazine, butyrophenone, and other psychotropic medication poisonings in children and adolescents. Journal of Toxicology—Clinical Toxicology 2000; 38(6):615–23.

560. Simeon JG, Ferguson HB: Alprazolam effects in children with anxiety disorders. Canadian Journal of Psychiatry 1987; 32(7):570–74.

561. Biederman J: Clonazepam in the treatment of prepubertal children with panic-like symptoms. Journal of Clinical Psychiatry 1987; 48 (Suppl. 10):38–41.

562. Kutcher SP, MacKenzie S: Successful clonazepam treatment of adolescents with panic disorder. Journal of Clinical Psychopharmacology 1988; 8(4):299–301.

563. Simeon JG, Ferguson HB, Knott V, Roberts N, Gauthier B, Dubois C, Wiggins D: Clinical, cognitive, and neurophysiological effects of alprazolam in children and adolescents with over anxious and avoidant disorders. Journal of the American Academy of Child and Adolescent Psychiatry 1992; 31(1):29.

564. Graae F, Milner J, Rizzotto L, Klein RG: Clonazepam in childhood anxiety disorders. Journal of the American Academy of Child and Adolescent Psychiatry 1994; 33(3):372–76.

565. Kutcher S, Williamson P, MacKenzie S, Marton P, Ehrlich M: Successful clonazepam treatment of neuroleptic-induced akathisia in older adolescents and young adults: a double-blind, placebo-controlled study. Journal of Clinical Psychopharmacology 1989; 9(6):403–6.

566. Kalachnik JE, Hanzel TE, Sevenich R, Harder SR: Benzodiazepine behavioral side effects: review and implications for individuals with mental retardation. American Journal of Mental Retardation 2002; 107(5):376–410.

567. Marrosu F, Marrosu G, Rachel MG, Biggio G: Paradoxical reactions elicited by diazepam in children with classic autism. Functional Neurology 1987; 2(3):355–61.

568. Wiley CC, Wiley JF: Pediatric benzodiazepine ingestion resulting in hospitalization. Journal of Toxicology—Clinical Toxicology 1998; 36(3):227–31.

569. Mahmood I, Sahajwalla C: Clinical pharmacokinetics and pharmacodynamics of buspirone, an anxiolytic drug. Clinical Pharmacokinetics 1999; 36(4):277–87.

570. Gammans RE, Stringfellow JC, Hvizdos AJ, Seidehamel RJ, Cohn JB, Wilcox CS, Fabre LF, Pecknold JC, Smith WT, Rickels K: Use of buspirone in patients with generalized anxiety disorder and coexisting depressive symptoms. A meta-analysis of eight randomized, controlled studies. Neuropsychobiology 1992; 25(4):193–201.

571. Zwier KJ, Rao U: Buspirone use in an adolescent with social phobia and mixed personality disorder (cluster A type). Journal of the American Academy of Child and Adolescent Psychiatry 1994; 33(7):1007–11.

572. Buitelaar JK, van der Gaag RJ, van der Hoeven J: Buspirone in the management of anxiety and irritability in children with pervasive developmental disorders: results of an open-label study. Journal of Clinical Psychiatry 1998; 59(2):56–59.

573. Pfeffer CR, Jiang H, Domeshek LJ: Buspirone treatment of psychiatrically hospitalized prepubertal children with symptoms of anxiety and moderately severe aggression. Journal of Child and Adolescent Psychopharmacology 1997; 7(3):145–55.

574. Niederhofer H: An open trial of buspirone in the treatment of attention-deficit disorder. Human Psychopharmacology 2003; 18(6):489–92.

575. Malhotra S, Santosh PJ: An open clinical trial of buspirone in children with attention-deficit/hyperactivity disorder. Journal of the American Academy of Child and Adolescent Psychiatry 1998; 37(4):364–71.

576. Gross MD: Buspirone in ADHD with ODD. Journal of the American Academy of Child and Adolescent Psychiatry 1995; 34:1260.

577. Sussman N: Anxiolytic antidepressant augmentation. Journal of Clinical Psychiatry 1998; 59 (Suppl. 5):42–48.

578. Thomsen PH, Mikkelsen HU: The addition of buspirone to SSRI in the treatment of adolescent obsessive-compulsive disorder. A study of six cases. European Child & Adolescent Psychiatry 1999; 8(2):143–48.

579. Arnsten AF: Genetics of childhood disorders: XVIII. ADHD, Part. 2: norepinephrine has a critical modulatory influence on prefrontal cortical function. Journal of the American Academy of Child and Adolescent Psychiatry 2000; 39(9):1201–3.

580. Connor DF, Fletcher KE, Swanson JM: A meta-analysis of clonidine for symptoms of attention-deficit hyperactivity disorder. Journal of the American Academy of Child and Adolescent Psychiatry 1999; 38(12):1551–59.

581. Jaselskis CA, Cook EHJ, Fletcher KE, Leventhal BL: Clonidine treatment of hyperactive and impulsive children with autistic disorder. Journal of Clinical Psychopharmacology 1992; 12(5):322–27.

582. Hunt RD, Arnsten AF, Asbell MD: An open trial of guanfacine in the treatment of attention-deficit hyperactivity disorder. Journal of the American Academy of Child and Adolescent Psychiatry 1995; 34(1):50–54.

583. Chappell PB, Riddle MA, Scahill L, Lynch KA, Schultz R, Arnsten A, Leckman JF, Cohen DJ: Guanfacine treatment of comorbid attention-deficit hyperactivity disorder and Tourette's syndrome: preliminary clinical experience. Journal of the American Academy of Child and Adolescent Psychiatry 1995; 34(9):1140–46.

584. Kemph JP, DeVane CL, Levin GM, Jarecke R, Miller RL: Treatment of aggressive children with clonidine: results of an open pilot study. Journal of the American Academy of Child and Adolescent Psychiatry 1993; 32(3):577–81.

585. Scahill L, Chappell PB, Kim YS, Schultz RT, Katsovich L, Shepherd E, Arnsten A, Cohen DJ, Leckman JF: A placebo-controlled study of guanfacine in the treatment of children with tic disorders and attention deficit hyperactivity disorder. American Journal of Psychiatry 2001; 158(7):1067–74.

586. Lustig SL, Botelho C, Lynch L, Nelson SV, Eichelberger WJ, Vaughan BL: Implementing a randomized clinical trial on a pediatric psychiatric inpatient unit at a children's hospital: the case of clonidine for post-traumatic stress. General Hospital Psychiatry 2002; 24(6):422–29.

587. Perry BD: Neurobiological sequelae of childhood trauma: PTSD in children, in Catecholamine Function in Posttraumatic Stress Disorder: Emerging Concepts (Progress in Psychiatry, No 42). Edited by Murburg MM. Washington, DC: American Psychiatric Press, 1994, pp. 223–55.

588. Pliszka SR, Greenhill LL, Crismon ML, Sedillo A, Carlson C, Conners CK, McCracken JT, Swanson JM, Hughes CW, Llana ME, Lopez M, Toprac MG: The Texas Children's Medication Algorithm Project: Report of the Texas Consensus Conference Panel on Medication Treatment of Childhood Attention-Deficit/Hyperactivity Disorder. Journal of the American Academy of Child and Adolescent Psychiatry 2000; 39(7):908–19.

589. McGrath JC, Klein-Schwartz W: Epidemiology and toxicity of pediatric guanfacine exposures. Annals of Pharmacotherapy 2002; 36(11):1698–1703.

590. Wilens TE, Biederman J, Spencer T: Clonidine for sleep disturbances associated with attention-deficit hyperactivity disorder. Journal of the American Academy of Child and Adolescent Psychiatry 1994; 33(3):424–26.

591. Prince JB, Wilens TE, Biederman J, Spencer TJ, Wozniak JR: Clonidine for sleep disturbances associated with attention-deficit hyperactivity disorder: a systematic chart review of 62 cases. Journal of the American Academy of Child and Adolescent Psychiatry 1996; 35(35):5.

592. Chandran KS: ECG and clonidine. Journal of the American Academy of Child and Adolescent Psychiatry 1994; 33(9):1351–52.

593. Dawson PM, Vander Zanden JA, Werkman SL, Washington RL, Tyma TA: Cardiac dysrhythmia with the use of clonidine in explosive disorder. DICP, The Annals of Pharmacotherapy 1989; 23(6):465–66.

594. Fleminger S, Greenwood RJ, Oliver DL: Pharmacological management for agitation and aggression in people with acquired brain injury. Cochrane Database of Systematic Reviews 2003; 1:CD003299.

595. Buitelaar JK, van der Gaag RJ, Swaab-Barneveld H, Kuiper M: Pindolol and methylphenidate in children with ADHD. Journal of Child Psychology and Psychiatry 1996; 37:587–95.

596. Vaiva G, Ducrocq F, Jezequel K, Averland B, Lestavel P, Brunet A, Marmar CR: Immediate treatment with propranolol decreases posttraumatic stress disorder two months after trauma. Biological Psychiatry 2003; 54(9):947–49.

597. Jarrar RG, Buchhalter JR: Therapeutics in pediatric epilepsy, Part 1: The new antiepileptic drugs and the ketogenic diet. Mayo Clinic Proceedings 2003; 78(3):359–70.

598. Robertson PJ, Hellriegel ET: Clinical pharmacokinetic profile of modafinil. Clinical Pharmacokinetics 2003; 42(2):123–37.

599. Ivanenko A, Tauman R, Gozal D: Modafinil in the treatment of excessive daytime sleepiness in children. Sleep Medicine 2003; 4(6):579–82.

600. Vastag B: Poised to challenge need for sleep, "wakefulness enhancer" rouses concerns. Journal of the American Medical Association 2004; 291(2):167–70.

601. Rugino TA, Samsock TC: Modafinil in children with attention-deficit hyperactivity disorder. Pediatric Neurology 2003; 29(2):136–42.

602. Levin ED, Rezvani AH: Nicotinic treatment for cognitive dysfunction. Current Drug Targets—CNS and Neurological Disorders 2002; 1(4):423–31.

603. Todd RD, Lobos EA, Sun LW, Neuman RJ: Mutational analysis of the nicotinic acetylcholine receptor alpha 4 subunit gene in attention deficit/hyperactivity disorder: evidence for association of an intronic polymorphism with attention problems. Molecular Psychiatry 2003; 8(1):103–8.

604. Wilens TE, Biederman J, Wong J, Spencer TJ, Prince JB: Adjunctive donepezil in attention deficit hyperactivity disorder youth: case series. Journal of Child and Adolescent Psychopharmacology 2000; 10(3):217–222.

605. Volkmar F, Cook EHJ, Pomeroy J, Realmuto G, Tanguay P: Practice parameters for the assessment and treatment of children, adolescents, and adults with autism and other pervasive developmental disorders. Journal of the American Academy of Child and Adolescent Psychiatry 2000; 39(7):938.

606. Willemsen-Swinkels SH, Buitelaar JK, Nijhof GJ, van England H: Failure of naltrexone hydrochloride to reduce self-injurious and autistic behavior in mentally retarded adults: double-blind placebo-controlled studies. Archives of General Psychiatry 1995; 52(9):766–73.

607. Hollister LE, Trevino ES: Calcium channel blockers in psychiatric disorders: a review of the literature. Canadian Journal of Psychiatry—Revue Canadienne de Psychiatrie 1999; 44(7):658–64.

608. Rosenberg D, Keshavan M, O'Hearn K, Dick E, Bagwell W, Seymour A, Montrose D, Pierri J, Birmaher B: Frontostriatal measurement in treatment-naive children with obsessive compulsive disorder. Archives of General Psychiatry 1997; 54 (September):824–30.

609. Garvey M, Perlmutter S, Allen A, Hamburger S, Lougee L, Leonard H, Witowski M, Dubbert B, Swedo S: A pilot study of penicillin prophylaxis for neuropsychiatric exacerbations triggered by streptococcal infections. Biological Psychiatry 1999; 45(12):1564–71.

610. van Harten J: Clinical pharmacokinetics of selective serotonin reuptake inhibitors. Clinical Pharmacokinetics 1993; 24(3):203–20.

611. Preskorn SH: Clinically relevant pharmacology of selective serotonin reuptake inhibitors: an overview with emphasis on pharmacokinetics and effects on oxidative drug metabolism. Clinical Pharmacokinetics 1997; 32 (Suppl. 1):1–21.

612. Preskorn SH: Introduction. Pharmacokinetics of psychotropic agents: why and how they are relevant to treatment. Journal of Clinical Psychiatry 1993; 54 (Suppl. 3–7):discussion 55–56.

613. Greenblatt D, Von Moltke L, Harmatz J, Ciraulo D, Shader R: Alprazolam pharmacokinetics, metabolism, and plasma levels: clinical implications. Journal of Clinical Psychiatry 1993; 54 (October supplement):4–11.

614. Feighner JP, Boyer WF: Paroxetine in the treatment of depression: a comparison with imipramine and placebo. Journal of Clinical Psychiatry 1992; 53 (Suppl.):44–47.

615. Boyer WF, Feighner JP: An overview of paroxetine. Journal of Clinical Psychiatry 1992; 53 (Suppl.):3–6.

616. Feighner JP, Boyer WF, Merideth CH, Hendrickson GG: A double-blind comparison of fluoxetine, imipramine and

Section IV: Principles of Treatment of Pediatric Neuropsychiatry

placebo in outpatients with major depression. International Clinical Psychopharmacology 1989; 4(2):127–34.

617. Feighner JP, Pambakian R, Fowler RC, Boyer WF, D'Amico MF: A comparison of nefazodone, imipramine, and placebo in patients with moderate to severe depression. Psychopharmacology Bulletin 1989; 25(2):219–21.

618. Riddle M, Scahill L, King R, Hardin M, Anderson G, Ort S, Smith J, Lechman J, Cohen D: Double-blind, crossover trial of fluoxetine and placebo in children and adolescents with obsessive-compulsive disorder. Journal of the American Academy of Child and Adolescent Psychiatry 1992; 31(6):1062–69.

619. DeVeaugh-Geiss J, Moroz G, Biederman JB, Cantwell D, Fontaine R, Greist J, Reichler R, Katz R, Landau P: Clomipramine hydrochloride in childhood and adolescent obsessive-compulsive disorder: a multi-center trial. Journal of the American Academy of Child and Adolescent Psychiatry 1992; 31(1): 45–49.

620. March JS, Johnston H, Jefferson JW, Kobak KA, Greist JH: Do subtle neurological impairments predict treatment resistance to clomipramine in children and adolescents with obsessive-compulsive disorder. Journal of Child and Adolescent Psychopharmacology 1990; 1(2):133–40.

621. Chavira DA, Stein MB: Combined psychoeducation and treatment with selective serotonin reuptake inhibitors for youth with generalized social anxiety disorder. Journal of Child and Adolescent Psychopharmacology 2002; 12(1):47–54.

622. Masi G, Toni C, Mucci M, Millepiedi S, Mata B, Perugi G: Paroxetine in child and adolescent outpatients with panic disorder. Journal of Child and Adolescent Psychopharmacology 2001; 11(2):151–57.

623. Mancini C, Van Ameringen M, Farvolden P: Serotonergic agents in the treatment of social phobia in children and adolescents: a case series. Depression and Anxiety 1999; 10(1):33–39.

624. Carlson JS, Kratochwill TR, Johnston HF: Sertraline treatment of 5 children diagnosed with selective mutism: a single-case research trial. Journal of Child and Adolescent Psychopharmacology 1999; 9(4):293–306.

625. Black B, Uhda T: Treatment of elective mutism with fluoxetine: a double-blind, placebo-controlled study. Journal of the American Academy of Child and Adolescent Psychiatry 1994; 33(7): 1000–6.

626. Oesterheld JR, Shader RI: Cytochromes: a primer for child and adolescent psychiatrists. Journal of the American Academy of Child and Adolescent Psychiatry 1998; 37(4):447–50.

Electroconvulsive Therapy in Pediatric Neuropsychiatry

28

C. Edward Coffey, MD

The past three decades have seen a remarkable resurgence of interest in electroconvulsive therapy (ECT). Indications have broadened; technical features are better understood, producing a safer and more effective therapy; and improved devices provide more effective electrical stimulation and better monitoring of seizures. What began as a treatment for adults, with emphasis on the elderly, is now finding an expanded application with adolescents and even children, including those with neurologic illness.

In this chapter, I review the history and clinical experience with ECT in children and adolescents; discuss guidelines and indications for its consideration; review physiological effects, treatment techniques, side effects, and patient attitudes; discuss theories of a mechanism of action; and call for greater flexibility in considering the use of ECT among children and adolescents with neuropsychiatric illness.

HISTORY

ECT was apparently first given to a child around 1941 (Hemphill & Walter, 1941) and to adolescents (two teenagers) in 1942 (Heuyer & Bour, 1942), approximately 4 to 5 years after the first administration of ECT to an adult. In 1943, Heuyer and colleagues (1943) reported the administration of ECT to 40 adolescents and children with various psychiatric diagnoses and found the treatment safe as well as effective for melancholia and (to a lesser extent) mania, but not for schizophrenia. In 1947, Bender (1947) reported that ECT improved the capacity of 96 of 98 children and adolescents with schizophrenia to deal with problems in living, and that treatment did not interfere with intellectual functioning or development, nor did it have any lasting effect on the electroencephalogram (EEG). In a follow-up of 32 of these patients, Clardy and Rumpf (1954) found that the effects of ECT were "temporary and resulted in no sustained improvement in the patterning of behavior" (p. 620).

These early reports were followed over the next several decades by additional case reports and small series involving scores of patients, which were reviewed by Bertagnoli and Borchardt (1990) and by Schneekloth et al. (1993). Despite numerous methodological limitations in these reports (Rey & Walter, 1997), ECT was found to be generally effective and free of serious side effects, including death. For patients with affective disorders or with catatonia, the results were described as "excellent" or it was stated that the subjects "recovered." In adolescent patients with schizophrenia, ECT elicited transient reductions in symptoms; however, those with severe character pathology or substance abuse had poor outcomes. An exception to these generally positive findings was the survey by Guttmacher and Cretella (1988) of 10 years of ECT experience at Strong Memorial Hospital. Only one of their four patients improved, and "prolonged seizures" occurred in three of the patients. The marked limitations of this report have been discussed by Abrams (2002).

CONTEMPORARY CLINICAL EXPERIENCE

The experience with ECT in adolescents and children has been limited by the philosophical view (now changing) that mental disorders in these age groups are largely caused by parenting and childhood psychosocial events, with biological contributions limited to a few conditions resulting from specific genetic defects or birth trauma. Perhaps because of this view, ECT has received scant consideration in textbooks of child and adolescent psychiatry. Consideration of ECT is also limited by concerns that seizures may damage the developing brain (Wasterlain, 1997; Camfield, 1997). An issue of *Lancet* carried a plea for a ban on the use of ECT in adolescents, arguing that adolescents cannot give informed consent for this treatment because they cannot competently assess the risks it poses to their learning and education (Baker, 1995). This negative public attitude toward the use of ECT in children and adolescents is also codified in legislation. In 1993, the Texas legislature banned the administration of ECT to persons younger than 16 years of age. Legislation in California (1974), Tennessee (1976), and Colorado (1977) prohibits the use of ECT in minors under 12, 14, and 16 years of age, respectively.

In a survey of the attitudes of child psychiatrists regarding the treatment of depression in young patients of various ages, 42% of the respondents opined that ECT was not useful in children, and 19% believed that ECT was not useful in adolescents for the treatment of psychotic depression, even when the condition was identical to that in adults (Parmar 1993). The respondents were unanimous, however, in their willingness to prescribe medications for these conditions.

In a 1978 survey of psychiatrists' attitudes toward ECT, only a small group felt that use of ECT in children and adolescents was acceptable, even in rare situations (American Psychiatric Association, 1978). A 1981 survey of child and adolescent psychiatrists in the United Kingdom revealed that less than 7% would consider using ECT in adolescents (Pippard and Ellam 1981). Ghaziuddin and colleagues (2001) surveyed a sample of members of the American Academy of Child and Adolescent Psychiatry (1998–1999) and found that the majority (70%) regarded ECT as a treatment of last resort. Yet, 54% indicated that they possessed minimal knowledge of ECT and 75% lacked confidence in providing a second opinion about ECT in children and adolescents. In a 2000 survey of the child psychiatrists in Australia and New Zealand, most (76%) approved of the use of ECT in adolescents (only 26% approved of its use in children), but only 41% felt confident about giving an opinion about its use if consulted (Walter & Rey, 2003b). The use of ECT in children and adolescents was not addressed in the 1985 National Institute of Mental Health (NIMH)-sponsored Consensus Development Conference on ECT (Consensus Conference, 1985). The American Psychiatric Association's Task Force on ECT did consider guidelines for the use of ECT in adolescents and children in both its 1990 (American Psychiatric Associ-

ation, 1990) and 2001 (American Psychiatric Association, 2001) reports, as did the Royal College of Psychiatrists in its 1995 book, *The ECT Handbook* (Freeman, 1995). The American Academy of Child and Adolescent Psychiatry has recently issued guidelines on the use of ECT in adolescents (2004). These reports are discussed below.

Electroconvulsive Therapy in Adolescents

Although there are no controlled data on the use of ECT in adolescents or children, since 1990 a growing clinical experience suggests that ECT may be very effective for adolescents with certain severe psychiatric illnesses (Table 28.1). Several of these reports represent methodological improvements over the earlier literature, with larger sample sizes, standardized diagnostic and outcome criteria, and more contemporary ECT technique. In general, the response rates (variously defined) to ECT ranged from approximately 50 to 90%, with higher rates for those patients with mood disorders or catatonia (Cohen et al., 1999; Ghaziuddin et al., 2002). These response rates are particularly noteworthy because almost all of the patients were severely ill (some had catatonia) and had failed to respond to multiple trials of medications and various psychotherapies. The number of treatments received was similar to that in adults.

Adverse effects from ECT were inconsistently sampled. In general, systemic side effects (headache, nausea, vomiting) were common, yet mild, transient, and responsive to symptomatic treatment. There were no fatalities. Prolonged or tardive seizures were described in some patients, but it remains unclear whether adolescents and children are at greater risk for such events than adults (Ghaziuddin et al., 2002; Walter and Rey, 1997).

Cognitive side effects (brief confusion, memory complaints) also appear to be common, mild, and temporary, but data are limited. Gurevitz and Helme (1954), examining cognitive and personality assessments in 16 children who had received bilateral sine-wave ECT, found no long-term impact on intellectual efficiency. Cognitive performance was reduced immediately after ECT but returned to baseline during the 5- to 27-month follow-up. Subjects' performance on simple cognitive and perceptual tests was unimpaired within 48 hours of the end of an ECT series. Two recent follow-up studies also provide encouraging findings. Cohen et al. (2000) assessed cognitive functioning in ten adolescents an average of 3.5 years after receiving successful bilateral ECT for severe mood disorders (nine were euthymic and one was mildly hypomanic), and compared the results to a group of psychiatric controls matched for age, gender, and diagnosis. There were no group differences on any of the measures, including the Mini-Mental State examination, the attention section of the Wechsler Memory Scale-Revised, and the California Verbal Learning Test. Although six of the ten patients treated with ECT complained of memory problems (Squire Subjective Memory Questionnaire) immediately after treatment, only one pa-

TABLE 28.1

SELECTED REPORTS OF ECT IN CHILDREN AND ADOLESCENTS SINCE 1990

Study	Subjects	ECT Technique	Findings
Paillere-Martinot et al. 1990	n = 9, 15–19 years old; Dx: schizophrenia (n = 2), delusional depression (n = 4), delusional mania (n = 3)	Sine waveform; Bitemporal X 9, 3X/week	Resolution of symptoms in 8 patients (89%); With continuation drug therapy (variable), 7 well at 3 months and 4 well at 6–12 months; Acute side effects: subjective memory disturbance (3), mania/hypomania (2), somnolence (2), headache (1)
Cook and Scott 1992	n = 5, all 17 years old, from Royal Edinburgh Hospital 1982–1992; Dx: schizophrenia (n = 3), depression (n = 1), bipolar depression (n = 1)	Not described	Not described
Schneekloth et al. 1993	n = 20 (10B, 10G), 13–18 years old, from Mayo Clinic 1983–1991; DSM-III-R schizophrenia/schizophreniform/schizoaffective (n = 10), depression (n = 5), bipolar (n = 4), "none" (n = 1)	Pulse waveform; bitemporal (n = 8), right unilateral (n = 9), mixed (n = 3); median 11.5 ECTs (range 8–21)	70% "improved"; "No residual adverse effects at discharge"
Kutcher and Robertson 1995	n = 16, 16–22 years old (mean = 19.6), over 8 years at Sunnybrook Health Science Center, Toronto; DSM-III-R bipolar mania (n = 8) or bipolar depression with psychosis (n = 8)	Pulse waveform; bitemporal (87% of treatments), right unilateral (13% of treatments) twice weekly for a mean = 10.4 ECTs (range 6–12)	Significant (70%) reduction in BPRS scores, and shorter length of stay than patients refusing ECT (74 vs. 176 days); 28% with "acute" side effects (headache, confusion, agitation, memory disturbance, vomiting)
Otegui et al. 1995	n = 29, 13–16 years old (median 15.1), Montevideo, Uruguay 1988–1995; DSM-III-R schizophrenia/schizophreniform/schizoaffective (n = 18), impulsive-aggressive disorder (n = 5), major depression with psychotic features (n = 2), bipolar manic (n = 1), obsessive compulsive disorder (n = 1)	Pulse (n = 13) or sine (n = 16) waveform; bitemporal (100%); median 8.4 ECTs (range 3–13)	83% "improved"; No "complications were observed"
Ghaziuddin et al. 1996	n = 11, 13–18 years old (mean 16.3), over 3 years at University of Michigan; DSM-III-R major depression (n = 9), bipolar depression (n = 1), organic mood disorder (n = 1)	Pulse waveform; right unilateral (n = 3), bi-temporal (n = 2), mixed (n = 6); thrice weekly for a mean 11 ECTs (range 7–15)	64% became euthymic (CDSR-R score ≤40); No change in MMSE; Acute side effects included headache (80%) and nausea/vomiting (64%)
Moise and Petrides 1996	n = 13 (11B, 2G), 16–18 years old (mean = 16.3), University Hospital Stony Brook, 1983–1993; DSM-III or III-R bipolar disorder (n = 4), schizophreniform disorder (n = 3), psychosis NOS (n = 2), catatonia (n = 2), schizophrenia (n = 1), major depression with psychosis (n = 1)	Pulse waveform; bitemporal (n = 8), right unilateral (n = 4), mixed (n = 1); thrice weekly for a mean 10.9 ECTs (range 3–20)	10 (77%) responded (remission of presenting symptoms for at least 1 month post ECT); No "complications"
Cohen et al. 1997	n = 21 (12B, 9G), 14–19 years old (mean = 17), Pitie-Salpetriere, Paris, 1984–1995; DSM-III-R major depression with psychosis (n = 10), schizophrenia/schizoaffective (n = 7), mania with psychosis (n = 4)	Sine waveform; bitemporal; thrice weekly for a mean 9.5 ECTs (range 3–15)	16 (76%) "improved"; 50% with mild side effects (headache, nausea, vomiting) or memory complaints
Hedge et al. 1997	n = 14, <16 years old (mean 12.4), NIMH Bangalore, India, 1990–1991; Dx: functional psychosis	Sine waveform; right unilateral; thrice weekly for 4–11 ECTs	13 (93%) "rated as markedly improved"

(continued)

TABLE 28.1

(continued)

Study	Subjects	ECT Technique	Findings
Rey and Walter 1997	Review of 60 studies comprising 396 patients; 7–18 years old with various diagnoses (information was incomplete)	Information incomplete	Of 154 patients with adequate data, 81 (53%) showed "marked improvement or recovery" (63% with depression, 80% for mania or catatonia, and 42% for schizophrenia); "adverse effects appeared similar in type and frequency to those in adults"
Walter and Rey 1997	n = 42 (24 B, 18G) patients received 49 courses of ECT; 14–18 years old, state of New South Wales, Australia, 1990–1996; DSM-IV major depression (n = 14 courses), major depression with psychosis (n = 14 courses), schizophrenia (n = 12 courses), schizoaffective disorder (n = 4 courses), mania (n = 3 courses), psychotic disorder NOS (n = 2 courses)	Pulse waveform; right unilateral (90%), bitemporal (11%), mixed (26%); Thrice weekly for a mean = 9.5 ECTs (range 4–21)	51% with "marked improvement or resolution of symptoms"; "minor side effects" (e.g., headache, memory complaints, nausea and vomiting) occurred in 65% of courses and were transient
Duffett et al. 1999	n = 12 (8G, 4B), 12–17 years old, United Kingdom, 1996; Dx: depressive illness (n = 8), manic illness (n = 2), schizoaffective (n = 1), and schizophrenia (n = 1)	No information	Of 11 patients with data, 8 (73%) were rated as "improved or very much improved"; side effects not reported
Strober et al. 1998	n = 10 (7G, 3B); 13–17 years old, UCLA 1978–1996; RDC major depression (n = 7) or bipolar depression (n = 3)	Pulse waveform; right unilateral (n = 2), bitemporal (n = 1), mixed (n = 7); Thrice weekly for a mean 12.1 ECTs (range 10–18)	60% "complete remission" and 40% "partial remission"; procedure was well tolerated, with headache in 50%
Bloch et al. 2001	n = 24 (15G, 9B); 13–19 years old, Shalvata Hospital, Israel, 1991–1995; DSM-III-R schizophrenia (n = 15), schizo affective (n = 4), major depression (n = 4), bipolar depression (n = 1)	Pulse waveform; bitemporal; 8–34 ECTs	58% "achieved remission"; "no serious adverse events"

All studies are retrospective.
BPRS = brief psychiatric rating scale; CDSR = children depression rating scale; RDC = research diagnostic criteria.

tient continued to complain of difficulty with memory at follow-up. Ghaziuddin et al. (2000) followed 16 adolescents for an average of 8.5 ($\pm$ 4.9) months after ECT. Although at 1 week after ECT the patients showed impairments in attention, concentration, verbal fluency, and verbal and visual delayed recall, their cognitive functioning had returned to pre ECT levels by the follow-up assessment (not every patient received every test).

Due to limitations in these reports, it is not possible to determine the relation of therapeutic response or cognitive side effects to technical parameters such as stimulus electrode placement and stimulus dosage.

Electroconvulsive Therapy in Children

The experience with children has also been positive, if much more limited. Carr and colleagues (1983) described the successful use of seven right unilateral ECT treatments to induce euthymia in a 12-year-old girl with medication-resistant mania and ventricular enlargement on brain computed tomography (CT) imaging. Black and colleagues (1985) described the successful treatment of a depressed 11-year-old boy with suicidal intent and severe head banging. The boy received 12 right unilateral ECT treatments, which resulted in remarkable improvement in his depressive symptoms. In the four cases reported by Guttmacher and Cretella (1988), the one patient who responded well was a 9-year-old boy. In another report, a 13-year-old prepubescent boy with depressive stupor was successfully treated with right unilateral ECT (Powell et al., 1988). This boy also exhibited dexamethasone suppression test changes that paralleled similar observations in depressed adults. More recently, Cizadlo and Wheaton (1995) described successful ECT (15 bilateral, then four right unilateral brief pulse treatments) in an 8-year-old girl in whom a severe catatonic stupor developed while she was taking antidepressant medication for DSM-III-R major depression; there were no observable deleterious side effects from the ECT. Hill and colleagues (1997) described two boys, 7 and 8 year olds, with DSM-IV mania, who responded well to brief pulse ECT (one received right unilateral electrode placement, the other both right unilateral and bilateral electrode placement). The treatments were associated with "minimal postictal confusion."

Electroconvulsive Therapy in Children and Adolescents With Associated Neurological Disease

In contrast to a growing literature on the use of ECT in adults with associated neurologic disease (Coffey & Kellner, 2000; Krystal & Coffey, 1997), there are only a small number of such reports in children or adolescents. An examination of the clinical descriptions of the "schizophrenic" children included in Bender's (1947) study suggests that at least some of these patients may have had brain disease (e.g., "encephalopathy beginning by age 2 years"). Most of Bender's patients were reported to have improved after sine-wave bilateral ECT. The successful use of ECT in three depressed patients with epilepsy has been reported, and in none was the experience described as adverse (Bender, 1947; Mansheim, 1983; Schneekloth et al., 1993). Indeed, the 17-year-old patient with epilepsy described by Mansheim (1983) also had meningomyelocele, hydrocephalus, and a functioning shunt, and responded to a course of seven right unilateral, brief pulse ECT treatments. Brief-pulse ECT was reported to be safe and effective in a male adolescent who had experienced a single spontaneous grand mal seizure immediately before the course of ECT (Schneekloth et al., 1993). As described previously, seven right unilateral brief-pulse ECT treatments produced euthymia in a 12-year-old girl with mania, a history of left posterior slowing on electroencephalogram (EEG), and enlarged lateral ventricles on brain CT scan (Carr et al., 1983). Depression was successfully treated with brief-pulse ECT in an adolescent with a septum pellucidum cyst (Schneekloth et al., 1993). Twelve ECT treatments lessened depressive symptoms in a 17-year-old girl with Kleine-Levin-Critchley syndrome (Jeffries & LeFebre, 1973). A 17-year-old girl with Down syndrome who had failed to respond to nortriptyline showed marked improvement in mood, behavior, and activities of daily living, and was actually able to return to school following 14 ECT treatments (Warren et al., 1989). Zaw and colleagues (1999) reported that brief pulse bifrontal ECT (13 treatments) was dramatically effective in treating severe catatonia in a 14-year-old boy with autism and depressive symptoms. Ghaziuddin and colleagues (2002) reviewed the effectiveness of ECT in adolescents and children with catatonia, and described the successful use of ECT for malignant catatonia in a 17-year-old girl with malignant neuroleptic syndrome (MNS). ECT was not effective in another adolescent with depression following traumatic head injury (Paillere-Martinot et al., 1990).

Electroconvulsive Therapy Utilization in Adolescents and Children

In adults the use of ECT appears to be increasing, although there is dramatic variation in such usage (from 0.4 to 81.2 patients per 10,000 population) across regions of the United States (Hermann et al., 1995; Rosenbach et al., 1997). The limited data that exist for adolescents and children suggest that the rate of ECT use is low. According to data from the National Institute of Mental Health, of 33,384 patients receiving ECT in the United States in 1980, only 500 (1.5%) were between the ages of 11 and 20 (Thompson & Blaine, 1987). Approximately 0.3% of all patients receiving ECT in California between 1977 and 1983 were younger than the age of 18 (Kramer, 1985). Rey and Walter (1997) reviewed the use of ECT in the state of New South Wales, Australia (population approximately six million) between 1990 and 1995 and found that only 42 (0.93%) patients were younger than 18 years old. These authors found similar rates (1.53/100,000 adolescents) in a follow-up study of ECT use in New South Wales between 1996 and 1999 (Walter & Rey, 2003a). Among those patients who received ECT, there was an increase in the proportion of girls hospitalized involuntarily from 1990 to 1995 and from 1996 to 1999. Chung (2003) reviewed a central database of ECT use in all public hospitals in Hong Kong from 2001 to 2002, and identified 14 patients (9% of the total sample) between the ages of 15 and 19. Scott and colleagues (2005) reported that while 2.5 patients per 100,000 people younger than 18 years had received ECT in Edinburgh from 1993 to 1998, no patient younger than 18 had received ECT in the ensuing 5 years (1999 to 2004).

THE PHYSIOLOGY OF ELECTROCONVULSIVE THERAPY

The physiology of ECT is well defined in adults. Because we have little information about any differences in physiological effect of ECT in children and adolescents, we infer the physiological effects from the available experience.

Cerebral Physiology

In convulsive therapy, a chemical (flurothyl or pentylenetetrazol) or an electrical stimulus elicits a generalized cerebral seizure. There appears to be no difference in the efficacy of treatments using electrical or chemical induction, and no theory of the mode of action assigns specificity to the electrical stimulus. How ECT seizures are propagated is not well understood. Bilateral ECT appears to lead to seizure generalization via direct stimulation of the diencephalon, whereas seizures induced with unilateral stimulation may begin focally in the stimulated cortex and then generalize via corticothalamic pathways (Brumback & Staton, 1982; Staton et al., 1981).

During the initial tonic motor phase of the convulsion, EEG activity is variable, consisting of low-voltage fast activity with polyspike rhythms. EEG activity rapidly evolves into the hypersynchronous polyspikes and waves that characterize the clonic motor phase. These regular patterns begin to slow and eventually disintegrate as the seizure ends, usually terminating abruptly in a "flat" EEG (Weiner & Krystal, 1993).

During the ECT course, cumulative changes are observed in the interictal EEG. Increasing predominance of theta and then delta activity varies with the number and frequency of ECT treatments given in the course (Weiner & Krystal, 1993). The interictal EEG typically returns to baseline within 30 days of completion of the ECT course.

An ECT-induced seizure is associated with increases in cerebral blood flow, cerebral blood volume (resulting in a transient rise in intracranial pressure), and cerebral metabolism of oxygen and glucose (Bolwig et al., 1977; Broderson et al., 1973; Prohovnik et al., 1986). The transient increase in intracranial pressure is rarely of clinical consequence, but anticipation of this increase is the reason that ECT is proscribed in patients with intracranial space-occupying lesions. Postictally, cerebral blood flow and metabolism decrease and remain low for at least several days after the seizure, but then return to normal values. ECT induces a temporary functional increase in cerebrovascular permeability. Disruption in blood-brain barrier permeability also occurs (Bolwig et al., 1977). Such changes may account for the short-lived increase in T1 relaxation times observed on brain magnetic resonance (MR) imaging after ECT (Mander et al., 1987; Scott et al., 1990).

Cardiovascular Physiology

ECT results in a marked activation of the autonomic nervous system, and the relative balance of parasympathetic and sympathetic nervous system activity determines the cardiovascular effects. Vagal (parasympathetic) tone, reflected in bradycardia or asystole, is sharply increased with the administration of the electrical stimulus. The cerebral seizure also activates the sympathetic nervous system, and this activation is expressed in increases in heart rate, blood pressure, and cardiac output (Webb et al., 1990). Peripheral sympathetic activation is manifested in piloerection and gooseflesh. Tachycardia and hypertension continue throughout the ictus but generally end with the seizure; these actions oppose the tendency to bradycardia and asystole. Shortly after the seizure terminates, there may be another period of increased vagal tone, possibly expressed as bradycardia and dysrhythmias, including the appearance of ectopic beats. As the patient awakens from anesthesia, increased heart rate and blood pressure may result from arousal (Welch & Drop, 1989).

The cardiovascular responses occurring during ECT combine to produce an increase in myocardial oxygen demand and a decrease in coronary artery diastolic filling time. Transient electrocardiogram (ECG) changes in the ST segment and the T waves may develop in some patients, although the relationship of these changes to myocardial ischemia is unclear. No corresponding increase in cardiac enzyme levels accompanies the ECG changes (Braasch & Demaso, 1980). A study that used echocardiographic monitoring during and after ECT reported transient regional heart-wall motion abnormalities more often in older adult patients with ST-T changes on ECG, suggesting the occurrence of a period of myocardial-demand ischemia in these patients (Messina et al., 1992).

THE PRACTICE OF ELECTROCONVULSIVE THERAPY IN ADOLESCENTS AND CHILDREN

ECT is a complex medical intervention in which generalized seizures are repeatedly elicited under anesthesia. It requires the coordinated skills of a psychiatrist, an anesthesiologist, and trained nursing and support personnel in a facility equipped to ensure patient safety and optimal ECT technique. The standards of ECT practice in Western countries are well documented (Abrams, 1997; American Psychiatric Association, 2001; Fink, 1988; Freeman, 1995).

Indications for Electroconvulsive Therapy

ECT has been developed and tested in the treatment of adults, and an extensive literature supports its use in adults of all ages, including the elderly (Abrams, 1997; American Psychiatric Association, 2001). ECT is an important treatment option, and may indeed be lifesaving, in patients with severely disturbed mood, suicidal ideation, agitation, restlessness, excitement, delirium, stupor, or catatonia. Not only do the mood aspects of these disorders respond, but psychosis, delirium, and abnormal motor activity (catatonia, parkinsonism, stupor), common accompaniments of the major mood disorders, also improve (Fink, 1993a).

Perhaps surprisingly, ECT is also a viable choice in patients whose thoughts have become so delusional as to interfere with normal living or whose despondency is accompanied by the vegetative turmoil of severe insomnia, anorexia, weight loss, inanition, perplexity, confusion, inability to concentrate, or "dementia." Such behaviors may arise without a defined biological cause, as occurs in the major mood or bipolar disorders, or may be a feature of a systemic disorder such as Parkinson's disease; they may also occur consequent to a cerebral stroke or result from metabolic or toxic derangement of brain functions. It is these abnormal behaviors, not the underlying pathology, that are the focus of treatment. For this reason, the decision to undertake ECT is defined not solely by the clinical diagnosis, the longitudinal history of malfunction, or the patient's age, but rather by the dominant cross-sectional clinical features, their duration, and their severity. ECT has the broadest spectrum of therapeutic activity of any modern biological treatment in neuropsychiatry.

Illnesses characterized by a lifelong history without specific acute onset of a defined psychopathology are not indications for ECT. Patients with only "psychoneuroses," situational maladjustments, character pathology, substance abuse, social pathology, or sexual identification syndromes are poor candidates for ECT. Although these caveats have been developed in the treatment of adults, it is likely that they are equally applicable to adolescents. None of the adolescents with only personality disorders in the Mayo Clinic sample responded to ECT (Schneekloth et al., 1993). The two nonresponders in the Stony Brook sample also had severe character pathology (Moise & Petrides, 1996).

There is also little merit in considering ECT unless the technical requirements for safe administration are available at the institution in which the patient is being treated, that is, trained and competent therapists and nursing personnel, knowledgeable collaborating anesthesiologists, modern technical equipment to induce and monitor seizures, established practice guidelines and privileging standards, and financial support to allow its use. The absence of such facilities in many state, municipal, and federal hospitals, as well as in many private and academic hospitals, is a principal impediment to the consideration of ECT (Hermann et al., 1995).

Given these considerations, both the American Psychiatric Association (2001) and the American Academy of Child and Adolescent Psychiatry (2004) have issued guidelines that specify indications for ECT in adolescents and children. Both organizations agree that adolescents and children must meet specific criteria regarding (1) diagnosis (specifically major depression, mania, schizoaffective disorder, schizophrenia, and neuroleptic malignant syndrome); (2) severity of illness (the patient's symptoms must be severe, persistent, and disabling); and (3) failure to respond to an adequate trial of drug therapy (the American Academy of Child and Adolescent Psychiatry specifies that the patient must have failed two adequate drug trials). Both organizations allow for ECT earlier in the patient's illness if the patient cannot safely take the medication, or if waiting for a response to the medication would endanger the youth.

Pretreatment Evaluation

Once the patient's treatment team has made the decision to treat with ECT, a consultation is required from at least one other psychiatrist (The American Psychiatric Association [2001] recommends the use of two additional consultants for children younger than the age of 13). This preECT evaluation should be performed by an individual privileged to administer ECT and experienced in the treatment of adolescents and children. The goals of the preECT evaluation are to (1) determine if ECT is indicated, (2) establish baseline measures of efficacy and cognitive side effects, (3) optimize the treatment of any active medical problems, (4) initiate the process of informed consent, and (5) begin preparation of the patient and family for the procedure

(Coffey, 1998). Of course, findings from the preECT evaluation should be documented in the clinical record.

The indications for ECT in adolescents and children were discussed previously. These indications are identified through a thorough and detailed neuropsychiatric history, interview, and examination. The historical review should include a review of the adequacy of previous pharmacologic and psychosocial treatments, as well as response to prior courses of ECT. A thorough mental status examination establishes the presence of signs of the mental disorder. Handedness is assessed for its relevance to the decision to use unilateral ECT with nondominant placement. A minority of left-handed patients and patients with mixed dominance may have language localized to the right hemisphere, an issue of importance when one is determining the nondominant hemisphere for unilateral treatment.

Most patients are referred for ECT after failing to respond to psychotropic medications, and the decision to try ECT is made while these medications are still being actively prescribed. An evaluation of such medications is required for optimal ECT (Fink, 1994; Kellner, 1993). Generally, all psychotropic medications are discontinued prior to ECT. Lithium taken in proximity to ECT has been linked to an increased incidence of delirium and seizures, and the customary practice is to discontinue lithium therapy. If the practitioner considers concurrent lithium to be beneficial, dosages are usually not given in the 24 hours before each ECT treatment so that lower serum lithium levels can be sustained during the seizure. Because some authors (e.g., Kellner, 1993) have described an impairment of seizure efficacy when benzodiazepines are administered, these drugs are usually discontinued before a course of ECT. An exception to this rule has recently been described in the management of patients with persistent or recurrent catatonia (Petrides et al., 1995). When benzodiazepine use is continued during ECT, adjustments are made in energy dosing and electrode placement to ensure adequate treatments.

Antidepressant medications are frequently discontinued prior to ECT, mainly because there is little evidence of synergism. Some practitioners are concerned that tricyclic antidepressant drugs may alter cardiac functions, especially in the elderly, and therefore discontinue antidepressant drugs in ECT patients with a history or evidence of cardiovascular disease. Anesthesiologists may be concerned that recent exposure to monoamine oxidase inhibitors (MAOIs) will interfere with the action of succinylcholine. Studies by El-Ganzouri and colleagues (1985), among others, find no basis for such concern, and ECT may be administered safely in the presence of MAOIs or even when their use has only recently been discontinued.

Antipsychotic medications may be continued, as there is evidence suggesting synergism of ECT with these drugs (Klapheke, 1993).

Objective data are essential for determining the outcome of the course of ECT. Baseline affective and cognitive status should be documented. The HAM-D or the Montgomery-

Asberg Depression Rating are standardized assessment instruments that are often used at intervals throughout the ECT course. Cognitive testing should focus upon memory and new learning ability. More extensive neuropsychological testing may be indicated in patients with certain neurologic illnesses. The American Academy of Child and Adolescent Psychiatry (2004) specifies that memory function should also be assessed "at an appropriate time after ECT treatment (usually between 3 to 6 months)."

Although ECT is among the safest medical treatments that require general anesthesia, the procedure does produce temporary, robust changes in cerebral and cardiac physiology, as described previously. As such, a thorough medical history and physical examination should be performed that focuses upon these two organ systems, as well as upon the pulmonary, dental, and musculoskeletal systems. A personal or family history of complications from previous anesthesia should be noted. Although there are no absolute contraindications to ECT, serious disease of the cardiovascular, central nervous, pulmonary, or musculoskeletal systems will require optimal treatment prior to ECT, and the ECT technique may need to be modified. Adjustments may be required in some medications (e.g., insulin, anticonvulsant medications). Consultation with anesthesia personnel is important because the provision of general anesthesia is associated with some (albeit small) medical risk. Indeed, an anesthesiologist experienced in ECT may also serve as the "medical" consultant and can greatly facilitate the medical evaluation of patients with systemic illness. Additional consultation from other specialists may occasionally be required. A limited laboratory evaluation is sufficient for most patients (ECG, serum potassium). All girls should have a pregnancy test unless pregnancy is not possible.

Initiating the process of informed consent is an essential element of the preECT workup. The consent process should include the patient and the family, and should provide information about the indication for ECT, the efficacy of ECT for that indication, alternative treatments to ECT, a description of the ECT procedure, expected routine side effects, less common side effects, and any condition that raises the risk of the procedure. Various written and video materials can facilitate the educational process. Written informed consent must be obtained, and The American Psychiatric Association's Task Force on ECT (2001) provides a model consent form which is an excellent template. The requirement that minors provide consent before receiving ECT varies by state, and practitioners must consider individual state laws governing the age at which a person can consent to psychiatric treatment and to ECT or surgical (i.e., anesthesia) procedures. In some states, the ages of consent may differ for the two procedures. If the patient is too young to give consent or is incompetent, a guardian provides consent. Surrogate (parental or guardian) consent is acceptable for noncompetent patients in some states; in others, however, a court proceeding is mandated.

Finally, the preECT evaluation affords the clinician an opportunity to establish important interpersonal relationships with the patient and family which are additionally therapeutic as well as personally rewarding to the clinician.

Electroconvulsive Therapy Procedure

In the United States, ECT is commonly administered as a series of single treatments on alternate mornings. Many adults now receive ECT on an outpatient basis, and this setting may be appropriate for many adolescents and children who meet appropriate criteria. The American Academy of Child and Adolescent Psychiatry (2004) recommends however, that ECT be administered to adolescents (and presumably children) on an inpatient basis. ECT is typically administered in either a special treatment suite or the recovery area of an operating room suite. Patients should have nothing to eat or drink for at least 8 hours prior to treatment.

In our experience with adolescents, we have found a remarkable equanimity and acceptance of ECT procedures by our patients once the need for the treatment is established and the procedures explained. Their physical tolerance of the procedures and rapid recovery from anesthesia allows them to participate in daily activities, including school classes, shortly after each treatment session.

The standard technique requires the establishment of a patent intravenous line. Electrodes for stimulation and for monitoring of the seizure are applied according to the appropriate technique. The medication sequence includes anticholinergic premedication (glycopyrrolate or atropine) to prevent vagal-mediated cardiac slowing (if indicated), followed by an anesthetic to induce amnesia (usually methohexital) and succinylcholine for muscle relaxation. Throughout the procedure, the patient is ventilated with 100% oxygen. Heart rate, blood pressure, and blood oxygen saturation are also monitored.

Once the patient is asleep and relaxed, a specially designed bite block is inserted into the mouth to protect the teeth from injury during jaw clenching as the electrical stimulus is applied. A predetermined electrical stimulus (see subsequent discussion on electrical stimulus dosing) is delivered, and, typically, a generalized seizure lasting from 30 to 90 seconds ensues. The seizure is monitored by observing brain electrical activity via EEG, and motor manifestations of the seizure via a blood-pressure cuff at the ankle (typically the right) inflated above systolic pressure to prevent access of succinylcholine to that extremity. Ventilatory support is continued until the patient breathes spontaneously, and further recovery is provided in a supportive environment. In addition, because the use of succinylcholine may be associated with an increased risk of malignant hyperthermia in children, patients should be monitored closely after each treatment for fever, muscular rigidity, and delirium (Welborn, 1996). The entire procedure takes approximately 20 minutes, and patients are often able to shower, dress, and have breakfast within an hour of the time of treatment. The American Academy of Child and Adolescent Psychiatry (2002) recommends that patients be monitored for 24 hours after an ECT treatment for the occurrence of tardive seizures.

A typical ECT course consists of six to 12 treatments, although occasional patients may require fewer or more treatments to achieve a full response. ECT is discontinued when the patient has achieved maximal clinical improvement or when side effects outweigh any further beneficial effects of the treatment. Special attention is given to continuation/maintenance treatment with either medication or ECT (see subsequent discussion on this topic).

Electrical Stimulus Dosing

The ECT stimulus should be delivered with a contemporary brief pulse, constant current device. Seizure threshold (the minimum amount of energy required to elicit an ECT seizure) increases with age (Coffey et al., 1995a; Sackeim et al., 1987); it is lowest in adolescents and children. Recent data in adult samples suggest an interaction of electrode placement, stimulus dosage, stimulus parameters and clinical efficacy so that threshold and barely suprathreshold stimulus intensities are clinically ineffective with unilateral nondominant electrode placements (Sackeim et al., 1993). Although ongoing studies are seeking to assess the parameters of this interdependence, data in adult samples suggest that stimulus dosages at multiples of four times or more of seizure threshold may be required to maximize the efficacy of unilateral ECT (McCall et al., 2000; Sackeim et al., 2000). Treatments with bilateral electrode placement, on the other hand, demonstrate less dependence on the strength of the electrical stimulus, so that stimulus dosing just above seizure threshold appears adequate for treatment efficacy.

Stimulus dosing is particularly important when unilateral nondominant electrode placement is selected. Some practitioners assess the seizure threshold by administering initial stimulations at a very low dosage and then increasing the dosage in a stepwise manner until a satisfactory seizure is elicited (Coffey et al., 1995a). This procedure is encouraged by the American Psychiatric Association Task Force on ECT (2001) and by the American Academy of Child and Adolescent Psychiatry (2004). However, such a procedure may be of limited usefulness in children and adolescents if the minimum stimulus dosage on the ECT device is at or above the seizure threshold in these age groups. My practice with adolescents is to estimate seizure threshold using a dosing titration protocol, then set the stimulus dosage for subsequent treatments at 1.5 times threshold for bilateral electrode placement and at 4 times initial seizure threshold for unilateral nondominant electrode placement.

As noted previously, the ECT seizure is monitored to ensure that it has ended and to estimate its therapeutic "adequacy." An adequate seizure may be defined as one that has a motor duration of at least 25 seconds and an EEG duration of more than 30 seconds, with well-defined periods of spike

and spike-and-wave ictal activity, and that terminates in a precise end point. If motor convulsion durations are less than 25 seconds, the EEG fails to show periods of defined spike and spike-and-wave activity, or the termination is imprecise, ECT is immediately repeated with higher stimulus dosage. Newer ECT devices provide quantitative estimates of these (and other) ictal EEG indices, but their routine clinical utility is limited at present by their sensitivity to EEG artifacts, variation in EEG lead placement, and inter- and intra-individual variation in the ictal EEG (Krystal, 1998).

Seizure threshold may rise during the course of treatment (Coffey et al., 1995b; Sackeim et al., 1987). As such, upward adjustments in stimulus dosage may be required to maintain efficacy. If an inadequate seizure is elicited, inductions are immediately repeated at a higher electrical dosage until an adequate seizure is obtained.

Occasionally, seizures persist beyond 180 seconds; such seizures are defined as "prolonged." They can be terminated by an intravenous bolus of methohexital or diazepam that is readministered if termination does not occur within 30 seconds and repeated at 30-second intervals until the seizure is clearly terminated.

Electrode Placement

The choice of stimulus electrode placement is complex. Unilateral nondominant ECT is associated with fewer cognitive side effects in adults, but unless stimulus dosing and electrode application are carefully prescribed and other medications restricted, treatment efficacy may be impaired with this placement. Bilateral (bitemporal) ECT may be more reliably effective in adults, but may be associated with greater cognitive side effects. The American Academy of Child and Adolescent Psychiatry (2004) recommends commencing with unilateral nondominant electrode placement given its favorable side effect profile, and switching to bitemporal placement if the response is not satisfactory. Treatment may begin with bitemporal electrode placement if the patient is critically ill and requires an urgent response. Potentially promising alternative electrode placements such as bifrontal (Baline et al., 2000), have not been studied in adolescents and children.

Continuation/Maintenance Treatment

Major depressive disorders are increasingly recognized as chronic, relapsing conditions (see Chapter 13). Some studies in adults with major depressive disorder have found 6-month relapse rates as high as 50% for patients initially responsive to antidepressants who are subsequently withdrawn from the medications (Prien & Kupfer, 1986). Relapse rates following successful pharmacotherapy are substantially reduced by continuation of antidepressant medication at full dosage (Frank et al., 1990). Similarly high rates of relapse have been noted in adults following ECT response when no form of follow-up therapy was given

(Jarvie, 1954). The risk of relapse after successful ECT is particularly high (especially in the first 4 months following ECT) in patients who were resistant to medication or who displayed psychotic symptoms during their index episode of illness (Grunhaus et al., 1995; Sackeim et al., 1993).

The American Psychiatric Association Task Force on ECT (2001) has defined *continuation therapy* as the ". . .provision of somatic treatment over the 6-month period after the onset of remission." Somatic treatment beyond 6 months that seeks to maintain euthymia is by convention defined as *maintenance treatment*. The usual clinical practice is to place patients with mood disorders on continuation therapy after a successful course of ECT, either with pharmacotherapy or with ECT. Recent controlled data suggest that continuation pharmacotherapy with nortriptyline and lithium is superior to nortriptyline alone, which is in turn superior to placebo in preventing relapse of major depression in adults who have responded to a course of ECT (Sackeim et al., 2001). We have less data to guide the choice of continuation pharmacotherapy after successful ECT for bipolar depression (a mood stabilizer plus an antidepressant are typically used), mania (a mood stabilizer plus possibly an antipsychotic are typically used), or schizophrenia (an antipsychotic is typically used).

Relapse rates remain high after successful index ECT, even in patients on continuation pharmacotherapy. As such, some practitioners recommend continuation therapy with ECT, particularly in patients with psychotic depression or those who were resistant to medication during the index episode. An evolving literature in adult samples indicates that continuation ECT (typically administered on an outpatient basis) is safe and effective in the prevention of depressive relapse following successful "index" ECT (American Psychiatric Association, 2001). Continuation/maintenance ECT typically involves single treatments administered on an ambulatory basis, initially at weekly intervals and then gradually reduced in frequency to every 4 to 8 weeks, as the patient's symptoms allow. The increased interval between treatments results in fewer cognitive side effects than during an "index" course of ECT; and this has led to the suggestion that bilateral electrode placement may be more acceptable for continuation/maintenance ECT. The logistical factors in ambulatory ECT are defined in the report by the Task Force on Ambulatory ECT of the Association for Convulsive Therapy (Fink et al., 1996).

There are no controlled data that assess the relative merits of continuation pharmacotherapy and continuation ECT. As of this writing, a four-site study is underway comparing the efficacy of continuation therapy with ECT versus lithium plus nortriptyline, after successful index ECT in depressed adults.

Based on the experience in adults, the American Academy of Child and Adolescent Psychiatry (2004) recommends continuation pharmacotherapy after successful ECT, although it acknowledges there may be a role for ECT in some cases. Although there are no controlled data in adolescents to inform these decisions, I recommend considering continuation ECT in those patients who were resistant to medications during the index episode.

ADVERSE EFFECTS AND THEIR MANAGEMENT

General Issues

The safety of ECT compares favorably with that of treatments requiring brief general anesthesia. ECT mortality in adults is reported as approximately 0.2 to 1.0 deaths per 10,000 patients (or approximately one per 80,000 treatments), about the same as mortality from general anesthesia for minor surgery (American Psychiatric Association, 2001; Kramer, 1985). Although there are no mortality data specifically for children and adolescents, the mortality risk from brief general anesthesia in this age group appears similar to (if not even lower than) that in healthy adults (Motoyama, 1996).

As noted previously, systemic side effects such as headache, nausea, and vomiting, are common during and shortly after the postECT recovery period. Headache may occur in as many as half of all patients, and although its etiology is not known, its throbbing character suggests a vascular mechanism. Nausea may affect up to 20% of patients, and may be secondary to headache or its treatment with narcotics, or as a side effect of the anesthesia. Generally, these symptoms are mild, transient, and quite responsive to symptomatic treatments. If these problems recur, prophylactic therapy may lessen their recurrence or severity. Some patients complain of muscle soreness after ECT, which is likely secondary to fasiculations induced by the depolarizing muscle relaxant. Symptoms tend to diminish after the first treatment (assuming muscle relaxation is adequate), but persistent soreness can be treated successfully with simple analgesics such as aspirin or acetaminophen.

Some patients experience an agitated emergent delirium immediately after a seizure on awakening from anesthesia. Such experiences are more often seen in the first or second treatment of a series and are readily treated with intravenous benzodiazepines (Fink, 1993b).

Cardiovascular Effects

As described previously, ECT results in a brief period of increased cardiac workload. This hemodynamic response should be well tolerated by the healthy older child or adolescent. If the presence of a preexisting heart condition raises a concern about such tolerance however, pharmacological blunting of the hemodynamic response may be indicated. The primary issues of concern are bradycardia, tachycardia, hypertension, and ventricular arrhythmia. Anticholinergic premedications (atropine, glycopyrrolate) are used to prevent vagally-induced bradycardia. Stimulus dosage titration to determine a patient's seizure threshold requires the administration of subconvulsive stimuli, which produces a vagal surge unaccompanied by the sympathetic outflow associated with a seizure. Such titrations require the routine use of anticholinergic premedication, especially in children, in whom resting vagal tone may be higher than that in adults (Welborn, 1996).

Clinically significant hypertension and tachycardia during ECT may be attenuated by short-acting intravenous adrenergic blockers such as labetalol or esmolol (Howie et al., 1990; Stoudemire et al., 1990). Beta-adrenergic blockers have anticonvulsant effects; their use during ECT may theoretically limit the intensity of the ECT seizure and, in turn, its therapeutic potency. Alternative treatments include sublingual nifedipine, hydralazine (an β-adrenergic antagonist), nitroglycerin (sublingual, transdermal, or intravenous), or the ganglionic blocking agent trimethaphan camsylate (Arfonad) (Maneksha, 1991; Petrides et al., 1996). Indiscriminate use of antihypertensive medication may lead to severe hypotension, and we do not routinely attempt to blunt cardiovascular responses to ECT in physically healthy patients unless such responses are extreme or are clearly associated with signs of cardiovascular compromise.

Cerebral Effects

There is no evidence that ECT causes structural brain damage (Devanand et al., 1994; Weiner, 1984). Carefully controlled, prospective brain-imaging studies in adults with follow-up durations up to 6 months have revealed no changes in brain structure after a course of ECT (Coffey, 1987; Coffey et al., 1991). Neuropathological studies in animals, including cell counts in regions thought to be at highest risk, have failed to find evidence of brain damage when seizures are induced under conditions approximating those used in standard clinical practice (i.e., when seizures are spaced, relatively brief, and modified by oxygenation and muscle relaxation). Furthermore, studies of the pathophysiology of seizure-induced structural brain damage in animals indicate that the conditions necessary for injury are not met in the modern practice of ECT.

Although it has been suggested that the developing brain may be more prone to the harmful effects of seizures, there are no data to support this contention as it applies to ECT. Indeed, an extensive clinical literature indicates that children and adolescents may sustain even multiple symptomatic seizures (e.g., secondary to toxic metabolic etiologies) without showing residual brain effects. Children with some types of epilepsy (e.g., Rolandic, absence) may eventually "outgrow" their epilepsy without demonstrating residual adverse cerebral effects. Finally, among the case descriptions of children and adolescents who have received ECT, there are no reports of brain injury from the treatment.

There are no reported cases of intracerebral hemorrhage with ECT or of ischemic stroke during ECT treatment.

Nonetheless, many clinicians fear the consequences of ECT in patients with cerebral disease and have described various intracranial processes as risk factors. Intracranial mass lesions and increased intracranial pressure are the most prominent of these purported risk factors. However, several cases of safe and effective ECT in adult patients with brain tumors have been described in which ECT was necessitated by the patients' mental state, and these case experiences provide guidelines for such treatment (Fried & Mann, 1988; Greenberg et al., 1988; Malek-Ahmadi & Sedler, 1989; Zwil et al., 1990). Patients with functioning intracranial shunts may also be treated safely, provided that normal intracranial pressure is maintained (Coffey et al., 1987; Mansheim, 1983). Subdural hematomas require evacuation prior to ECT (Abrams, 1997).

Cognitive Effects

The cognitive side effects of ECT include acute postictal confusion/delirium, and interictal impairments in attention, concentration, and memory (American Psychiatric Association, 2001). Other neuropsychological functions are generally unaffected by ECT. These ECT side effects have not been systematically studied in adolescents and children. In adults, the severity of these effects varies with age, electrical stimulus waveform, electrode placement, stimulus dosing, and frequency of treatments (Abrams, 1997; American Psychiatric Association, 2001; Fink, 1979). The cognitive side effects of the procedure in adults, and likely in adolescents and children as well, may be minimized by modern use of brief-pulse currents, selective electrode placement and stimulus dosing, and varied frequency of treatments.

Most patients experience disorientation immediately upon awakening during the postECT recovery process (Calev et al., 1993; Summers et al., 1979). The duration and severity of this disorientation is particularly sensitive to age, being extended in the elderly but remarkably short (e.g., 1 hour or less), in our experience, in adolescents. Impairments in attention and concentration are also common after a course of ECT, but are typically mild and resolve shortly after completion of the treatment.

ECT selectively results in anterograde and retrograde amnesia, particularly for episodic memory. Such effects are generally mild. The former typically resolves within weeks of completing the treatments, while the time course for resolution of the latter is often more gradual. Any residual memory gaps are usually mild and limited to the period of illness and treatment. Although it has been feared that children and adolescents may be at greater risk for these cognitive side effects as a result of the relative immaturity of their brains, no studies or case reports exist that support such a concern. Indeed, in my experience, the remarkably rapid recovery of adolescents after each treatment and their resistance to the development of measurable cognitive side effects make it unlikely that such concerns have merit. As discussed above, the studies by Ghaziuddin and colleagues

(2000) and Cohen and colleagues (2000) of follow ups ranging from 8 months to 3.5 years, provide additional reassurance that the cognitive effects of ECT in adolescents are similar to (and no worse than) those in adults.

With additional ECT treatments, the EEG shows progressive slowing of frequencies, increased amplitudes, and well-defined burst formations during interictal recording (Fink, 1979; Fink & Kahn, 1957). These manifestations are sensitive to age, being more common in the elderly. Such EEG slowing may be associated with confusion, disorientation, and impairment of immediate recall. Generally with adolescents, such interictal confusion is rare, despite marked slowing of EEG frequencies.

PSYCHOSOCIAL ISSUES

In addition to its biological effects, ECT elicits strong intrapsychic and interpersonal responses. It should not be surprising that a treatment involving passage of an electrical current through a patient's head while asleep is perceived as powerful and mysterious. ECT arouses fears and fantasies in patients, parents, family members, and peers alike. Patients may feel quite vulnerable as they lie partially disrobed on a stretcher, waiting for treatment to commence, and this experience can raise issues of trust and personal bodily autonomy, especially in patients with a history of trauma. These fears can be minimized by providing ongoing education, ensuring that the treatment team members are well known to the patient and are experienced in ECT, and by paying careful attention to the anxieties and concerns of the patient and family.

Patient attitude surveys in adults have found that although ECT is typically poorly understood, the experience is not considered frightening (Benbow, 1988; Cowley, 1985; Fox, 1993; Hughes et al., 1981; Pettinati et al., 1994; Pettit, 1971). In fact, in the experience of some patients, it has been regarded as no more upsetting than a trip to the dentist (Malcolm, 1989). Similar studies are badly needed in the young.

MECHANISM OF ACTION OF ECT

Despite considerable research, the mechanism of action of ECT remains a mystery. ECT produces a number of changes in brain chemistry, endocrinology, and electrophysiology. Current hypotheses of the mechanism of action of ECT focus on changes in hypothalamic neuroendocrine status (Fink, 1990), changes in brain neurotransmitters (these are similar but not identical to those seen with antidepressant drug therapy) (Nutt et al., 1993), or increases in seizure threshold (Sackeim, 1999) over the course of the treatment. It remains unclear however, whether any of these neurobiological changes accounts for the clinical effects of ECT, or whether they represent merely epiphenomena.

OTHER BRAIN STIMULATION THERAPIES

A number of other brain stimulation therapies are currently under investigation for treatment of mood disorders in adults, including rapid transcranial magnetic stimulation, deep brain stimulation, and magnetic seizure therapy (Lisanby, 2002). Vagus nerve stimulation has recently been approved by the FDA for treatment-refractory depression in adults; there are no data on this procedure in children and adolescents with mood disorders.

CONCLUSION

A growing clinical experience suggests that ECT may be an effective treatment for severe mood disorders and other selected psychiatric disorders in adolescents and possibly children. These response rates are particularly noteworthy because almost all of the patients were severely ill (some had catatonia) and had failed to respond to multiple trials of medications and various psychotherapies. Recent guidelines from the American Psychiatric Association (2001) and the American Academy of Child and Adolescent Psychiatry (2004) now endorse the use of ECT, although there remains an emphasis (unnecessarily restrictive?) on its role as a treatment of "last resort." The improved safety of contemporary ECT constitutes a compelling argument for its increased consideration in the treatment of adolescents with acute mental illness, especially when the illness is severe enough to require hospital care and is complicated by psychosis, inanition, suicidality, catatonia, delirium, or stupor.

An urgent need exists for more research on the efficacy, side effects, treatment technique, and mechanism of action of ECT in children and adolescents. We also need studies that clarify the attitudes and experiences of patients and their parents to the experience of ECT. Equally compelling is the need for education to promote a heightened understanding of ECT by child and adolescent psychiatrists.

REFERENCES

Abrams R. (2002). *Electroconvulsive Therapy.* 4th Ed. New York: Oxford University Press.

American Academy of Child and Adolescent Psychiatry. (2004). Summary of the practice parameter for use of electroconvulsive therapy with adolescents. *J Am Acad Child Adolesc Psychiatry* 43:119–122.

American Psychiatric Association. (1978). *Electroconvulsive Therapy* (Task Force Report No. 14). Washington, D.C.: American Psychiatric Association.

American Psychiatric Association. (1990). *The Practice of Electroconvulsive Therapy: Recommendations for Treatment, Training and Privileging.* Washington, D.C.: American Psychiatric Association.

American Psychiatric Association. (2001). *The Practice of Electroconvulsive Therapy: Recommendations for Treatment, Training and Privileging.* 2nd Ed. Washington, D.C.: American Psychiatric Association.

Baker T. (1995). ECT and young minds (letter). *Lancet* 345:65.

Baline SH, Rifkin A, Kayne E, et al. (2000). Comparison of bifrontal and bitemporal ECT for major depression. *Am J Psychiatry* 157:121–123.

Benbow SM. (1998). Patients' views on electroconvulsive therapy on completion of a course of treatment. *Convuls Ther* 4:146–162.

Bender L. (1947). One hundred cases of childhood schizophrenia treated with electric shock. *Trans Am Neurol Assoc* 72:165–169.

Bertagnoli MW, Borchardt CM. (1990). A review of ECT for children and adolescents. *J Am Acad Child Adolesc Psychiatry* 29:302–307.

Black DWG, Wilcox JA, Stewart M. (1985). The use of ECT in children: case report. *J Clin Psychiatry* 46:98–99.

Bloch Y, Levcovitch Y, Bloch AM, et al. (2001). Electroconvulsive therapy in adolescents: similarities to and differences from adults. *J Am Acad Child Adolesc Psychiatry* 40:1332–1336.

Bolwig TG, Hertz MM, Paulson OB, et al. (1977). Blood-brain barrier during electroshock seizures in man. *Eur J Clin Invest* 7:87–93.

Braasch ER, Demaso DR. (1980). Effect of electroconvulsive therapy on serum isoenzymes. *Am J Psychiatry* 137:625–626.

Broderson P, Paulson OB, Bolwig TG, et al. (1973). Cerebral hyperemia in electrically induced epileptic seizures. *Arch Neurol* 28:334– 338.

Brumback RA, Staton RD. (1982). The electroencephalographic pattern during electroconvulsive therapy. *Clin Electroencephalogr* 13:148–153.

Calev A, Pass HL, Shapira B, et al. (1993). ECT and memory. In: Coffey CE, ed. *The Clinical Science of ECT*. Washington, D.C.: American Psychiatric Press, pp 125–142.

Camfield PR. (1997). Recurrent seizures in the developing brain are not harmful. *Epilepsia* 38:735–737.

Carr V, Dorrington C, Schrader G, et al. (1983). The use of ECT for mania in childhood bipolar disorder. *Br J Psychiatry* 143:411–415.

Chung KF. (2003). Electroconvulsive therapy in Hong Kong: Rates of use, indications, and outcome. *J ECT* 19:98–102.

Cizadlo BC, Wheaton A. (1995). ECT treatment of a young girl with catatonia: a case study. *J Am Acad Child Adolesc Psychiatry* 34:332–335.

Clardy ER, Rumpf EM. (1954). The effect of electric shock on children having schizophrenic manifestations. *Psychiatr Q* 28:616–623.

Coffey CE. (1987). Structural brain imaging and electroconvulsive therapy. In: Coffey CE, ed. *The Clinical Science of ECT*. Washington, D.C.: American Psychiatric Press, pp 73–92.

Coffey CE. (1998). The pre-ECT evaluation. *Psychiat Ann* 28:506–508.

Coffey CE, Hoffman G, Weiner RD, et al. (1987). Electroconvulsive therapy in a depressed patient with a functioning ventriculo-atrial shunt. *Convuls Ther* 3:302–306.

Coffey CE, Weiner RD, Djang WT, et al. (1991). Brain anatomic effects of ECT: a prospective magnetic resonance imaging study. *Arch Gen Psychiatry* 48:1013–1021.

Coffey CE, Lucke J, Weiner RD, et al. (1995a). Seizure threshold in electroconvulsive therapy, I: initial seizure threshold. *Biol Psychiatry* 37:13–20.

Coffey CE, Lucke J, Weiner RD, et al. (1995b). Seizure threshold in electroconvulsive therapy, II: the anticonvulsant effect of ECT. *Biol Psychiatry* 37:777–788.

Coffey CE, Kellner CH. (2000). Electroconvulsive therapy in geriatric neuropsychiatry. In: Coffey CE, Cummings JL, eds. *Textbook of Geriatric Neuropsychiatry*. 2nd Ed. Washington D.C.: American Psychiatric Press, pp 829–859.

Cohen D, Cottias C, Basquin M. (1997). Cotard's syndrome in a 15-year-old girl. *Acta Psychiatr Scand* 95:164–165.

Cohen D, Flament M, Dubos PF, et al. (1999). Case series: catatonic syndrome in young people. *J Am Acad Child Adolesc Psychiatry* 38:1040–1046.

Cohen D, Taieb O, Flament M, et al. (2000). Absence of cognitive impairment at long-term follow-up in adolescents treated with ECT for severe mood disorder. *Am J Psychiatry* 157:460–462.

Consensus Conference. (1985). Electroconvulsive therapy. *JAMA* 254:2103–2108.

Cook A, Scott A. (1992). ECT for young people. *Br J Psychiatry* 161:718–719.

Cowley PN. (1985). An investigation of patients' attitudes to ECT by means of Q-analysis. *Psychol Med* 15:131–139.

Devanand DP, Dwork AJ, Hutchinson ER, et al. (1994). Does ECT alter brain structure? *Am J Psychiatry* 151:957–970.

Duffett R, Hill P, Lelliott P. (1999). Use of electroconvulsive therapy in young people. *Br J Psychiatry* 175:228–230.

El-Ganzouri AR, Ivankovich AD, Braverman B, et al. (1985). Monoamine oxidase inhibitors: should they be discontinued preoperatively? *Anesth Analg* 64:592–596.

Fink M. (1979). *Convulsive Therapy: Theory and Practice*. New York: Raven.

Fink M. (1988). Convulsive therapy: a manual of practice. In: Frances AJ, Hales RE, eds. *American Psychiatric Press Review of Psychiatry*, Vol 7. Washington, D.C.: American Psychiatric Press, pp 482–497.

Fink M. (1990). How does convulsive therapy work? *Neuropsychopharmacology* 3:73–82.

Fink M. (1993a). Who should get ECT? In: Coffey CE, ed. *The Clinical Science of Electroconvulsive Therapy*. Washington, D.C.: American Psychiatric Press, pp 3–16.

Fink M. (1993b). Post-ECT delirium. *Convuls Ther* 9:326–330.

Fink M. (1994). Combining electroconvulsive therapy and drugs: a review of safety and efficacy. *CNS Drugs* 1:370–376.

Fink M, Kahn RL. (1957). Relation of EEG delta activity to behavioral response in electroshock: quantitative serial studies. *Arch Neurol and Psychiatry* 78:516–525.

Fink M, Abrams R, Bailine S, et al. (1996). Ambulatory ECT: report of the Association of Convulsive Therapy Task Force. *Convuls Ther* 12:42–55.

Fox HA. (1993). Patients' fear of and objection to electroconvulsive therapy. *Hosp Commun Psychiatry* 44:357–360.

Frank E, Kupfer DJ, Perel JM, et al. (1990). Three-year outcomes for maintenance therapies in recurrent depression. *Arch Gen Psychiatry* 47:1093–1099.

Freeman CP, ed. (1995). *The ECT Handbook: The Second Report of the Royal College of Psychiatrists' Special Committee on ECT*. London: Royal College of Psychiatrists.

Fried D, Mann JJ. (1988). Electroconvulsive treatment of a patient with a known intracranial tumor. *Biol Psychiatry* 23:176–180.

Ghaziuddin N, King CA, Naylor MW, et al. (1996). Electroconvulsive treatment in adolescents with pharmacotherapy-resistant depression. *J Child Adolesc Psychopharmacol* 6:259–271.

Ghaziuddin N, Laughrin D, Giordani B. (2000). Cognitive side effects of electroconvulsive therapy in adolescents. *J Child Adolesc Psychopharmacol* 10:269–276.

Ghaziuddin N, Kaza M, Ghazi N, et al. (2001). Electroconvulsive therapy for minors: experiences and attitudes of child psychiatrists and psychologists. *J ECT* 17:109–117.

Ghaziuddin N, Alkhouri I, Champine D, et al. (2002). ECT treatment of malignant catatonia/NMS in an adolescent: a useful lesson in delayed diagnosis and treatment. *J ECT* 18:95–98.

Greenberg LB, Mofson R, Fink M. (1988). Prospective electroconvulsive therapy in a delusional depressed patient with a frontal meningioma: a case report. *Br J Psychiatry* 153:105–107.

Grunhaus L, Dolberg O, Lustig M. (1995). Relapse and recurrence following a course of ECT: reasons for concern and strategies for further investigation. *J Psychiatr Res* 29:165–172.

Gurevitz S, Helme WH. (1954). Effects of electroconvulsive therapy on personality and intellectual functioning of the schizophrenic child. *J Nerv Ment Dis* 120:213–226.

Guttmacher LB, Cretella H. (1988). Electroconvulsive therapy in one child and three adolescents. *J Clin Psychiatry* 49:20–23.

Hedge GR, Srinath S, Sheshadri AP, et al. (1997). More on ECT (letter). *J Am Acad Child Adolesc Psychiatry* 36:446–447.

Hemphill RE, Walter WG. (1941). The treatment of mental disorders by electrically induced convulsions. *J Ment Sci* 87:256–275.

Hermann RC, Dorwart RA, Hoover CW, et al. (1995). Variation in ECT use in the United States. *Am J Psychiatry* 152: 869–875.

Heuyer G, Bour F. (1942). Electrochoc chez des adolescents. *Ann Med Psychol* (Paris) 2:75–84.

Heuyer G, Bour F, Leroy R. (1943). L'electrochoc chez les enfants. *Ann Med Psychol* (Paris) 2:402–407.

Hill MA, Courvoisie H, Dawkins K, et al. (1997). ECT treatment of intractable mania in two prepubertal male children. *Convuls Ther* 13:74–82.

Howie MB, Black HA, Zvar AD, et al. (1990). Esmolol reduces autonomic hypersensitivity and length of seizures induced by electroconvulsive therapy. *Anesth Analg* 71: 384–388.

Hughes J, Barraclough BM, Reeve W. (1981). Are patients shocked by ECT? *J R Soc Med* 74:283–285.

Jarvie H. (1954). Prognosis of depression treated by electric convulsive therapy. *BMJ* 1:132–134.

Jeffries JJ, LeFebre A. (1973). Depression and mania associated with Kleine-Levin-Critchley syndrome. *Can Psychiatr J* 18:439–444.

Kellner C, ed. (1993). ECT and drugs: concurrent administration. *Convuls Ther* 9:237–351.

Klapheke MM. (1993). Combining ECT and antipsychotic agents: benefits and risks. *Convuls Ther* 9:241–255.

Kramer BA. (1985). Use of ECT in California, 1977–1983. *Am J Psychiatry* 142:1190–1192.

Krystal AD. (1998). The clinical utility of ictal EEG seizure adequacy models. *Psychiatric Annals* 28:3035.

Krystal AD, Coffey CE. (1997). Neuropsychiatric considerations in the use of electroconvulsive therapy. *J Neuropsychiatry Clin Neurosci* 9: 283–292.

Kutcher S, Robertson HA. (1995). Electroconvulsive therapy in treatment-resistant bipolar youth. *J Child Adolesc Psychopharmacol* 5: 167–175.

Lisanby SH. (2002). Update on magnetic seizure therapy: a novel form of convulsive therapy. *J ECT* 18:182–188.

Malcolm K. (1989). Patients' perceptions and knowledge of electroconvulsive therapy. *Psychiatr Bull* 13:161–165.

Malek-Ahmadi P, Sedler RR. (1989). Electroconvulsive therapy and asymptomatic meningioma. *Convuls Ther* 5:168–170.

Mander AJ, Whitfield A, Kean DM, et al. (1987). Cerebral and brain stem changes after ECT by nuclear magnetic resonance imaging. *Br J Psychiatry* 151:69–71.

Maneksha FR. (1991). Hypertension and tachycardia during electroconvulsive therapy. *Convuls Ther* 7:28–35.

Mansheim P. (1983). ECT in the treatment of a depressed adolescent with meningomyelocele, hydrocephalus, and seizures. *J Clin Psychiatry* 44:385–386.

McCall WV, Reboussin DM, Weiner RD, et al. (2000). Titrated moderately suprathreshold vs fixed high-dose right unilateral electroconvulsive therapy. *Arch Gen Psychiatry* 57:438–444.

Messina AG, Paranicas M, Katz B, et al. (1992). Effect of electroconvulsive therapy on the electrocardiogram and echocardiogram. *Anesth Analg* 75:511–514.

Moise FN, Petrides G. (1996). Case study: electroconvulsive therapy in adolescents. *J Am Acad Child Adolesc Psychiatry* 35:312–318.

Motoyama EK. (1996). Safety and outcome in pediatric anesthesia. In: Motoyama EK, Davis PJ, eds. *Smith's Anesthesia for Infants and Children.* St. Louis, MO: CV Mosby, pp 897–908.

Nutt DJ, Gleiter CH, Glue P. (1993). Neuropharmacological aspects of ECT: in search of the primary mechanism of action. *Convuls Ther* 5: 250–260.

Otegui JT, Lyford-Pike A, Zurmendi P, et a1. (1995), Electroconvulsive therapy in adolescents and children in private hospitals in Montevideo (Uruguay) (abstract). *Convuls Ther* 11:73.

Paillere-Martinot M-L, Zivi A, Basquin M. (1990). Utilization de l'ECT chez l'adolescent. *Encephale* 16:399–404.

Parmar R. (1993). Attitudes of child psychiatrists to electroconvulsive therapy. *Psychiatr Bull* 17:12–13.

Petrides G, Bush G, Francis AJ. (1995). Combined lorazepam and ECT to treat catatonia (NR490). In: *New Research Program and Abstracts: American Psychiatric Association 148th Annual Meeting,* Miami, FL, May 1995. Washington, D.C.: American Psychiatric Association, pp 186–187.

Petrides G, Maneksha F, Zervas I, et al. (1996). Trimethaphan (Arfonad) control of hypertension and tachycardia during electroconvulsive therapy: a double-blind study. *J Clin Anesthesia* 8:104–109.

Pettinati HM, Tamburello TA, Ruetsch CR, et al. (1994). Patient attitudes toward electroconvulsive therapy. *Psychopharmacol Bull* 30: 471–475.

Pettit DE. (1971). Patients' attitudes toward ECT-not the "shocker" we think? *Can Psychiatr Assoc J* 16:365–366.

Pippard J, Ellam L. (1981). *Electroconvulsive Treatment in Great Britian.* London: Headley Brothers Ltd. The Invicta Press.

Powell JC, Silviera WR, Lindsay R. (1988). Pre-pubertal depressive stupor: a case report. *Br J Psychiatry* 153:689–692.

Prien R, Kupfer DJ. (1986). Continuation drug therapy for major depressive episodes: how long should it be maintained? *Am J Psychiatry* 143:18–23.

Prohovnik I, Sackeim HA, Decina P, et al. (1986). Acute reductions of regional cerebral blood flow following electroconvulsive therapy. Interactions with modality and time. *Ann NY Acad Sci* 462:249–262.

Rey JM, Walter G. (1997). Half a century of ECT use in young people. *Am J Psychiatry* 154:595–602.

Rosenbach ML, Herman RC, Dorwart RA. (1997). Use of electroconvulsive therapy in the Medicare population between 1987 and 1992. *Psychiatr Serv* 48:1537–1542.

Sackeim HA. (1999). The anticonvulsant hypothesis of the mechanisms of action of ECT: current status. *J ECT* 15:5–26.

Sackeim HA, Decina P, Prohovnik I, et al. (1987). Seizure threshold in electroconvulsive therapy: effects of sex, age, electrode placement, and number of treatments. *Arch Gen Psychiatry* 44:355–360.

Sackeim HA, Prudic J, Devanand DP, et al. (1993). Effects of stimulus intensity and electrode placement on the efficacy and cognitive effects of electroconvulsive therapy. *N Engl J Med* 328:839–846.

Sackeim HA, Prudic J, Devanand DP, et al. (2000). A prospective, randomized, double-blind comparison of bilateral and right unilateral electroconvulsive therapy at different stimulus intensities. *Arch Gen Psychiatry* 57:425–434.

Sackeim HA, Devanand DP, Lisanby SH, et al. (2001). Treatment of the modal patient: does one size fit all? *J ECT* 17:219–231.

Schneekloth D, Rummans A, Logan KM. (1993). Electroconvulsive therapy in adolescents. *Convuls Ther* 9:158–166.

Scott AI, Douglas RH, Whitfield A, et al. (1990). Time course of cerebral magnetic resonance changes after electroconvulsive therapy. *Br J Psychiatry* 156:551–553.

Scott AI, Gardner M, Good R. (2005). Fall in ECT use in young people in Edinburgh. *J ECT* 21:50.

Staton RD, Hass PJ, Brumback RA. (1981). Electroencephalographic recording during bitemporal and unilateral nondominant hemisphere (Lancaster position) electroconvulsive therapy. *J Clin Psychiatry* 42:264–269, 337.

Stoudemire A, Knos G, Gladson M, et al. (1990). Labetalol in the control of cardiovascular responses to electroconvulsive therapy in high-risk depressed medical patients. *J Clin Psychiatry* 51:508–512.

Strober M, Rao U, DeAntonia M, et al. (1998). Effect of electroconvulsive treatment in adolescents with severe endogenous depression resistant to pharmacotherapy. *Biol Psychiatry* 43:335–338.

Summers WK, Robins E, Reich F. (1979). The natural history of acute organic mental syndrome after bilateral electroconvulsive therapy. *Biol Psychiatry* 14:905–912.

Thompson JW, Blaine JD. (1987). Use of ECT in the United States in 1975 and 1980. *Am J Psychiatry* 144:557–562.

Walter G, Rey JM. (1997), An epidemiological study of the use of ECT in adolescents. *J Am Acad Child Adolesc Psychiatry* 36:809–815.

Walter G, Rey JM. (2003a). Has the practice and outcome of ECT in adolescents changed? Findings from a whole-population study. *J ECT* 19:84–87.

Walter G, Rey JM. (2003b). How fixed are child psychiatrists' views about ECT in the young? *J ECT* 19:88–92.

Warren AC, Holroyd S, Folstein MF. (1989). Major depression in Down's syndrome. *Br J Psychiatry* 155:202–205.

Wasterlain CG. (1997). Recurrent seizures in the developing brain are harmful. *Epilepsia* 38:728–734.

Webb MC, Coffey CE, Saunders WR, et al. (1990). Cardiovascular response to unilateral electroconvulsive therapy. *Biol Psychiatry* 28: 758–766.

Weiner R. (1984). Does electroconvulsive therapy cause brain damage? *Behav Brain Sci* 7:1–53.

Weiner R, Krystal AD. (1993). EEG monitoring of ECT seizures. In: Coffey CE, ed. *The Clinical Science of ECT.* Washington, D.C.: American Psychiatric Press, pp 93–109.

Welborn LG. (1996). Pediatric outpatient anesthesia. In: Motoyama EK, Davis PJ, eds. *Smith's Anesthesia for Infants and Children.* St. Louis, MO: Mosby, pp 709–725.

Welch CA, Drop LJ. (1989). Cardiovascular effects of ECT. *Convuls Ther* 5:35–43.

Zaw FKM, Bates GDL, Murali V, et al. (1999). Catatonia, autism, and ECT. *Dev Med Child Neurol* 41:843–845.

Zwil AS, Bowring MA, Price TRP, et al. (1990). Prospective electroconvulsive therapy in the presence of intracranial tumor. *Convuls Ther* 6:299–307.

Genetic Evaluation, Counseling, and Treatment

29

Carol E. Anderson, MD

Information from the Human Genome Project (Venter et al., 2001; Sachidanandam et al., 2001) is being applied in virtually all medical subspecialties to study, understand, diagnose, and treat human disorders. Initial application of linkage analysis and positional cloning was successful in identifying the gene alterations (genotype) responsible for over 1,000 single gene disorders (most often ones with a secure *phenotype*, a change or changes observed on examination, radiograph, or biochemical testing that allow diagnosis reflecting the effects or manifestations of the changed genotype or genotypes.) Single gene syndromes including complex, heterogeneous phenotypes, such as breast cancer (Miki et al., 1994; Wooster et al., 1995) or colorectal cancer (Nishisho et al., 1991), offer insights into the pathogenesis of these disorders. With knowledge of the interaction of multiple genes to result in genetic susceptibility (as well as the environmental triggering factors) comes the possibility of presymptomatic measurement of genetic susceptibility, with subsequent manipulation of contributing molecular and environmental factors. However, the ability to perform such measurement and manipulation carries a heavy price of responsibility and raises difficult questions about the future role of gene testing and therapy in the treatment of human disease.

The first part of this chapter provides a brief overview of the history of genetics and introduce some of the various molecular biological techniques used in genetic research. The next section outlines the known categories of inheritance, including examples of the disorders associated with each. An approach to clinical genetic evaluation and genetic counseling is outlined. In the final section of the chapter I introduce current approaches to the treatment of genetic disorders, and touch briefly on the future possibilities of gene therapy in neuropsychiatry.

HISTORY OF GENETICS

The history of genetics as a scientific discipline is only a little more than a century old. Gregor Mendel published his studies of breeding in peas in 1866. Based on his observations, he suggested that discrete *elements*, or *genes*, explain the inheritance of traits from generation to generation (Mendel, 1866/1965). In the early 1900s, these concepts were rediscovered and applied to understanding the inheritance of human characteristics. It was only as recently as 1956 that techniques for visualizing human chromosomes confirmed that the normal human diploid number was 46. Lyon's (1968) hypothesis regarding X-inactivation allowed a better understanding of the role of the one remaining active X chromosome in development. The introduction of special banding techniques in the 1970s permitted a more detailed analysis of portions of specific chromosomes, and somatic cell hybridization began to enable the mapping of human genes.

Since Watson and Crick in 1953 first proposed the structure of DNA as the basis of inheritance, a proliferation of molecular techniques based on the *one gene–one protein* model has allowed for the identification and manipulation of individual genes as well as the elucidation of their structure, function, and pathology. It is estimated that the human genome contains approximately 30,000 genes. McKusick's *Online Mendelian Inheritance in Man* (OMIM) surpassed 10,000 entries in December, 1998, and included over 14,000 entries in January, 2004. Only a small proportion of human disorders have been fully understood at the gene level. The following section briefly reviews some of the techniques used to identify and study genes.

MOLECULAR BIOLOGICAL TECHNIQUES

Techniques in molecular biology are based on our understanding of how deoxyribonucleic acid (DNA) underlies inheritance. At the heart of the Watson–Crick hypothesis was the precept that complementary strands of DNA form the basis of DNA replication, transcription, and translation into protein. Following the rules of base pairing (i.e., adenine pairing with thymine and cytosine with guanine), DNA polymerase adds bases to the template of each of two parental strands to form two identical offspring strands. In transcription, the DNA serves as a basis for the formation of messenger RNA (mRNA, in which uridine takes the place of thymine). The single-stranded mRNA contains sequences that are translated into protein (exons), together with intervening sequences (introns) that are spliced from the mRNA before nuclear transport and subsequent translation into a protein on the ribosomes. The genetic code involved in the translation of the mRNA sequence into protein is the three-nucleotide unit (codon) that specifies insertion of a particular amino acid in sequence into the protein. Thus, for example, AAA or AAG in genomic DNA specifies phenylalanine. The AUG codon for methionine is part of the initiation sequence of every mRNA molecule. The ACT codon in genomic DNA functions as a stop signal. There are numerous transcriptional, translational, and posttranslational controls on the process by which a gene or sequence of nucleotides specifies a protein. Whereas a mutation or change in the DNA sequence in the coding region may result in an altered protein product, with possible loss or gain of function of that protein, mutations in the regulatory regions may alter the quantity of protein made.

Recombinant DNA Technology

Because the Watson–Crick rules describe how base pairs hybridize, a complementary sequence of DNA, called a *probe*, can be used to show whether a given gene is present in a sample of DNA. Hybridization with the gene sequence of interest can be indicated by radioactive labeling of the probe. If the mRNA for a given protein can be isolated and purified, reverse transcriptase can be used to generate that protein's cDNA (complementary DNA) molecule. This probe will hybridize only with the translated (not the genomic)

sequences, including both the exons and the introns. If a probe for a protein is available, the gene for that protein product can be cloned and introduced into a bacterial species, where it can be produced in quantity, allowing subsequent characterization or manipulation. This procedure is the basis of recombinant DNA technology. The probe is used to identify which colonies of the bacteria carry the desired gene, so that they can be selected and grown in quantity. The gene can be sequenced to determine the exact order of bases, and this sequence of bases can then be compared with sequences of other known genes in computer databases to look for homology. The sequencing procedure is illustrated in Figure 29.1, which shows how a point mutation yields a protein with altered function, resulting in disease.

Southern Blotting

Molecular techniques have made possible the diagnosis of many genetic disorders. One such technique, Southern blotting, is based on digestion of DNA by restriction enzymes.

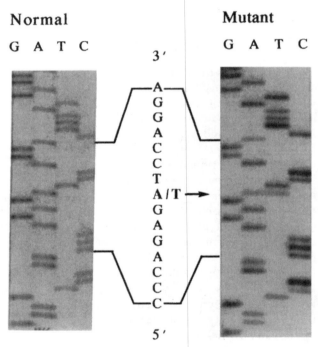

Figure 29.1 An autoradiograph of a portion of two DNA-sequencing gels. Each gel is produced according to the method of Sanger: DNA is added to each of four tubes, together with enzyme, reaction mixture, and a radioactive label specific for one of the four nucleic acids (guanine, adenine, thymine, or cytosine). DNA sequences are terminated at each position occupied by the nucleic acid studied in that tube, and a label is attached to the terminal nucleic acid position. After electrophoresis, the gel is exposed to x-ray film. For comparison, the normal sequence from a portion of "control" hexosaminidase is shown at left to illustrate a point mutation in the "mutant" sample shown at right. An adenine-to-thymine change is illustrated.
Source: Figure courtesy of Eugene Grebner, PhD, and Jerzy Tomczak, DVM, Tay-Sachs Laboratory, Jefferson Medical College, Philadelphia, PA.

More than 100 of such restriction enzymes have been characterized. These endonucleases cleave DNA at specified base-pair sequences, termed *recognition sites*, generating DNA fragments whose lengths are determined by the distance between recognition sites. After separation of the fragments according to length on gel electrophoresis, the DNA is transferred to a nitrocellulose filter. With radioactively-labeled probes, the fragments containing the gene (or portion of the gene) are shown by autoradiography. A decrease in size (deletion) or an increase in size (insertion or duplication) of the gene can be determined in this way.

Polymerase Chain Reaction Analysis

Another revolutionary technique, which requires relatively small amounts of biological material and greatly speeds analysis, is polymerase chain reaction (PCR) analysis. Knowledge of the base sequence in the region around the DNA of interest is required. Oligonucleotide probes complementary to the two ends of the sequence to be amplified must be constructed. Each probe hybridizes and then acts as a primer for a thermophilic DNA polymerase that uses nucleotide precursors to produce two copies of the sequence to be amplified. Successive cycles (determined by temperature changes) of denaturation, annealing (primer hybridization), and synthesis result in orders-of-magnitude amplification of the sequence of interest in less than a day. Direct visualization of the PCR-amplified sequence by ultraviolet fluorescence yields rapid results.

Linkage Analysis

If a mutation of interest alters a specific restriction site, Southern blotting, or PCR analysis can be used to show the difference in length that results after restriction enzyme digestion. In instances where the mutation is not known, linkage analysis will identify other inherited variations in nearby restriction sites to indirectly indicate whether a DNA segment of interest is present. Because alteration of the restriction sites results in sequences of varying length after digestion with the appropriate restriction enzyme, and because these restriction-length patterns are inherited according to Mendelian modes, such restriction fragment length polymorphisms (RFLPs) can be used as markers in linkage analysis. Variable-number tandem repeats (VNTRs) represent a special case of the RFLP category; these highly polymorphic markers have proved extremely useful in family studies. Finally, the sequencing of the human genome has made it possible to use single-nucleotide polymorphisms (SNPs) for linkage and association studies.

Linkage analysis is a tool used for gene mapping as well as molecular diagnosis. Such analysis is based on family studies and the physical presence of two loci located very close together on the same chromosome. Assumptions underlying linkage analyses include the gene model (e.g., single-gene, multifactorial), the mode of inheritance

(e.g., autosomal dominant, autosomal recessive, X-linked), and the penetrance. When loci are inherited together, they are said to be *linked*. The greater the distance between the two loci, the less linked they will appear, as the result of meiotic recombination secondary to formation of chiasmata, crossing over, and recombination. Thus, if the genes are on different chromosomes or are sufficiently far apart on the same chromosome, they will appear to assort independently in families and will not appear to be linked as they pass from one generation to the next. *Genetic distance*, the percentage of recombinants, is related to the physical distance between loci, but not in a one-to-one manner. Genetic distance is expressed in centimorgans (cM), where 1 cM represents 1% recombination.

Through linkage analysis, a marker with a known mode of inheritance can be used to locate another gene whose location was previously unknown. A *lod score* of 3 is usually required as proof of linkage (the lod score is a logarithmic expression; the logarithm of 3 means that the odds of linkage at a given distance between the two loci is 1,000 [103] times greater than that of no linkage). Calculation of the lod score is usually performed by computer program and is based on the principle of maximum likelihood analysis. This kind of analysis (based on the known mode of inheritance) was used to locate the genes for Huntington's disease (see Chapter 21), cystic fibrosis, and neurofibromatosis. Linkage analysis has also been used in certain family situations for presymptomatic or prenatal diagnosis of disorders, such as Duchenne's muscular dystrophy or hemophilia A (Antonarakis, 1989).

Good reviews have been written on the statistical basis of linkage analysis (Ott, 1991) as well as on the difficulties in applying the technique to behavioral disorders (Gershon & Cloninger, 1994), because for complex human diseases there is not a simple mode of genetic inheritance and accurate categorization as to who is affected and who is not proves difficult.

The techniques described have been applied to dissection of DNA changes, especially as they relate to the etiology of human conditions; that is, genomics. An alternative but complementary approach is proteomics, the application of techniques such as two-dimensional gel electrophoresis or mass spectroscopy to the analysis of the gene products, proteins. Proteomics can be applied to analyze the response of cells in culture exposed to specific states, such as inflammation, drugs, or toxins, and to look at pathways and signaling networks involved in the response to those conditions. It is possible, based on genetic code, to work backward, from the protein of interest to identify the genes involved in the cellular response. For example, if it were possible to look at a patient's response to stress, differences might be discerned between patients with depression from those without. Thus, it is hoped that the joint disciplines of genomics and proteomics can be applied to understand the pathophysiology of many poorly understood human conditions.

CATEGORIES OF INHERITANCE

Categories of inheritance include classical Mendelian modes (i.e., single-gene mutations), chromosomal mechanisms, multifactorial modes, and nonclassical mechanisms (i.e., mitochondrial mutation, genetic imprinting, and unstable repeat sequences).

Classical (Mendelian) Modes of Inheritance

Single-Gene Disorders

A single-gene disorder occurs when there is a mutation from the wild type allele at one locus (on one or both members of a pair of chromosomes) that results in an observable phenotypic change. Inheritance of the phenotype generally follows the Mendelian rules of inheritance: autosomal dominant, autosomal recessive, or X-linked. Based on population studies, it is estimated that the incidence of single-gene disorders is between 2 and 3% by 1 year of age but is closer to 5% by age 25 years (Baird et al., 1988). These percentages do not include disorders with potentially later onset or identification, such as Huntington's disease, spinocerebellar ataxia, neurofibromatosis, and bipolar depression. Patients with single-gene disorders are those most likely to be referred to a genetics clinic for evaluation or counseling because of a family history of the disorder.

With *autosomal dominant* inheritance of a phenotype, one dose of the altered gene results in some degree of expression of the phenotype. Thus, a parent with one mutated copy and one normal copy has a 50% chance of passing on the mutated gene to any offspring. The expression is variable. In general, there are few human examples of homozygosity for autosomal dominant mutations. Where such homozygosity has been proven (as in the case of a double dose of the mutation for achondroplasia), the phenotypic effects are more severe than those resulting from a single copy of the abnormal gene. The gender of the individual does not determine whether he or she will receive the altered gene, although gender may affect gene expression. Autosomal dominant traits pass from generation to generation (so-called vertical transmission), affecting on the average about half of the offspring of any affected individual.

In contrast, *autosomal recessive* inheritance of a disorder requires two doses of the mutant allele for any phenotypic effect. A single dose of a gene (i.e., carrier status) may pass through many generations without two carrier parents having any affected offspring. Only when both parents are carriers is there a 25% risk that an offspring will inherit a double dose of the mutant allele. Thus, more than one sibling of either gender may be affected within the same generation (so-called horizontal inheritance) with no family history. The rarer the gene, the more likely it is that consanguinity, the sharing of genes identical by descent, is present. Hence, many of the metabolic disorders included in newborn screening were described in the inbred Amish and Mennonites (Morton et al., 2003).

Finally, in *X-linked* inheritance, the female carrier is in general less severely affected than the hemizygous males. For *X-linked recessive* traits, the female carrier is usually unaffected. Half of her daughters on the average will be carriers, and half of her sons will be affected. Thus, the trait may appear to skip generations but will always be inherited through the maternal side. In contrast to autosomal dominant inheritance, in which vertical transmission may also occur, there will never be male-to-male transmission in X-linked recessive inheritance. A male with an X-linked recessive disorder will have no affected sons, but all of his daughters will be carriers. *X-linked dominant* traits are occasionally seen in which female carriers are more mildly affected than the hemizygous males in the family.

Variability and Heterogeneity

Several key concepts in clinical genetics should give rise to caution in the interpretation of family histories.

It is important to realize that for any of the three major single-gene categories of inheritance, affected individuals may have a negative family history for the disorder in question. For autosomal dominant and X-linked inherited traits, there may be a new mutation (in general, such new mutations are correlated with advanced age in the father of the affected individual). For recessive disorders, a negative family history is common unless there is inbreeding.

Another reason that phenotypes may appear not to follow Mendelian rules of inheritance has to do with *variability of expression*. For dominantly inherited traits in particular, there may be great variability in the nature and severity of the symptoms of the disorder, even within a single family (where presumably all of the affected members carry the same mutation). When there is variation in age at onset, earlier age at onset is taken to be an indicator of greater severity.

Finally, because of *genetic heterogeneity*, one phenotype can turn out to be related to many different genotypes. Tuberous sclerosis provides an example of this genetic heterogeneity. Linkage of tuberous sclerosis (see Chapter 22) with chromosome 9 was initially reported in the United Kingdom (Fryer et al., 1987). A report of positive linkage with chromosome 11 then came from the United States (Smith et al., 1990), although this linkage has not been extensively confirmed. Subsequently, the majority of families studied have shown linkage with chromosome 16 (Kandt et al., 1992). No clear phenotypic differences are observed among the families showing linkage to the different loci, other than the concurrence of infantile polycystic kidney disease with tuberous sclerosis pointing to the chromosome 16 locus where these genes are contiguous. Thus, to conduct a linkage analysis to determine which locus is responsible for the phenotype in a given family, sufficient numbers of affected and unaffected informative individuals must be alive and willing to cooperate with the studies. Only then could linkage analysis be used; for example, in a prenatal diagnosis. Detection of the putative allele would not allow prediction of the severity of the effects.

Another example of heterogeneity with even greater complexity is Alzheimer's disease. Only approximately 10% of Alzheimer's cases are inherited in an autosomal dominant fashion. There are no clear clinical differences between the familial and the sporadic cases. Furthermore, among the early onset familial cases, some are related to changes in an amyloid precursor protein (APP) gene on chromosome 21 (St. George-Hyslop et al., 1987) and others are related to a gene on chromosome 14 (St. George-Hyslop et al., 1992). Late-onset familial cases have been linked to chromosome 19 (Pericak-Vance et al., 1991), a finding that points to a possible role for the apolipoprotein E gene in sporadic cases of late-onset Alzheimer's disease (Corder et al., 1993). Familial cases constitute only a small portion, less than 10% of all patients with Alzheimer's disease, but they have contributed to understanding of the truly multifactorial majority of cases.

Occasionally, linkage analysis will demonstrate *allelic heterogeneity;* that is, different alleles within the same gene giving rise to slightly different phenotypes. For example, both the Duchenne and the Becker types of muscular dystrophy are linked to the dystrophin gene on the X chromosome. The Becker form of muscular dystrophy has a later onset and a milder course. Different areas within the gene represent deletional hot spots for the two disorders (Forrest et al., 1987; Monaco & Kunkel, 1987). Another gene in which linkage analysis revealed that different mutations or alleles gave rise to very different disorders is the Ll cell adhesion molecule gene (L1 CAM), which was found to be related to X-linked complicated spastic paraplegia, the MASA (mental retardation, aphasia, shuffling gait, and adducted thumbs) syndrome, and X-linked hydrocephalus associated with aqueductal stenosis (Fryns et al., 1991; Kenwrick et al., 1996; Rosenthal et al., 1992; Vits et al., 1994). Apparently because of the extensive role of the L1 CAM in brain development, alterations in different areas of the gene give rise to a variety of developmental brain anomalies.

Chromosomal Abnormalities

Chromosomes are the structures in which the genes are packaged. They are visible at the time of cell division. The normal diploid (2n) number of human chromosomes is 46. Twenty-two pairs of chromosomes are designated *autosomes,* with the remaining pair (the X and the Y) constituting the *sex chromosomes.* In general, just as one member of each pair of genes is inherited from each parent, one member of each chromosome pair is inherited from each parent. It is a matter of chance which member of the pair is inherited.

It is estimated that approximately 1 in 200 live newborns will have a chromosome abnormality. The frequency is even greater in perinatal deaths, in which the rate of chromosomal abnormality ranges from 5 to 10%. The frequency of chromosome disorders in first-trimester miscarriages is estimated to be approximately 50%. In general, chromosome disorders occur when there is either an excess or a deficiency of chromosomal material, both of which can arise either through a change in chromosome number or a rearrangement of chromosome structure.

Changes in chromosome number are of two types. In *polyploidy,* there is an abnormal multiple of the haploid number 23 (e.g., in triploidy, there are 69 chromosomes). In *aneuploidy,* the numerical deviation from normal is a discrete number of chromosomes. Deficiency of one chromosome (*monosomy*) is usually lethal; the most common monosomy compatible with survival is Turner syndrome (45,X). *Trisomy* refers to the presence of one extra chromosome; the most common live-born example of this deficiency is Down syndrome. The International System for Human Cytogenetic Nomenclature (ISCN) designation (Mitelman, 1995) for a male with trisomy 21 is 47,XY,+21.

Partial monosomy or trisomy can also arise by means of *structural rearrangements of chromosomes,* including deletion, duplication, translocation (reciprocal or Robertsonian), isochromosome formation, and inversion. Such rearrangements have been used to identify gene loci for single gene disorders such as Duchenne muscular dystrophy and neurofibromatosis, type I.

Cytogenetics is the study and analysis of chromosomes for structural abnormalities. Chromosomes are microscopically viewed in growing tissues where cells are dividing. For the sake of convenience, white cells from a heparinized blood sample are generally grown in tissue culture for diagnostic purposes. Colchicine is added to stop the process of mitosis at the metaphase stage. Hypotonic solution lyses the nuclear membrane, allowing the chromosomes from one cell to spread just far enough apart so that they can be stained, visualized with a microscope, and analyzed. Initially, chromosomes were homogeneously stained with Giemsa stain. With the development of special staining techniques in the 1970s, however, it became possible to evaluate chromosomes in greater detail. Pretreatment of the chromosome material with a protease (generally trypsin) allows for visualization of G-bands, and other stains identify different bands (e.g., Q-bands, R-bands, C-bands). *Preparing a karyotype* means arranging the pairs of chromosomes from one cell according to the lengths of the arms.

By standard G-banding, metaphase chromosomes contain between 200 and 550 bands. These bands allow for detailed analysis of rearrangements, but even the smallest visible deletion would involve 1 to 2% of a chromosome—anywhere from a few to 100 genes. In certain clinical situations in which a recognized multiple-malformation syndrome is suspected on the basis of a change involving one chromosome, *high-resolution chromosome analysis* is used to determine whether a *microdeletion*, that is, a deletion not usually detectable with standard G-banding, might account for the features observed in the affected individual. One of the best-known microdeletion syndromes is Prader-Willi syndrome, which is characterized by neonatal hypotonia, small hands and feet, distinctive facial features, short stature, mental retardation, and central obesity secondary to hyperphagia. About half of cases of Prader-Willi syndrome are related to a microdeletion in the long arm of chromosome 15 (Ledbetter et al., 1981).

High-resolution analysis of prometaphase chromosomes (which contain between 500 and 1,000 bands) is more difficult than standard G-banding of metaphase chromosomes. For this reason, this technique is usually reserved for situations in which a particular deletion is suspected based on clinical evidence. The laboratory conducting the analysis is dependent on information about the patient to know where to look for a potential chromosomal abnormality.

In addition to prometaphase cytogenetic techniques, a new technique, *fluorescent in situ hybridization (FISH) analysis*, allows for definition of submicroscopic deletions or cryptic rearrangements. DNA probes for the critical region-specific genetic sequences are tagged with fluorescent dyes. When these FISH probes hybridize with the chromosome preparations, they confirm the presence or absence of the segment under the fluorescent microscope in cases where the deletions are too small to see even with prometaphase methods. Figure 29.2 depicts a standard G-banded chromosome preparation, which appears to be that of a normal

female (46,XX); however, in Figure 29.3, a FISH study of the same subject indicates the presence of two number-15 chromosomes with deletion of the Prader-Willi syndrome critical area.

Microdeletion syndromes are being studied in an attempt to determine which of the contiguous genes in the missing region contributes to the phenotype. Thus, for example, in a patient with a deletion of one copy of the Prader-Willi syndrome critical area, if the single remaining dose carries an altered recessive gene, such as the P gene for type II oculocutaneous albinism, the patient's syndrome will manifest oculocutaneous albinism secondary to the one copy of the altered gene (Hamabe et al., 1991). In this way, the identity of other deleted genes contributing to the mental retardation or behavioral phenotype in Prader-Willi syndrome may be uncovered. No clear neuropathological correlates of the hyperphagia and food-seeking behavior have been found, although such correlates have been sought in neuropathological studies of the hypothalamus. Individuals with Prader-Willi syndrome may display temper tantrums, compulsivity, and aggression with regard to food (Dykens & Cassidy, 1995).

The number of known microdeletion syndromes is continually expanding (Table 29.1). Although there is

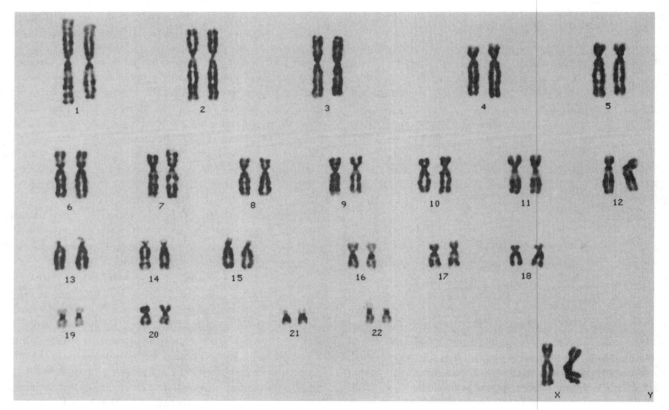

Figure 29.2 Standard G-banded human karyotype, with chromosomes arranged in pairs by size. The International System for Human Cytogenetic Nomenclature (ISCN) designation for this normal female karyotype would be 46,XX.
Source: Figure courtesy of Marge Sherwood, Cytogenetics Laboratory, Division of Medical Genetics, Jefferson Medical College, Philadelphia, PA.

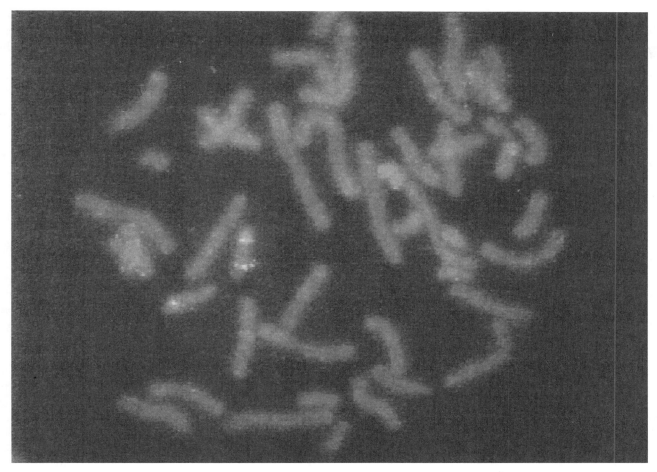

Figure 29.3 A fluorescent in situ hybridization (FISH) study on a metaphase spread. The chromosomes look orange when viewed under the fluorescent microscope. Fluorescein-tagged probes appear yellow. The metaphase preparation has been hybridized with a mixture of two cosmid probes. One identifies 15g11g12, the Prader-Willi syndrome/Angelman's syndrome (PWS/AS) critical region. The other probe hybridizes to the 15q22 area to identify the fact that there are two number-15 chromosomes. The analysis reveals two number-15 homologues but only one copy of the PWS/AS critical region. This microdeletion was not visible on prometaphase spreads. (For color detail, see full color insert.)
Source: Figure courtesy of Jolla Gibas, Cytogenetics Laboratory, Division of Medical Genetics, Jefferson Medical College, Philadelphia, PA.

theoretically no limit on the number of different chromosome abnormalities that can occur, syndromes defined by multiple cases have been catalogued in a number of comprehensive sources (Borgaonkar, 1991; DeGrouchy & Turleau, 1984; Gardner & Sutherland, 1989; Schinzel, 2001).

Multifactorial Conditions

The term *multifactorial inheritance* implies not only that single-gene inheritance has been ruled out but also that the familial aggregation noted for a trait accords with a series of predictions that follow from the hypothesis of multiple genes interacting with environmental factors to produce the trait. Examples of such traits include height and dermatoglyphic ridge counts.

The multifactorial model was developed by Carter in the 1960s specifically to describe his observation that

isolated birth defects (i.e., a single malformation that is not accompanied by other malformations suggestive of a syndrome or other disorder with single-gene inheritance) aggregate in families. Examples of such isolated malformations include neural tube defects and cleft lip (with or without cleft palate), each of which has a population incidence on the order of 1 in 1,000. In general, once the first family member is affected, the risk of the defects occurring in close relatives will be much greater than that in the general population (depending on the degree of relationship, or the number of genes shared in common); that is, approximately 5% for first-degree relatives. More distant relatives (who have fewer genes in common as well as fewer shared environmental exposures) will have a risk that is slightly higher than the population risk. When the ratio of affected individuals is skewed toward one gender, the risk to relatives will be greater when the index

TABLE 29.1

MICRODELETION SYNDROMES

AHD	arteriohepatic dysplasia (Alagille syndrome) (del 20pl l.23pl2.2)
ATMR	hemoglobin H/alpha-thalassemia-mental retardation (del 16pl3.3)
CDCR	choroideremia, deafness, clefting, and retardation (del Xg21)
DGS	DiGeorge/velocardiofacial syndrome (del 22g11)
DMD	Duchenne's muscular dystrophy and contiguous genes (del Xp21)
GCPS	Greig cephalopolysyndactyly (del 7p13)
HOLO	holoprosencephaly (one form) (del 7q34)
KAL	Kallmann's syndrome and contiguous genes (del Xp22.8)
MDS	Miller-Dieker syndrome (del 17p13)
PWS/AS	Prader-Willi syndrome/Angelman's syndrome (del 15q12)
RB	retinoblastoma (del 13g14.11)
RTS	Rubinstein-Taybi syndrome (del 16pl3.3)
SMS	Smith-Magenis syndrome (del 17pll.2)
STS	Steroid sulfatase deficiency (del Xp22.3)
TRP	trichorhinophalangeal/Langer-Giedion syndrome (del 8g24.1)
WS	Williams syndrome (del 7q11.23)
WAGR	Wilms' tumor, aniridica, genital abnormalities, and retardation (del llpl3)

Note: If one of these microdeletion syndromes is suspected, the clinician must convey specific clinical concerns to the molecular cytogenetics laboratory so that the appropriate prometaphase studies, fluorescent in situ hybridization studies, or uniparental disomy studies can be initiated. It is also important to understand the heterogeneity of these conditions, because for some syndromes only a portion of truly affected patients will show any positive diagnostic results. In these instances, the clinician should clearly communicate to the family that a negative result does not rule out the syndrome.

individual is the less frequently affected gender, as in the example of pyloric stenosis, in which the male-to-female ratio is 5 to 1, and the risk to the offspring of affected females is greater than that to the offspring of affected males. The greater the number of family members affected or the more severe the defect, the greater the risk to relatives. Once a trait's pattern of occurrence has been shown to accord with multifactorial predictions in a given population, empirical, or observed, risk estimates may be used for members of that population.

In practice, because of the possibility of genetic heterogeneity, family histories and medical examination results must be inspected for associated abnormalities. Teratological exposures must also be assessed, because, for example, a mother on an anticonvulsant who has a child with cleft lip will be more likely in future pregnancies to have a similarly affected child if her exposure to the drug continues. Because adequate studies do not exist for all relationships in all populations, empirical estimates must be offered with caution, as the best estimates available, but not as certain as Mendelian risk estimates (Bartley & Hall, 1978).

One example of a behavioral disorder with familial aggregation that does not fit Mendelian modes of inheritance is schizophrenia (see also Chapter 10). Whereas the lifetime risk of schizophrenia in the general population is roughly 1%, the risk is ten times greater in siblings or offspring (but slightly lower in parents) of an affected individual. If more relatives are affected, the risk increases from 9 to 10% with one sibling affected, to 16 to 30% when both a parent and a sibling already have the disorder.

Twin studies have been used in the attempt to unravel the nature-versus-nurture question for schizophrenia. Monozygotic twins have 100% of their genes in common; dizygotic twins have, on average, 50% of their genes in common. Thus, if genes have an important role in the etiology of a disorder, one would expect to see a higher concordance in monozygotic than in dizygotic twins. Adoption studies of schizophrenia have also been conducted to further delineate the separate contributions of nature and nurture. The results of these studies have supported the role of genes (as opposed to shared environment) in the disorder, because the pattern of occurrence was found to be related more to the diagnosis in the biological parents than to that in the adoptive parents.

However, identifying the genes predisposing to schizophrenia raises difficult methodological issues. In general, linkage analyses depend on the initial assumptions as to mode of inheritance of a single gene. Efforts to search the genome for genetic markers in extended families have been undertaken in the attempt to identify genes that may contribute to the multifactorial category of schizophrenia. However, initial positive results (Sherrington et al., 1988) have not been replicated in subsequent studies (McGuffin et al., 1990). Not only may there be multiple susceptibility genes contributing to diagnoses in large families, but there are possible difficulties with diagnostic categories. For example, if one family member has the disorder according to the most rigorous criteria and another has a milder disorder that might be related, how should the latter case be classified? Is it possible that the more mildly affected individual will develop the full-blown syndrome over time? Linkage analysis is sensitive to misclassification of who is affected and who is not.

Some of these methodological difficulties might be overcome with population-based, collaborative studies in large numbers of nuclear families, but agreement regarding classification is a critical prerequisite to such research (Cloninger, 1994). Alternative statistical approaches to linkage analysis might also be used, including the affected sibpair approach, which is not as sensitive to misclassification errors associated with nonaffected individuals who subsequently develop the syndrome or disorder (Risch, 1990). Studies attempting to detect multiple simultaneous genetic effects or environmental triggers are also needed, given the compelling evidence for genetic susceptibility (Gershon & Cloninger, 1994). Perhaps it should not be surprising that complicated phenotypes such as behaviorally defined neuropsychiatric disorders are so difficult to unravel. There are comorbid conditions that may affect different members of the same family, as in the overlapping predisposition to schizophrenia and bipolar disorder in the 22q critical region for DiGeorge/Velocardiofacial syndrome (Berrettini, 2003). Another multifactorial disorder is autism (Spence 2001) where speech delay maps to 7q, one of the several regions identified in genomewide scans contributing to autism. The search for putative genes is actively being pursued (Bonora et al., 2002).

Nonclassical Mechanisms of Inheritance

Nonclassical mechanisms of inheritance include mitochondrial mutation, genetic imprinting, and unstable repeat sequences.

Mitochondrial Mutation

The finding of strictly maternal transmission of Leber's hereditary optic neuropathy led to the first documentation of inheritance due to a mitochondrial DNA (mtDNA) mutation (i.e., because mtDNA is transmitted via the egg, not the sperm) (Wallace et al., 1988). Table 29.2 provides a partial list of the classical mitochondrial disorders; for additional documentation of the variety of responsible mutations in mtDNA, the reader is referred to the new section on mitochondrial disorders in McKusick's *Mendelian Inheritance in Man* (12th Edition, 1998).

Human mtDNA is a small (16.5 kb), circular, double-stranded molecule that contains 13 structural genes for proteins involved in oxidative phosphorylation. Other genes coding for the balance of proteins involved in oxidative phosphorylation reside in the nuclear DNA. Body tissues vary in the extent to which they are sensitive to changes in energy metabolism secondary to oxidative

TABLE 29.2

MITOCHONDRIAL DISORDERS HEADD: HYPOTONIA, EPILEPSY, AUTISM, AND DEVELOPMENTAL DELAY

LHON	Leber's hereditary optic neuropathy
MELAS	Mitochondrial encephalopathy, lactic acidosis, and stroke-like events
MERRF	Myoclonic epilepsy with ragged red fibers
MNGIE	Myoneurogastrointestinal encephalopathy syndrome
KSS	Kearns-Sayre syndrome (chronic progressive external ophthalmoplegia)
NARP	Neuropathy, ataxia, and retinitis pigmentosa
Leigh disease	
Diabetes with sensorineural hearing loss	
Pearson syndrome	

phosphorylation defects. Besides tissue-specific variation, there are also age-related effects. In fact, it has been suggested that cumulative oxidative damage to mitochondrial DNA contributes to aging in general. With reference to neurodegenerative diseases, it is hypothesized that changes in mitochondrial DNA could contribute to Alzheimer's disease and Parkinson's disease (Shigenaga et al., 1994). Interestingly, other systemic manifestations of mitochondrial disease may be depression (Johns, 1995) or autism (Graf et al., 2000; Pons, 2004).

Genetic Imprinting

Genetic imprinting occurs when the phenotypic effect of a gene mutation depends on which parent transmitted it. In classical Mendelian inheritance, phenotypic expression is the same regardless of which parent contributed the gene. However, animal models have provided evidence that in some instances the phenotype could depend on which parent contributed the altered gene; or, conversely, on which parent did *not* contribute a *normal copy* of genetic material.

One of the best-known human examples of imprinting is the critical region on the long arm of chromosome 15 (15g11g13), which, as previously described, has been found to be deleted in about half of patients with Prader-Willi syndrome. In all of these patients, the deletion occurred in the chromosome 15 inherited from the father, leaving a single copy of the genetic material inherited from the mother. Alternatively, if the deletion were inherited from the mother (leaving only one normal copy from the father), the offspring would be affected with a different disorder, Angelman's syndrome (formerly known as the "happy puppet syndrome") (Magenis et al., 1987).

Deletion of one copy of the critical region for these two syndromes can occur either de novo (as a result of a translocation) or by the mechanism of *uniparental disomy,* in which both members of a given chromosome pair are inherited from one parent, with no contribution from the other parent. Uniparental disomy for chromosome 15 has been observed for Prader-Willi syndrome and, less frequently, for Angelman's syndrome (Malcolm et al., 1991; Nicholls, 1993). If both copies of chromosome 15 come from the mother (i.e., none from the father), Prader-Willi syndrome results; conversely, if both copies come from the father (i.e., with none from the mother), Angelman's syndrome results. Cases have been reported in which a trisomy for chromosome 15 observed on chorionic villus sampling in the first semester had changed to uniparental disomy (i.e., secondary to the loss of the one copy of chromosome 15 from the father) by follow-up amniocentesis at 16 weeks, with the net result being Prader-Willi syndrome (Cassidy et al., 1992). Thus, for region 15g11g13, normal contributions from both parents are required for normal human development. The frequency with which genetic imprinting or uniparental disomy occurs, as well as the biological significance of these inheritance mechanisms, is under investigation.

Unstable Repeat Sequences

The mechanism of unstable repeat sequences was discovered in relation to fragile X–linked mental retardation (see Chapter 8), the most common inherited form of retardation (affecting approximately one in 1,600 boys). A cytogenetic marker, an apparent fragile site at Xq27.3, was first described by Lubs (1969) in a family with X-linked mental retardation in which the affected males had the fragile site but the nonaffected males did not. Using the culture medium TC199, Sutherland (1977) clarified the role of low levels of folic acid and thymidine in induction of the fragile site. Subsequent experience with the fragile X marker showed it to be present in kindreds in which the males exhibited the phenotype described by Martin and Bell (1943); namely, moderate-to-severe retardation with long faces; prognathism; large, everted ears; and large testicles. The fragile X marker was not found in other forms of X-linked mental retardation. A number of features inconsistent with simple X-linked recessive inheritance began to be noted, such as transmission by normal males and an increased risk of retardation in the offspring of mentally impaired females (Sherman et al., 1985).

Cloning of the *FMR-1* gene allowed molecular techniques to be applied to elucidation of the mechanisms underlying the fragile site and enabled improved diagnosis of conditions related to this marker (Oberle et al., 1991; Verkerk et al., 1991). The basis for the fragile site turned out to be a GCC triplet repeat sequence that normally codes for a series of arginines in the EMR-1 protein. That sequence is inherited in stable form when there are fewer than 43 repeats. However, if the number of triplet repeats increases to the range of 50 to 70 (sometimes termed the *unstable range*, or premutation), instability during maternal meiosis results, usually with an increase in the number of repeats. Transmitting males with 50 to 70 repeats do not show any phenotypic effect or fragile sites, but their daughters have an increased risk of affected sons as a result of disruption of *FMR-1* gene function by even larger repeat sequences. When 200 or more GCC repeats are present, the fragile site may be seen. This increased number of repeats is termed a *full mutation*. *Somatic mosaicism*, the presence of repeat sequences numbering in the thousands in some tissues, is occasionally observed in affected males. In general, the size of the repeat sequence correlates positively with the severity of the developmental delay in affected males. Females do not show such a straightforward correlation, given lyonization (X chromosome inactivation in females) and the presence of another normal allele.

Interestingly, other diseases associated with unstable repeat sequences are also frequently related to neurological dysfunction. Besides the fragile X A site at Xq27.3, the fragile X E site nearby is apparently related to a milder form of retardation. Two other fragile sites (fragile X F and fragile X 16 A) are also related to increases in the number of CGG repeats and hypermethylation of the nearby CpG island, but these sites are not known to be associated with mental retardation. Another category of unstable repeats is associated with six neurodegenerative disorders: Huntington's disease, spinobulbar muscular dystrophy, type I spinocerebellar atrophy, dentarubral-pallidoluysian atrophy, the allelic Haw River syndrome, and Machado-Joseph disease. All of these disorders are dominantly inherited, progressive neurodegenerative disorders with later onset (although one measure of their severity is age at onset, which can be as early as childhood). All are related to increased numbers of CAG repeats, with possible gain of function conferred on the gene product. Presymptomatic testing for Huntington's disease is now possible and consists of determining the number of CAG repeats. In contrast to the fragile X dynamic mutation, in which the instability occurs only during maternal meiosis, the instability in Huntington's disease occurs during paternal meiosis.

The phenomenon of *anticipation* (i.e., worsening phenotype with successive generations), which has been clinically reported in myotonic dystrophy, correlates with progressively larger expansions of a CTG repeat through the maternal line. The congenital form of myotonic dystrophy, characterized by expansion to more than 1,000 repeats, occurs mainly in the offspring of affected mothers (Harley et al., 1992; Hunter et al., 1992). Apparent anticipation has also been described in analyses of pedigrees for bipolar affective disorder (McInnis et al., 1993; Nylander et al., 1994), which suggests that repeat sequences may also have a role in that disorder.

CLINICAL GENETICS: GENETIC EVALUATION AND COUNSELING

Formal genetic evaluation of a family can be undertaken either at the family's request or upon referral by a physician. However, the timing of the evaluation—and, more importantly, of the counseling—should be considered carefully with regard to how circumstances may influence the family's ability to understand the information provided. For example, if a serious disorder has just been diagnosed in a family member, the ensuing emotions may make it difficult for the family to absorb and understand complicated information. On the other hand, if such a diagnosis is made during another family member's pregnancy, there may be urgency to providing information and helping the family to understand options. To evaluate the possible genetic basis of a disorder, complete information must be gathered, including a detailed medical history (prenatal, birth, and subsequent illnesses and events), a detailed general medical and neuropsychiatric examination, or documentation of such relevant evaluations, and appropriate laboratory testing.

Genetic evaluation always includes a family history. This analysis can be presented in shorthand form with the use of standard pedigree symbols (Bennett et al., 1995) (Fig. 29.4). In the genetic counseling situation, the individual

Pedigree Symbols

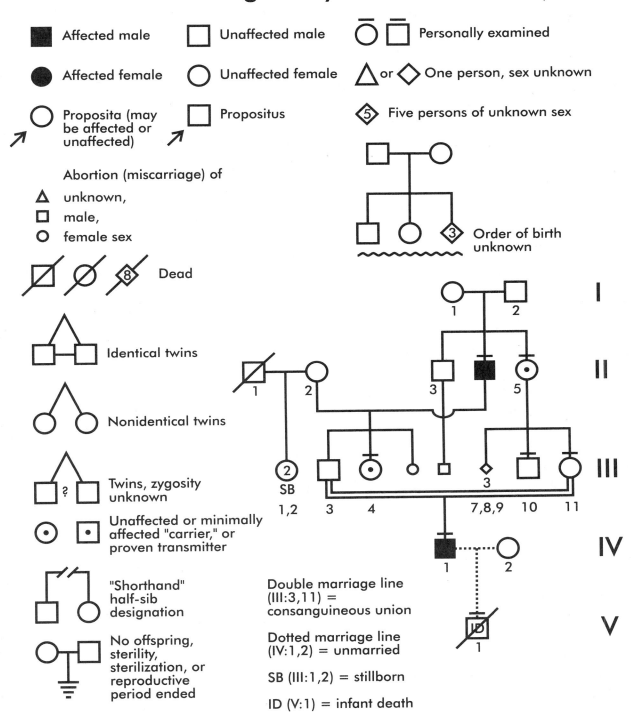

Figure 29.4 Pedigree symbols. Reprinted from "Instructions for Contributors." American Journal of Medical Genetics (Neuropsychiatric Genetics) 67:120, 1996. Copyright 1996, John Wiley & Sons, Inc. Used with permission.

seeking genetic information or testing, designated the "consultand", is indicated with an arrow. The first affected family member coming to medical attention is called the *proposita/propositus*, *proband*, or *index case*. (Figure 29.4 is from a medical journal, where [in contrast to the genetic counseling situation] the proposita/propositus rather than the consultand is of primary interest and thus receives the arrow indicator.) A key indicates what each filled-in circle or square denotes. If additional family members are affected, these are indicated by filling in the appropriate squares or circles (depending on the sex of the individual).

The value of a pedigree depends on the completeness and care with which the information is gathered. The parents and siblings of the affected individual should be included, starting with the oldest individual on the left and proceeding to the youngest in each generation. Usually grandparents, aunts, and uncles are included as well. Deceased individuals are designated by a slanted line through the square or circle, with an indication of age at death and cause. This information may be important to determine whether that individual lived long enough to manifest a late-onset disorder. If age rather than date of birth is noted below the symbol for each person, the recorder will need to indicate the date that the pedigree was taken. Later adjustments can be made (births, deaths, changes in relationships, and new diagnoses) in subsequent visits.

Numbers within a circle, square, or diamond shape (indicating unknown gender) denote the number of unaffected siblings or offspring. It may be important to indicate whether individuals in the pedigree were ever formally assessed or tested for the condition under evaluation. Review of medical records may be necessary to verify the results, because the family member providing the information may not be aware of all the relevant details or tests performed.

The pedigree may include sensitive information not available to all family members (e.g., nonpaternity, infertility, or test results not meant to be available to insurance companies or employers). Thus, confidentiality should be respected and careful thought given to what information should be included.

Open-ended questions can be very helpful in eliciting information about more distant relatives who may not have been initially included in the pedigree. Opinions within the family regarding affected or unaffected individuals can be indicated as such. For example, family members may attribute an individual's retardation to a "difficult birth." This information can be included without prejudgment as to its validity. Also, related historical details, such as late language development, poor school performance, or behavioral difficulties, can be recorded without assigning diagnoses.

In a genetics clinic, it is often the genetic counselor who gathers information, including the pedigree, medical records, and the list of questions the family wants answered. Because correct diagnostic information is the cornerstone of accurate genetic counseling, the counselor may enlist the aid of a clinical geneticist for review of the records, examination of affected family members, and, possibly, additional testing. In turn, the clinical geneticist may consult colleagues in other subspecialties for any help needed in interpreting the records.

The actual process of communicating risks and options to a family is complex and is influenced by many factors. The family members' backgrounds, education, religious beliefs, and life experiences affect their questions and perceptions. If a medical diagnosis has been made in a family member, the family's information may be limited to the problems exhibited by that individual. Some family members may not be familiar with the natural history, treatment possibilities, and range of outcomes for the disorder. The nature of the diagnosis, including whether it can be treated or prenatally diagnosed, may also influence the family's feelings.

The psychological issues are many. The attitudes and perceptions of family members regarding the genetic condition may vary, depending on their relationship to the affected individual. For a parent, guilt related to a child's diagnosis with a genetic disorder might be overwhelming, whereas a sibling may resent the amount of care and attention received by the affected child. If two parents or members of a couple disagree on important issues, such as the burden or severity of a particular disorder, the significance of the risks (high versus low), or the acceptability of prenatal diagnosis and termination of pregnancy, it may be hard for them to cope and to make decisions about future reproduction.

In general, the genetic counselor should strive to be nondirective, to be as clear as possible about risks and options, and to support the family in its response to the information provided and decisions regarding how this information might affect future plans for reproduction or testing. The goal is to promote autonomy, individual responsibility, and informed decision making. Follow-up can be critical in regard to providing reinforcement of the risk figures given (i.e., since many studies show that a large portion of families do not retain accurate information about recurrence risks) as well as clarification of other issues and communication of new information or testing results that may change the risk information provided or the options available. Additional family members may also need genetic evaluation, testing, or counseling.

Referral to family support groups may be helpful; information about such groups may be found online through the Alliance of Genetic Support Groups as well as in online websites offered by individual disease-specific support groups. Referral for individual psychological counseling, marital counseling, or family therapy may benefit some individuals.

The supportive role of the genetic counselor is emphasized in the definition of genetic counseling formulated by an ad hoc committee of the American Society of Human Genetics (Fraser 1974, p. 63):

[Genetic counseling is] a communication process which deals with the human problems associated with occurrence, or risk of occurrence of a genetic disorder in a family. This process involves an attempt by one or more appropriately trained persons to help the individual or family to (1) comprehend the medical facts including the diagnosis, the probable course of the disorder, and the available management; (2) appreciate the way heredity contributes to the disorder and the risk of recurrence in specified relatives; (3) understand the options for dealing with the risks of recurrence; (4) choose the course of action which seems appropriate to them in view of their risk and their family goals, and act in accordance with that decision; and (5) make the best possible adjustment to the disorder in an affected family member and/or to the risk of recurrence of that disorder.

Efforts have been made to develop counseling models that integrate psychological, philosophical, and ethical principles (Kessler, 1979). Certainly there are ethical aspects to genetic testing, as, for example, regarding the testing of presymptomatic young people for late-onset untreatable disorders. Although there seems to be some consensus within the genetics community that persons younger than 18 years of age should not be tested for Huntington's disease (American Society of Human Genetics/ American College of Medical Geneticists, 1995), situations exist in which the issue must be carefully considered. Despite the fact that most clinical geneticists eschew any eugenic approach, some clinicians acknowledge their desire to reduce the frequency of the Huntington's disease gene in the population and thereby prevent much individual suffering (Harper, 1984). Notwithstanding, all clinicians are troubled when recalling the complicity of geneticists in Nazi Germany in the sterilization of individuals with genetic diseases.

TREATMENT OF GENETIC DISEASE

Progress continues in elucidating the metabolic basis of inherited disease (Scriver et al., 2001). The success of newborn screening and treatment for disorders such as phenylketonuria and beta-thalassemia illustrates how an understanding of the metabolic basis of a disorder can lead to effective therapy.

In the case of classic phenylalanine hydroxylase deficiency, modification of the infant's diet to control blood levels of phenylalanine prevents much of the brain damage that occurs with accumulation of substrate in the absence of effective enzyme. Screening programs for phenylketonuria that used careful follow-up have allowed identification of phenylketonuria variants, dihydropteridine reductase (DHPR) deficiency and impaired tetrahydrobiopterin (BH4) metabolism, that do not respond to dietary limitation of phenylalanine (Kaufman, 1985). In these disorders, cofactor therapy may be helpful, as has been the case in certain other metabolic disorders.

Another therapeutic approach for treating metabolic disease is providing a "somatic" source of the missing enzyme; as, for example, with renal transplantation in cystinosis (Ehrich et al., 1991). Similarly, bone marrow transplantation for beta-thalassemia (Lucarelli et al., 1991) replaces the deficient hemoglobin with effective hemoglobin. Of course, there are many factors to consider with this type of therapy, such as financial costs, morbidity, mortality, the limited availability of human leukocyte antigen (HLA)-identical donors, and the age of the recipient. In southern Italy, the incidence of beta-thalassemia was reduced by the combined approach of population screening and prenatal diagnosis (Cao et al., 1981), as had been done for Tay-Sachs disease in the United States (Kaback et al., 1977). However, although a similar approach is theoretically possible for other metabolic disorders, the success of population-level programs depends on the public perception of the burden of the disease and whether families are willing to undertake prenatal diagnosis to prevent the disorder. The experience with cystic fibrosis suggests that many families do not find prenatal diagnosis (especially with consequent pregnancy termination) to be an acceptable preventive approach.

Gene Therapy

For single-gene disorders in which the molecular pathogenesis is known, the strategy of inserting a normal gene (or appropriately modified nucleic acids) directly into the genome of the affected individual to correct the disorder has been actively pursued. Because the goal is to achieve gene expression in the correct intracellular location, attempts have been aimed at somatic modification rather than germline modification. Ethical guidelines have included the precept that gene transfer attempts should target significant medical illnesses only, not genetic characteristics that might be considered cosmetic or trivial. The first human gene therapy trial occurred in 1989. By the end of 1994, more than 80 clinical trials involving gene transfer (enlisting more than 200 participants) had been approved by the National Institutes of Health (NIH) Recombinant DNA Advisory Committee (RAC) (Ledley, 1995), despite opposition from some groups to recombinant DNA research of any kind. These trials focused not only on rare, single-gene disorders (e.g., cystic fibrosis, Duchenne's muscular dystrophy) but also on disorders as common as cancer, acquired immunodeficiency syndrome (AIDS), and arthritis. By the year 2004, over 900 clinical trials were either completed, ongoing, or approved throughout the world (Edelstein et al., 2004). Over 100 distinct genes had been transferred. Though most trials were found to be safe, some were discontinued because of side-effects and unforeseen risks. The entire approach to gene therapy was re-evaluated after the death of Jesse Gelsinger in 1999 in a phase I trial to treat his ornithine transcarbamylase deficiency. Research in gene therapy continues, with particular attention to the need for safety.

A variety of approaches to gene therapy have been used. One approach, which involves harvesting and cultivating cells from the affected individual, introducing the recombinant genes into those cells in culture, and then reintroducing the altered cells into the patient, has met with some success for disorders in which the deficiency affects mainly the cells in the bloodstream, such as adenosine deaminase (ADA) deficiency, the first genetic disease to be approved by the RAC for a gene therapy trial. ADA deficiency is particularly deleterious to the immune cells, especially the T-lymphocytes. It accounts for about one-half of the cases of autosomal recessive severe combined immunodeficiency. After the first affected child in a family is identified, subsequent siblings could be screened for the disease either prenatally or at birth. Previous therapy for the disorder involved repeated transfusions with irradiated blood, which provided enough ADA to temporarily meet the needs of the individual (adequate immune-system function can be achieved with less than the full normal levels of ADA). In a more recent therapeutic approach, the ADA gene was inserted into the blood of two affected patients by means of a retroviral vector. The genetically engineered cells were then reinfused back into the patients, thus bypassing the risks of autologous transfusion. The results were encouraging in that both patients subsequently responded to immunological challenges (Morgan & Anderson, 1993). Additional research is in progress.

For some disorders, simply achieving normal levels of a deficient protein is not enough to correct the underlying defect. For example, in cystic fibrosis, a double dose of the cystic fibrosis transmembrane regulator (CFTR) gene decreases chloride transport across epithelial cell membranes in the pancreas, lung, and sweat glands, resulting in the complex pulmonary and pancreatic symptoms characteristic of the disorder. However, to restore normal chloride transport and viscosity of secretions, the therapeutic gene must be introduced at the correct transmembrane position in the affected glands. Altered adenovirus sprayed in aerosolized form has been investigated in animal models, but the results were complicated by varying degrees of inflammatory response. An initial study that used a similar approach in a small number of cystic fibrosis patients was not markedly successful in incorporating the CFTR gene into nasal epithelial cells (Knowles et al., 1995). There was also considerable inflammatory response. However, continuing work on alteration of the virus and possibly even alteration of the immune response to the virus is in progress.

Animal models are not always entirely predictive of the human experience. The difficulties in transferring techniques from the laboratory to the bedside were illustrated in a study that attempted to transmit normal dystrophin into boys affected with Duchenne's muscular dystrophy by transplanting myoblasts. Whereas animal studies had demonstrated efficient incorporation of human myoblasts into mouse muscle, the boys in this study showed poor incorporation of the myoblasts and little clinical improvement (Mendell et al., 1995). Although these preliminary attempts were not successful, their results should not be viewed as definitive; rather, such trials constitute an important part of the investigative process into the means of achieving successful gene incorporation into appropriate tissues. As these and similar efforts continue, longterm evaluation of the impact of such transfer approaches on participating human subjects is essential.

One of the great challenges in the treatment of neuropsychiatric disorders, assuming that the predisposing genes can be found and the pathogenesis understood, is crossing the blood-brain barrier. This barrier effectively protects the human brain from infection, but it also prevents direct transfer of viral vectors from the bloodstream into the central nervous system. Thus, for gene therapy of a disorder such as Tay-Sachs disease, efficacy would depend on targeting the tissue affected by the hexosaminidase deficiency. For multifactorial psychiatric conditions, vector therapies using conditional expression systems induced by the same environmental triggers that exacerbate psychiatric symptoms would be theoretically desirable (Sapolsky, 2003).

One "gene therapy" success story is the treatment of the nonneuronopathic form of Gaucher's disease. This most common form of Gaucher's disease is characterized by accumulation of lipid-laden white cells and platelets in the reticuloendothelial system, giving rise to enlargement of the liver and spleen. Targeting the deficient enzyme (glucocerebrosidase) by exposing the normally covered N-acetylglucosamine and mannose residues on the enzyme produces low but sufficient levels of enzyme in those cells. Use of a commercial product (Ceredase) in patients with type I Gaucher disease has resulted in decreased spleen size, increased platelet counts, and ultimately but very gradually, a decrease in bone pain (Barton et al., 1991; Beutler, 1991). Although the cost of the therapy is high, it represents a successful targeting strategy. Such innovation might ultimately be successful in bypassing the blood-brain barrier, although there is no way to predict how many years of research with animal models would be required to achieve that end. In addition, postnatal gene therapy would not be effective to addressing disorders that result from the interaction of multiple genes during development. Thus, it is only fair to be realistic with patients' families about the lack of imminence of such a breakthrough. As knowledge of the genetic contributions to neurologic and psychiatric disorders continues, however, it will be important for clinicians to become familiar with the knowledge gained by genetic epidemiologic and genomic research. Tools that have become available from the study of single-gene conditions, the human genome, and multifactorial conditions may be applied in creative ways first the understanding of the pathogenesis of pediatric neuropsychiatric disorders, but also hopefully to the prevention and treatment of such disorders.

REFERENCES

Alliance of Genetic Support Groups (http://www.geneticalliance.org/):

American Society of Human Genetics/American College of Medical Geneticists: Points to consider: ethical, legal, and psychosocial implications of genetic testing in children and adolescents (report). Am J Hum Genet 57:1233–1241, 1995.

Antonarakis SA: Diagnosis of genetic disorders at the DNA level. N Engl J Med 320:153–163, 1989.

Baird P, Anderson TW Newcomb HB, et al: Genetic disorders in children and young adults: a population study. Am J Hum Genet 42:677–693, 1988.

Bartley JA, Hall BD: Mental retardation and multiple congenital abnormalities of unknown etiology: frequency of occurrence in similarly affected sibs of the proband. Birth Defects 14:127–137, 1978.

Barton NW, Brady RO, Dambrosia JM, et al: Replacement therapy for inherited enzyme deficiency: macrophage-targeted glucocerebrosidase for Gaucher's disease. N Engl J Med 324:1464–1470, 1991.

Bennett RL, Steinhaus KA, Uhrich SB, et al: Recommendations for standardized human pedigree nomenclature. Am J Hum Genet 56:745–752, 1995.

Beutler E: Gaucher's disease. N Engl J Med 325:1354–1369, 1991.

Berrettini W: Evidence for shared susceptibility in bipolar disorder and schizophrenia. Am J Med Genet 123C:59–64, 2003.

Bonora E, Bacchelli E, Levy ER, et al (International Molecular Genetic Study of Autism Consortium IMGSAC): Mutation screening and imprinting analysis of four candidate genes for autism in the 7q32 region. Mol Psychiatry 76:289–301, 2002.

Borgaonkar DS: Chromosomal Abnormalities and Anomalies, 6th Ed. New York: Wiley-Liss, 1991.

Cao A, Furbetta M, Galanello R, et al: Prevention of homozygous beta-thalassemia by carrier screening and prenatal detection in Sardinia. Am J Hum Genet 33:592–605, 1981.

Cassidy SB, Lai L-W Erickson RP, et al: Trisomy 15 with loss of the paternal 15 as a cause of Prader-Willi syndrome due to maternal disomy. Am J Hum Genet 51:701–708, 1992.

Cloninger CR: Turning point in the design of linkage studies of schizophrenia. Am J Med Genet (Neuropsychiatric Genetics) 54:83–92, 1994.

Corder EH, Saunders AM, Strittmatter WJ, et al: Gene dose of apolipoprotein E type 4 and the risk of Alzheimer's disease in late-onset families. Science 261:921–923, 1993.

DeGrouchy J, Turleau E: Clinical Atlas of Human Chromosomes, 2nd Ed. New York: Wiley, 1984.

Dykens E, Cassidy S: Correlates of maladaptive behavior in children and adults with Prader-Willi syndrome. Am J Med Genet (Neuropsychiatric Genetics) 60:546–549, 1995.

Edelstein ML, Abedi MR, Wixon J, et al: Gene therapy clinical trials worldwide 1989-2004—an overview. J Genet Med 6:597–602, 2004.

Ehrich JHH, Brodehl J, Byrd DI, et al: Renal transplantation for childhood cystinosis. Pediatr Nephrol 5:707–714, 1991.

Forrest SM, Cross GS, Speer A, et al: Preferential deletion of exons in Duchenne and Becker muscular dystrophies. Nature 329:638–640, 1987.

Fraser FC: Genetic counseling. Am J Hum Genet 26:636–659, 1974.

Fryer AE, Chalmers A, Connor J, et al: Evidence that the gene for tuberous sclerosis is on chromosome 9. Lancet 1:659–661, 1987.

Fryns JP, Spaepen A, Cassiman JJ, et al: X-linked complicated spastic paraplegia, MASA syndrome and X-linked hydrocephalus owing to congenital stenosis of the aqueduct of Sylvius: variable expression of same mutation at Xq28 (letter). J Med Genet 28:429–431, 1991.

Gardner RJM, Sutherland GR: Chromosome Abnormalities and Genetic Counseling. New York: Oxford University Press, 1989.

Gershon ER, Cloninger CR (eds): Genetic Approaches to Mental Disorders. Washington, D.C.: American Psychiatric Press, 1994.

Graf WD, Marin-Garcia J, Gao HG, et al: Autism associated with the mitochondrial DNA G8363A transfer RNA (Lys) mutation. J Child Neurol. 15:357–361, 2000.

Hamabe J, Fukushima Y, Harda N, et al: Molecular study of the Prader-Willi syndrome: deletion, RFLP and phenotype analysis of 50 patients. Am J Med Genet 41:54–63, 1991.

Harley HG, Brook JD, Rundle SA, et al: Expansion of an unstable DNA region and phenotypic variation in myotonic dystrophy. Nature 355:545–546, 1992.

Harper P: Practical Genetic Counselling, 2nd Ed. Bristol, UK: Wright, 1984.

Hunter A, Tsilfidis C, Metter G, et al: The correlation of age of onset with CTG trinucleotide repeat amplification in myotonic dystrophy. J Med Genet 29:774–779, 1992.

Johns DR: Seminars in Medicine of the Beth Israel Hospital in Boston: mitochondrial DNA and disease. N Engl J Med 333:638–644, 1995.

Kaback MM, Rimoin DL, O'Brien JS (eds): Tay Sachs Disease: Screening and Prevention. New York: Alan R. Liss, 1977.

Kandt RS, Haines JL, Smith M, et al: Linkage of an important gene locus for tuberous sclerosis to chromosome 16 marker for polycystic kidney disease. Nat Genet 2:37–41, 1992.

Kaufman S: Hyperphenylalaninemia caused by defects in tetrahydrobiopterin deficiency. J Inherit Metab Dis 8:20–27, 1985.

Kenwrick S, Jouet M, Donnai D: X linked hydrocephalus and MASA syndrome. J Med Genet 33:59–65, 1996.

Kessler S (ed): Genetic Counseling: Psychological Dimensions. New York: Academic Press, 1979.

Knowles MR, Hohneker KW Zhou Z, et al: A controlled study of adenoviral vector mediated gene transfer in the nasal epithelium of patients with cystic fibrosis. N Engl J Med 333:823–831, 1995.

Ledbetter DH, Riccardi V Airharts SD, et al: Deletions of chromosome 15 as a cause of Prader-Willi syndrome. N Engl J Med 304:325–329, 1981.

Ledley RD: After gene therapy: issues in long-term clinical care. Adv Genet 32:1–15, 1995.

Lubs HA: A marker X chromosome. Am J Hum Genet 21:231–244, 1969.

Lucarelli G, Galimberti M, Polchi P, et al: Bone marrow transplantation in thalassemia. Hematol Oncol Clin North Am 5:549–556, 1991.

Lyon M: Chromosomal and subchromosomal inactivation. Ann Rev Genet 2:31–52, 1968.

Magenis RE, Brown MG, Lacy DA, et al: Is Angelman syndrome the alternate result of del(15) (qII-q13)? Am J Med Genet 28:829–858, 1987.

Malcolm S, Clayton-Smith J, Nichols M, et al: Uniparental disomy in the Angelman syndrome. Lancet 337:694–697, 1991.

Martin JP, Bell J: A pedigree of mental defect showing sex-linkage. J Neurol Psychiatry 6:154–157, 1943.

McGuffin P, Sargeant M, Hett G, et al: Exclusion of a schizophrenia gene from the chromosome 5gl1-q13 region: new data and a re-analysis of previous reports. Am J Hum Genet 47:524–535, 1990.

McInnis MG, McMahon FC, Chase GA, et al: Anticipation in bipolar affective disorder. Am J Hum Genet 53:385–390, 1993.

McKusick V: Mendelian Inheritance in Man: A Catalog of Human Genes and Genetic Disorders, 12th Ed. Baltimore, MD: Johns Hopkins University Press, 1998.

Mendel G: Experiments in Plant Hybridisation (1866). Translated by the Royal Horticultural Society of London. Cambridge, MA: Harvard University Press, 1965.

Mendell JR, Kissel JT, Amato AA, et al: Myoblast transfer in the treatment of Duchenne muscular dystrophy. N Engl J Med 33:832–838, 1995.

Miki Y, Swensen J, Shattuck-Eidens D, et al: A strong candidate for the breast and ovarian cancer susceptibility gene BRCA1. Science 266:66–71, 1994.

Mitelman F (ed): An International System for Human Cytogenetic Nomenclature. Basel, Switzerland: Karger, 1995.

Monaco AP, Kunkel LM: A giant locus for the Duchenne and Becker muscular dystrophy gene. Trends Genet 3:33–37, 1987.

Morgan RA, Anderson WF: Human gene therapy. Am Rev Biochem 62:191–217, 1993.

Morton DH, Morton CS, Strauss KA, et al: Pediatric medicine and the genetic disorders of the Amish and Mennonite People of Pennsylvania. Am J Med Genet Part C (Semin Med Genet) 121C: 5–17, 2003.

Nicholls RD: Genomic imprinting and uniparental disomy in Angelman and Prader-Willi syndromes: a review. Am J Med Genet 46:16–25, 1993.

Nishisho I, Nakamura Y, Miyoshi Y et al: Mutations of chromosome 5q21 genes in FAP and colorectal cancer patients. Science 253:665–669, 1991.

Nylander P, Engstrom C, Chotai J, et al: Anticipation in Swedish families with bipolar affective disorders. J Med Genet 31:686–689, 1994.

Oberle I, Rousseau F, Heitz D, et al: Instability of a 550 base-pair DNA segment and abnormal methylation in fragile X syndrome. Science 252:1097–1102, 1991.

Online Mendelian Inheritance in Man, OMIM ™. McKusick-Nathans Institute for Genetic Medicine, Johns Hopkins University (Baltimore, MD) and National Center for Biotechnology Information, National Library of Medicine (Bethesda, MD), 2000. Available at: http://www.ncbi.nlm.nih.gov/omim/.

Ott J: Analysis of Human Genetic Linkage, 2nd Ed. Baltimore, MD: Johns Hopkins University Press, 1991.

Pericak-Vance MA, Bebout JL, Gaskell PC, et al: Linkage studies in familial Alzheimer disease: evidence for chromosome 19 linkage. Am J Hum Genet 48:1034–1050, 1991.

Pons R, Andreu AL, Checcarelli N, et al: Mitochondrial DNA abnormalities and autistic spectrum disorders. J Pediatr 144:81–85, 2004.

Risch N: Linkage strategies for genetically complex traits, III: the effect of marker polymorphism analysis on affected sib pairs. Am J Hum Genet 46:242–253, 1990.

Rosenthal A, Jouet M, Kenwick S: Aberrant splicing Ll CAM mRNA associated with X-linked hydrocephalus. Nat Genet 2:107–112, 1992.

Sachidanandam R, Weissman D, Schmidt SC et al: A map of human genome sequence variation containing 1.4 million single nucleotide polymorphisms. Nature 409:928–933, 2001.

Sapolsky R M: Gene therapy for psychiatric disorders. Am J Psychiatry 160: 208–220, 2003.

Schinzel A: Catalogue of Unbalanced Chromosome Aberrations in Man, 2nd Ed. Berlin: deGruyter, 2001.

Scriver CR, Beaudet AL, Sly WS, et al. (eds): The Metabolic and Molecular Basis of Inherited Disease, 8th Ed, Vols 1–4. New York: McGraw-Hill, 2001.

Sherman SL, Jacobs PA, Morton NE, et al: Further segregation analysis of the fragile X syndrome with special reference to transmitting males. Hum Genet 69:289–299, 1985.

Sherrington R, Brynjolfson J, Petursson H, et al: Localization of a susceptibility locus for schizophrenia on chromosome 5. Nature 336:164–167, 1988.

Shigenaga MK, Hagen TM, Ames BN: Oxidative damage and mitochondrial decay in aging. Proc Natl Acad Sci USA 91:10771–10778, 1994.

Smith M, Smalley S, Cantor R, et al: Mapping of a gene determining tuberous sclerosis to human chromosome 11g14–11g23. Genomics 6:105–114, 1990.

Spence MA: The genetics of autism. Curr Opin Pediatr 13:561–565, 2001.

St. George-Hyslop P, Tanzi RE, Polinsky RJ, et al: The genetic defect causing familial Alzheimer's maps on chromosome 21. Science 235:885–890, 1987.

St. George-Hyslop P, Haines J, Rogaev E, et al: Genetic evidence for a novel familial Alzheimer's disease locus on chromosome 14. Nat Genet 2:330–334, 1992.

Sutherland GR: Fragile sites on human chromosomes: demonstration of their dependence on the type of tissue culture medium. Science 197:265–266, 1977.

Venter, JC, Adams MD, Myers EW et al: The sequence of the human genome. Science 291:1304–1351, 2001.

Verkerk AJ, Peiretti M, Sutcliffe JS, et al: Identification of a gene (*FMR-1*) containing a CCG repeat coincident with a breakpoint cluster region exhibiting length variation in fragile X syndrome. Cell 65:905–914, 1991.

Vits L, VanCamp G, Coucke P, et al: MASA syndrome is due to mutations to the neural cell adhesion gene L1 CAM. Nat Genet 7:408–413, 1994.

Wallace DC, Singh G, Lott MT, et al: Mitochondrial DNA mutation associated with Leber's hereditary optic neuropathy. Science 242:1424–1430, 1988.

Watson JD, Crick FHC: The molecular structure of nucleic acids: a structure of deoxyribose nucleic acid. Nature 171:737–738, 1953.

Wooster R, Bignell G, Lancaster J, et al: Identification of the breast cancer susceptibility gene. BRCA2. Nature 378:789–792, 1995.

Psychological and Behavioral Interventions

30

Robert T. Ammerman, MD   Mariah E. Coe, MD

Historically, the prominence of behavioral and psychological interventions as frontline treatments of neuropsychiatric disorders in children has waxed and waned. In the 1950s and 1960s, the rise of behavior therapy was driven in part by the emergence of innovative therapies for mentally retarded and developmentally disabled children. Viewed as untreatable by most psychoanalysts, children with the significant cognitive limitations often associated with neuropsychiatric disorders were typically institutionalized and provided with few treatment options. For these children, behavior therapy offered new approaches for decreasing psychopathological behaviors that impeded integration into the community and allowed for the teaching of social, educational, and vocational skills that further enhanced mental health and overall well-being. Simultaneously, the corresponding emphasis on empirical demonstration of treatment effectiveness (which is one of the core tenets of behavioral therapy) called into question accepted approaches and contributed to the demand that these approaches also provide scientific evidence for their therapeutic impact. Accordingly, psychoanalytic and

psychodynamic models (some of which erroneously attributed certain developmental disabilities to parental dysfunction) and the overuse of nonspecific pharmacotherapeutic approaches fell into disfavor.

In the 1970s and 1980s, scientific investigations into the etiology of neuropsychiatric disorders delineated the neuropathological and genetic contributions to such conditions. New pharmacotherapies, which were developed in tandem with advances in cognitive neuroscience, further added to the armamentarium of the clinician. Moreover, neuropsychiatry matured quickly, growing beyond issues of localization of brain function and its clinical correlates to more sophisticated conceptualizations of neurological organization involving the interactions of neurological, physiological, and environmental systems. Indeed, the biopsychosocial model is now the only scientifically tenable approach to the design and implementation of comprehensive interventions in child neuropsychiatry and psychology.

Paradoxically, the biological revolution has contributed to a misperception that there is a conceptual dichotomy between somatic (e.g., pharmacotherapy, electroconvulsive therapy [ECT]) approaches to treatment and their psychological and behavioral counterparts. In some treatment settings, psychological and behavioral approaches to the treatment of child neuropsychiatric disorders are marginalized or are not integrated into the overall treatment plan. Likewise, in settings where behavioral interventions predominate (e.g., special education), neuropsychiatric

Acknowledgments:
This chapter was written with the partial support of Grant No. H133G000134 from the National Institute in Disability and Rehabilitation Research, U.S. Department of Education, Grant No. RO1 MH53703-05 from the National Institute on Mental Health, and by USPHS GCRC Grant #M01 RR 08084 from the National Center for Research Resources, NIH.

resources may be absent or tangential. Such disjunctive practices perpetuate the unjustified stereotypes of neuropsychiatrists as solely dispensers of medications and of the psychologists as unappreciative of neurological and genetic contributions to psychopathology.

Truly effective care of children with neuropsychiatric conditions can occur only in multidisciplinary, integrated treatment settings. Within these settings, interventions that have as their goals reduction of psychopathology and enhancement of skills that promote mental health and longterm adjustment should work in tandem. Scientific credibility and a strong linkage between etiological understanding and subsequent intervention are the common denominators of effective treatment, regardless of the clinician's therapeutic orientation or professional training.

In this chapter we present an overview of psychological and behavioral approaches to the treatment of neuropsychiatric disorders in childhood. These approaches are referred to as *child psychotherapy* or more generally, as *psychological interventions*. In keeping with the requirement of scientific credibility, we first review and consider research evidence for the effectiveness of child psychotherapy. Following a general survey of psychotherapeutic issues relevant to work with developmentally disabled children, we address principles and practices of behavioral assessment and treatment. We close the chapter with a discussion of family issues.

EFFICACY OF PSYCHOLOGICAL TREATMENTS FOR CHILDREN AND ADOLESCENTS

What is child psychotherapy? How effective is it? What factors and characteristics are associated with positive outcomes? These questions have generated considerable debate over the past half-century and have been the subject of several reviews in the last decade (Kazdin, 2000). There is a consensus that research on child and adolescent psychotherapy is nascent in comparison with that on adult psychotherapy. However, there has also been a strong drive in recent years to take stock of the child and adolescent psychotherapy literature both to examine the overall effectiveness of such interventions and to identify mechanisms and moderators of positive outcome. The overall effectiveness of psychological interventions with children is relevant to pediatric neuropsychiatry in that, to the extent that such interventions have been empirically shown to be effective, they become viable treatment options for neuropsychiatric disorders as well.

Critical Reviews and Meta-Analyses

The first question, What is psychotherapy? defies a simple answer. Kazdin (1991, 2000) has estimated that there are more than 230 approaches to child psychotherapy, which he broadly defined as

> An intervention designed to decrease distress, psychological symptoms, maladaptive behavior or to improve adaptive and psychosocial functioning. These ends are sought primarily through interpersonal sources of influence such as learning, persuasion, counseling, and discussion integrated into a specific treatment plan. The focus is on some facet regarding how clients feel (affect), think (cognition), and act (behavior). (Kazdin, 1991, p. 785)

Early reviews (e.g., Levitt, 1957) argued against the effectiveness of child psychotherapy relative to no treatment, although the literature on which these conclusions were based was scant and characterized by serious methodological limitations, including absence of control groups, unclear or poor delineation of subject populations, use of vague treatment protocols, failure to monitor treatment integrity, and application of inappropriate assessment strategies. In many of the investigations conducted to date there has been the lack of statistical power to detect significant differences between treatments (as opposed to between treatment and no-treatment control conditions). Since then, there has been considerable improvement in the methodological rigor of child psychotherapy outcome research, particularly in the last decade (Kazdin, 2003). Evidence for the effectiveness of child psychotherapy has emerged from meta-analyses of the expanded literature, which by conservative estimates includes over 1,500 controlled studies (Kazdin, 2003). The maturity of the field is further demonstrated by the dissemination of *empirically-based psychological treatments* for children by the American Psychological Association (Task Force on Promotion and Dissemination of Psychological Procedures, 1995).

The advent of meta-analysis (Mann, 1990) has permitted quantitative examination of treatment outcome research. In meta-analysis, studies are aggregated and rated according to predetermined criteria, and main effects across studies are derived. Specifically, each study is quantified in such a way as to generate an effect size, which is defined as the difference between the means of the treatment and control groups divided by the standard deviation of the control group. The effect size reflects overall treatment effectiveness and is used to delineate factors associated with treatment outcome (e.g., type of treatment, subject characteristics, contextual influences). The advantage of meta-analysis is that it is an objective approach to examining multiple studies rather than one that relies primarily on subjective judgment and opinion, as do more traditional reviews. However, meta-analysis is a correlation procedure and thus does not remove the effects of within-study methodological limitations; all studies have equal weight in a meta-analysis, regardless of their design limitations, although such factors can be empirically examined in meta-analyses (Wilson and Lipsey, 2001).

Meta-analyses conducted in the past decade (Casey and Berman, 1985; Durlak, et al., 1991; Weisz, et al., 1987;

Weisz, Weiss, Han, Granger, & Morton, 1995) have sought to determine the overall effectiveness of child and adolescent psychotherapy and to identify factors associated with positive outcomes. In the first of these meta-analyses, Casey and Berman (1985) examined 75 studies (published between 1952 and 1983) of psychotherapy outcome in children and adolescents 3 to 15 years of age. Specific goals of the meta-analysis were to determine (1) whether some forms of psychotherapy were superior to others, (2) whether the efficacy of psychotherapy varied as a function of the outcome measures used, and (3) which subject characteristics mediated outcome. Studies reviewed had an average sample size of 42 subjects at posttreatment, examined children who were primarily male (60%) with a mean age of 8.9 years, and included treatment durations averaging 9.5 weeks (range = 1 to 37 weeks). Behavior therapy was the treatment most often represented (56%); other studies evaluated cognitive behavior therapy (21%), client-centered therapy (28%), and psychodynamic therapy (9%).

The results of this analysis indicated an overall effect size of 0.71 for child psychotherapy (Casey and Berman 1985). In other words, the outcomes of children receiving psychotherapy were more than two thirds of a standard deviation better than those of subjects in a control condition. This effect size is consistent with results of meta-analyses of adult psychotherapy (e.g., Shapiro and Shapiro 1982; Stevens, Hynan, and Allen, 2000). Behavioral interventions were more effective than nonbehavioral ones (effect sizes of 9.91 and 0.40, respectively). No differences were found for play versus nonplay therapies, individual versus group approaches, parent-involved versus child-only interventions, or as a function of age. Treatment effectiveness was greater in children who displayed impulsivity, phobia, and somatic problems (these three symptoms were also most likely to be targeted in the studies that evaluated behavior therapy); problems of social adjustment were less responsive to treatment.

Casey and Berman's (1985) finding of superior efficacy for behavioral psychotherapy is consistent with the results of Shapiro and Shapiro's (1982) meta-analysis of adult studies. However, in their conclusions, Shapiro and Shapiro argued that the relative superiority of behavior therapy was tempered by the fact that behavioral and nonbehavioral treatment outcome studies tended to target different problems. Moreover, these authors contended that assessment measures used in behavioral studies were often directly linked to treatment targets, as opposed to the more global indices of functioning used in nonbehavioral studies. When these therapy-specific measures (which Shapiro and Shapiro believed led to an artificially inflated effect size for behavioral therapy) were excluded from the analysis, behavioral therapy was no longer superior to nonbehavioral interventions.

In a second meta-analysis, Weisz and colleagues (1987) examined 105 outcome studies (see Weiss and Weisz, 1990) of behavioral and nonbehavioral interventions with children and adolescents 4 to 18 years of age. Studies were selected only if they contrasted a treatment condition with a nontreatment or minimal-treatment (i.e., attention) control condition. Like Casey and Berman (1985), the authors sought to examine overall treatment effectiveness as well as correlates of positive treatment outcome. However, contrary to the conclusions of Shapiro and Shapiro (1982), Weisz and coworkers (1987) argued that the direct link between assessment approaches and treatment targets in most behavioral evaluations does not necessarily represent a confounding factor in determining the effect size of behavioral versus nonbehavioral interventions. They pointed out that, for example, in the case of phobia, the most clinically meaningful indication of fear and its reduction is approach to the feared stimulus (a measure typically used to assess behavioral interventions for phobia). For such a condition, therefore, global measures of child adjustment would be tangentially rather than primarily relevant. In their meta-analysis, Weisz and associates (1987) distinguished between outcome "measures similar to the training procedures [that] are appropriate and necessary for a fair test of treatment success" (p. 546) and those assessments intricately linked to treatment, which were deemed "unnecessary."

Findings by Weisz and colleagues (1987) revealed a mean effect size of 0.79 for treatment-versus-control comparisons. Once again, behavior therapy was found to be more effective than nonbehavioral interventions (0.88 versus 0.44). This superiority remained when appropriate and necessary assessments were retained (0.93 versus 0.45), but it disappeared when all therapy-specific measures were eliminated. Overall effect size did not significantly change as a function of problem type (i.e., overcontrolled versus undercontrolled behavioral disorders). Children (ages 4 to 12 years) were more likely to improve than were adolescents (ages 13 to 18 years). Also, investigations that used nonclinical samples obtained findings equivalent to those that recruited subjects from clinics. Finally, treatment gains were likely to be maintained at 6-month follow-up.

In a third meta-analysis, Weisz and colleagues (1995) examined 150 studies published between 1967 and 1993 that were nonoverlapping with their previous meta-analyses. These included multiple presenting disorders (aggression, delinquency, anxiety, depression, somatic problems) treated with varying interventions (behavior therapy, relaxation, social skills training, cognitive therapy, insight oriented approaches). As in previous meta-analyses, child treatment exhibited sizable effects (0.71). Additional findings included a superiority of behavioral over nonbehavioral strategies, increased effectiveness in females over males, and greater effectiveness in adolescents over children (in contrast to Casey and Berman), and equivalent effectiveness with internalizing and externalizing disorders.

Although the body of literature on psychotherapy for children and youth with developmental disabilities is smaller than that for children with emotional and behavioral disorders, there is a growing consensus that a range of treatments are potentially beneficial for this population as well. Prout and Nowak-Drabik (2003) reviewed 92 studies and case reports of psychological treatments for persons with mental retardation (26% of studies involved children and adolescents; 5% included mixed samples of children and adults). Although the methodological rigor of this sample was highly variable, expert ratings of treatment outcomes indicated moderate effects overall. An effect size of 1.09 was derived for 9 studies sufficiently controlled to permit meta-analysis. As with the aforementioned meta-analyses of the larger child treatment literature, behavioral treatments were superior to their nonbehavioral counterparts; although nonbehavioral treatments are infrequently used or studied in this population (Beail, 2003).

These meta-analyses yielded several important conclusions. First, psychotherapy is an effective intervention for a variety of social, emotional, and behavioral problems in children and adolescents with psychiatric disorders. Moreover, treatment effects are durable, being maintained at shortterm follow-up. Second, behavior therapy is a particularly effective type of intervention. And third, similar effect sizes are found in meta-analyses of the child and the adult treatment literatures.

A frequent complaint among clinicians is that the experimental research literature has limited generalizability to actual clinical cases. There are potential limitations to evidence-based treatments (e.g., Levant, 2004), and, indeed, the limited outcome research in natural clinic settings (without the methodological control of laboratory studies) has yielded less positive results than have more empirically rigorous evaluations (although there is disagreement about the extent of differences between clinic-based and laboratory-based outcomes; see Shadish, Navarro, Matt, and Phillips, 2000). Weisz, et al. (1995) explored 10 hypotheses regarding why such disparities exist between laboratory and clinical findings. Their meta-analysis revealed that research treatment differed from clinic treatment in that clinical samples were more pathologically disturbed, research settings had superior resources, and behavior therapy (which is more likely to be part of research studies but less likely to be employed by the clinical community as a whole (Kazdin, 2000)) is more effective than nonbehavioral treatments. The analysis by Weiss and colleagues (1995) did not support other hypotheses (e.g., that recent research uses superior methodologies, research clinicians are superior to community researchers, research therapists receive more rigorous training, research psychotherapy is more circumscribed in terms of clinical presentations, research therapy is more highly structured). Although much work clearly remains to be done in bridging the gap between treatment provided in clinical settings and that provided in research evaluations (Weisz, et al., 1995), the evidence for the superiority of behavior therapy relative to alternative psychological interventions for children and adolescents is compelling.

Guidelines for Empirically Supported Treatments

The emergence of an empirical foundation for psychological interventions in childhood disorders has spawned efforts to develop clinician guidelines and decision trees in selecting treatments for specific disorders (Herschell, McNeil, and McNeil, 2004). The American Psychological Association's Task Force on Promotion and Dissemination of Psychological Procedures (1995) established criteria for categorizing treatments as well established or probably efficacious based on multiple efficacy trials, clear procedural guidelines (i.e., treatment manuals), and independent replications. These, in turn, were applied to different childhood disorders and reviewed and summarized in a series of articles in *The Journal of Clinical Child Psychology* in 1998. Well-established treatments included behavioral parent training for Conduct Disorder, Oppositional Defiant Disorder, and Attention Deficit/Hyperactivity Disorder (ADHD); and modeling and reinforced practice for phobias. A number of additional treatments, all cognitive and behavioral in approach, were also identified as probably efficacious. These included, but are not limited to, cognitive behavior therapy for depression and anxiety, Multisystemic Therapy, Parent-Child Interaction Therapy for conduct problems, and behavior therapy for obesity. The establishment of these clinical guidelines reflects the maturing state of the still evolving literature on psychological treatments for childhood disorders.

The *American Journal on Mental Retardation* published results of an expert consensus panel on the treatment of behavioral and psychiatric disorders in persons with mental retardation (Rush and Frances, 2000). The purpose of this effort was to establish best practices in the treatment of children and adults with mental retardation. Guideline 3, Psychosocial Treatment, reports on consensus treatment recommendations based on severity of mental retardation, and type of disorder/behavior problem. The degree of consensus was high. Specifically, three psychosocial interventions consistently emerged as recommended or treatment of choice for a variety of disorders and behavior problems: applied behavior analysis (operant and classical conditioning procedures), managing the environment, and client and family education. It is noteworthy that, for most specific behavior problems in this population, several psychosocial treatments were recommended.

PSYCHOLOGICAL TREATMENT IN NEUROPSYCHIATRIC DISORDERS

Although the meta-analyses described above suggest that behavior therapy and its derivatives are the psychological treatments of choice for neuropsychiatric disorders in childhood, basic principles of psychotherapy are applicable to this population as well. Indeed, the cornerstones of psychotherapy, establishment of a therapeutic alliance, empathy, and unconditional acceptance; use of effective listening, are equally relevant to behavior therapy, despite the erroneous stereotype of behavior therapy as cold and overly clinical. Such relationship and process variables, although not viewed by behavior therapists are etiologically crucial or as the primary mechanisms through which treatment success is achieved, are nonetheless the sine qua non of positive outcomes (Beutler, et al., 2003).

Ironically, behavior therapy flourished in the 1960s because of its success with children who were thought to be poor candidates for psychoanalysis or other relationship-based interventions. This previously ignored population became the focus of a rapidly emerging and highly effective technology of behavior modification and change. Recently, however, there has been increased recognition of the emotional and interpersonal needs of neuropsychiatrically impaired children and youth. This awareness has occurred in tandem with (1) the acknowledgement that developmentally disabled children can exhibit a variety of psychopathologies, including internalizing disorders, in addition to the overt behavioral anomalies inherent to their primary disabilities; and (2) a greater appreciation for the diversity of developmental abilities and outcomes in children with neuropsychiatric disorders.

Accordingly, some authors (Harris 1995; Prout, Thompson and Douglas, 1998) have called attention to the importance of psychotherapeutic interventions with neuropsychiatrically impaired children and adults. A number of factors can undermine such children's self-esteem, self-efficacy, and sense of well-being (typically viewed as aspects of functioning that are targeted for change in psychotherapy). Relative ineffectiveness in one's environment, social isolation, and emotional abuse by peers are but some of the variables that can lead to anxiety, dysphoria, and demoralization. Communication limitations can interfere with obtaining needed social attention or tangible assistance, thereby contributing to frustration and learned helplessness. Dependence on others to provide for basic needs and the requirements of daily living can further engender feelings of helplessness and inferiority. Such feelings can intensify upon reaching developmental stages when independence and emancipation are expected (e.g., adolescence). Although these experiences will vary from child to child based on the type and severity of disability and the degree to which the child's family and other caregivers (e.g., educators, mental health professionals) are supportive and sensitive to the child's needs, they remain clinically significant features of the lives of virtually all children with neuropsychiatric impairments.

Harris (1995) has conceptualized psychotherapy in individuals with developmental disabilities from an attachment perspective. Attachment theory, first articulated by Bowlby (1969) and later expanded by Ainsworth (1969) and Sroufe and Rutter (1984), holds that establishment of the affective bond between infant and caregiver is the first and most important stage of social and emotional devel-

opment. Secure attachment emerges from reciprocal interactions of infant and caregiver, consisting of sensitivity to infant cues on the part of the caregiver and of socially reinforcing behaviors on the part of the infant. Insecure attachment, most often resulting from maladaptive parenting, can lead to avoidant, passive, or disorganized behavioral and emotional response patterns in infants. Insecure attachment in infancy, the crucial first stage of emotional and social development, is likely to lead to failure to master subsequent developmental challenges in these domains, even extending into adulthood.

Attachment is an especially relevant construct in neuropsychiatric disorders. Several features of these disorders interfere with the development of a secure attachment relationship. First, some neuropsychiatric disorders have social and interpersonal dysfunction as primary features of the diagnosis (e.g., autism). Second, central nervous system abnormalities inherent in many neuropsychiatric conditions may interfere with mechanisms responsible for the regulation of emotional processes (e.g., in head-injured youth) or other aspects of psychological and behavioral functioning (e.g., inattention, behavioral dysregulation, language disorders). Third, children with congenital abnormalities or early onset of neuropsychiatric conditions may exhibit characteristics that prevent formation of or undermine the attachment bond, or that are especially challenging for caregivers. For example, irritability, screaming, maladaptation to changes in routine or setting, or other behavioral sequelae of neuropsychiatric disorders in infants, can negatively affect the infant–caregiver relationship, particularly when the parent's ability to effectively identify infant cues and respond to them quickly and sensitively is already compromised (Ammerman and Patz, 1996). And fourth, social isolation and peer rejection interfere with socialization in neuropsychiatrically impaired children over and above the limitations imposed by the extent and severity of neurological dysfunction. Essentially, there are only a limited number of social and life experiences from which children may learn developmentally appropriate social and interpersonal skills. To the extent that attachment and subsequent socialization are undermined across the life span, neuropsychiatrically disturbed children are at increased risk for developing other forms of internalizing and externalizing disorders.

Some authors have argued that language-based psychotherapy is appropriate and potentially beneficial for persons with developmental disabilities if adaptations are made to simplify language, focus on more modest goals, and utilize strategies that are more effective given intellectual challenges (Prout, Thompson, and Douglas 1998). In conducting psychotherapy with individuals with developmentally disabilities, Hurley (1989) has recommended six adaptations to the practices implemented with their cognitively intact counterparts: (1) use a directive approach, (2) involve family and caregiving staff in treatment, (3) alter the intervention to the individual's cognitive and developmental level, (4) recognize and acknowledge the individual's interpersonal distortions and biases, (5) be flexible in selecting and applying interventions, and (6) assist the individual in accepting his or her disability. Treatment is facilitated by acknowledging the emotional and interpersonal needs of the child and by building into the treatment plan the means by which those needs can be met.

PRINCIPLES OF BEHAVIORAL PSYCHOLOGY

Behavioral psychology has its roots in the early years of both experimental and clinical psychology. The application of classical conditioning paradigms found its early expression in the work of Watson (1924) and M.C. Jones (1924) in the treatment of childhood fears. Watson, in particular, is credited with establishing behavioral psychology's emphasis on empiricism and observable phenomena, a radical departure from the intrapsychic approach of psychoanalysis and the introspective tradition of early experimental psychology. Operant conditioning flourished under the leadership of its leading exponent and most prolific researcher, B.F. Skinner (1953). By the 1950s, experimental research with operant conditioning and classical conditioning paradigms had led, both directly and indirectly, to the design and evaluation of clinical interventions. Today, a considerable array of clinical procedures based on behavioral psychology is available to clinicians (Kazdin, 2001).

In this section we provide a brief overview of the basic principles of behavioral psychology. Many of these principles were originally identified in the laboratory with animal models, although their applicability to humans in general and to neuropsychiatrically impaired children in particular has been established. A thorough understanding of these principles is essential to the effective implementation of behavioral treatments. Indeed, a cookie cutter approach to behavior therapy, in which a series of techniques is indiscriminantly applied to targeted behavioral psychopathologies independent of a careful conceptualization, is unlikely to work. Instead, treatment should emerge from an understanding of the variables that cause and maintain maladaptive behavior patterns, as well as an appreciation for how environmental manipulations can alter these patterns.

Operant Conditioning

Operant conditioning forms the basis of the majority of behavioral interventions used in pediatric neuropsychiatry. In operant conditioning, a behavior is followed by a consequence that either increases or decreases the probability that the behavior will occur in the future. *Reinforcement* increases the likelihood that a behavior will recur, whereas punishment decreases that likelihood. In *positive reinforcement* a pleasurable stimulus (e.g., praise, food) is presented, while in *negative reinforcement* an aversive stimulus is withdrawn

(e.g., escape from an unpleasant activity). Punishment consists of either the presentation of a noxious stimulus (e.g., yelling) or the removal of a pleasant stimulus (e.g., taking away a favorite toy). Temporal contiguity between the behavior and the consequence is critical: the interval must be short, often only a few seconds. Determining which stimuli are reinforcing or punishing is an empirical issue that can only be resolved by observing a stimulus' effect on the behavior (i.e., an increase or decrease in the probability of recurrence). *Intensity* of reinforcers and punishers is equally critical. Reinforcers that are intense and delivered to individuals in a relative state of deprivation will lead to a more robust and durable behavioral response. Likewise, if the individual is satiated, the effect of the reinforcer will be diminished. Punishers, too, must be intense in order to be effective. This phenomenon is one of the reasons that punishment is rarely used in clinical practice: ethical concerns preclude administration of aversive stimuli of sufficient intensity to significantly suppress an undesirable behavior. Moreover, the side effects of intense punishment are highly negative (e.g., pain, anger, anxiety, fearfulness).

Schedules of reinforcement pertain to the rules, or *contingencies*, under which reinforcers are delivered. In *continuous reinforcement*, a reinforcer is delivered each time a behavior occurs. *Intermittent reinforcement*, on the other hand, involves delivery of the reinforcer after the emission of more than one occurrence of the behavior or within a particular time frame. For example, ratio schedules require delivery of a reinforcer after a specific number of behaviors, and *interval schedules* dictate the delivery of reinforcers after a specific period of time has elapsed. Reinforcer delivery can be fixed (i.e., after every 10th response or after a 1-minute interval) or variable (i.e., after an average of every 10 responses or after an average interval of 1 minutes). Two variations of the above schedules of reinforcement are *differential reinforcement of other behavior* and *differential reinforcement of incompatible behavior* schedules, in which a reinforcer is delivered after an interval of time during which a particular behavior is *not* emitted. Differential reinforcement of other behavior and differential reinforcement of incompatible behavior schedules are widely used with neuropsychiatrically disturbed children who exhibit aggressive or self-injurious behaviors.

A final aspect of reinforcement is *fading*. In fading, the contingencies for delivering reinforcers are gradually shifted to require more responses (in ratio schedules) or a greater time interval (in interval schedules) between reinforces. Fading creates a more durable response pattern and decreases the labor needed to deliver frequent reinforcers.

When the contingencies change so that a reinforcer is no longer delivered after a response, *extinction* will occur. The pattern of responding during extinction varies as a function of the reinforcement schedule previously in place. If responses were continuously reinforced, responding decreases quickly and eventually ceases. With intermittent reinforcement schedules, responding is more durable, taking a longer time to drop off. Often, a significant increase in responding (i.e., an extinction "burst") occurs when reinforcement is first withdrawn. For example, a preschooler's tantrums that are reinforced by a parental attention may initially increase in frequency and intensity when the parent begins to ignore them.

Other important features of operant conditioning are *stimulus discrimination* and *generalization*. Discrimination describes the degree to which the individual distinguishes between specific features of the stimuli present in the setting where the reinforcer is delivered (e.g., a child is noncompliant with parents but not with teachers). Stimulus generalization is said to occur if the child is noncompliant in all settings in which demands are placed. When operant methods are used to increase positive behaviors (e.g., social initiation in a withdrawn child), generalization is desirable, that is, it is hoped that skills learned in the hospital unit will generalize to school and the playground. However, generalization rarely occurs unless it is specifically built into the treatment plan (Edelstein, 1989).

Shaping is the process by which complicated behaviors are taught by means of positive reinforcement. In shaping, *successive approximations* of the desired behavior are reinforced, with the criteria for receiving the reinforcer made progressively more stringent. In the case of the social withdrawal, a child may initially receive positive reinforcement for leaving his room in a hospital unit, then for gathering with other children, and finally for talking with them. Children with significant cognitive impairments will require a much finer breakdown of the behaviors to be subsequently shaped. A *task analysis* specifies the sequence of steps required to perform the targeted behaviors (e.g., brushing teeth). Task analyses are most often used with autistic and/or mentally retarded children.

Classical Conditioning

Classical conditioning is a form of learning in which two or more stimuli become associated. It is generally viewed as a more passive form of learning than operant conditioning in that the targets to be altered are reflexive and autonomic responses rather than overt behaviors (operants). In classical conditioning, an unconditioned stimulus initially elicits an unconditioned response. For example, an individual may experience a traumatic event (unconditioned stimulus) and become extremely anxious (unconditioned response). A stimulus temporally contiguous with the unconditioned stimulus, referred to as the conditioned stimulus, subsequently elicits a conditioned response that is topographically similar to the unconditioned response. For example, the individual may experience anxiety in settings similar to those in which the traumatic event occurred. Therefore, classical conditioning involves the learned association between a conditioned stimulus and an unconditioned stimulus, which in turn leads to a conditioned response.

The conditioned stimulus must precede the unconditioned stimulus. Essentially, the conditioned stimulus alerts the individual that an unconditioned stimulus is coming. As in operant conditioning, the time interval between the conditioned stimulus and the unconditioned stimulus must be brief (i.e., 1 to 2 seconds). The only exception to this requirement is for *conditioned taste aversion*, in which the interval can be several hours. The conditioned response is strengthened by repeated pairings of the conditioned stimulus and the unconditioned stimulus. If the conditioned stimulus is intense, fewer pairings (or even only one paring) will be needed to bring about a conditioned response. Presentation of the conditioned stimulus without the unconditioned stimulus results in extinction and a weakening of the conditioned response. Passage of time has little effect on the strength of the conditioned response. Stimulus discrimination and generalization (in which the conditioned response may be elicited by stimuli similar but not identical to the conditioned stimulus) also occur in classical conditioning.

Classical conditioning is important in the development or maintenance of several anxiety disorders, including specific phobias, posttraumatic stress disorder, social phobia, and obsessive-compulsive disorder. *Systematic desensitization* and *exposure* are two widely used behavioral interventions of anxiety disorders that are also based on classical conditioning. In pediatric neuropsychiatry, in which developmental disorders predominate, there are relatively fewer applications for classical conditioning. However, there has been a recent convergence of assessment and treatment approaches in the literatures on children with developmental disabilities and children with emotional and behavioral problems such that there is increasing overlap in implementation and outcomes (Clarke, Dunlap, and Stichter, 2002).

Social Learning Theory

Unlike operant and classical conditioning, in which environmental factors predominate as determinants of behavior, social learning theory assigns a prominent role to cognition in the etiology of child psychopathology. *Modeling* is an important form of learning (Bandura, 1977) whereby children acquire knowledge by observing others. Attributions are also critical; self-efficacy, or the child's belief that he or she is a competent person, promotes effective social behavior and is associated with overall well-being and mental health. The tenets of social learning theory are consistent with the cognitive focus of developmental psychopathology, developmental models of socialization and emotional regulation, and cognitive therapy. An important advance in social learning theory has been in our understanding of development of antisocial behavior in children and adolescents (e.g., Patterson, 1997). Because of its cognitive focus, social learning theory is less applicable to children with neuropsychiatric disorders who are nonverbal or cognitively limited.

BEHAVIORAL ASSESSMENT AND TREATMENT

Behavioral Assessment

Behavioral assessment operates under several assumptions. First, behavior is primarily controlled by environmental contingencies, and the functional relationship between environmental variables and specific target behaviors is the primary focus of assessment. Second, target behaviors must be operationally defined, observable, and measured reliably. Third, because behavior is likely to differ across settings, it is necessary to gather data from multiple venues in the child's life. And fourth, assessment and treatment are intricately linked, such that treatment plans should emerge from assessment data and should be periodically altered to reflect changes in patterns of behavior. Thus, unlike more traditional psychological assessments, in which measures are administered discretely before and after treatment, behavioral assessment is ongoing and continuous.

Behavioral assessment also takes into account the numerous factors that influence the child's clinical presentation (MacDonald, 2003). These factors include the child's physical health, genetic liability to psychiatric disorder, neurological impairment, family system, and growth and psychosocial development.

What is categorized under the rubric of behavioral assessment techniques has expanded greatly over the years. Originally, *direct observation of behavior* in the natural environment was the defining feature of behavioral assessment, and this method remains the cornerstone of data gathering. With this approach, target behaviors are operationally defined, clear criteria for their occurrence are stipulated, and exploratory samplings are conducted during which the behavior is measured. Behaviors can be counted (e.g., number of hostile verbalizations) and timed (e.g., number of minutes spent mouthing an object in a given hour), or a behavior can be recorded as having occurred or not occurred during a specific time interval (e.g., out of seat at any time during 5-minute intervals). *Antecedents* (events that precede the emission of the behavior) and *consequences* (responses to the behavior) are also recorded. Reliability checks are conducted to ensure that data are being collected in an accurate and consistent manner. Data are collected prior to (baseline) and during treatment.

Single-case experimental designs (Tervo, Estrem, Bryson-Brockmann, and Symons, 2003) are used to evaluate an intervention's effectiveness. Examples of such methodologies include the *alternate-treatments design* (A-B-A-B), in which the intervention is alternately introduced and removed, with the expectation that the behavior will change in the predicted direction as a function of the intervention, and the *multiple-baseline design*, in which the intervention is introduced sequentially across classes of behavior or across settings.

Observation can also be conducted in analog fashion; examples include simulated social interactions (role-play tests) and clinician-directed parent–child interactions (i.e., asking a parent to place a demand on the child so that their interactions can be observed). Behavioral assessment also measures products of treatment, such as body weight (in a weight-loss program), physiological arousal (in an anxiety-reduction intervention), or number of items correct on a test (in a program for ADHD).

Most behavior therapists incorporate additional forms of measurement in their assessments, including self-report questionnaires, semistructured and structured interviews, symptom checklists, personality assessments, functional skills inventories, diagnostic interviews, cognitive and developmental functioning tests, and family functioning indices, to name but a few. This broadening of the definitions of behavioral assessment is viewed by most behavior therapists as a positive development in that it brings together approaches to data gathering that have as their common feature a reliance on empirical methods for instrument development.

Behavioral Treatments

General Issues

Before specific behavioral interventions are addressed, we note several implementation issues critical to the successful outcome of behavior therapy.

First, behavior therapy involves considerable effort on the part of the clinicians and caregivers. Restructuring environmental contingencies requires the participation of parents, teachers, and others in the child's life. Indeed, the time commitment required may discourage families and clinicians from embarking on behavioral treatment plans. However, considerable evidence exists of the shortterm and longterm benefits of behavior therapy, and caregivers frequently underestimate the amount of time they already spend responding (usually without positive effect) to psychopathological behavior in their children.

A second issue is *consistency in carrying out behavioral interventions*. Behavioral programs are extremely sensitive to inconsistent implementation, which typically results in failure. For example, if a reinforcement program is administered correctly by the child's mother but incorrectly by the father, the intervention is likely to collapse. A general rule of thumb is that clinicians should enlist the active cooperation and involvement of caregivers before proceeding with the intervention. Toward this end, therefore, behavior therapy requires a partnership between families and clinicians. A corollary to this rule is that it is best not to begin a behavioral intervention until the family's active and full participation has been enlisted; otherwise, the plan will fail, and the family will attribute that failure to the specific intervention, thereby undermining future attempts by other professionals to use behavioral approaches.

A third issue is the ethical and legal imperative to *use the least restrictive intervention possible* when designing and carrying out treatments (Spreat and Jampol, 1997). This principle means that interventions should be as unintrusive as possible, provide maximum freedom and choice to the patient, and be conducted in settings that are open and uncontrolling. Failure in these settings justifies interventions that are more restrictive in nature, although it is imperative that such failure be well documented before alternative settings or treatments are pursued. In the case of behavior therapy, it is virtually universally recognized that positive approaches to behavior change are preferable to punishment, and that, should aversive interventions be used, a positive behavioral program should be part of the overall treatment package.

A fourth consideration is *concurrent implementation of behavior therapy with other treatments.* It is generally believed that behavior therapy is a less restrictive form of treatment than some kinds of pharmacotherapy and thus should be tried before medications are prescribed. In practice, however, the use of behavior therapy prior to pharmacotherapy is the exception rather than the rule. Although the underuse of behavior therapy can be partly attributed to lack of training in or appreciation of behavior therapy as an efficacious treatment on the part of mental health practitioners, it is also the case that severe psychopathologies, particularly those involving aggression or self-injury, often require multiple interventions, and that such combined interventions are more likely to lead to a rapid treatment response. Thus, concurrent use of behavioral and somatic treatments is often desirable. Although the literature on concurrent use of medications and behavioral treatments in children is sparse, preliminary evidence suggests that these approaches may have additive or synergistic effects (see Pelham, et al., 2000). There are few scenarios in which such combined treatments are contraindicated, except perhaps in the anxiety disorders (e.g., the use of anxiolytics in patients with specific phobias may interfere with extinction of conditioned anxiety).

Behavioral Techniques

Specific behavioral interventions should emerge from the *functional assessment,* in which the antecedents and consequences of targeted behaviors are identified. Patterns of behavior are examined to establish contextual parameters in which the behavior is likely to occur. During this stage, potential reinforcers are also identified by observing the child and interviewing the child and caregivers. For children who are nonverbal or who have profound cognitive impairments, identifying an array of potential reinforcers can be quite challenging. Creativity is often required to generate toys, objects, smells, or tactile stimuli that might be reinforcing. *Reinforcement sampling* (Patel, Carr, Kim, Robles, and Eastridge, 2000) refers to the process whereby simple behaviors are shaped by introducing a variety of potential reinforcers in an effort to identify those stimuli with the strongest reinforcing properties. In this paradigm, potentially reinforcing stimuli are first presented to the child in an effort to determine their relative pleasantness

(approach) or unpleasantness (avoidance). To evaluate their strength, stimuli that appear to be reinforcing are then used to teach the child simple tasks. In this way, a menu of reinforcers is created that can be used in more complicated behavioral programming. Assumptions should not be made about what stimuli might or might not be reinforcing; social praise may mean little to an autistic child, and a neurologically impaired child may be overstimulated by physical touch and find such stimuli aversive.

For most children with neuropsychiatric disorders, it will be desirable both to decrease negative behaviors (i.e., aggression, defiance, noncompliance, inattention, self-abuse) and to increase positive behaviors (e.g., social initiation, social skills, recreational skills, problem-solving skills, self-control skills). Positive behavioral programming (Gresham, et al., 2004) encompasses behavioral interventions that are based on positive reinforcement and that are minimally restrictive in nature.

The first step in behavioral interventions is to *structure the environment.* The functional assessment will have revealed stimuli or settings in which the behavior problem is most likely to occur. Changes in these settings or in the child's routine may be the most effective (and certainly the least intrusive) way of reducing maladaptive behaviors. For example, many autistic children react negatively to changes in routine or transitions during the day. Ample advance warning about upcoming transitions, or ensuring that such changes are not abrupt and unexpected, may prevent negative reactions.

Positive reinforcement is the centerpiece of any behavior program. Positive reinforcement is not only a less restrictive intervention; in addition, because it has as its focus the learning of new behaviors, it has the potential to enhance the behavioral functioning of the child rather than simply suppressing an undesirable behavior. Reinforcing stimuli are identified through the functional analysis conducted during behavioral assessment as well as through reinforcement sampling. Behavioral interviews with the family and child (if possible) are also sources of information about reinforcing stimuli. Differential reinforcement of other behavior and differential reinforcement of incompatible behavior schedules are implemented to decrease aggressive or self-abusive behaviors; other reinforcement schedules are used when new behaviors are to be learned. With differential reinforcement of other and differential reinforcement of incompatible behavior schedules, reinforcement is delivered contingent upon a behavior's absence.

Differential reinforcement of appropriate response schedules target specific behaviors for reinforcement that are directly incompatible with the aberrant behavior and that serve to enhance the child's overall functioning. Initially, contingencies should be structured so that the child is highly likely to earn rewards. Effort on the part of the clinician, staff, and family is greatest at this point.

Prompting, manual guidance, and *shaping* are critical approaches in the early implementation stages of reinforcement programs for teaching new skills and behaviors. As the child receives reinforcers and successfully adapts to the program, the contingencies are gradually made more stringent (*fading*). To promote *generalization* of learned behaviors to other settings or with other caregivers, the program is then expanded to these areas. Failure to actively promote generalization will likely result in rapid deterioration after discontinuation of treatment. Using reinforcers that are likely to occur in the child's natural environment is the best way to facilitate generalization.

For behavior problems that are reinforced in the child's natural environment (e.g., tantrums reinforced by parental attention), *extinction* is often employed. In this procedure, the reinforcing stimuli are withdrawn in the hope that the behavioral problem will decrease or disappear if it is not reinforced. As previously mentioned, a brief increase in intensity of the behavior (the extinction "burst") is to be expected when the reinforcing stimuli are first withdrawn. Extinction should never be the sole intervention used, for the simple reason that it is an approach that is almost impossible to implement consistently. Almost invariably, someone in the child's environment will inadvertently reinforce the negative behavior, thereby providing intermittent reinforcement and strengthening the behavior's resistance to extinction. Extinction is more likely to be effective if used in conjunction with other behavioral interventions.

For self-stimulatory or self-abusive behaviors, which are often controlled by internally-based reinforcers rather than environmental ones, *sensory extinction* is a variable treatment. In this procedure, the reinforcing aspects of the behavior are reduced or eliminated (e.g., a desk is padded with soft material for a child who head-bangs on that surface). Such an intervention can be quite effective in combination with differential reinforcement of other behavior, differential reinforcement of incompatible behavior, and differential reinforcement of appropriate response schedules. Under controlled conditions, extinction has been found to be an effective intervention. For example, Iwata and colleagues (1990) used extinction to treat hand biting, face hitting, and head banging in seven children and adolescents with mild to profound mental retardation. Withdrawal of reinforcing stimuli (e.g., escape from demand, attention) results in clinically significant reductions in self-injury.

Functional communication (e.g., Kahng, Hendrickson, and Vu, 2000) has recently emerged as a major treatment option for neuropsychiatrically disturbed children who are nonverbal or who have limited language abilities. This approach derives from the assumption that aggressive, self-abusive, and self-stimulatory behaviors occur partly as a result of frustration secondary to ineffectiveness in one's environment and problems in communicating needs and wants. Accordingly, teaching children alternative ways of communicating ("I need help" or "I want a break") by using assistive devices or sign language should reduce frustration and lead to decreases in aberrant behavior. Functional communication also teaches children alternative

ways (e.g., other than acting out) to escape aversive situations, thereby circumventing the negative-reinforcement contingencies that can maintain aggressive and self-stimulatory behaviors.

Punishment paradigms should be used only 1) when positive reinforcement methods have been tried and have failed, 2) in conjunction with positive reinforcement programs, 3) when the clinical consequences of the behavior problem are seriously detrimental to the child or others, and 4) after being appropriately reviewed by the treatment team or an independent body (e.g., human rights committee) (National Institutes of Health, 1991). Depending on the setting, state and federal regulations typically mandate extensive restrictions on the use of aversive approaches. *Response cost* is a relatively mild aversive procedure in which reinforcers are withdrawn contingent upon the emission of a targeted negative behavior. Essentially, it involves a penalty used in the context of a positive reinforcement program. Response cost procedures may bring about a more rapid treatment response; these have been found to be especially helpful in children with disruptive behavior disorders (Musser, Bray, Kehle, and Jenson, 2001). *Overcorrection* involves requiring the child to undo or correct (i.e., make restitution for) the damage resulting from an aggressive behavior (e.g., throwing objects) and then to carry out a series of steps (e.g., using the object appropriately) incompatible with the acting-out behavior (positive practice). *Time-out* is a procedure whereby the child is removed from a setting in which negative behaviors are being reinforced to an area where no such reinforcement is possible. The time-out may involve moving to the corner of a classroom away from the group (exclusionary time-out) or being isolated in a separate room with the door closed (seclusionary time-out). In most settings, types and durations of time-out are quite restricted. Time-out is most effective if it is quickly implemented, of short duration, used with behavior problems maintained by social reinforcers (which are absent in the time-out situation), and not in itself reinforcing (i.e., positively reinforcing by attracting attentions, or negatively reinforcing by allowing the child to escape an unpleasant task).

In general, punishment should be used sparingly. As previously noted, the side effects of punishment (e.g., fear, anger) are undesirable, and punishment procedures do not by themselves teach the child alternative behaviors. Moreover, these approaches are easily abused. The role of punishment in the treatment of neuropsychiatrically impaired children is still a matter of debate, however, and some advocate its use for cases of severe self-injury in which other interventions have been ineffective.

Token Economy

Token economics emerged in the 1960s as an important approach to behavioral change in developmentally disabled and neuropsychiatrically disturbed children.

Essentially, a token economy is a system in which contingencies are established for the earning of objects or symbols that in turn are exchanged for reinforcers. The rules for earning, losing, and exchanging tokens, as well as the types of reinforcers that can be earned, are established by the clinician. Because the token economy is designed to influence groups of people, it is employed in closed and controlled settings such as classrooms, inpatient units, and group homes.

Tokens have no reinforcing properties by themselves; they usually consist of chips, paper cutouts, or points on a card. Williams, Williams, and McLaughlin (1989) noted that, to be effective, tokens should be easily dispensed, easy to carry and exchange, draw little attention away from the task at hand when distributed, and have an understandable exchange value. Tokens are secondary reinforcers, that is, they gain their reinforcing qualities by their association with primary reinforcers. To the extent that the primary reinforcers are salient and powerful, the tokens will also take on those features. As with all reinforcement programs, success is dependent upon establishing a menu of desirable reinforcing stimuli with which tokens are paired. If the child does not find the stimuli to be reinforcing, the token system will deteriorate and fail. Likewise, if the contingencies for earning tokens are too stringent and difficult for the child, motivation will decrease and the system will not work. If the child has several reinforcers from which to choose, the token system is more likely to be effective. Thus, a good economy has an array of reinforcing stimuli and allows the child to earn tokens readily.

Tokens are typically used for group management. For example, inpatient units may have a levels system whereby privileges are earned through points awarded contingent upon maintenance of self-control and participation in ward programs. There also exists a sizable literature documenting the use of token economies as primary treatment modalities (Martin and Pear, 2002). Indeed, token economies were originally developed to treat, rather than simply manage, behavior problems. Examples of treatment targets include social initiation, compliance, delusional verbalizations, and language acquisition.

Token economies have several advantages over other interventions. Tokens are effective reinforcers, and provision of a menu of reinforcers decreases the likelihood of satiation. Moreover, a token economy is a relatively less restrictive form of intervention, tokens can be paired with social reinforcers (e.g., praise) to enhance their reinforcing strength, and tokens can be used to promote generalization of learned behaviors to other settings.

Paradoxically, despite the demonstrated effectiveness of token economies, their use has decreased, and they are rarely established for reasons other than group management. A number of factors are responsible for this decline, including concerns about cost, the labor required to set up and maintain a token system, potential problems arising from the use of extrinsic rewards for social behaviors, legal limitations on what can and cannot be administered to individuals contingently, and problems with generalization. However, token economies are cost effective, run smoothly when implemented properly, and can be easily manipulated to fade reliance on tangible reinforcers and promote generalization to other settings (Martin and Pear, 2002). For these reasons, they should be considered a viable and highly successful approach to behavior change.

Summary of Behavioral Assessment and Treatment

It is clear that behavior therapy encompasses a series of approaches and techniques embedded within a theoretical conceptualization of how aberrant behavior originates and how it can be altered. Haphazard application of behavioral strategies in the absence of a careful case formulation is almost certain to fail. Rather, for behavior therapists, assessment and treatment are tightly woven together, each influencing the other in a dynamic manner.

Table 30.1 presents a summary (grouped by type of approach) of the behavioral interventions outlined in this section in order to articulate a step-by-step approach to behavioral assessment and treatment. It should be emphasized that the selection of appropriate interventions must arise from the assessment. Moreover, the choice of treatment may change as the ongoing assessment reveals new functional relationships and areas in need of intervention.

Assessment begins with the *behavioral interview*. This interview differs somewhat from other clinical interviews in that its primary goals are to identify factors relevant to behavioral intervention. Thus, in addition to gathering information on interpersonal, family, and school functioning, the behavioral interview focuses on specific parameters of problem behaviors (severity and frequency), antecedents and consequences of behaviors, settings in which the behaviors may be better or worse, skills that the child may have, and potential reinforcers that may maintain or increase negative behaviors or that may subsequently be used in a reinforcement program. From the beginning, then, information gathering focuses on features that will be incorporated into treatment.

Behavior therapists also employ *standardized assessments*, which are useful in comparing the child's behavior with that of relevant normative or control groups. Moreover, specific items on some standardized measures may lead to a better understanding of factors contributing to the behavior and controlling its expression. As in any clinical assessment, collection of information from multiple sources is imperative. Nonetheless, such measures are not integral to treatment selection and treatment effectiveness monitoring; rather, they supplement the behavioral measures articulated earlier in this chapter.

Direct observation is the cornerstone of behavioral assessment. Recording the occurrence and parameters of

TABLE 30.1

SUMMARY OF BEHAVIORAL ASSESSMENT AND TREATMENT APPROACHES TO BEHAVIORAL DISORDERS IN PEDIATRIC NEUROPSYCHIATRY

Assessment

Steps	Approach	Objectives
1.	Behavioral interview	Obtain information from patient, family, and other caregivers regarding frequency and severity of behavior problem, antecedents and consequences, stimulus control, social skills, coping skills, cognitive style, and reinforcers.
2.	Self-report and report by others	Using standardized instruments and checklists, gather information about behavior problems and overall psychosocial functioning.
3.	Direct observation	Directly monitor and record parameters of behaviors, and related variables of interest (e.g., antecedents and consequences).
4.	Functional assessment	Manipulate environmental factors to determine functional relationships between such factors and behavior.
5.	Additional assessments	Conduct additional assessments that may be etiologically important or have implications for treatment selection and effectiveness (e.g., neuropsychological evaluation, neuroimaging studies).

Treatment

Behavioral Intervention Approaches	Illustrative Strategies
Operant conditioning	Positive reinforcement programs, contingency management, token economy, skills training, relaxation training
Classical conditioning	Systematic desensitization, flooding, other counterconditioning interventions
Cognitive approaches	Cognitive therapy

behavior problems in the environments in which they are exhibited is essential both for documenting the severity of these problems and for monitoring changes resulting from intervention. Direct observation also permits identification of antecedents, consequences, and environmental stimuli that may influence the behavior.

The *functional assessment* involves manipulation of environmental factors to observe their impact on the expression of behavior. In this way, the functional relationship between environmental variables and behavior can be ascertained, and changes can be made in those variables associated with an increase in aberrant behavior.

Finally, information gathered from *other assessment approaches* may be critical to understanding the etiology and treatment of behavioral disorders. *Imaging studies* may implicate specific neurological contributions. Likewise, *neuropsychological evaluations* may identify neurocognitive impairments and learning difficulties. Because such phenomena may interfere with learning, behavioral interventions may need to be adapted for optimal effectiveness.

FAMILY ADAPTATION AND INTERVENTION

Historically, the family was viewed as the primary etiological influence in child neuropsychiatry and psychology.

Psychopathology and behavioral disturbances in children were attributed to dysfunctional family systems in general, and to inappropriate parenting practices in particular. Another widespread belief was that raising a child with a disability led to longterm family distress and, in some cases, psychopathology in family members. In other words, a disabled child results in a disabled family.

More modern research, however, has largely dispelled the myths that neuropsychiatrically impaired children necessarily emerge from dysfunctional families and that all families fail to adapt to childhood disabilities (Quittner and DiGirolamo, 1998). Instead, it is increasingly apparent that the etiologies of neuropsychiatric disorders are multidetermined and frequently involve processes that are out of the direct control of family members (e.g., genetic anomalies, neurological damage) (Schuntermann, 2002).

Most recently, research has started to track resiliency factors; those aspects of the family environment and interpersonal traits that increase the likelihood of positive adaptation. Resiliency, simply defined, is the presence of adequate social resources and coping strategies to allow the family to successfully adapt to the added strain of disability. In other words, the presence of positive family traits may more than compensate for the presence of family pathology in adaptation (Hastings and Taunt, 2002). This is not to say that dysfunctional family systems play no role in the etiology, maintenance, or exacerbation of child psychopathology. On the contrary, a rich and growing scientific literature is documenting such relationships and evaluating effective treatments for children and their families (Henggeler, Schoenwald, and Pickrel, 1995). But current models of family adaptation to children with disabilities in general and neuropsychiatric disorders in particular, highlight the importance of mediating factors, both positive and pathological, as critical determinants of functioning. These variables shift in their relevance, intensity, and influence, resulting in changes in family responding over time. Adaptation, therefore, is best characterized as a continuous process, rather than static, and an interactive, reciprocal process rather than linear.

Although virtually all children with neuropsychiatric disorders can be said to place strain on the family, the manifestation of stressors will vary from child to child depending upon the neuropsychiatric impairment. Numerous features of the child's disability have been implicated in family adaptation, including functional limitations, impact on language, externalizing symptoms, additional time required to care for the child, depletion of tangible resources, and disruptions in routine. Strain, in general, is exacerbated by the lack of predictability that may accompany certain neuropsychiatric disorders, such as epilepsy and traumatic brain injury (Cohen, 1993; Franks, 2003). This lack of predictability manifests as everyday, daily hassles of living that are more important stressors than intermittent negative life events in producing strain on the family, as is the inability to establish and maintain daily routines due to the fluctuating demands of the disability.

Family and social support are primary resiliency factors, as they can buffer the impact of caring for a difficult-to-manage child regardless of the type of neuropsychiatric disability. A distinction is made between *social support* (in which the family has someone on whom it can rely for emotional and tangible assistance) and *social network* (the number of contacts with others). Social support, or *quality*, of interpersonal contacts, appears to be more important than social network, or *quantity*, of contacts, for psychological health (Perlesz, Kinsella, and Crowe, 1999), although the two are clearly related. Respite care is an important resource for giving parents a break from caring for their child as well as an opportunity to increase their social networks and to build supportive relationships outside of professional care systems.

Families of children with disabilities often have limited social networks as the result of the particular features of the child's disability. Others may not wish to associate with them because of the stigma of neuropsychiatric disorders, such as with seizures in epilepsy or the lowered cognitive functioning in a child with developmental delay (Ellis, Upton and Thompson, 2000; Melnyk, Feinstein, Moldenhouer, and Small, 2001). Both adults and children may experience difficulties in relating to or being around children that fail to reciprocate in social interactions; for example, the child with autism. The child with ADHD may be impulsive and behave with other children in such a way that limits the ability to successfully make friends. Also, curtailed mobility of the child (e.g. wheelchair reliant) may limit access to social networks and more normative family activities and interactions.

Adding to family stress is the realization that, even with appropriate therapies and interventions, features of the disability may be present lifelong (Majovski, 2000; Perlesz, et al., 1999). When parenting a child without disabilities, parents recognize the time-limited nature of the child's lack of abilities, such as walking and talking. As children undergo normal development, these stressors subside; as when a child learns to walk, so increases the mobility of the family, or when a child learns to use language to make requests, relieving the parent of the responsibility of trying to ascertain the needs of and speaking for the child. Conversely, the families of children with neuropsychiatric disabilities may anticipate a lifelong responsibility for a child with restricted mobility or who lacks the cognitive functioning to successfully use language to express basic needs.

Children with less physically impairing disabilities may still place strain on the family in other ways. For example, children with ADHD are, overall, more impaired in educational settings. They are more likely to be suspended or expelled from school, to underachieve academically, and to be held back a grade than children without a disability. While these traits create longterm challenges for the individual as he or she moves into young adulthood, the family feels the strain during the childhood years; parents may spend considerable extra time in contact with school staff.

Other stressors in the family may also undermine adaptation. Financial hardship, family violence, inadequate housing, and neighborhood violence further add to family stress. Coping styles of individual family members and the family unit as a whole moderate the impact of stress and foster resiliency. Parents with effective problem-solving skills and optimist cognitive styles are more likely to cope effectively with adversity or the daily stressors of raising a neuropsychiatrically impaired child. Families with limited cognitive abilities or few psychosocial resources will be less effective in coping with stressors (Sloper and Turner, 1993).

Family adaptation is also influenced by parental expectations and attributions. Excessively high expectations about the child's abilities, rigid beliefs about how children should behave, and erroneous attributions of a child's behavioral dysfunction to purposeful intent erode the parent–child relationship and contribute to family dysfunction. This effect points to the need for parental education about the particular disability as an intervention to aid in the family's successful adaptation to and parenting of a child with a developmental trajectory and pattern of behavior unique to their particular disability (Schuntermann, 2002).

Family adaptation is affected by features of the parent–child relationship. Failure of a child to establish a secure attachment with caregivers will negatively affect family adaptation. This is particularly challenging with neuropsychiatrically impaired children, such as those with autism, who are less able to reciprocate in interpersonal relationships thus resulting in less attachment. Temperamental mismatches between a parent and a child with a disability may also be implicated in family distress. Parental premorbid functioning also contributes to family adaptation. Family functioning can be negatively affected by parental psychiatric disorder, particularly substance abuse and other disorders that lead to family instability (e.g., psychoses).

As is the case with psychological and behavioral treatment of children, family-based interventions should emerge from a comprehensive assessment. Numerous measures are available that can be used to assess aspects of family functioning (e.g., communication, rituals, relationships), social support, parental psychiatric status, and parents' attitudes toward their children. From this assessment, a range of intervention options can be constructed. Some families will require greater community resources, such as self-help groups or respite programs. Others will require extensive education about their child's disorder or will need instruction on child development and basic child care. Still others will require more intensive therapeutic intervention to remediate dysfunctional aspects of family interactions and relationships, including help in facilitating the adjustment of other children (without disabilities) in the family. In certain cases, it will be desirable for the parents to receive treatment for psychiatric disorders.

In order for behavioral interventions for children to be successful, parents must be partners in implementing these programs. *Parent training* involves instructing parents in how to implement behavioral programs for their children. Although parent training is essential for parents with deficient parenting skills, it is typically provided to all parents who are required to carry out behavioral interventions at home. An added therapeutic benefit of such training is that it empowers parents and families to actively work toward the remediation of the child's behavioral problems. Parents are taught specific behavioral skills (e.g., reinforcement, contingency contracting) to improve child management, reduce reliance on physically punitive strategies, and increase nurturing and relationship-enhancing behaviors. Although several widely used parent-training protocols exist (e.g., Baker, 1989), they all share several features. First, they are highly structured and didactic. Second, they involve the extensive use of in-clinic training with at-home practice. And third, they use behavioral training principles, including modeling of skills by therapists, practice through simulated role-playing and/or in-clinic analogs, and feedback provided to parents by therapists.

SUMMARY

The comprehensive treatment of neuropsychiatric disorders in children requires an integrated approach that incorporates both psychological and somatic interventions. Assessment involves measurement of social, emotional, behavioral, cognitive, neurological, neurophysiological, and other medical domains of functioning. Although a variety of psychological interventions for behaviorally disturbed children are available, recent meta-analyses have supported the superior effectiveness of behavior therapy. Behavioral strategies have special relevance for children with developmental disabilities or neuropsychiatric impairments, including those with significant cognitive limitations.

Core features of psychotherapy (e.g., establishing a therapeutic alliance) must be altered to maximally benefit children and adolescents with developmental disabilities and neuropsychiatric disorders. Within the larger assessment of clinical psychopathology and child functioning, behavioral assessment is carried out to identify functional relationships that serve to maintain or exacerbate behavioral dysfunction. Interventions are developed on the basis of this assessment. Principles of learning are applied to increase social and other skills and to decrease maladaptive behaviors. Ongoing observational assessment provides data regarding the effectiveness of the intervention and guides needed alterations in the intervention. In general, treatments pursued should be the least restrictive possible and should incorporate interventions based on positive reinforcement. Treatment necessarily requires family participation, although some families will need additional intervention. Families with few social and psychological resources are those at greatest risk for maladaptive responses to raising a neuropsychiatrically impaired child.

REFERENCES

Ainsworth, M. D. (1969). Object relations, dependency, and attachment: a theoretical review of the infant-mother relationship. *Child Development*, 40: 969–1025.

Ammerman, R. T., & Patz, R. (1996). Determinants of child abuse potential: contribution of parent and child factors. *Journal of Clinical Child Psychology*, 25: 300–307.

Baker, B. L. (1989). *Parent training and development disabilities*. Washington, DC: American Association on Mental Retardation.

Bardura, A. (1977) *Social Learning Theory*. Englewood Cliffs, NJ: Prentice Hall.

Beail, N. (2003). What works for people with mental retardation? Critical commentary on cognitive-behavioral and psychodynamic psychotherapy research. *Mental Retardation*, 41: 468–472.

Beutler, L. E., Malik, M., Alimohamed, S., Harwood, T. M., Talebi, H., Noble, S., et al. (2003). Therapist variables. In M. J. Lambert (Ed.), *Handbook of psychotherapy and behavior change* (5th ed., pp. 227–306). New York: Wiley.

Bowlby, J. (1969). *Attachment and loss: Vol. 1*. New York: Basic Books.

Casey, R. J., & Berman, J. S. (1985). The outcome of psychotherapy with children. *Psychological Bulletin*, 98: 388–400.

Clarke, S., Dunlap, G., & Stichter, J. P. (2002). A descriptive analysis of intervention research in emotional and behavioral disorders from 1980 through 1999. *Behavior Modification*, 26: 659–683.

Cohen, M. H. (1993). The unknown and the unknowable: managing sustained uncertainty. *Western Journal of Nursing Research*, 17: 77—96.

Durlak, K. A., Fuhrman, T. & Lampman, C. (1991). Effectiveness of cognitive-behavior therapy for maladapting children: A meta-analysis. *Psychological Bulletin*, 110:204-214.

Edelstein, B.A. (1989). Generalization: terminological, methodological and conceptual issues. *Behavior Therapy*, 20: 311–324.

Ellis, N., Upton, D., & Thompson, P. (2000). Epilepsy and the family: a review of current literature. *Seizure*, 9: 22–30.

Franks, R. P. (2003). Psychiatric issues of childhood seizure disorders. *Child and Adolescent Psychiatric Clinics of North America*, 12: 551–565.

Gresham, F. M., McIntyre, L. L., Olson-Tinker, H., Dolstra, L., McLaughlin, V., & Van, M. (2004). Relevance of functional behavioral assessment research for school-based interventions and positive behavioral support. *Research in Developmental Disabilities*, 25: 19–37.

Harris, J. C. (1995). *Developmental neuropsychiatry: Assessment, diagnosis, and treatment of development disorders Vol. 2*. New York: Oxford University Press.

Hastings, R. P., & Taunt H. M. (2002). Positive perceptions in families of children with developmental disabilities. *American Journal of Mental Retardation*, 107: 116–127.

Henggeler, S. W., Schoenwald, S. K., & Pickrel, S. G. (1995). Multisystemic therapy: bridging the gap between university- and community-based treatment. *Journal of Consulting and Clinical Psychology*, 63: 709–717.

Herschell, A. D., McNeil, C. B., & McNeil, D. W. (2004). Clinical child psychology's progress in disseminating empirically supported treatments. *Clinical Psychology, Science and Practice*, 11: 267–288.

Hurley, A. D. (1989). Individual psychotherapy with mentally retarded individuals: a review and call for research. *Research in Developmental Disabilities*, 10: 261–275.

Iwata, B. A., Pace, G. M., Kalsher, M. J., Cowdery, G.E., & Cataldo, M.F. (1990) Experimental analysis and extinction of self-injurious escape behavior. *Journal of Applied Behavior Analysis*, 23:11-27.

Jones, M. C. (1924). A laboratory study of fear: the case of Peter. *Journal of Genetic Psychology*, 31: 308–315.

Kahng, S. W., Hendrickson, D. J., & Vu C. P. (2000). Comparison of single and multiple functional communication training responses for the treatment of problem behavior. *Journal of Applied Behavior Analysis*, 33: 321–324.

Kazdin, A. E. (1991). Effectiveness of psychotherapy with children and adolescents. *Journal of Consulting and Clinical Psychology*, 59: 785–798.

Kazdin, A. E. (2000). *Psychotherapy for children and adolescents: Directions for research and practice*. New York: Oxford University Press.

Kazdin, A. E. (2001). *Behavior modification in applied settings* (6th ed.). Belmont, CA: Wadsworth.

Kazdin, A. E. (2003). Psychotherapy for children and adolescents. *Annual Review of Psychology*, 54: 253–276.

Levant, R. F. (2004). The empirically validated treatments movement: a practitioner/educator perspective. *Clinical Psychology: Science and Practice*, 11: 219–224.

Levitt, E. E. (1957). The results of psychotherapy with children: an evaluation. *Journal of Consulting Psychol*, 21: 189–196.

MacDonald, E. K. (2003). Principles of behavioral assessment and management. *Pedriatic Clinics of North America*, 50: 801–816.

Majovski, L. V. (2000). Selected neurodevelopmental delay syndromes and their impact on adult neuromaturation and adjustment. *Seminars in Clinical Neuropsychiatry*, 5: 171–176.

Mann, C. (1990). Meta-analysis in the breech. *Science*, 249: 476–480.

Martin, G. L., & Pear, J. (2002). *Behavior modification: What it is and how to do it* (7th ed.). Saddle River, NJ: Prentice Hall.

Melnyk, B. M., Feinstein, N. F., Moldenhouer, Z., & Small, L. (2001). Coping in parents of children who are chronically ill: strategies for assessment and intervention. *Pediatric Nursing*, 27: 548–558.

Musser, E. H., Bray, M. A., Kehle, T. J., & Jenson, W. R. (2001). Reducing disruptive behaviors in students with serious emotional disturbance. *School Psychology Review*, 30: 294–305.

National Institutes of Health. (Sept 1991). Consensus development conference on the treatment of destructive behaviors in person with development disabilities. (NIH Publ No 91-2410). Washington, DC: U.S. Department of Health and Human Services, Public Health Service.

Ollendick, T. H. (Ed.): J Clin Ch Psychol, 28

Patel, M. R., Carr, J. E., Kim, C., Robles, A., & Eastridge, D. (2000). Functional analysis of aberrant behavior maintained by automatic reinforcement: assessments of specific sensory reinforcers. *Research in Developmental Disabilities*, 21: 393–407.

Patterson, G. R. (1997). A developmental model for late-onset delinquency. *Nebraska Symposium on Motivation*, 44: 119–177.

Pelham, W. E., Gnagy, E. M., Greiner, A. R., Hoza, B., Hinshaw, S. P., Swanson, J. M., et al. (2000). Behavioral versus behavioral and pharmacological treatment in ADHD children attending a summer treatment program. *Journal of Abnormal Child Psychology*, 28: 507–525.

Perlesz, A., Kinsella, G., & Crowe, S. (1999). Impact of traumatic brain injury on the family: a critical review. *Rehabilitaton Psychology*, 44: 90–105.

Prout, H. T., & Nowak-Drabik, K. M. (2003). Psychotherapy with persons who have mental retardation: an evaluation of effectiveness. *American Journal of Mental Retardation*, 108: 82–93.

Prout, H. T. (1998). Issues in mental health counseling with persons with mental retardation. *Journal of Mental Health Counseling*, 20: 112–120.

Quittner, A. L., & DiGirolamo, A. M. (1998).Family adaptation to childhood disability and illness. In R. T. Ammerman & J. V. Campo (Eds.), *Handbook of pediatric psychology and psychiatry, Vol. 2* (pp. 70–102). Boston, MA: Allyn & Bacon.

Rush, A. J., & Frances, A., (eds.). (2000). Expert consensus guideline series: Treatment of psychiatric and behavioral problems in mental retardation. *American Journal of Mental Retardation*, 105: 159–226.

Schuntermann, P. (2002). Pervasive developmental disorder and parental adaptation: previewing and reviewing atypical development with parents in child psychiatric consultation. *Harvard Review of Psychiatry*, 10: 16–27.

Shadish, W. R., Navarro, A. M., Matt, G. E., & Phillips, G. (2000). The effects of psychological therapies under clinically representative conditions: a meta-analysis. *Psychological Bulletin*, 126: 512–529.

Shapiro, D. A., & Shapiro, D. (1982). Meta-analysis of comparative therapy outcome studies: a replication and refinement. *Psychological Bulletin*, 92: 581–604.

Skinner, B. F. (1953). *The behavior of organisms*. New York: Macmillan.

Sloper, P., & Turner, S. (1993). Risk and resistance factors in the adaptation of parents of children with severe physical disability. *Journal of Child Psychology and Psychiatry*, 34:167–188.

Spreat, S., & Jampol, R. C. (1997). Residential services for children and adolescents. In R. T. Ammerman & M. Hersen (Eds.), *Handbook of preventions and treatment with children and adolescents* (pp. 106–133). New York: Wiley.

Sroufe, L. A., & Rutter, M. (1984). The domain of developmental psychopathology. *Child Development*, 55: 17–29.

Stevens, S. E., Hynan, M. T., & Allen, M. (2000). A meta-analysis of common factor and specific treatment effects across domains of the phase model of psychotherapy. Clinical Psychology: Science and Practice, 7: 273–290.

Task Force on Promotion and Dissemination of Psychological Procedures, Division of Clinical Psychology, American Psychological Association. (1995). Training in and dissemination of empirically-validated psychological treatments: report and recommendations. *The Clinical Psychologist*, 48: 3–23.

Tervo, R. C., Estrem, T. L., Bryson-Brockmann, W., & Symons, F. J. (2003). Single-case experimental designs: applications in developmental-behavioral pediatrics. *Journal of Developmental and Behavioral Pediatrics*, 24: 438–448.

Watson, J. B. (1924). *Behaviorism*. New York: People's Publishing.

Weiss, B., & Weisz, J. R. (1990). The impact of methodological factors on child psychotherapy outcome research: a meta-analysis for researchers. *Journal of Abnormal Child Psychology*, 18: 639–670.

Weisz, J. R., Weiss, B., Alicke, M. D., Klotz, M.L., et al. (1987). Effectiveness of psychotherapy with children and adolescents: a meta-analysis for clinicians. *Journal of Consulting and Clinical Psychology*, 55: 542–549.

Weisz, J. R., Weiss, B., Han, S. S., Granger, D. A. A., & Morton, T. (1995). Effects of psychotherapy with children and adolescents revisited: a meta-analysis of treatment outcome studies. *Psychological Bulletin*, 117: 450–468.

Williams, B. F., Williams, R. L., & McLaughlin, T. F. (1989). The use of token economies with individuals who have developmental disabilities. In E. Cipani (Ed.), *The treatment of severe behavior disorders: Behavior analysis approaches* (pp. 3–18). Washington, DC: American Association on Mental Retardation.

Wilson, D. B. & Lipsey, M. W. (2001). The role of method in treatment effectiveness research: Evidence from meta-analysis. *Psychological Methods*, 6:413-429.

31

Psychoeducational Interventions in Pediatric Neuropsychiatry

Jeffrey A. Miller, MD   Stephen Bagnato, EdD   Carl J. Dunst, PhD
Hillary Mangis, MSEd

Brain injury or malfunctioning occurs all too frequently in children and adolescents (Annegers, 1983; Frankowski, Annegers, and Whitman, 1985; Langlois and Gotsch, 2001; Moyes, 1980; Snow and Hooper, 1994). Two broad areas of science—the biological and the behavioral—have contributed substantially to our understanding of the causes and sequelae of brain disorders. Research in the neurosciences generally and in neuropsychiatry specifically has advanced our knowledge of brain–nervous system–behavioral disorder linkages, while research in neuropsychology, psychology, and education has enhanced our understanding of the behavioral manifestations of neurological impairments and of how environmental interventions can influence these behaviors in an adaptive manner. According to Mrazek and Haggerty (1994), there is an "increasing tendency within the biological and behavioral sciences to appreciate the complexity and interplay of genetic and environmental interactions" (p. 498). This renewed appreciation reflects an increased recognition of the environment's vital role in influencing both brain functioning and the behavioral characteristics associated with brain disorders.

In this chapter we discuss a number of themes and critical elements of emerging best practice in one domain of environmental influence, psychoeducational interventions. Our purpose is not to describe in detail specific kinds of psychoeducational interventions; such detailed discussions can be found elsewhere (e.g., Cohen, 1991; Eslinger, 2002; Ewing-Cobbs, et al., 1986; Glang, et al., 1992; Semrud-Clikeman, 2001; Snow and Hooper, 1994). Rather, our intention is to present a framework that pediatric neuropsy-

chiatrists can use to ensure that appropriate educational interventions are developed and implemented for children and adolescents with neuropsychiatric disorders. More specifically, it is our goal in this chapter to provide pediatric neuropsychiatrists with information they can use to bridge neuropsychiatric diagnoses with environmental interventions that have a high probability of producing positive, socially adaptive outcomes and to identify facilitators and inhibitors for success of these environmental interventions.

The chapter is divided into six sections. In the first, we briefly discuss the importance of both neurobehavioral markers and behavioral characteristics of neuropsychiatric disorders in children and adolescents and show how these markers and characteristics can inform the use of appropriate psychoeducational interventions. In the second section, we describe several assessment and classification systems used in psychology, special education, developmental disabilities, and related interdisciplinary fields. These systems are important because their purposes, functions, and methods differ from those of the system used almost exclusively by professionals in the neuropsychiatric community, the *Diagnostic and Statistical Manual of Mental Disorders-Fourth Edition-Text Revision* (DSM-IV-TR) (American Psychiatric Association, 2000). In the third section of this chapter, we outline the characteristics of psychoeducational intervention approaches best suited for children and adolescents with neuropsychiatric disorders. These characteristics are ones that collectively define emerging best practice in terms of those psychoeducational interventions having the greatest potential to produce positive benefits. In the fourth section, we address the broader-based context of physician–family–school relationships, including the current call for adoption of family-centered approaches to neurobehavioral problems. Family-centered interventions have emerged as a philosophy and approach for ensuring that family members are supported and meaningfully involved in the diagnostic and care processes so that they in turn can interact with their children in ways that support the children's behavioral and developmental progress. In the final two brief sections intervention effectiveness research is examined and a case example provided in which the seven elements of psychoeducational interventions are highlighted.

NEUROBEHAVIORAL MARKERS AND PATTERNS OF BEHAVIOR IN CHILDREN WITH BRAIN DISORDERS

Researchers in a number of basic science and applied fields (e.g., early intervention, developmental disabilities, developmental pediatrics, developmental neuropsychology, medicine, neuropsychiatry) have become increasingly interested in brain–behavior relationships and how those relationships influence behavioral and developmental outcomes in children with brain disorders (e.g., Johnson, 1993). Whereas neuropsychiatrists may focus on the particular mechanisms that lead to brain disorders, including the defining characteristics of specific types and subtypes of psychiatric or neurological conditions, psychoeducational interventionists focus primarily on the behavioral consequences of brain disorders and the environmental conditions best suited to promoting adaptive functioning in individuals with such disorders. Psychoeducational interventionists differentiate between the *antecedents* (i.e., risk markers) of specific kinds of disabilities and the behavioral characteristics that represent the *consequences* of these conditions. This distinction is an important one, because it is the latter (i.e., the *patterns of behavior* associated with a disability or impairment) that are the focus of psychoeducational interventions.

Risk Markers

Problems accompanying brain injury or malfunction are often correlated with particular behavioral markers; that is, specific risk factors associated with the onset, severity, and patterns of particular neurodevelopmental problems or behaviors. For example, the onset of pervasive developmental disorders, including autism and childhood schizophrenia, is often preceded by signs such as unusual eye movements. According to Mrazek and Haggerty (1994), such signs *mark*, or identify the potential for, different kinds of problems or unfavorable outcomes. However, although for psychoeducational intervention a risk marker may indicate the *need for intervention*, it may not necessarily be the *target* of such intervention. Rather, as indicated above, the consequences are the typical targets of psychoeducational interventions.

Specific risk markers have been found to be associated with both congenital and acquired brain injury and malfunctioning. For example, young children who subsequently manifest developmental delays and disabilities are often found to have had early disturbances in areas of self-regulatory functioning related to sleep patterns, feeding, attention/activity, arousal, sensory organization, coping with environmental changes, and control of emotional behavior (DeGangi, 1991; Neisworth, Bagnato, and Salvia, 1995). Many of these self-regulatory problems are also found in children who have been prenatally exposed to drugs, who have sustained subtle brain insults prenatally or postnatally, who have difficult temperament styles, or who have particular kinds of congenital syndromes (Bagnato and Campbell, 1993; Coie, et al., 1993; Drotar and Strum, 1991; Yeates, Ris, Taylor, 2000). Acquired brain damage, whether resulting from injury or disease, has been found to be correlated with various kinds of risk markers that can be used both in diagnosis and in decisions about the need for intervention (Snow and Hooper, 1994).

From a psychoeducational perspective, the importance of risk markers is rather straightforward. The presence of markers known to be associated with brain-related problems signals the need for interventions to prevent or deter the emergence of maladaptive functioning and to promote and enhance adaptive behavior and competence (DeGangi, 1991). In general, the more risk markers present, the higher the probability of adverse consequences and thus the greater the need for intervention. For example, intrauterine growth retardation is associated with as many as eight biological risk markers (Harel, et al., 1991) in addition to related physical and behavioral risk signs (Harel, et al., 1993). Similarly, children who have experienced brain trauma often manifest a number of symptoms and complications that collectively indicate the presence and severity of brain damage and the need for intervention (Semrud-Clikeman, 2001; Snow and Hooper, 1994).

Behavioral Characteristics and Templates

As previously noted, combinations of risk markers and other neurobehavioral indicators are often used to diagnose brain disorders. Emerging evidence reveals that many neurological disorders are presaged by specific signs and markers, and that certain disorders are associated with specific clusters of behavioral characteristics (Hertzig, 1983; Miller and Ramer, 1990; Rourke, et al., 2002; Thompson, 1989; Whitney and Thoman, 1993). Although individuals with different disorders often manifest similar behavioral characteristics, it is nonetheless possible to construct neurobehavioral templates that can be used to differentiate disorders with similar presentations, to select the optimal targets and approaches for psychoeducational interventions, and to anticipate the emergence of intervention targets over the developmental period. For example, Table 31.1 shows behavioral characteristics associated with four different brain disorders. Delineating such disorder-specific neurobehavioral characteristics is an important prerequisite to identifying and differentiating the antecedents from the consequences of the disorder (as previously emphasized, it is the latter that become the targets of psychoeducational interventions).

TABLE 31.1
PATTERNS OF BEHAVIOR ASSOCIATED WITH SELECTED BRAIN DISORDERS

Fragile X Syndrome

Deficits in social play skills
Gaze avoidance
Repetitive motor behaviors
Social communication deficits
Hyperactivity/attention deficits
Object mouthing
Excessive tantrums
Self-injury
Hyperreactivity to new events

Autistic Spectrum Disorder

Absence of pretend play
Imitative deficits
Sensory hypersensitivities
Poor adjustment to change
Disorganized play
Hyperactivity
Self-stimulation
Social communication deficits

Rett Syndrome

Normal development for first 6 months
Head-growth decline
Loss of purposeful hand skills
Decline of neuromotor, language skills
Stereotyped midline hand movements:
    wringing/squeezing/clapping/tapping/mouthing/washing/
    rubbing
Breath holding
Teeth grinding
Facial tics
Torso tremors
Seizures/staring

Early Brain Injuries

Neuromotor deficits
Sensory and affective hypersensitivities
Response latencies
Social communication deficits
Motor planning problems
Disorganized play routines
Low physical endurance
Poor goal-directed behavior
Attention and memory deficits
Easy frustration
Variable alertness and awareness

Both researchers and practitioners have found early identification and specification of the behavioral clusters associated with particular brain disorders to be helpful in detecting problems, and designing and evaluating psychoeducational interventions (Bagnato and Neisworth, 1999a; Baumgardner, et al., 1995; Miller and Ramer 1990; Neisworth, et al., 1995; Rourke, et al., 2002). For example, among older individuals (8+ years to adult) with fragile X syndrome (Baumgardner, et al., 1995), researchers have identified a cluster of neurobehavioral characteristics—hyperactivity, stereotyped and self-injurious behavior, inappropriate speech, and coping difficulties—that have been used as the targets of psychoeducational interventions. Such behavioral templates can help practitioners to recognize behaviors that could be responsive to intervention. Also, the Temperament and Atypical Behavior Scale (TABS) (Neisworth, et al., 1999) uses an authentic assessment approach and parent–professional observations to identify clusters of related concerns which detect types of self-regulatory behavior problems in young children. The TABS identifies atypical aspects of temperament and self-control, and evidence-based interventions in four major behavior clusters: Detached; Hypersensitive/Active; Underreactive; and Dysregulated. The TABS is endorsed by the American Academy of Pediatrics for use by pediatricians in the early identification of behavior problems in infants, toddlers, and preschoolers. Several assessment systems useful for identifying intervention targets are briefly described in the following section.

FUNCTIONAL ASSESSMENT AND CLASSIFICATION SYSTEMS

Professionals who work with children and adolescents with or at risk for neurodevelopmental disorders often employ functional approaches to assessment that directly link assessment with intervention practices. The term "functional" is used in this chapter to refer to the ability to perform various functions within the context of real life situations. Functional assessment and classification systems are especially useful from a psychoeducational perspective because they rely on methods that directly lead to the selection of intervention targets and approaches. Such systems are used to ascertain specific capabilities of children and adolescents rather than global indices such as behavioral traits, intelligence, or personality, because it is these capabilities that constitute the targets of psychoeducational interventions.

Functional approaches to assessment and classification often used with children and adolescents with brain disorders include the *International Classification of Functioning, Disability and Health* (ICF) (World Health Organization, 2001); the Adaptive Behavior Assessment System-Second Edition (ABAS-II) (Harrison & Oakland, 2003) that closely aligns with the American Association on Mental Retardation classification system (American Association on Mental Retardation, 2002); Functioning After Brain Injury (FABI) (Smith, et al., 2004), and the System to Plan Early Childhood Services (SPECS) (Bagnato & Neisworth, 1990). Each of these systems includes methods for ascertaining the presence and severity of neurodevelopmental disorders. More importantly, each system assists in identifying intervention targets and approaches for effecting behavioral and developmental change. That is, because these assessment systems emphasize identification of the behavioral consequences of disorders and disabilities, they contribute to decisions and practices that can be used to strengthen existing competencies and to promote acquisition of new, adaptive capabilities.

International Classification of Functioning, Disability, and Health (ICF)

The International Classification of Impairments, Disabilities, and Handicaps (ICIDH) (World Health Organization, 1980) was originally created to emphasize behaviors associated with specific disorders and the behavior–environment relationships that account for variations in behavioral functioning. More specifically, the ICIDH assessed (1) how diseases, injuries, and disorders result in impairments in behavioral functioning; (2) how these impairments translate into disabilities in terms of incapacity to perform specific activities; and (3) how both impairments and disabilities influence outcome in terms of impeding the affected individual's access to social, economic, and other opportunities. Complimentary to the *ICD-10th Revision* (World Health Organization, 1992) and part of the World Health Organization Family of International Classifications (WHO-FIC), the ICF (World Health Organization, 2001) has replaced the ICIDH. The ICF is designed to describe how health conditions impact individuals' lives. It covers a variety of domains within each of four components: body functions and structures, activities and participation, environmental factors, and personal factors. A domain "is a practical and meaningful set of related physiological functions, anatomical structures, actions, tasks, or areas of life" (World Health Organization, 2001, p. 3). The first component covers mental functions and body structures and includes domains such as mental functions and the nervous system. This first component is used to describe changes to the individual as a result of disease or injury. The next two components (activities and participation; environmental factors) are most relevant to setting functional goals for psychoeducational interventions and examining environmental facilitators or inhibitors to their success. The activities and participation domains are learning and applying knowledge; general tasks and demands; communication; mobility; self-care; domestic life; interpersonal interactions and relationships; major life areas; and community, social and civic life. The environmental domains, organized from the individual's most proximal environment to the most global, are products and technol-

ogy; natural environment and human-made changes to environment; support and relationship; attitudes; and services, systems and policies. The last component, personal factors, includes internal influences not part of the health condition such as gender, habits, and past life events. Personal factors, however, are not coded in the ICF.

The system allows professionals to determine and classify the severity of an individual's behavioral problems in functional terms and to grade the impact of those problems on the individual's performance and social integration. Also, there is a strong focus on individual and environmental strengths that facilitate successful adaptation. The ICF includes methods for assessing behavioral changes resulting from interventions and for evaluating the potential for recovery in several neurodevelopmental domains of functioning.

Adaptive Behavior Assessment System-Second Edition

The *Adaptive Behavior Assessment System-Second Edition* (ABAS-II) (Harrison and Oakland, 2003) is a norm-referenced, cross-informant assessment system that closely aligns with the 10 adaptive skills areas specified by the *Diagnostic and Statistical Manual of Mental Disorders-Fourth Edition-Text Revision* (DSM-IV-TR) (American Psychiatric Association, 2000) and the current guidelines for the diagnosis of mental retardation from the recently revised *Mental Retardation: Definition, Classification, and Systems of Support-Tenth Edition* (American Association on Mental Retardation (AAMR), 2002). The skill areas assessed using the teacher and parent forms of the ABAS-II are communication, community use, functional preacademics, school/home living, health and safety, leisure, self-care, self-direction, social, and work. For younger children, motor skills replaces work skills. Difficulties identified in each area represent functional goals for psychoeducational intervention.

The ABAS-II also assesses the three clusters of adaptive skills identified by the American Association on Mental Retardation (2002) for the diagnosis of mental retardation. Historically, the AAMR emphasized assessment of intellectual functioning and two aspects of adaptive skills: personal independence and social responsibility (Harrison and Oakland, 2003). These aspects of adaptive skills have been revised by the AAMR to cover conceptual (money concepts and academic skills), social (responsibility and social competence), and practical (activities of daily living and occupational skills) adaptive skills. The skill areas measured by the ABAS-II can be organized into these three general aspects of adaptive functioning. This organization is important to plan and monitor psychoeducational interventions, as well as to make the diagnosis of mental retardation. Currently, according to AAMR, two criteria are used for making a diagnosis of mental retardation: the individual must concurrently demonstrate significant limitations in intellectual functioning and in adaptive behavior as expressed in conceptual, social, and practical adaptive skills. More importantly, because intellectual and adaptive strengths and weaknesses are assessed for the individual in the context of specific community and cultural environments, such assessment can lead directly to identification of the kinds of individualized supports, educational interventions, and instructional practices that are needed to promote a child's competence.

Functioning after Brain Injury

The Functioning After Brain Injury (FABI) (Smith, et al., 2004) is a clinical performance measure for traumatic and nontraumatic pediatric brain injury, suited for both inpatient and home aftercare settings. It was designed to align closely with the *International Classification of Functioning, Disability and Health* (ICF) (World Health Organization, 2001). The FABI is the successor to the *Pediatric Evaluation of Disabilities Inventory* (PEDI), a standardized, norm-referenced instrument designed to provide a functional appraisal of the capabilities of young children with sensory, neuromotor, brain-related, and other types of developmental problems (Haley, et al., 1992). The FABI allows assessment of the following major domains: Physical Activities, Cognitive/Behavioral Activities, and Readiness for Community Functioning. Each domain has several dimensions. The scales are designed to identify intervention targets and assess behavioral outcomes from treatment as well as other important predictors. First, the system uses an algorithm to predict expected levels of functioning at discharge based on a combination of injury-related and personal factors (comparable to the ICF). Second, it was devised to be amenable to correlational study with biochemical markers of severity to determine signs closely indicative of brain recovery.

System to Plan Early Childhood Services (SPECS)

The SPECS employs collaborative team assessment and a decision-making format that links assessment information directly with intervention targets and approaches (Bagnato and Neisworth, 1990). This system is designed for use with young children between 2 and 6 years of age, who have, or who are at risk for, developmental delays or disabilities. This functional assessment system integrates data from multiple sources and settings across occasions and instruments to enable a team of parents and professionals to profile a child's needs in 19 functional domains. It also includes procedures that lead to consensus about the severity of neurodevelopmental problems. Additionally, the SPECS generates information that aids in decision making about appropriate intervention modes and team collaboration regarding the specific details of an intervention plan, including the intensities of intervention, in the following behavioral and developmental areas: early education,

adaptive needs, behavior therapy, speech/language therapy, physical therapy, occupational therapy, vision and hearing services, medical services, and transition services.

Although these four approaches differ in their purposes and methods of assessment and classification, they share several common features: (1) they emphasize the identification of behaviors that establish the presence of a disorder or disability; (2) they specify those aspects of behavior that become the focus of psychoeducational interventions; (3) they inform practice in terms of influencing which procedures, methods, and supports will be used to effect change in positive, socially adaptive functioning; and (4) they provide a repeatable metric for assessing outcomes of psychoeducational interventions.

KEY ELEMENTS OF PSYCHOEDUCATIONAL INTERVENTIONS

Children and adolescents with congenital or acquired brain disorders are most likely to benefit from psychoeducational interventions that are characterized by an integrated functional approach to promoting adaptive capabilities (i.e., emphasize the acquisition of practical life skills in the context of daily living) (Bagnato and Mayes, 1986; Bagnato and Neisworth, 1985). Such intervention strategies differ from traditional educational approaches, in which various school personnel (e.g., regular and special education teachers, speech/language therapists, occupational and physical therapists, nurses) tend to perform their respective functions in an isolated, nonintegrative manner. The importance of an integrated approach derives from the fact that interventions are more likely to be functional and implemented *consistently* across settings and people when they are implemented collaboratively (Anderson, et al., 1993). An integrated intervention approach is especially important for working with two special populations: (1) children with congenital brain disorders, who need a range of interventions in order to receive optimal benefit; and (2) children and adolescents reentering school after traumatic brain injury, who require creative, flexible, individualized, and ever-changing psychoeducational interventions to help them navigate this difficult process (Ylvisaker, Feeney, Maher-Maxwell, et al., 1995; Ylvisaker, Feeney, & Mullins, 1995).

Psychoeducational intervention approaches are characterized by the following seven principles and elements: (1) functional intervention goals, (2) a developmental perspective on change, (3) functional assessment/intervention linkages, (4) functional instructional strategies, (5) functional contexts and settings, (6) integrated support services, and (7) collaborative teamwork. Collectively, intervention practices characterized by these features increase the likelihood that psychoeducational interventions will have optimal benefits (see Bagnato and Mayes, 1986; Bagnato and Neisworth, 1985, 1999b; Dunst, 2002; Dunst, et al., 2002; Neel and Billingsley, 1989; Wellman, 2001).

Functional Goals

According to Wolery (1989), functional intervention goals are those that (1) are immediately useful, (2) enable a child to be as independent as possible, (3) allow the child to learn other, more complex skills, (4) allow the child to function in the least restrictive environment possible, and (5) enable family members and others to more easily care for the child. Neel and Billingsley (1989) have similarly noted that functional goals are ones that permit a child to have greater control over environmental events and consequences.

White (1980) made a useful differentiation between behavioral form and behavioral function that has important implications for developing psychoeducational goals: *form* refers to the observable behavior to be taught, whereas *function* refers to the effect of the behavior on the child's social and nonsocial environments. According to Wolery (1996), "for some goals, the form (behavior) is important, as in the case of self-feeding; for other goals, the effect is more important, as in the case of initiating social interactions with peers or requesting a drink" (p. 505).

Generally, functional instructional goals are ones that specify observable and purposeful behaviors across many major developmental domains or behavioral areas: cognition, preacademic/academic, motor, language, social communication, and self-regulatory behavior. For example, the goal of getting across the room with decreasing reliance on others might be an appropriate one for helping an individual in a wheelchair to increase his or her independence, whereas the goals of communicating personal needs and initiating social interactions might be appropriate for helping a child acquire better communication skills.

Developmental Perspective

A developmental perspective of psychoeducational interventions maintains that the form and function of behavior change across time. Such change is, in part, a result of the reinforcing consequences of an individual's acquisition of socially adaptive competencies (Dunst and McWilliam, 1988). In contrast with adults, children have not mastered fundamental developmental milestones of normal development. So, as the child recovers competencies lost due to a disability the child must concurrently achieve normal developmental competencies making for additional challenges that must be considered for intervention planning (Dennis, 2000; Thomson and Kerns, 2000). Accordingly, the goals of psychoeducational interventions must be ordered (sequenced) and promoted in a manner that permits progressively more complex socially adaptive capabilities to be acquired over time as well as meet the vicissitudes of development, thus enabling a child to become involved in or to reenter a variety of environments. Consequently, psychoeducational interventions are most likely to be effective if they have sequential functional goals, link the child's assessed capabilities with these goals and methods, include

procedures for monitoring improvement as a function of intervention type, and modify strategies and practices in response to behavioral and developmental change in the child (Bagnato and Campbell, 1993; Bagnato and Mayes, 1986; Bagnato and Neisworth, 1985; Dennis, 2000).

Assessment/Intervention Linkages

A functional approach to assessment and intervention directly links assessment information with the selection of intervention plans and instructional goals and practices. That is, the information obtained by gathering assessment data leads to a better appreciation of the environmental conditions, situations, and contexts that will optimize the socially adaptive benefits resulting from psychoeducational interventions (Miller, Tansy, and Hughes, 1998). Unlike traditional assessment methods, which tend to focus on a child's level of functioning in terms of an intelligence (IQ) or social quotient (SQ) or some other global index, functional assessment methods examine the form and function of behavior across and within settings and environments, with particular emphasis on the environmental conditions associated with variations in behavioral form and function. For example, the SPECS (Bagnato and Neisworth, 1990) pools assessment information from multiple informants (e.g., parents, teachers, therapists) to reach a consensus about a child's capabilities, determines intervention needs and selects appropriate priorities, and monitors progress toward desired goals. The approach to functional behavioral assessment for individuals with disabilities by Miller et al. (1998) employs a similar approach of directly linking eight domains of functioning (affective regulation/emotional reactivity, cognitive distortion, reinforcement, modeling, family issues, physiological/constitutional, communicate need, and curriculum/instruction) with instructional goals and methods.

Functional Instructional Strategies

According to Neel and Billingsley (1989), "increasing control over the environment is the major goal of instruction" (p. 15). The achievement of this goal draws upon a number of different methods and procedures for promoting a child's acquisition of socially adaptive competence. Although functional instructional strategies may deploy any number of different intervention practices, all share one feature: they contribute to change in the form and function of socially adaptive capabilities as a result of the experiences and opportunities afforded the child (McClean, Wolery, & Bailey, 2003).

Wolery (1996) has described a useful framework for examining how differences in the form and function of a child's behavior might lead to different intervention approaches. For example, when behavioral form is adequate but function is limited (e.g., a child has a rich topography of gestures but does not use them for communicative purposes), the emphasis of instruction would be to "teach new functions using existing forms and promote maintenance of existing functions" (Wolery, 1996, p. 506). In contrast, when behavioral function is multiple but form is limited (e.g., a child uses only hand gestures to communicate a variety of needs, desires, and wishes), the focus would be to "teach new forms for existing functions and promote maintenance of existing forms" (Woolery, 1996, p. 506). It should be readily apparent from these examples that a child cannot be fitted to one instructional method; on the contrary, instructional practices must fit and match the child's unique learning needs.

Although the term *instruction* has generally been used to refer to techniques employed by a teacher or therapist to teach a child specific behavioral goals and objectives, the term in a broader sense refers to any practices that contribute to changes in the form or function of a child's socially adaptive capabilities. Such practices include direct teaching, responsive teaching, programmed instruction, making available materials that evoke desired behavior, scheduling activities in ways that increase behavioral responding, arranging the environment so that it facilitates adaptive behavior, and providing access to different environmental settings and conditions, all of which, either individually or in combination, can be used to promote and enhance behavioral competence and developmental change.

Regardless of the particular methods employed, effective psychoeducational interventions share certain key features (Wolery 1996):

1. Promote student participation in classroom activities and routines, as well as independence and mastery of the environment.
2. Address functional goals many times throughout the student's day.
3. Address as many goals as possible within the same activities and routines.
4. Use a functional goal-by-activity/routine framework (matrix) to determine which goals can be addressed in which activities and routines.
5. Adapt the student's activities and routines as necessary to promote acquisition of identified goals and behaviors.
6. Monitor (i.e., evaluate) the effects of the instructional practices used to achieve identified goals/outcomes so that appropriate changes and/or modifications can be made as needed.

Instructional practices that adhere to these guidelines are more likely to produce desired effects and developmental changes in both the form and the function of behavior. When deciding among instructional practices that equally meet Wolery's (1996) criteria, Brown, Odom, and Conroy (2001) recommend that the most appropriate interventions are ones that are (1) effective for children with similar markers or behaviors (i.e., evidence-based); (2) efficient (i.e., least demanding on service providers); and (3) normalized (i.e., authentic and naturalistic to the individual's environment)

Functional Settings and Contexts

Because of the importance of the environments in which children and adolescents must learn to function adaptively and independently, instructional settings and contexts deserve to be considered as a separate element of psychoeducational interventions (Neel and Billingsley, 1989; Wolery, Bashers, and Neitzel, 2002). Functional instructional practices are ones in which instruction occurs in the settings and contexts that a child directly experiences in daily living. That is, functional instruction must occur in environments that have meaning to the child, not in isolated or contrived locations that bear no resemblance to real life settings (Ware, 1990). This principle is especially relevant for instructional support services, which we describe next.

Integrated Instructional Support Services

Instructional support services, including sensory, communication, and neuromotor therapies, for children with neurological or other developmental disorders have traditionally been provided in a pull-out fashion. For example, physical therapy for a child with cerebral palsy may be offered once weekly in a 45-minute session in a school building therapy room or a hospital-based clinic. These kinds of pull-out services, however, are costly, and their effectiveness is as yet undetermined. Moreover, these approaches often disrupt one of the most important predictors of a child's learning potential: time on task (i.e., engagement in functional learning activities/environments) (Greenwood, 1991; McWilliam and Bailey, 1992; Rosenshine, 1978). Finally, because they occur apart from classroom routines, pull-out services do not address generalization of specific functional skills (e.g., Cole, et al., 1989; Giangreco, 1986, 2000).

Instructional support services include communication, speech/language, physical, occupational, and other kinds of therapies and supportive interventions (e.g., adaptive equipment and augmentative devices) (Ried, et al., 1995) that are used integratively and that adhere to the previously identified key features of functional instructional strategies. Thus, psychoeducational and support service personnel must communicate and work together on an ongoing basis if this kind of integration is to become a reality (Weist, et al., 2003).

Collaborative Teamwork

The likelihood that these first six key elements of psychoeducational interventions will be operationalized in a consistent fashion is increased considerably if collaborative teams are used to identify functional goals and settings and to implement instructional practices (see Bagnato and Mayes, 1986; Bagnato and Neisworth, 1985, 1999b; Campbell, 1987; Miller, et al., 1998; Walther-Thomas, Korinek, and McLaughlin, 1999; West and Cannon, 1988). Appropriate team members include school personnel, other professionals working with the child and his or her family (e.g., neuropsychiatrists), the child's parents, and, when appropriate, the child himself or herself. Collaborative teamwork encourages consensus decision making, flexible judgments regarding the child's capabilities, and identification of the most creative and appropriate ways to deliver services. Further, Walther-Thomas and colleagues (1999) identified the features supportive of collaboration including shared leadership, family involvement, cohesive school vision, comprehensive program planning, provision of adequate resources, sustained implementation, and ongoing performance evaluation and improvement. In order for collaborative team efforts to work and the identified functional goals to be attained, team members must be flexible and define their roles in terms of what is best for the child. In many instances, achieving the necessary flexibility may require staff members to function in a consultative rather than a direct service capacity and to use a transdisciplinary team model in which all team members integrate their knowledge and expertise into a more functional instructional approach (Campbell 1987; West and Cannon, 1988). These properly distributed professional responsibilities allow for opportunities for all team members to contribute to the well-being of the individual and to have ownership in the process of treating children with disabilities (Walther-Thomas, et al., 1999).

All of these key components of psychoeducational interventions are implemented in the context of broader based environmental influences, several of which we describe next.

PHYSICIAN–FAMILY–SCHOOL RELATIONSHIPS

Building strong physician–family–school relationships can be accomplished by bringing together the knowledge, competence, and expertise needed to inform psychoeducational practices and to ensure that other needed supports and resources are available to children and adolescents with brain disorders. According to ecological theory (Bronfenbrenner, 1979, 1992), different settings (e.g., hospital, school, home) and people within these settings are characterized by different degrees of linkages and levels of reciprocal relationships, respectively. In settings in which relationships (linkages) are strong, information sharing and collaboration among participants are more likely to occur in ways that serve supportive functions. For example, parents' knowledge and understanding of their child can help inform both neuropsychiatric and psychoeducational practices; neuropsychiatric expertise can inform psychoeducational practice and vice versa; and both neuropsychiatric and psychoeducational knowledge and expertise can be supportive of parents' efforts to care for their child with a brain disorder.

Two emerging systems practices (described below) hold special promise for forging and strengthening physician–family–school relationships. The first of these, school-based health clinics/school-linked services, specifically aim to promote integration of educational, medical, mental health, therapeutic, and other kinds of services and supports. Such integration has the explicit purpose of bringing important resources to bear on the development and implementation of interventions for children with brain-related and other kinds of developmental disabilities. The second of these promising practices is family-centered interventions, which specifically aim to promote the flow of different kinds of resources in ways that strengthen the family. Such systems interventions are premised on a new larger body of evidence indicating that social-support networks involving reciprocal transactions among network members are associated with positive effects in multiple areas of child, parent, and family functioning (Dunst, Trivette, and Jodry, 1997).

School-Based Collaboration

The basic argument for instituting school-based collaboration is that it will result in increased access to treatment. School-based collaboration offers promise in bridging the gap between service need and service utilization (Ambruster and Lichtman, 1999). Hacker and Wessel (1998) list seven qualities critical for effective school-based collaboration: (1) clarification of roles and redefinition regarding integration and collaboration, (2) strong leadership, (3) emphasis on shared ownership of the program, (4) training, (5) continued education, (6) creative compromise, and (7) mutual respect and support.

Several innovative service-delivery projects have recently been instituted to facilitate school-based collaboration among medical, educational, and mental health professionals. An example of school-based collaboration is HealthyCHILD (Collaborative Health Interventions for Learners With Differences) (Bagnato, 1999; Bagnato, et al., 2004), a school-linked developmental health care service serving young children (0 to 8 years) with chronic health conditions, neurodevelopmental disabilities, or behavioral health (e.g., self-regulatory behavior) problems and their families in public school settings.

The predominant mission of HealthyCHILD is to plan, deliver, and monitor the impact and outcomes of a transagency model for providing developmental health care resources and support in naturalistic school or agency environments such as early childhood classrooms and family child care settings. In the context of these naturalistic environments, resources and support are provided to teachers, parents, and their children with developmental delays/disabilities, chronic medical conditions, and challenging behaviors (e.g., extremes in temperament and problems in social and self-regulatory behaviors). This program began as a collaborative effort involving a major children's hospital, an urban public school system, a university-based psychiatric facility, a county mental health department, and a number of primary care pediatricians and family practitioners. HealthyCHILD uses a mobile, transdisciplinary team composed of a teacher, a psychologist, and a pediatric nurse practitioner, with consultation from a developmental pediatrician, who collectively provide direct support to children, parents, and teachers, and programmatic consultation and mentoring to personnel in public school settings, Head Start programs, early intervention programs, and early care and education centers. A developmental health care plan serves as the protocol for generating consensus goals by the family, teachers, and allied health professionals and for forging supportive linkages between the primary care pediatrician and the school staff. For example, the nurse, psychologist, teacher, and parent collaborate to produce individualized interventions for delivering health care services on-site in the classroom setting for children with asthma, diabetes, seizure disorders, and various neurodevelopmental disabilities including fragile X syndrome, Autism Spectrum Disorder, and Traumatic Brain Injury. The interventions target jointly the medical and developmental conditions and the impact on the functional early learning needs of such children, as well as the priorities of the families.

The HealthyCHILD model demonstration program research was funded originally by federal and foundation research grants from the U.S. Department of Education, Office of Special Education and Rehabilitative Services (OSERS), School-Linked Services for Better Outcomes competition, (1994 to 1998, PR award HO23D40013) and the Jewish Healthcare Foundation of Pittsburgh (1995 to 1997). The evidence-based practices for the HealthyCHILD model were established during this phase (Bagnato, 1999) and undergo current research and refinements with each new interagency contractual venture beyond the original research phase.

Currently, HealthyCHILD is administered by the Early Childhood Partnerships program of Children's Hospital of Pittsburgh and the UCLID Center at the University of Pittsburgh and is directed by one of the the authors, S. J. Bagnato, with a full-time transagency coordinator. It has evolved into a school-linked or agency-linked developmental health care consultation venture funded by contracts with school districts, early intervention programs, and Head Start grantees across Pennsylvania and in West Virginia. Currently, HealthyCHILD employs one full-time nurse, three psychologists, 12 full-time developmental health care consultants, and one full-time interagency liaison to coordinate and deliver collaborative support services to nearly 4,000 children and families and over 300 teachers and staff under six interagency contracts. Bagnato (2001) studied the service quality and behavioral outcomes for children served under the HealthyCHILD model during the 2000 to 2001 school year. Results indicated that service providers showed significant increases in their skill level to work with

children with medical and behavioral difficulties, increases in the level of support they were provided through the model, and increased opportunity to team with professionals from multiple disciplines in the service of the children. Children served under the HealthyCHILD model showed significantly increased social skill acquisition and decreased behavior problems (Bagnato, 2001).

In another example of a school-based collaborative project, Costello-Wells and colleagues (2003) developed a multisite, school-based mental health center called InteCare. The focus of the Indianapolis coalition of four mental health clinics is building on the strengths of the family by allowing them to search for expectations and discover their own possibilities. This approach is in contrast to focusing on the weaknesses that tend to overwhelm individuals, families, and service providers. In this program, the psychiatrist conducted initial evaluations; led clinical staffings with psychologists, nurses, and therapists; reviewed treatment plans; prescribed medication; and reevaluated clients progress quarterly. Qualitative data from the study found that school-based collaboration resulted in greater parental involvement in school and their children's education, less reports of problematic behaviors, lower incidence of children running out of medicine, improved support for personnel, and family reports of feeling more comfortable with receiving treatment from the school rather then services in a traditional outpatient setting.

Family-Centered Care

Although historically the idea of family-centered care can be traced to the early 1960s, its potential value was more recently articulated in 1987 by then-Surgeon General C. Everett Koop at a conference jointly sponsored by the American Academy of Pediatrics and the U.S. Department of Health and Human Services. In the report of the proceedings of this conference (Koop, 1987), Dr. Koop described new ways to improve both access to health care and related services and the quality of life of children with special healthcare needs. The contents of this report in part formed the basis for a new approach to delivering health care, education, and early intervention services to children and adolescents with medically related and other developmental problems, one based in the community and centered on families.

An emphasis on a family-centered approach to service delivery has emerged in the federal special education law *Individuals With Disabilities Education Act* (IDEA, 1997) (see Chapter 32). Many children served by the neuropsychiatrist will be covered under IDEA since medical conditions and traumatic brain injury are qualifying conditions. In IDEA, professionals are expected to recognize the family's expertise, guide and facilitate the family's understanding of and adherence to IDEA, and provide family training (Miller & Gallagher, 1997).

Dunst (2002) has defined family-centered care as: beliefs and practices that treat families with dignity and respect; individualized, flexible, and responsive practices; information sharing so that families can make informed decisions; family choice regarding any number of aspects of program practices and intervention options; parent–professional collaboration and partnerships as a context for family-program relations; and the provision and mobilization of resources and supports necessary for families to care for and rear their children in ways that produce optimal child, parent, and family outcomes (p. 139)

Shelton and colleagues (Shelton, 1999; Shelton and Stepanek, 1994; Shelton, Jeppson, and Johnson, 1987) developed eight elements of family-centered care that operationalize a philosophy of care for use in day-to-day practices across a variety of programs, settings, and situations (see Table 31.2). Both individually and collectively, intervention strategies that incorporate these elements of care increase the probability that other kinds of interventions (e.g., neuropsychiatric and psychoeducational) will have *value-added benefits*; that is, outcomes produced beyond those attributable to more traditional clinical practices.

Dunst and colleagues (Dunst and Trivette, 1996; Dunst, et al., 2002), for example, summarize evidence indicating that professional helpgiving practices that foster family choice and decision making and the active involvement of parents in helping relationships produce better outcomes, compared with traditional clinical practices. This result seems to be the case because family-centered care brings to bear supports and resources from many sources to flexibly and responsively deliver an array of individualized services to children and adolescents and their families. Unfortunately, family-centeredness has only taken hold in early childhood intervention programs and has yet to extend into elementary and secondary settings (Dunst, 2002).

EFFECTIVENESS OF PSYCHOEDUCATIONAL AND SYSTEMS INTERVENTION

The methods typically used to ascertain the effectiveness of psychoeducational interventions are quite different from those used by medical researchers (i.e., double-blind clinical trials). Psychoeducational evaluation methods include studies that contrast different interventions designed to produce similar effects, compare different features of the same intervention, and examine those conditions of specific interventions that produce desired effects, as well as the processes that contribute to the implementation of intervention practices as planned and intended (Eslinger & Oliveri, 2002). Studies of this kind were cited throughout earlier sections of this chapter.

Studies examining the effectiveness of psychoeducational interventions in children with disabilities or those at risk for poor outcomes and their families currently focus on questions of the following sort: To what extent do specific aspects of interventions have similar or different effects on children and families differing according to child or family characteristics, or both? These second generation studies differ from first generation studies, which were concerned with questions about efficacy (e.g., did the intervention work?). This shift has occurred because second generation but not first generation research *directly* informs practice in the ways described in this chapter. Thus, if we know which

---

TABLE 31.2
KEY ELEMENTS OF FAMILY-CENTERED CARE

- Incorporate into policy and practice the recognition that the family is the constant in a child's life, while the service systems and support personnel within those systems fluctuate
- Facilitate family/professional collaboration at all levels of hospital, home, and community care:
  — care of an individual child
  — program development, implementation, evaluation, and evolution
  — policy formation
- Exchange complete and unbiased information between families and professionals in a supportive manner at all times
- Incorporate into policy and practice the recognition and honoring of cultural diversity, strengths, and individuality within and across all families, including ethnic, racial, spiritual, social, economic, educational, and geographic diversity
- Recognize and respect different methods of coping and implement comprehensive policies and programs that provide developmental, educational, emotional, environmental, and financial supports to meet the diverse needs of families
- Encourage and facilitate family-to-family support and networking
- Ensure that hospital, home, and community service and support systems for children needing specialized health and developmental care and their families are flexible, accessible, and comprehensive in responding to diverse family-identified needs
- Appreciate families as families and children as children, recognizing that they possess a wide range of strengths, concerns, emotions, and aspirations beyond their need for specialized health and developmental services and support

Source: Reprinted with permission from Shelton, T. L., & Stepanek, J. S. (1994). *Family centered care for children needing specialized health and developmental services.* Bethesda, MD: Association for the Care of Children's Health.

aspects of an intervention produce what kinds of effects with what kinds of children and families under what conditions, we can be specific about making informed, empirically-based recommendations. The pursuit of data and supporting evidence, both direct and corroborative, about intervention effectiveness for children with specific aptitudes or characteristics is just emerging and an is need of further study.

With respect to first generation studies, a number of meta-analyses have been conducted examining the effectiveness of various psychoeducational interventions. In a summary of these meta-analyses Forness (2001) found that interventions such as mnemonic strategies, reading comprehension strategies, behavior modification, and direct instruction consistently evidenced large effect sizes. Interventions found to have medium effect sizes included cognitive behavioral therapy, psychotherapy, stimulant medication, computer-assisted instruction, and peer tutoring. Based on these findings, Forness (2001) concluded that best practices "include monitoring students' progress and providing positive consequences for improvement; teaching cognitive-behavioral self-management; and, at least in the case of children with ADHD, considering a systematic course of stimulant medications" (p. 194).

CASE EXAMPLE

This case involves Amy, an 8-year-old girl with a complicated medical history including congenital heart failure and seizure disorder. She had to be resuscitated twice during her first weeks of life and a pacemaker was implanted. She has taken antiepileptic medication since approximately 3 years of age after experiencing several generalized tonic–clonic seizures. Most recently, she underwent surgery to repair a vertebral arteriovenus fistula. Educationally, Amy's current teacher is quite rigid and does not reinforce her successes. Children in her class have begun teasing her with respect to academic failures by calling her stupid. She becomes easily frustrated and upset when she does not do well on academic tasks. Her parents are divorced and her father is only peripherally involved. In fact, visits to the father often exacerbate her adjustment problems. Her mother appears to lack confidence in parenting and becomes frustrated with Amy quite easily.

Cognitive testing revealed that Amy's verbal reasoning ability is in the low average range, perceptual reasoning ability is in the below average range, working and long-term memory are in the below average range, executive functions such as the ability to shift mental sets are in the well below average range, basic reading and reading comprehension were at grade level, spelling was at grade level, and mathematics skills were well below grade level. Taken together Amy has relative strengths in verbal reasoning

and language-based academics. However, the significance of these strengths would be moderated if one adopts a developmental perspective on change. That is, although she has a relative strength in language-based academics, her cognitive functioning is at best within the low average range. As a second grader, the level of challenge with respect to language-based academics is relatively low. She will need to be closely monitored through the developmental period to ensure that her reading and writing skills do not begin to lag significantly behind her age-mate peers as academic expectations increase. Overall, test results indicate she has significant difficulties in memory, executive control, and mathematics. Adaptive testing using the ABAS-II (Harrison and Oakland, 2003) (described previously) indicated that Amy has significant functional difficulties in the areas of home/school living, self-care, self-direction, and social functioning. These areas of difficulty fall within the practical and social domains of the ABAS-II.

Difficulties in the cognitive areas of memory and executive control, the academic areas of mathematics, and the adaptive functioning areas of home/school living, self-care, self-direction, and social function are the consequences of Amy's conditions and therefore are the targets for intervention. Interventions are then planned for Amy and her environment to promote adaptive functioning with respect to each of the intervention targets. Further, the psychoeducational interventions are implemented in an integrated manner in which the neuropsychiatrist leads a team of professionals that conduct or supervise interventions in the school, home, and community.

The neuropsychiatrist involved Amy's mother in both the planning and intervention stages to ensure that she could help monitor consistency of treatment across settings and to directly improve her ability to care for Amy. The psychoeducational intervention plan also included members of the school instructional support team so that Amy's services were not dependent on a single school professional, namely the teacher. Rather, the school psychologist, counselor, nurse, teacher, and special education teacher were included at the planning and intervention stages. School personnel worked with the parent so that both settings (home and school) would become more responsive to Amy's needs and to indications that she was struggling. Specific psychoeducational interventions recommended for Amy included direct instruction in metacognitive strategies such as mnemonics, note-taking, and listening skills to increase memory and reduce cognitive demands. She was provided with individual counseling using cognitive-behavioral techniques in school to help with her coping, frustration tolerance, and social functioning. Her mother and teacher were informed and educated about these cognitive-behavioral techniques so they could be practiced in the home and in the classroom. Amy was provided itinerant support in the classroom for mathematics. Her teacher was provided with classroom management techniques to help reduce the impact of teasing on Amy. Finally, through a partnership between the neuropsychiatrist and the primary physician her antiepileptic medication and general physical health continued to be monitored.

CONCLUSION

In this chapter we have described the major features of functional psychoeducational approaches to intervention and practice for children and adolescents with neuropsychiatric disorders, and have placed these practices within the broader context of two different but complementary systems-level interventions, school-based services and family-centered care. Our goal is to provide professionals with a framework for understanding the key characteristics of effective psychoeducational interventions in pediatric neuropsychiatry, which they can use for informing these children and adolescents and their families about what they should look for in obtaining effective educational and related services. Consequently, the contents of the chapter, and especially the seven principles and elements described in the key elements of psychoeducational interventions section of this chapter, can be used as a checklist for determining the appropriateness of educational practices used with children and adolescents with brain disorders. At a minimum, emerging best practice psychoeducational interventions are ones that focus on the form and function of behavior, as well as the environmental conditions that contribute to optimal, socially adaptive outcomes. To the extent that neuropsychiatrists incorporate these elements in their treatment recommendations to family members and other professionals, they will make a major contribution toward bettering the lives of children and adolescents with brain disorders and disabilities.

REFERENCES

Ambruster, P., Lichtman, J. (1999). Are school based mental health services effective? Evidence from 36 inner city schools. *Community Mental Health Journal*, 35: 493–504.

American Association on Mental Retardation. (2002). *Mental retardation: Definition, classification, and systems of supports*, (10th ed.). Washington, DC: American Association on Mental Retardation.

American Psychiatric Association. (2000). *Diagnostic and statistical manual of mental disorders, 4th edition, text revision*. Washington, DC: American Psychiatric Association.

Anderson, J. L., Albin, R. W., Mesaros, R. A., et al. (1993). Issues in providing training to achieve comprehensive behavioral support. In: J. Reichle & D. P. Wacker, (Eds.), *Communicative Alternatives to Challenging Behavior: Integrating Functional Assessment and Intervention Strategies* (pp. 363–406). Baltimore, MD: Paul H Brookes.

Annegers, J. F. (1983). The epidemiology of head trauma in children. In: K. Shapiro (Ed.), *Pediatric head trauma* (pp. 1–10). Mount Kisco, NY: Futura.

Bagnato, S. J. (1999). *Efficacy of collaborative developmental healthcare support in inclusive early childhood programs: Final research report of HealthyCHILD* (Grant Award HO23D40013). Pittsburgh, PA: Early Childhood Partnerships and Children's Hospital of Pittsburgh/University of Pittsburgh, US Department of Education, Office of Special Education and Rehabilitative Services.

Bagnato, S. J. (2001). Profiles of the Quality and Outcomes of HealthyCHILD in Allegheny Intermediate Unit Head Start. Available at http://www.uclid.org:8080/uclid/pdfs/HealthyCHILD_Outcome_Report.pdf. Accessed September 6, 2005.

Bagnato, S. J., Blair, K., Minzenberg, B., et al. (2004). Developmental healthcare partnerships in inclusive early childhood intervention settings: The HealthyCHILD model. *Infants and Young Children*, 17: 78–98.

Bagnato, S. J., & Campbell, T. F. (1993). Comprehensive neurodevelopmental evaluation of children with brain insults. In G. Miller & J. Ramer, (Eds.), *Static Encephalopathies of Infancy and Childhood* (pp. 28–43). New York: Raven.

Bagnato, S. J., & Mayes, S. D. (1986). Patterns of developmental and behavioral progress for young brain-injured children during interdisciplinary intervention. *Developmental Neuropsychology*, 2: 213– 244.

Bagnato, S. J., & Neisworth, J. T. (1985). Efficacy of interdisciplinary assessment and treatment for infants and preschoolers with congenital and acquired brain injury. *Analysis and Intervention in Developmental Disabilities*, 5: 107–128.

Bagnato, S. J., & Neisworth, J. T. (1990). *System to Plan Early Childhood Services (SPECS): Manual for a team assessment/intervention system*. Circle Pines, MN: American Guidance Service.

Bagnato, S. J., & Neisworth, J. T. (1999a). Normative detection of early regulatory disorders and Autism: Empirical confirmation of DC: 0–3. *Infants and Young Children*, 12: 98–106.

Bagnato, S. J., & Neisworth, J. T. (1999b). Collaboration and teamwork in assessment for early intervention. *Child and Adolescent Psychiatric Clinics of North America*, 8: 347–363.

Baumgardner, T. L., Reiss, A. L., Freund, L. S., et al. (1995). Specification of the neurobehavioral phenotype in males with fragile X syndrome. *Pediatrics*, 95: 711–752.

Bronfenbrenner, U. (1979). *The ecology of human development: Experiments by nature and design*. Cambridge, MA: Harvard University Press.

Bronfenbrenner, U. (1992). Ecological systems theory. In R. Vasta (Ed). *Six theories of child development: Revised formulations and current issues* (pp. 187–249). London, England: Jessica Kingsley.

Brown, W. H., Odom, S. L., & Conroy, M. A. (2001). Intervention hierarchy for promoting young children's peer interactions in natural environments. *Topics in Early Childhood Special Education*, 21: 162– 175.

Campbell, P. H. (1987). The integrated programming team: an approach for coordinating professionals of various disciplines in programs for students with severe and multiple handicaps. *The Journal of the Association for Persons with Severe Handicaps*, 12: 107–116.

Cohen, S. B. (1991). Adapting educational programs for students with head injuries. *Journal of Head Trauma Rehabilitation*, 6: 56–63.

Coie, J. D., Wat, N. F., West, S. G., et al. (1993). The science of prevention: A conceptual framework and some directions for a national research program. *The American Psychologist*, 48: 1013–1022.

Cole, K. N,. Harris, S. R., Eland, S. F., et al. (1989). Comparison of two service delivery models: in-class and out-of-class therapy approaches. *Pediatric Physical Therapy*, 1: 49–54.

Costello-Wells, B., McFarland, L., Reed, J., et al. (2003). School-based mental health clinics. *Journal of Child and Adolescent Psychiatric Nursing*, 16: 60–70.

DeGangi, G.A. (1991). Assessment of sensory, emotional, and attentional problems in regulatory disordered infants, part 1. *Infants and Young Children*, 3: 1–8.

Dennis, M. (2000). Childhood medical disorders and cognitive impairment: biological risk, time, development, and reserve. In K. O. Yeates, M. D. Ris, H. G. Taylor, (Eds.), *Pediatric neuropsychology: Research, theory, and practice* (pp. 3–22). New York: The Guilford Press.

Drotar, D., & Strum, L. (1991). Mental health intervention with infants and young children with behavioral and developmental problems. *Infants and Young Children*, 4: 1–11.

Dunst, C. J. (2002). Family-centered practices: Birth through high school. *The Journal of Special Education*, 36: 139–147.

Dunst, C. J., Boyd, K., Trivette, C. M, et al. (2002). Family-oriented program models and professional help giving practices. *Family Relations*, 51: 221–229.

Dunst, C. J., & McWilliam, R. A. (1988). Cognitive assessment of multiply handicapped young children. In T. D. Wachs, R. Sheehan, (Eds.), *Assessment of young developmentally disabled children* (pp. 213–238). New York: Plenum.

Dunst, C. J., & Trivette, C. M. (1996). Empowerment, effective helpgiving practices and family centered care. *Pediatric Nursing*, 22: 334–337.

Dunst, C. J., Trivette, C. M., & Jodry, W. (1997). Influences of social support on children with disabilities and their families In M. J. Guralnick, (Ed.), *The effectiveness of early intervention: Directions for second generation research* (pp. 499–522). Baltimore, MD: Paul H Brookes.

Eslinger, P. J. (2002). *Neuropsychological interventions*. New York: The Guilford Press.

Eslinger, P. J., & Oliveri, M. V. (2002). Approaching interventions clinically and scientifically. In P. J. Eslinger, (Ed.), *Neuropsychological interventions* (pp. 3–15). New York: The Guilford Press.

Ewing-Cobbs L, Fletcher J. M., Levin H. S.: Neurobehavioral sequelae following head injury in children: educational implications. Journal of Head Trauma Rehabilitation 1:57-60, 1986.

Forness, S. R. (2001). Special education and related services: What have we learned from meta-analysis? *Exceptionality*, 94, 185–197.

Frankowski, R. F., Annegers, J. F., & Whitman, S. (1985). Epidemiological and descriptive studies, part I: The descriptive epidemiology of head trauma in the United States. In D. P. Becker & J. T. Povlishock, (Eds.), *Central nervous system trauma status report—1985* (pp. 33–43). Bethesda, MD: National Institute of Neurological and Communicative Disorders and Stroke: National Institutes of Health.

Giangreco, M. F. (1986). Effects of integrated therapy: a pilot study. *The Journal of the Association for Persons with Severe Handicaps* 11: 205–208.

Giangreco, M. F. (2000). Related services research for students with low-incidence disabilities: Implications for speech-language pathologists in inclusive classrooms. *Language, Speech, and Hearing Service in Schools*, 31: 230–239.

Glang, A., Singer, G., Cooley, E., et al. (1992). Tailoring direct instruction techniques for use with elementary students with brain injury. *Journal of Head Trauma Rehabilitation*, 7: 93–108.

Greenwood, C. (1991). Longitudinal analysis of time, engagement, and achievement in at-risk versus non-risk students. *Exceptional Children*, 58: 521–535.

Hacker, K., & Wessel, G. L. (1998). School-based health centers and school nurses: Cementing the collaboration. *Journal of School Health*, 68: 409–414.

Haley, S., Coster, W., Ludlow, B., et al. (1992). *Pediatric Evaluation of Disability Inventory (PEDI)*. Boston, MA: Pediatric Evaluation Research Group.

Harel, S., Kutai, M., Tomer, A., et al. (1993). Intrauterine growth retardation: diagnosis and neurodevelopmental outcome. In N. Anastasion & S. Harel, (Eds.), *At-Risk Infants* (pp. 145–160). Baltimore, MD: Paul H Brookes.

Harel, S., Tal-Posener, E., Kutai, M., et al. (1991). Intrauterine growth retardation and brain development, part I: Pre- and perinatal diagnosis. *International Pediatrics*, 6: 109–120.

Harrison, P., & Oakland, T. (2003). *Adaptive Behavior Assessment System-Second Edition Manual*. San Antonio, TX: The Psychological Corporation.

Hertzig, M. E. (1983). Temperament and neurological status. In M. Rutter, (Ed.), *Developmental neuropsychiatry* (pp. 164–180). New York: Guilford.

Individuals with Disabilities Education Act, 20, U.S.C, & Sect. 1400, et. seq. (I.D.E.A. 1997)

Johnson, M. J. (Ed.). (1993). *Brain development and cognition*. Cambridge, MA: Blackwell.

Koop, C. E. (1987). *Surgeon general's report. Children with special health care needs: Commitment to family centered, coordinated care for children with special health needs*. Washington, DC: U.S. Department of Health and Human Services, U.S. Government Printing Office.

Langlois, J., & Gotsch, K. (2001). *Traumatic brain injury in the United States: Assessing outcomes in children*. Atlanta, GA: National Center for Injury Prevention and Control, Centers for Disease Control and Prevention.

McLean, M., Wolery, M., & Bailey, D. B. (2003). *Assessing infants and preschoolers with special needs*, (3rd Ed.). New Jersey: Prentice Hall.

McWilliam, R. A., & Bailey, D. (1992). Promoting engagement and mastery. In D. Bailey & M. Wolery, (Eds.). *Teaching infants and preschoolers with disabilities*, (2nd Ed., pp. 229–255). Englewood Cliffs, NJ: Merrill/Prentice Hall.

Miller, G., & Ramer, J. (Eds.). (1990). *Static encephalopathies of infancy and childhood*. New York: Raven.

Miller, D. T., & Gallagher, P. A. (1997). Early intervention for children with disabilities: A role for family and consumer sciences. *Family and Consumer Sciences Research Journal*, 89: 52–54.

Miller, J. A., Tansy, M., & Hughes, T. L. (1998). Functional behavioral assessment: The link between problem behavior and effective intervention in schools. *Current Issues in Education* 1, Available at: http://cie.ed.asu.edu/volume1/number5/. Accessed September 8, 2005.

Moyes, C. D. (1980). Epidemiology of serious head injuries in childhood. *Child: Care, Health and Development*, 6: 1–6.

Mrazek, P., & Haggerty, R. (Eds.). (1994). *Reducing risks for mental disorders*. Washington, DC: National Academy Press.

Neel, R. S., & Billingsley, F. F. (1989). *A functional curriculum handbook for students with moderate to severe disabilities*. Baltimore, MD: Paul H Brookes.

Neisworth, J. T., Bagnato, S. J., & Salvia, J. (1995). Neurobehavioral markers for early regulatory disorders. *Infants and Young Children*, 8: 8–17.

Neisworth, J. T., Bagnato, S. J., Salvia, J. D., et al. (1999). *Temperament and Atypical Behavior Scale: Early childhood indicators of developmental dysfunction*. Baltimore, MD: Paul H Brookes.

Ried, S., Strong, G., Wright, L., et al. (1995). Computers, assistive devices, and augmentative communication aids: Technology for social inclusion. *Journal of Head Trauma Rehabilitation*, 10: 80–90.

Rourke, B. P., Ahmad, S. A., Collins, D. W., et al. (2002). Child clinical/pediatric neuropsychology: Some recent advances. *Annual Review of Psychology*, 53: 309–339.

Rosenshine, B. (1978). Academic engagement, content covered, and direct instruction. *Journal of Education*, 160: 38–99.

Semrud-Clikeman, M. (2001). *Traumatic brain injury in children and adolescents: Assessment and intervention*. New York: The Guilford Press.

Shelton, T. L. (1999). Family-centered care in pediatric practice: When and how? *Journal of Developmental and Behavioral Pediatrics*, 20: 117–119.

Shelton, T. L., & Stepanek, J. S. (1994). *Family centered care for children needing specialized health and developmental services*. Bethesda, MD: Association for the Care of Children's Health.

Shelton, T. L., Jeppson, E. S., & Johnson, B. H. (1987). *Family-centered care for children with special health care needs*. Washington, DC: Association for the Care of Children's Health.

Smith, K. W., Haley, S. M., Coster, W. J., et al. (2004, in press). *Functioning After Brain Injury (FABI)*. Watertown, Mass.: New England Research Institutes, Inc.

Snow, J., & Hooper, S. (1994). *Pediatric traumatic brain injury*. Thousand Oaks, CA: Sage.

Thompson, R. J. (1989). *Behavior problems of children with developmental and learning disabilities*. Ann Arbor, MI: University of Michigan Press.

Thomson, J. B., & Kerns, K. A. (2000). Mild traumatic brain injury in children. In S. A. Raskin & C. A. Mateer, (Eds.), *Neuropsychological management of mild traumatic brain injury* (pp. 233–253). New York: Oxford.

Walther-Thomas, C., Korinek, L., & McLaughlin, V. (1999). Collaboration to support student's success. *Focus on exceptional children*, 32: 1–18.

Ware, J. (1990). Designing appropriate environments for people with profound and multiple learning difficulties. In W. I. Fraser, (Ed.), *Key issues in mental retardation research* (pp. 316–326). New York: Routledge.

Wellman, P. (2001). *Life beyond the classroom: Transition strategies for young people with disabilities*. Baltimore, MD: Paul Brookes.

West, J. F., & Cannon, G. S. (1988). Essential collaborative consultation competencies for regular and special educators. *Journal of Learning Disabilities*, 21: 56–63.

Weist, M. D., Goldstein, A., Morris, L., et al. (2003). Integrating expanded school mental health programs and school-based health centers. *Psychology in the Schools*, 40: 297–308.

White, O. R. (1980). Adaptive performance objectives: Form versus function. In W. Sailor & B. Wilcox, (Eds.). *Methods of instruction for severely handicapped students* (pp. 47–69). Baltimore, MD: Paul H Brookes.

Whitney, M. P., & Thoman, E. B. (1993). Early sleep patterns of premature infants are differentially related to later developmental disabilities. *Journal of Developmental and Behavioral Pediatrics*, 14: 71–80.

Wolery, M. (1989). Using assessment information to plan instructional programs. In D. Baily & M. Wolery, (Eds.), *Assessing infants and preschoolers with handicaps* (pp. 478–495). Englewood Cliffs, NJ: Merrill/Prentice Hall.

Wolery, M. (1996). Using assessment information to plan intervention programs. In M. McLean, M. Bailey, & M. Wolery, (Eds.),

Assessing infants and preschoolers with special needs, (2nd ed., pp. 491– 518). Englewood Cliffs, NJ: Merrill/Prentice Hall.

Wolery, M., Bashers, M. S., & Neitzel, J. C. (2002). Ecological congruence assessment for classroom activities and routines: identifying goals and intervention practices in childcare. *Topics in early childhood special education,* 22: 131–142.

World Health Organization. (1980). *International classification of impairments, disabilities, and handicaps.* Geneva, Switzerland: World Health Organization.

World Health Organization. (1992). *International statistical classification of diseases and health related problems (The) ICD-10 Volume 1.* Geneva, Switzerland: World Health Organization.

World Health Organization. (2001). *International classification of functioning, disability, and health.* Geneva, Switzerland: World Health Organization.

Yeates, K. O., Ris, M. D., & Taylor, H. G. (Eds). (2000). *Pediatric neuropsychology: Research, Theory, and Practice* (pp. 3–22). New York: The Guilford Press.

Ylvisaker, M., Feeney, T., Maher-Maxwell, N., et al. (1995). School entry following severe traumatic brain injury: guidelines for educational planning. *Journal of Head Trauma Rehabilitation,* 10: 25–41.

Ylvisaker, M., Feeney, T., & Mullins, K. (1995). School reentry following mild traumatic brain injury: a proposed hospital-to-school protocol. *Journal of Head Trauma Rehabilitation,* 10: 42–49.

Selected Legal Issues

32

Peter S. Latham, JD   *Patricia H. Latham, JD*

It is important that medical and legal professionals understand enough of each other's disciplines to ensure that both provide the best professional services of which they are capable. It is our intent in this chapter to foster such an understanding.

Specifically, in this chapter, we provide a legal overview of various pertinent laws, discuss standards for determining whether a disorder is covered under each of the laws, address entitlements under the laws, explain documentation requirements from a legal perspective, discuss the professional report, and provide an overview of the concept of confidentiality under the law.

BASIC PRINCIPLES

The Constitution

The government of the United States of America is a limited one. It has those powers expressly granted it by the United States Constitution and no others. The Tenth Amendment to the United States Constitution provides:

> The powers not delegated to the United States by the Constitution, nor prohibited by it to the states, are reserved to the states respectively, or to the people.

The powers of the federal government may be exercised through legislation which is authorized by, and enacted pursuant to, specific provisions of the Constitution. As a result, the federal legal rights accorded individuals with disabilities must be found in the Constitution of the United States, or those statutes which Congress has enacted pursuant to its provisions. There are three relevant Constitutional provisions: the Commerce Clause, the Spending

Clause, and the Fourteenth Amendment. Disability legislation must be authorized by one or more of these provisions in order to be valid. Each of these laws, and the Constitutional provisions which authorize them, will be discussed next. In contrast, the states have all powers *not* specifically delegated to the federal government. These powers are, in many cases, far broader than the federal ones and permit states to enact legislation which the federal government cannot.

The Statutory Overview

To protect individuals with disabilities, Congress enacted three key federal statutes: the Rehabilitation Act of 1973 (RA) (1), the Education for All Handicapped Children Act, now called the Individuals with Disabilities Education Act (IDEA) (2), and in 1990, the Americans with Disabilities Act (ADA) (3).

The ADA and RA are civil rights statutes that outlaw discrimination but do not necessarily provide funds for the activities mandated by them. The IDEA goes beyond the civil rights objective of a ban on disability-based discrimination; it provides funding for the provision of a free appropriate public education to students whose needs are such that they require special education and related services to learn. What follows is an overview of these laws. Each statute is discussed in greater depth subsequently.

The Rehabilitation Act of 1973

The Rehabilitation Act of 1973 (RA) made discrimination against individuals with disabilities unlawful in three areas: (1) employment by the executive branch of the federal government, (2) employment by most federal government contractors, and (3) activities that are funded by federal subsidies or grants. The last mentioned category includes all public elementary and secondary schools and most post-secondary institutions. The section of the statute that prohibits discrimination in grants and other forms of financial

---

This chapter has been adapted and updated by the authors from their texts, including *Learning Disabilities and the Law,* published by JKL Communications.

assistance was numbered 504 in the original legislation, and the Rehabilitation Act is often referred to simply as Section 504. Other sections, for example, create a limited requirement for affirmative action in the hiring of individuals with disabilities by the executive branch of the federal government and most federal government contractors.

The RA applies to state agencies, local governmental agencies, and private firms because those entities have agreed that it should apply. Agreement to the terms of the Rehabilitation Act is required in order to receive federal financial support and funding. The courts have given the nondiscrimination provisions of Section 504 a broad reach by finding the existence of federal financial support and funding in circumstances in which the interpretation of receipt of such funding is far from immediately obvious.

The RA is authorized by the Spending Clause of the United States Constitution which provides that "The Congress shall have Power to lay and collect Taxes. . .to. . . provide for the. . .general Welfare of the United States. . . ." (4). Under this authority the federal government provides funding for good purposes, such as education, which it could not provide directly itself. It accomplishes this through the use of grants, which are much like contracts. Any contract, by definition, requires the agreement of the parties, and so the question becomes, what have the states agreed to when they receive grants authorized under the Spending Clause? Sometimes states are found to have agreed to waive immunity to suits by private parties. On the other hand, the Supreme Court has held that the States have *not*, for example, agreed to accept liability for punitive damages for violations of the RA (see *Barnes v. Gorman* (2002) (5)). Nor have they agreed to liability for violation of the myriad of regulations issued pursuant to the RA in suits brought by private parties (see *Alexander v. Sandoval* [2001]) (6). However, the RA does clearly prohibit states from engaging in intentional discrimination against persons with disabilities and that states are not immune from private suits based upon intentional discrimination.

The Individuals With Disabilities Education Act

In 1975, the Congress enacted a statute titled the Education for All Handicapped Children Act. That statute, now called the Individuals with Disabilities Education Act (IDEA), which was reauthorized in December, 2004, provides funds to state and local elementary and secondary schools for the education of children with disabilities. It provides for a free appropriate public education (FAPE) and represents a unique approach to civil rights in that the IDEA provides at least a part of the funds which enable these school systems to comply with federal disability-based civil rights laws. Comparable financing does not exist for compliance with race-based and gender-based civil rights laws. Under the IDEA, the school is responsible for identifying and evaluating students with disabilities, who by reason thereof, need special education and related services and then, for providing to them such education and services under an Individualized Education Program (IEP). These services are to be provided in the least restrictive environment (LRE), appropriate to the needs of the child. In other words, to the extent appropriate in terms of the needs of the child, the child should be integrated with other children, with and without disabilities, and still receive special services. This is sometimes referred to as inclusion. A child found ineligible under the IDEA still may be eligible for services under Section 504 of the RA.

The IDEA is authorized by the Spending Clause. The states have validly consented to its provisions.

The Americans with Disabilities Act of 1990

In 1990, the Congress enacted the Americans with Disabilities Act (ADA). This Act extended the concepts of Section 504 to (1) employers with 15 or more employees (Title I), (2) all activities of state and local governments, including but not limited to employment and education (Title II), and (3) virtually all places which offer goods and services to the public, termed "places of public accommodation" (Title III). In addition, ADA standards apply to employment by the Congress.

Two constitutional provisions authorize the ADA. First, Titles I and III are authorized by the Commerce Clause, which provides that Congress has the authority "To regulate Commerce. . .among the several States. . . ." (7). Title II is authorized by the Fourteenth Amendment which provides in pertinent part that:

> No state shall make or enforce any law which shall. . .deprive any person of life, liberty, or property, without due process of law; nor deny to any person within its jurisdiction the equal protection of the laws. . . .

Note that the Fourteenth Amendment applies to states and not to the federal government. The Fifth Amendment applies to the federal government and contains the prohibition against deprivation "of life, liberty, or property, without due process of law. . . ." While the Fifth Amendment does not contain the equal protection guarantees, in practice, the Fifth Amendment has been interpreted to include it. Note also that the Fourteenth Amendment provides for the enactment of implementing legislation.

The Fourteenth Amendment prohibits only intentional discrimination. For this reason, the Americans with Disabilities Act of 1990 is limited in its application to states. We will discuss intentional discrimination further in this chapter.

Social Security

The Social Security Act, in Titles II and XVI, provides for the payment of benefits and Supplemental Security Income (SSI) to disabled persons. To obtain SSI benefits, an individual must (1) be disabled and (2) have income and resources that do not exceed the prescribed maximums (8).

Entitlement must be established through the presentation of evidence supported by acceptable medical sources (e.g., appropriately qualified medical personnel). The validity of many of the claims for SSI benefits is decided on the basis of evidence presented by the treating sources (i.e., by those actually treating the patient). Other forms of evidence are medical reports and results from consultative examinations. The content of medical reports is specified by regulation. Essentially, a medical report is one that involves all the elements of a standard examination in the applicable medical specialty (9). The Social Security Act is authorized by the Commerce Clause.

State Law

Most states have enacted laws prohibiting discrimination against individuals with disabilities. Their coverage, in some cases, exceeds that of the federal statutes we will be discussing. The laws of each state should be consulted in dealing with any particular issue.

Children and adults also may be entitled to services under state statutes authorizing the furnishing of social services and education to individuals with disabilities. In *Mullins v. North Dakota Department of Human Services* (10), individuals with attention-deficit/hyperactivity disorder (ADHD) were held to be developmentally disabled persons entitled to social services under statutory language similar to that used in the federal statutes and regulations. In reaching this decision, the court disregarded an administrative manual used by the state agency that, while purporting to provide administrative guidance, in fact narrowed the class of potential recipients.

In *In re Richard M.* (11), the Supreme Court of New Hampshire ruled that a brain injury resulting from an automobile accident may result in a "specific learning disability" under a state statute providing for social services for the developmentally disabled. The court also held that a state regulation limiting the application of the term *developmental disability* to those individuals with onset of the disability before age 18 years was invalid under the statutory definition. (It should be noted that the New Hampshire statute in question used the IDEA definition of disability.)

WHO IS A QUALIFIED INDIVIDUAL WITH A DISABILITY?

The Rehabilitation Act or the ADA may apply when a *physical or mental impairment* exists that *substantially limits a major life activity*. In order to obtain the protections of the Rehabilitation Act or the ADA, a patient is required to establish that the Rehabilitation Act or the ADA applies and that he or she (1) is an "individual with a disability," (2) is "otherwise qualified," *and* 3) was denied a job, education, or other benefit by reason of that disability (12).

Impairments Covered

The Rehabilitation Act or ADA apply to any "individual with a disability," which includes one who "has a physical or mental impairment which substantially limits one or more of such person's major life activities" (13). The term "individual with a disability" includes individuals with ADHD, specific learning disabilities, autism, other neurological impairments, and neuropsychiatric disorders that substantially limit a major life activity. Alcoholism is covered, but current illegal drug use is not. A recovering drug user who has been drug free for a reasonable period is, in all likelihood, covered as having an impairment under the ADA. Conditions such as left-handedness and lack of familiarity with the English language are not covered, even though they may interfere with learning and working.

Substantially Limits

The impact of the impairment must be severe enough to result in actual substandard performance or in significant restriction of the manner in which a major life activity is performed. The regulations use the term "substantially limits," by which is meant that an individual *either* (1) is "[u]nable to perform a major life activity that the average person in the general population can perform" or (2) is "[s]ignificantly restricted as to the condition, manner or duration" of the major life activity in question, when measured against the abilities of the "average person in the general population" (13).

Who is the average person, and what is the general population? How do you measure the severity of an impairment? Do you consider the beneficial effects of coping strategies and medication? The Supreme Court addressed these questions in a series of cases.

Prior to 1999, most courts held that, under the ADA, the severity of an impairment is to be measured *without* considering the effects of a person's coping strategies, medication, or prosthetic devices. In *Sutton v. United Air Lines, Inc.* (1999) (14), the Supreme Court rejected those cases.

Karen Sutton and her twin sister, Kimberly, had "severe myopia," which was *correctable* to "20/20 or better" with glasses or contact lenses. Without these, however, both sisters "effectively" could not "see to conduct numerous activities such as driving a vehicle, watching television or shopping in public stores." Nonetheless, the sisters applied to United Airlines for employment as commercial pilots. They were rejected because United's policy required 20/20 vision without the corrective effects of glasses or contact lenses. They sued under the ADA and, having lost at trial and on appeal, petitioned the Supreme Court which affirmed the dismissal of their case. The Supreme Court concluded that Congress never intended the ADA to protect, as disabled, those who, like the sisters, were able to "function identically to individuals without a similar impairment," when employing "mitigating measures such as medicines, or assistive or prosthetic devices." The Court reached the same result with respect to medication (*Murphy v. United Parcel Service, Inc.* (1999) (15), and compensatory strategies (*Albertsons, Inc. v. Kirkingburg* (1999)) (16).

Major Life Activities

An impairment must substantially limit a "major life activity" before it can be considered a "disability" under the law. The major life activities are considered to be "caring for oneself, performing manual tasks, walking, seeing, hearing, speaking, breathing, learning, and working" (17). The Equal Employment Opportunity Commission (EEOC) has added: *thinking, concentrating, and interacting with others as well as sleeping* to the list of major life activities its investigators will recognize. Whether, and to what extent, the courts will agree with the EEOC is uncertain. Note: Some courts hold that reading and writing are separate major life activities, but these appear to be minority views. It should be noted that the regulations specify that *learning and working* are major life activities, and these are the ones that most concern us. However, working is treated differently from all other major life activities for purposes of considering whether an individual with an impairment is substantially limited thereby. To be considered to represent a substantial limitation on *working*, the individual's impairment must bar him or her from significant *classes* of jobs, not just from a *particular* job. Only disabilities with the former (and broader) impact are considered to substantially limit working. *Whitlock v. Mac-Gray, Inc.* (18).

Under the ADA, the impairment must *substantially limit* a major life activity. In *Toyota Motor Manufacturing, Kentucky, Inc., v. Williams* (2002) (19), the United States Supreme Court considered the level of severity required. That case involved a suit by an automobile assembly worker who experienced pain in her neck and shoulders and was eventually diagnosed with carpal tunnel syndrome and other disorders. However, while her carpal tunnel syndrome limited her "ability to perform the range of manual tasks associated with an assembly line job," it did not limit her ability to perform isolated, nonrepetitive manual tasks over a short period of time, such as tending to her personal hygiene or carrying out personal or household chores. She was placed on "a no-work-of-any-kind restriction" by her treating physicians. Toyota then terminated her employment, and she sued under the ADA, claiming that she was disabled because she was substantially limited, among other things, in the major life activities of performing manual tasks and working.

The United States Supreme Court ruled that Williams was not an individual with a disability because she could not meet the "demanding standard for qualifying as disabled" created by the ADA. It ruled that to be "substantially limited" in a "major life activity":

> an individual must have an impairment that prevents or severely restricts the individual from doing activities that are of central importance to most people's daily lives. The impairment's impact must also be permanent or long-term.

Applying this reasoning to the case at hand, the Supreme Court noted that repetitive work with hands and arms extended at or above shoulder levels for extended periods of time, "is not an important part of most people's daily lives." Williams' ability to perform household chores, bathing, and brush her teeth were, because these "are among the types of manual tasks of central importance to people's daily lives, and should have been part of the assessment of whether [Williams] was substantially limited in performing manual tasks." The case was then returned to the court of appeals for further proceedings.

Lower federal courts have applied similar reasoning in cases involving the ADA and RA. One case, involving a public high school student with learning disabilities, ADD, and epilepsy, is *Costello v. Mitchell Pub. Sch. Dist.* (20). The court found that the student was not substantially limited in any major life activity compared to the general population. While the student may have had a more difficult time learning compared to her peers, any limitations she had did not prevent her from moving to the next grade level. Note, however, that the application of state law may produce radically different results. California, for example requires only that an impairment limit participation in a major life activity. Proof of substantial limitation is not required (21).

Otherwise Qualified

Under both the Rehabilitation Act and the ADA, an "individual with a disability" must be one who is "otherwise qualified." An "otherwise qualified" individual is one who, although possessed of a disability, would be eligible for the education, job, or program benefit, with or without, a reasonable accommodation. It should be noted that in public elementary and secondary schools, a student is presumed to be qualified for public education. Thus, it is not necessary to prove that the student is otherwise qualified.

The RA and ADA requirement that an individual with a disability be otherwise qualified will exclude many individuals with neuropsychiatric impairments from educational programs and the workplace because it is difficult to show that one is both substantially limited in a major life activity such as learning and is also qualified for the educational program or job. The facts that prove substantial limitation also show a lack of qualification. Conversely, a person whose neuropsychiatric impairments do not disqualify him or her is unlikely to be considered disabled under federal law. In *Robertson v. Neuromedical Center* (22), for example, the Fifth Circuit upheld the termination of a neurologist with ADHD. Holding that there was no duty to accommodate Robertson in his medical practice, the Court found that he was not otherwise qualified to practice medicine, because he was a threat to the "basic medical safety" of his patients, saying:

> Robertson posed a 'direct threat' to the health and safety of others in the workplace. Robertson's short-term memory

problems had already caused various mistakes to be made in patients' charts and in dispensing medicine. Most significantly, Robertson voiced his own concerns about his ability to take care of patients, stating that it was only a matter of time before he seriously hurt someone.

The Central Dilemma of the ADA

The ADA and RA pose a central dilemma: to prove that one has a disability under the ADA/RA, one must show an impairment which both substantially limits a major life activity but (despite its severity) does not render one unqualified for the job or educational program. A great many plaintiffs with neuropsychiatric conditions find that they are either: (1) qualified, but not disabled or (2) disabled, but not qualified.

THE RIGHT TO BE FREE FROM DISCRIMINATION

Illegal discrimination exists in two senses, intentional discrimination and a refusal to accommodate. Intentional discrimination is illegal whether done by governmental or private entities. Refusals to accommodate are illegal only when done by private parties. We will consider each below.

Equal Protection and Intentional Discrimination

The Fourteenth Amendment provides in part that "No state shall. . .deny to any person within its jurisdiction the equal protection of the laws. . . ." In the context of disabilities, equal protection of the laws is denied when intentional discrimination occurs. Intentional discrimination consists of a baseless and unlawful difference in the treatment of individuals by reason of their race, gender, or disability characteristics. Whether a difference in treatment is unlawful depends on whether it has a rational basis. Distinctions based on race or gender are *presumed* to have no rational basis and are, for all practical purposes, unlawful. *Nevada Department of Human Resources v. Hibbs*, (U.S.S.C. 2003) (23).

Differences in treatment on the basis of disability may or may not have a rational basis; it all depends on the facts of each case. There is no presumption against different treatment. (See *City of Cleburne, Texas v. Cleburne Living Center, Inc.* (1985) and *Kimel v. Florida Bd. of Regents* (2000) (24) For example, it would be unlawful for a government to bar African Americans or females from employment as bus drivers. There can be no reason for such a distinction. However, a prohibition against the employment as bus drivers of persons who lack the ability to see has a rational basis even though it involves a difference in the treatment accorded persons with a disability. Under the Constitution, there is no duty to provide individuals with disabilities accommodations, reasonable or otherwise. Failure to provide accommodations does not constitute intentional discrimination.

In *University of Alabama v. Garrett* (2001) (25), the United States Supreme Court said:

> States are not required by the Fourteenth Amendment to make special accommodations for the disabled, so long as their actions towards such individuals are rational.

In *Garcia v. S.U.N.Y. Health Sciences Ctr. of Brooklyn* (26), the court held that a medical student dismissed from a state university could not maintain a suit for monetary damages against the university under either the ADA or Section 504 of the RA, unless the university violated the Fourteenth Amendment by committing intentional discrimination (not simply failure to accommodate a disability), and, as to Section 504, unless the state knowingly waived its sovereign immunity from suit when it accepted federal funds. In *Garcia*, the court found that the state had not waived its sovereign immunity.

However, where the discrimination by a state government is intentional, both the Constitution and the ADA, as well as the RA, provide available remedies. In the case of *Olmstead v. L. C.* (1999) (27), the Supreme Court held that the ADA's "proscription of discrimination" may require placement of persons with mental disabilities in community settings rather than in institutions. The persons in question were two women, both of whom were mentally retarded. In addition, one of the two, L.C. suffered from schizophrenia, and the other, E.W., a personality disorder. Community placement, found the Court, is "in order when the State's treatment professionals have determined that community placement is appropriate, the transfer from institutional care to a less restrictive setting is not opposed by the affected individual, and the placement can be reasonably accommodated, taking into account the resources available to the State and the needs of others with mental disabilities." The Court considered the applicability of these rules:

"Unjustified isolation, we hold, is properly regarded as discrimination based on disability."

L.C. and E.W. were entitled to liberty, the maximum reasonable freedom, under the Fourteenth Amendment. Anything less was illegal segregation. In this case, the discrimination consisted of intentional segregation and violated the Fourteenth Amendment as well as the ADA.

In the context of elementary and secondary public education, it is often meaningful access to education. In *Padilla v. School District No. 1* (28), the Court held that the parents had alleged facts which, if true, would constitute a valid claim of intentional discrimination. The facts follow. Between 1992 and 1997, a school district failed to provide a special education student "with the behavioral programming, augmentative communication, and tube feeding services identified in her IEP." The school district also repeatedly "placed her in a windowless closet, restrained in a stroller without supervision," contrary to her IEP. During one of these incidents "she tipped over and hit her head on the floor, suffering serious physical injuries, including a skull fracture and exacerbation of a seizure disorder, which kept her from attending school for the remainder of the term." Being locked in a closet and physically abused deprives one of access to education.

In *Davis v. Monroe County Board of Education* (1999) (29), the United States Supreme Court considered what types of access deprivation might be actionable. The Court noted that the "most obvious example" of deprivation "would thus involve the overt, physical deprivation of access to school resources." Conduct which prevented "students from using a particular school resource—an athletic field or a computer lab, for instance" would give rise to liability. It "is not necessary, however, to show physical exclusion to demonstrate that students have been deprived. . .of an educational opportunity." Conduct "that is so severe, pervasive, and objectively offensive, and that so undermines and detracts from the victims' educational experience, that the victim-students are effectively denied equal access to an institution's resources and opportunities," is actionable. Note that, while the Court was discussing sexual harassment, the same principles apply in the area of disabilities. (See *Gebser v. Lago Vista Independent School Dist* (30) and *Rees v. Jefferson School District)* (30a). Intentional discrimination must also be proved under the RA (see *Alexander v. Sandoval*) (31). Following *Sandoval*, the Court was careful to point out that its rulings were not based on regulations. In *Jackson v. Birmingham Board of Education*, 544 U.S. __ (2005), the court held that a private party may sue a school that receives federal funds in a case in which the private party (a male coach) alleges acts of retaliation against him for reporting discrimination against girls on a girls' sports team "based on sex." Following *Alexander v. Sandoval*, the court refused to base its holding on the Department of Education's regulations. The court said:

> We do not rely on regulations extending Title IX's protection beyond its statutory limits: indeed, we do not rely on the Department of Education's regulations at all, because the statute itself contains the necessary prohibition.

Due Process and Intentional Discrimination

The test of what constitutes intentional discrimination is different when due process is concerned. The Fourteenth Amendment also provides that "No state shall. . .deprive any person of life, liberty, or property, without due process of law. . . ." That is because due process requirements apply when the government seeks to require something of the individual. In *Tennessee v. Lane*, 541 U.S. 509 (2004) (31a), the U. S. Supreme Court considered Title II of the ADA in a case involving the issue of physical access by persons with paraplegia to the courts. The Court ruled in a 5–4 decision that private parties could sue states for monetary damages under Title II of the ADA where fundamental due process rights, such as access to the courts, are at issue. Applied in this manner, the ADA "is congruent and proportional" to the congressional "object of enforcing the right of access to the courts." Put another way, if a court has the authority to take actions against individuals by holding them liable,

then due process requires that those subject to the courts have the ability to use them effectively. For this reason, the United States Supreme Court held the ADA to be constitutional as applied in *Lane*, but not in *Garrett* (25).

Duty to Accommodate

Intentional discrimination consists of a baseless and unlawful difference in the treatment of individuals by reason of their race, gender, or disability characteristics. In the ADA/RA, the concept has been expanded to include a refusal to provide reasonable accommodations. For example, the ADA provides with respect to employment that "No covered entity shall discriminate against a qualified individual with a disability because of the disability of such individual. . . ." Discrimination is defined to include "not making reasonable accommodations to the known physical or mental limitations of an otherwise qualified individual with a disability. . . ." (32). Similar prohibitions are applicable to places of public accommodation, including private schools.

It should be noted at the outset that states and their agencies, including public educational institutions are barred only from engaging in intentional discrimination. There is no duty to provide reasonable accommodations in the public classroom. Reasonable accommodations are alterations in *nonessential* testing requirements (33), delivery of course materials (34), or job requirements (35) that will enable a child or adult with a disability to perform the *essential* or *fundamental* tasks involved. Modifications that would require alteration of the fundamental nature of a test, course of study, or job or that would cause an undue hardship are not reasonable and are not required (36) (see *Zukle v. Regents*) (37).

The requirement for reasonable accommodation affects virtually all educational institutions, regardless of whether they are elementary, secondary, or postsecondary, in three principal areas:

- Testing (for admissions, evaluation of academic performance, and graduation)
- Delivery of course materials
- Nonacademic benefits of school or college life (e.g., sports, dormitory living)

The bases for these common requirements vary, depending on whether the educational institution is public or private, elementary or postsecondary. Special education and services in *public* elementary and secondary education are governed by the IDEA (38). The Rehabilitation Act and ADA also apply, but in many cases their coverage is less comprehensive than the IDEA's coverage (39).

Accommodations in *private* elementary and secondary education are governed only by the Rehabilitation Act and the ADA. Accommodations in postsecondary institutions, including colleges, graduate schools, and institutions that prepare individuals to take entrance examinations and professional licensing examinations or that administer such examinations, are governed by the Rehabilitation Act and the ADA (40). As previously noted, the Rehabilitation Act would not apply unless the school receives federal funding, and the ADA would not apply to religiously controlled schools.

Examinations must be structured in such a way that their results "accurately reflect the individual's aptitude or achievement level or whatever other factor the examination purports to measure" (41).

In general, entrance and other examinations may not reflect "the individual's impaired sensory, manual, or speaking skills" unless (1) the purpose of the test is to measure those factors and (2) the measurement of those factors has a valid educational purpose. Testing that relies on a single criterion is unlawful where that criterion can be shown to be an inaccurate predictor of performance and the use of that criterion has no compelling justification.

Examinations are generally required to be modified (1) in the "length of time permitted for completion" and (2) in the "manner in which the examination is given" (42). Auxiliary aids and services must be provided. Modifications are not required where they will alter the fundamental nature of the course or pose an undue hardship. The U.S. Department of Education has stated that in making undue hardship determinations, the primary consideration will be the size and budget of the institution in comparison with the cost of the requested aids, and not the amount of tuition paid by the student (43).

An educational institution must provide equal access to classroom and other educational materials. This duty is described in the regulations as an obligation to provide auxiliary aids and services (44). The auxiliary aids and services must "recognize individual communications needs" and must provide "contemporaneous communication" of the entire educational experience, including class participation, being offered. Their selection is to be guided primarily by a consultative process with the student and not just made unilaterally by the institution (45).

The requirement for reasonable accommodation generally applies in the workplace as well. Again, *nonessential* testing and job performance requirements must be modified. Modifications that would require fundamental job alterations or undue hardship are not required. These requirements apply to federal executive (46) and congressional (47) branch employment, federal funding recipients (48), federal government contractors (49), state and local governments, and most private employers.

THE RIGHT TO EDUCATIONAL ASSISTANCE—IDEA

Thus far we have discussed the right to be free from discrimination by reason of disability. However, some impairments are sufficiently serious that more proactive measures are required. In the case of education, these measures are contained in the Individuals with Disabilities Education Act (IDEA). The IDEA applies to "children with disabilities," which the *United States Code Annotated* (U. S.C.A.) defines as children:

(i) with mental retardation, hearing impairments including deafness, speech or language impairments, visual impairments including blindness, serious emotional disturbance, orthopedic impairments, autism, traumatic brain injury, other health impairments, or specific learning disabilities; and

(ii) who, by reason thereof, need special education and related services (50).

It should be noted that to be eligible, a child must (1) have a listed disability and (2) "by reason thereof, need special education and related services."

The IDEA has been interpreted to cover ADHD under the categories of "specific learning disabilities," "other health impairments," and "serious emotional disturbance." (See Chapter 11 for discussion of ADHD.) Mood disorders, schizophrenia, anxiety, and other psychiatric illnesses could be covered under the emotional disturbance category. (See Chapter 13 for discussion of mood disorders, Chapter 14 for anxiety disorders.) Autism and Asperger's Syndrome are also covered.

The IDEA is implemented by the *Code of Federal Regulations* (12), which repeats the terms of the U.S.C.A. definition. The disability definitions in the IDEA are interpreted to be consistent with those that appear in the regulations issued under the Rehabilitation Act and the ADA. For example, the IDEA's definition of "specific learning disability" governs the interpretation of the term "specific learning disability" as it appears in the regulations issued under the Rehabilitation Act and the ADA (13).

The special education and related services are delivered by means of an *individualized education program* (IEP), which reflects agreement between the school district and the parents as to the specific services that will be delivered during the academic year. Failure to agree triggers a requirement for a due process hearing whose purpose is to create an IEP based on evidence from a variety of sources, including classroom teachers, parents, and professionals.

The IDEA applies only to those disorders and impairments that are sufficiently severe to require special education and related services. Many states give great weight to a "2-year" rule-of-thumb for assessing the impact of a learning disability. Specifically, they refuse to find that a child needs special education and related services unless the child is 2 years behind in his or her academic progress. Thus, a child who puts forth a Herculean effort to perform at grade level in achievement may in effect work his or her way out of qualifying for special education and related services. In some states, the applicable state law may bring about a result more favorable to students with learning disabilities. For example,

Massachusetts requires special education services to develop successfully each child's educational potential. Many states have used a "severe discrepancy" test in deciding whether a specific learning disability exists. The 2004 IDEA, 20 U.S.C. §1414(b)(6)(50a), provides that "when determining whether a child has a specific learning disability. . . a local educational agency shall not be required to take into consideration whether a child has a severe discrepancy between achievement and intellectual ability in oral expression, listening comprehension, written expression, basic reading skill, reading comprehension, mathematical calculation, or mathematical reasoning." The local educational agency may, of course, consider such a discrepancy as a factor in its assessment.

Special education and related services are delivered under the IDEA by means of an IEP, which reflects agreement between the school district and the parents as to the specific services that will be delivered during the academic year. As noted earlier, failure to agree triggers a requirement for a due process hearing whose purpose is to create an IEP based on evidence to be supplied from a variety of sources (e.g., classroom teachers, parents, professionals) (51). Services must be delivered in the *least restrictive environment* appropriate to the needs of the child.

An issue currently of concern is the exclusion for misconduct of elementary and secondary public school students with behavioral and mental impairments. Children with disabilities who are receiving services in public school under the IDEA may not be expelled or suspended for more than 10 days for misconduct arising out of their disabilities, except if maintaining the student in the current placement is substantially likely to cause injury, in which case proper procedures must be followed. Generally, rather than exclude the student from the school program, the school should use the IEP process to determine what additional services may be appropriate to address the disability-related behavior.

A suspension for more than 10 days constitutes a change in placement and triggers a notice and the right to a due process hearing. During these proceedings, the child remains in the original placement. Students who bring firearms to school are treated differently. Such students may be suspended for up to 45 days and may be maintained in an interim placement pending completion of any hearings requested by their parents. Even when a child is excluded from a program because of misconduct, the child is entitled under the IDEA to continuing services.

Students with disabilities who are receiving services under Section 504 of the Rehabilitation Act are also entitled to procedural safeguards in the event of misconduct. However, in contrast with the IDEA, Section 504 has been interpreted to permit the school to cease providing educational services during periods of disciplinary exclusion from school.

THE RIGHT TO CARE: SOCIAL SECURITY

The Social Security Act (SSA) provides for financial support to certain persons with disabilities. To obtain SSI benefits, an individual must have 1) a qualifying disability and 2) income and resources that do not exceed the prescribed maximums (52). A child's disability is measured in terms of what would disable an adult. In other words, a child's ability to function as other children of the same age do must be impaired to a degree comparable to that required of adults. Other statutes provide for *social services* to individuals with disabilities. Individuals with disabilities are also covered by the Fair Housing Act (53).

The SSA (54) applies when a *physical or mental impairment* exists that *effectively precludes* an individual from working and/or caring for himself or herself. A *disability* for purposes of SSI is "the inability to do any substantial gainful activity by reason of any medically determinable physical or mental impairment which can be expected to result in death or which has lasted or can be expected to last for a continuous period of not less than 12 months" (55). The degree of impairment required by this test is greater than that required by the Rehabilitation Act and the ADA.

The following impairments are those specifically covered for children:

- Multiple-body-system impairments, which include "acquired disorders" that create "significant interference with age-appropriate major daily or personal care activities" (56).
- Organic mental disorders ("abnormalities in perception, cognition, affect, or behavior associated with dysfunction of the brain") (57).
- Neurological impairments, including seizure disorders (58).
- Mental retardation, defined as "dependence on others for personal needs" and as having a "valid verbal, performance, or full scale IQ of 60 through 70" accompanied by "impairment imposing additional and significant limitation of function" (59).
- Autistic disorder and other pervasive developmental disorders (60).
- ADHD (61).
- "Developmental and emotional disorders of newborn and younger infants" (62).

THE RIGHT TO PROTECTION: CRIMINAL AND CIVIL COMMITMENT

Criminal Justice System

A disability such as schizophrenia may constitute an *excuse* that requires a finding of *not guilty by reason of insanity*. A disorder may preclude a witness from testifying when its severity is such that the individual is not a *competent* witness. A disability may be a factor that reduces the severity of an offense for which an individual may be convicted. A disability also may require a lesser or a modified sentence or may influence the approach to rehabilitation.

Two cases may serve as examples of the increasing interplay between disability-based requirements and the criminal law.

In a case involving a motor vehicle accident, *Jackson v. Inhabitants of Sanford, Me* (63). Jackson, the plaintiff, had been jailed for operating a motor vehicle while under the influence of alcohol or drugs. The evidence of his alleged alcohol-based or drug-based impairment consisted of certain physical difficulties, including partial paralysis and slurred speech. However, Jackson succeeded in establishing that these conditions resulted not from alcohol or drug use but from a prior stroke. The court held that the Town of Sanford, Maine, was liable for discriminatory arrest in violation of Title II of the ADA.

In *State v. Woody* (64), the defendant had been arrested for driving under the influence of alcohol. The principal proof against him was his blood alcohol results. However, the court held these test results inadmissible because the arresting officer had not provided the defendant, who was deaf, with a qualified sign language interpreter from the human resources department at the time the tests were made, as required by state statutes.

The right to adequate physical and mental *health treatment* in prison is evolving. Suffice it to say that although the *existence* of such a right is theoretically established (i.e., by the Eighth Amendment's prohibition against cruel and unusual punishment), the *scope* of that right is disputed, and the enthusiasm with which it is recognized by correctional institutions varies (65). The applicability of the Rehabilitation Act (because of federal law enforcement moneys) and the ADA (because of Title II, which prohibits disability-based discrimination by state and local governments) may lead to improved care.

The right to *education* for children and adolescents who would be entitled to it under the IDEA were they not incarcerated stands on a more substantial footing. In general, the IDEA requires such education, and the various jurisdictions have made progress in implementing these requirements.

Civil Commitment

Involuntary civil commitment involves compelling individuals with mental illnesses or mental impairments to receive care and treatment. States have various standards for involuntary commitment, one of which is *danger to self or others*. Over the past 20 years, there has been increasing recognition of the importance of less restrictive alternatives to longterm institutional care. Most states provide for an initial commitment period for observation. An individual may not be held beyond that initial period without a hear-

ing. Longer-term commitment without periodic review is unlawful (66). Usually, commitment is to an inpatient institution. Sometimes, involuntary outpatient commitment is an alternative option.

Almost all states have voluntary admission procedures under which an individual may initiate admission for treatment. Minor children with parents or legal guardians have less due process protection than adults. The United States Supreme Court has held that an admitting physician's determination is sufficient for children to be committed to state hospitals by their parents (67).

Treatment Approaches and Legal Rights

Patients in institutions have legal rights, which may include legal rights to treatment and habilitation, to basic necessities, to refusal of treatments, and to treatment in the least restrictive environment. The courts have held that patients with mental disabilities have a constitutional right to treatment and habilitation (68). Competent individuals have the right to refuse medication for psychiatric conditions, although such medication may be forcibly administered in an emergency situation. In the case of persons who are ruled incompetent to stand trial, antipsychotic medication may be forcibly administered, consistent with due process (69).

The law governing electroconvulsive therapy (ECT) in most states is that before ECT can be administered, the individual, when competent, must give knowing and voluntary consent. In one case, a court honored the declaration of a patient, made prior to her incapacity, withdrawing her consent to further ECT (70). (See Chapter 28 for discussion of ECT.)

The United States Supreme Court has established a restrictive institutional liability standard. Generally, for liability to be imposed, it must be demonstrated that a "substantial departure from accepted professional judgment, practice, or standards" occurred (71). A federal court in Pennsylvania has held that the professional judgment standard should be applied in an action brought by the U.S. Department of Justice under the Civil Rights of Institutionalized Persons Act (CRIPA). The Department alleged that residents of an institution for persons with mental retardation were deprived of adequate basic and medical care and were unduly restrained. The court found that most of the institution's practices, while not necessarily the most desirable practices, did meet minimal constitutional requirements (72).

DOCUMENTATION

Individuals with neuropsychiatric disabilities or their parents or guardians seek evaluations for a variety of reasons. Increasingly, evaluations are sought to determine eligibility for benefits, services, or accommodations under a number of laws. Documentation of the disability is vital to establishing eligibility. Ordinarily, documentation is based on history, testing, and personal interview and medical examination.

Components of Documentation

History

Compilation of a personal history can be of critical importance in making well documented diagnoses and recommendations. The following areas ordinarily should be considered:

- Obstetrical history
- Developmental history
- Medical history
- School history
- Family history

The patient and his or her family are an essential source of information. However, when disorders such as ADHD and learning disabilities and other psychiatric disorders are at issue, the individual's early family and school experiences may be highly relevant from a clinical viewpoint. When possible, interviews with family members, schoolteachers, and medical advisers can be invaluable in confirming the existence of these disabilities. Additionally, school and medical records can provide important information.

Testing

The purpose of IQ testing is to measure intelligence. Psychoeducational testing is undertaken to assess the individual's proficiency in performing academic tasks, and neuropsychological testing is undertaken to assess the functioning of relevant brain regions.

Results from prior testing can be useful. However, because certain disorders, such as ADHD, may lessen in severity or impact with age, a childhood diagnosis of ADHD may not in itself be persuasive when one is attempting to document an adolescent or adult case of that disorder. Similarly, some learning disabilities may have a lessened impact in adulthood because of compensations developed over the years and the greater freedom adults have in selecting activities that are a good match. Therefore, in order to be persuasive, the testing and evaluations undertaken should be recent enough to be clearly relevant to the individual at his or her present stage of life. Recent testing and a prior record of these disabilities are, when occurring together, highly persuasive.

The same is true of school records. A record of accommodation in elementary school, by itself, is probably insufficient evidence to establish the existence of an adult disability and entitlement to accommodations. When combined with results from recent testing, however, such a record is highly persuasive.

Personal Interview/Medical Examination

The patient is, of course, the focus of the evaluation. The personal interview and medical examination are of fundamental importance in arriving at well-documented diagnoses and recommendations. (See Chapters 3 and 4.)

Sufficiency of the Documentation

Determining how much testing and evaluation is enough is a matter of professional judgment and depends on the use to which the results will be put. At one end of the spectrum is the individual who has sought testing to gain self-knowledge and treatment recommendations. In such a case, the amount of documentation is simply that which a responsible medical practitioner would require in order to make a diagnosis, prescribe medication, and select appropriate additional treatment. At the other end of the spectrum is the individual with disabilities who has sought testing in connection with the assertion of a legal right. A school or employer might be resistant to the request for accommodations or services. Probably the best strategy is to proceed on the assumption that the individual may one day desire to request accommodations or services, even if they are not needed now, and to provide appropriate documentation.

Reasonableness of the Documentation

Determining the amount and type of documentation that is reasonable is a medical and legal exercise. The medical professional documenting a neuropsychiatric disability may have to function both as a scientist and as an advocate. Essential medical terms in documentation and their corresponding legal terms under the Rehabilitation Act and the ADA are presented in Table 32.1. Testing, observation, medical examinations, and interviews support the diagnosis. When the purpose of the diagnosis is to assist an individual in obtaining services or academic adjustments in school or accommodations in the workplace, the diagnosis must also support the legal finding that the patient is

TABLE 32.1
MEDICAL–LEGAL TRANSLATOR

Medical		Legal
Diagnosis	=	Impairment
Impact	=	Substantially limits a major life activity compared to the average member of the population, considering all the beneficial and negative effects of strategies, coping mechanisms and medication
Recommendations	=	Reasonable accommodations for an otherwise qualified individual

"otherwise qualified" (although this is presumed in public elementary and secondary school) and is an "individual with a disability" as those terms appear in the law.

As a practical matter, then, the medical practitioner must "document" the patient's disability by presenting that amount of evidence necessary to persuade the individuals with whom the practitioner is dealing, or, in the event that more formal proceedings become necessary, by proving entitlement by "a preponderance of the evidence." This legal language means essentially that the practitioner's evidence must be more convincing than that of his or her "opponent." Since the practitioner can never know for certain when he or she will be called on to support the patient's case with testimony, the documentation should be developed with care.

The practitioner may testify as an expert witness. Under the *Federal Rules of Evidence,* he or she may be "qualified as an expert by knowledge, skill, experience, training, or education" to do so (73). As such, the practitioner may offer testimony concerning "scientific, technical, or other specialized knowledge," provided that it will "assist" the judge or jury "to understand the evidence or to determine a fact in issue" (74). The practitioner's opinion may be based on "facts or data in the particular case," which are "those perceived by or made known to" the practitioner "at or before the hearing." The "facts or data need not be admissible in evidence" if they are "of a type reasonably relied upon by experts in the particular field in forming opinions or inferences upon the subject" (75).

Documentation of the Disability in a Report

Elements of Documentation

Using as an example the Rehabilitation Act and the ADA, we noted that persons with impairments that substantially limit a major life activity are considered "individuals with disabilities" under those laws. To obtain their protections, an individual may be required to *document* his or her disability. There are three basic elements to proper disability documentation: (1) diagnosis, (2) impact evaluation, and (3) recommendations.

A *diagnosis* is what its name suggests: an *authoritative* opinion by one qualified to assert it, concluding that a specific disability is present. Legally speaking, the diagnosis also establishes the existence of an *impairment* under the Rehabilitation Act and the ADA. Some courts appear to prefer diagnoses that refer to the current edition of the American Psychiatric Association's *Diagnostic and Statistical Manual of Mental Disorders,* now in its fourth edition (DSM-IV) (76).

An *impact evaluation* demonstrates how the diagnosed *impairment* affects the individual. Legally speaking, it must show that in the individual case the impairment *substantially limits a major life activity,* such as learning or working, compared to the average member of the population. It must consider the positive and negative effects of pros-

thetic devices, medications, and compensatory strategies employed by the individual, together with an assessment of the impact of the impairment on the individual's day-to-day tasks. In this regard, it must also address the question of whether and to what extent the impairment was life long.

Recommendations suggest reasonable accommodations appropriate for the individual.

The Report

The professional's findings are set forth in a report, which usually consists of at least three sections:

- Introductory material
- Fact section (describing history, interview, medical examination, and testing)
- Opinion section (setting forth diagnosis, evaluation of impact, and recommendations)

Some Dos and Don'ts

The medical professional's report is central to the patient's future. A well-supported and well-reasoned report can persuade the school, college, or employer with which the practitioner is dealing. The report can make further advocacy and litigation unnecessary. A poorly reasoned and unsupported report can lead to a refusal to grant the patient's request and may increase the chances of a dispute and possibly litigation. Here are a few common errors to avoid.

- *Writing the report for the wrong purpose.* A patient may want an evaluation and report for (1) self-knowledge, (2) the development of skill-building strategies or compensatory strategies, or (3) requests for benefits, services, or reasonable accommodations. It is important that both the practitioner and his or her patient know which purpose is intended.
- *Including inaccurate information to avoid offending the patient.* Accuracy can be painful. As a compassionate professional, the practitioner may want to minimize the severity of a disorder so that the patient will not feel discouraged. Such kindness can be harmful, however. In one case, a competent psychologist, having concluded that an auditory processing problem lay at the root of a patient's academic problems, hastened to add that no learning disability was present. This comment was as harmful as it was kind, for the report suggested that certain of the patient's academic problems did not result from a disability. Consequently, the university in question had no duty to provide certain of the reasonable accommodations requested.
- *Providing raw data with no explanations.* When writing a report dealing with benefits, special education, services, or reasonable accommodations, the practitioner is writing for a *legal* as well as a *scientific* purpose. The practitioner should remember that his or her medical conclusions support corresponding legal conclusions, as shown in

Table 32.1. Thus, the practitioner must explain the significance of the raw data in terms of the purpose of the report.

- *Including irrelevant information.* A report written for the development of *personal strategies* must necessarily focus on those strategies. An emphasis on those strategies may not be appropriate in a report in the which the purpose is to discuss reasonable accommodations. A discussion of certain personal strategies may mistakenly convey the impression that reasonable accommodations would not be necessary if more effective personal strategies were followed. The use of effective personal strategies is not required by law; provision of reasonable accommodations is so required.

- *Using an obsolete edition of a textbook or test.* The practitioner should be sure that he or she cites to the most current edition of the *Diagnostic and Statistical Manual of Mental Disorders* and uses the most current edition of the tests he or she administers. At best, the use of an earlier edition or of superseded texts or tests can sharply diminish the credibility of one's work; at worst, it could, under certain circumstances, constitute malpractice. In a North Carolina case, for example, a psychologist's professional license was revoked for a number of professional deficiencies, including that in one case his professional opinions were based on test results from an obsolete (and inappropriate) intelligence test (77).

- *Misjudging when legal advice is appropriate.* An attorney's advice often is not necessary. However, when the practitioner is uncertain as to whether the report is legally sufficient, or when he or she anticipates opposition to the recommendations in the report, legal complications are probable, and the patient may benefit by consulting with an attorney.

Confidentiality

Confidentiality may be a major concern for individuals with disabilities. There are several sources of requirements that define when and on what terms confidential information must be protected. Generally, information is public unless its dissemination is *prohibited* by one or more of the following:

- Contract
- Constitutional law
- Statutory provisions and their implementing regulations
- Court decisions

Of these, two that are important for pediatric neuropsychiatrists are contractual agreements and state law statutory provisions applicable to the practice of neuropsychiatry in a particular state.

Arrangements with patients and their families as to confidentiality should be clear and, of course, adhered to in a professional manner.

States have laws that require confidentiality for information furnished to certain professionals. These laws carry with them criminal penalties for unauthorized disclosure. Violations, by professionals, of these laws may also be punished by suspension or revocation of professional licenses. Each state has its own definition of the classes of professionals whose patient–client communications are considered privileged. Virtually all states recognize as confidential communications made to clergy, medical doctors, and lawyers. Psychologists are frequently also included. However, professionals who are not listed in the statutes of a particular state but who perform functions similar to those of listed professionals may *not* be covered. Thus, in *Thompson v. State* (78), the court held that communications made to a "crisis intervention specialist" were *not* protected under a statute creating a psychotherapist–patient privilege.

The psychotherapist–patient privilege is not absolute. Cases have upheld the duty of a psychiatrist, when the patient is a danger to another, to use reasonable care to protect an intended victim. The privilege did not block enforcement of subpoenas issued to psychiatrists during an insurance fraud investigation in which the requested information pertained to patient identities and treatment lengths (79).

Federal laws provide confidentiality protections for children and adults with disabilities. The IDEA provides for confidentiality of school records concerning students with disabilities (80). Regulations provide that these records may be retained permanently by the school unless the parents request that the records be destroyed. The only records that need not be destroyed following such a request are the student's name, address, and telephone number; grades; attendance record; grade level completed; and year completed (81).

At the college level, the IDEA does not apply, but protections are provided by the Family Educational Rights and Privacy Act (FERPA), also known as the Buckley Amendment, which was passed in 1974. It affords students the right to have access to their educational records, requires their consent to release of records to third parties, and allows them to challenge information in their records. The FERPA applies to all colleges that receive federal funds. However, FERPA can no longer be enforced by private law suits. The Supreme Court has ruled that the states have not agreed to liability for suits by private parties to enforce the confidentiality provisions of the Family Educational Rights and Privacy Act of 1974 (20 U.S.C. § 1232g; FERPA (81a). (See *Gonzaga University v. Doe* (2002)) (82). The only remedy left for disappointed students and their parents are the administrative remedies available from the Department of Education.

Statutes and regulations establish rules of general applicability. On a showing of necessity, courts may authorize or prohibit the release of records based on the factual necessities of the case.

SUMMARY

The task of the medical professional has broadened in recent years to include advocacy on behalf of patients who wish to use medical information to support legal claims. To accomplish this purpose, the medical professional must understand, in general terms, what legal elements have to be proven, how the medical facts may assist in this demonstration, and what information should be contained in the files of patients who are asserting legal claims and may therefore be subject to disclosure in the course of potential litigation.

REFERENCES

1. 29 U.S.C.A. § 701 *et seq.*
2. 20 U.S.C.A. § 1400 *et seq.*
3. 42 U.S.C.A. § 12101 *et seq.*
4. Constitution, Art I, §8; Cl. 1.
5. *Barnes v. Gorman*, Docket No. 01-682 (U.S.S.C. June 17, 2002).
6. *Alexander v. Sandoval*, 532 U.S. 275 (2001).
7. Constitution, Art I, §8; Cl. 4.
8. 42 U.S.C.A. § 402 *et seq.* (1995); 42 U.S.C.A. §§ 1381, 1382c(a)(3).
9. Disability Evaluation Under Social Security (U.S. Department of Health and Human Services Sept. 1994).
10. *Mullins v. North Dakota Department of Human Services*, 483 N.W2d 160 (N.D. 1992).
11. *In re Richard M.*, 497 A.2d 1200 (N.H. 1985).
12. 29 U.S.C.A. § 706(8)(b)(i) (1995); see also 42 U.S.C.A. § 12102(2); *Fitzgerald v. Green Valley Area Education Agency*, 589 F. Supp. 1130 (S.D. Iowa 1984).
13. 29 C.F.R. § 1630.2(j)(1)(i)-(ii) (1995).
14. *Sutton v. United Air Lines, Inc.*, 527 U.S. 1031 (1999).
15. *Murphy v. United Parcel Service, Inc.*, 527 U.S. 516 (1999).
16. *Albertsons, Inc. v. Kirkingburg*, 527 U.S. 555 (1999).
17. 29 C.F.R. § 1630.2(i) (1995).
18. *Whitlock v. Mac-Gray, Inc.*, Docket No. 02-2568 (1st Cir. Oct 6, 2003).
19. *Toyota Motor Manufacturing, Kentucky, Inc., v. Williams*, Docket No. 00-1089 (U.S.S.C. January 8, 2002).
20. *Costello v. Mitchell Pub. Sch. Dist.*, 266 F.3d 916 (8th Cir. 2001).
21. *Colmenares v. Braemar Country Club, Inc.*, Docket No. S098895 (CA Feb. 20 2002).
22. *Robertson v. Neuromedical Center*, Docket No. 97-31169 (5th Cir. December 3, 1998), *cert. denied*, Docket No. 98-1377 (May 3, 1999).
23. *Nevada Department of Human Resources v. Hibbs*, Docket No. 01-1368 (U.S.S.C. May 27, 2003).
24. *City of Cleburne, Texas v. Cleburne Living Center, Inc.*, 473 U.S. 432 (1985); *Kimel v. Florida Bd. of Regents*, 528 U.S. 62 (2000).
25. *University of Alabama v. Garrett*, 531 U.S. 351 (2001).
26. *Garcia v. S.U.N.Y. Health Sciences Ctr. of Brooklyn*, 2001 WL 1159970 (2nd Cir. Sept. 26, 2001).
27. *Olmstead v. L. C.*, 527 U.S. 581 (1999).
28. *Padilla v. School District No. 1*; (Docket Nos. 99-1061;99-1345 (10th Cir. Dec. 5, 2000).
29. *Davis v. Monroe County Board of Education*, Docket No. 9-843 (U.S.S.C. May 24, 1999).
30. *Gebser v. Lago Vista Independent School Dist.*, 524 U.S. 274 (1998); *Rees v. Jefferson School District*, Docket No. 99-3554314J (9th Cir. March 9, 2000).
31. *Alexander v. Sandoval*, 532 U.S. 275 (2001).
31a. *Tennessee v. Lane*, 541 U.S. 509 (2004).
32. 42 U.S.C.§ 12112(b)(5)(A).
33. *Stutts v. Freeman*, 694 F.2d 666 (11th Cir. 1983).
34. *United States v. Becker C.P.A. Review*, 1993 WL 632257 (D.D.C. 1993).
35. *Lynch v. Department of Education*, 52 M.S.PR. 541 (1992); but see *Bolstein v. Reich*, 1995 WL 46387 (D.D.C.), aff'd, 1995 WL 686236 (D.C. Cir. 1995) [DOL attorney with depression that prevented him from performing independent, unsupervised high-level legal analysis, research, and writing is not otherwise qualified when these skills are essential features of his job.]
36. United States Equal Employment Opportunity Commission: The Americans With Disability Act: Your Rights as an Individual (EEOC-BK 18). Washington, DC, U.S. Equal Employment Opportunity Commission, 1991.
37. *Zukle v. Regents of the University of California*, 166 F.3d 1041 (9th Cir. 1999).
38. 20 U.S.C.A. § 1400 *et seq.* (1995).
39. See, e.g., 34 C.F.R. §§ 104.33, 10435–10436 (1995).
40. *United States v. Becker C.P.A. Review*, 1993 WL 632257 (D.D.C. 1993).
41. 28 C.F.R. § 36.309(b)(1)(i) (1995).
42. 28 C.F.R. § 36.309(b)(2) (1995).
43. Letter from W Smith, Acting Assistant Secretary for Civil Rights, U.S. Department of Education, to Neill Stern, Executive Vice President, Parker College of Chiropractic, March 6, 1990, at 3–4.
44. 28 C.F.R. § 36.309 *et seq.* (1995).
45. *United States v. Becker C.P.A. Review*, 1993 WL 632257 (D.D.C. 1993).
46. The Rehabilitation Act of 1973, 29 U.S.C.A. § 701 *et seq.* (1995); Civil Service Reform Act of 1978, 5 U.S.C.A. § 2302 *et seq.* (1995).
47. The Americans With Disabilities Act of 1990, 42 U.S.C.A. § 12209 (1995).
48. 29 U.S.C.A. § 794 *et seq.* (1995) [This section is often informally referred to as "Section 504," its designation in the Public Law that Congress originally enacted.]
49. 29 U.S.C.A. § 793 *et seq.* (1995).
50. 20 U.S.C.A. § 1401(a)(1)(A) (1995) 12. 34 C.F.R. § 300.530 *et seq.* (1995).
50a. 20 U.S.C. § 1414(b)(6).
51. 20 U.S.C.A. § 1415 (1995).
52. 42 U.S.C.A. § 402 *et seq.* (1995).
53. See, generally, 24 C.F.R. § 8.4 *et seq.* (1995).
54. 42 U.S.C.A. § 402 *et seq.* (1995).
55. 20 C.F.R. § 404.1505(a) (1995).
56. 20 C.F.R. § 404, Subpt. P, App. 1 § 110.00 (1995).
57. 20 C.F.R. § 404, Subpt. P, App. 1, § 112.02 (1995).
58. 20 C.F.R. § 404, Subpt. P, App. 1, § 111.00, A-B (1995).
59. 20 C.F.R. § 404, Subpt. P, App. 1, §§ 112.05 B, D (1995).
60. 20 C.F.R. § 404, Subpt. P, App. 1, § 112.10 (1995).
61. 20 C.F.R. § 404, Subpt. P, App. 1, § 112.11 (1995).
62. 20 C.F.R. § 404, Subpt. P, App. 1, § 112.12 (1995).
63. *Jackson v. Inhabitants of Sanford, Me.*, 63 U.S.L.W 2351 (D. Me. 1994).
64. *State v. Woody*, 449 S.E.2d 615 (Ga. App. 1994).
65. *Vaughan v. Lacey*, 49 F.3d 1344 (8th Cir. 1995) ; but see *J.E.W v. State*, 349 S.E.2d 713 (Ga. 1986).
66. *Wyatt v. King*, 773 F. Supp. 1508 (M.D. Ala. 1991).
67. *Parham v. J.R.*, 442 U.S. 584 (1979).
68. *Wyatt v. Stickney*, 325 F. Supp. 781 (M.D. Ala. 1971).
69. *United States v. Charters*, 863 F.2d 302 (4th Cir. 1988), *cert. denied*, 494 U.S. 1016 (1990).
70. *In re Rosa M.*, 16 MPDLR 46 (N.Y Sup. Ct. 1991).
71. *Youngberg v. Romeo*, 457 U.S. 307, 323 (1982).
72. *United States v. Pennsylvania*, 902 F. Supp. 565 (WD. Pa. 1995).
73. Fed. R. Evid. 702.
74. Fed. R. Evid. 702.
75. Fed. R. Evid. 703.
76. *Pandazides v. Virginia Board of Education*, 804 F. Supp. 794, 803 (E.D. Va. 1992); *reversed on other grounds*, 13 F.3d 823 (4th Cir. 1994)
77. *White v. North Carolina State Board of Examiners of Practicing Psychologists*, 388 S.E.2d 148 (N.C. App. 1990).
78. *Thompson v. State*, 615 So.2d 737 (Fla. Dist. Ct. App. 1993).
79. *In re Zuniga*, 714 F.2d 632 (6th Cir.), *cert. denied*, 464 U.S. 983 (1983).
80. 20 U.S.C.A. § 1417(c) (1995).
81. 34 C.F.R. § 300.573 (1995).
81a. 20 U.S.C. § 1232g; FERPA.
82. *Gonzaga University v. Doe*, Docket No. 01-679 (U.S.S.C. June 20, 2002).

Index